D1067830

Editors

WILLIAM S. HAUBRICH, M.D.

Clinical Professor of Medicine, University of California,
San Diego; Senior Consultant, Division of Gastroenterology,
The Scripps Clinic and Research Foundation, LaJolla

MARTIN H. KALSER, M.D., Ph.D.

Professor of Medicine and Chief, Division of Gastroenterology,
University of Miami, Florida

JAMES L. A. ROTH, M.D., Ph.D.

Professor of Clinical Medicine, School of Medicine,
University of Pennsylvania; Director, Institute of Gastroenterology,
Presbyterian-University of Pennsylvania Medical Center

FENTON SCHAFFNER, M.D.

George Baehr Professor of Medicine and Professor of Pathology;
Chief, Division of Liver Disease, Mount Sinai School of Medicine
of City University of New York

Editorial Consultant

FRANCISCO VILARDELL, M.D., D.Sc.

Director, Escuela de Patologia Digestiva, Universidad Autonoma
de Barcelona, Spain

Editorial Associate

DANIEL PELOT, M.D.

Associate Professor of Medicine, University of California, Irvine

Volume 3

Bockus

GASTROENTEROLOGY

Fourth Edition

Editor-in-Chief

J. EDWARD BERK, M.D., D.Sc.

Distinguished Professor of Medicine
University of California, Irvine

W. B. SAUNDERS COMPANY 1985

Philadelphia London Toronto Mexico City Rio de Janeiro Sydney Tokyo

W. B. Saunders Company: West Washington Square
Philadelphia, PA 19105

1 St. Anne's Road
Eastbourne, East Sussex BN21 3UN, England

1 Goldthorne Avenue
Toronto, Ontario M8Z 5T9, Canada

Apartado 26370—Cedro 512
Mexico 4, D.F., Mexico

Rua Coronel Cabrita, 8
Sao Cristovao Caixa Postal 21176
Rio de Janeiro, Brazil

9 Waltham Street
Artarmon, N.S.W. 2064, Australia

Ichibancho, Central Bldg., 22-1 Ichibancho
Chiyoda-Ku, Tokyo 102, Japan

Library of Congress Cataloging in Publication Data

Bockus, Henry L. (Henry Le Roy), 1894–1982

Bockus GASTROENTEROLOGY.

1. Digestive organs—Diseases. 2. Gastrointestinal system—Diseases. I. Berk, J. Edward (Jack Edward) II. Title. [DNLM: 1. Gastrointestinal diseases. WI 100 B665g]

RC801.B663 1985 616.3 83–20120

ISBN 0–7216–1777–8

Listed here is the latest translated edition of this book together with the language of the translation and the publisher.

Italian (*2nd Edition*)—Editrice Universo, Rome, Italy

Spanish (*2nd Edition*)—Salvat Editores, Barcelona, Spain

Spanish (*3rd Edition*)—Salvat Editores S.A., Barcelona, Spain

Volume 1 ISBN 0-7216-1778-6
Volume 2 ISBN 0-7216-1779-4
Volume 3 ISBN 0-7216-1780-8
Volume 4 ISBN 0-7216-1781-6
Volume 5 ISBN 0-7216-1782-4
Volume 6 ISBN 0-7216-1783-2
Volume 7 ISBN 0-7216-1784-0
Bockus Gastroenterology 7 Volume set ISBN 0-7216-1777-8

Last digit is the print number: 9 8 7 6 5 4 3 2 1

Contributors
VOLUME 3

SIAMAK A. ADIBI, M.D., Ph.D.
Professor of Medicine and of Clinical Nutrition, University of Pittsburgh School of Medicine; Chief, Clinical Nutrition Unit, Montefiore Hospital, Pittsburgh, Pa.

JAMIE S. BARKIN, M.D.
Associate Professor of Medicine, University of Miami School of Medicine; Coordinator of Endoscopy, Veterans Administration Medical Center, Miami, Fla.

ELIZABETH BARRETT-CONNOR, M.D.
Professor of Community and Family Medicine and of Medicine, University of California, San Diego, School of Medicine, San Diego, Calif.

STANLEY BAUM, M.D.
Eugene P. Pendergrass Professor and Chairman of the Department of Radiology, School of Medicine, University of Pennsylvania, Philadelphia, Pa.

BENGT BORGSTRÖM, M.D., Ph.D.
Professor of Physiological Chemistry, Medical Faculty, University of Lund, Lund, Sweden.

JAY L. COHEN, M.D.
Attending Physician, John F. Kennedy Memorial Hospital, Palm Beach, Fla.

ISIDORE COHN, Jr., M.D.
Professor and Chairman of the Department of Surgery, Louisiana State University School of Medicine; Surgeon-in-Chief, LSU Surgical Service, Charity Hospital of Louisiana, New Orleans, La.

W. T. COOKE, M.D.
Hon. Consultant Physician and Gastroenterologist, The General Hospital, Birmingham, England.

F. SCOTT CORBETT, M.D.
Clinical Fellow in Gastroenterology, University of Miami School of Medicine, Miami, Fla.

SIDNEY CYWES, M.Med. (Surgery)
Professor and Head of the Department of Paediatric Surgery, University of Cape Town; Chief Paediatric Surgeon, Red Cross War Memorial Children's Hospital, Cape Town, South Africa.

WILLIAM O. DOBBINS, III, M.D.
Professor of Internal Medicine, University of Michigan Medical School; Associate Chief of Staff for Research, Veterans Administration Medical Center, Ann Arbor, Mich.

HERBERT L. DuPONT, M.D.
Professor of Medicine and Director, Program in Infectious Diseases and Clinical Microbiology, University of Texas Health Science Center, Houston, Texas.

ROBERT H. GALLAVAN, Jr., Ph.D.
Research Assistant Professor of Surgery, University of Cincinnati College of Medicine, Cincinnati, Ohio.

CEDRIC GARLAND, Dr.P.H.
Assistant Professor-in-Residence, Department of Community and Family Medicine, University of California, San Diego, School of Medicine, San Diego, Calif.

SHERWOOD L. GORBACH, M.D.
Professor of Medicine and Microbiology, Tufts University School of Medicine; Chief, Infectious Diseases Division, New England Medical Center Hospitals, Boston, Mass.

SCOTT M. GRUNDY, M.D., Ph.D.
Professor of Internal Medicine and Biochemistry, and Director of the Center for Human Nutrition, University of Texas Health Sciences Center at Dallas, Dallas, Texas.

JAMES B. HAMMOND, M.D.
Associate Professor of Medicine and Chief of the Division of Gastroenterology, Chicago Medical School; Chief, Gastroenterology Section, Medical Service, Veterans Administration Medical Center, North Chicago, Ill.

STEPHEN B. HANAUER, M.D.
Assistant Professor of Medicine, Section of Gastroenterology, University of Chicago Pritzker School of Medicine, Chicago, Ill.

ALBERT M. HARARY, M.D.
Clinical Assistant Professor of Medicine (Gastroenterology), New York Medical College; Attending Physician, Lenox Hill Hospital, New York, N.Y.

WILLIAM S. HAUBRICH, M.D.
Clinical Professor of Medicine, University of California, San Diego, School of Medicine; Senior Consultant, Division of Gastroenterology, Scripps Clinic and Research Foundation, La Jolla, Calif.

HANS HERLINGER, M.D.
Professor of Radiology, School of Medicine, University of Pennsylvania, Philadelphia, Pa.

G. K. T. HOLMES, M.D.
Consultant Physician and Gastroenterologist, Derbyshire Royal Infirmary, Derby, England.

DEXTER H. HOWARD, Ph.D.
Professor and Vice Chairman of the Department of Microbiology and Immunology, University of California, Los Angeles, School of Medicine, Los Angeles, Calif.

EUGENE D. JACOBSON, M.D.
Professor of Physiology and Biophysics, University of Cincinnati College of Medicine, Cincinnati, Ohio.

JOSEF P. JANSSENS, M.D.
Associate Professor of Medicine, University of Leuven; Assistant Head, Division of Gastroenterology, University Hospital St. Rafael, Leuven, Belgium.

HUGH A. JORDAN, M.B.
Visiting Assistant Professor of Radiology, School of Medicine, University of Pennsylvania, Philadelphia, Pa.

MARTIN H. KALSER, M.D., Ph.D.
Professor of Medicine and Chief, Division of Gastroenterology, University of Miami School of Medicine; Chief of the Division of Gastroenterology, Jackson Memorial Medical Center, Miami, Fla.

GERALD T. KEUSCH, M.D.
Professor of Medicine, Tufts University School of Medicine, Boston, Mass.

CHARLES E. KING, M.D.
Associate Professor of Medicine, Division of Gastroenterology and Nutrition, University of Florida College of Medicine, Gainesville, Fla.

SUMNER C. KRAFT, M.D.
Professor of Medicine and Committee on Immunology, University of Chicago Pritzker School of Medicine, Chicago, Ill.

IGOR LAUFER, M.D.
Professor of Radiology, School of Medicine, University of Pennsylvania; Chief of Gastrointestinal Radiology, Hospital of the University of Pennsylvania, Philadelphia, Pa.

MICHAEL D. LEVITT, M.D.
Professor of Medicine, University of Minnesota School of Medicine; Associate Chief of Staff for Research, Veterans Administration Medical Center, Minneapolis, Minn.

CHARLES J. LIGHTDALE, M.D.
Associate Professor of Clinical Medicine, Cornell University Medical College; Director, Diagnostic Gastrointestinal Unit, Memorial Sloan-Kettering Cancer Center, New York, N.Y.

ARMAND LITTMAN, M.D., Ph.D.
Professor of Medicine, Loyola University Stritch School of Medicine; Chief, Medical Service, Edward Hines Jr. Veterans Administration Hospital, Hines, Ill.

JAN H. LOUW, M.D., Ch.M.
Emeritus Professor of Surgery, University of Cape Town; Hon. Consultant Surgeon, Groote Schuur Hospital, Cape Town, South Africa.

CHARLES M. MANSBACH, II, M.D.
Associate Professor of Medicine, Duke University School of Medicine, Durham, N.C.

HOWARD D. MANTEN, M.D.
Assistant Professor of Medicine, University of Miami School of Medicine, Miami, Fla.

JOHN B. MARSHALL, M.D.
Clinical Assistant Professor of Medicine, University of South Dakota School of Medicine, Rapid City, S.D.

SIDNEY NEIMARK, M.D.
Clinical Instructor in Medicine, Thomas Jefferson University School of Medicine, Philadelphia, Pa.; Chief of Gastrointestinal Endoscopy, Veterans Administration Medical and Regional Office Center, Wilmington, Del.

ELIMELECH OKON, M.D.
Senior Lecturer, Hebrew University Hadassah Medical School; Chief Physician, Department of Pathology, Hadassah University Hospital, Jerusalem, Israel.

ROBERT J. PAULEY, Ph.D.
Assistant Professor of Microbiology and Immunology, University of Miami School of Medicine, Miami, Fla.

FREDERICK F. PAUSTIAN, M.D.
Professor of Internal Medicine and Physiology/Biophysics, Associate Dean for Continuing and Graduate Medical Education, University of Nebraska Medical Center, Omaha, Neb.

B. D. PIMPARKAR, M.D.
Emeritus Professor, Seth G. S. Medical College; Hon. Physician, Nanavati Hospital, Bombay, India.

DANIEL RACHMILEWITZ, M.D.
Associate Professor of Medicine, Hebrew University Hadassah Medical School; Head, Department of Gastroenterology, Hadassah University Hospital, Jerusalem, Israel.

ARVEY I. ROGERS, M.D.
Professor of Medicine, University of Miami School of Medicine; Chief of the Gastroenterology Section, Veterans Administration Medical Center; Director of Medical Services, University of Miami Hospitals and Clinics, Miami, Fla.

THOMAS W. SHEEHY, M.D.
Professor of Medicine, University of Albama, Birmingham, School of Medicine; Chief of Medicine, Veterans Administration Medical Center, Birmingham, Ala.

PAUL SHERLOCK, M.D.
Professor and Vice Chairman of the Department of Medicine, Cornell University Medical College; Chairman, Department of Medicine, Memorial Sloan-Kettering Cancer Center, New York, N.Y.

MARGOT SHINER, F.R.C.(Path.), D.C.H.
Consultant Gastroenterologist, Clinical Research Centre, Northwick Park Hospital, and Central Middlesex Hospital, London, England.

PHILLIP P. TOSKES, M.D.
Professor of Medicine and Director of the Division of Gastroenterology and Nutrition, University of Florida College of Medicine, Gainesville, Fla.

ERNEST URBAN, M.B.B.S.
Associate Professor of Medicine, Division of Gastroenterology and Nutrition, University of Texas Health Sci-

ences Center at San Antonio; Assistant Chief, Medical Service, Audie L. Murphy Veterans Administration Medical Center, San Antonio, Texas.

GASTON R. VANTRAPPEN, M.D.
Professor of Medicine, University of Leuven; Head, Department of Medicine and Division of Gastroenterology, University Hospital St. Rafael, Leuven, Belgium.

THOMAS A. WALDMANN, M.D.
Chief, Metabolism Branch, National Cancer Institute, National Institutes of Health, Bethesda, Md.

RICHARD R. P. WARNER, M.D.
Associate Clinical Professor of Medicine, Mount Sinai School of Medicine of the City University of New York, New York, N.Y.

ELLIOT WESER, M.D.
Professor and Deputy Chairman of the Department of Medicine, University of Texas Health Sciences Center at San Antonio; Chief, Medical Service, Audie L. Murphy Veterans Administration Medical Center, San Antonio, Texas.

Contents

VOLUME 3

Intestine, Part One. Small Intestine; Vascular Disorders; Specific Infectious Diseases

SECTION 12. THE INTESTINE

Bockus

GASTROENTEROLOGY

VOLUME 3

Intestine, Part One

Small Intestine; Vascular Disorders; Specific Infectious Diseases

Chapter 87

Embryology and Anomalies of the Intestine

Jan H. Louw • Sidney Cywes

Embryology of the Intestines[1-4]

The formation of the digestive system is initiated within 2 weeks of fertilization by the development of the ectodermal amniotic cavity and the entodermal yolk sac within the blastocyst. At the close of the second week, the floor of the amnion sac (ectoderm) and the roof of the yolk sac (entoderm) come to lie in apposition to constitute an oval plate, the embryonic disc, which, together with the amnion and yolk sac, is attached to the primitive chorion by a bridge of cells, the body stalk (Fig. 87–1). At this stage, a diverticulum of the yolk sac, the allantois, pushes into the body stalk toward the chorion, while the primitive streak originates as a thickened band of ectoderm in the midplane of the embryonic disc and establishes the longitudinal axis of the embryo. Proliferation from the primitive streak gives rise to the mesoderm of the embryo proper. The head end of the primitive streak enlarges into a primitive knot (Hensen's node), out of which a rodlike extension of mesoderm grows forward between the ectoderm and entoderm to form the future notochord. *If the ectoderm and entoderm become adherent in the midline at any point, the notochord will split around this point and give rise to various malformations, including duplications of the foregut or hindgut associated with vertebral anomalies.*[5, 6]

During the third and fourth weeks the flat embryonic disc is transformed into a cylindrical embryo attached to the yolk sac by a narrow stalk. This change is brought about by a process of folding, resulting in the formation of head, tail, and lateral folds. The entoderm, destined to become the primitive gut, participates in this folding process. Pushing into the head end and then into the tail end of the embryo, the entodermal layer assumes the form of 2 blind tubes, the foregut and the hindgut. The blind ends of the foregut and hindgut come into direct contact with the ectoderm on the ventral surface of the embryo, and the fused plates thus produced are named the pharyngeal membrane and the cloacal membrane, respectively. The intermediate region communicates freely with the yolk sac and forms the midgut, which is converted into a tube by the formation of the lateral body folds. Further growth and folding constrict the communication with the yolk sac into a narrow vitellointestinal duct. Very early in the growth of the embryo, shortly after the appearance of the allantoic diverticulum, the blind end of the hindgut dilates to form a cloaca or reservoir. The latter communicates with the rest of the hindgut dorsally and the allantois ventrally. The cloacal membrane occupies the midventral surface of this cloaca and extends along the allantois as the infraumbilical membrane (Figs. 87–1 and 87–2). At the 5 mm stage (4 weeks) the angle between the allantois and hindgut forms a distinct fold, the urorectal septum (Fig. 87–2*A*).

The ultimate derivations of the 3 sections of the primitive gut are as follows: (1) *foregut*—pharynx, respiratory tract, esophagus, stomach, and duodenum proximal to entry of bile duct; (2) *midgut*—duodenum distal to entry of bile duct, liver, pancreas, jejunum and ileum, appendix, and colon proximal to its midtransverse segment; and (3) *hindgut*—colon distal to its midtransverse segment, rectum, and most of the urogenital system (from the allantois).

Development of the Rectum and Anus[7–9]

Separation of the urogenital and anorectal derivatives of the cloaca occurs during the fifth to eighth weeks of development. The simplest concept of these events is that the urorectal septum grows from above downward, like a coronally placed curtain, until it impinges on the cloacal membrane, thus dividing the cloaca into ventral (urogenital sinus) and dorsal (an-

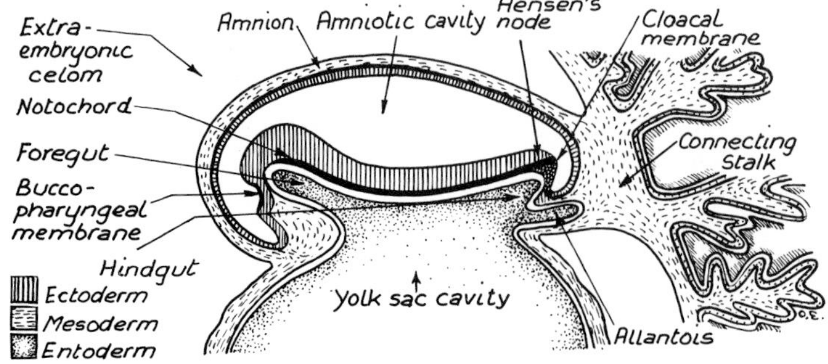

Figure 87–1. Diagrammatic longitudinal section of a human embryo at about 2 weeks illustrating early development of the head and tail folds and the formation of the foregut and hindgut.

orectal) components. The subdivision of the cloaca, however, is not as simple and depends upon at least 4 interrelated embryologic processes (Fig. 87–2):

1. Some downgrowth of the urorectal fold does occur, but only as far as the line of Müller's tubercle, just cephalad to the openings of the mesonephric ducts (Fig. 87–2*A*). If development is arrested at this stage, the rectum will open into the urogenital sinus at the site of Müller's tubercle. *Such developmental arrest will result in high or supralevator anorectal anomalies.*

2. Further subdivision of the cloaca is brought about by caudal migration of the rectal orifice in the dorsal wall of the cloaca toward the cloacal membrane (Fig. 87–2*B*). *Failure of this migration will result in supralevator and intermediate anorectal anomalies.*

3. *The third major event is subdivision of the remaining portion between the urorectal septum and the cloacal membrane (Fig. 87–2C).* This is effected by an inward surge of mesenchyme from the lateral aspects of the embryo, indenting the sides of the cloacal cavity until they meet and fuse with each other in the midline, with the urorectal septum above and the cloacal membrane below. *Errors in development during this phase will result in intermediate anorectal anomalies* (see later section on Anorectal Malformations).

4. The final separation of the urogenital and anorectal systems is associated with the development of the external cloaca and genitalia (Fig. 87–2*D*). By the end of the seventh week, the external cloaca has separated into anal and urethral regions, corresponding to the anorectal and urogenital components of the internal cloaca and separated from them by the cloacal membrane. Following this, the ventral and dorsal components of the cloacal membrane rupture and disappear and the division of the cloaca is concluded. *Premature dehiscence of the cloacal membrane and its allantoic extension is probably responsible for exstrophy of the cloaca.*[2, 10, 11] *Abnormal development of the external cloaca will result in low or translevator anorectal anomalies.*

Formation of the Abdominal Cavity and Mesenteries

Even before the entodermal disc becomes a tube, layers of mesoderm intervene from either side between the amnion above and the yolk sac below. A split in these layers results in lateral spaces (intraembryonic coeloms) running the length of the primitive gut (Fig. 87–3). The mesodermal layer eventually becomes the mesothelium, connective tissue, and muscle lining the pleural, pericardial, and peritoneal cavities. The body folds close ventrally to form the anterior chest and abdominal walls, thereby sealing

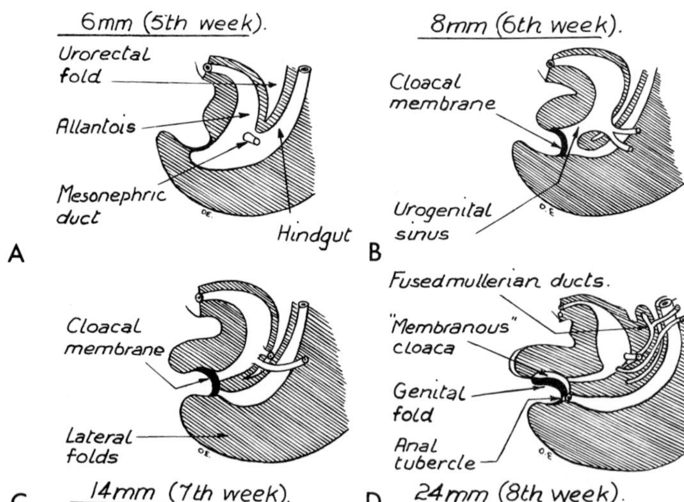

Figure 87–2. Subdivision of the cloaca (see text).

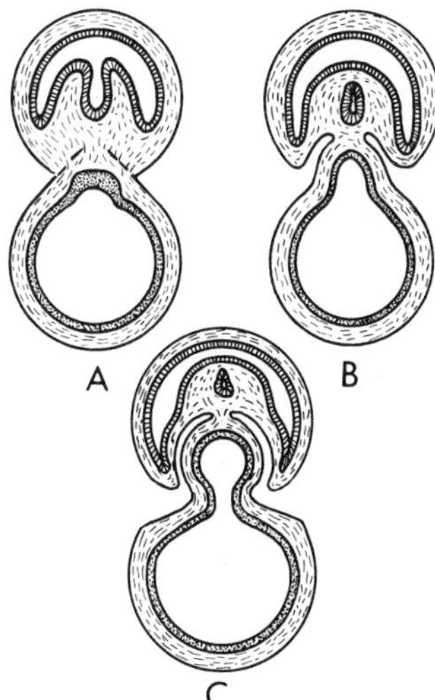

Figure 87–3. Transverse diagrams of the development of the abdominal cavity of the early embryo. *A,* Intervening mesoderm splits between the amnion above and the yolk sac below. *B,* Lateral spaces form around the archenteron. *C,* The lateral body walls extend inferiorly and medially to seal off the intraembryonic celoms.

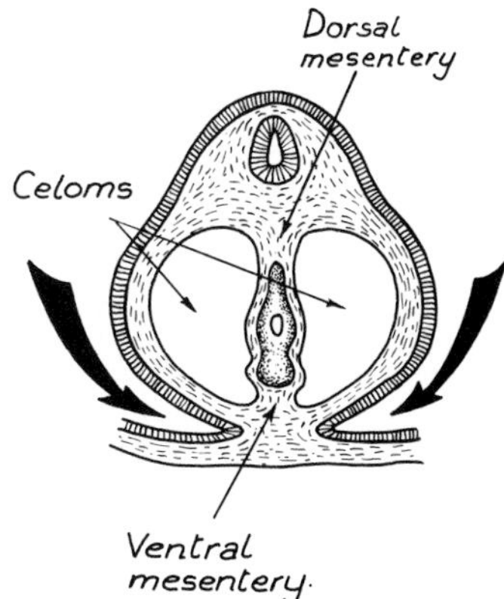

Figure 87–4. The inferior and medial extensions of the lateral body walls seal off the intraembryonic celoms and also assist in the formation of the ventral mesentery and the dorsal mesentery and the dorsal mesentery in which the primitive gut and its appendages are enveloped.

off the intraembryonic coeloms from the cavity of the chorion except at the umbilical attachment to the yolk sac. A transverse septum arises from the body wall ventral to the foregut to form part of the diaphragm and demarcates the future thoracic and abdominal cavities. At first the future pleural and peritoneal cavities communicate freely by means of the paired pleuroperitoneal canals, but in the fifth week pleuroperitoneal membranes appear. These encroach on the canals during the seventh week and close them off shortly afterward. Following this closure, the costal components of the diaphragm are muscularized by ingrowth of mesenchyme dorsally (to form the crura) and anterolaterally. The triangular space where these 2 muscle groups join forms the lumbocostal trigone with its apex at the site of the pleuroperitoneal membrane.[2] *Failure of closure of a pleuroperitoneal canal is associated with failure of adequate muscularization of the adjacent lumbocostal trigone and results in a common type of diaphragmatic hernia (congenital posterolateral hernia, or Bochdalek's hernia).*[12–14]

In the abdominal cavity the upper layer of the mesoderm becomes the parietal peritoneum, while the lower layer envelops the gut to form the mesenteries and provide the muscular wall of the gut. Envelopment by the mesoderm results in longitudinal attachments of the gut both from above (dorsally) and from below (ventrally) (Fig. 87–4). The caudal ventral attachment disappears early, the abdominal coelomic cavities become confluent, and the primitive intestine is suspended only by its persistent dorsal attachment. The ventral attachment persists cranially; within it, the liver and a ventral component of the pancreas form. Along the free edge of this ventral attachment runs the single umbilical vein. In the adult, the ventral attachment of the liver persists as the falciform ligament, while the course of the erstwhile umbilical vein is marked by the round ligament of the liver (ligamentum teres hepatis).

Early Development of the Intestinal Tract

Active growth of the various components of the digestive tube commences during the fourth week, corresponding to the time when the embryo acquires its own circulation.

Foregut. The beginning of the stomach can be detected toward the end of the fourth week as an asymmetric, spindle-shaped, proximal dilatation at the level of segments C3 to C5.[2] At the same time the duodenum can be identified by the appearance of the hepatic and ventral pancreatic diverticula on the ventral aspect of the bowel and the dorsal pancreatic diverticulum on its dorsal aspect (Fig. 87–5). Soon afterward, the celiac axis, which supplies these organs, can be recognized. During the sixth to seventh weeks, the forward growth of the head end of the embryo results in elongation of the foregut cephalad to the gastric dilatation to form the esophagus. There is also an apparent "descent" of the stomach to its permanent location in the abdomen.[2] At the same time the entire organ increases in length and rotates through 90° about its long axis so that the greater curvature lies on the left and the lesser curvature on the right. By the sixth week, the dorsal primordium of the developing pancreas extends into and causes bulging of the dorsal mesentery of the duodenum, while the ventral pancreatic primordium is shifted to a dorsal position by rapid growth of the left half of the duodenal circumference. As a result of these developments, the duodenum "rotates" to the right to assume its normal curvature, and its proximal part becomes fixed posteriorly. Concomitantly, the ventral pancreas migrates to the right and ultimately dorsally to form the peripheral part of the head and the uncinate process of the pancreas (Fig. 87–5). *Failure of this migration may be responsible for an annular pancreas.*[1, 2]

From the fifth week onward, there is considerable epithelial activity within the duodenum. By the eighth

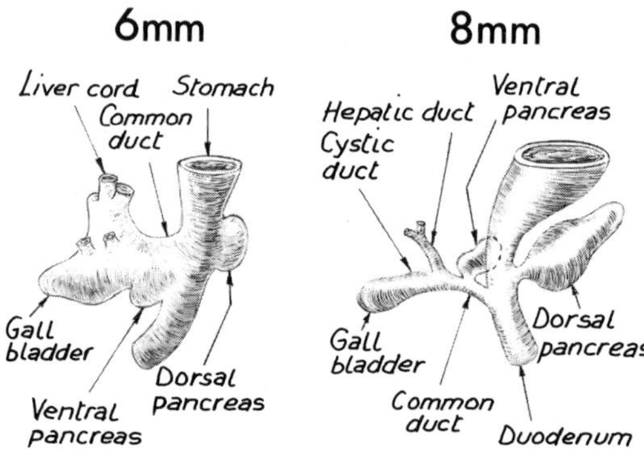

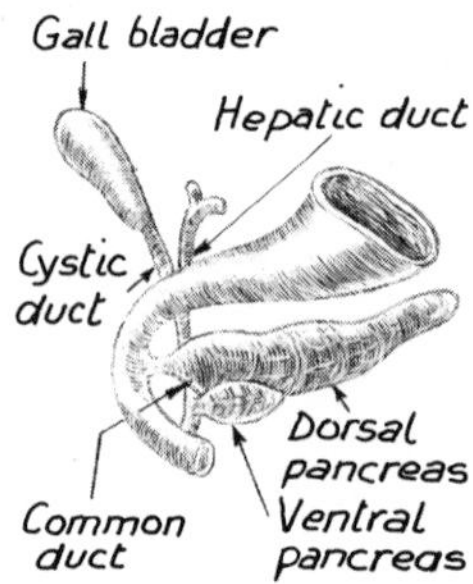

Figure 87–5. Development of the human pancreas (after Arey[1]).

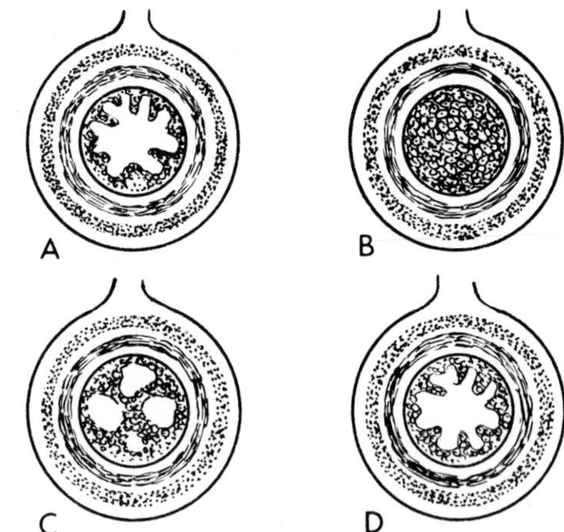

Figure 87–6. The duodenum of a normal human embryo illustrating the solid stage that exists between the 5th and 8th weeks. *A,* Before epithelial proliferation. *B,* Solid stage with concrescence of epithelial surfaces. *C,* Later stage with development of isolated vacuoles. *D,* Re-establishment of a continuous lumen.

week, its lumen becomes almost filled by epithelial cells. Indeed, in about one third of embryos the lumen is obliterated, thus converting the duodenum into a solid organ. During the eighth week, rapid regression of the epithelial hyperplasia commences and, by a process of vacuolization, the lumen is restored by the tenth week (Fig. 87–6). *Failure of recanalization may result in intestinal atresia and stenosis, while irregular vacuolization may be responsible for a localized type of duplication.*[15, 16]

Mid- and Hindgut. At the beginning of the fifth week, the arteries supplying the other parts of the digestive tube can be recognized, e.g., superior mesenteric to the midgut and inferior mesenteric to the hindgut. At the point where the mid- and hindgut join, the intestine becomes fixed to the posterior abdominal wall by a condensed part of the dorsal mesentery to form the so-called colic angle. The extremities of the midgut are thus firmly anchored by the fixed proximal duodenum above and the fixed colic angle below. These 2 points are quite close together, forming the duodenocolic isthmus.

Active growth of the mid- and hindgut begins during the fifth week, reaches a peak during the eighth week, and slows down again about the tenth week. Rapid elongation of the midgut causes it to bend ventrad in the midplane to form a U-loop with the yolk stalk attached to its apex (Fig. 87–7). The superior mesenteric artery forms the axis of this loop as it runs forward through the duodenocolic isthmus to the yolk stalk. The segments of bowel above and below the yolk stalk are designated the cranial (prearterial) and caudal (postarterial) limbs of the intestinal loop, respectively. As the loop increases in length, the superior mesenteric artery becomes tautly stretched like a cord from beginning to termination.

At this stage the bud for the cecum and appendix appears on the postarterial segment, thus demarcating the boundary between the future small and large bowel. The midgut elongates so rapidly that the intraembryonic coelom is too small to hold it, and part of the loop is extruded into the umbilical cord, forming a temporary physiologic hernia (Fig. 87–7). At the sharply curved extremity of the intraumbilical loop, the omphalomesenteric (vitellointestinal) duct communicates with the shrinking yolk sac. Normally, this duct disappears when the yolk sac becomes obliterated (seventh week), but *vestiges may persist as Meckel's diverticulum and related anomalies.*[17]

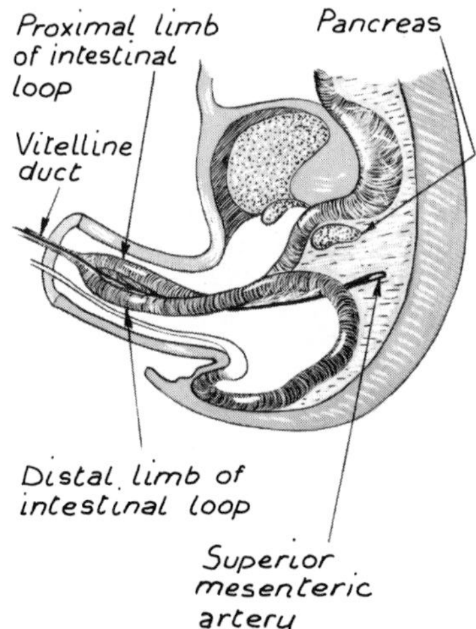

Figure 87–7. Sagittal diagram of a 6-week embryo. The midgut loop has been extruded into the umbilical cord.

Succeeding changes include enlargement, elongation, and rotation of the intestine and its final placement and fixation. Early in development, the caliber of the small intestine exceeds that of the colon, but the colon increases more rapidly in diameter to bring about the adult proportions. On the other hand, the small bowel elongates much more rapidly than the large bowel. No marked epithelial hyperplasia occurs distal to the duodenum, but in occasional embryos the hyperplasia may be sufficient to cause temporary occlusion of the proximal jejunum or colon during the sixth and seventh weeks. *Irregular vacuolization may lead to intramural duplications or atresias.*[15, 18, 19]

Rotation of the Midgut

The chronology of rotation of the midgut loop is conveniently divided into 3 stages[2, 20, 21]:

First Stage (Fig. 87–8*A*). This takes place while the loop is being extruded and is maintained while it lies in the umbilical cord between the fifth and tenth weeks. It is brought about largely by the development of the liver. The great growth of its right lobe carries the liver downward and to the right, taking the left umbilical vein (ligamentum teres) with it. This produces pressure on the base of the prearterial segment of the midgut loop, pushing it to the right and caudad. Since the pre- and postarterial segments lie side by side within the narrow confines of the umbilical cord, the movement of the prearterial portion down and to the right forces the postarterial segment to the left and cephalad. The net result is that the ends of the midgut loop have rotated through 90° in an anticlockwise direction (as one views the embryo from the ventral side).

Dott[20] believed that this completed the first stage of rotation, but most recent studies indicate that further elongation and realignment of the small bowel occur within the umbilical hernia, resulting in an additional 90° anticlockwise rotation before return of the bowel to the abdomen.[2, 21] When this has happened, the mesentery of the prearterial segment is caudad to the omphalomesenteric vessels, while the mesentery of the postarterial segment is cephalad to them.

Second Stage (Fig. 87–8*B*). By the tenth week, the abdominal cavity has increased sufficiently in size to accommodate the intestine, and the midgut loop starts returning to the abdomen from the umbilical cord. This process occurs very rapidly (perhaps in only a few seconds).[21] The bowel, being too bulky to be returned en masse, retreats in a definite sequence. The order of this sequence is determined by the retention of the cecum in the sac until the remaining gut has reduced. This depends on the bulk of the cecum in relation to the size of the umbilical ring. If the ring is abnormally large, the cecum may return unduly early, thus upsetting the sequence and causing consequent abnormal rotation. The prearterial portion returns first, commencing with its proximal portion, i.e., the distal duodenum. The returning small gut enters the abdomen to the right of the superior mesenteric artery. The space there, however, is too limited, and so the first coils are pushed across to the left *behind* the taut artery by those following. By their passage to the left, the coils of small bowel displace the dorsal mesentery of the hindgut (which occupies the midline) before them. Consequently, the descending colon comes to occupy the left flank, and the colic angle is pushed cephalad to form the future splenic

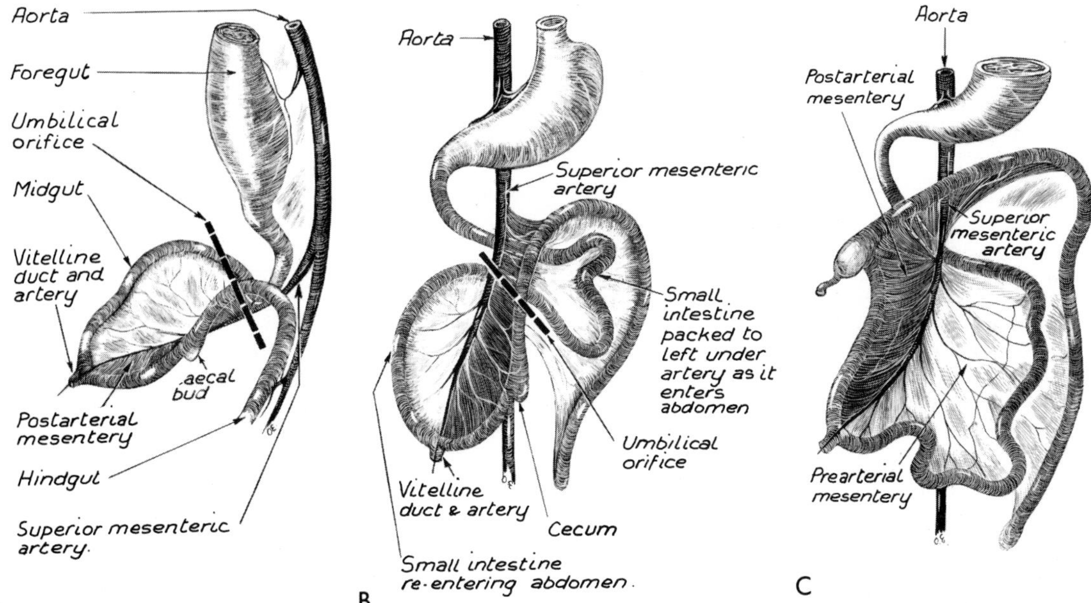

Figure 87–8. Rotation of midgut (after Dott[20]). *A*, First stage. The loop has rotated 90° counterclockwise. *B*, Second stage. The physiologic umbilical hernia is reducing. The small gut is re-entering the abdomen on the right of the superior mesenteric vessels and passing to the left side of the abdomen behind the vessels. The cecum still lies outside the umbilicus. *C*, Completion of second stage. The cecum is in contact with the posterior abdominal wall in the right loin. Midgut loop has rotated 270° counterclockwise.

flexure. The last coil of ileum carries the termination of the superior mesenteric artery with it as it is reduced. The cecum and ascending colon, which have become relatively larger than the small bowel, are the last to reduce; they pass upward and to the right and cross in front of the small bowel and origin of the superior mesenteric artery. Thus, the cecum comes to lie in the right upper quadrant under the liver, and subsequent elongation of the colon pushes it into the right loin. This completes the second stage of rotation.

At this time (eleventh week), the midgut loop has undergone a further 90° anticlockwise rotation that, added to the previous rotation of 180°, makes a total of 270° rotation on the axis of the superior mesenteric artery (Fig. 87–8C). The superior mesenteric artery thus comes to lie anterior to the third portion of the duodenum and posterior to the transverse colon, i.e., the essentials of the permanent disposition of the viscera have been attained.

Third Stage. This commences in the eleventh week and continues until shortly before birth. The cecum descends further to reach the right iliac fossa, and as the liver decreases in relative size and "retreats" cephalad, a hepatic flexure appears in the originally oblique proximal limb of the colon. This flexure becomes increasingly sharper. There next follows fixation of various parts of the gut to the posterior abdominal wall by fusion of their mesenteries with the posterior parietal peritoneum.

The dorsal mesentery of the duodenum, which has swung to the right, is almost completely resorbed. As a result, the second, third, and fourth parts of the duodenum become retroperitoneal. The blood vessels and ducts, originally within the dorsal mesentery, therefore enter the duodenum from the left or medial aspect of the duodenal curve. This arrangement permits the adult duodenum to be mobilized safely from the right along the plane of fusion.

The uppermost root of the small intestinal mesentery comes to be situated just to the left of the second lumbar vertebra. Since the cecum has carried the terminal ileum to the right lower abdomen, the attachment of its mesentery is shifted from its original straight, longitudinal line to a diagonal line from the left above to the right below at the level of the fourth or fifth lumbar vertebra.

The postarterial mesentery of the transverse colon persists as the transverse mesocolon, which fuses with the overlying greater omentum (derived from the dorsal mesogastrium). The mesenteries of the cecum, ascending colon, hepatic and splenic flexure, and the entire hindgut, except the pelvic colon, become completely obliterated by fusion with the posterior parietal peritoneum. The mesentery of the pelvic colon persists as the future pelvic mesocolon. The development of the colon permits the surgeon to safely mobilize the ascending and descending segments of the colon by dissecting from their lateral margins along the planes of fusion toward the midline.

Anomalies of the Intestines

Intestinal Atresia and Stenosis.[22–28] Congenital intestinal atresia and stenosis are common causes of intestinal obstruction in the newborn. During the period 1959 through 1978 we encountered 163 cases of intestinal atresia and stenosis at the Red Cross War Memorial Children's Hospital in Cape Town, South Africa.[22, 27] These accounted for almost one third of all infants presenting with neonatal intestinal obstruction (excluding anorectal malformations) during that period.

The term "atresia" denotes complete intrinsic occlusion of the intestinal lumen as a result of anomalous development of its walls. The term "stenosis" refers to incomplete occlusion. Clinically, there is ample justification for not making too sharp a demarcation between atresias and stenoses and for grouping them together as intrinsic obstructions of the intestine. However, certain etiologic and pathologic aspects make it desirable to recognize standard types of occlusion. Thus, in 1889, Bland-Sutton described 4 standard types (Fig. 87–9):

1. *Stenosis or incomplete occlusion.* A localized narrowing in the caliber of the bowel or a diaphragm (membrane) with a small perforation. Most stenoses are so severe that symptoms develop during the neonatal period.

2. *Atresia type 1.* A thin diaphragm or membrane. The bowel is normal in length.

3. *Atresia type 2.* Blind ends joined by a band. Only rarely is there a corresponding defect in the mesentery when the length of the bowel may be subnormal.

4. *Atresia type 3.* Disconnected blind ends with a gap in the mesentery and often a considerably shortened small bowel.

This simple morphologic classification has stood the test of time. However, since early mortality of patients born with intrinsic intestinal occlusions has declined, the long-term prognosis, which is related not only to the surgical procedure but also to the extent of intrauterine damage to the fetal small bowel, has become increasingly more relevant. For this reason we have adopted a revised classification[22, 27]:

1. *Stenosis and atresia types 1 and 2.* As before.
2. *Atresia type 3.* This is subdivided into:
   a. *Type 3a.* Blind ends with a simple gap. Loss of tissue of both bowel and mesentery has occurred and the length of the small bowel, although always subnormal, is variable. The unaffected intestine has an anatomically normal blood supply.

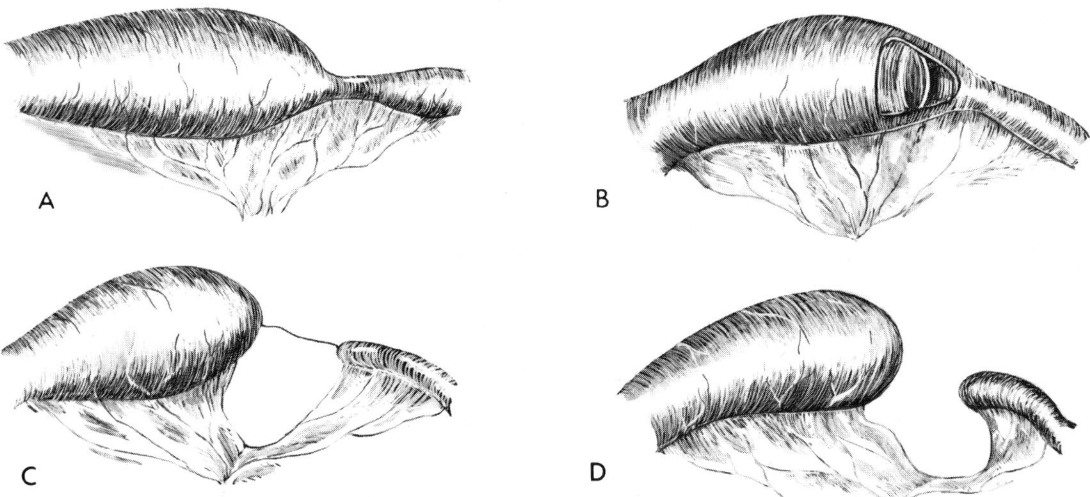

Figure 87–9. Intestinal stenosis and atresia—standard types (see text).

   b. *Type 3b.* "Apple peel" or "Christmas tree" atresia. Extensive jejunal atresia with an associated gross mesenteric defect due to an extensive infarction of the fetal midgut secondary to a proximal superior mesenteric arterial occlusion. The distal ileum remains viable and receives its blood supply via an abnormal arterial collateral source from the main arterial supply to the right colon. A significant loss of intestinal length always accompanies this type of atresia, and the unused distal bowel tends to be coiled around the feeding artery. (Fig. 87–10).

3. *Atresia type 4.* Multiple intestinal occlusions. This type includes 2 or more occlusions (atresias and stenoses) of the same or varying types, giving the appearance of a string of sausages or a Christmas tree, with multiple interruptions in the distal small bowel. There may be considerable shortening of the bowel.

In our series of 163 cases, the lesions were distributed as follows: duodenum 45%, jejunum 26%, ileum 15%, colon 1.5%, and multiple 12.5%. Multiple lesions were limited to the jejunoileum and, in fact, accounted for 20% of jejunoileal occlusions. One patient, however, had an associated duodenal atresia and 2 had associated colonic atresias.[22, 27] Stenotic and membranous lesions were particulary common in the duodenum and accounted for 70% of the duodenal occlusions. In contrast, blind ends were much more common in the jejunum and ileum and accounted for 56% of the jejunoileal occlusions. These findings conform to those of a survey by the American Academy of Pediatrics in 1967[23, 24] and of Nixon and Tawes.[28]

Prematurity and coexistent malformations are common in infants with atresia and stenosis. Here too, however, there is a striking difference between infants with duodenal occlusions and those with other types. We found that approximately 60% of the babies with duodenal occlusions weighed less than 2.3 kg and 51% had coexistent severe malformations, mostly of other systems (20% suffered from Down's syndrome). The corresponding figures for jejunoileal occlusions were 44% and 18%, respectively, and all the severe coexisting anomalies were limited to the abdomen. The Academy survey revealed that 48% of infants with duodenal occlusions had serious associated anomalies (Down's syndrome in 30%),[24] whereas only 7% of infants with jejunoileal lesions suffered from coexistent extra-abdominal malformations.[23] These differences suggest that the pathogenesis of duodenal atresia may differ from that of atresia of the rest of the bowel.

Pathogenesis. In 1900 Tandler first demonstrated that the human duodenum passes through a solid stage between the fifth and eighth weeks of embryonic life. He suggested that arrest of development during this stage was responsible for intestinal atresia (see Fig. 87–6). Johnson[29] and others have confirmed his observations.[18, 30, 31] Failure of recanaliza-

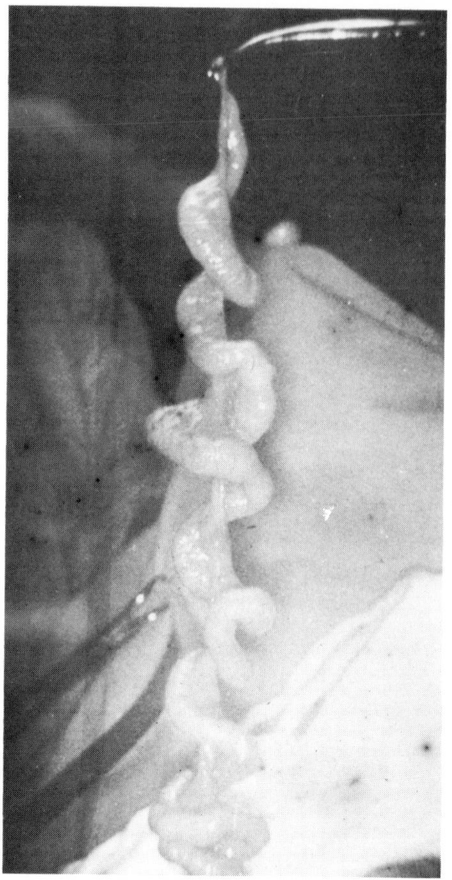

Figure 87–10. "Apple peel" or "Christmas tree" atresia (see text).

tion could, theoretically, leave a diaphragm or a stenotic area (the common types of duodenal occlusion) or even a solid segment, but it is difficult to conceive how this process could account for disconnected blind ends. Moreover, this solid stage occurs in the duodenum of only about one third of human embryos and is rarely seen in the proximal jejunum and colon. The factors responsible for arrest of growth during the solid stage have not been elucidated. The frequent coexistence of other malformations with duodenal atresia, however, suggests an insult affecting the embryo as a whole at an early stage of embryogenesis. Such an insult would especially affect the areas of active growth at the time,[32] and during the seventh and eighth weeks the duodenum is the most actively growing part of the gastrointestinal tract.[33]

Atresia of the rest of the small bowel and the colon is not as easily explained on the basis of Tandler's theory. However, in many cases there is evidence that the atresia might result from infarction of the bowel late in fetal life. In our series, there was evidence of a "fetal accident" (volvulus, intussusception, snaring at the umbilical ring) in 30% of infants with jejunoileal occlusions. The Academy series revealed a probable cause (malrotation, volvulus, gastroschisis, intussusception) in 25% of infants and meconium ileus with intrauterine perforation or volvulus in 9%.[23] In our series, the anomalies associated with jejunoileal occlusions were mostly of such a type as to predispose to strangulation of the fetal bowel, e.g., omphalocele, gastroschisis, meconium peritonitis, and malrotation with midgut volvulus. In addition, 34% of the infants had a rotational anomaly or defective intestinal fixation that would predispose to volvulus and intussusception.[22, 27]

By experimental work on pregnant dogs, we have proved conclusively that interruption of the blood supply to a loop of fetal bowel late in pregnancy may produce all the varieties of intestinal atresia found in human infants.[33, 34] This work, which has been confirmed by others in dogs,[5, 35] rabbits,[36] sheep,[37] and chickens,[36, 38] also accounts for the apparent impairment of the blood supply to the blind ends frequently encountered at surgery. Moreover, a localized vascular accident occurring late in fetal life, rather than a more generalized insult during earlier embryogenesis, explains the low incidence of coexistent abnormalities of extra-abdominal organs in infants suffering from jejunoileal and colonic atresias. It should also be noted that in fully 30% of patients with jejunoileal atresias, meconium (containing epithelial squames and/or bile) is present in the stools. Since bile is not secreted until the eleventh week of embryonic life and the skin has no squames until the third month, such atresias must obviously have occurred late in fetal life after the solid stage (eighth week) and, indeed, after the third month. (Tibboel et al.[36, 38] have shown that atresia in chick embryos may also follow intestinal perforation with meconium peritonitis at a somewhat earlier stage.)

Clinical Manifestations. Ultrasound evaluation of the fetus during the last 3 months of pregnancy has sharply advanced the recognition of intestinal obstruction in the fetus. The obstructed and dilated fetal intestine is fluid-filled and therefore most suitable for assessment by this technique. Reports are now appearing in which accurate diagnosis of fetal intestinal obstruction has been made prenatally.[39–44] This may occur incidentally during an investigation carried out to determine the biparietal diameter of the fetal skull or to assess the fetus in a pregnancy complicated by polyhydramnios. Indeed, between 20% and 30% of mothers carrying fetuses with high small intestinal obstructions develop polyhydramnios during the last trimester.[23] During the past 2 years we have treated 8 infants with intestinal atresia diagnosed prenatally by ultrasonography (Fig. 87–11). In all of them, polyhydramnios was the indication for the investigation, which we now consider essential whenever this complication of pregnancy occurs. Forewarned is forearmed, and the infant born with a congenital intestinal obstruction diagnosed in utero must have a better prognosis than the unfortunate patient whose diagnosis is missed for a number of days after birth. Indeed, it may be feasible in the future to correct the problem by intrauterine surgery before birth.[45]

Polyhydramnios is the most important prenatal clue to atresia. The family history is also of some benefit. Familial forms have been described in which siblings have had intestinal atresias due to fetal intussusceptions.[46] Intestinal atresia may complicate mucoviscidosis,[47, 48] and familial forms associated with anomalies of intestinal rotation and/or fixation have also been reported.[49] A positive family history, therefore, may indicate the need for early diagnostic amniocentesis. Although most jejunoileal and colonic atresias apparently occur during the second or third trimester, many duodenal atresias occur early (eighth week); some of the more distal occlusions may occur during the fifth to eleventh week owing to snaring of the intestine within the extra-abdominal coelom. Increased bile salt concentration and disaccharide activity in the amniotic fluid may indicate the presence of intestinal obstruction.[50] Amniofetography may confirm this suspicion, but the effect of iodide contrast dyes on the fetal thyroid is not yet known.

In all atresias and the majority of stenoses, symptoms develop within the first 1 or 2 days of life. In less severe stenoses, symptoms may be delayed for weeks, months, or even years. The classic features are neonatal vomiting, varying abdominal distention, and inadequate evacuation of meconium. Dehydration and fever soon become manifest and aspiration pneumonia is common in neglected cases. Non-hemolytic jaundice occurs

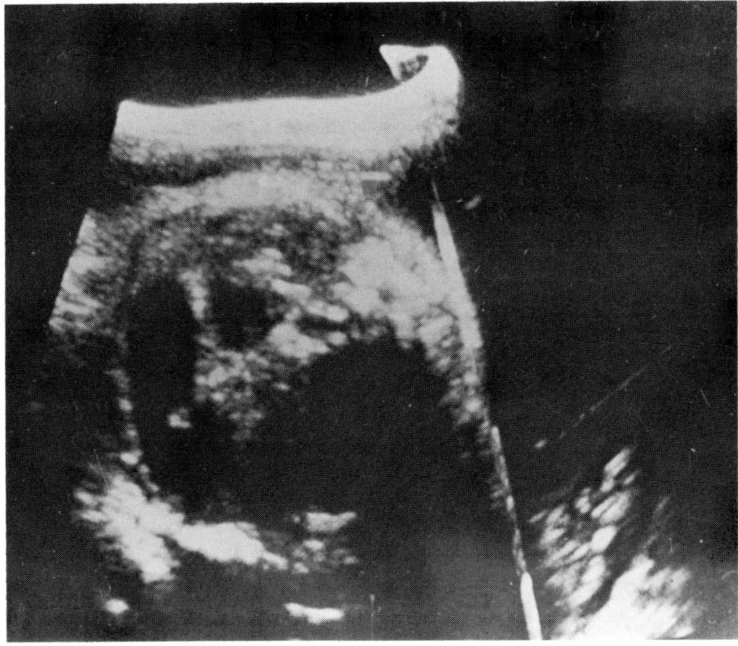

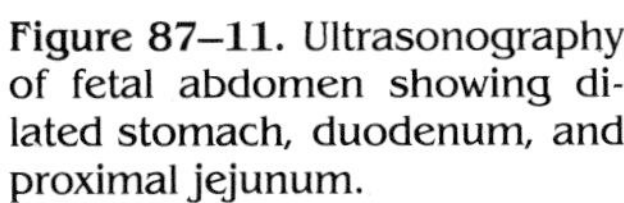

Figure 87–11. Ultrasonography of fetal abdomen showing dilated stomach, duodenum, and proximal jejunum.

in approximately 40% of duodenal occlusions, 30% of jejunal occlusions, and 20% of ileal occlusions.

Vomiting is the most constant and usually the first symptom. In duodenal occlusions it is bile-stained in 75% of the infants (in supra-ampullary lesions no bile is present unless there is splitting of the choledochus). In jejunoileal and colonic lesions the vomitus is usually, but not necessarily, bile-stained. Bilious vomiting in a neonate is always a danger signal. In the absence of an obvious medical explanation to account for it, prompt investigation to exclude intestinal obstruction is required.

Distention is not a prominent sign in duodenal lesions, being present in only 30% of cases. It progressively increases with more distal lesions and is present in 98% of infants with ileal occlusions.

Absolute constipation is not a constant feature but most of the infants fail to evacuate meconium adequately within the first 48 hours after birth. Some meconium is passed by approximately 50% of infants with duodenal occlusions (mainly stenoses and supra-ampullary atresias) and by 30% of those with jejunoileal occlusions. Although the meconium may appear normal, the "stools" are usually small and hard and delayed beyond 24 hours. On the other hand, they may be bile-stained and contain squames even when there is complete discontinuity of the bowel. Farber's test[51] for identification of squames in the meconium is therefore not always helpful in differentiating complete from incomplete obstruction.

Diagnosis. A nasogastric tube should be passed at birth in all infants considered to be at risk. These include neonates in whom prenatal ultrasonography provided a positive result, all babies born of a pregnancy complicated by polyhydramnios, and those who manifest an obvious congenital abnormality of surrounding parietal structures enclosing the abdominal viscera. Dysmorphic anomalies of this type, which may be complicated by intestinal atresia, include omphalocele, gastroschisis, and posterolateral diaphragmatic hernia. The largest firm red rubber catheter that can be introduced through the nostril should be used. This maneuver is carried out first and foremost to exclude esophageal atresia. If no esophageal anomaly is encountered, emptying the stomach of its content may provide useful information. An aspirate in excess of 25 ml is regarded as indicative of a pathologic lesion. A bile-stained aspirate may suggest the presence of a high but postampullary complete small intestinal obstruction. In such cases, a small amount of air should be injected through the nasogastric tube to act as a contrast and the patient referred for radiologic investigation.

Abdominal radiographs are imperative in all infants presenting with the postnatal warning signs just outlined. A diagnosis of obstruction can usually be confirmed by plain radiographs of the abdomen taken with the infant in the erect and inverted positions. These will reveal dilated, gas-filled loops of bowel with fluid levels, and the pattern may indicate the site of the obstruction. However, if the obstructed bowel is completely filled with fluid, air-fluid levels may be absent. The gastric contents should be aspirated in these instances and a small amount of air injected through the nasogastric tube; this will produce the typical picture.[52]

In *duodenal atresia,* the erect film usually shows the classic double bubble (attributable to air-fluid levels in the dilated stomach and first part of the duodenum) with absence of gas beyond the duodenum (Fig. 87–12). A contrast enema will demonstrate a narrow, unused "microcolon," unless the obstruction

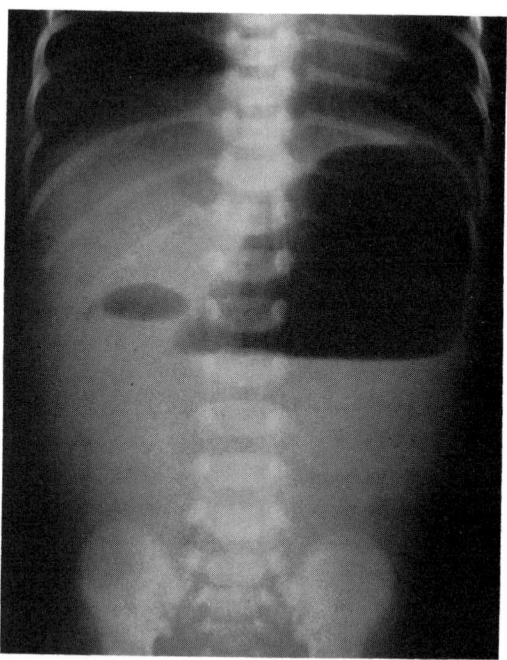

Figure 87–12. The typical "double bubble" of duodenal atresia (see text).

is supra-ampullary. In this case, the colon may be normally distended by the passage of biliary and pancreatic secretions. In *duodenal stenosis,* a double bubble may or may not be seen, depending on the severity of the obstruction. Small quantities of gas will also be visible in the distal bowel. Sometimes it may be necessary to inject air or a small quantity of barium through the nasogastric tube to confirm a duodenal stenosis.[52]

In *jejunoileal occlusions,* the plain films will reveal multiple air-fluid levels, sometimes with a particularly large loop immediately proximal to the obstruction (Fig. 87–13). Ileal occlusions may be difficult to differentiate from colonic obstructions and therefore a contrast enema is necessary. This may also reveal a "microcolon" in infants with complete small bowel occlusion (Fig. 87–14), an associated colonic atresia or stenosis, and/or associated malrotation.

Treatment. Surgical intervention is mandatory and should await only decompression of the proximal gastrointestinal tract by nasogastric catheter and adequate correction of fluid and electrolyte derangements. The tiny baby tolerates operative intervention all the better with a few hours of preoperative supportive care and should not be taken to the operating room until an optimum condition has been reached.

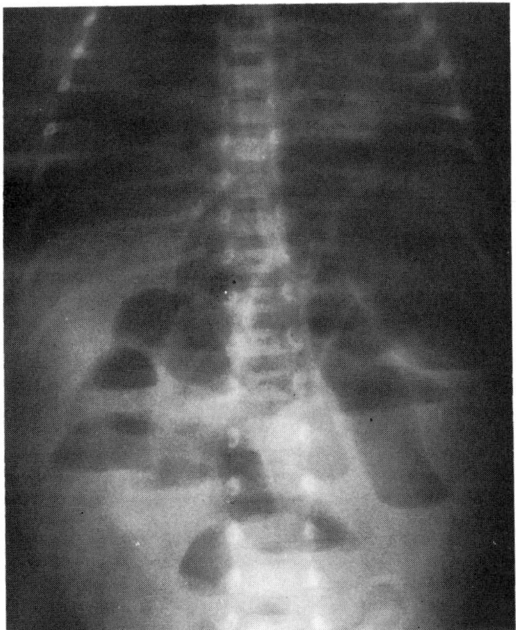

Figure 87–13. Multiple fluid levels in an infant with ileal atresia.

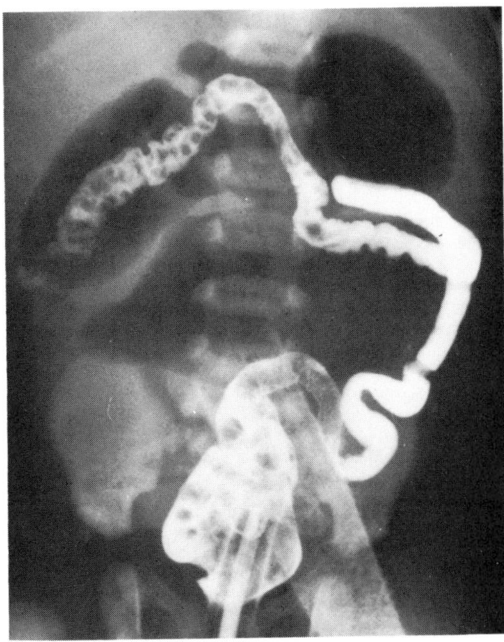

Figure 87–14. "Microcolon" in an infant with jejunal atresia.

When the diagnosis is made during the first 3 days of life and the obstruction is not complicated by perforation of the bowel or aspiration pneumonia, little preparation is necessary. Nevertheless, an IV drip should always be set up to rehydrate the infant, to correct metabolic acidosis, and to facilitate blood transfusion during operation. When the bowel has perforated (as a result of postnatal necrosis of the ischemic blind ends in jejunoileal occlusions), the infants are usually in severe shock with gross distention, enlarged veins, and abdominal tenderness. This requires energetic fluid therapy. If abdominal distention causes respiratory distress, intermittent positive pressure breathing is often lifesaving. Needle puncture may even be necessary to relieve the intra-abdominal pressure.

The choice of operation can be made only when the abnormal anatomy has been defined. It is essential in all cases to look for additional atretic areas and coexistent malrotation with obstructive bands. The procedure of choice in duodenal occlusions is a direct oblique duodenoduodenostomy to avoid a blind loop, although a duodenojejunostomy may be necessary for technical reasons. The anastomosis should be supplemented by a gastrostomy for decompression and the insertion of a transanastomotic Silastic feeding tube. In jejunoileal and colonic occlusions, liberal resection of the proximal dilated, atonic, and ischemic blind end is essential, and limited resection of the distal blind end is advisable. Resection in high jejunal atresias may have to be limited up to the duodenal flexure. Tailoring of the proximal dilated segment in the form of a duodenojejunoplasty is then advised.[53] A similar procedure may be necessary in other lesions when the length of remaining bowel is critical. (In our opinion the surgeon should aim at leaving not less than 75 cm of small bowel, and in distal ileal lesions the ileocecal valve should be preserved if possible.) Direct anastomosis of blind ends and simple puncture or excision of membranous lesions should be avoided. An oblique end-to-end (end-to-back) single-layer anastomosis is the best, although variations may be necessary. In high jejunal occlusions, a supplementary gastrostomy with transanastomotic feeding tube is advisable. In distal ileal lesions complicated by perforation or meconium peritonitis in poor-risk infants, a Bishop-Koop[54] decompressive anastomosis may be preferable. In neglected colonic atresias, a simple loop colostomy may be lifesaving.

Results of Treatment. Survival statistics in pediatric surgery are of little significance unless the type of patient operated upon is taken into account. Three "risk" groups, designated A (good), B (intermediate), and C (poor), and based on weight and the presence of associated abnormalities are recognized. In general, the mortality in group C cases can be expected to remain very high.[28]

For duodenal occlusions, Nixon and Tawes[28] report 88% survival in groups A and B and 21% in group C. Because of the high incidence of associated malformations, 40% of their patients were placed in group C, which brought the overall survival down to 61%. In the American Academy of Pediatrics survey,[24] the overall survival rate for duodenal atresia and stenosis was 64%; in our series the figure was 75%.

For jejunoileal occlusions, Nixon and Tawes[28] report 81% survival for groups A and B and 32% for group C, with an overall survival rate of 62%. In our series, the survival rates were 95% for A and B, 73% for C, and 88% for all cases. Nixon and Tawes have also found that the survival rate is less favorable in proximal lesions, e.g., high jejunal 55%, mid small intestinal 66%, and terminal ileal 78%. In the Academy series, the survival was 58% for jejunal and 72% for ileal atresias.[23] Paradoxically, the prognosis in colonic atresias seems to be poorer. However, the condition is so rare that no single surgeon has been able to report a large recently treated series.

In general, the survival of infants with congenital atresias has increased appreciably during recent years. Associated malformations, especially congenital heart disease, are still responsible for a significant mortality in duodenal occlusions. In jejunoileal occlusions, respiratory complications, sepsis, functional obstruction at the anastomosis, and especially the short bowel syndrome following resection for "apple peel" and multiple atresias preclude universally satisfactory results.

Duplications of the Alimentary Tract.[2, 48, 55–60] The term "duplications of the alimentary tract," which was introduced by Ladd[57] in 1937, signifies spherical or tubular structures firmly attached to, and sometimes communicating with, a part of the alimentary tract anywhere from the mouth to the anus. These structures have a well-developed coat of smooth muscle and an epithelial lining resembling gastrointestinal mucosa. They are invariably situated on the mesenteric side of the digestive tract and share the same blood supply. Previously these structures were referred to as enterogenous cysts, enteric cysts, or diverticula.

From the point of view of embryogenesis, duplications are conveniently classified into 3 broad varieties: (1) localized abdominal duplications, (2) duplications associated with malformations of the spinal cord, and (3) complete duplication of the colon.[2]

Localized Abdominal Duplications. These are most frequent in the ileum but also occur in the duodenum, jejunum, ileocecal region, colon, and rectum. They may present as spherical cysts projecting into the lumen of the gut or closely attached to its mesenteric border, or they may be of the tubular type (Fig. 87–15). Symptoms are caused by intraluminal intestinal obstruction, intussusception, or volvulus. Occasionally, duplications reach such enormous proportions that they may compress the bowel or compromise its blood supply. They are frequently lined by gastric mucosa, and if there is a communication with the adjacent bowel, peptic ulceration, complicated by perforation or hemorrhage, may occur.

These duplications seem to be the result of

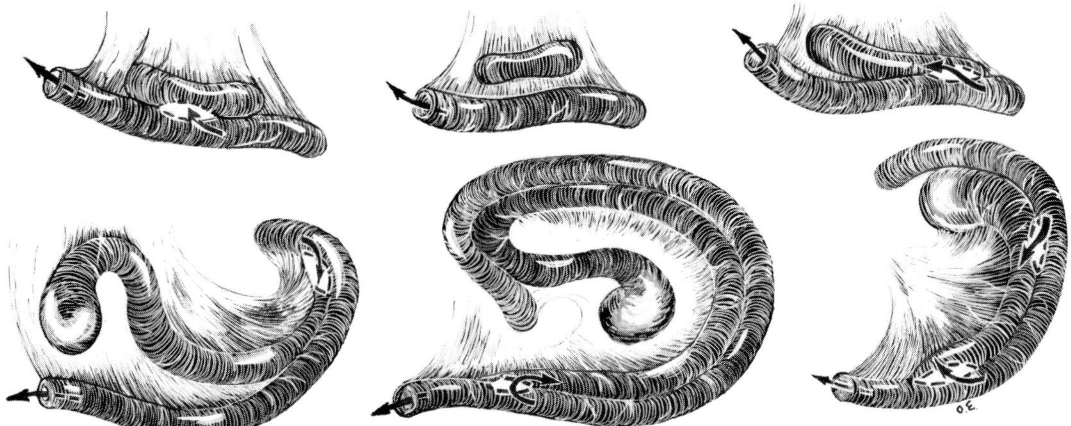

Figure 87–15. Various types of localized intestinal duplications. Note the bulbous ends in several of the specimens (redrawn from Bremer[15]).

localized faults in the development of the gut. Bremer[19] first attributed them to overgrowth of intestinal buds or diverticula, which, according to Lewis and Thyng,[61] develop around the circumference of the bowel of animal and human embryos of 4 to 23 mm (Fig. 87–16*A*). Although this theory may account for the spherical cysts, it fails to explain their frequent location on the mesenteric border of the gut and cannot explain tubular malformations. Bremer[15] therefore suggested that the latter originated from abnormal persistence of the vacuoles that are normally formed in the process of recanalization of the solid stage of the intestine. These vacuoles tend to form in longitudinal chains and then to coalesce with each other to re-form the lumen of the gut. If such chains of fused vacuoles retain their form, they could cause intestinal duplications (Fig. 87–16*B*). However, this theory fails to explain the location of the duplications on the mesenteric border of the bowel and the presence of a complete muscular coat.

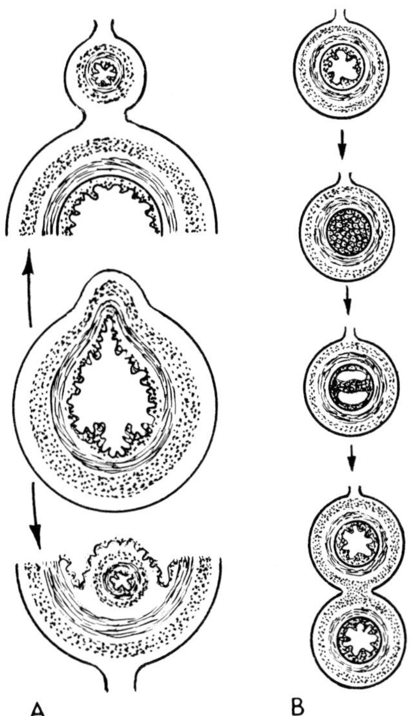

Figure 87–16. Two theories of duplication. *A*, Budding diverticula may become isolated as cysts within the mesentery or when failing to penetrate the muscle coats as intraluminal duplications. *B*, Incomplete coalescence of vacuoles during recanalization of the solid stage may result in duplicate lumina (redrawn from Bremer[15]).

Duplications Associated with Vertebral and Other Anomalies. In 1943, Saunders[62] pointed out that thoracic duplications situated in the posterior mediastinum often extended caudally through the diaphragm into the abdomen where they ended blindly or communicated with the duodenum or jejunum. He also found that they were frequently associated with malformations of the cervical and upper thoracic vertebrae and that some were attached to a vertebral body or communicated with the spinal canal. These findings have been confirmed by others.[5, 6] There have also been descriptions of anterior spina bifida traversed by coils of gut and of intestinal fistulas penetrating a dorsal vertebra. Similar anomalies of the sacrum associated with duplications of the rectum have been described,[63] and Rickham[64] and Johnston[10] have suggested that the same might apply to some duplications of the small bowel.

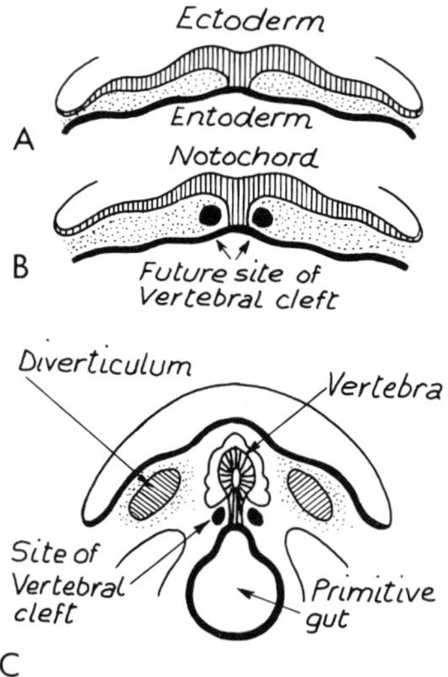

Figure 87–17. The split notochord theory (after McLetchie et al.[59]). *A,* Adhesions between ectoderm and entoderm. *B,* Duplication of notochord. *C,* Formation of intestinal duplication with malformation of vertebra.

These anomalies are probably due to splitting of the notochord.[5, 59, 62] This theory postulates that abnormal adhesion of the primitive ectoderm and entoderm prevents ingrowth of mesodermal cells, thus rendering ventral closure of the spinal column impossible (Fig. 87–17). It explains the association of vertebral anomalies and alimentary tract duplications as well as the occurrence of entodermal remnants inside the spinal canal.[59]

Complete Duplication of the Colon. Complete doubling of the colon with multiple associated anomalies of the lower half of the body is a rare variant of duplication.[48, 60, 65] It usually forms part of the syndrome known as exstrophy of the cloaca (vesicointestinal fissure), first described in detail by Sir Arthur Keith in 1908.[66] Although variations occur, the majority of cases show the same basic pattern.[64, 67-69] There is exstrophy of the urinary bladder, which is bifid. Between the 2 halves is a zone of intestinal mucosa with an upper orifice leading into the terminal ileum (which often prolapses) and a lower orifice leading into a shortened colon that ends in front of the sacrum. The exposed bowel is the cecum. The latter may be duplicated, often with double appendices. The blind colon may also be duplicated, as are the external genitalia. The rectum and anus are absent, and there are often associated upper urinary tract anomalies, omphalocele, and spina bifida with meningomyelocele.

The fundamental fault in the genesis of this anomaly is failure of the primitive mesoderm to invade the allantoic extension of the cloacal membrane (infraumbilical membrane), so that ectoderm and entoderm remain in abnormal contact in the developing lower abdominal wall. Because of the absence of intervening mesoderm, this extension is liable to dehisce and to disintegrate, just like the cloacal membrane itself. According to Johnston,[10] exstrophy of the cloaca is caused by premature dehiscence of the cloacal membrane as well as its infraumbilical extension before formation of the urorectal septum at the 5 mm stage.

Duplications of the colon occasionally exist without the other anomalies just mentioned. A number of cases have been recorded in which the condition was associated with anorectal agenesis and rectourethral fistula.[48, 60, 68] Griess et al.[65] reported a case of complete duplication of the colon in a woman who was in good health at the age of 30 years. These anomalies appear to be similar in origin to the localized abdominal duplications involving shorter segments of bowel.

Uncommon Congenital Diverticula.[2, 48, 70] Apart from Meckel's diverticulum, congenital diverticula of the gastrointestinal tract are rare. They should be distinguished from duplications and particularly from the relatively common acquired diverticula of various parts of the bowel.

Duodenal diverticula are commonly seen as an incidental finding during barium meal examinations. They are rare before the age of 30 years, but the incidence rises rapidly after the age of 50. About 70% occur in the second part of the duodenum on its concavity in close proximity to the entry of the common duct; they are also found in the third and fourth parts at the points of entry of blood vessels. The diverticula may be multiple and more than 30% of patients have concomitant diverticula of the colon (Chapter 85).

The findings just mentioned, coupled with the fact that the walls of these diverticula usually consist of mucosa alone, strongly suggest that they are not congenital but are secondary to pulsion through a weakened area in the duodenal wall; however, some may be congenital. In 1932, Boyden[71] pointed out that in some embryos the hepatic bud bifurcates soon after its appearance during the fourth week. He postulated that subdivision of the bud at this period, when growth changes are extremely rapid, offers an explanation for the occasional occurrence of double common bile ducts in man. MacGregor and duPlessis[72] have gone further and suggested that persistence of the proximal part of one of these ducts may be responsible for the development of a congenital duodenal diverticulum. The so-called vaterian and perivaterian duodenal diverticula may also be congenital.[72] In the former, the ampulla of Vater is dilated into a considerable diverticulum with a narrow orifice resembling the extramural dilated ampulla of certain animals, such as seals and guinea pigs. In the latter, the pancreatic and common bile ducts open into the apex of a wide-mouthed duodenal diverticulum not unlike that of elephants and whales. In both types, heterotopic pancreatic tissue may be present in the diverticulum.

Diverticula of the small bowel are uncommon. Most are of the acquired type, occurring close to the mesenteric attachment where mucosa herniates through the point of entry of a blood vessel (Chapter 111). Diverticula, probably of congenital origin, have occasionally been found in the small intestine. They are usually solitary, with walls composed of all the coats of the intestine. Unlike duplications and acquired diverticula, they are most often seen on the antimesenteric border. Their pathogenesis is unknown, but it is possible that they represent persistence of the embryonic diverticula described by Lewis and Thyng.[61]

Diverticula of the colon are acquired and are discussed elsewhere (Chapter 135). The solitary diverticulum of the cecum, however, is probably congenital.[73] It is usually situated on the medial wall near the ileocecal junction and often contains a fecolith. Unless complicated, it is symptomless and its presence is disclosed as a chance finding on barium enema examination. Diverticulitis may occur and tends to develop before the age of 40 years. The acute cases are usually diagnosed as acute appendicitis or Crohn's disease. Subacute inflammation of the diverticulum may produce an ulcer. Indeed, there are good reasons for believing that the so-called solitary ulcers of the cecum are, in fact, examples of cecal diverticulitis.[73]

Meckel's Diverticulum.[2, 48, 60, 72, 74, 75] Failure of complete obliteration of the yolk stalk (vitelline or omphalomesenteric duct) may be responsible for several anomalous conditions. Of these, Meckel's diverticulum is by far the most common and most significant (Fig. 87–18*A*). The defect represents persistence of the intra-abdominal portion of the vitelline duct and was first correctly described by Johann Friedrich Meckel, the younger, in 1809.[17] The diverticulum arises from the antimesenteric border of the ileum. In adults, it is usually situated about 60 cm, but sometimes up to 130 cm, from the ileocecal junction. In infants, the maximum distance is 40 cm. Most frequently, it exists as a simple diverticulum approximately 5 cm in length (range 1 to 11 cm), but it may have loculations. The diameter is usually slightly less than that of the ileum but considerably

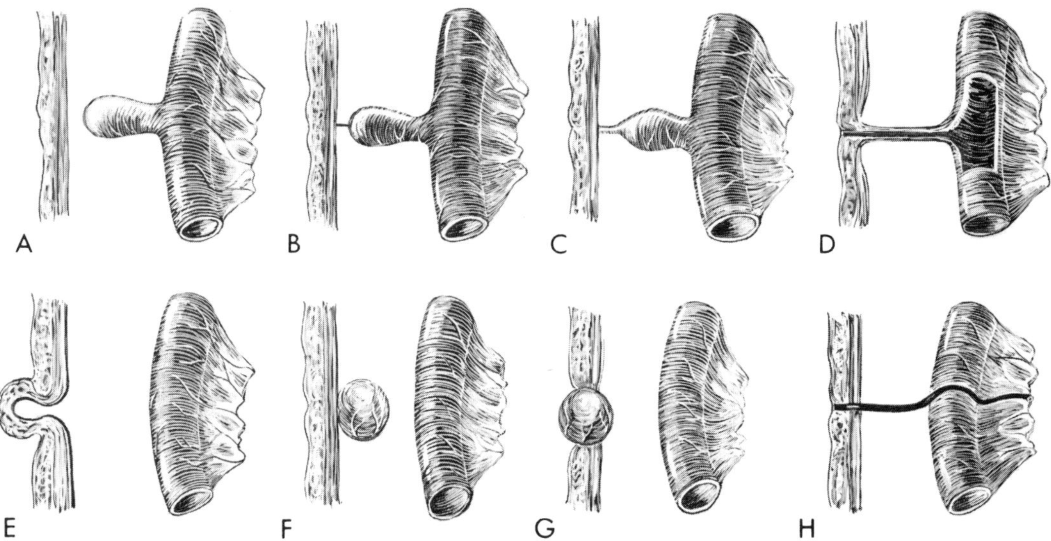

Figure 87–18. Anomalies of the vitello-intestinal duct (see text).

greater than that of the appendix. Its blood supply is derived from the right vitelline artery, which arises as an end artery from the superior mesenteric artery and reaches the diverticulum in a mesodiverticular fold. A fibrous cord may be attached to the apex of the diverticulum, and the distal end of this cord may be free or attached to the posterior aspect of the umbilicus (Fig. 87–18*B*), to the mesentery, or to other structures. Rarely there may be a fistulous tract between Meckel's diverticulum and the umbilicus (Fig. 87–18*C*).

These diverticula possess all 3 coats of the intestinal wall. The mucosal lining is similar to that of the adjacent ileum, but ectopic tissue is present in more than 50% of resected specimens. About 70% to 80% of the ectopic tissue is gastric and the remainder includes pancreatic, duodenal, jejunal, and even biliary and colonic tissue.

Meckel's diverticula occur in approximately 2% of the population, and necropsy figures reveal an equal sex distribution. The vast majority remain uncomplicated, to be discovered as an incidental finding at laparotomy or necropsy. In 1962 Weinstein et al.[75] found that 70% of Meckel's diverticula resected at the Mayo Clinic were incidental findings.

Complications. These tend to occur more frequently in infants and young children; approximately one third develop in the first year of life and another one third in the succeeding 2 years. An interesting finding is that complications are much more common in males, especially during childhood. In 1969 Androulakis et al.[74] reported the male preponderance of complicated Meckel's diverticulum as 8 to 1 in children and 2 to 1 in adults. At the Red Cross War Memorial Children's Hospital, Cape Town, the male to female ratio is 3 to 1.

The principal complications are intestinal obstruction, peptic ulceration, and acute inflammation. Their relative frequency is related to the age of the patient. In children, acute intestinal obstruction is the most common, with peptic ulceration a close second; in adults, diverticulitis heads the list. All other complications are uncommon.

OBSTRUCTION. Obstruction may be caused by a variety of mechanisms: *Intussusception,* with the diverticulum forming the apex of the intussusception, is the most common cause of obstruction. A short diverticulum with a broad base and a bulbous apex (owing to the presence of inflamed heterotopic tissue) predisposes to this complication. *Volvulus* may occur around the attachment of a Meckel's diverticulum to the back of the umbilicus or to other intra-abdominal structures. The obstruction is of the closed loop variety with its attendant risks of early necrosis and gangrene. *Snaring* of a loop of intestine is not uncommon. It may be caused by a fibrous band connecting a Meckel's diverticulum to the abdominal wall, the mesentery, or other structures; by the mesodiverticular fold carrying the vitelline artery; or by an abnormal attachment of a long Meckel's diverticulum to some other viscus. The obstruction also tends to be of the closed loop variety. Very rarely, a long diverticulum may form a true *knot* around a loop of intestine. In the few cases reported, the diverticula had large bulbous ends owing to ectopic tissue. Meckel's diverticulum may find its way into a hernial sac and may become obstructed and strangulated *(Littre's hernia).* In most of the reported cases, an inguinal hernia has been involved, but the condition has been found in umbilical, ventral, femoral, and even sciatic and lumbar hernias.

PEPTIC ULCERATION. The heterotopic gastric mucosa within a Meckel's diverticulum may be responsible for peptic ulceration in the diverticulum itself or in the ileum distal to it. The ulceration is subject to the usual complications of hemorrhage, which may be massive (particularly in children under the age of 3 years); perforation, and cicatricial stenosis. Since Meckel's diverticulum is relatively mobile and unprotected within the abdomen, perforation is usually complicated by rapidly spreading peritonitis.

INFLAMMATION. Acute Meckel's diverticulitis may occur. This change is relatively much less common than acute appendicitis because Meckel's diverticula are usually short, with a wide base that allows free passage of the fecal stream. Long diverticula with a narrow base, however, are prone to infection, which may be complicated by perforation and spreading peritonitis.

Chronic inflammation of the diverticulum with the development of concretions containing calcium has been reported, as have tuberculosis and Crohn's disease.

FOREIGN BODY PERFORATION. Less than 50 cases have been reported. Fish bones are most commonly responsible. Cocktail sticks and pine needles have also been found.

TUMORS. These are also extremely rare. The

tumors most frequently encountered have been carcinoids, sarcomas, and carcinomas.

UMBILICAL PATHOLOGY. A Meckel's diverticulum associated with patency of the distal part of the vitellointestinal duct may be responsible for a fecal discharge from the umbilicus.

Clinical Manifestations. Meckel's diverticula are symptomless unless complicated. The presenting symptoms depend on the complication.

INTESTINAL OBSTRUCTION. Acute intestinal obstruction presents with the usual picture of colicky abdominal pain, vomiting, distention, and constipation. Intussusception is the common type of obstruction in children, and typical "red currant jelly" stools may be passed. Obstruction by volvulus, snaring, and Littre's hernia is often associated with symptoms and signs of strangulation. Symptoms of chronic intestinal obstruction may develop as a sequel to stenosis of the ileum because of chronic peptic ulceration.

BLEEDING PER RECTUM. This is a sequel to peptic ulceration and is usually painless. The blood varies in amount and appearance. It is usually fairly copious and intermediate in color between the bright red of colonic lesions and the melena of upper gastrointestinal tract disease. In brisk hemorrhages, fresh blood may be passed per rectum. Hematemesis has also been reported,[60] but we have not observed this symptom. Chronic blood loss with the development of iron deficiency anemia is rare.

ABDOMINAL PAIN. The clinical picture of acute Meckel's diverticulitis is almost indistinguishable from that of acute appendicitis, although the symptoms and signs of the former tend to be localized around and below the umbilicus. Failure to demonstrate an inflamed appendix at laparotomy demands a search for a Meckel's diverticulum. Perforation of Meckel's diverticulum by a peptic ulcer or a foreign body may also be responsible for acute abdominal pain. The early onset of generalized peritonitis should suggest this diagnosis.

"Dyspepsia meckeli," due to peptic ulceration or subacute Meckel's diverticulitis, has been described in children. It is said to be characterized by feeding difficulties and bouts of abdominal pain occurring 15 to 30 minutes after meals and subsiding after about an hour when the food has reached the ileum.

Diagnosis. Most Meckel's diverticula are found by chance. In infants and children with abdominal complaints, a diagnosis of Meckel's diverticulum must always be entertained. It is the usual cause of massive, painless rectal bleeding in this age group and an important cause of intestinal obstruction and peritonitis.

A calcified concretion in a Meckel's diverticulum may be seen on a plain radiograph and will provide a clue to the diagnosis. Demonstration of a Meckel's diverticulum by barium meal is possible, although seldom achieved; the use of a bolus of barium provides more positive results. Unfortunately, when the information is most needed it is least available because the inflamed or obstructed diverticulum cannot be filled with barium. Jewett et al.[76] reported in 1970 that Meckel's diverticula that contain gastric mucosa could be readily identified by the use of ^{99m}Tc-pertechnetate. This has been confirmed by us in recent cases (Fig. 87–19). The success of the method depends upon the affinity of the isotope for the parietal cells of the gastric glands, but it is of questionable value during active bleeding. Angiography has also been used to visualize a bleeding Meckel's diverticulum.[77]

Treatment. The treatment of a complicated Meckel's diverticulum is excision. If the adjacent ileum is affected by a complicating lesion, e.g., peptic ulceration, inflammation, or strangulation, it should be removed with the diverticulum. Most surgeons agree that if a Meckel's diverticulum is encountered as

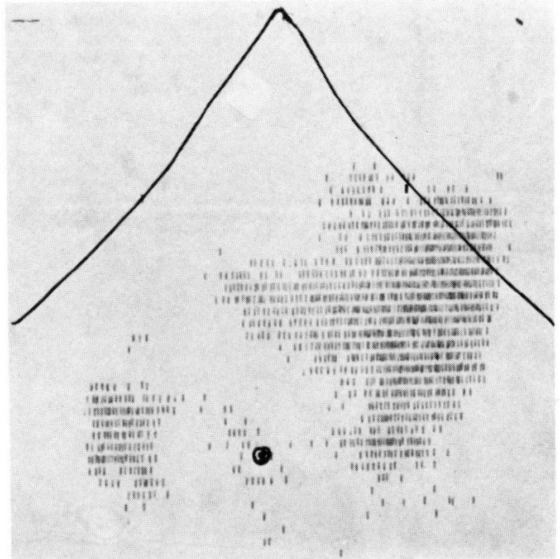

Figure 87–19. ^{99m}Tc-pertechnetate scan showing uptake of the isotope in the stomach and in a Meckel's diverticulum.

an incidental finding at laparotomy, it should be removed, provided the primary pathology and the condition of the patient permit further surgery.

Other Vitelline Remnants.[2, 48, 60, 72] A *patent vitelline duct* (Fig. 87–18*D*) represents complete failure of obliteration of the duct. An umbilical fistula exists that communicates directly with the ileum or with the apex of a Meckel's diverticulum. Usually the tract is narrow, with discharge of only small quantities of feces at the umbilicus. Occasionally there may be a wide tract with a profuse fecal leak and even prolapse of ileum through the patent duct, resulting in a complicated variety of intussusception.

An *umbilical sinus (enterotoma)* (Fig. 87–18*E*) results from persistence of the umbilical end of the vitelline duct. Because it is turned inside out by intra-abdominal pressure, it has the appearance of a raspberry-red tumor in the umbilicus.

Vitelline cysts (enterocystocele and cyst of the umbilicus) (Fig. 87–18*F* and *G*) occur when the vitelline duct has closed at both ends but part of the intermediate portion has remained patent. This part enlarges to form a cyst situated intra-abdominally behind the umbilicus (enterocystocele) or within the umbilicus.

A fibrous band (Fig. 87–18*H*), representing the remains of the vitelline duct or its vessels, may extend from the umbilicus to some part of the mesentery or to the ileum and cause intestinal obstruction by snaring or volvulus.

Meconium Ileus.[48, 60, 68, 78, 79] In this disorder the small bowel is obstructed by tenacious meconium. It is a complication of mucoviscidosis, a generalized condition, transmitted as an autosomal recessive trait, in which the fundamental abnormality is the formation of abnormal mucus by the mucus-secreting glands of many parts of the body—lungs, pancreas, gastrointestinal tract, biliary system, and salivary glands. The mucus is excessively viscid and blocks the pulmonary bronchioles, pancreatic acini, bile canaliculi, and intestinal mucous glands. The pathologic changes are most pronounced in the pancreas where the secretory cells are gradually replaced by fibrous tissue and fat (fibrocystic disease of the pancreas).

Lack of pancreatic enzymes causes the meconium in the lower intestine to change from its normal semifluid consistency to a putty-like mass. In addition, the abnormal viscid mucus secreted by the intestinal glands causes the meconium to stick to the intestinal walls and in 10% to 15% of patients leads to acute intestinal obstruction (meconium ileus). The distal ileum in these cases is usually small and contracted and contains firm grayish pebble-like particles of meconium. The mid-ileum becomes enormously dilated and contains grayish-black tenacious material. The abnormal meconium adheres firmly to the mucosal surface of the small intestine. The small unused colon, often erroneously called a microcolon, contains some inspissated mucus or grayish meconium. In about 50% of infants suffering from meconium ileus, the condition is complicated by volvulus, meconium peritonitis, intestinal atresia, or colonic perforation.

The clinical manifestations of meconium ileus are those of neonatal intestinal obstruction, i.e., vomiting of bile, abdominal distention, and failure to pass meconium. Plain films of the abdomen reveal multiple dilated loops of bowel, but the erect films show a comparative lack of fluid levels because of the tenacious nature of the meconium. Sometimes, masses of meconium containing small air bubbles may give the appearance of coarse, granular, "ground-glass" shadows (Fig. 87–20). A contrast enema will reveal a minute, ribbon-like colon, and if the terminal ileum should be filled during the examination, meconium pellets may be visualized (Fig. 87–21).

The differential diagnosis from other types of low intestinal obstruction in neonates, such as ileal and colonic atresia, long segment Hirschsprung's disease, the small left colon syndrome, and the meconium plug syndrome, may be impossible without a contrast enema. Of particular importance is the differentiation from the *meconium plug syndrome.*[68] In this condition the infant usually presents with the symptoms and signs of low intestinal obstruction during the first few days of life. No meconium is passed, but a small amount of pale, yellowish mucus may be evacuated. The obstruction may be felt on rectal examination, and thereafter the characteristic plug is often passed, followed by flatus. The length of the plug varies from 5 to 30 cm; it tapers from a blunt distal end and is dark green in color, except for the end, which is often chalky, granular, and pale yellow. If the plug is not released, an immediate meglumine diatrizoate (Gastro-

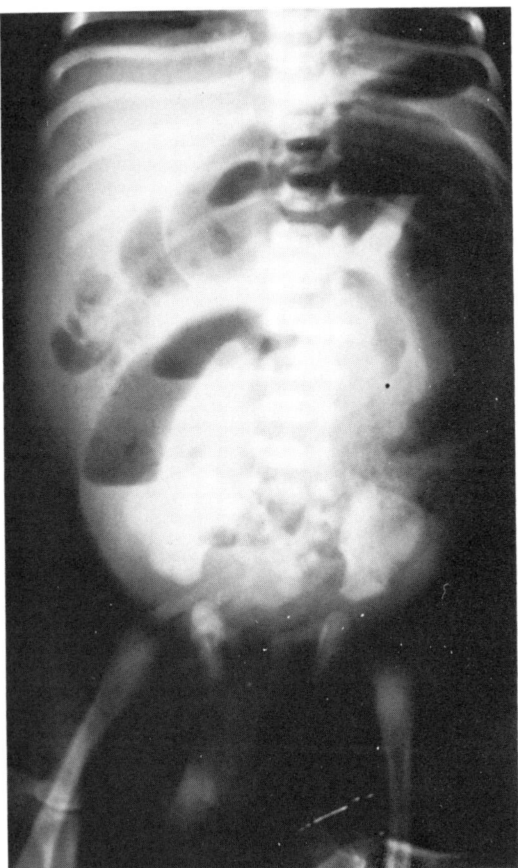

Figure 87–20. Plain radiograph of an infant with meconium ileus. Note the comparative lack of fluid levels and the coarse, granular ground-glass appearance in the left iliac fossa.

grafin) enema should be performed. This will not only confirm the diagnosis but usually will also dislodge the plug. However, the syndrome is frequently found in infants with Hirschsprung's disease. Hence, further observation and radiologic examinations are essential.

A positive preoperative diagnosis of meconium ileus is usually possible after assessing the clinical and radiologic features and obtaining a family history of cystic fibrosis. Absence of tryptic activity in meconium or duodenal aspirate is not a constant finding, and the sweat test to detect excessive quantities of sodium and chloride is inappropriate in newborn infants because sufficient sweat cannot be collected.[48] Once a diagnosis has been made, it is important to distinguish between simple and complicated meconium ileus since the obstruction in the former may be relieved by nonoperative means.

Uncomplicated meconium ileus can be treated successfully by Gastrografin enema,[48, 79–81] which is particularly useful in infants with marginal pulmonary reserve. In cases selected for non-operative treatment, it is important to exclude other forms of distal intestinal obstruction by means of a diagnostic barium enema study. Equally important is exclusion of complications. During the procedure, the infant must be given adequate fluid IV and electrolyte replacement. The success of the method depends largely on the enthusiasm of the operator; Helen Noblett, who introduced it in 1969, has achieved remarkable results.[48] The procedure is not without its own dangers, and a surgical consultation is essential before it is undertaken.

When obstruction persists after Gastrografin enema, surgical exploration is necessary. Surgery is mandatory in complicated meconium ileus. Numerous surgical procedures have been employed. In uncomplicated cases, enterotomy and intraoperative irrigation with saline, hydrogen peroxide,

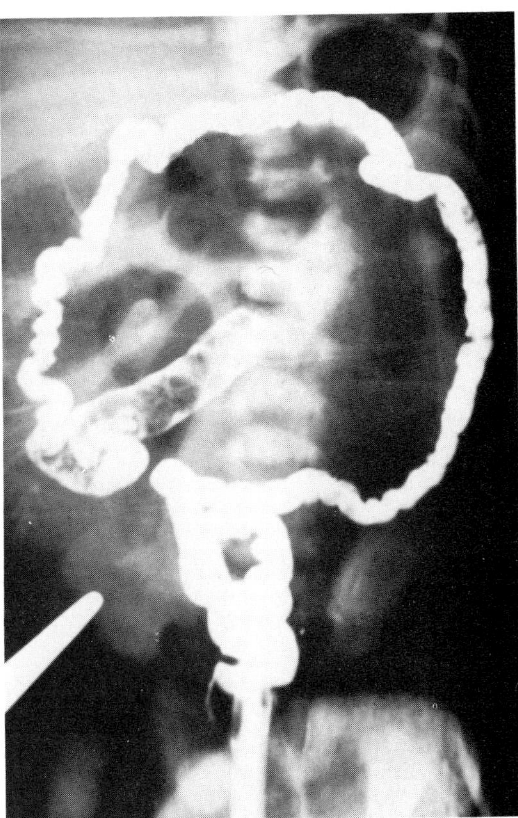

Figure 87–21. Contrast enema in the same infant shown in Figure 87–20. Note the microcolon and "pellets" in the terminal ileum.

acetylcysteine, and pancreatic enzymes have been tried with varying success. Simple enterostomy and postoperative irrigation with pancreatic enzymes have met with less success, but the use of a T-tube has achieved more favorable results.[80] Intraoperative clearance of the sticky meconium by means of Gastrografin introduced by enema and use of the nasogastric tube combined with T-tube enterostomy are safer than intraoperative needle puncture to introduce the Gastrografin. Many surgeons prefer resection of the dilated segment of bowel and the creation of either a Mikulicz double-barreled enterostomy or some modification such as that of Bishop and Koop.[54] The latter consists of resection of the dilated bowel, Roux-en-Y ileostomy, exteriorization of the distal limb, and postoperative irrigation with pancreatic enzymes or Gastrografin. Resection with primary anastomosis after dispersal of the meconium has some advocates. Resection is necessary in most cases of complicated meconium ileus and should be followed by enterostomy, preferably of the Bishop-Koop type.

Survival rates approaching 80% in simple and 60% in complicated meconium ileus are now being reported.[48]

Omphalocele (Exomphalos).[2, 48, 82] Omphalocele is a midline defect in the abdominal wall through which the intestines and other abdominal viscera protrude. The viscera are always covered by a membranous sac consisting of peritoneum and amniotic membrane identical to the Wharton's jelly of the umbilical cord. In some cases the sac ruptures during or soon after birth, but remnants are always noted. As a rule, the umbilical cord emerges from the top of the sac (Fig. 87–22) and the abdominal wall defect is often large.

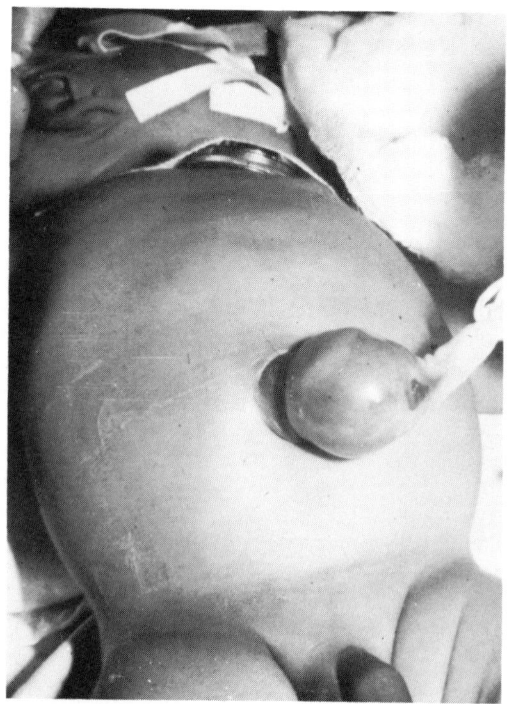

Figure 87–22. Newborn infant with small omphalocele.

An omphalocele is embryologically a "celosomia," i.e., a persistent extraembryonic coelom (physiologic hernia of the fetus), and arises from failure of normal formation of the body folds. This failure occurs in most cases at the level of the lateral folds, and the umbilical ring does not form normally but remains widely patent (middle celosomia). In rare cases the defect extends upward into a sternal, diaphragmatic, and pericardial defect with ectopia cordis and cardiac anomalies (cephalic or upper or epigastric celosomia, sometimes referred to as Cantrell's pentalogy). This is due to early failure of formation of the head fold. In other rare cases the defect extends downward to communicate with an exstrophied urinary bladder. This situation is usually associated with agenesis of the hindgut and exstrophy of the cecum (vesicointestinal fissure) due to failure of formation of the tail fold and referred to as lower or caudal or hypogastric celosomia.

Omphaloceles are also classified according to the size of the orifice into type 1 (less than 2.5 cm), type 2 (2.5 to 5 cm), and type 3 (greater than 5 cm). This classification is of some value from the therapeutic and prognostic points of view but should not be rigid because a great deal depends on the size of the infant, the size of the sac, and the contents of the sac, especially if it contains the liver. Another important factor concerns the presence of associated congenital anomalies, which are extremely common. Some are part of specific syndromes, e.g., the upper midline and lower midline syndromes previously mentioned and the Beckwith-Wiedemann or EMG syndrome (exomphalos, macroglossia, and gigantism).[48, 83] Several abnormalities are encountered in the latter. There is overgrowth of somatic and visceral tissues (a large baby with a large tongue,[84] sometimes hemihypertrophy of the limbs, enlarged kidneys and adrenals, and hyperplasia of endocrine organs, e.g., islet cells of the pancreas and adrenal cortex). There is also a predisposition to the development of nephroblastoma and adrenocortical carcinoma. The most important abnormality is the development of hypoglycemia, which should be kept in mind in all infants suffering from omphaloceles. Apart from the recognized syndromes, associated cardiovascular anomalies occur in about 15% of infants suffering from omphaloceles. The most common entity is tetralogy of Fallot. Other common abnormalities are rotational anomalies of the midgut and intestinal atresia.

The diagnosis of omphalocele is self-evident. Ruptured omphaloceles, however, have to be differentiated from gastroschisis, in which there is a defect to the side (usually the right) of a normally inserted umbilical cord. In gastroschisis there is no sac, and the prolapsed midgut, which is often nonrotated and abnormally short, is usually grossly thickened, edematous, and covered by exudate with gross impairment of peristaltic activity.

The treatment of omphaloceles depends on factors such as the size of the defect, the sac, and the infant; the severity of associated abnormalities; and the integrity of the sac. Surgical treatment is mandatory in all ruptured omphaloceles. In small omphaloceles (type 1), excision of the sac with closure of the umbilical defect presents no problems, even when other congenital anomalies are present. In intermediate omphaloceles (type 2), excision of the sac and primary closure are still possible but can be achieved only after the colon and upper gastrointestinal tract have been emptied and the lateral abdominal muscles forcibly stretched. If the underdeveloped peritoneal cavity cannot accommodate the herniated gut after excision of the sac, a staged repair may be attempted, as advocated by Gross.[56, 85] Better still is Schuster's method[86] of suturing a Silastic bag to the margins of the defect to contain the intestine. The herniation is gradually reduced over the next 5 to 7 days, when delayed closure of the defect is possible.

In the very large or giant omphaloceles (type 3), and also in type 2 defects associated with severe abnormalities of other organs, conservative treatment is preferable to a Schuster pouch. Provided there is no associated intestinal obstruction, the condition may be treated conservatively by converting the sac into an eschar, as first described by Grob,[87] using 2% merbromin (Mercurochrome). This produces a good and strong eschar, but mercuric intoxication is a real danger with 2% solutions, especially when the Mercurochrome is dissolved in alcohol and repeatedly painted on the sac. We therefore use a 1% aqueous solution and apply it only for 24 hours. Thereafter, we combat infection by applying povidone-iodine (Betadine) and promote drying by using 0.5% silver nitrate if necessary. Epithelialization starts soon proceeding from the edges inward; in 1 to 2 months the omphalocele is covered. The remaining large hernia may be dealt with electively at a later date. The method is not without its own problems, however. The underlying bowel tends to adhere to the drying membrane, and adhesive intestinal obstruction may necessitate operative intervention before complete epithelialization has occurred.

For a further discussion of anomalies involving the umbilicus, consult Chapter 228.

Anomalies of Rotation and Fixation of the Gut[2, 20, 21, 48, 58, 60, 72]

First Stage of Rotation. The first stage of rotation is seldom interfered with. *Complete failure of rotation* is rare but has been observed in infants with exomphalos. In such cases the small and large intestines have a common longitudinal mesentery running vertically downward in the midline of the posterior abdominal wall. *Non-rotation affecting only the duodenum* may be discovered as an incidental finding. The duodenum fails to rotate to the right and takes a spiral course from the second to the third part. The anomaly per se is unimportant.

Second Stage of Rotation. The principal errors during the second stage of rotation are:

Non-rotation (Fig. 87–23). This occurs when an abnormally lax umbilical ring has allowed the midgut to return en masse without rotating. The first and second parts of the duodenum are situated normally, but the third and fourth parts descend vertically downward along the right side of the superior mesenteric artery. The small bowel lies chiefly to the right side of the midline, and the colon, doubled on itself, is confined to the left side of the abdomen. Although the gut may become fixed in these abnormal positions, there is often failure of fixation, so that the entire midgut loop may be suspended in the abdominal cavity by an extremely narrow pedicle, which is, in fact, the primitive duodenocolic isthmus.

Since the cecum and appendix are situated in the left iliac fossa, the condition may be confused with ***situs inversus.*** In the latter condition, however, the disposition of the viscera is a mirror image of the normal location; rotation has occurred, but clockwise instead of counterclockwise.

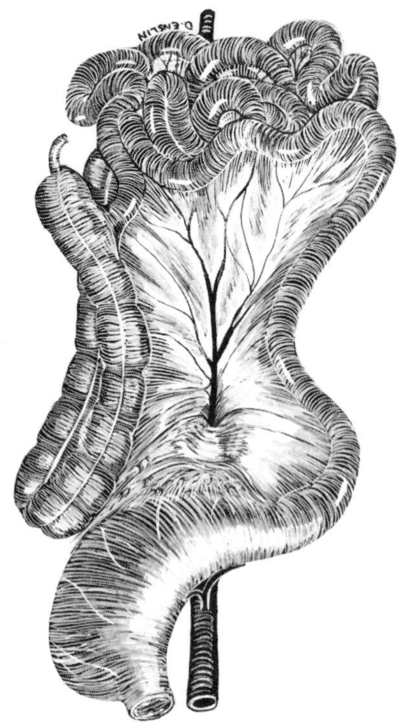

Figure 87–23. Non-rotation (see text).

Reversed Rotation (Fig. 87–24). The cecum and colon have reduced first and passed behind the superior mesenteric vessels, while the small bowel has reduced in front of the vessels. The transverse colon therefore crosses behind the superior mesenteric artery, and the duodenum crosses in front of it.

Malrotation (Fig. 87–25). This occurs when the normal process of rotation is arrested or deviated at varying stages. The best known example is nondescent of the cecum, in which this structure remains in the subhepatic position attained toward the end of the second stage of rotation. The clinical importance of a truly undescended subhepatic cecum lies in problems that arise when patients who have the anomaly develop acute appendicitis. First is the diagnostic problem of differentiating between acute appendicitis and acute cholecystitis. Second is the difficulty of appendectomy through a lower abdominal incision.

In some patients, non-descent of the cecum is associated with anomalous fixation of the gut. First, bands (Ladd's bands) may form across the duodenum, extending from the cecum and right colon to the right upper quadrant of the abdomen (Fig. 87–25*A*).[88] These bands tend to obstruct the duodenum to a variable extent and may be responsible for acute duodenal obstruction in the neonate at the one extreme and chronic duodenal "ileus" in adults at the other.[89] Second, there is often associated failure of the normal fixation of the mesentery. As a result, the common mesentery of the small bowel and right colon is attached only by the narrow area in the region of the superior mesenteric artery, setting the stage for midgut volvulus (Fig. 87–25*B*). Third, bands may form between the right colon and duodenum, drawing them together to create a narrow pedicle, which enhances the tendency toward volvulus. It should also be noted that in infants who present with acute duodenal obstruction due to Ladd's bands, there may be an associated intrinsic membrane. Less commonly, the colon is crowded into and lies doubled on itself in the left side of the abdomen, while the duodenum crosses in front of the artery, where it has become fixed. The jejunum swings to the right. Frequently there is also abnormal fixation of its proximal part with acute kinks at the duodenojejunal junction and beyond (Fig. 87–25*C*).

Third Stage of Rotation. Derangements of the third stage of rotation include delayed or deficient fixation and premature fixation, which is often excessive. ***Delayed fixation*** results in hyperdescent of the cecum, which comes to lie in the pelvis (pelvic or low cecum). This common developmental anomaly of the colon occurs when "descent" of the ascending colon and cecum during the third stage of rotation carries the cecum well below the right iliac fossa into the pelvis. This was regarded in the past as a cause of local and systemic symptoms due to stasis, but there is no statistically significant evidence to support this.[90] The only problem that is associated with the anomaly arises in connection with the development of appendicitis.[21]

Deficient fixation of the duodenum causes abnormal mobility of this organ between the fixed pylorus proximally and the fixed duodenojejunal junction distally. This results in abnormal sagging of the duodenum in the upright position with acute kinking at the duodenojejunal junction. The obstruction so caused may result in abnormal elongation and dila-

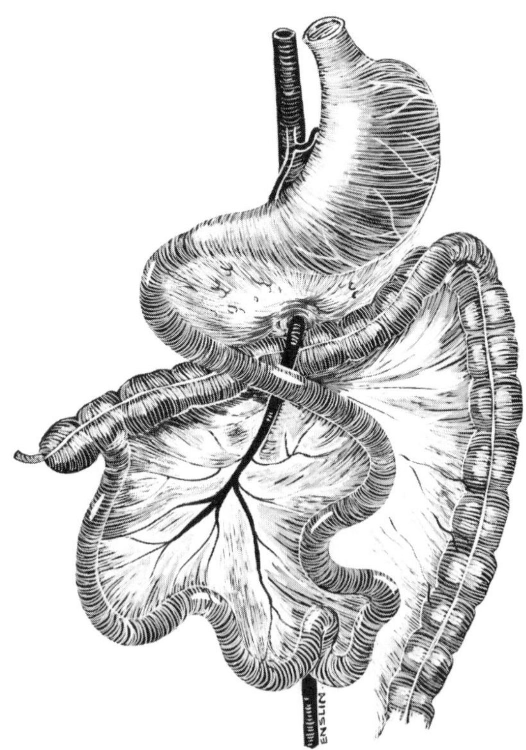

Figure 87–24. Reversed rotation (see text).

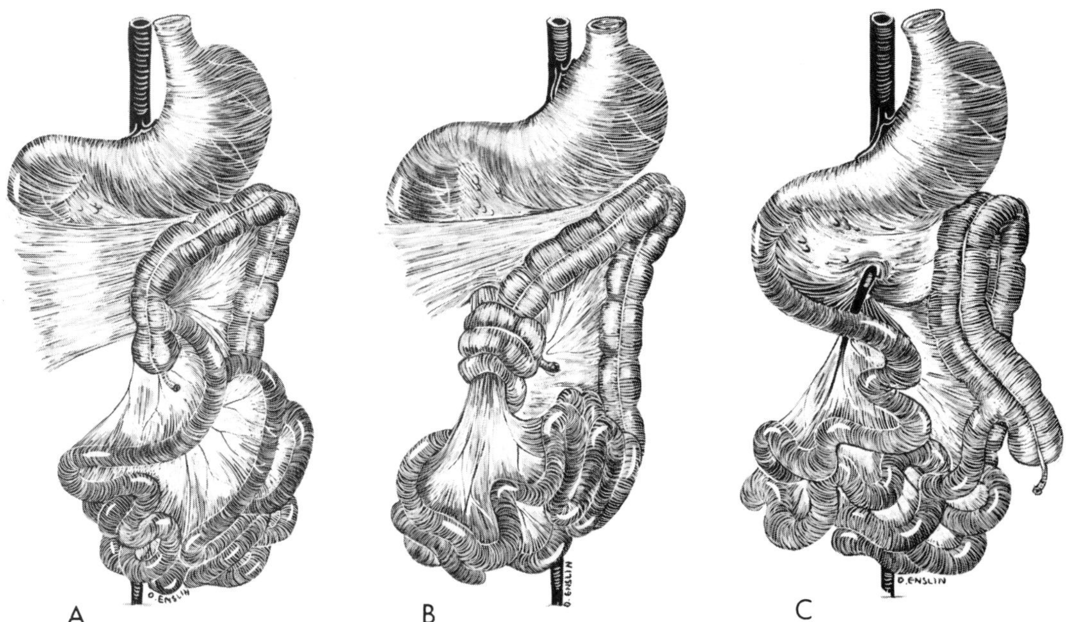

Figure 87–25. Malrotation. *A,* Ladd's bands with duodenal compression. *B,* As in *A,* plus midgut volvulus. *C,* Duodenum anterior to artery and large bowel in left side of abdomen.

tation of the duodenum and the development of duodenal ileus (Chapter 83).[89]

Lack of fixation of the mesentery of the small bowel and right colon is responsible for the so-called universal mesentery (mesenterium commune) attached only by a narrow area at the origin of the superior mesenteric artery. This anomaly, which often coexists with rotational abnormalities but may occur on its own, predisposes to midgut and cecal volvulus and intussusception.

Inadequate fixation of various parts of the colon used to be incriminated as a cause of various vague abdominal symptoms. There is no evidence, however, that hypermobility of any part of the colon is a frequent cause of gastrointestinal or systemic symptoms. A possible exception is a hypermobile cecum, which may cause right lower abdominal pain[90] and predispose to cecal volvulus or volvulus of the small intestine.[21]

A particular group of anomalies, which are now believed to be the result of incomplete fixation of the mesentery, are the so-called *internal hernias.* Hansmann and Morton[91] compiled an impressive list of internal hernias (Fig. 87–26), the most common of which are the paraduodenal and pericecal varieties. These hernias were first thought to be caused by the entry of a loop of bowel into one of the numerous fossae in the peritoneal cavity. Andrews[92] suggested rather that these hernias represent anomalies of intestinal rotation in which the small bowel is trapped behind the mesocolon as the cecum rotates from the left to the right; the trapped bowel eventually becomes incarcerated when the mesocolon fuses with the posterior peritoneum. Estrada[21] believes that the fossae in the vicinity of the duodenum are formed when there is a defect in the dorsal mesentery and that the internal hernia develops during the sec-

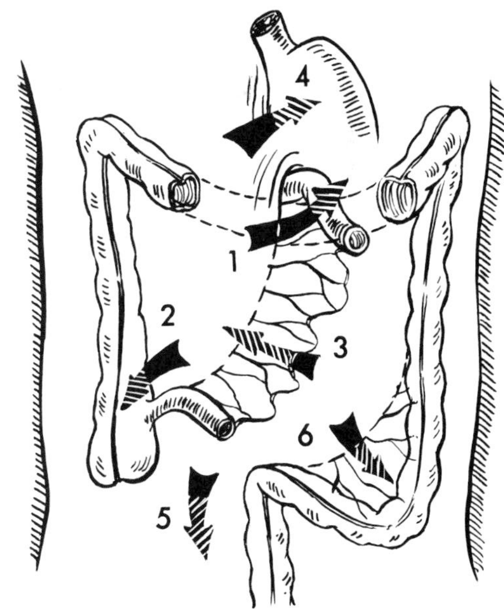

Figure 87–26. Sites of internal hernias (after Hansmann and Morton[91]).

ond stage of rotation. Most of the internal hernias remain uncomplicated, but there may be partial or complete intestinal obstruction, frequently of the strangulating type.

Baker[93] has pointed out that the origin of the so-called *mesocolic cysts* is somewhat similar to that of internal hernias, i.e., failure of fusion of localized areas of the mesocolon with the posterior parietal peritoneum. The enclosed space so created may become distended with peritoneal fluid to form a localized cyst. These cysts have to be differentiated from the more common lymphogenous mesenteric cysts.

Premature or excessive fixation may be responsible for a number of significant anomalies. Non-descent of the cecum associated with the formation of Ladd's bands that compress the duodenum, and the occurrence of similar bands with kinking of the duodenojejunal junction in cases of malrotation, has already been mentioned. Occasionally, abnormally situated membranous bands or ligamentous folds of peritoneum are encountered at laparotomy that may appear to restrain or encroach or impinge on the intestine. Their functional or anatomic significance, however, is probably negligible.

Incomplete descent of the cecum from the right loin to the right iliac fossa is the result of premature fixation during the third stage of rotation. In contrast to a true subhepatic cecum, which is rare, incomplete descent is found in 5% of the population.[94] In some of these cases, the ascending colon has continued to grow after fixation of the cecum and has caused festooning of a loop of colon into the right iliac fossa. The cecum in this circumstance usually points cephalad with the appendix directed upward or to the sides, i.e., an upside-down cecum (Fig. 87–27). The clinical importance of the inverted cecum rests on the difficulty of appendectomy and the possibility of volvulus of the small intestine. There may also be diagnostic problems in differentiating acute appendicitis from acute cholecystitis.[90]

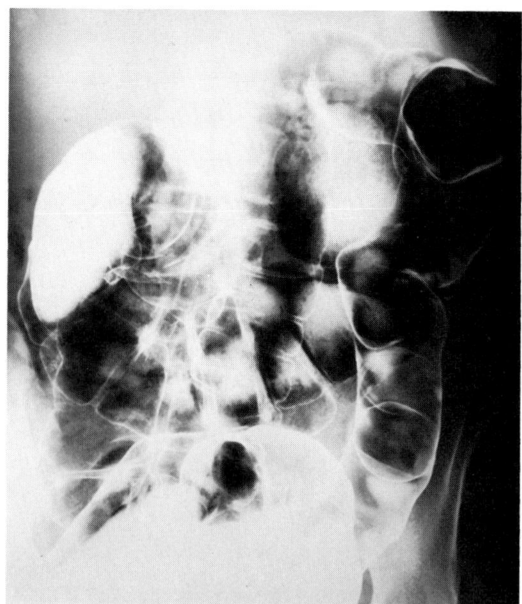

Figure 87–27. Upside-down cecum fixed in subhepatic region.

Clinical Manifestations of Anomalous Rotation. The pathologic effects of anomalous rotation of the gut arise from interference with mobility, compression, or kinking of the bowel and predisposition to volvulus, torsion, intussusception, and ptosis. Abnormal rotation also predisposes to volvulus by reducing the duodenocolic isthmus to a narrow pedicle. The most common type of volvulus involves the whole of the midgut. Since it tends to occur during the first few days of life, it is known as volvulus neonatorum.

It must be emphasized that no functional disturbance may result from abnormal rotation or fixation.[90] In patients who develop obstruction, vomiting (usually containing some bile) and some distention tend to occur early. About half of the patients present during the neonatal period, many of them within the first few days of life. Most of the rest present during early childhood; it is rare for symptoms to appear for the first time in adult life.

In the classic Ladd's syndrome (undescended cecum, malfixation of the mesentery, and bands constricting the duodenum), the clinical features in the neonate are indistinguishable from those of duodenal stenosis. Moreover, plain films will reveal a double bubble with some gas in the bowel. However, a barium enema examination may show the cecum in its undescended position in the upper abdomen (Fig. 87–28). In about half of these patients, the anomaly is complicated by midgut volvulus. In such instances, abdominal distention is more pronounced and the plain films reveal a paucity of gas shadows in the abdomen associated with a dilated stomach; sometimes air-fluid levels are seen in a centrally placed gut (Fig. 87–29). A barium enema examination may reveal devia-

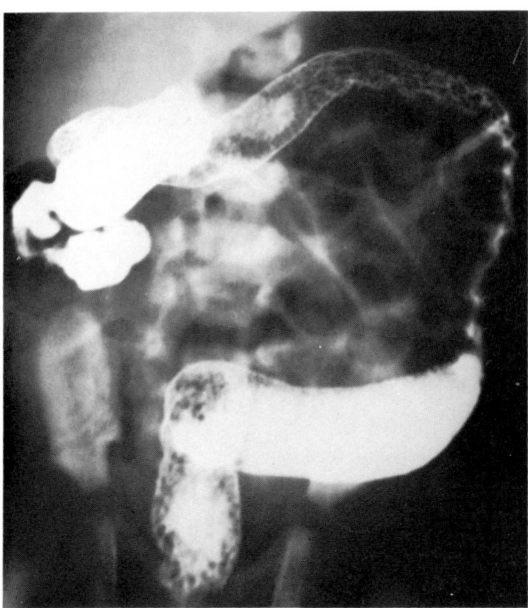

Figure 87–28. Barium enema showing undescended cecum.

tion of the transverse colon and obstruction of the ascending colon.

Older children often have a history of repeated attacks of vomiting, sometimes misdiagnosed as "cyclic" vomiting. These attacks are probably the result of recurrent partial volvulus that corrects itself but may eventually lead to considerable dilatation of the duodenum and chronic duodenal ileus. Indeed, it would appear that many cases of chronic duodenal ileus are the result of duodenal compression and kinking by abnormal bands consequent to anomalies of rotation and fixation of the midgut loop. Ladd's bands may occasionally be responsible, but more often there is constriction at the duodenojejunal flexure due to excessive fixation by fibrous bands. The latter cause kinking of the bowel at the flexure, which is aggravated by sagging of the duodenum with the passage of years.

Most of the internal hernias are asymptomatic and are discovered incidentally at operation or autopsy. When symptoms are produced, they are usually those of acute intestinal obstruction, often with strangulation. The patient is usually an adult, and a correct diagnosis can be made provided the condition is borne in mind and a palpable mass can be detected. Barium meal studies for vague abdominal distress or recurring intestinal obstruction sometimes reveal the presence of a hernia. A barium enema examination may show distortion of the colon as it encircles the loculated small bowel mass.

Treatment of Anomalous Rotation. In patients with Ladd's syndrome and related anomalies associated with obstruction, operative relief is essential. In neonates who may have complicating volvulus, it is a matter of urgency. The principles of the operative procedure, first described by Ladd in 1936,[58, 88] are reduction of the midgut volvulus when present, release of the restraining peritoneal bands holding the colon in its abnormal position, relief of any restricting bands binding the duodenum to the mesocolon and small bowel mesentery, and replacement of the bowel in the position of nonrotation. An associated intrinsic membrane, which occurs in about 15% of patients, must be excluded. The results of surgery are excellent in the neonate but may be compromised by the presence of other congenital anomalies. In older children and adults with chronic dila-

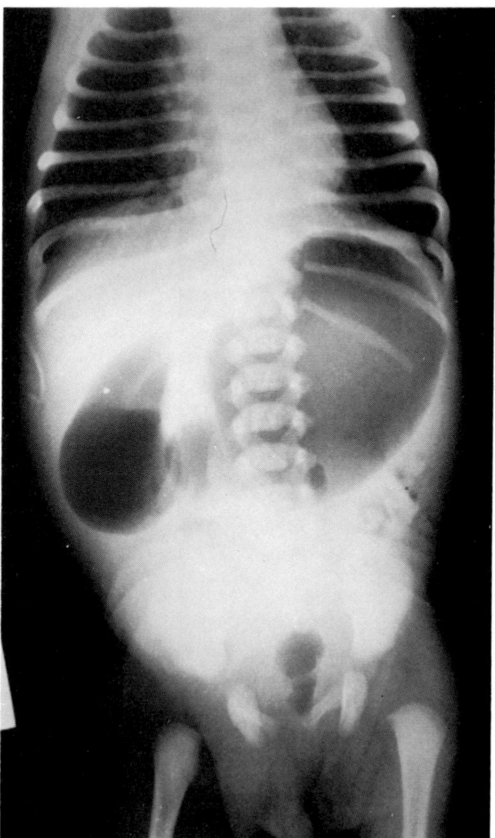

Figure 87–29. Midgut volvulus. Note the distended stomach and duodenum and paucity of gas shadows in the rest of the abdomen.

tation of the duodenum, the procedure should be combined with a duodenojejunostomy.

Early surgical intervention is mandatory in internal hernias with intestinal obstruction, particularly if strangulation is suspected. The condition must be distinguished at operation from other internal obstructions, especially prolapse of the small bowel through a congenital defect in one of the mesenteries and snaring by a congenital band or cord. In dealing with such incarcerated hernias, the intestine must be retrieved without incising the hernial orifice, which often contains vital mesenteric vessels.

Meconium Peritonitis.[48, 53, 68, 95, 96] Meconium peritonitis is an aseptic chemical peritonitis that results from perforation of the fetal gut with escape of sterile meconium into the peritoneal cavity during the last trimester of pregnancy.

The perforation is usually secondary to an obstructive lesion of the small bowel, most commonly atresia or meconium ileus but also volvulus, mesenteric hernia, congenital bands, and intussusception. Less common causes include a perforated appendix, Meckel's diverticulum, duodenal ulcer, duplications, and even puncture by amniocentesis needles.[38] Tibboel et al.[36, 38] have produced the condition in chick embryos by division or puncture of the bowel on the sixteenth day of hatching. In a small percentage of infants, no definite cause can be demonstrated, and in such cases vascular insufficiency or "enteritis" has been implicated[48, 96] on rather flimsy evidence.

The meconium that escapes is sterile but highly irritating and evokes a considerable inflammatory reaction. This may seal off the perforation before the infant is born and may even lead to stenosis and atresia of the bowel at the site of the leakage.[36, 38] The outcome depends upon the timing and extent of the perforation.[96] If the perforation occurs only a few days before birth, the infant presents with *meconium ascites.* The perforation may have sealed off but the abdomen is distended with viscid meconium-stained ascitic fluid. Fine stippled calcification may be present on the peritoneum. Adhesions between loops of bowel are fibrinous rather than fibrous, and the calcium has not had time to become deeply enmeshed in the tissues. If the perforation occurs earlier and is sealed, most of the fluid will have been absorbed at birth, and dense vascular adhesions form between the loops of bowel, which become matted together and distended. This gives rise to the generalized *fibroadhesive meconium peritonitis.* The perforation is often not obvious, and a feature of this condition is the calcification that occurs on the surface of the bowel in the extravasated meconium.

When the extravasation has occurred earlier in gestation or the perforation is minute, a dense fibrous membrane may develop around the area, forming a *meconium pseudocyst.* Loops of intestine may be involved in the wall but most of the peritoneal cavity is generally free of adhesions. The wall of the pseudocyst may contain dense calcium and yet the perforation may not have sealed before birth. A fourth type, *infected meconium peritonitis,* has been described[38] but should not be included in the syndrome of meconium peritonitis. It occurs in neonates in whom the perforation remains patent until birth, at which time the original sterile peritonitis is soon infected. This produces postnatal bacterial peritonitis, which is often associated with pneumoperitoneum.

Infants with meconium peritonitis usually present with symptoms and signs of neonatal intestinal obstruction. Abdominal distention is often considerable, especially in the ascitic variety and in those types with superimposed septic peritonitis and pneumoperitoneum. The adhesive variety is occasionally not associated with obstruction and is discovered later as an incidental finding or as a cause of subsequent obstruction. Pseudocysts are usually palpable, and sometimes a fluid inguinal hernia (communicating hydrocele) may be present.

Plain radiographs will usually point to the correct diagnosis because of the presence of extraluminal calcification and distended gas-filled loops of bowel. Calcification that is observed radiographically generally means that the perforation occurred at least 10 days prior to birth. It may be extremely faint but is usually dense enough to outline the walls of the peritoneal cavity. Sometimes the calcification may even extend along a patent processus vaginalis and show up in the scrotum (Fig. 87–30).

The indications for operation in meconium peritonitis are intestinal obstruction and evidence of postnatal patency of the perforation. These complications are usually clearly indicated on plain radiographs of the abdomen as multiple air-fluid levels within or outside the bowel. Meconium-stained ascites, an enlarging abdominal mass, cellulitis of the abdominal wall, and other evidence of sepsis are also indications for surgery. On the other hand, the mere presence of the typical calcification of meconium peritonitis does not necessarily constitute an indication for operation. In infants who do require surgery, a lengthy and difficult procedure is often necessary and the mortality remains high, especially in those with superimposed postnatal septic peritonitis.

Annular Pancreas.[48, 58, 72, 97] In this comparatively rare anomaly, a ring of pancreatic tissue surrounds the second part of the duodenum. It results from persistence of a por-

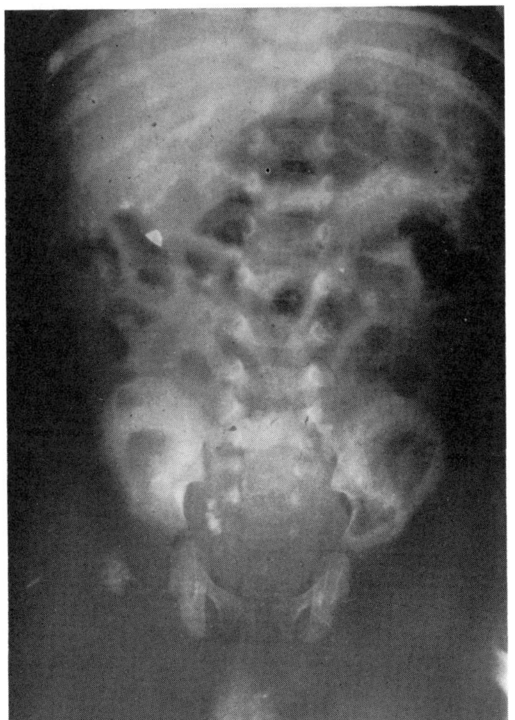

Figure 87–30. Plain radiograph of an infant with meconium peritonitis. Note the speckled calcifications, particularly in the right upper quadrant and also in the scrotum.

tion of the ventral pancreatic anlage, which maintains its ventral position instead of migrating to the dorsal aspect of the duodenum.[72] The rest of the ventral pancreas containing the anlage of the main pancreatic duct migrates with the hepatic anlage to fuse with the dorsal pancreatic anlage. Connection with the nonrotated portion is retained, but the duct structure is often anomalous and a major duct may be present in the portion that embraces the duodenum circumferentially.

Drey[97] has found it useful to classify annular pancreas into neonatal and adult types. The former is usually associated with duodenal obstruction, thought to be the result of extrinsic compression. However, all our cases and most of those described in the literature have been associated with intrinsic duodenal atresia or stenosis. It is tempting to suggest that these intrinsic lesions might be the result of ischemia caused by the constricting pancreas, but the frequent coexistence of other malformations, especially those associated with Down's syndrome, suggests that both malformations are the result of a more generalized insult during the first few weeks of intrauterine life.

The adult type of annular pancreas usually remains asymptomatic and may be discovered as an incidental finding at laparotomy or autopsy. Among 62 cases collected by Drey,[97] epigastric discomfort was described in 56 and vomiting in 38 patients, including 7 with hematemesis. A majority had symptoms for more than 5 years. The pancreatic tissue is grossly indistinguishable from that of the normal pancreas and pancreatic function tests are usually normal. However, it is conceivable that a pancreas with an annular anomaly may be more susceptible to pancreatitis because of the aberrant duct system.

The symptoms and signs in infants are those of acute or subacute duodenal obstruction and the diagnosis is made only at laparotomy. In adults, the diagnosis may be made by barium meal with or without hypotonic duodenography. Dodd and Nafis[98] have pointed out that eccentric narrowing of the duodenum, focal effacement of the mucosal pattern, or localized medial retraction of the descending segment is characteristic of annular pancreas. The differential diagnosis includes duodenal distortion by postbulbar peptic ulcer, pericholecystitis, intraluminal neoplasm, and pancreatitis.

The need for treatment depends upon the symptoms. Urgent surgery to overcome the acute obstruction is necessary in infants and duodenoduodenostomy is the procedure of choice. In adults, the incidental finding of an annular pancreas without evidence of obstruction probably does not warrant treatment because the encroachment on the duodenum is not progressive. When there are obstructive symptoms and signs, however, something should be done. Division of the annular portion is not recommended because of the risk of dividing a large duct, whereas gastrojejunostomy often fails to correct the proximal duodenal stasis. The consensus is clearly in favor of duodeno-duodenostomy or duodeno-jejunostomy.[48, 58]

Heterotopia and Hamartomas[99]

Heterotopia. This may be defined as misplacement of tissue, i.e., tissue of an organized adult structure appears in an area in which it does not normally belong.[99] Usually the condition is congenital in origin and results from some abnormal differentiation in the primitive ectoderm or entoderm. Heterotopia of the digestive tube is of entodermal origin, and the cell differentiation is confined almost without exception to derivatives of the foregut. This includes gastric mucosa in a Meckel's diverticulum and pancreatic tissue in the stomach, duodenum, and jejunum.

Heterotopic pancreas is not exceptionally

susceptible to neoplasia or inflammation and is usually asymptomatic and devoid of clinical interest. However, the nodule of tissue may provide the leading point of an intussusception, especially when located in a Meckel's diverticulum.

Hamartoma. According to Willis,[99] hamartoma denotes a congenital malformation of tissue masses indigenous to the part in which it is located. Usually the various tissues of a part are present in improper proportions or distribution, with prominent excess of one particular tissue. Although not neoplastic in origin, they may become so. Hamartomas of the intestine are not common and when they do occur, there are usually similar malformations elsewhere, especially in the skin.

Anomalies of Size and Length of the Colon[48, 90, 100, 101]

Megacolon (Chapter 133). Congenital lesions are responsible for most of the cases seen. *Hirschsprung's disease* results from congenital absence of ganglion cells in the terminal bowel. Fully 80% of the cases are currently diagnosed during the neonatal period. Indeed, colonic aganglionosis is one of the most common causes of neonatal intestinal obstruction. *Acquired organic megacolon* is often secondary to anorectal malformations. In *functional megacolon* the history often begins in early childhood, and in some cases a congenital anomaly, such as dolichocolon, may be responsible. However, the possibility of short segment aganglionosis should always be excluded.

Microcolon. This is an unfortunate term that suggests that the colon is structurally diminished in size and length, a state of affairs that probably never exists. Microcolon actually refers to the small, unused colon found in infants suffering from complete occlusion of the proximal bowel, e.g., atresia and meconium ileus. If the proximal obstruction is incomplete, as in stenosis and malrotation, or is located above the biliary papilla, sufficient quantities of meconium are propelled into the colon to dilate it. In total colonic aganglionosis the colon is also smaller and often shorter than normal.

It was not realized in the past that the small, contracted colon would assume normal dimensions after relief of the proximal obstruction. However, it is now known that the condition is not pathologic but is simply a manifestation of a colon that has not been used in fetal life. Indeed, the presence of a microcolon is today considered an important diagnostic radiologic feature of complete proximal intestinal occlusion. Barium enema examinations are intentionally performed in many centers in infants with neonatal intestinal obstruction primarily to determine the presence or absence of an unused colon and to exclude associated lesions, such as colonic atresia or malrotation.[52]

Deficient Length of Colon. Shortening of the colon is a constant feature in vesicointestinal fissure. The shortening in this condition is caused by gross restriction in longitudinal growth of the bowel distal to the vitelline duct. Shortening is also seen in some cases of colonic atresia and rectal atresia, in which it is the result of infarction of segments of the fetal colon. Rarely, the whole or a large part of the colon may be absent (colonic agenesis). This is usually associated with other serious malformations, and the anus is virtually always absent.[102–105]

SHORT COLON MALFORMATION. Short saccular colonic dilatation with absence of the normal formation of part of the large bowel resulting in a short colon is a very rare anomaly associated with anorectal malformation. Most of these patients have been reported from India.[106–109] The anomaly is characterized by an anorectal malformation and severe abdominal distention. Diagnosis is based on the typical radiographic appearance of a large gas shadow occupying practically the whole of the pelvis with a colonic fluid level greater than half the abdominal girth (Fig. 87–31). A fistulous communication with the bladder in the male and with the urogenital complex in the female is invariably seen at laparotomy. The dilated pouch is thin walled without any obvious colonic characteristics.

Treatment may be difficult. A colostomy or ileostomy is required in the first instance, followed later by resection of this dilated sac and a pull-through procedure.

APLASIA. Aplasia of the colon, i.e., a condition in which the continuity of the bowel is uninterrupted but no differentiation into the colon has occurred, is even less common. Bennington and Haber[110] described a patient in whom only 75 cm of bowel of uniform caliber extended from the pylorus to the anus.

SMALL LEFT COLON SYNDROME. This terminology was coined by Davis et al.[100] to describe a syndrome, previously recognized by others,[111] consisting of intestinal obstruction

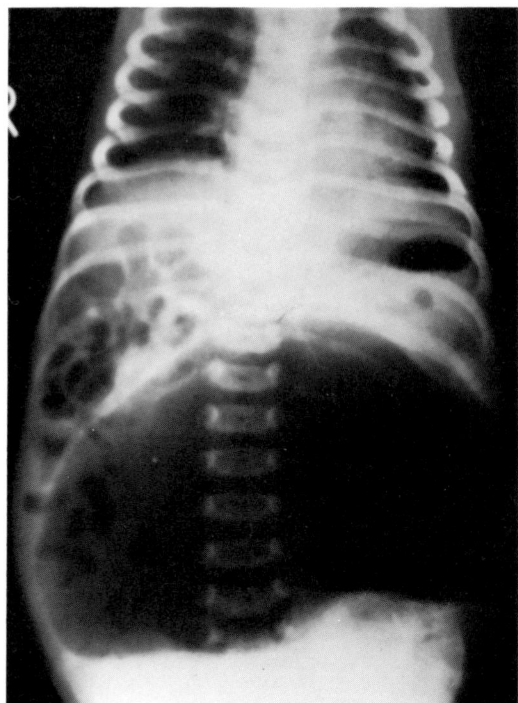

Figure 87–31. Short colon malformation. Note the enormously distended colon occupying the pelvis and lower abdomen. The fluid level is wider than half the abdominal girth.

in the newborn with disturbance of bowel motility, normal ganglion cells and, characteristically, a transition zone at the splenic flexure as seen on contrast enema examination (Fig. 87–32). Most of these infants are born to diabetic mothers. Conversely, approximately 40% of infants born to diabetic mothers have this syndrome in varying degrees.[101] Hirschsprung's disease and meconium plug syndrome may produce the same clinical and radiologic features.

The theory that patients with small left colon syndrome have a relative increase in immature ganglion cells[100] has not been confirmed. It has also been suggested that glucagon production might be increased in these patients, producing a decrease in bowel motility.

Treatment entails continuation of the diagnostic contrast enema with a second enema of Gastrografin under fluoroscopic control. This is followed with saline irrigations in the ward. In the majority of these patients, the obstruction will be relieved.

The main complication is cecal perforation. Thus, there should be no hesitation in performing a colostomy if the obstruction is not relieved by the washouts. A rectal suction biopsy should be taken in all these patients to rule out congenital aganglionosis.

Dolichocolon (Redundancy).[90, 94] This is a syndrome in adults characterized by a long, redundant colon. The entire colon or only a segment may be redundant. The pelvic colon, including the sigmoid region, is most commonly involved. Constipation is the major symptom and may date in some cases from early life. Laxative and/or enema abuse is commonly associated. Not infrequently, the patient will note that the water from an enema is not expelled.

Colon redundancy is almost universally present in patients with volvulus of part of the colon (Chapter 122). Conversely, volvulus is an infrequent sequela of redundancy of the colon, considering the prevalence of dolichocolon.

Therapy involves treatment of the constipation (Chapters 7 and 134). Surgical intervention is ordinarily not indicated in the absence of volvulus.

Anorectal Malformations.[8, 9, 48, 52, 112] Malformations of the rectum and anus are among the most common serious congenital abnormalities encountered. They include a wide spectrum of defects, ranging from minor aberrations of the anus to the most complex and serious anomalies of the rectum and

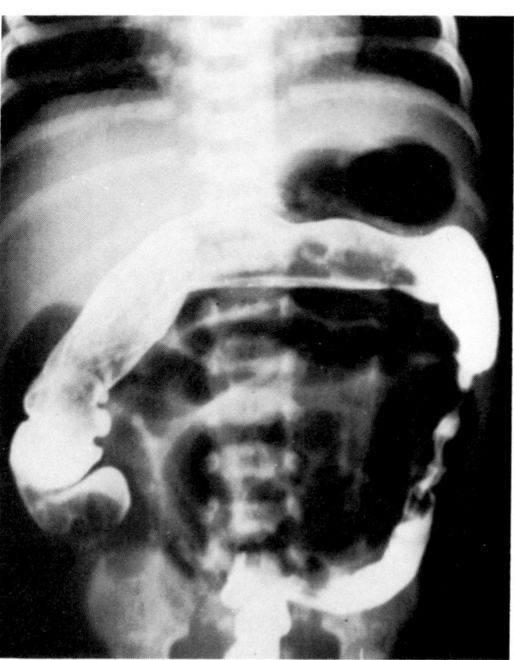

Figure 87–32. Small left colon syndrome. Note the foreshortened and narrowed left colon with a "transitional zone" at the splenic flexure.

anus. They are also often associated with other major congenital abnormalities.

A detailed description of the various anomalies is beyond the scope of this chapter. Suffice it to say that the crucial factor, from the therapeutic and prognostic standpoints and to a certain extent also from the anatomic and embryologic aspects, is the relationship of the terminal bowel to the levator ani muscle—in particular to the puborectalis component of this muscle. During the Centenary Paediatric Surgical Congress of the Royal Children's Hospital, Melbourne, in 1970, an ad hoc committee of international participants was formed to standardize nomenclature (Chapter 143). The classification decided upon is shown in Table 87–1, and a discussion of the terms used, with accompanying diagrams, follows.

Table 87–1. CLASSIFICATION OF ANORECTAL MALFORMATIONS*

- I. *High or Supralevator Deformities*—in which the bowel ends above the pelvic floor (40%)
  - A. Anorectal agenesis
    - 1. Without fistula
    - 2. With fistula
      - a. Males:
        - Rectovesical
        - Rectourethral
      - b. Females:
        - Rectovesical
        - Rectocloacal
        - Rectovaginal (high)
  - B. Rectal atresia
- II. *Intermediate Deformities* (15%)
  - A. Anal agenesis
    - 1. Without fistula
    - 2. With fistula
      - a. Males:
        - Rectobulbar
      - b. Females:
        - Rectovaginal (low)
        - Rectovestibular
  - B. Anorectal stenosis
- III. *Low or Translevator Deformities*—in which the bowel ends below the pelvic floor and is embraced by the puborectalis muscle (40%)
  - A. At normal site
    - 1. Covered anus
    - 2. Anal stenosis
  - B. At perineal site
    - 1. Anocutaneous fistula
    - 2. Anterior perineal anus
  - C. At vulvar site
    - 1. Vulvar anus
    - 2. Anovulvar fistula
    - 3. Anovestibular fistula
- IV. *Miscellaneous* (5%)

*The percentages shown indicate the frequency of the various anomalies in our experience with almost 500 cases.

In the diagnosis and management of any particular case, it is important to determine the relationship of the terminal bowel to the puborectalis muscle. This is often possible from the clinical presentation alone, but sometimes radiologic assessment is required for a diagnosis. Radiologic diagnosis is based primarily on the position of the gas in the terminal bowel as seen on lateral films of the inverted infant, but contrast studies (loopograms and fistulograms) may be necessary for accuracy. Stephens[113] has pointed out that a line drawn from the pubic bones to the sacrococcygeal junction on the radiograph (P–C line) approximates the level of the levator ai muscle. We have found that the level of the puborectails portion of the levator ani muscle is somewhat further caudad than the pubococcygeal line (Fig. 87–33) and prefer to relate the terminal gas shadow to the inferior border of the ischium, i.e., Kelly's I point.[114]

High or Supralevator Deformities (Fig. 87–34). These anomalies accounted for 40% of our cases. They represent an arrest in development of the rectum at a very early stage of subdivision of the cloaca, before the down-

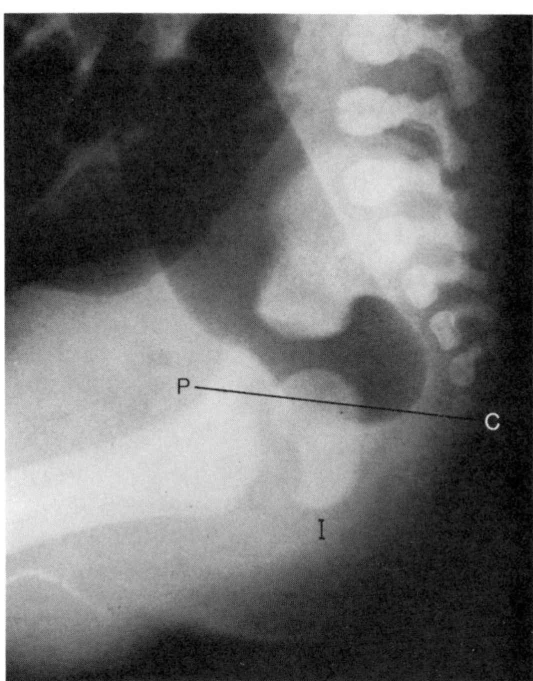

Figure 87–33. Lateral inverted film showing pubic bones, sacral vertebrae, and ischium. P—C = pubococcygeal line. I = lower border of ischium. In this infant with a supralevator anomaly the terminal gas shadow is above (cephalad to) the I point. Note the gas in the bladder.

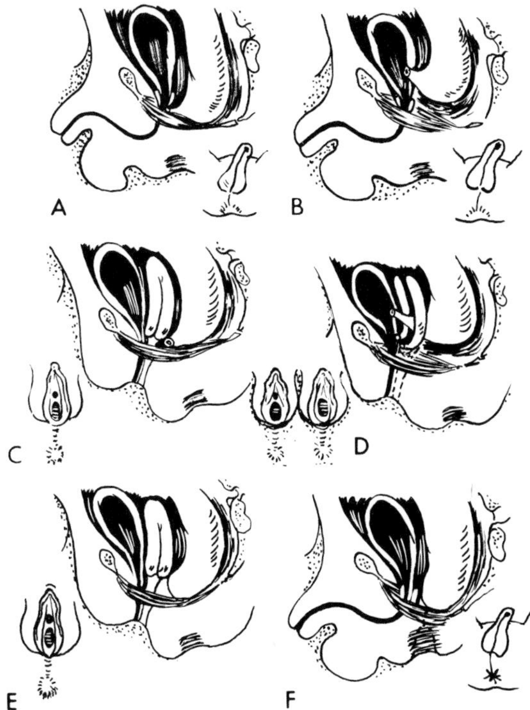

Figure 87–34. High or supralevator deformities (see text).

growth of the urorectal fold and caudad migration of the rectal orifice in the dorsal wall of the cloaca. In addition, growth of the anal canal is also arrested. These deformities are always serious because, despite the usual presence of a fistulous opening, there is almost always *severe obstruction that must be treated by colostomy soon after birth.* Associated abnormalities of the vertebrae and upper urinary tract are common, and innervation of the pelvic musculature is often defective. The provision of adequate muscular control involves complicated and difficult surgical reconstruction by a sacro-abdominoperineal approach to ensure that the colon is pulled through within the sling fibers of the puborectalis muscle. This reconstruction is best deferred for 6 to 12 months. During the waiting period, the anatomy of the deformities can be more accurately studied by loopograms.[52]

ANORECTAL AGENESIS (Fig. 87–34). This is the usual high anomaly and is much more common in boys than in girls. In both sexes a fistula is almost always present.

In the common variety in *boys,* there is a rectourethral fistula (Fig. 87–34*A*). The clinical features are early obstruction, no opening in the perineum, and the passage of meconium in the urine. On plain roentgenograms the gas shadow is above the I point (Fig. 87–33). Less commonly there is a rectovesical fistula (Fig. 87–34*B*). The clinical features are similar, although obstruction may not be as severe. Plain films may show air in the bladder (Fig. 87–33). Rarely there is no fistula in association with complete obstruction and no meconium in the urine.

In the common variety in *girls,* there is a fistula into the vault of the vagina (Fig. 87–34C). The clinical features are early obstruction, no opening in the perineum, and the passage of meconium per vaginam. On separation of the labia, only 2 openings are visible, i.e., the vagina and urethra, as the fistula is not visible. A plain roentgenogram may reveal a terminal gas shadow above the I point if the obstruction is severe.

Less commonly, the anatomy is more primitive and a cloaca is present with a fistula into either the cloacal canal or the bladder (Fig. 87–34*D*). In these cases, obstruction is always severe and the external genitalia have a masculine appearance. Meconium is seldom passed. On separation of the labia, either a single orifice (the cloacal canal) is seen or 2 orifices (cloaca and urethra); the rectal fistula is not visible.

Rarely, no fistula is present (Fig. 87–34*E*). Obstruction occurs at an early stage and no meconium is passed. On separation of the labia, 2 orifices (urethra and vagina) are seen and a plain film shows a terminal gas bubble above the I point.

RECTAL ATRESIA (Fig. 87–34*F*). This very rare anomaly (2% of our cases) occurs in both boys and girls. An anal canal is present but the rectum ends blindly above the pelvic floor. Obstructive symptoms develop early. The diagnosis may be missed, however, because of the presence of an apparently normal anal canal. Simple roentgenograms show a terminal gas bubble well above the I point and at a considerable distance from the tip of a thermometer inserted into the anus.

Low or Translevator Deformities (Fig. 87–35). These accounted for 40% of our cases and are generally not serious. Obstruction is seldom severe and usually transient. Associated anomalies are not common, the pelvic nerves are intact, and *reconstruction usually involves only a simple perineal operation.* However, unwarranted operations may have disastrous consequences.

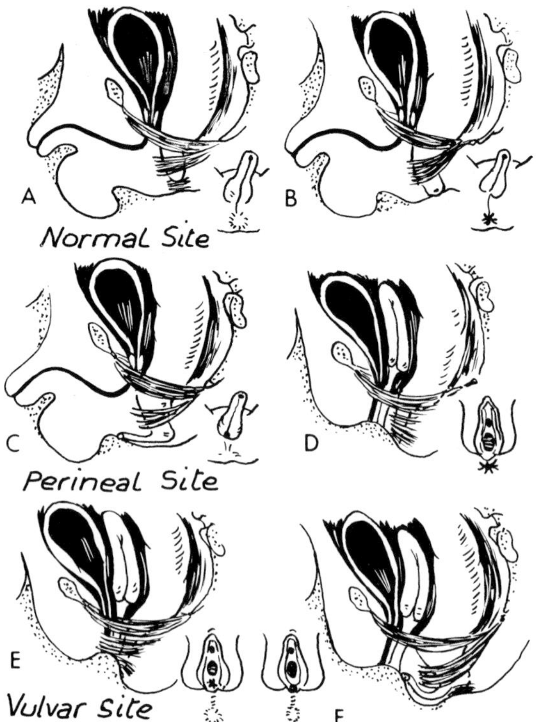

Figure 87–35. Low or translevator deformities (see text).

The rectum is present and normal in these infants and is embraced by the puborectalis muscle. The anus, however, is abnormal and may be situated at the normal site, in the perineum anterior to the normal site, or, in girls, in the vulva. An orifice is almost always present but is usually stenosed.

AT NORMAL ANAL SITE. These anomalies are rare (5% of our cases) and include *covered anus* and *anal stenosis.* The latter is mostly a variant of covered anus (the pinhole anus described by Browne[112]). Both types are more common in boys than in girls. In covered anus (Fig. 87–35*A*) the meconium will be seen shining through the skin at the anal site. In anal stenosis (Fig. 87–35*B*) the skin has ruptured, leaving a tiny opening through which meconium exudes. A plain roentgenogram will reveal a terminal gas bubble well below the I point. The diagnosis can be confirmed by injecting Gastrografin into the bowel through the perineum, but this is usually unnecessary.

AT PERINEAL SITE. *Covered anus with anocutaneous fistula* is much more common in boys (Fig. 87–35C). The diagnosis is self-evident because meconium can be seen tracking beneath the skin in the midline from the site of the normal anus to the point of exit in the perineum; it may even extend farther forward to the raphe of the scrotum or the ventral surface of the penis. In girls, the track of meconium is less easily identified; a probe passed into the orifice in the perineum goes directly backward immediately subcutaneously. Further investigations are unnecessary, but a fistulogram will confirm the diagnosis.

The *anterior perineal anus* is simply a slightly stenosed but normal anus placed forward of the normal site. In girls, this gives the typical "shotgun perineum" appearance described by Browne[112] (Fig. 87–35*D*).

AT VULVAR SITE. An opening into the vulva close to the fourchette occurs in a number of low anomalies in girls. The *vulvar anus,* also known as the vestibular anus or vulvar etopic anus, looks like a normal anus (Fig. 87–35*E*). The *anovulvar fistula* is a variant of the covered anus, and the opening has a ragged appearance (Fig. 87–35*F*). In the *anovestibular fistula* the bowel has passed through the puborectalis muscle but an anal canal has not formed. The terminal bowel communicates with the vestibule through a small fistula.

In all 3 varieties a probe inserted into the orifice passes somewhat dorsally and not cephalad, as in certain intermediate anomalies. A fistulogram may be necessary for accurate diagnosis.[52]

Intermediate Deformities (Fig. 87–36). This group accounted for 15% of our cases and occurred in both boys and girls. It embraces a number of anomalies that, in the past, have been included with the high anomalies by some and with the low anomalies by others. Those viewing the lesions as high anomalies tended to use a sacro-abdominoperineal approach for the reconstruction; those regarding them as low anomalies have preferred a simple perineal anoplasty. *We believe the initial treatment should be colostomy, and we have used an abdominoperineal approach for the reconstruction at a later date.*

ANAL AGENESIS. *Anal agenesis without fistula* (Fig. 87–36*A*) is rare (3%) in both boys and girls. The clinical presentation is similar to that of anorectal agenesis without fistula, an even rarer anomaly (see earlier discussion). Plain roentgenograms will reveal the terminal gas shadow below the I point.

Anal agenesis with fistula is also rare. In *boys,* the fistula opens into the bulbous part of the

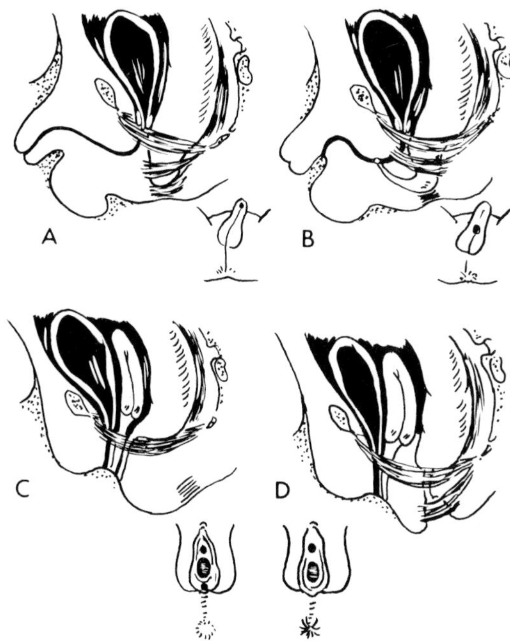

Figure 87–36. Intermediate deformities (see text).

urethra (Fig. 87–36*B*). Clinically, it presents exactly like anorectal agenesis with rectourethral fistula, i.e., early obstruction, no orifice on the perineum, and the passage of meconium in the urine. However, there is almost always an associated hypospadias. Plain films will reveal the terminal gas bubble at the I point. In *girls,* the fistula may open in the vagina. In this case it has to be differentiated from anorectal agenesis with fistula. This depends on visualizing the opening on colposcopy, but a fistulogram or subsequent loopogram is often necessary for accurate diagnosis. Less commonly, a narrow fistula opens into the vestibule (Fig. 87–36C). The clinical presentation then is similar to that of the various low anomalies with an opening at the vulvar site. However, a probe introduced into the orifice will pass cephalad and not dorsally. Fistulograms or subsequent loopograms are essential for diagnosis.

ANORECTAL STENOSIS (Fig. 87–36*D*). This is also rare (3%) but important because it may be confused with anal stenosis. The stenosis involves the anus as well as the lower rectum and therefore abdominoperineal reconstruction is necessary. Fistulograms or subsequent loopograms are essential for diagnosis.

Miscellaneous Lesions. Miscellaneous lesions collectively accounted for less than 5% of our cases, and only imperforate anal membrane and anal membrane stenosis warrant mention. Both are extremely rare.

The clinical presentation of an *intact anal membrane* is similar to that of rectal atresia, i.e., early obstruction with the presence of an apparently normal anus. Frequently, the membrane has already ruptured when the baby is first seen, but the opening may be too small for adequate decompression *(anal membrane stenosis).* A finger or thermometer inserted into the anal canal meets with obstruction low down. Plain roentgenograms show a terminal gas shadow below the I point and impinging on the tip of the thermometer inserted into the anus. The membrane can be seen through a proctoscope, and it may be possible to pass a catheter through the opening of a ruptured membrane. Contrast enema done in patients with a ruptured membrane will reveal the changes.

Treatment is simple excision of the membrane with subsequent dilatations of the anal canal.

References

1. Arey LB. Developmental Anatomy. A Textbook and Laboratory Manual of Embryology. 7th Ed. Philadelphia: WB Saunders, 1974.
2. Gray SW, Skandalakis JE. Embryology for Surgeons. (The Embryological Basis for the Treatment of Congenital Defects.) Philadelphia: WB Saunders, 1972.
3. Hamilton WJ, Boyd JD, Mossman HW. Human Embryology (Prenatal Development of Form and Function). 4th Ed. Cambridge: W Heffer & Sons, 1972.
4. Patten BM. Human Embryology. 3rd Ed. New York: McGraw-Hill, 1968.
5. Beardmore HE, Wiglesworth FW. Vertebral anomalies and alimentary duplications: Clinical and embryological aspects. Pediatr Clin North Am 1958; 5:457–74.
6. Bentley JFR, Smith JR. Developmental posterior enteric remnants and spinal malformations. The split notochord syndrome. Arch Dis Child 1960; 35:76–86.
7. Bill AH, Johnson RJ. Failure of migration of the rectal opening as the cause for most cases of imperforate anus. Surg Gynecol Obstet 1958; 106:643–51.
8. Louw JH. Congenital Abnormalities of the Rectum and Anus. Current Problems in Surgery. Chicago: Year Book Medical Publishers, 1965.
9. Stephens FD, Smith ED. Ano-rectal Malformations in Children. Chicago: Year Book Medical Publishers, 1971.
10. Johnston TB. Extroversion of the bladder complicated by the presence of intestinal openings on the surface of the extroverted area. J Anat 1913; 48:89–106.
11. Wilson PM. Observations on some aspects of vesico-intestinal fissure. S Afr Med J 1967; 41:712–8.
12. Müntener M. Contribution to the knowledge of the development of the human diaphragm. Z Klin Chir 1968; 5:350.
13. Wells LJ. Development of the human diaphragm and pleural sacs. Contrib Embryol Carnegie Inst Wash 1954; 35:107–34.
14. White JJ, Suzuki H. Hernia through the foramen of Bochdalek; a misnomer. J Pediatr Surg 1972; 7:60–1.
15. Bremer JL. Congenital Anomalies of the Viscera: Their Embryological Basis. Cambridge, Mass: Harvard University Press, 1957.

16. Tandler J. Zur Entwicklungsgeschichte des menschlichen Duodenums im fruhen Embryonalstadien. Morphol Jb 1902; 29:187–216.
17. Meckel JF. Manual of Pathological Anatomy. London: E. Henderson, 1938 (Translation).
18. Boyden EA, Cope JG, Bill AH. Anatomy and embryology of congenital intrinsic obstruction of the duodenum. Am J Surg 1967; 114:190–202.
19. Bremer JL. Diverticula and duplications of the intestinal tract. Arch Pathol 1944; 38:132–40.
20. Dott NM. Anomalies of intestinal rotation. Br J Surg 1923; 11:251–86.
21. Estrada RL. Anomalies of Intestinal Rotation and Fixation. Springfield, Ill: Charles C Thomas, 1958.
22. Cywes S, Davies MRQ, Rode H. Congenital jejuno-ileal atresia and stenosis. *In*: Persaud TVN, ed. Advances in the Study of Birth Defects. Vol 6. Lancaster: MTP Press, 1982.
23. deLorimier AA, Fonkalsrud EW, Hays DM. Congenital atresia and stenosis of the jejunum and ileum. (A review compiled by the members of the Surgical Section of the American Academy of Pediatrics). Surgery 1969; 65:819–27.
24. Fonkalsrud EW, deLorimier AA, Hays DM. Congenital atresia and stenosis of the duodenum. (A review compiled by the members of the Surgical Section of the American Academy of Pediatrics). Pediatrics 1969:43:79–83.
25. Hays DM. Intestinal Atresia and Stenosis. Current Problems in Surgery. Chicago: Year Book Medical Publishers, 1969.
26. Louw JH. Jejunoileal atresia and stenosis. J Pediatr Surg 1966; 1:8–23.
27. Louw JH, Cywes S, Davies MRQ, Rode H. Congenital jejuno-ileal atresia: Observations on its pathogenesis and treatment. Z Kinderchir Grenzgeb 1981; 33:1–17.
28. Nixon HH, Tawes R. Etiology and treatment of small intestinal atresia: Analysis of a series of 127 jejuno-ileal atresias and comparison with 62 duodenal atresias. Surgery 1971; 69:41–51.
29. Johnson FP. The development of the mucous membrane of the oesophagus, stomach and small intestine in the human embryo. Am J Anat 1910; 10:521–61.
30. Lynn HB, Espinas EE. Intestinal atresia: An attempt to relate location to embryologic processes. Arch Surg 1959; 79:357–61.
31. Moutsouris C. The "solid stage" of congenital intestinal atresia. J Pediatr Surg 1966; 1:446–50.
32. Tedeschi CG, Ingalls TH. Vascular anomalies of mice fetuses exposed to anoxia during pregnancy. Am J Obstet Gynecol 1956; 71:16–28.
33. Louw JH. Congenital intestinal atresia and stenosis in the newborn. Observations on its pathogenesis and treatment. Ann R Coll Surg Engl 1959; 25:209–34.
34. Louw JH, Barnard CN. Congenital intestinal atresia: Observations on its origin. Lancet 1955; 2:1065–7.
35. Bernstine RL, Coran AG. Surgical techniques in the study of canine fetal physiology. J Pediatr Surg 1971; 6:466–73.
36. Tibboel D, Molenaar JC, van Nie CJ. New perspectives in foetal surgery: The chicken embryo. J Pediatr Surg 1979; 14:438–40.
37. Abrams JS. Experimental intestinal atresia. Surgery 1968; 64:185–91.
38. Tibboel D. De Atresien van het Jejunum, het Ileum en het Colon en de Meconiumperitonitis. Thesis for the degree of Doctor of Medicine at the Vrije Universiteit, Amsterdam. Meppel, Krips Repro, 1979.
39. Duenhoelter JH, Santos-Ramos R, Rosenfeld CR, Coln CD. Prenatal diagnosis of gastrointestinal tract obstruction. Obstet Gynecol 1976; 47:618–20.
40. Fletman, D, McQuown D, Kanchanapoom V, Gyepes MT. 'Apple peel' atresia of the small bowel: Prenatal diagnosis of the obstruction by ultrasound. Pediatr Radiol 1980; 9:118–9.
41. Fogel SR, Katragadda CS, Costin BS. New ultrasonographic finding in a case of fetal jejunal atresia. Tex Med 1980; 76:44–5.
42. Lee TG, Warren BH. Antenatal ultrasonic demonstration of fetal bowel. Radiology 1977; 124:471–4.
43. Loveday BJ, Barr JA, Aitken H. The intrauterine demonstration of duodenal atresia by ultrasound. Br J Radiol 1975; 48:1031–2.
44. Touloukian RJ, Hobbins JC. Maternal ultrasonography in the antenatal diagnosis of surgically correctable fetal abnormalities. J Pediatr Surg 1980; 15:373–7.
45. Louw JH. Whither paediatric surgery? S Afr Med J 1974; 48:1597–8.
46. Mishalany HG, Najjar FB. Familial jejunal atresia: Three cases in one family. J Pediatr 1968; 73:753–5.
47. Blanck C, Okmian L, Robbe H. Mucoviscidosis and intestinal atresia. A study of four cases in the same family. Acta Paediatr Scand 1965; 54:557–65.
48. Ravitch MM, Welch KJ, Benson CD, Aberdeen E, Randolph JG. Pediatric Surgery. Vol 2, 3rd Ed. Chicago: Year Book Medical Publishers, 1979.
49. Guttman FM, Braun P, Garance PH, Collin PP, Dallaire L, Desjardins JG, Perreault G. Multiple atresia and a new syndrome of hereditary multiple atresias involving the gastrointestinal tract from stomach to rectum. J Pediatr Surg 1973; 8:633–40.
50. Délèze G, Sidiropoulus D, Paumgartner G. Determination of bile acid concentration in human amniotic fluid for prenatal diagnosis of intestinal obstruction. Pediatrics 1977; 59:647–50.
51. Farber S. Congenital atresia of the alimentary tract: Diagnosis by microscopic examination of meconium. JAMA 1933; 100:1753–4.
52. Cremin BJ, Cywes S, Louw JH. Radiological Diagnosis of Digestive Tract Disorders in the Newborn. A Guide to Radiologists, Surgeons and Paediatricians. London: Butterworth & Co, 1973.
53. Thomas CG. Jejunoplasty for the correction of jejunal atresia. Surg Gynecol Obstet 1969; 129:545–6.
54. Bishop HC, Koop CE. Management of meconium ileus. Ann Surg 1957; 145:410–4.
55. Forshall I. Duplication of intestinal tract. Postgrad Med J 1961; 37:570–89.
56. Gross RE. The Surgery of Infancy and Childhood. Philadelphia: WB Saunders, 1953.
57. Ladd WE. Duplications of the alimentary tract. South Med J 1937; 30:363–71.
58. Ladd WE, Gross RE. Abdominal Surgery in Infancy and Childhood. Philadelphia: WB Saunders, 1951.
59. McLetchie NGB, Purvis JK, Saunders RL. The genesis of gastric and certain intestinal diverticula and enterogenous cysts. Surg Gynecol Obstet 1954; 99:135–41.
60. Mustard WT, Ravitch MM, Snyder WH Jr, Welch KJ, Benson CD. Pediatric Surgery. Vols 1 and 2. 2nd Ed. Chicago: Year Book Medical Publishers, 1969.
61. Lewis FT, Thyng FW. The regular occurrence of intestinal diverticula in embryos of the pig, rabbit and man. Am J Anat 1907; 7:505–19.
62. Saunders RL. Combined anterior and posterior spina bifida in a living neonatal human female. Anat Rec 1943; 87:255–78.
63. Ravitch MM. Hindgut duplication—doubling of colon and genital urinary tracts. Ann Surg 1953; 137:588–601.
64. Rickham PP. Vesico-intestinal fissure. Arch Dis Child 1960; 35:97–102.
65. Griess DF, Dixon CF, Bargen JA. Complete duplication of the large intestine: Report of a case. Proc Staff Meet Mayo Clin 1947; 22:141–4.
66. Keith A. Three demonstrations of malformations of the hind end of the body. I. Specimens illustrating malformations of the rectum and anus. Br Med J 1908; 2:1736.
67. Johnston JH, Penn IA. Exstrophy of the cloaca. Br J Urol 1966; 38:302–7.
68. Rickham PP, Lister J, Irving IM. Neonatal Surgery. 2nd Ed. London: Butterworth & Co, 1978.
69. Soper RT, Kilger K. Vesico-intestinal fissure. J Urol 1964; 92:490–501.
70. Jones FA, Gummer JWP. Clinical Gastroenterology. Oxford: Blackwell Scientific Publications, 1960.
71. Boyden EA. The problem of the double ductus choledochus. (An interpretation of an accessory bile duct found

attached to the *pars superior* of the duodenum.) Anat Rec 1932; 55:71–93.
72. MacGregor AL, duPlessis DJ. A Synopsis of Surgical Anatomy. 10th Ed. Bristol: John Wright & Sons, 1969.
73. Goligher JC. Surgery of the Anus, Rectum and Colon. 3rd Ed. London: Bailliere, Tindall & Cassel, 1975.
74. Androulakis JA, Gray SW, Lionakis B, Skandalakis JE. The sex ratio of Meckel's diverticulum. Am Surg 1969; 35:455–60.
75. Weinstein EC, Cain JC, ReMine WH. Meckel's diverticulum: 55 years of clinical and surgical experience. JAMA 1962; 182:251–3.
76. Jewett TC, Duszynski DO, Allen JE. The visualization of Meckel's diverticulum with ^{99m}Tc-pertechnetate. Surgery 1970; 68:567–70.
77. Faris HC, Whitley JE. Angiographic demonstration of Meckel's diverticulum. Radiology 1973; 108:285–6.
78. Bodian M. Fibrocystic Disease of the Pancreas in Infants and Children. Springfield, Ill: Charles C Thomas, 1954.
79. Noblett HR. Treatment of uncomplicated meconium ileus by Gastrografin enema. J Pediatr Surg 1969; 4:190–7.
80. Harberg FJ, Senekjian EK, Pokorny WJ. Treatment of uncomplicated meconium ileus via T-tube ileostomy. J Pediatr Surg 1981; 16:61–3.
81. Kalayoglu M, Sieber WK, Rodnan JB, Kiesewetter WB. Meconium ileus: A critical review of treatment and eventual prognosis. J Pediatr Surg 1971; 6:290–300.
82. Noordijk JA. Omphalocoele and gastroschisis. *In*: Persaud TVN, ed. Advances in the Study of Birth Defects. Vol 6. Lancaster: MTP Press, 1982.
83. Beckwith JB, Wang CI, Donnell GN, Gwinn JL. Hyperplastic fetal visceromegaly with macroglossia, omphalocele, cytomegaly of adrenal frontal cortex, postnatal somatic gigantism, and other abnormalities. Proceedings of the American Pediatric Society, Seattle, Washington, June 16–18, 1964 (Abstract 41).
84. Irving IM. Exomphalos with macroglossia: A study of eleven cases. J Pediatr Surg 1967; 2:499–507.
85. Gross RE. A new method for surgical treatment of large omphaloceles. Surgery 1948; 24:277–92.
86. Schuster SR. A new method for the staged repair of large omphaloceles. Surg Gynecol Obstet 1967; 125:837–50.
87. Grob M. Conservative treatment of exomphalos. Arch Dis Child 1963; 38:148–50.
88. Ladd WE. Surgical diseases of the alimentary tract in infants. N Engl J Med 1936; 215:705–8.
89. Louw JH. Intestinal malrotation and duodenal ileus. J R Coll Surg Edinb 1960; 5:101–26.
90. Bockus HL. Minor developmental anomalies of the colon: Clinical aspects. *In*: Bockus HL, ed. Gastroenterology. Vol 2, 3rd Ed. Philadelphia: WB Saunders, 1976.
91. Hansmann GH, Morton SA. Intra-abdominal hernia: Report of a case and review of literature. Arch Surg 1939; 39:973–86.
92. Andrews E. Duodenal hernia—a misnomer. Surg Gynecol Obstet 1923; 37:740–50.
93. Baker AH. Developmental mesenteric cysts. Br J Surg 1961; 48:534–40.
94. Kantor JL. Common anomalies of duodenum and colon: Their practical significance. JAMA 1931; 97:1785–90.
95. Forshall I, Hall EG, Rickham PP. Meconium peritonitis. Br J Surg 1952; 40:31–40.
96. Lorimer WS, Ellis DG. Meconium peritonitis. Surgery 1966; 60:470–5.
97. Drey NW. Symptomatic annular pancreas in the adult. Ann Intern Med 1957; 46:750–72.
98. Dodd GD, Nafis WA. Annular pancreas in the adult. Am J Roentgenol Rad Ther Nucl 1956; 75:333–42.
99. Willis RA. Pathology of Tumours. London: Butterworth & Co, 1948.
100. Davis WS, Allen RP, Favara BE, Slovis TC. Neonatal small left colon syndrome. Am J Roentgenol Rad Ther Nucl Med 1974; 120:322–9.
101. Davis WS, Campbell JB. Neonatal small left colon syndrome: Occurrence in asymptomatic infants of diabetic mothers. Am J Dis Child 1975; 129:1024–7.
102. Ashcraft KW, Holder TM. Congenital megaileocolon (basket-ball bowel) with teratoma. J Pediatr Surg 1966; 1:178–83.
103. Blunt A, Rich GF. Congenital absence of the colon and rectum. Am J Dis Child 1967; 114:405–6.
104. Trusler GA, Mestel AL, Stephens CA. Colon malformation with imperforate anus. Surgery 1959; 45:328–34.
105. Zaidi ZH. Congenital absence of most of colon: Anomaly associated with imperforate anus, syndactylism and polydactylism. Am J Dis Child 1959; 98:385–7.
106. Agarwal S, Patnaik R. Review of cases of short colon. Presented at the World Congress of Pediatric Surgery, Bombay, February 1980.
107. Pathak IC, Mitra SK, Yadav K, Bhattacharyya NC. Short colon. Presented at the World Congress of Pediatric Surgery, Bombay, February 1980.
108. Singh A, Singh R, Singh A. Short colon malformation with imperforate anus. Presented at the World Congress of Pediatric Surgery, Bombay, February 1980.
109. Vaezzadeh K, Gerami S, Kalani P. Short colon associated with imperforate anus. A plan for definitive treatment by colonorrhaphy. Presented at the World Congress of Pediatric Surgery, Bombay, February 1980.
110. Bennington JL, Haber SL. The embryologic significance of an undifferentiated intestinal tract. J Pediatr 1964; 64:735–9.
111. Berdon WE, Slovis TL, Campbell JB, Baker DH, Haller JO. Neonatal small left colon syndrome: Its relationship to aganglionosis and meconium plug syndrome. Radiology 1977; 125:457–62.
112. Browne D. Some congenital deformities of the rectum, anus, vagina and urethra. Ann R Coll Surg Engl 1951; 8:173–92.
113. Stephens FD. Congenital imperforate rectum, rectourethral and rectovaginal fistulae. Aust NZ J Surg 1953; 22:161–72.
114. Kelly JH. The radiographic anatomy of the normal and abnormal neonatal pelvis. J Pediatr Surg 1969; 4:432–44.

Chapter 88

Gross Anatomy of the Small Intestine

William S. Haubrich

The Duodenum **The Jejunum and Ileum**

The Duodenum

The name duodenum (a Latin derivation from the Greek *dodekadaktulon,* 12 fingers) was applied to the most proximal segment of the small intestine because of its length—12 fingers' breadth. In German it is called the "zwölffingerdarm." The shortest, widest, and most fixed segment of the small intestine, its length ranges between 20 and 30 cm, and its diameter varies from 3 to 5 cm. Its shape is generally that of a horseshoe as applied to the posterior abdominal wall, with the open end directed up and to the left. The duodenum is conveniently subdivided into 4 portions: the first or superior portion, which corresponds to the radiologist's designation of duodenal cap or bulb; the second, or vertical or descending portion; the third, the horizontal or transverse portion; and the fourth, the oblique or ascending portion (Fig. 88–1).

The *first portion,* the "cap" or "bulb," is shaped as a hollow cone, with its base resting on the pylorus and its apex usually pointing cephalad, to the right, and slightly posteriorly. In the more familiar 2-dimensional radiographic picture, the duodenal cap appears as a triangle and is best demonstrated in oblique projections. It is remarkable that over 90% of all duodenal peptic ulcers, among the most common lesions of the digestive system, occur in this first 5-cm portion of the duodenum.

In order to describe disease in this segment more accurately, specific names have been given to each point and side of the duodenal cap (Fig. 88–2.) The first portion of the duodenum is almost completely enveloped by peritoneum and, hence, is the most mobile segment. Posteriorly, a fold of peritoneum forms a small omental bursa between the first portion of the duodenum and the pancreas. Over the upper aspect, the anterior and posterior layers of peritoneum join together and proceed cephalad as the hepatoduodenal ligament. Within this ligament is situated the important triad of the portal vein, hepatic artery, and common bile duct. The free margin of this ligament, facing to the right, constitutes the anterior border of the foramen of Winslow. To the left and proximally, the hepatoduodenal ligament is continuous with the gastrohepatic ligament, which forms the anterior wall of the lesser omental space. Immediately above the first portion of the duodenum is the quadrate lobe of the liver and the gallbladder; the latter normally can impinge on the lesser curve of the cap to produce a smooth concavity in radiographs. Behind and below, the first portion of the duodenum is adjacent to the head of the pancreas. Because of this relation, the

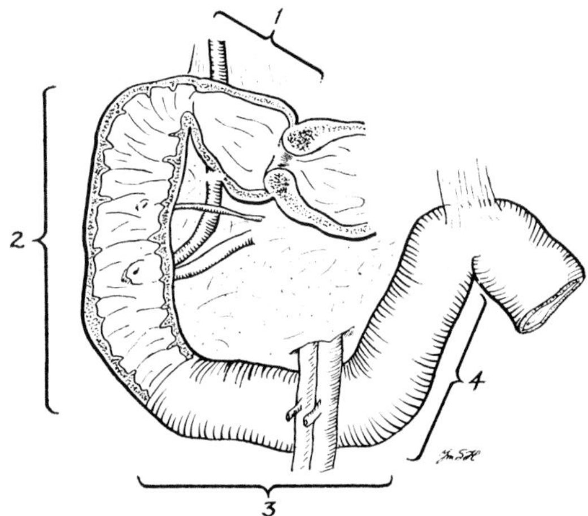

Figure 88–1. Schematic drawing of the duodenum delineating the 4 portions described in the text and illustrating the duodenum's relation to the common bile duct and to the superior mesenteric artery and vein. The first and second portions are depicted as opened to illustrate the difference in mucosal patterns.

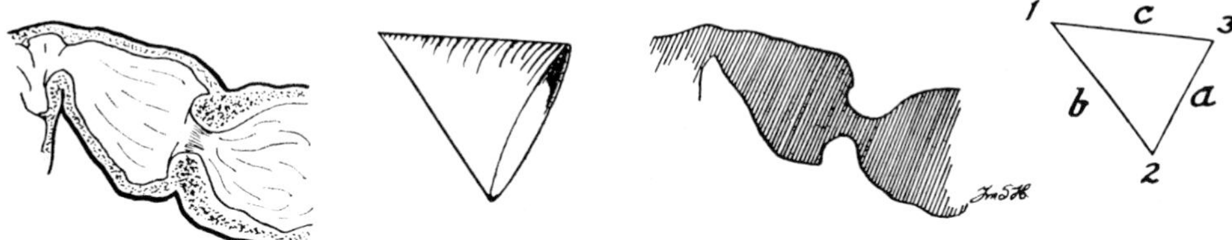

Figure 88–2. Diagrams of the first portion or duodenal bulb. In 3 dimensions it resembles a hollow cone. In 2 dimensions, as seen in radiographs, its shape is a triangle. In the figure at the far right, the sides are: *a,* base; *b,* greater curve; and *c,* lesser curve (taken from the corresponding aspects of the stomach); the points are: *1,* apex; *2,* greater recessus; and *3,* lesser recessus. Peptic ulcer deformity often leads to the appearance of pseudodiverticula at *2* or *3.*

pancreas is the commonest site of confined perforation by a duodenal ulcer.

The *second or descending portion* of the duodenum descends vertically at the right of the midline from the apex of the cap, usually at the level of the first lumbar vertebra, to the second flexure of the duodenum, usually at the level of the third lumbar vertebra. Its course is slightly concave to the right as it hugs the head of the pancreas. Occasionally, a carcinoma or inflammatory mass in the head of the pancreas can efface the mucosal pattern along the medial aspect of the descending duodenum. The descending segment is retroperitoneal. Horizontally across its midpoint, folds of peritoneum come together from above and below to form the mesocolon (see Fig. 131–7). Congenital diverticula of the duodenum are commonly seen extending from the medial aspect of the second portion. Also, approximately at its midpoint along the medial aspect, the main pancreatic duct (of Wirsung) joins the common bile duct to form an ampulla which projects into the duodenum as a papilla (of Vater). About 2.5 cm superiorly may occur the orifice of the accessory pancreatic duct (of Santorini). Blood vessels supplying the descending segment are situated along its *medial* aspect; hence, the Kocher procedure for mobilization of the duodenum begins by incising the peritoneal attachment along its *lateral* aspect.

The *third or transverse portion* of the duodenum turns to the left and crosses the midline horizontally at about the level of the third lumbar vertebra. It is almost wholly retroperitoneal except at a point two-thirds along its course where the peritoneum folds out to form the root of the mesentery of the small intestine. This mesentery carries the superior mesenteric artery, vein, and nerve plexus *anterior* to the third portion of the duodenum; posteriorly run the aorta and inferior vena cava. In a rare individual, usually of an asthenic habitus, the superior mesenteric vessel sheath may impinge on the third portion of the duodenum and produce chronic intermittent *arteriomesenteric occlusion* of the duodenum (Chapter 83). Another unusual cause of obstruction along the second or third portion of the duodenum is represented by congenital ligamentous bands (of Harris), which may descend from the liver or gallbladder to a firm attachment in the mesocolon.

The *fourth or ascending portion* of the duodenum passes in front and to the left of the aorta and ascends obliquely to about the level of the second lumbar vertebra where it turns abruptly forward and downward to continue as the jejunum. The intimacy of the duodenum and aorta can lead to a dire complication of aortic grafting, wherein the graft erodes the duodenal wall; the result can be massive intestinal hemorrhage. The duodenojejunal junction is fixed by a fibromuscular ligament (of Treitz), which is composed of 2 parts: (1) a slip of striated muscle extending downward from the right crus of the diaphragm, and (2) a fibromuscular band that extends from the duodenum to blend with pericoeliac connective tissue.[1] Occasionally, in radiographs of the barium-filled stomach and duodenum, the gastric angulus appears at the level of the duodenojejunal junction. A barium outline of the small bowel then may be superimposed on the barium outline of the lesser curve of the stomach to erroneously suggest an additive defect in the stomach.

Immediately above the fourth portion of the duodenum is the body of the pancreas, in which a space-occupying lesion may displace the duodenum downward. As a result of the secondary fixation of the mesentery of the descending colon to the posterior abdominal wall, just to the left of the duodenojejunal junction, there are one or more recesses which vary considerably in size and depth from one individual to another. The significance of these *duodenal fossae* is that they may contain hernias of jejunum or ileum. Usually such hernias extend to the left of the fourth portion of the duodenum.

It is helpful to know that the mucosal pattern of the first portion or duodenal cap can be distinguished radiographically and endoscopically from that of the remaining duodenum. In the cap, relatively shallow folds run longitudinally and often are obliterated as the cap is distended or compressed. Beginning abruptly at the junction between the first and second portions of the duodenum, one sees the deeper, permanent transverse *valvulae conniventes* (folds of Kerckring) characteristic of the small intestine.

The course of the duodenum is susceptible to distortion by intrinsic or extrinsic disease, of which several examples have been cited. At the same time it must be appreciated that there can be considerable normal variation in the configuration of the duodenum (Fig. 88–3). These variations can appear quite startling in radiographs but should not be mistaken for disease.

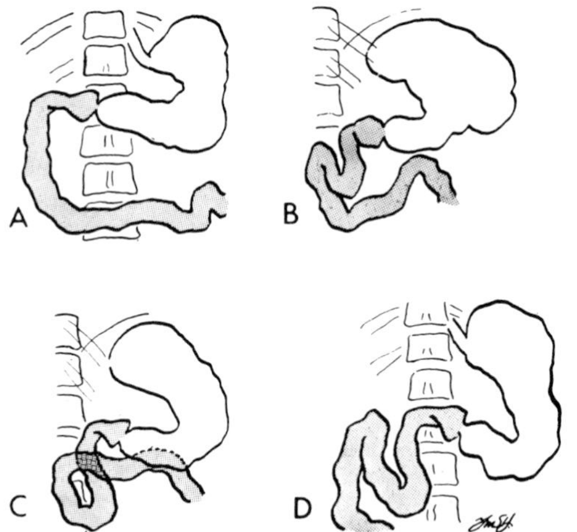

Figure 88–3. Examples of variations in configuration of the duodenum as a result of anomalous fixation and usually not associated with symptoms: *A,* Absence of the fourth portion, with low duodenojejunal attachment (if the third portion is absent, i.e., if the jejunum takes off to the right of the vertebrae, then malrotation of the entire intestine is likely). *B,* Redundant superior and descending segments. *C,* Reversed duodenal loop. *D,* Redundancy with duodenojejunal junction to the right of the midline; this configuration almost invariably is associated with anomalous non-rotation in which the small intestine, including the distal duodenum, and the colon share a common mesentery (Chapter 87).

The Jejunum and Ileum

The length of the mesenteric small intestine is about 6 meters (20 feet). It tends to be slightly longer in men than in women and varies with the height of the subject.[2, 3] A precise measurement is illusory, as the living intestine is capable of elongation and shortening. In fact, a 3-meter aspirating tube will usually pass from the patient's mouth to the cecum or beyond. Also, a surgically removed segment of the small intestine will contract markedly on resection and by almost half when fixed in formalin.[3] The proximal two-fifths of the mesenteric small intestine is customarily referred to as *jejunum* (from the Latin, meaning "empty"), and the distal three-fifths is designated as *ileum* (from the Greek *eilein,* "to roll or twist").

The division between jejunum and ileum is arbitrary, there being no sharp demarcation. There is, however, a gradual and significant change in structure by which the 2 segments can be distinguished. The wall of the jejunum is thicker and its lumen is wider. There is also a gradual diminution in caliber of the small intestine from the duodenum to the distal ileum. Because of its narrower lumen, the ileum is more susceptible to obstruction either by obturation, as in gallstone ileus, or by intrinsic disease, as in regional enteritis.

There is a characteristic distinction in the mesentery of the jejunum and ileum which is useful to the surgeon as he examines the small intestine at laparotomy (Fig. 88–4): the fat is thicker in the ileal mesentery and extends fully to the intestinal attachment. It is of interest that in chronic regional enteritis (as in Crohn's disease) the thickened mesenteric fat encroaches further beneath the serosa of the small intestine, occasionally almost enveloping its circumference (Chapter 127).

The mesentery is richly seeded with lymph nodes disposed along a rich network of lymphatic channels. The wall of the small intestine normally is infiltrated by lymphocytes and other mononuclear cells occurring singly and accumulated in solitary nodules. The

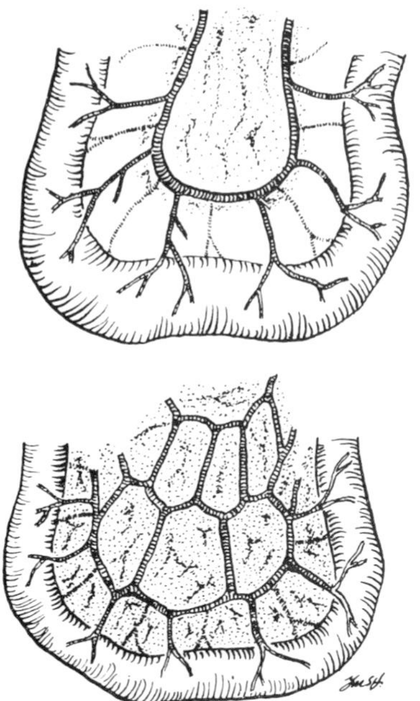

Figure 88–4. Comparative diagrams of the mesentery of the jejunum *(above)* and of the ileum *(below)* illustrating the differences in extent of the mesenteric fat and in vascular patterns.

solitary lymphocyte nodules are particularly well developed in the ileum, where they can be seen as elliptical plaques (Peyer's patches) along that aspect of the ileal wall opposite the mesenteric attachment.

The most striking distinction between the jejunum and ileum is in the vascular pattern within the supporting mesentery[4] (Chapter 115). The jejunum and ileum are served by 12 or more branches of the superior mesenteric artery which fan out between the peritoneal layers of the mesentery to form extensive loops or arcades. From these arcades, straight arterial branches run to the intestinal wall. For most of the jejunum, the arterial arcades are single and the straight branches are longer. For the ileum, the arcuate pattern becomes progressively complex, with 2, 3, and 4 arcades toward the ileocecal junction; the straight arterial branches are consequently shorter. It is noteworthy that the straight arterial branches are, for the most part, end-arteries, i.e., there is little, if any, direct communication between the terminal twigs. Therefore, if a straight arterial branch is severed or occluded, that segment of bowel which it supplies may be precariously dependent on capillary anastomoses.

As one views the opened abdomen, the loops of small intestine appear to be disposed almost at random. In general, the jejunum occupies the left upper portion of the abdominal cavity, and the ileum occupies a part of the pelvis and the right lower abdomen.[5] This disposition is accounted for by the situation of the mesentery. It is remarkable that, although the small intestine is 6 meters long, only about 15 cm separate the duodenojejunal junction and the ileocecal valve. This distance of 15 cm represents the extent of the root of the mesentery, which begins at the left of the second lumbar vertebra and extends diagonally downward to the right of the fourth or fifth lumbar vertebra. The distance from the root of the mesentery to its attachment on the small bowel varies from 12 to 25 cm along the jejunum and proximal ileum, then diminishes to about 5 cm at the terminal ileum.[6] If one grasps the root of the mesentery between the fingers of both hands and draws his hands toward the intestine, one can immediately identify the polarity of any given segment of small intestine. Regrettably, it is not possible to apply this maneuver to radiographs.

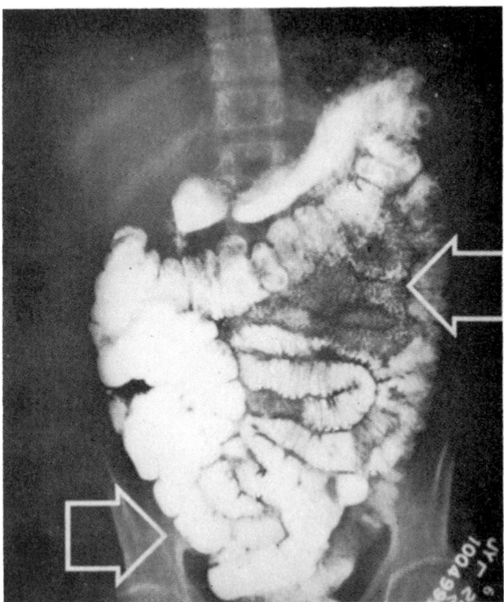

Figure 88–5. Barium outlining simultaneously the stomach, small intestine, and most of the colon. The fine, feathery mucosal pattern of the jejunal loops in the upper abdomen *(upper arrow)* contrasts with the sausage-shaped ileal loops in the right lower abdomen and pelvis *(lower arrow).* The valvulae conniventes are clearly seen in the intermediate loops.

The mucosa in the proximal and distal segments of the small intestine is grossly distinguishable. In the jejunum, as they are in the duodenum, the transverse folds of Kerckring (valvulae conniventes) are thick, tall, and numerous. When the bowel is contracted, they tend to be tortuous. In the ileum the transverse folds are progressively fewer and less prominent. Because of this difference, the radiographic patterns of the barium-filled jejunum and ileum are normally distinctive (Fig. 88–5). The transverse folds may not completely encircle the lumen but extend about two-thirds around the circumference, where an individual fold may branch to join its neighbor; some folds may appear as spirals.[1]

References

1. Williams PL, Warwick R. Gray's Anatomy, 36th ed. Philadelphia: WB Saunders, 1980.
2. Underhill BML. Intestinal length in man. Br Med J 1955; 2:1243–6.
3. Jit I, Grewel SS. Lengths of the small and large intestine in North Indian subjects. J Anat (India) 1975; 24:89–100.
4. Anderson JE. Grant's Atlas of Anatomy, 7th ed. Baltimore: Williams & Wilkins, 1978: 2–91.
5. Figge FHJ. Sobotta Atlas of Anatomy, 9th ed. New York: Hafner Press, 1974: 126–9.
6. Hollinshead WH. Anatomy for Surgeons. Vol II, 2nd ed. New York: Harper & Row, 1971: 460–70.

Chapter 89

Microscopic Anatomy of the Small Intestine

Margot Shiner

The 4 coats of the cylindrically shaped bowel wall are, from within outward: mucosa, submucosa, muscular layers, and subserosa and serosa.

The *mucosa* is thrown into circular or convoluted folds known as the folds of Kerckring or valvulae conniventes. These are redder, thicker, taller, and more numerous in the jejunum than in the ileum. They run in a transverse direction to the longitudinal axis of the bowel and interdigitate. Each of these folds is covered by fingerlike projections, the intestinal villi, which are taller in the jejunum than in either the duodenum or the ileum. It follows that the jejunum presents a greater surface area to the bowel lumen than the other parts of the small intestine, and this is no doubt of great importance for luminal absorption and food digestion. The total mucosal thickness of the normal jejunum varies between 530 and 900 μ (average 696.9 μ) and the villous height between 300 and 780 μ (average 525.4 μ). The mucosa is separated from the submucosa by a layer of smooth muscle, the muscularis mucosae.

The *submucosa* is composed of a network of loose connective tissue rich in small blood vessels, lymphatics, and nerve plexuses of Meissner. It is situated between the muscularis mucosae and the muscular layers.

The *muscular layers* consist of 2 coats of smooth or nonstriated muscle, the inner circular and the outer longitudinal layer. The circular muscle is much thicker than the longitudinal. Both layers are thickest in the duodenum and gradually diminish in thickness down the small intestine. The myenteric plexus (of Auerbach), a ganglionated plexus of non-myelinated nerve fibers, and also a plexus of lymph vessels lie between the 2 muscle layers.

The *serosa,* or serous coat, is formed by peritoneum derived from the mesentery. It covers the duodenum incompletely and the jejunum and ileum almost completely. The serosa forms the outermost coat of the bowel except for a narrow strip posteriorly at the junction of visceral and mesenteric peritoneum. The subserosa is a fine layer of loose connective tissue between the longitudinal muscle coat and the serosa.

Mucosal Histology

The duodenum, jejunum, and ileum share, in general, a common morphologic layout. In addition, certain features such as Brunner's glands of the duodenum and Peyer's patches of the ileum are confined largely to specific parts of the small intestine. This chapter describes the common histologic appearances first, followed by the specific and regional features.

The villi facing the lumen of the bowel are lined by a single layer of tall columnar cells (Fig. 89–1) containing oval-shaped nuclei, which are situated toward the lower pole of the cells. The cells, derived from the junction of crypt and villi, are tallest and best developed in the middle third of the villus.[4, 18] Toward the tip of the villus the epithelial cells are often irregular; this is the site from which they are ultimately shed into the lumen. Apart from the mature absorptive epithelial cell, which forms the majority of cells of the villi, there are 3 other cell types to be found: the goblet cell, the theliolymphocyte, and the cells of the gut neuroendocrine system, also known as the APUD (amine precursor uptake and decarboxylation) cells. The peptides within the APUD cells may be broadly classified as mucosal (endocrine-paracrine) peptides and neuropeptides.

At the luminal end of the villous epithe-

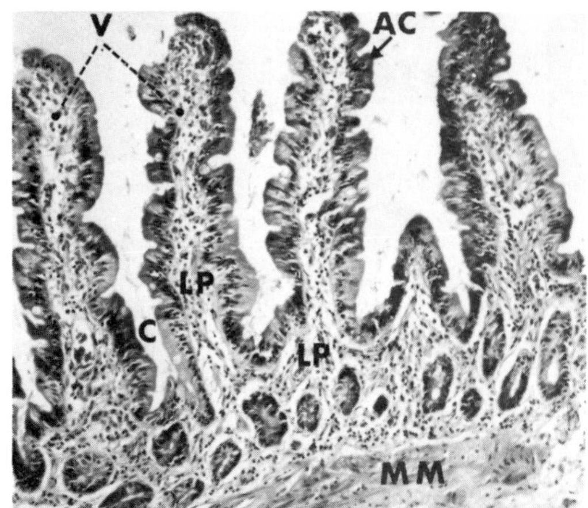

Figure 89–1. Light micrograph of the normal jejunal mucosal villi (V); absorbing cell (AC); crypt (C); muscularis mucosae (MM); and lamina propria (LP) (× 1500).

lium is the brush border, which is composed of tall, closely packed microvilli through which absorption takes place. At the lower pole of the absorbing epithelium and exterior to the cell membrane, the basal lamina or basement membrane forms a fine reticular layer between the cells and the connective tissue filling the core of the villi. The connective tissue or lamina propria is a loose coat of predominantly reticular fibers, containing most important structures of different types. There are thin fibers of smooth muscle radiating from the muscularis mucosae beneath and extending toward the tips of the villi, thus enabling the latter to contract. Small blood vessels, which represent terminal ramifications and central lacteal vessels, are found in abundance in the connective tissue and are in intimate contact with the basal laminae of the absorbing cells. The lamina propria is also rich in nerve fibrils and may contain occasional lymph nodules. At all times the connective tissue is infiltrated by inflammatory cells, of which the lymphocytes and plasma cells are the most numerous. Other cells types include eosinophils, macrophages, and occasional mast cells. The connective tissue is replenished by fibrocytes situated within the lamina propria.

The mucosal glands or *crypts of Lieberkühn* occupy the area of the lamina propria between the villi and the muscularis mucosae. The glands are short and tubular and several of them can, in a 3-dimensional view, be seen to surround a single villus[18] (Chapter 47). The columnar crypt cells are in direct continuity with the villous absorbing cells and are also derived from the area at the junction of crypts and villi—the junctional zone. They can be divided into undifferentiated and differentiated cells. The former are seen mainly in the upper parts of the crypts and are of 2 types—the immature cells rich in ribosomes and the undifferentiated cell proper characterized by an abundance of mitochondria and endoplasmic reticulum. The differentiated cells are the Paneth cells, the goblet cells, and the APUD cells.

The *Paneth cells* are the exocrine secretory cells situated near the base of the crypts and are recognized by their intensely staining eosinophilic granules. They are most numerous in the ileum, jejunum, and duodenum, in that order, but may also be found in the normal appendix.[22] Under pathologic conditions they may be found in the stomach and colon.[16] Their turnover is slower than any other crypt cell with the exception of the APUD cells.[8] The granules are discharged by a merocrine-type of secretory process.[22]

The chemical composition of the Paneth cell granules is a carbohydrate-protein complex.[17] The cells are rich in enzymes, principally lysosomal enzymes[28] (non-specific acid phosphatases and E 600–resistant esterases), as well as monoamine oxidases and ubiquinone, and contain important trace elements such as zinc and calcium, which may act as activators and stabilizers of lysozyme.[22]

The *goblet cells* are most numerous in the lower parts of the crypts and decrease on their way upward toward the villi. They produce an exocrine secretion rich in acid mucopolysaccharide and glycoproteins.[26] In the mature goblet cells the secretory granules appear large and pale, occupying the cytoplasm above the nucleus. The origin of the goblet cells is uncertain, but they may be derived from the same cell type that forms the columnar absorbing cells.

The *theliolymphocytes* were first described by Fichtelius[10] in 1968. These cells, resembling lymphocytes, are found throughout the small intestinal interepithelial spaces formed by the separation of lateral intercellular membranes. In the normal mucosa they are recognized at the light microscopic level by their small, densely staining nuclei surrounded by light-colored cytoplasm, with counts of less than 30 cells/100 epithelial cells.[2] Immunologic studies have shown that they are T cells with both suppressor and cytolytic activity.[1] Hence, they may function as effector cells.

Ultrastructurally, they are composed of both small and large lymphocytes as well as "blast" lymphocytes and have been shown to undergo cell division.[20] Since they can be seen mainly in the distal parts of the interepithelial spaces and often dissect the epithelial cell basal lamina, it has been assumed that they traffic in and out between these spaces and the lamina propria. Some theliolymphocytes resemble macrophages with large, indented nuclei and numerous cytoplasmic organelles, including mitochondria, rough and smooth endoplasmic reticulum, Golgi vesicles, and a few dense granules.

The *APUD cells* represent a diffuse system of cells which connect the central nervous system (hypothalamo-pituitary region and the pineal gland) with the gastro-entero-pancreatic endocrine cells and probably a number of other organs (Chapter 241). Their classification and characterization are difficult. Although at present over 40 different peptide series are known, it has been possible to identify only 18 specific cell types (Santa Monica 1980 classification).[30] Those mucosal endocrine cells located among the small intestinal epithelial cells of the mucosal villi or crypts contain secretion granules.[28] They can be divided into: (1) peptides with specific endocrine function (such as gastrin in the G and IG cells and secretin in the S cells) and (2) peptides functioning as circulatory hormones (gastric inhibitory polypeptide (GIP) in the K cells, motilin in the Mo cells, and probably cholecystokinin (CCK) in the I cells). Some peptides are released by food components, such as neurotensin from N cells situated in the lower small intestine, enteroglucagon from L cells, and somatostatin from D cells.[34]

Of the mucosal endocrine cells, the enterochromaffin (EC) cells are among the oldest identified cell types because of their argentaffinity and their characteristic ultrastructure. The EC cell usually occupies a basal position within the crypts and is rarely seen in the villi. Its secretory granules are situated infranuclearly, facing the basal lamina. These granules are smaller than those of the Paneth cells and stain positively by all silver staining techniques. They secrete 5-hydroxytryptamine and are probably the source of serotonin.

The *cells containing neuropeptides* are mainly situated deeper in the intestinal wall and are intimately associated with the nerve plexuses of Meissner and Auerbach, as well as with the small blood vessels surrounding these plexuses. Some neuropeptides, however, are also found within the mucosal endocrine cells, which may thus contain more than one specific peptide.[30] Examples of such heterogeneity are gastrin, somatostatin, and cholecystokinin.

Among the other neuropeptides identified are vasoactive intestinal polypeptides (VIP), substance P, bombesin, enkephalins, and thyrotropin-releasing hormone (TRH).[27] Many of these peptides are also found in the brain. Their physiologic role has been determined: (1) they act on gut muscle either as constrictors (substance P) or relaxers (VIP); (2) they reduce gastric and intestinal motility and secretion (enkephalins and TRH); (3) they act as vasodilators (VIP, substance P); (4) they block release of gastrointestinal hormones (somatostatin, TRH); (5) they act as neurotransmitters (substance P, enkephalins, CCK, gastrin, bombesin, and TRH); or (6) they have specific actions on pancreatic secretion, gallbladder tone, and water and electrolyte secretion in the gut.

Epithelial cell renewal in the human intestinal mucosa has been studied by serial peroral biopsies with techniques using mitotic counts or radioactive isotopes and microautoradiography. These studies have revealed a zone of cell proliferation occupying the greater part of the crypts of Lieberkühn.[6] These cells are the precursors of the mature villous epithelium and are the only cells with mitotic activity. The tritium-labeled thymidine used in these studies is incorporated into the deoxyribonucleic acid (DNA) of proliferating crypt cells, and the position of labeled and unlabeled cells permits an estimate of the removal of labeled cells and thus of cell renewal. Cell removal and cell renewal are interdependent, so that the faster the cell renewal, the greater the cell turnover is likely to be. Estimates of the migration time of cells from the proliferative zone in the crypts to the tips of the villi and ultimately to the lumen of the small intestine have varied from 2 to 6 days.[3, 6, 15, 19] Cell removal has been estimated at 1 to 2 cells/100 cells/hour.[15]

Brunner's glands, like Peyer's patches, lie mainly in the submucosa but often extend into the mucosal layers. They occur in the duodenum of all mammals. Brunner's glands begin at the junction of gastric and duodenal mucosa and extend distally to a variable degree, even beyond the duodenojejunal flexure. They appear to decrease with age.

The glands occur as aggregates in the proximal duodenum and become more scattered distally. Microscopically they are composed of branching tubules into which acini open. Their long ducts pass through the whole thickness of the mucosa to open on the surface or into the crypts of Lieberkühn. The acinar cells are flattened epithelial structures containing a clear mucuslike substance, but other "dense" or "dark" nonsecretory cells have been described. Their nuclei are basally situated. The functional aspect of Brunner's glands in man has not been adequately studied. It is known that in other mammals a mucinlike substance secreted by the acinar cells stains positively with periodic acid–Schiff (PAS). A metachromatic reaction obtained with toluidine blue and related dyes suggests the presence of sulfated mucin.[13] Food induces a response to acinar secretion, but the actual stimulation occurs through a humoral mechanism. Glucagon[11], and secretin[31] have been found to stimulate secretion of the glands.

Peyer's patches are aggregates of lymph nodules found mainly in the ileum. They are normally confined to the submucosa but may encroach upon the mucosa and the mucosal villi. Peyer's patches are situated opposite the mesenteric attachment and are identified by their oval shape. Their longitudinal axis coincides with that of the intestinal wall. Each aggregated nodule is composed of a group of solitary lymphoid nodules surrounded by lymphatic plexuses or sinuses. The nodules are more numerous in the lower half of the ileum and decrease with age.[5] The number of patches found varies between 40 and 100 and their length between 0.3 and 28.0 cm. Animal investigations have suggested that the general pattern of lymphoid tissue is laid down early in fetal life and that removal of Peyer's patches after birth is not followed by compensatory new formation of lymphoid tissue at other sites. In human fetuses Peyer's patches can be identified as early as 24 weeks of gestation. They increase in size and number throughout the second half of fetal life and continue to do so up to 10 years of age. Peyer's patches behave immunologically like peripheral lymph nodes. They may be composed of both thymus-derived and bursa-derived types of lymphoid cells and may contain IgM and IgG "memory" cells which have migrated from the spleen.[9]

Scanning electron microscopic studies of Peyer's patches show smooth, round mounds of tissue surrounded by groups of villi.[23] The epithelial cells of the mound have microfolds on their surface which distinguish them from the microvilli of surrounding villous epithelial cells. They were thus termed the *M cells*. Transmission electron microscopy further characterized the M cells by their thin bridges of cytoplasm of greater electron density than that of the surrounding lymphocytes and by their interdigitating processes which join onto other M cells or villous epithelial cells by tight and desmosomal junctions. Short, thick microfolds of the M cells face the lumen of the bowel, and lymphocytes (presumably derived from the underlying lymphoid follicles) occupy the spaces between adjacent interdigitating cells. These cells appear at times to be extruded into the bowel lumen. The remarkable M cell was seen as a fully specialized cell with transport activity for substances derived from the bowel lumen which, by virtue of the intimate relationship to lymphocytes from underlying lymphoid follicles, induces immune stimulation.

Mucosal Ultrastructure[32, 33, 35]

The villous epithelium of the small intestine has the typical fine structural appearances of absorbing cells throughout the body. Such a cell is shown diagrammatically in Figure 89–2 and ultrastructurally in Figure 89–3. The most characteristic feature of the villous

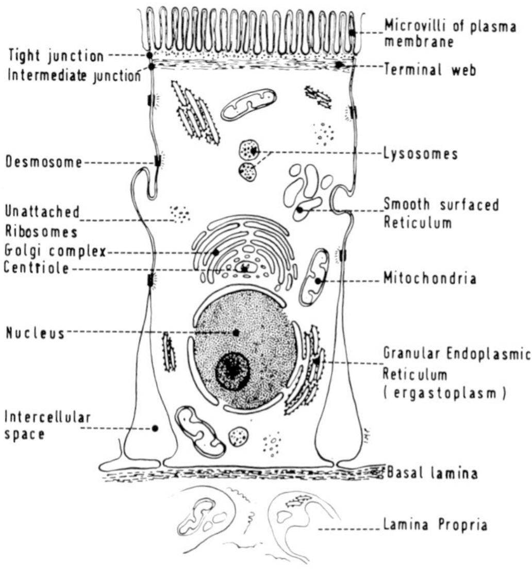

Figure 89–2. Schematic drawing of the fine structure of a columnar absorbing cell at the middle third of a villus.

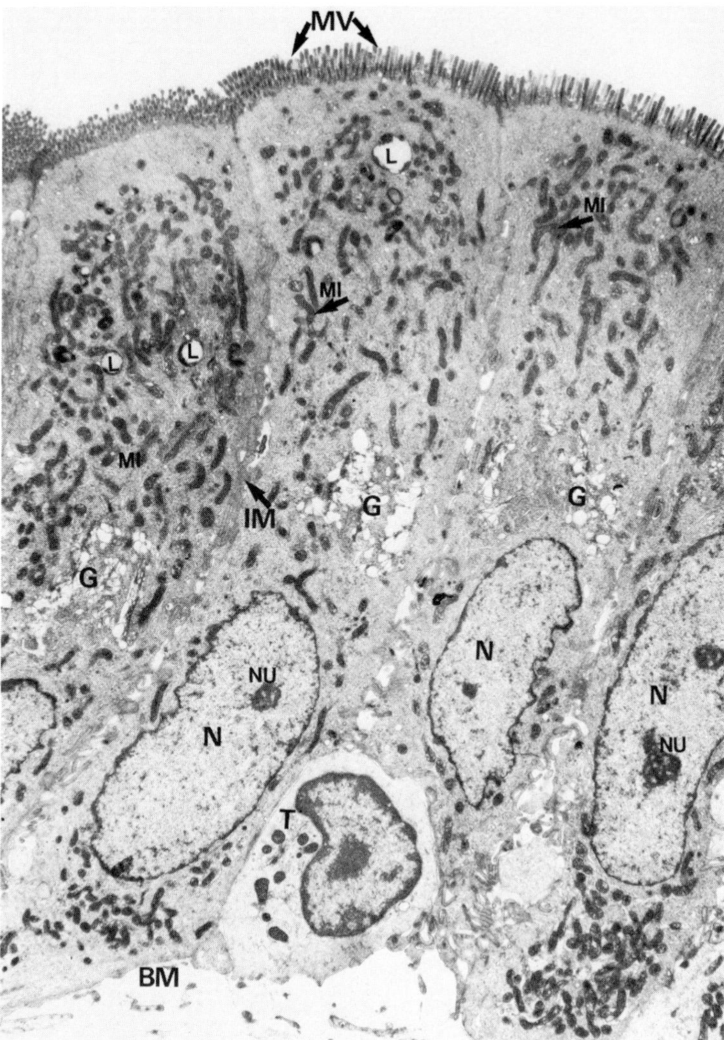

Figure 89–3. Several mature absorbing epithelial cells from the middle third of a normal villus showing microvilli (MV) at their luminal end, a fine basal lamina (BM) at the lower pole, and lateral intercellular membrane (IM). The IM is in part separated, and the intercellular space thus created is occupied by a theliolymphocyte (T). Within the cytoplasm is a basally situated nucleus (N) with nucleoli (NU), dilated Golgi vesicles (G), mitochondria (MI), and lysosomes (L) (× 2200).

absorbing epithelium is the brush border at the luminal surface of the absorbing cell. This consists of about 3000 microvilli/cell composed of tall fingerlike structures, average length 1.0 μ and width 0.08 μ (Fig. 89–4). The *microvilli* are surrounded by the 2 layers of the plasmalemma, or plasma membranes, which are part of and continuous with those of the lateral and basal membranes of the epithelial cell. The interior of the microvilli shows a core of fine longitudinal fibrils (arrow) which continue into the upper part of the cellular cytoplasm known as the terminal web (TW). This area terminates laterally at the terminal bar where the junctional complexes (JC) are found (Fig. 89–4).

The *plasma membrane* covering the microvilli, the lateral and the basal surfaces of the absorbing cell, is a triple-layered structure with 2 outer and more electron-dense leaflets enclosing a central and electron-lucent zone. Applied to the outer leaflet of the apical plasma membrane is a fine filamentous coat rich in acid mucopolysaccharides known as the glycocalyx. The lateral plasma membranes of adjacent absorbing cells show abundant interdigitations. They are held together by various junctional complexes, from above downward (Fig. 89–4): the zonula occludens (ZO) or tight junction, the zonula adherens (ZA) or intermediate junction, and the desmosomes or macula adherens (MA). The ZO and ZA are found only in the area of the terminal bar, whereas desmosomes are seen at all levels between the lateral cell membranes of adjacent cells. The ZO remains apposed at all times, but the ZA and the desmosomes show a space between the apposing membranes even in the resting phase of the cell. According to Brunser and Luft,[4] an amorphous material surrounds the ZO and ZA and extends from the terminal bar into the terminal web. It may function as a cement and may explain the adherence of the terminal web and bar to the microvilli during attempted disruptions of the cell, resulting in "brush border preparations."[21] The desmosomes, on the other hand, possess fine fibrils which are most dense at their junctional attachment and extend as a loose network, the desmosomal web, into the cellular cytoplasm. They permit separation of the lateral plasma

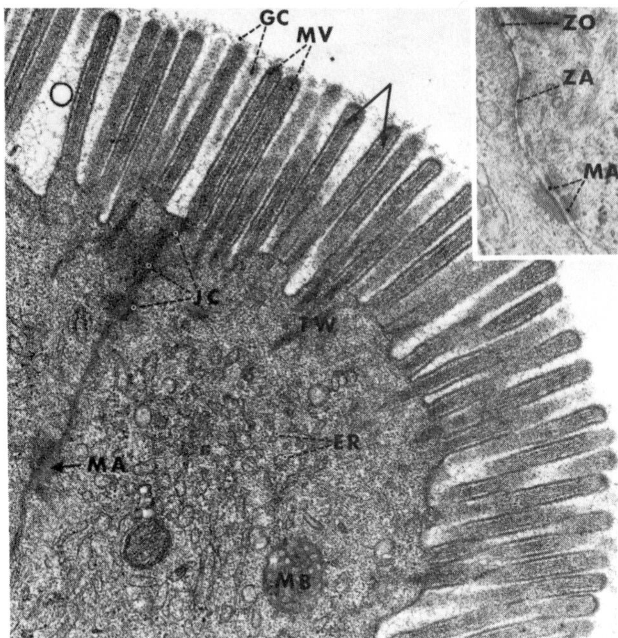

Figure 89–4. Electron micrograph of upper third of absorbing cells showing microvilli (MV); glycocalyx (GC); terminal web (TW); junctional complexes (JC); smooth endoplasmic reticulum (ER); and multivesicular body (MB) (× 30,000).

Inset shows the three types of junctional complexes: zonula occludens (ZO); zonula adherens (ZA); and macula adherens (MA) (× 55,000).

membranes below the ZO and the ZA during absorption. The theliolymphocytes are located in the intercellular spaces thus formed (Fig. 89–5).

Within the cytoplasm of the absorbing cell a variety of organelles are found below the level of the terminal web. Prominent among these is the *endoplasmic reticulum* (ER) or ergastoplasm, which is particularly well developed in the absorbing type of epithelium. It consists of tubular or parallel lamellar membrane-limited interconnecting systems extending throughout the cytoplasm (Figs. 89–4 and 89–6). The granular or rough surface ER (RER) contains ribosomes attached to the outer surface of the membranes, whereas the agranular or smooth surface ER is devoid of ribosome granules. The mature absorbing cells are characterized by relatively sparse numbers of free-lying ribosomes, most of these being attached to ER. The *mitochondria* are numerous and in the resting phase are situated mainly around the nucleus. During absorption they are found throughout the cytoplasm. They are usually elongated or ovoid in shape but may also appear branched. They are membrane-limited structures containing numerous membrane-bound partitions, the cristae mitochondriales. One of their principal functions is oxidative phosphorylation.

Whereas the mitochondria are surrounded by a 2-leaflet membrane, the *Golgi complex* or *apparatus* is composed of a system of single-layered, membrane-bound sacs or cisternae, situated above the nucleus (Fig. 89–7). In the resting phase of the absorbing cell, the Golgi cisternae are collapsed, but during absorption the cisternae dilate and appear to be involved in various metabolic processes such as concentrating absorbed material or the formation of zymogen granules (e.g., in the Paneth cells) and possibly of lysosomes.

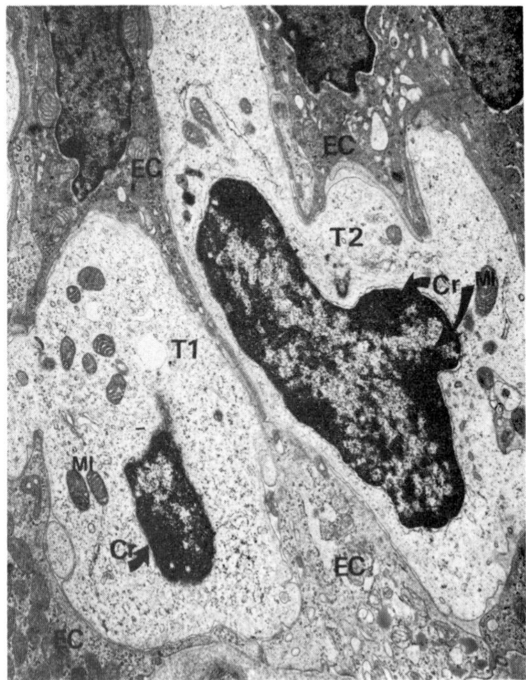

Figure 89–5. The theliolymphocytes (T1 and T2) with dense nuclear chromatin (Cr) and light background cytoplasm in which ribosomes predominate but a few mitochondria (MI), Golgi vesicles (G), ER, RER, and dense bodies *(arrow)* are seen. They are in the intercellular spaces between villus epithelial cells (EC) (× 3900).

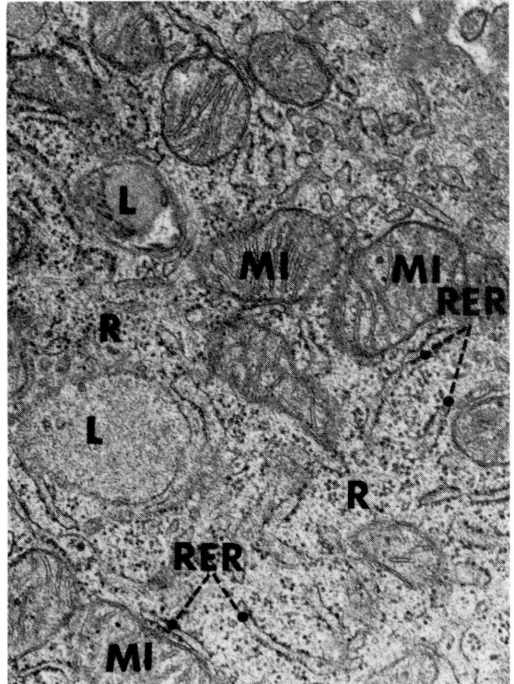

Figure 89–6. Electron micrograph through the middle third of an absorbing cell showing the intimate relationship of rough endoplasmic reticulum (RER) to mitochondria (MI). Some ribosomes (R) are unattached to ER. Two lysosomes (L) are also seen (× 30,000).

Lysosomes are normally found in the absorbing epithelium but become more numerous in pathologic states. They are found in the upper part of the cytoplasm and are saclike structures bound by a single membrane containing hydrolytic enzymes (Fig. 89–6). They are therefore the main components of an intracellular digestive system and may be either primary lysosomes, containing newly formed hydrolases that have not yet been involved in digestive processes, or secondary lysosomes within which the digestive functions are performed.[7] Substrates of lysosomal digestion may be either exogenous objects engulfed by endocytosis (heterophagy) or endogenous material such as small portions of cytoplasm (autophagy). Another form of autophagy is that of membrane fusion of lysosomes with other organelles, e.g., secretory granules (crinophagy).

Fine narrow *microtubules* (Fig. 89–8) of unknown function are seen within absorbing cells. Other cytoplasmic organelles are the *centrioles* (Fig. 89–8) situated at the apical pole of the nucleus in a central position with respect to the cell. They are seen in pairs, each consisting of a series of hollow cylinders which are closed at one end.

The *nucleus* (see Fig. 89–3) of the absorbing cell is situated in the lower half of the cell and is elliptical or irregularly rounded, with shallow indentations. It is surrounded by 2 membranes which are discontinuous at sites known as fenestrations. The most easily identified structures within the nucleus are the chromatin granules and often the nucleolus (Figs. 89–3 and 89–7).

The *basal lamina* (basement membrane) (see Fig. 89–2) is a part of the basal membrane of the absorbing cell and is situated on its outer side. It is a moderately thin band of fine filaments, chemically identified as collagen, which is embedded in an amorphous matrix composed of acid mucopolysaccharide. Beyond this layer lie the fibrils of the connective tissue, which include a limited number of collagen and smooth muscle fibers (Fig. 89–9). Embedded in these fibers are the fibroblasts, fibrocytes, and reticulum cells, the cells arising from the reticuloendothelial system (plasma cells, lymphocytes, mast cells, eosinophils, and macrophages) (Figs. 89–10 and 89–11), Schwann cells (Fig. 89–12), nonmyelinated nerve fibrils, and the endothelium forming the walls of capillaries and lymphatics. The *capillary endothelium* is composed of long, thin cytoplasmic processes of single cells (Fig. 89–13) increasing in diameter only in the region of the nucleus. The membranes are interrupted by porelike fenestrations which distinguish them from those of the lymphatic endothelium, which are uninterrupted. Both types of endothelia are surrounded by a basal lamina which is more clearly identified around the capillaries.

The *crypt epithelium* is composed of a variety of cell types with distinct fine structural appearances. Most of the single layer of cells possess a short brush border at their apices. At their lower pole a fine basal

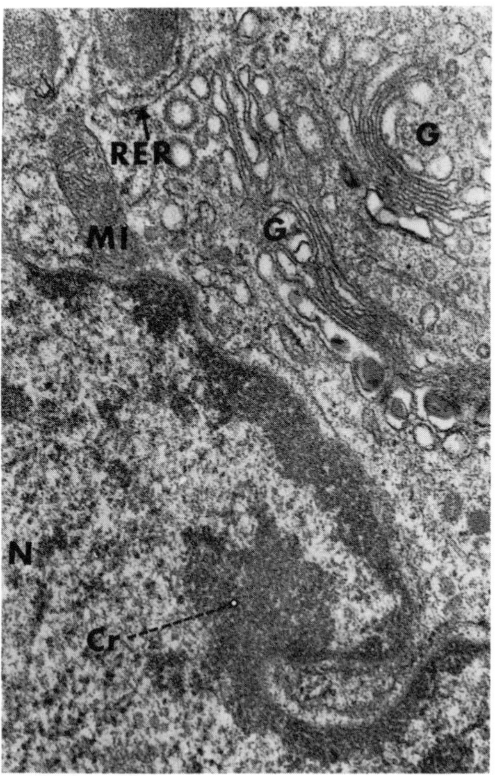

Figure 89–7. Electron micrograph at nuclear and supranuclear level of an absorbing cell showing part of the nucleus (N) and the membrane and the Golgi complex (G). (See text.) Cr = chromatin, RER = rough endoplasmic reticulum, MI = mitochondria (× 30,000).

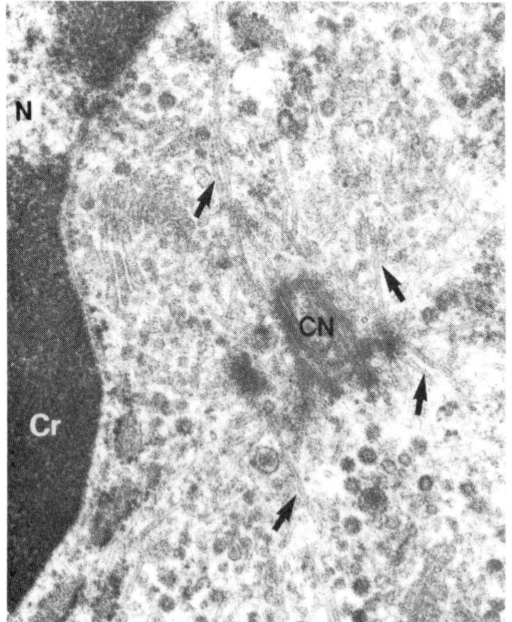

Figure 89–8. A centriole (CN) surrounded by microtubules *(arrows)* in the cytoplasm of an absorbing cell. Note its close relation to the nucleus (N). Cr = chromatin (× 18,000).

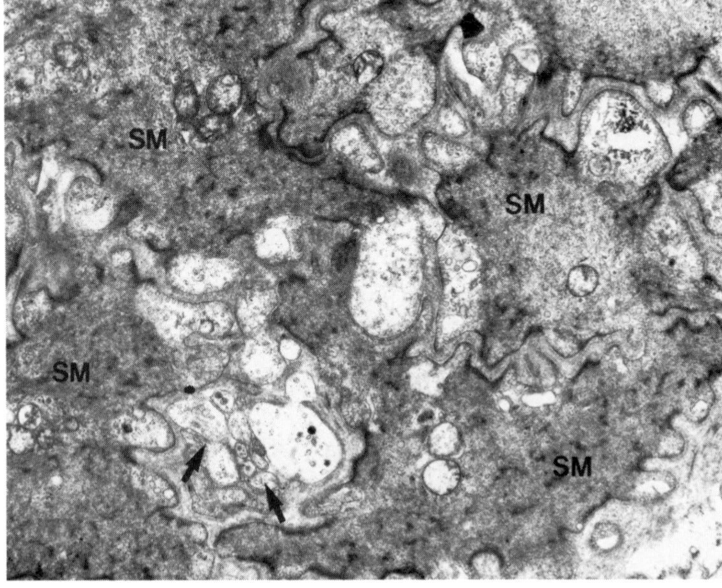

Figure 89–9. Smooth muscle fibers (SM) of the muscularis mucosae in which are embedded bundles of nerve axons *(arrows)* forming a plexus (× 7300).

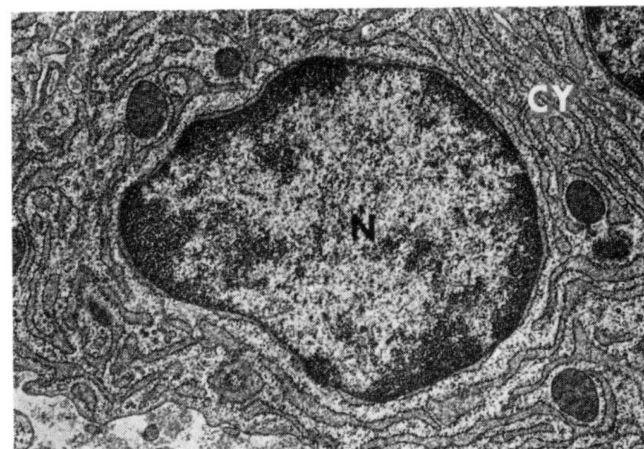

Figure 89–10. A plasma cell with its nucleus (N) and numerous cytoplasmic cisternae (CY) (× 8000).

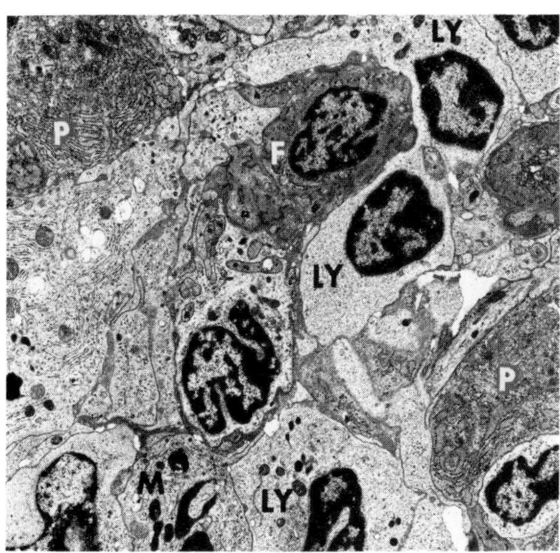

Figure 89–11. Various cell types in the mucosal connective tissue. F = fibrocyte, Ly = lymphoblast or lymphocyte, P = plasma cell, M = macrophage (× 4000).

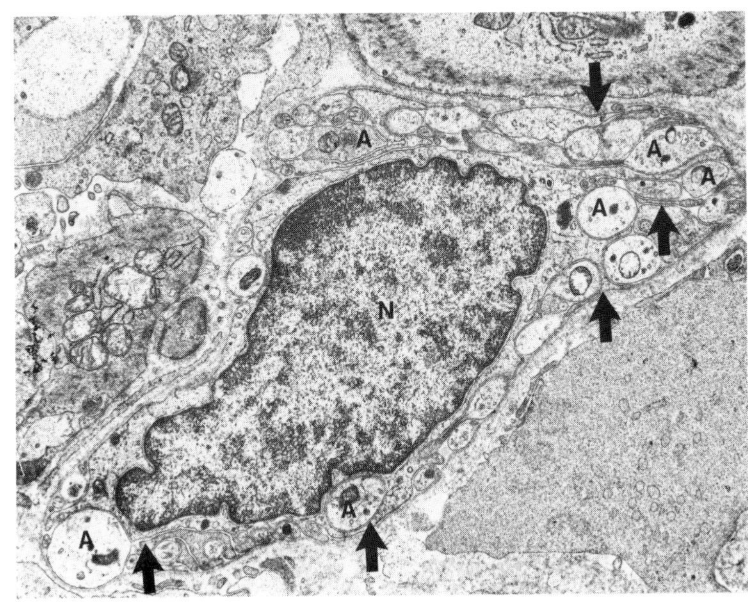

Figure 89–12. Cross section of several axons (A) surrounded by a sheath *(arrows)* derived from the Schwann cell with its nucleus (N). The axoplasm of the axons contains small dense bodies, neurotubules, and neurofibrils (× 10,500).

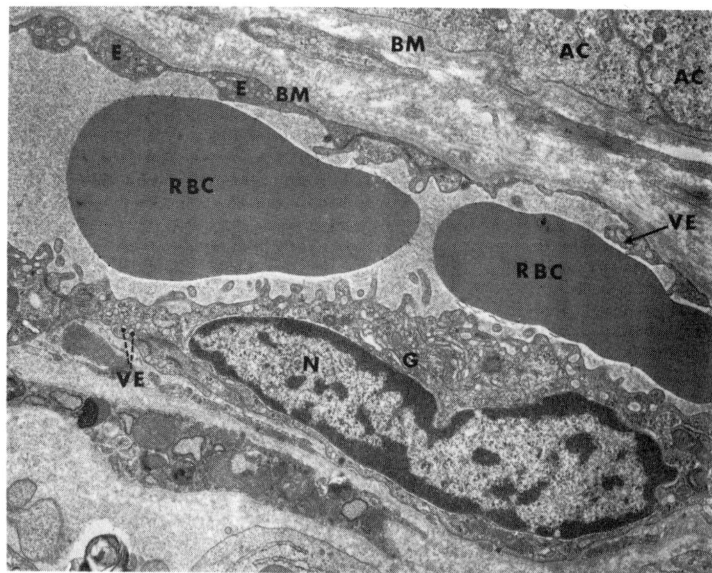

Figure 89–13. Electron micrograph of a small blood vessel lying in the connective tissue immediately below the villous absorbing cells. The endothelium (E) consists of flattened cells which are wider in the area surrounding the nucleus (N). The cells contain numerous pinocytotic vesicles (VE). A basement membrane (BM) or basal lamina surrounds the endothelium and is also shown below the lower limiting membrane of absorbing cells (AC). RBC = red blood cell, G = Golgi complex (× 16,500).

lamina separates the epithelium from the lamina propria.

The immature cell (IC) (Fig. 89–14) is situated basally within the crypt and appears to reach the crypt lumen only at a somewhat later stage in development (1 and 2 in Fig. 89–14) when sparse microvilli can be seen on its luminal surface. The characteristic features of the immature cells are their round shape, a large centrally situated nucleus, an abundance of free-lying ribosomes, sparse ER, and rather few mitochondria. It is not known whether they are the precursors of the structurally more developed cells known as the undifferentiated cells (UD) (Fig. 89–15). These are elongated cells with basally situated nuclei and a more or less well developed brush border facing the crypt lumen. They can be distinguished from the immature

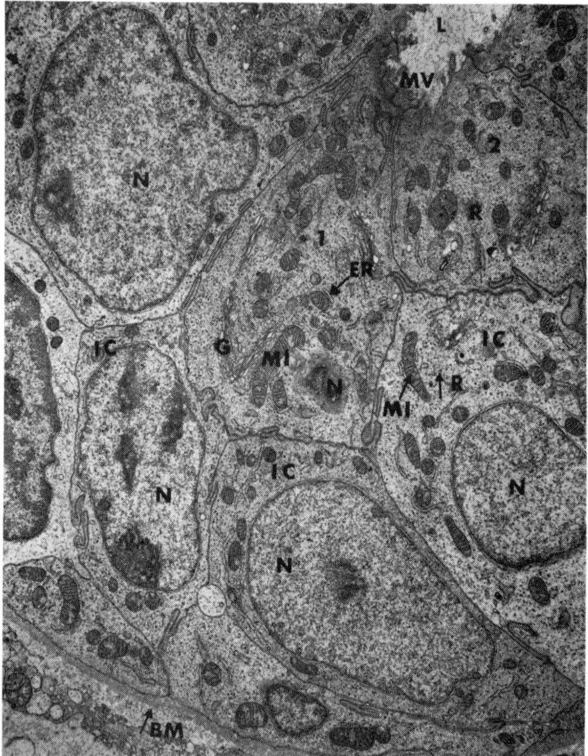

Figure 89–14. Electron micrograph through several crypt cells showing the more basally situated immature cells (IC) and two maturing cells (1, 2) with microvillous surfaces (MV) facing the crypt lumen (L). BM = basement membrane, ER = endoplasmic reticulum, MI = mitochondria, N = nucleus, G = Golgi complex (× 8250).

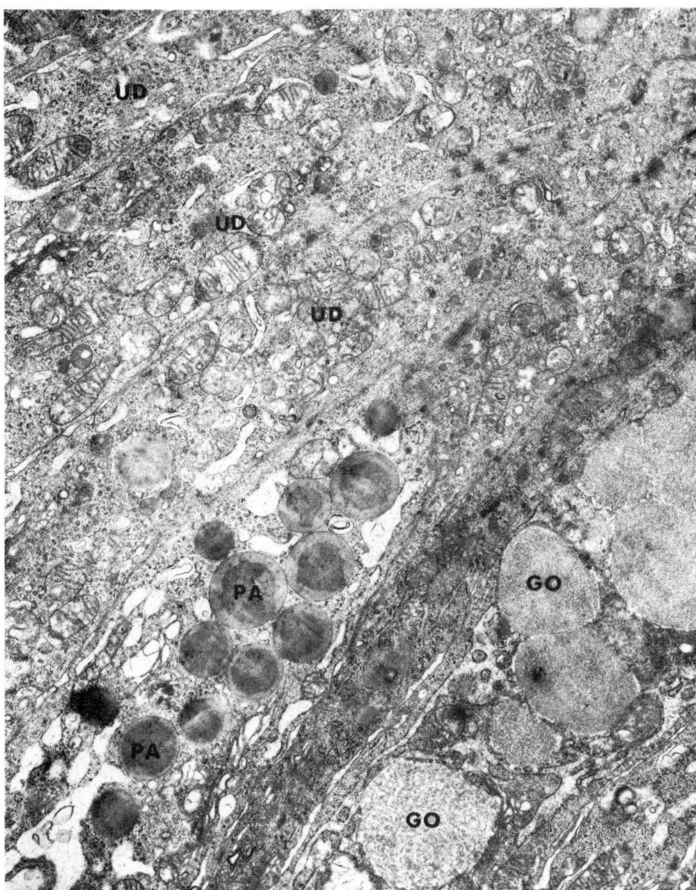

Figure 89–15. Electron micrograph through several crypt cells near the lower end of the crypt, showing 3 undifferentiated cells (UD) at the top end of the print, a Paneth cell with its large dense droplets (PA) in the center, and a goblet cell and its less dense droplets (GO) toward the lower and right-hand corner (× 17,500).

cell by an abundance of RER and ER, numerous mitochondria, and usually dilated cisternae of the Golgi complex, and the cytoplasm appears more electron dense than that of most other crypt cells. Secretory granules of greater or lesser density may be seen in some of the undifferentiated cells; it can be assumed that these are the precursors of either Paneth or goblet cells.

The *Paneth cells* (Fig. 89–15) are highly differentiated cells found in groups at the lower pole of the crypts. Their distinguishing features are the large membrane-bound secretory droplets, varying in size between 50 and 200 Å and appearing denser as they approach the apical cell surface. The RER is particularly well developed and of similar appearance to the pancreatic acinar cell. The cisternae of the RER and Golgi are dilated and intimately involved in the elaboration of secretory material. A short brush border or microvillous surface faces the crypt lumen. The nucleus is basally situated.

The *goblet cell* (Fig. 89–15) is the second type of exocrine secretory cell and is found not only at all levels of the crypts but also among the villous absorbing epithelium. It possesses a short luminal microvillous border and a nucleus which at the height of the cellular activity is squashed into an extreme basal position. The secretory granules of the goblet cell appear less electron dense than those of the Paneth cell. Their translucency and the goblet-type shape of the cells, in general, distinguish them from the Paneth cell. The size of the membrane-bound granules is again very variable and comparable to that of the Paneth cells. Both cell types show an elaborate system of elongated cisternae lined by RER, and the smooth vesicles of the Golgi complex situated in the supranuclear region are also actively dilated. The mitochondria become fewer with greater maturity of the cell.

The cells belonging to the APUD system may or may not possess a microvillous surface. The typical enterochromaffin cell (EC) is a basally situated cell without a brush border. It is distinguished by its small, intensely electron-dense, membrane-bound granules situated in the basal cytoplasm of the cell (Fig. 89–16). These are variable in size and shape. The nucleus is found in the apical part. Other and larger types of APUD cells have also been defined ultrastructurally, some of them showing a brush border and opening to the crypt lumen. They can be distinguished from

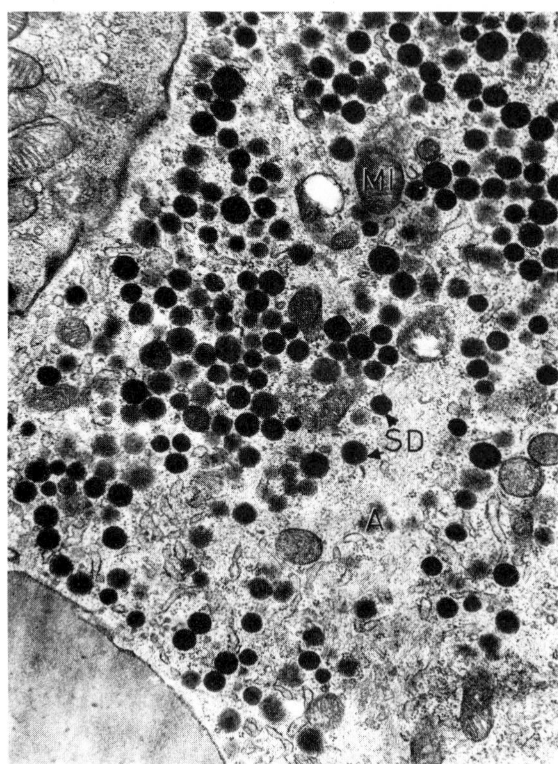

Figure 89–16. Electron micrograph of an APUD cell (A) showing the intensely dense-staining secretory droplets (SD), which are smaller than those of either Paneth or goblet cells. MI = mitochondria (× 22,000).

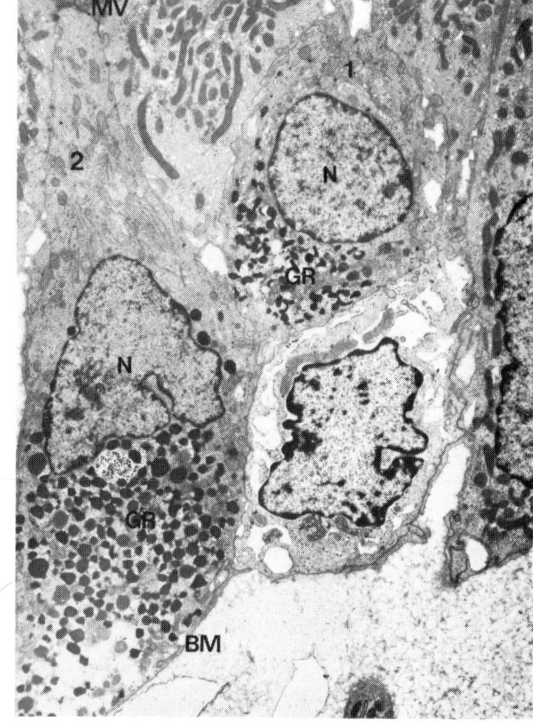

Figure 89–17. Two APUD cells (1 and 2) with dense secretory granules (GR), situated below the nucleus (N) and facing the basal laminae (BM). Cell 2 extends to the lumen and has microvilli (MV) (× 2000).

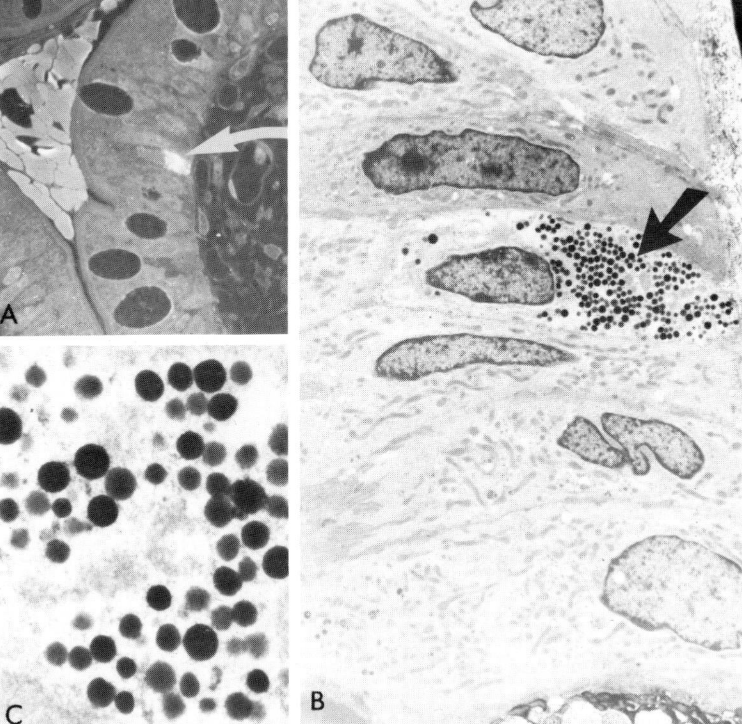

Figure 89–18. *A,* A semi-thin (500 nm) section showing a neurotensin-immunoreactive cell *(arrow)* (× 500). *B,*, A serial thin (60 nm) section of the same area, with the immunostained cell indicated by the arrow (× 5000). *C,* Higher magnification of the cell, revealing details of the secretory granules (× 30,000). (Courtesy of Dr. J. M. Polak.)

the smaller and basally situated enterochromaffin cells by the varying sizes and shapes of their secretory granules (Figs. 89–16 to 89–18).

Much is unknown about the cytomorphology of the various cell types of the small intestinal mucosa and their detailed function. This mucosa is a complex structure of absorbing, metabolizing, secreting (both exocrine, and endocrine), and immunologically active components, with a cell renewal rate second only to that of the hemopoietic system. It deserves active study and continuing interest.

References

1. Arnaud-Battandier F, Bundy B, O'Neill M, Bienenstock JJ, Nelson DL. Cytotoxic activities of gut mucosal lymphoid cells in guinea pigs. J Immunol 1978; 121:1059–65.
2. Asquith P. Cell mediated immunity in coeliac disease. *In:* Hekkens WThJM, Pena AS, eds. Coeliac Disease: Proceedings of the Second International Coeliac Symposium. Leiden: 1974: 242–60.
3. Bertalanffy FD, Nagy KP. Mitotic activity and renewal rate of the epithelial cells of human duodenum. Acta Anat 1961; 45:362–70.
4. Brunser O, Luft JH. Fine structure of the apex of absorptive cells from rat small intestine. J Ultrastruct Res 1970; 31:291–311.
5. Cornes JS. Number, size and distribution of Peyer's patches in the human small intestine. I. The development of Peyer's patches. Gut 1965; 6:225–9.
6. Creamer B. The turnover of the epithelium of the small intestine. Br Med Bull 1967; 23:226–30.
7. DeDuve C. The lysosome in retrospect. Front Biol 1969; 14A:3–40.
8. Deschner EE. Observations on the Paneth cell in human ileum. Exp Cell Res 1967; 47:624–8.
9. Henry C, Faulk WP, Kuhn L, Yoffey MD, Fudenberg HH. Peyer's patches: Immunological studies. J Exp Med 1970; 131:1200–10.
10. Fichtelius KE. The gut epithelium—a first level lymphoid organ? Exp Cell Res 1968; 49:87–104.
11. Himal HS, Moetaderi F, Dreiling DA, Kark AE, Rudick J. Glucagon stimulates Brunner's gland secretion. Nature 1970; 228:767–8.
12. Ito S. The enteric surface coat on cat intestinal microvilli. J Cell Biol 1965; 27:475–91.
13. Jennings MA, Florey HW. Autoradiographic observations on the mucous cell of the stomach and intestine. Q J Exp Physiol 1956; 41:131–52.
14. Leblond CP, Stevens CE, Bogoroch R. Histological localization of newly formed deoxyribonucleic acid. Science 1948; 108:531–3.
15. Lewin K. The Paneth cell in health and disease. Ann R Coll Surg Eng 1969; 44:23–37.
16. Lipkin M, Sherlock P, Bell B. Cell proliferation kinetics in the gastrointestinal tract of man. II. Cell renewal in stomach ileum, colon and rectum. Gastroenterology 1963; 45:721–9.
17. Liu HY, Baker BL. The influence of technique and hormones on histochemical demonstration of enzymes in intestinal epithelium. J Histochem Cytochem 1963; 11:349–64.
18. Loehry CA, Creamer B. Three-dimensional structure of the human small intestinal mucosa in health and disease. Gut 1969; 10:6–12.
19. McDonald WC, Trier JS, Everett NB. Cell proliferation and migration in stomach, duodenum and rectum of man: Radioautographic studies. Gastroenterology 1964; 46:405–17.

20. Marsh MN. Studies of intestinal lymphoid tissue. Scand J Gastroenterol 1981; 70(Suppl 16):87–106.
21. Miller D, Crane RK. The digestive function of the epithelium of the small intestine. II. Localization of disaccharide hydrolysis in the isolated brush border portion of the intestinal epithelial cells. Biochim Biophys Acta 1961; 52:293–8.
22. Otto HF. The intestinal Paneth cell. Veroffentlichungen aus der morphologischen Pathologie, Heft *94*. Stuttgart: Gustav Fischer Verlag, 1973; 1–25.
23. Owen RL, Jones AL. Epithelial cell specialization within human Peyer's patches: An ultrastructural study of intestinal lymphoid follicles. Gastroenterology 1974; 66:189–203.
24. Padykula HA, Strauss EW, Ladman AJ, Gardner FH. A morphologic and histochemical analysis of the human jejunal epithelium in nontropical sprue. Gastroenterology 1961; 40:735–65.
25. Pearse AGE, Coulling I, Weavers B, Friesen S. The endocrine polypeptide cells of the human stomach, duodenum and jejunum. Gut 1970; 11:649–58.
26. Peterson M, Leblond CP. Synthesis of complex carbohydrates in the Golgi region, as shown by radioautography after injection of labeled glucose. J Cell Biol 1964; 21:143–8.
27. Polak JM, Bloom SR. Distribution, origin and pathology of the gut peptidergic innervation. *In:* Grossman MI, Brazier MAB, Lechago J, eds. Cellular Basis of Chemical Messengers in the Digestive System. New York: Academic Press, 1981: 267–82.
28. Riecken EO, Pearse AGE. Histochemical study on the Paneth cell in the rat. Gut 1966; 7:86–93.
29. Selby WS, Janossy G, Jewell, DP. Immunohistological characterization of intraepithelial lymphocytes of the human gastrointestinal tract. Gut 1981; 22:169–76.
30. Solcia E, Breutzfeldt W, Falkmer S, Fujita T, Greider MH, Grossman MI, Grube D, Hakanson R, Larsson LI, Lechago J, Lewin K, Polak JM, Rubin W. Human gastroenteropancreatic endocrine-paracrine cells: Santa Monica 1980 Classification. *In:* Grossman MI, Brazier MAB, Lechago J, eds. Cellular Basis of Chemical Messengers in the Digestive System. New York: Academic Press, 1981: 159–65.
31. Stening GF, Grossman MI. Hormonal control of Brunner's glands. Gastroenterology 1969; 56:1047–52.
32. Trier JS. Structure of the mucosa of the small intestine as it relates to intestinal function. Fed Proc 1967; 26:1391–1404.
33. Trier JS. Studies on small intestinal crypt epithelium. I. The fine structure of the crypt epithelium of the proximal small intestine of fasting humans. J Cell Biol 1963; 18:599–620.
34. Walsh JH. Nature of gut peptides and their possible functions. *In:* Grossman MI, Brazier MAB, Lechago J, eds. Cellular Basis of Chemical Messengers in the Digestive System. New York: Academic Press, 1981:3–11.
35. Zetterquist H. The Ultrastructural Organization of the Columnar Absorbing Cells of the Mouse Jejunum. Stockholm: Aktiebolaget Godvil, 1956.

Chapter 90

Small Bowel Motility

Gaston R. Vantrappen • Josef P. Janssens

The main function of the small intestine is digestion and absorption of nutrients. In this process the role of small bowel motility is to mix food products with the digestive enzymes, to promote contact of chyme with the absorptive cells over a sufficient length of bowel, and finally to propel remnants into the colon. Segmentation and propulsion are the appropriate motor actions to perform this function. It has become clear recently that well organized motility patterns occur in the fed as well as in the fasting state. During fasting, a cyclic motor phenomenon consisting of alternating periods of activity and rest is present throughout the small intestine. This motility pattern is called the *migrating motor complex* because it originates in the gastroduodenal area and slowly migrates down the small intestine. Although the contractile pattern becomes more uniform after meals, different food substances seem to produce different motor patterns. The importance of these motility patterns is apparent from the dysfunctions that occur when they are absent or disordered.

Methods

Several methods have been used to study small bowel motility, such as radiocinematography, intraluminal pressure measurements, transit studies, and recording of electrical activity from muscles and nerves.[1–4] The problem, however, is that these different methods focus on different aspects of motility, and it is not always possible to transpose results from one method to the other.

Radiocinematography. *Fluoroscopic studies* with contrast material, initially used in 1896 by Cannon, have been replaced today by radiocinematography. Cannon showed that *segmentation* is the dominant motor pattern of the small intestine and more recent observations confirm this. Segmentation is brought about by stationary ring contractions that divide the intraluminal content into several segments. The segments are then, in turn, divided by other ring contractions to create new segments. These movements primarily mix the bowel contents, but segmenting stationary contractions can result in some propulsion if the resistance is lower in the aboral direction or if the number of contractions is higher orally. Sometimes, aborally progressing peristaltic contractions are observed that propel the intraluminal contents over a shorter or longer distance. In humans studied by radiocinematography, 2 types of clearly propulsive contractions have been observed: (1) Annular contractions. These move in a peristaltic fashion at a fast speed of about 1.2 cm/second in the upper small bowel and strip the content over a considerable length of bowel. (2) Rhythmic contractions. These move aborally at a much slower speed of 7 cm/minute and push the bowel content ahead of them.

Intraluminal Pressure. *Intraluminal pressure measurements* have been used extensively to study small bowel motility. According to their shape and duration, the pressure waves are usually divided into *phasic (type 1)* and *tonic (type 3)* waves. Type 1 waves are single waves with a duration between 2.5 and 5 seconds; type 3 waves consist of an elevation of the baseline pressure upon which a series of type 1 waves may be superimposed. Combined manometric and radiocinematographic studies indicate that type 1 activity is produced by ring contractions that may be stationary (segmentary contractions) or progressive (propulsive contractions). The function of type 3 waves is not quite clear.

Transit. *Transit studies* have been carried out by means of perfusion using chemical or radioisotopic markers or by administering food containing radiopaque or radioisotopic markers. Studies by these methods of the effect of drugs on transit time in the jejunum and ileum have yielded valuable results. Transit studies have also been correlated with intraluminal pressure measurements during the different phases of the migrating motor complex (to be discussed).

Electrical Activity. Important information has come from the recording of the *electrical activity* of the small intestinal muscle wall and of the myenteric plexus. This has been accomplished with the use of intracellular electrodes as well as extracellular recording techniques. The findings have led to new concepts of the myogenic and neural control of small intestinal motility.

Control Mechanisms

Several control mechanisms cooperate to produce the various motility patterns observed in the small intestine in the fasting and fed states.

Myogenic Control.[5–7] Intracellular microelectrode recordings indicate that smooth muscle fibers are polarized. The resting membrane potential, about 40 to 50 mv, fluctuates rhythmically with cyclic depolarizations and repolarizations of 3 to 15 mv. This phenomenon has been variously termed slow waves, basic electrical rhythm, pace-setter potentials, and electrical control activity. *Slow waves* are continuously present, whether or not obvious muscle contractions are observed. When one or more rapid depolarizations (spikes, action potentials, electrical response activity) occur superimposed upon the slow wave, the smooth muscle contracts more or less vigorously, depending on the size and number of spikes (Fig. 90–1). The mechanism that gives rise to slow waves is still controversial. According to some, the rhythmic membrane depolarizations are due to an electrogenic ion transport system, probably a sodium-potassium pump. Others consider periodic changes in membrane conductance and resistance to be the basis for the slow waves.

It is generally believed that the slow waves of the small intestine originate in the longitudinal muscle layer and spread electronically into the circular layer.[8] The highly ramified intestinal cells of Cajal lying in the interval between the longitudinal and circular muscle layer may be the origin of the slow waves.[9] The longitudinal muscle layer can transmit the slow waves aborally because single smooth muscle cells are electrically connected to contiguous cells by tight junctions. At least 2 kinds of tight junctions have been described in the small bowel: (1) the *nexus,* which is a partial fusion of a small segment of the cell membrane of 2 adjacent

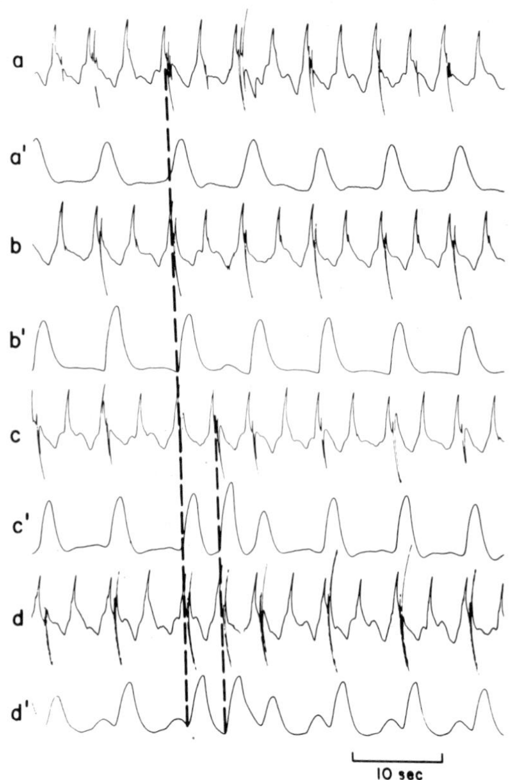

Figure 90–1. Spontaneous electrical (a–d) and corresponding mechanical (a′–d′) activity recorded from 4 loci situated 2 cm apart in the jejunum of a cat. The dashed line on the left, connecting the onset of contractions at each point, indicates propagation from point "a" to point "d." The line also passes through corresponding slow waves, indicating that they propagate at the same velocity as the contractions. The dashed line to the right indicates more localized (segmental) contractions. All contractions are preceded by spikes. The slow wave is partially differentiated owing to the short time constant (0.1 second) of the amplifier. (From Bortoff A, Sacco J. *In*: Daniel EE, ed. Fourth International Symposium on Gastrointestinal Motility. Vancouver: Michell Press, 1974: 55. Reproduced with permission.)

muscle cells; and (2) *gap junctions,* which are quite similar to the nexus, except that a narrow gap remains between the 2 cells.[10]

Slow waves are probably purely myogenic in origin. They occur in excised and thus extrinsically denervated bowel segments, persist after nerve blockade with tetrodotoxin, and are also detected in chick amnion that is devoid of nervous tissue.

The rhythm of the slow waves decreases aborally along the small intestine (small intestinal frequency gradient). The decrease is not continuous but stepwise, giving rise to the so-called *frequency plateaus.* In the small intestine of man, the frequency of the duodenal slow waves is about 11 to 12 cycles/minute, with a plateau extending from the duodenum to 10 to 15 cm beyond the angle of Treitz. From there on, plateaus are less well defined. In the ileum, the slow wave rhythm is 8 to 9 cycles/minute. Transection of the small bowel at any level produces a drop in slow wave frequency below the cut. *Each segment of the small bowel has its own intrinsic slow wave frequency and this frequency decreases along the tract.* Because of the electrical coupling that exists between the smooth muscle cells, the intrinsic frequency is pulled up by the higher frequency of the orad segment.

Many of the characteristics of the slow wave frequency along the small intestine can be simulated by computers. The best model consists of a series of bilaterally coupled relaxation oscillators.[11] The oscillator with the highest intrinsic frequency occupies the most proximal site, that with the lowest frequency the most distal site. When an oscillator is isolated from the chain, it oscillates at its own intrinsic frequency. When coupled in a chain, the oscillator with the highest frequency controls the frequency of the others over a considerable length along the chain (the plateau), depending on the tightness of the coupling. The better the coupling, the longer the plateau will be. At the end of the plateau, either the coupling is insufficient or the frequency of the driving oscillator is too high for the next oscillator to follow. The factors that determine the strength of the coupling are not well known. In hyperthyroid patients, the first plateau extends far into the jejunum, indicating a tighter coupling in patients with this disease. In a frequency plateau, the slow waves are phase-locked with a given phase lag. Owing to the phase lag, the slow waves appear to move aborally throughout the length of the plateau. This polarity is preserved after reversal of a jejunal segment.

It is not known why the intrinsic frequency decreases along the small bowel. One factor may be the diameter of the smooth muscle cells, which are smaller in the jejunum. Clustering of the mitochondria near the cell membrane in the jejunum, but not in the ileum, may also have a role.[12] The rhythm of the slow waves at any given level of intestine is reasonably constant and is influenced by only few factors. One of these is temperature, the rhythm being temperature-dependent. In the dog, the frequency varies according to the temperature, with a $Q_{10} = 2.34$. Stabilization occurs in the range of 33 to 37°C. The frequency of the slow waves is increased in hyperthyroidism and decreased in hypothyroidism. Cerulein and serotonin decrease the frequency. Electrical pacing can increase the slow wave frequency, but only within certain limits.[13]

When the smooth muscle cell is partially depolarized during the slow wave cycle, the cell membrane can elicit spike potentials. Spikes are rapid changes in membrane potential that initiate smooth muscle contraction. They do so by affecting the process of excitation-contraction coupling by stimulating actomyosin adenosine triphosphatase (ATPase) activity through the release of troponin inhibitors. The factors that determine the occurrence of spike potentials, and thus of contractions, are not clearly understood. Nervous responses to stimulation of chemo- and mechanoreceptors in the gut wall appear to play a major role. Gastrointestinal hormones may also affect the occurrence of contractions.

Action potentials are conducted over only short distances in smooth muscle. Therefore, a contraction can be a very localized phenomenon. Ring contractions can be less than 2 cm long, with neighboring regions remaining quiescent or contracting independently in time. Spike potentials occur with a reasonably constant phase relationship to the slow wave. Therefore, slow waves determine the moment when a contraction may occur and the maximal rate of contractions and their propagation characteristics. During phase 3 of the migrating motor complex, every slow wave has spike potentials. The ensuing rhythmic contractions move aborally in a peristaltic fashion at the progression velocity of the slow wave and are therefore highly propulsive.

The electrical activity of the human small intestine can be recorded with intraluminal suction electrodes.[14, 15] Slow waves, as well as spike potentials, can be recorded and the tracing is almost identical to that obtained with surgically implanted electrodes. These studies may provide additional information about intestinal electrophysiology in health and disease.

Nervous Control. The nervous control system of the small intestine is located at various levels: the intrinsic nerve plexuses in the intestinal wall, the extrinsic nerves and autonomic ganglia, and the control centers in the central nervous system.

Intrinsic Nerve Plexuses. Numerous neurons, nerve endings, and receptors lie in the intestinal wall. These nerve elements tend to be concentrated in nerve plexuses, the most prominent of which is the myenteric plexus of Auerbach between the longitudinal and the circular muscle layers. All intramural nerves are nonmyelinated. Axonal fibers run freely between smooth muscle cells and secrete their chemical transmitters at the level of several varicosities along the nerve fibers. The relative number of axons is low as compared with the number of smooth muscle cells. The neurons in the plexus receive input from several sources, including receptors in the mucosa and in the muscle wall, from other neurons in the plexus, and from extrinsic nerves. They form an important neural control center acting in effect as a "little brain" of the gut.

From a neuropharmacologic viewpoint, 4 types of efferent nerves are involved in this control: cholinergic excitatory; adrenergic inhibitory; nonadrenergic, noncholinergic inhibitory; and, probably, noncholinergic excitatory nerves.[16]

A great deal of our understanding of the function of the plexus has come from electrical recordings from single neurons within the plexus.[17–19] In extracellular recordings, 3 types of neuronal units may be distinguished on the basis of patterns and properties of action potential discharge: (1) Mechanosensitive units, of which 3 types have been observed thus far: fast adapting mechanoreceptors, slowly adapting mechanoreceptors, and tonic-type mechanosensitive units that, once activated, discharge prolonged trains of spikes for up to 40 msec (Fig. 90–2); (2) single spike units, which probably are not dependent on synaptic input; and (3) burst-type units, which discharge periodic bursts of spike potentials with silent interburst intervals. Some burst-type units (erratic bursters) require synaptic input, whereas others (steady bursters) are independent and seem to have an endogenous pacemaker mechanism.

The plexus contains both unipolar and multipolar ganglion cells. Interestingly, the properties of the cell soma and of the attached processes of these multipolar cells are distinctly different. The processes are markedly more excitable than the somal mem-

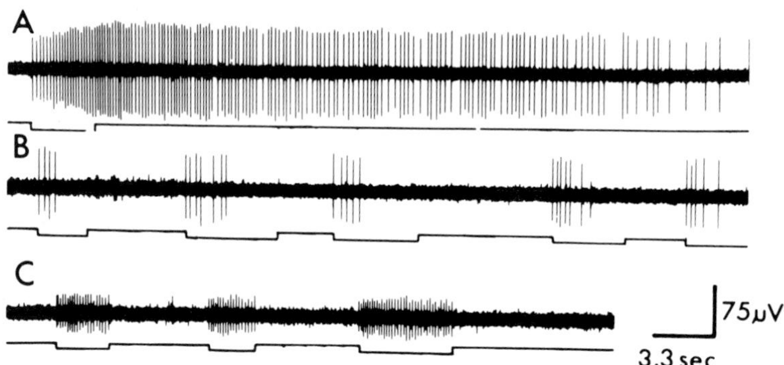

Figure 90–2. Enteric mechanosensitive units recorded extracellularly. *A*, Long-lasting train of spikes discharged by an AH/type 2 myenteric neuron from cat small intestine. *B*, Fast-adapting mechanosensitive neuron in myenteric plexus of cat small intestine. *C*, Slowly adapting mechanoreceptor in myenteric plexus of dog small intestine. The lower trace of each record indicates application of stimulus. (From Wood JD. *In*: Wienbeck M, ed. Motility of Digestive Tract. New York: Raven Press, 1982: 33. Reproduced with permission.)

brane. In this way, independent spike initiation is possible in each of the cell processes, with the soma acting as electrical insulation in between. One neuron, therefore, may function as if it consisted of several different neurons, depending on the number of processes. AH/type 2 neurons (classification of Hirst[17] and of Nishi and North[18] on the basis of intracellular recording) belong to the group of multipolar cells. They have a high resting membrane potential and a low input resistance relative to the other types of neurons (S/type 1 neurons). They also discharge only 1 or 2 spikes at the onset of a prolonged depolarizing current, and their action potentials are followed by prolonged hyperpolarizing after-potentials. However, under certain conditions, as in the presence of slow excitatory postsynaptic potentials (EPSPs) (which can be recorded in AH/type 2 neurons after electrical stimulation of interganglionic connections), the somal membrane of the multipolar cells assumes a state of augmented excitability. Consequently, all processes fire synchronously, and the cell responds with repetitive spike discharges for a prolonged period after the termination of the stimulus. This type of electrical discharge closely corresponds to the tonic-type mechanosensitive units identified by extracellular recordings. The function of these neurons probably is the production of a prolonged excitation at the neuronal or neuroeffector junction within the small intestinal wall. Serotonin is probably the chemical neurotransmitter of the slow EPSPs. Fast EPSPs also occur in AH/type 2 neurons, but they are most prominent in S/type 1 neurons. The specialized properties of the AH/type 2 neurons and their synaptic input thus provide a mechanism whereby in one functional state, excitation is restricted to a short, limited distance (the length of one cell process), whereas, in the other, the neuronal excitation spreads to adjacent ganglia, thus providing a neuronal basis for propagated peristaltic events.

Inhibitory postsynaptic potentials (IPSPs) have been recorded in the myenteric as well as in the submucous nerve plexus. Both stimulus-evoked and spontaneously occurring IPSPs have been observed. They provide a pathway for descending inhibition in the plexus and may check the spread of neural information along the bowel. It is not always possible to transpose results of such neurophysiologic data to what happens at the level of the contracting smooth muscle layer. In any event, control of the responsiveness of the muscle cells to the pacemaker slow waves and control of spread of excitation within the elctrical syncytium of the muscle wall require modulation by continuously active inhibitory innervation. The presence of the latter explains why each slow wave does not elicit a muscle contraction of maximal strength, as is the case after neural blockade, and why excitation usually does not spread over a great distance.

In 1899 Bayliss and Starling recognized that distention of the small intestine elicits contraction above and relaxation below. This phenomenon was called the *peristaltic reflex*. More recent work by Hirst and McKirdy[17] provided evidence for a possible neural pathway for this reflex within the plexus. They showed that distention of a balloon elicited 2 distinct patterns of fast EPSPs in neurons of the longitudinal strip aboral to the balloon. One group of neurons showed a transient burst of EPSPs within 0.2 to 1.2 seconds after balloon distention, corresponding in time with the occurrence of transient inhibitory junction potentials in the circular muscle. A second population of neurons showed EPSPs with a much longer latency (2 to 11 seconds), corresponding in time with excitatory junction potentials in both longitudinal and circular muscle. Above the site of distention, excitatory junction potentials were elicited almost simultaneously with the distention.

Numerous studies have tried to elucidate the neurotransmitters involved in the intrinsic innervation of the gut. Of the neurons that are in direct contact with the smooth muscle cells, those that are excitatory are clearly cholinergic. The inhibitory neurons are noncholinergic and nonadrenergic, but the exact nature of the transmitter is still debated. Among the candidates are adenosine triphosphate (ATP) and peptides such as vasoactive intestinal polypeptide (VIP) and cholecystokinin (CCK).[20] Immunofluorescence and histochemical studies have shown that somatostatin, enkephalins, serotonin, and probably also substance P are present in some neurons of the plexus. Whether they are interneurons and what their exact function may be remain unknown.

Extrinsic Innervation and Central Control. The extrinsic innervation to the small bowel is provided by the vagal and splanchnic nerves.[21, 22] The vagus carries 4 groups of nerve fibers. The *first* group consists of preganglionic cholinergic nerves synapsing with intramural excitatory cholinergic neurons. The *second* group are preganglionic cholinergic nerves synapsing with intramural noncholinergic, nonadrenergic inhibitory neurons. These preganglionic inhibitory fibers have a smaller diameter and hence a slower conduction velocity than the excitatory fibers. The *third* type are sympathetic noradrenergic fibers originating from the cervical ganglia. The *fourth* type are fibers originating from different receptors within the gut wall. The *splanchnic nerves* contain preganglionic sympathetic and postganglionic sympathetic and sensory fibers for the transmission of pain sensation. The noradrenergic innervation is unusual in that the cell bodies of the noradrenergic neurons reside entirely outside the gut itself. Extrinsic denervation, therefore, removes all traces of noradrenergic terminals from the small intestinal wall.[23] The action of the sympathetic transmitter is probably dual: it inhibits the excitatory ganglionic transmission by axo-axonic interaction at the cholinergic axon terminal; it also acts directly on smooth muscle.

The role of the extrinsic innervation in small bowel motility under normal physiologic conditions is largely unknown. Small intestinal motor activity is essentially unaffected by either vagotomy or splanchnicectomy. However, stimulation of the cut distal end of the vagus produces peristaltic contractions. It has also been demonstrated that the vagus carries information for the onset of phase 3 of the migrating motor complex in the gastroduodenal area and that small bowel paralysis during postoperative ileus is due to an overwhelming activity of the splanchnic sympathetic outflow. Physiologically, the extrinsic nerves only modulate small bowel motility. In this respect, it is important to note that several mechano-, chemo-, and even thermoreceptors have been described in the small intestine that send their information to the central nervous system via vagal afferent nerves.[24] The central connections between afferent impulses from and efferent impulses to the bowel have not been studied in depth. It has been shown, however, that they are not limited to the brain stem and the spinal cord. The fastigial nucleus of the cerebellum clearly influences small bowel motility, probably via the sympathetic intestinal nerve supply.[25] The extrinsic innervation is involved in some reflex patterns, such as the inhibitory intestino-intestinal reflex, the inhibitory ileo-gastric reflex, and the inhibitory intestino-colic reflex. Some of these long-distance reflexes may act through the prevertebral ganglia without passing via the central nervous system.

Humoral Control. Many endogenous chemical agents and peptides may affect small bowel motor activity. Alpha as well as beta adrenergic agents generally inhibit motility. The inhibitory effect of beta-stimulating agents is brought about primarily by way of β_1-receptors. Alpha adrenergic receptors, although inhibitory in several species (including man), may have an excitatory effect in others (opossum). Part of the inhibitory effect of sympathomimetic agents is due to a decrease in the release of acetylcholine by the myenteric plexus.[26]

Serotonin induces contraction of intestinal smooth muscle through a dual mechanism: (1) stimulation of serotoninergic receptors on excitatory neurons in the plexus, and (2) a direct effect on the smooth muscle itself. However, serotonin also activates nonadrenergic, noncholinergic intrinsic inhibitory neurons. Serotonin is probably the neurotransmitter of a population of enteric interneurons.[27, 28] *Prostaglandins* $F_{1\alpha}$ and $F_{2\alpha}$ generally cause contraction of both longitudinal and circular muscle layers of isolated intestine of man. Prostaglandins E_1 and E_2 cause contraction of the longitudinal muscle, but usually inhibit the circular muscle.[29] Indomethacin, which selectively inhibits prostaglandin synthesis, causes a loss of tone and a decrease of spontaneous activity in longitudinal strips of human ileum, but increases or initiates spontaneous activity in circular muscle strips. The in vivo effects of prostaglandins are less clear. Intravenous administration of prostaglandin $F_{2\alpha}$ (0.8 μg/kg/ minute) was reported to inhibit segmental activity of the human small intestine owing to relaxation of the circular muscle coat. However, some progressive contractions were also recorded. In these experiments the ileum was more sensitive than the jejunum.[30] In the canine ileum, however, the same agent (1 μg/kg/minute) markedly stimulated longitudinal and circular muscle contractions.

Several polypeptide hormones have a pronounced effect on small bowel motility.[31] In general, cholecystokinin-like peptides increase motor activity, whereas secretin-like peptides decrease it. *Gastrin* stimulates segmentary contractions, probably by increasing the release of acetylcholine from the myenteric plexus. *CCK* (and *cerulein)* has almost the same effect, although the duodenum seems less reactive to CCK. *Motilin* stimulates small intestinal motor activity, particularly the duodenum. *Secretin* clearly inhibits small intestinal motility. The inhibitory effect of *glucagon* is even more pronounced. *Endogenous opioids* may also be involved in the modulation of small bowel contractile activity inasmuch as many studies have shown a dose-dependent inhibition of motility by enkephalins.

It is not quite clear whether the effect of these agents on bowel motility is due to physiologic or pharmacologic action. It is also not known how they are involved in normal small intestinal motor function. Moreover, their effect on muscle strips is sometimes markedly different from their effect on small bowel motility patterns.

Small Bowel Reflexes

Intestino-intestinal Inhibitory Reflex.[51] Inhibition of tonus and motility of the small bowel occurs when the peritoneum is stimulated or there is abnormal distention of a segment of small bowel, provided the extrinsic sympathetic nerves and spinal cord below T6 are intact. The reflex is mediated through the thoracolumbar sympathetic pathways. Both sensory and motor fibers traverse these pathways. The center for the reflex is in the spinal column, T7 to L6. The longer the segment of distended bowel, the smaller the increase in intraluminal pressure necessary to inhibit motility. Repeated episodes of distention facilitate this reflex, whereas spinal anesthesia interrupts it.

This reflex has clinical applications. If there is distention of a small segment as the result of either mechanical obstruction or paralytic ileus, motility and tonus of adjacent areas are decreased. These, in turn, become distended and cause the same phenomena in contiguous regions. The distention therefore spreads, and the reflex is perpetuated in a vicious circle. If, however, a tube is passed and the intestine is decompressed, the stimulus may be removed and the reflex may be inhibited. Vagal fibers do not influence this reflex.

Gastroileal Reflex.[52] This reflex is independent of extrinsic innervation and may represent, at least in part, a true physiologic effect of gastrin increasing small bowel motility. In this reflex, there is a response to feeding or introduction of food into the stomach. This is manifested as a rapid and prolonged motor response in the ileum. The reflex persists after vagotomy.

Migrating Motor Complex

In 1969, Szurszewski[32] identified an electrical complex in the small intestine of fasting dogs. This complex is characterized by a front of intense spiking activity that migrates down the entire small bowel; as the front reaches the terminal ileum, another front develops in the gastroduodenal area and progresses down the intestine. The phenomenon has been called the *interdigestive migrating myoelectrical complex* or the *migrating motor complex.* Feeding interrupts the cycle and changes the interdigestive fasting pattern into a pattern of irregular spiking activity called the *fed pattern.*

A complex closely resembling that of the dog also exists in man.[33] It consists of 4 different phases (Fig. 90–3). During *phase 1,* the bowel is almost quiescent. During *phase 2,* the intestinal motor activity becomes gradually more and more intense; the contractions may occur quite irregularly or may be arranged in bursts appearing with intervals of 1 or 2 minutes (the minute rhythm). *Phase 3,* also called the activity front, is characterized by the sudden onset of intense rhythmic contractions; during this phase the intestine is contracting at its maximal frequency, which is equal to its basal electrical rhythm (Fig. 90–4). Phase 3 is usually followed by a short *phase 4,* characterized by a period of rapidly decreasing contractile activity. Following the last phase, a new phase 1 begins. Each phase of the cycle moves sequentially along the gastrointestinal tract; therefore, each phase is present at some point along the small intestine at any one time. The duration of the cycle in man is about 90 to 130 minutes. As in dogs, feeding interrupts the complex and changes the fasting pattern to a fed one. The migrating motor complex is not limited to the stomach and the small intestine, but involves the lower esophageal sphincter as well.

The migrating motor complex has been observed in several animal species. In some species, a fasting pattern may persist in the nonfasting state, depending on the feeding habits of the animal. When pigs, rabbits, or

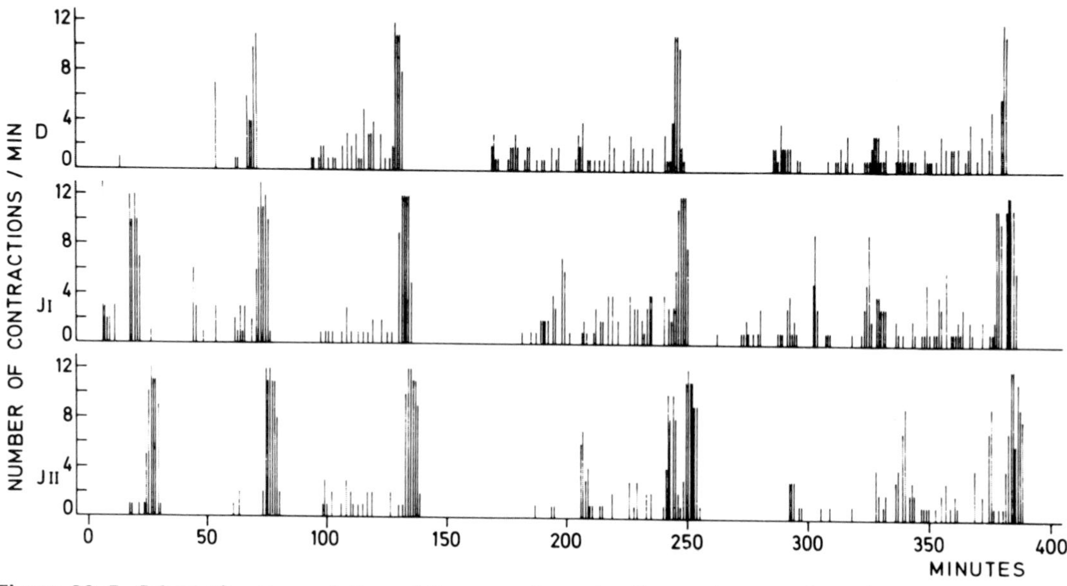

Figure 90–3. Schematic representation of 5 consecutive migrating motor complexes in a normal subject. Displayed are the number of contraction waves/minute throughout a 400 minute recording period at 3 different levels of the upper small intestine: D, duodenum; JI, jejunum I (± 15 cm below the angle of Treitz); JII, jejunum II (± 40 cm below the angle of Treitz). (From Vantrappen G et al.[37] Reproduced with permission.)

sheep are fed ad libitum (i.e., eat more or less continuously), the complex recycles continuously throughout the day without disruption by eating. When the animals take food only once or twice daily, the migrating motor complex occurs only during the fasting state and is disrupted by feeding. However, it was shown that although dogs normally have distinct fasting and feeding motility patterns, continuous intraduodenal tube feeding induces the feeding pattern for a limited period of time. After several hours of continuous feeding, a fasting-like migrating motor complex again becomes apparent in the small bowel.

The different phases of the complex greatly influence intestinal transit and absorption. *Transit* is more rapid during phase 3, slowest in phase 1, and intermediate during phase 2. *Absorption* is greatest during phase 1 and least during phase 3. However, absorption is greater postprandially than during any phase of fasting, although transit time is similar to phase 2. Simultaneous manometric and radiocinematographic studies in dogs and man have shown that the consecutive peristaltic contractions of the activity front of the migrating motor complex are highly propulsive. They clear the bowel of food remnants and desquamated cells, thereby preventing creation of a medium favorable to bacterial overgrowth in the small intestine.[33, 34]

The migrating motor complex is accompanied by secretory phenomena as well. Phase 3 in the duodenum is preceded by an increase in gastric acid secretion, pepsin out-

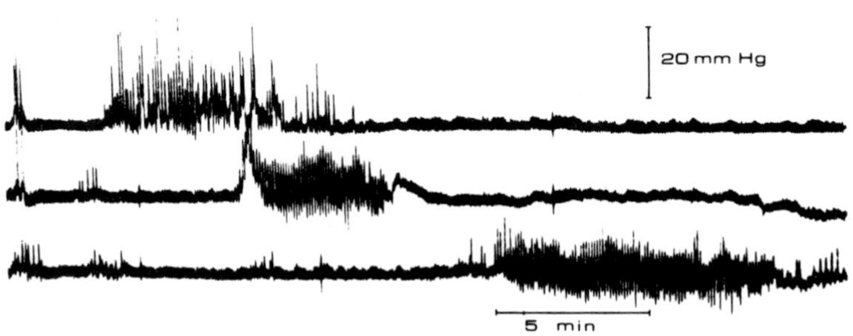

Figure 90–4. Manometric recordings in the duodenum, the jejunum 15 cm below the angle of Treitz, and the jejunum 40 cm below the angle of Treitz. The activity front of the interdigestive motor complex is characterized by a burst of rhythmic contraction waves that progress down the intestine. (From Vantrappen G et al. J Clin Invest 1977; 59:1158–60. Reproduced with permission.)

put, and bile acid production and is followed by a peak of bicarbonate and amylase secretion. There is some evidence that small intestinal secretion is also modulated by the complex. The accompanying secretory phenomena have been called the *secretory component of the migrating motor complex.*[35]

A correlation exists between sleep stage changes and the various phases of the migrating motor complex. This correlation supports the concept that an oscillator, possibly central in location, influences several functions, including the migrating motor complex periodicity.[36]

Regulating Mechanisms. Several studies have tried to elucidate the mechanisms that regulate the migrating motor complex.[37-39] It seems probable that the initiation of the complex, its progression, and its disruption by food are produced by different mechanisms.

Initiation of the Migrating Motor Complex. The capability of generating a migrating motor complex appears to be a basic characteristic of the small intestine, provided the myenteric nerve plexus is intact. Indeed, autotransplanted (extrinsically denervated) jejunal segments generate complexes. These complexes, however, are not coordinated with those in the main intestine, indicating that their initiation cannot be regulated by circulating hormones.[40]

The migrating motor complex in the intact animal usually starts in the gastroduodenal area and travels down the small intestine in a well coordinated manner. Hormones must be involved in the initiation of the complex in the stomach. This assumption is based on the fact that the autotransplanted fundic pouch, in contrast with an autotransplanted small intestinal segment, generates complexes in phase with those in the remainder of the stomach.[41] Even if the pouch and the main stomach had an intrinsic biologic clock with the same frequency, the 2 rhythms would become out of phase after some time unless a hormonal factor coordinated them. Motilin, pancreatic polypeptide, and somatostatin plasma levels all fluctuate in accordance with the different phases of the complex; the levels are highest during late phase 2 and during phase 3. The motilin and pancreatic polypeptide peaks occur somewhat earlier than the somatostatin peak. Exogenous infusions of motilin in doses resembling spontaneously occurring motilin peaks are able to initiate complexes that start in the stomach and migrate down the small bowel.[42] Infusions of pancreatic polypeptide lower endogenous motilin levels and inhibit the occurrence of the complex in the stomach; however, normal complexes continue to occur in the small intestine during the infusion, even at high plasma pancreatic polypeptide levels.[43] Exogenous somatostatin infusions that provoke plasma somatostatin increments within the physiologic range also inhibit endogenous motilin and the occurrence of complexes in the stomach. However, they induce migrating motor complexes in the human small bowel at a much higher frequency than normally present. Somatostatin-induced complexes exhibit only phase 1 and 3 and lack phase 2.[44]

These data are compatible with the concept that spontaneously occurring plasma motilin peaks trigger phase 3 in the stomach. This induces an increase in plasma somatostatin, which, in turn, facilitates the occurrence of phase 3 in the duodenum. The mechanism that induces the cyclic variations of plasma motilin, however, remains unknown. The accompanying pancreatic polypeptide peak is not involved in the regulation of the motor component of the migrating motor complex. Other gastrointestinal hormones, such as gastrin, secretin, CCK, glucagon, VIP, gastric inhibitory peptide (GIP), and substance P do not fluctuate with the different phases of the complex and have no apparent role in its initiation during the fasting state.

Several other chemical agents are known to affect the migrating motor complex. Morphine initiates premature activity fronts, whereas enkephalins inhibit phase 3. Histamine (H_1) agonists stimulate the occurrence of the front. Prostaglandins E_2 and I_2 decrease the frequency of occurrence of complexes, whereas prostaglandin $F_{2\alpha}$ has the opposite effect. The physiologic significance of these effects, if any, remains to be determined.

Progression of the Migrating Motor Complex. It is unlikely that circulating hormones are involved in the orderly progression of the migrating motor complex along the small intestine because every phase of the complex is always present somewhere along the tract. Nerves, however, clearly participate in this regulation. Both the intrinsic and the extrinsic innervation seem to be important.

The *extrinsic nervous system,* although not required for the initiation of the complex in the small intestine, takes part in the regulation of its progression. Therefore, the activity front in a Thiry-Vella (isolated) loop is better coordinated with the complex in the main intestine than it is in an autotransplanted jejunal segment; the complex in the latter occurs at its own independent rhythm.[45] This explains why in the studies of Aeberhard et al.[46] (in which jejunal and ileal segments of dog small intestine were interchanged with their extrinsic innervation remaining intact) the jejunal activity front preceded the ileal one as if the 2 segments were still in their normal location. After 3 to 4 weeks, the transplanted segments adapted to their new anatomic location and became integrated into a normal aboral sequence.

The effect of sympathectomy and/or bilateral vagotomy remains controversial. Acute blocking by cooling of the vagosympathetic trunk in the neck of dogs eliminates the activity front in the lower esophageal sphincter and stomach; but not in the small intestine.[47]

The role of the intrinsic nervous plexus in the progression of the migrating motor complex was studied by Sarna et al.[48] Atropine applied locally to a small segment of bowel through intra-arterial injection not only inhibited the complex at that level, but also prevented its distal progression. Transection with reanastomosis of the small bowel at 3 different levels (with intact extrinsic nerves) has been observed to disorganize the propagation of the migrating complex from one segment to the other. Indeed, so thorough is the interruption that it was concluded that the intrinsic nerve plexus must be the more important regulatory factor for the orderly progression of the complex.

Disruption of the Migrating Motor Complex by Food. In most animal species and in man, the migrating motor complex is disrupted whenever a large meal is taken. The duration of the disruption is related not only to the amount of calories taken, but also to the nature of the food products, with fats producing the longest disruption.

The mechanism responsible for the conversion of the motility pattern from the fasting to the fed state is poorly understood. Regulation by hormones is an attractive hypothesis. Hormones are undoubtedly involved in the disruption of the migrating motor complex in the stomach because feeding abolishes the complex in an autotransplanted fundic pouch. Feeding raises the plasma levels of almost all gastrointestinal hormones, and exogenous infusions of gastrin, insulin, CCK, glucagon, and secretin have all been reported to disrupt the complex. However, it is not clear whether this disruption represents a physiologic or a pharmacologic action of the hormone. Intravenous infusion of neurotensin in man inhibited the occurrence of the activity front and changed the fasting motility pattern into a fed type. The inhibition occurred at plasma neurotensin levels below those obtained after a meal.[49]

Several studies have pointed to the importance of the extrinsic innervation in the disruption of the migrating motor complex after feeding. Vagotomy delays the time of onset of the disruption and increases the amount of food required to induce the fed pattern. As previously mentioned, when the vagosympathetic nerve trunk in the neck of dogs is blocked by cooling during the feeding state, this pattern changes into a fasting pattern with reappearance of activity fronts in the duodenum and jejunum, but not in the lower esophageal sphincter and stomach. It has also been shown that feeding no longer disrupts the migrating motor complex in an extrinsically denervated (autotransplanted) jejunal segment. The stimulus for the interruption originates from the gastrointestinal tract, inasmuch as parenteral alimentation is unable to disrupt the complex. The disruption can be triggered not only from the stomach, but also from the duodenum and ileum.

The seemingly irregular pattern of motor activity characteristic of feeding may not be as irregular as it initially appears.[50] Analysis of the digestive activity as a sequence of periods of activity alternating with periods of rest has clearly shown that different food products produce different patterns of digestive activity. How different food products can induce different motility patterns is unknown.

In summary, hormonal mechanisms are important for the initiation of migrating motor complexes as well as for their disruption by feeding in the lower esophageal sphincter and stomach. They may even facilitate the progression of phase 3 from the stomach to the small bowel. In the small intestine, however, nervous mechanisms predominate for the initiation of the complex, its progression, and its disruption by food. Much remains to be done to elucidate fully the regulation of the migrating motor complex.

References

1. Christensen J. The physiology of gastrointestinal transit. Med Clin North Am 1974; 58:1165–80.
2. Davenport HW Physiology of the Digestive Tract, An Intro-

ductory Text. Motility of the Small Intestine. Chicago: Yearbook Medical Publishers, 1982:58–71.

3. Farrar JT. Motility of the small intestine. *In:* Sircus W, Smith AN, eds. Scientific Foundations of Gastroenterology. London: William Heinemann, 1980::445–50.
4. Cohen S, Long WB, Snape WJ Jr. Gastrointestinal Motility. *In:* Crane RK, ed. International Review of Physiology, Gastrointestinal Physiology III, Vol 19. Baltimore: University Park Press, 1979:107–49.
5. Bortoff A. Myogenic control of intestinal motility. Curr Topics Physiol 1976; 56:418–34.
6. Code CF, Marlett JA, Szurszewski JH, Kelly KA, Smith IB. A concept of control of gastrointestinal motility. *In:* Code CF, ed. Handbook of Physiology, Section 6: Alimentary Canal, Vol V: Motility. Washington, DC: American Physiological Society, 1968: 2881–96.
7. Becker JM, Duff M, Moody FG. Myoelectric control of gastrointestinal and biliary motility: A review. Surgery 1980; 89:466–77.
8. Connor JA, Mangel AW, Nelson B. Propagation and entrainment of slow waves in cat small intestine. Am J Physiol 1979; 237:C 237–46.
9. Thuneberg L, Rumessen JJ, Mikkelsen HB. The interstitial cells of Cajal: Intestinal pacemaker cells? *In:* Wienback M, ed. Motility of the Digestive Tract. New York: Raven Press, 1982: 115–22.
10. Daniel EE, Duchon G, Henderson R. The ultrastructural bases for coordination of intestinal motility. Am J Dig Dis 1972; 17:289–98.
11. Sarna SK, Daniel EE, Kinkma YJ. Simulation of slow-wave electrical activity of small intestine. Am J Physiol 1971; 221:166–75.
12. Job DD, Griffing WJ, Rodda BE. A possible origin of intestinal gradients and their relation to motility. Am J Physiol 1974; 226:1510–15.
13. Collin J, Kelly KA, Phillips SF. Increased canine jejunal absorption of water, glucose and sodium with intestinal pacing. Am J Dig Dis 1978; 23:1121–4.
14. Christensen J, Schedl HP, Clipton JA. The small intestinal basic electrical rhythm (slow wave) frequency gradient in normal men and in patients with a variety of diseases. Gastroenterology 1966; 50:309–15.
15. Fleckenstein P, Oigaard A. Electrical spike activity in the human small intestine. Dig Dis 1979; 23:776–80.
16. Bennett A, Stockley HL. The intrinsic innervation of the human alimentary tract and its relation to function. Gut 1975; 16:443–53.
17. Hirst GDS, McKirdy HC. A nervous mechanism for descending inhibition in guinea-pig small intestine. J Physiol (London) 1974; 238:129–44.
18. Nishi S, North RA. Intracellular recording from the myenteric plexus of the guinea-pig ileum. J Physiol (London) 1978; 231:471–91.
19. Wood JD. Intrinsic neural control of intestinal motility. Ann Rev Physiol 1981; 43:33–51.
20. Gillespie JS. Non-adrenergic non-cholinergic inhibitory control of gastrointestinal motility. *In:* Wienback M, ed. Motility of the Digestive Tract. New York: Raven Press, 1982; 51–66.
21. Gonella J. La motilité digestive et sa régulation nerveuse. J Physiol (Paris) 1978; 74:131–40.
22. Gershon MD, Erde SM. The nervous system of the gut. Gastroenterology 1981; 80:1571–94.
23. Furness JB, Costa M. The adrenergic innervation of the gastrointestinal tract. Engeb Physiol 1979; 69:1–15.
24. Mei N. Mécanorécepteurs vagaux digestifs chez le chat. Exp Brain Res 1970; 11:502–14.
25. Martner J. Influences on colonic and small intestinal motility by the cerebellar fastigial nucleus. Acta Physiol Scand 1975; 94:82–94.
26. Kazié T. Effect of adrenergic factors on peristalsis and acetylcholine release. Eur J Pharmacol 1971; 16:367–73.
27. Vizi VA, Vizi ES. Direct evidence for acetylcholine releasing effect of serotonin in the Auerbach plexus. J Neural Trans 1978; 42:127–38.
28. Costa M, Furness JB. The site of action of 5-HT in nerve muscle preparations from guinea-pig small intestine and colon. Br J Pharmacol 1979; 65:237–48.
29. Eley KG, Bennett A, Stockley HL The effects of prostaglandins E_1, E_2, $F_{1\alpha}$, and $F_{2\alpha}$ on guinea-pig ileal and colonic peristalsis. J Pharm Pharmacol 1977; 29:276–80.
30. Cummings JH, Newman A, Misiewicz JJ, Milton-Thompson GJ, Billings JA. Effect of intravenous prostaglandin $F_{2\alpha}$ on small intestinal function in man. Nature 1973; 243:169–71.
31. Onyang A, Cohen S. Effects of hormones on gastrointestinal motility. Med Clin North Am 1981; 65:1111–27.
32. Szurszewski JH. A migrating electric complex of the canine small intestine. Am J Physiol 1969; 217:1757–63.
33. Vantrappen G, Janssens J, Hellemans J, Ghoos Y. The interdigestive motor complex of normal subjects and patients with bacterial overgrowth of the small intestine. J Clin Invest 1977; 59:1158–66.
34. Code CF, Schlegel JF. The gastrointestinal interdigestive housekeeper: Motor correlates of the interdigestive myoelectric complex of the dog. *In:* Daniel EE, ed. Proceedings of the 4th International Symposium on Gastrointestinal Motility. Vancouver: Mitchell Press, 1974:631–4.
35. Vantrappen G, Peeters TL, Janssens J. The secretory component of the interdigestive migrating motor complex in man. Am J Dig Dis 1979; 24:497–500.
36. Finch PM, Ingram DM, Henstridge JD, Catchpole BN Relationship of fasting gastroduodenal motility to the sleep cycle. Gastroenterology 1982; 83:605–12.
37. Vantrappen G, Janssens J, Peeters TL. The migrating motor complex. Med Clin North Am 1981; 65:1311–29.
38. Wingate DL. Backwards and forwards with the migrating complex. Dig Dis Sci 1981; 25:641–66.
39. Itoh Z, Aizawa I, Sekiguchi T. The interdigestive migrating complex and its significance in man. Clin Gastroenterol 1982; 11:497–521.
40. Sarr MG, Kelly KA. Myoelectric activity of the autotransplanted canine jejunoileum. Gastroenterology 1981; 81:303–10.
41. Thomas PA, Kelly KA. Hormonal control of interdigestive motor cycles of canine proximal stomach. Am J Physiol 1979; 237:E192–7.
42. Vantrappen G, Janssens J, Peeters TL, Bloom SR, Christofides ND, Hellemans J. Motilin and the interdigestive motor complex in man. Dig Dis Sci 1979; 24:497–500.
43. Janssens J, Hellemans J, Adrian TE, Bloom SR, Peeters TL, Christofides N, Vantrappen G. Pancreatic polypeptide is not involved in the regulation of the migrating motor complex in man. Reg Peptides 1982, 3:41–9.
44. Peeters TL, Janssens J, Vantrappen G. Somatostatin and the interdigestive migrating motor complex in man, Gastroenterology 1981; 80:1250.
45. Carlson GM, Bedi BS, Code CF. Mechanism of propagation of intestinal interdigestive myoelectric complex. Am J Physiol 1972; 222:1027–30.
46. Aeberhard PF, Magnenat LD, Zimmermann WA. Nervous control of migratory myoelectric complex of the small bowel. Am J Physiol 1980; 238:G102–8.
47. Diamant NE, Meri H, El-Sharkawy TY, Hall K. The vagus controls lower esophageal sphincter and gastric components of the migrating complex in the dog. Gastroenterology 1972; 76:1122.
48. Sarna S, Stoddard C, Belbeck L, McWade D. Intrinsic nervous control of migrating myoelectric complexes. Am J Physiol 1981; 241:616–23.
49. Thor K, Rosell S, Rökaeus A, Kager L. [Gln^4]-Neurotensin changes the motility pattern of the duodenum and proximal jejunum from a fasting-type to a fed type. Gastroenterology 1982; 83:569–74.
50. Eeckhout C, Vantrappen G, Hellemans J, Janssens J, De Wever I. Patterns in digestive myoelectrical activity. *In:* Weinbeck M, ed. Motility of the Digestive Tract. New York: Raven Press, 1982: 433–6.
51. Youmans WB. Innervation of the gastrointestinal tract. *In:* Code CF, ed. Handbook of Physiology. Section 6, Vol 4. Washington, DC: American Physiological Society, 1968: 1655–64.
52. Kosterlitz HW. Intrinsic and extrinsic nervous control of motility of the stomach and intestines. *In:* Code CF, ed. Handbook of Physiology. Section 6, Vol 4. Washington, DC: American Physiological Society, 1968: 2147–72.

Chapter 91

Principles of Absorption

Martin H. Kalser

In the normal physiologic state, the gastrointestinal tract is a finely integrated system geared to carry out assimilation of ingested foodstuffs. *Assimilation* (the process by which ingested foods reach body fluids) consists of 2 stages: *digestion* (the breakdown of large molecules into their component smaller molecules) and *absorption* (the transport across the intestinal mucosa to body fluids). The total process is intertwined and interdependent.

Each type of foodstuff is assimilated in its own unique manner. The major source of digestive enzymes for hydrolysis of fat, protein, and carbohydrate is the pancreas, but the stomach contributes to protein digestion (pepsin) and enzymes of the intestinal mucosal brush border are essential for complete hydrolysis of polypeptides and disaccharides prior to absorption. While carbohydrates must be completely digested to monosaccharides before being transported across the intestinal membrane, some amino acids are transported as di- or tripeptides. Dietary fat, long-chain triglycerides, are only partially hydrolyzed to 2 molecules of free fatty acids and the remaining to monoglyceride. Assimilation of fat is the most complex of all the foodstuffs, requiring a functioning pancreas, liver, biliary tract, and jejunal and ileal intestinal mucosal cells.

Almost all substances are absorbed at a rate that is independent of extraintestinal factors, with the exceptions of iron and calcium. The rate of absorption of iron is dependent upon the body stores of iron. If serum-ionizable calcium concentrations are low, a mechanism is begun to increase absorption of calcium from the gut.

Structural Function (Table 91–1)

Stomach. The main function of the stomach in assimilation is a mixing action on the chyme. The mixing action breaks ingested fat into an emulsion, which consists of smaller particles of fat mixed with water. The emptying action of the stomach is such that the chyme is released in small amounts, with a hypertonic meal being brought toward isotonicity by gastric secretion. The secretion of pepsin starts the digestion of protein, while the secretion of intrinsic factor (IF) is essential to the absorption of vitamin B_{12}.

Duodenum. Major physiologic actions in the duodenum are the release of the hormones cholecystokinin-pancreozymin (CCK-PZ) and secretin from the duodenal mucosa when the chyme leaves the stomach and is in contact with the mucosa. These hormones result in secretion of bicarbonate and enzymes from the pancreas and contraction of the gallbladder with bile salts being excreted through the biliary tract. All of these are essential for the proper digestion of fats, carbohydrates, and protein. Mixing of the chyme with these secretions begins in the duodenum. Absorption also begins in the duodenum, and the maximum rates of absorption of iron and calcium occur in the duodenum.

Jejunum. In the normal intact gut, the jejunum is the site of maximum absorption of all ingested foodstuffs, including carbohydrates, fats, protein, vitamins (except for vitamin B_{12}), and a great proportion of water and minerals. The jejunal mucosa is such that hypertonic contents are quickly brought to isotonicity by rapid absorption of solute and by secretion of a hypotonic fluid. This rapid transfer of solute and water results from the large-sized pores of the intercellular spaces of 7.5 Å as compared with the smaller size of 3.5 Å within the ileum. Thus, the jejunum is a highly permeable membrane with large movement of solute by passive transfer (see later).

Ileum. Conjugated bile salts and vitamin

Table 91–1. INTEGRATED ASSIMILATION FUNCTION OF THE GASTROINTESTINAL TRACT

Stomach
Mixing
Emulsion formation
Controlled emptying into the duodenum
Protein digestion (pepsin)
Intrinsic factor secretion (vitamin B_{12} absorption)
Duodenum
Secretin and cholecystokinin-pancreozymin release from mucosa
Mixing of chyme with bile and pancreatic enzymes
Iron and calcium absorption
Jejunum
Highly permeable to passive absorption
Brush border enzymes for hydrolysis of disaccharides and oligopeptides
Protein, fat, and carbohydrate completely absorbed
Large proportion of water, minerals, ions, and vitamins (except for vitamin B_{12}) absorbed
Ileum
Conserving membrane
Less permeable to passive absorption
Sodium actively absorbed
Conjugated bile salt absorption receptors in distal 100 cm of ileum
Vitamin B_{12} absorption
Colon
Least permeable to passive absorption
Most efficient water and sodium absorption
Potassium secreted
Pancreas
Primary organ for synthesis and secretion of enzymes for digestion
Liver
Synthesis and secretion of conjugated bile salts
Biliary Tract
Delivery of conjugated bile salts

B_{12} are absorbed at a maximum rate by specific receptors in the distal ileum. This is the only effective site for transport of these substances. Loss or serious dysfunction of the terminal 100 cm or more of ileum seriously impairs the transport of these substances, resulting in subsequent deficiencies (Chapter 108) and potentially serious consequences.

The ileum is also a conserving membrane, conserving sodium and water. Because of its relatively small pores, there is less net secretion into the ileum. Absorption of sodium is by an active process (see later), assuring more complete absorption of the sodium. Thus, the ileum is a relatively impermeable membrane as compared with the jejunum, with transfer of solute primarily by an active mechanism rather than the passive transfer in the jejunum.

Colon. The colon is the most impermeable and conserving membrane for solute transfer. It has the smallest pore size (2.5 Å), as compared with the jejunum and ileum, and is hence most resistant to passive transfer (discussed later in section on Transport). Sodium is actively absorbed, while potassium is secreted into the lumen, resulting in stool possessing a higher concentration of potassium than of sodium.

Intestinal Integration

Fat Assimilation. Because the process of fat assimilation demonstrates the integrated system of a complex process, it is summarized here for illustrative purposes (a more extensive and detailed discussion of fat absorption is found in Chapter 92).

When the emulsified fatty meal passes into the duodenum, several important events happen almost simultaneously. The hormones CCK-PZ and secretin are released from the duodenal mucosa. When they reach the pancreas by way of the blood stream, synthesis and secretion of pancreatic enzymes in an alkaline solution are initiated, with passage of this solution into the duodenum. Here, hydrolysis of triglycerides to free fatty acids and β-monoglyceride occurs. At the same time, CCK-PZ causes gallbladder contraction, and bile salts in high concentration enter the duodenum through the common bile duct. The high concentrations of conjugated bile salts form mixed micelles with the monoglyceride and fatty acids. This phase is essential for fat assimilation. While the fatty acids and monoglyceride are absorbed into the intestinal mucosal cell, the bile salts travel down the gut to the distal ileum where they are absorbed into the ileal mucosa. Within the jejunal intestinal mucosal cell, the fatty acids and monoglyceride are resynthesized to triglyceride and extruded into the lymph system. The bile salts are then absorbed by the distal ileal mucosa and are returned to the gallbladder by way of the enterohepatic circulation. Thus, normal fat assimilation requires integration between the stomach, duodenal mucosa, pancreas, liver, biliary tract, jejunal mucosa, and an intact lymph system (Chapter 92).

Enterohepatic Circulation. The total body pool of conjugated bile salts circulates several times each day from the gut to the liver. Vitamin D metabolites also undergo enterohepatic circulation. Between meals, the bile salts are stored in the gallbladder. After contraction of the gallbladder on eating a meal, these molecules form mixed micelles in the gut, consisting of fat and lipid-soluble molecules, and during this phase fats are absorbed in the jejunum. The conjugated bile salts are absorbed by specific receptors in the distal 100 cm of ileum; only a very small fraction flows into the colon and is excreted with feces. After absorption from the ileum, the bile salts circulate in the portal blood to the liver, where they are picked up and secreted into the bile. They then are either stored in the gallbladder until the next meal or, if the meal is still in progress, are secreted directly into the duodenum. The enterohepatic circulation, therefore, is dependent upon: (1) a functioning and intact distal ileal mucosa, (2) an intact portal venous system, (3) normal hepatic function, and (4) a patent biliary tract. The enterohepatic circulation is not affected by cholecystectomy.

Secretion. Although the gut is primarily an *absorbing* organ, considerable secretion occurs physiologically and in disease states. Normally, an individual ingests about 2 liters of fluid per day. This adds to the secretion of 7 liters from various parts of the gut into the lumen (Table 91–2). Once secreted into the gut lumen, the fluid and solute are handled the same as exogenous material requiring assimilation. Thus, endogenous secretions add considerably to the load of the gut.[1]

Bacterial toxins, neoplastic hormones, and extraintestinal diseases can convert the intestine from a net water-absorbing organ to a net secretory organ productive of a watery diarrhea that may be severe. Classic examples are cholera toxin and the hormone vasoactive intestinal peptide (VIP).

Pathologic States. Loss of the jejunum results in minimal overall absorptive difficulty

Table 91–2. ENDOGENOUS SECRETION INTO THE GASTROINTESTINAL TRACT DAILY

From	ml
Salivary glands	1500
Stomach	2500
Liver	500
Pancreas	1500
Intestine	1000
Total	7000

as compared with resection of a large amount (over 100 cm) of the distal ileum and the ileocecal valve (Chapter 108). The major factor is the loss of bile salt absorptive receptors. This loss, in turn, results in diminution of the bile salt pool and consequently in impaired assimilation of fat and fat-soluble vitamins. Deconjugation by colonic bacteria of the bile salts that are enabled to enter the colon as a result of the ileal resection further impairs fat assimilation (Chapter 107).

Transport

Transport across the intestinal mucosa from the lumen of the gut to the body fluids at the serosal surface is accomplished by several mechanisms,[2,3] including *active* and *passive transport*. Passive transport can be by (1) *diffusion* along a chemical *concentration gradient* or an *electrical gradient*, or (2) solvent drag (convection). The mechanism of transport varies with the specific substance being transported, its concentration and ion charge, and the part of the intestine involved. An example of this is sodium transport. In the jejunum, when there is a high concentration of glucose, sodium is absorbed by *passive* transport, i.e., solvent drag, secondary to the absorption of glucose. In the ileum and colon, however, because of the different membrane characteristics, sodium is absorbed by an *active* mechanism.[4]

Transfer from the lumen of the gut to body fluids can occur directly through the *pores* or intercellular spaces or indirectly by way of the intestinal mucosal cell. Passive transfer takes place primarily through the intercellular spaces, while active transport occurs only by way of the intercellular pathway. The intracellular pathway, in turn, is composed of 2 steps: (1) *uptake*, which carries the absorbed substance across the cellular membrane into the cell and may involve a *carrier*, and (2) *extrusion* of the substance from the cell at the serosal surface.

Active Transport (Fig. 91–1). This is transport against an electrochemical gradient. It is an "uphill" transport from an area of low concentration to one of high concentration and concomitantly against an electrical gradient or *potential difference* (PD) (see later). The latter exists between the luminal and serosal surfaces when a cation is transported from the electrically negative luminal surface to the electrically positive serosal surface.

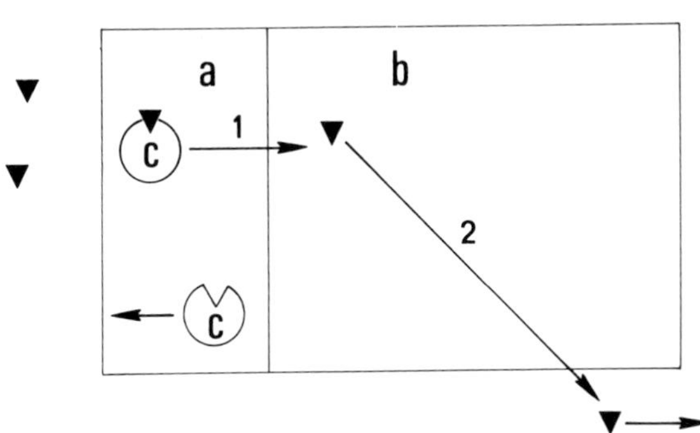

Figure 91–1. Schematic representation of *active transport* through the intestinal mucosal cell. At the luminal side of the brush border (a), the carrier first (1) picks up the substance to be absorbed and carries it to the interior of the cell (b) where the absorbed substance is released. The carrier returns to the luminal side of the brush border and the absorbed substance is then released at the serosal surface (2).

Active transport, as noted, is a 2-step process involving uptake into the cell and extrusion from the cell at the serosal surface. Either step may be an active process, or both may be active. Requirements for active transport are *cellular energy* and *molecular structural specificity*. Active transport is most efficient at low luminal concentrations. In most cases, a specific *carrier* is needed to transport the substance across the cellular membrane.

The rate of active transport of a given substance increases along an hyperbolic curve as its concentration is increased; when maximum concentration is reached, there is complete saturation of the transport mechanism. This is referred to as "saturation" kinetics (Michaelis-Menten kinetics) in comparison with passive transfer in which the rate of transfer varies directly with concentration at all concentrations.

Carrier (Fig. 91–1). It is postulated that a "carrier" is part of the active transport process of certain molecules across the luminal intestinal mucosal cell membrane. The carriers are believed to be proteins that combine reversibly with a given substance. The carrier has a high affinity for the transported substance at the luminal surface and a low affinity at the interior cellular surface, so that the transported substance is released into the cell and the carrier is available again for transport at the luminal surface of the cell membrane. The same carrier may be involved with several molecules of similar structure, with 1 molecule having greater affinity. Hence, there may be competition between similar molecules for a given carrier. Also, a carrier for 1 molecule may require another ion in order to effect transport. This is postulated for the glucose carrier, which requires sodium ion to transport glucose.

An ion and a hexose are theoretically necessary in a common carrier for transport. This theorization is fostered by the demonstration that sodium ion is needed for glucose transport across the intestinal mucosa *in vitro*. The basic mechanism in this transport is believed to be the *sodium pump*, in which there are receptor sites in the carrier for both sodium and glucose. These are transported by the carrier to the interior of the cell from the brush border. Once inside the cell, the sodium and glucose are dissociated from the carrier and the sodium is actively *pumped* out of the cell at the lateral border by an active energy-requiring mechanism.

Passive Absorption (Fig. 91–2). This form of transport occurs along a chemical or elec-

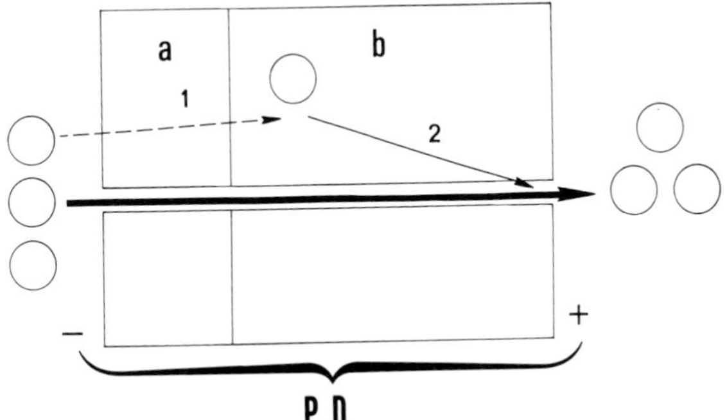

Figure 91–2. Schematic representation of *passive absorption*. This is transport along a concentration or electrical gradient. The major pathway is through the intercellular aqueous channels *(heavy arrow)*. Passive transfer also occurs through an intracellular pathway (1, 2) to a much lesser extent (a = luminal side of the brush border; b = interior of the cell; P.D. = potential difference).

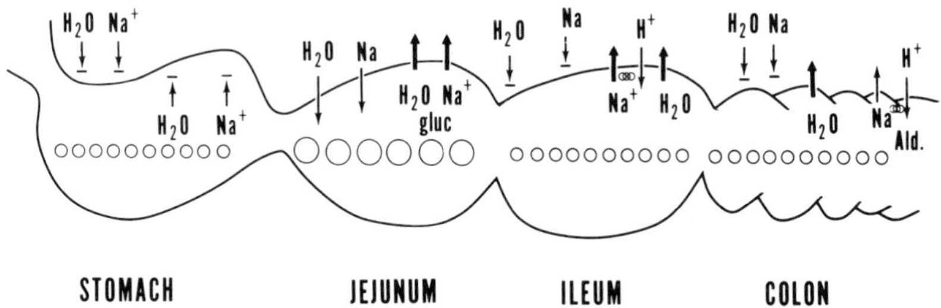

Figure 91–3. This is a representation of water and sodium unidirectional flow between blood and gut lumen, and vice versa in the stomach, jejunum, and colon. The stomach has small pores as compared with the jejunum and, therefore, the bulk flow of water in either direction is relatively slow; there is little absorption of sodium and water and, conversely, there is little dilution of a hypertonic meal. There is a relative "block" to sodium and water transport. The jejunum has rather large pores, so that the bulk flow of water occurs rapidly to dilute a hypertonic meal. There is rapid absorption of glucose, and sodium is passively absorbed in the jejunum along with the water as "solvent drag." The ileum and the colon have small pores and therefore are "tight" membranes. Because of the small pores, little secretion of water and sodium occurs into the lumen. Sodium absorption is active and very efficient, with a coupled hydrogen exchange. Thus, this part of the gut is a "conserving" membrane, conserving sodium and water. In the colon, sodium absorption is influenced by aldosterone (Ald).

trical gradient or by the process of *solvent drag* (see next paragraph). Transport occurs primarily in the "pores" or intercellular spaces; cellular energy is not required. The rate of transfer is directly related to concentration and does not have a maximal limit (Fick kinetics). Passive absorption is related to size of the intercellular pores as well as the intraluminal concentration of the given substance being absorbed. The highest intraluminal concentration of most substances is in the jejunum and the largest pores are also in the jejunal mucosa, as compared with the ileum and colon. Thus, passive absorption is greatest in the jejunum.

Solvent Drag (Fig. 91–3). This occurs primarily in the jejunum and minimally in the ileum or colon, because of the larger pore diameter in the jejunum. The classic example is the absorption of glucose in the jejunum that carries along sodium ions that are in solution in the water. Sodium ions are in effect "dragged" along with the solvent (water). Solvent drag of sodium ions occurs when glucose either is absorbed passively along a concentration gradient or is actively absorbed against a concentration gradient. Solvent drag also occurs when the jejunal luminal contents are hypotonic as compared with interstitial fluid; the hypotonic fluid moves inward through the intercellular spaces from a region of lower to one of higher osmolality.

Aqueous Channels (Table 91–3). The intestinal mucosal cell has a lipoidal cell membrane that is relatively impermeable to water, but aqueous channels exist on the lateral surfaces between cells. The diameter of these intercellular aqueous channels determines the passive transport characteristics. The jejunum with large pores (7.5 Å to 8.0 Å) is most favorable for this type of transport; the ileum with smaller pores (3.0 Å to 3.5 Å) is less favorable, and the colon (2.0 Å to 2.5 Å) is least favorable. Jejunal mucosa is referred to as a "loose" membrane, adapted for very rapid transfer of fluid and solute. In contrast, the ileum, and more so the colon, are "tight" membranes. Since the passive flow of solvent and solute is bidirectional (see subsequent discussion of Flux) from serosa to lumen as well as from lumen to serosal surface through the aqueous channels, passive flow from serosa to lumen is also greatest in the jejunum.

Table 91–3. MUCOSAL MEMBRANE CHARACTERISTICS

	Jejunum	Ileum	Colon
Aqueous channel (mean radius Å)	7.5–8.0	3.0–3.5	2.0–2.5
Resting potential (mV)	3–6	5–15	15–30
Solvent drag	Large	Moderate	Minimal

Facilitated Absorption. This is a specific form of passive transport in which energy is not required, but specificity of molecular structure is necessary. Facilitated absorption may be carrier-mediated, although it is not active absorption. An example is the transport of fructose.

Potential Difference (PD). A potential difference is present between the lumen and serosal surfaces. As mentioned earlier, the mucosal surface has a negative charge and the serosal surface a positive one. Resting PD is lowest in the jejunum and highest in the colon, varying inversely with mean pore size (Table 91–3).

PD increases with ion absorption. Because of the luminal negative charge, cations, such as potassium (K^+), will tend to diffuse into the lumen. In the steady state (Nernst equation), the chemical concentration of the anion will balance the existing electrical gradient so that the K^+, which is passively transported, maintains a higher concentration in the jejunal lumen than in the serum. Luminal concentration of potassium is highest in the lumen of the colon, where the PD is highest.

Flux (Fig. 91–3). There is a simultaneous flow of water and solute from the serosal surface to the lumen, as well as from the lumen to the serosal surface. The rate of the unidirectional flow per unit of mucosal area is defined as "*flux*." The flux from lumen to blood is inward (*insorption*), while the reverse flux is outward (*exsorption*) from blood to gut. *Net absorption* occurs when the inward exceeds the outward flux. *Net secretion* occurs when the outward flux from blood to lumen exceeds the inward flux. The jejunal mucosa with its larger aqueous channel pores has the highest unidirectional flow rates as compared with ileum and colon.

References

1. Field M. Secretion of electrolytes and water by mammalian small intestine. *In*: Johnson LR, ed. Physiology of the Gastrointestinal Tract. New York: Rowen Press, 1981.
2. Moore EW. Physiology of intestinal water and electrolyte absorption. *In*: Undergraduate Teaching Project VII A, American Gastroenterological Association. Timonium, Md: Milner-Fenwick, 1981.
3. Wilson TH. Fluid movement across the wall of the small intestine. Am J Physical 1956; 187:244–50.
4. Schultz GS. Salt and water absorption by mammalian small intestine. *In*: Johnson LR, ed. Physiology of the Gastrointestinal Tract. New York: Rowen Press, 1981.

Chapter 92

Fat Assimilation

Bengt Borgström

Fat in the chemical and physical form in which it exists in food is unavailable for absorption. For normal assimilation by the intestinal tract, fat must undergo chemical changes catalyzed by enzymes delivered at different levels of the intestinal tract. These chemical conversions involve transformation from less polar to more polar compounds. The latter interact with the bicarbonate of pancreatic juice and the different constituents of bile to produce a system that can be efficiently taken up by the enterocyte membrane.

Most important among the dietary lipids are the long chain triacylglycerols, the triglycerides (TG). These lipids make up the bulk of the dietary fat and provide approximately 40% of the energy (corresponding to about 100 g a day). They are also important because absorption of the minor lipid components is highly dependent on the simultaneous digestion and absorption of TG fat. The minor lipid components of the diet are the phospholipids (PL) (1.5 to 2 g a day), the sterols (0.4 to 0.6 g), the fat-soluble vitamins, and several mostly nonpolar compounds in minor amounts. Included among the latter are insecticides, herbicides, fungicides, biota, and industrial pollutants. In the diet, these minor lipids principally occur dissolved in the TG fat.

The physical form of dietary fat is chiefly a more or less finely dispersed emulsion that is stabilized by and covered at the interface by the more polar lipids and by proteins. Membrane lipids (primarily phospholipids) comprise another typical form of the dietary lipids.

Several publications review fat digestion and intestinal lipid absorption in great detail.[1, 2] The reader with particular interest in these processes may wish to refer to these reviews.

Intraluminal Phase (Fig. 92–1)

Lipolysis. Four well recognized enzymes and one cofactor are involved in the degradation of the dietary fat: (1) *lingual lipase;* (2) classic *pancreatic lipase* with its cofactor, *colipase;* (3) *pancreatic carboxylester hydrolase,* which is given many names; and (4) *pancreatic phospholipase* A_2.

Lingual lipase has recently drawn attention.[3] It is secreted by glands on the back of the tongue and most probably is responsible for the activity of the so-called gastric lipase. It hydrolyzes dietary triglycerides (TG) in the stomach content and is responsible for the presence of 15% to 20% of free fatty acids in fat recovered from the stomach content. Lingual lipase is stable and functions at the acid pH of the gastric contents. The products are mainly protonated fatty acids and diglycerides still in the emulsified form.[4] These gastric lipolysis products are likely of great importance to the next step in the digestive cycle, duodenal digestion, which is concerned with the activity of pancreatic lipase/colipase.

Pancreatic lipase is an enzyme that by itself is capable of hydrolyzing triglyceride fat to 2-monoglyceride and fatty acid. The probable reason for its inability to hydrolyze the ester bond in the middle or 2-position of the triglyceride is that this ester bond never becomes available at the water/lipid interface of the emulsion particles, the substrate for lipase.[5] The fact that the monoglycerides are spared from lipolysis appears of great importance for the intricate physical chemistry of fat assimilation.

Under conditions normally prevailing in the intestinal contents, pancreatic lipase cannot compete favorably for the glyceride interface, the substrate on which it acts.[6] A prerequisite is that the bile salts clear the interface of the glyceride substrate of interfering substances. This, in turn, is complicated by removal of lipase as well, thus physically separating this lipolytic enzyme from its substrate and actually inactivating it. It is here that the function of the relatively newly discovered lipase cofactor, colipase, begins.[7] *Colipase,* a polypeptide with a molecular weight of 11,000, is secreted in the pancreatic juice. It binds to lipase and probably changes its molecular conformation, enabling the lipase to compete favorably with the bile salts and PL for the substrate interface. Colipase has been shown to be secreted into the pancreatic juice in a pro-form that is activated by trypsin analogous to the proenzymes of the juice.[8] Deficiency of colipase has been reported to lead to malabsorption of fat.[9] An important function of bile salts in lipid digestion is to act as a detergent that cleans the interface of the dietary fat from amphiphilic substances that would hinder the function of lipase. Bile salts have a reputation for emulsifying the dietary fat, but are, in fact, poor emulsifiers of fat. Another important function of the bile salts is to interact physically with the products of lipolysis (see below). Bile salts, furthermore, serve to stabilize lipase in the presence of colipase.

There is a second lipid-splitting enzyme in pancreatic juice that, similar to lipase, can be classified as a carboxylic ester hydrolase. This enzyme has been given names such as *bile salt–stimulated lipase, cholesterol ester hydrolase, monoglyceride lipase,* and *nonspecific lipase.* It catalyzes the hydrolysis of different types of neutral lipid substrates, including the fat-soluble vitamin esters, but which lipid constitutes its main substrate is unknown. An immunologically identical enzyme, which has recently been shown to be present in human milk and the milk of some primates, is considered important in the digestion of dietary fat, especially in the premature infant.[10]

Phospholipase A_2 is secreted in the pancreatic juice in a pro-form and is activated by trypsin. It catalyzes the hydrolysis of PL, chiefly phosphatidylcholine or lecithin, to their lyso-form and a free fatty acid. The action of this enzyme extends to both the dietary PL and the quantitatively more important biliary PL.[11]

Bicarbonate contained in pancreatic juice is also important in the fat digestion process. The primary products formed as a result of the lipolytic process are protonated fatty acids, which stay in the lipid phase and do not interact with water to any extent. The bicarbonate of the pancreatic juice is also important in the fat digestion process, as it interacts with the fatty acids, partly ionizing them and thereby changing their physical properties and interactions with water. Complete transformation to soaps never occurs in the intestinal contents, as the pH, in spite of pancreatic bicarbonate, seldom goes above 7.

Gastric contents are fractionally delivered to the duodenum over a period of time, the length depending on the composition of the meal.[12] The concentration of pancreatic lipase in duodenal contents is about 1000 tributyrin units/ml^{-1} (0.10 mg of lipase/ml^{-1}) during the digestion of a test meal.[13] The total volume of duodenal contents passing per meal is about 2000 ml,[14] so that approximately 200 mg of lipase is mixed with a meal. This amount of lipase (specific action against long chain TG = 3000 μmol/$minute^{-1}$/mg^{-1}) is capable of hydrolyzing 0.6 mol or 540 g of TG to diglyceride in 1 minute. Since the amount of TG in a mixed meal is about 30 g and since relatively unimpaired digestion and absorption of fat take place with lipase activity in intestinal contents as low as 10% of normal,[15] there is obviously more than enough lipase in the duodenal contents to hydrolyze dietary fat in a very short time. Yet, it has been repeatedly observed that it is difficult to substitute effectively for the lipase needed per meal (at least 20 mg) to fully hydrolyze dietary TG in patients with severe pancreatic insufficiency.[16, 17]

Physicochemical Transformation. The end product of lipolysis generated by the enzymes just discussed are fatty acids (partly ionized), 2-monoacylglycerol, and lysophospholipids dispersed in bile salt solution. Physically, these products form mixed micellar solutions in a process that is dynamic. One of the most interesting developments of recent years is the study of the time sequence of these interactions. By observing the lipo-

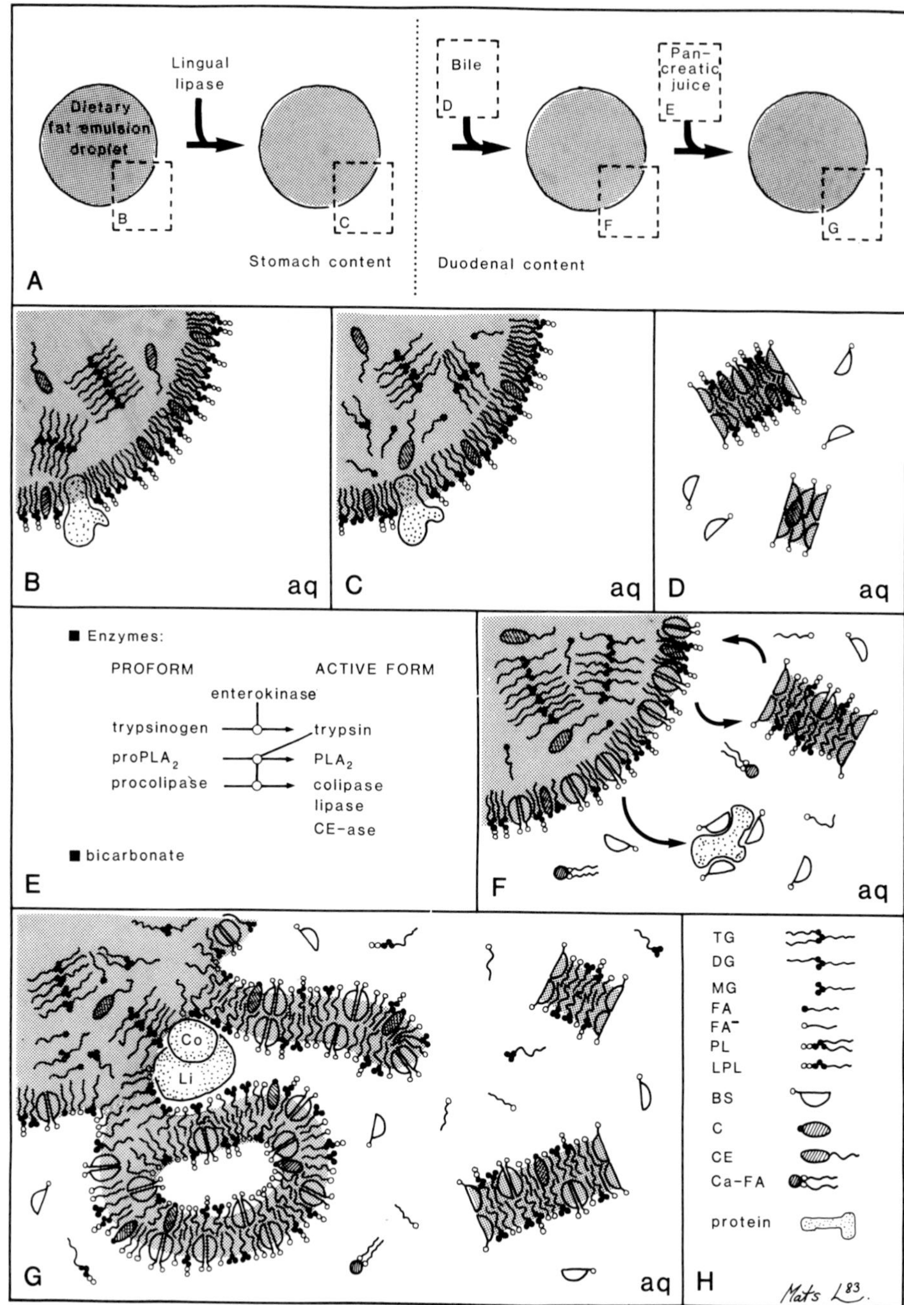

Figure 92–1. *See legend on opposite page*

lytic process microscopically, Patton and Carey[18] identified at least 2 new product phases produced under physiologic conditions: (1) a crystalline phase of calcium soaps, and (2) a liquid crystalline phase of mostly monoglyceride and protonated fatty acids. These clearly visible phases can be dispersed by an excess of bile salts into the micellar form. These phases may be of importance physiologically at the high lipase and relatively low bile salt concentrations that exist in intraduodenal content in man during digestion.[19]

During the active phase of lipid digestion in the duodenal lumen, therefore, at least 5 enzyme product phases may exist in dynamic equilibrium: (1) an oil phase, (2) a crystalline soap phase, (3) a liquid crystalline phase, (4) a micellar phase, and (5) a molecular dissolved phase. Studies[20] indicate that bile contains mixed bile salt–lecithin micelles with a diameter of ≃ 60 Å coexisting with simple bile salt–cholesterol micelles and monomeric bile salts. Upon dilution of the bile in the duodenal contents, much larger disc-shaped micelles appear (diameter up to ≃ 1000 Å). When these micelles meet the dietary fat, an interface exchange can be expected to take place. The aggregates become even larger as lipolysis products are formed, folding into unilamellar liposomal vesicles. The simple micelles are used to build up the aggregates, and the so-called intermicellar concentration (monomeric + simple micelles) of bile salt decreases. During actual fat digestion in the duodenal contents, therefore, no simple micelles can be expected to exist. The importance of these physical phases for fat assimilation by the enterocyte is not clear at the present time. So far, experimental evidence for an important role exists only for the molecular and the micellar phases.

Uptake (Fig. 92–2). It was suggested as part of the micellar hypothesis for fat absorption that the micellar content was taken up as a unit. This was based on the finding that 2 components of a mixed bile salt micelle, mono-olein and oleic acid, were taken up in the same ratio as they were present in the micelle. Later, this was found to be a coincidence and not a general trend.[2] The micelles are thought to dissociate during fat absorption.

The process of uptake that takes place with the different components in molecular solution is now better understood as a result of studies done by Westergaard and Dietschy.[21,22] In most biologic systems there are 2 barriers to uptake into a cell: (1) a diffusion barrier of unstirred water, and (2) the cell membrane. The unstirred layer resists transport from the bulk phase of the intestinal content to the cell membrane. Flux across the unstirred water layer is a function of the concentration gradient over the layer times the permeability of the layer, the latter being

---

Figure 92–1. *A,* General outline of the lipid digestion process (see text).

B, Structure of dietary fat. The oil phase (shaded) contains mainly triglyceride in an unordered structure. The interphase between oil and water is covered by a monolayer of mainly phospholipid and interdigitated cholesterol. Triglyceride is also present at the interphase; it has been estimated as about 3% of the interphase.

C, Triglyceride is converted to diglyceride and fatty acid by lingual lipase. The diglyceride stays to a large extent at the interface with the phospholipids. At the pH of stomach content, fatty acids that are set free are largely nonionized and stay in the oil phase with remaining tri- and diglyceride.

D, The lipid components of the bile are present as simple bile salt micelles and mixed bile salt–lecithin–cholesterol micelles in equilibrium with monomeric bile salt. As the bile is diluted in the duodenal content, the micelles enlarge and the monomer concentration decreases.

E, Bicarbonate, enzymes, and coenzymes are mixed into the duodenal content.

F, Complex interactions occur when lipid products from the stomach are mixed with bile and pancreatic juice in the duodenal content. Bile is diluted and the micelles enlarge. An exchange of components also occurs between the bile micelles and the interface of the dietary fat. Bile salts penetrate the interface and by increasing the surface pressure displace the protein adhering to it. Some phospholipid is also exchanged. The fatty acids are ionized and go into the interphase and the aqueous phase, where they may interact with the mixed micellar phase.

G, The colipase/lipase complex binds to the interface and hydrolyzes, remaining tri- and diglyceride. Interfacial micellar uptake of lipolysis products saturates the micelles and large mixed disk-shaped micelles form, which fold into vesicles. The monomeric bile salt concentration decreases further with no simple micelles existing and a low bile salt monomer concentration.

H, Key to molecular symbols. *Abbreviations:* PLA_2, pancreatic phospholipase A_2; CE-ase, cholesterol esterase; aq, aqueous; Co, colipase; Li, lipase; TG, triglyceride; DG, diglyceride; MG, monoglyceride; FA, un-ionized fatty acid; FA^-, ionized fatty acid; PL, phospholipid; LPL, lysophospholipid; BS, bile salt; CE, cholesterol ester; C, cholesterol; Ca–FA, calcium–fatty acid. (Drawing courtesy of Dr. Mats Lindström.)

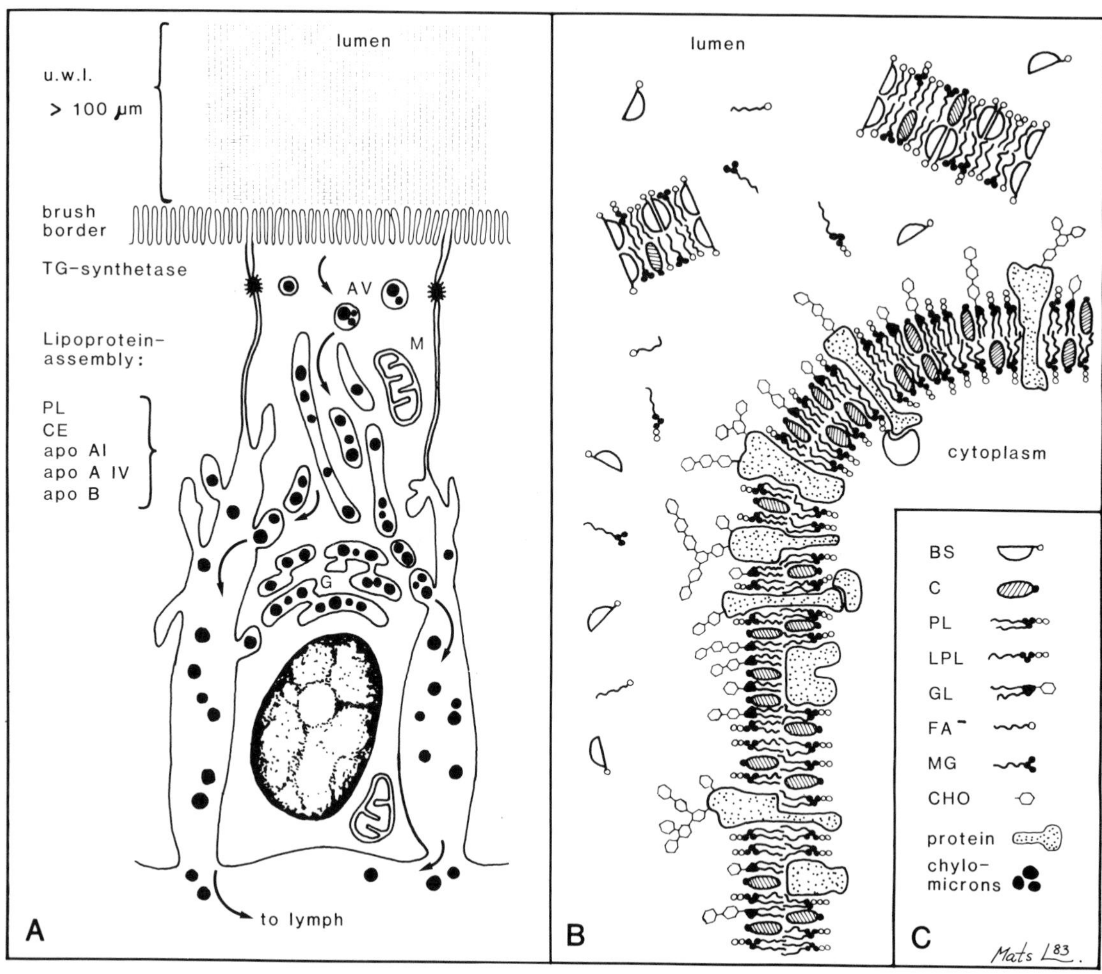

Figure 92–2. Schematic presentation of the uptake and further metabolism of the product phases from the digestion of the dietary fat. The brush border is approximately 10,000 Å thick; the unstirred water layer covering it is at least 10 times as thick and contains structural components (the glycocalix) of unknown importance.

A, The enterocyte with the different synthetic reactions leading to the assembly of the chylomicrons, which are fed into the intercellular space.

B, Section of the brush border membrane at high magnification absorbing luminal digestion product phases.

C, Key to molecular symbols. *Abbreviations:* TG, triglyceride; PL, phospholipid; CE, cholesterol ester; apo, apoprotein; AV, apical vesicle; M, mitochondrion; G, Golgi apparatus; u.w.l., unstirred water layer; CHO, carbohydrate; GL, glycolipid; BS, bile salt; C, cholesterol; LPL, lysophospholipid; FA⁻, ionized fatty acid; MG, monoglyceride. (Drawing courtesy of Dr. Mats Lindström.)

determined by the effective thickness of the layer and the aqueous diffusion coefficient of the molecule in question. Flux through the membrane is similarly determined by the gradient over the membrane and the permeability factor. Total resistance to the transport of a molecule passing from the bulk phase of the lumen into the cell is the sum of the resistances of the separate phases, and their relative contributions determine the concentration profile. This means that when diffusion is limited by the membrane, flux is proportional to the permeability of the membrane. The other extreme is the condition that occurs when the rate of penetration of the solute through the membrane is much faster than its rate of diffusion over the unstirred water layer. In these circumstances, flux is proportional to the aqueous diffusion constant of the molecule for any given concentration in the bulk phase and the thickness of the unstirred layer.

The major conclusion to be drawn from these considerations and experimental in vitro work is that the unstirred water layer and not the microvillus membrane is rate limiting to the uptake of long chain fatty acids and other nonpolar compounds, such as cholesterol. Experimental results were also obtained to define the polarity of the villus membrane. The rate of passive penetration of a cell membrane is determined by the membrane/water partition coefficient for the molecule in question. The microvillus membrane could be characterized as relatively polar, more polar than bulk isobutanol.[22]

The thickness of the unstirred water layer overlying the upper villi has been calculated to vary from 115 to 334 μm.[21] This rather enormous and seemingly unphysiologic depth of the unstirred water layer, compared with the approximately 25 μm height of the absorptive cell, has prompted search for another possible interface diffusion barrier. Experimental evidence indicates that the intestinal mucous coat constitutes such a barrier.[23]

The effect of bile salts on the rate of uptake of nonpolar lipids such as long chain fatty acids and cholesterol has been studied by varying the solute concentration in the bulk phase at constant or changing bile salt concentration as compared with a change of both in parallel. These studies indicate that the nonpolar solute is absorbed through a monomer phase in equilibrium with the micelle and that the principal role of the micelle in facilitating lipid absorption is "to overcome the resistance of the unstirred layer."[2] By this is meant that the presence of mixed bile salt micelles will maintain a maximal monomer concentration at the aqueous-membrane interface. It is not definitely known where the mixed micelle dissociates, but it is likely that this occurs after diffusion into the unstirred water layer close to the membrane. Assumed as part of this model is that the main part of the bile salts is not absorbed in vivo at the same level of the intestine as are the split products of dietary fat.[24] The latter are absorbed beginning in the proximal jejunum, whereas the hydrophilic bile salts are absorbed in the ileum by an active process that shows saturation kinetics, is susceptible to metabolic inhibitors, and is sodium-dependent[25] (Chapter 97).

The mechanism of fat assimilation as pictured by Westergaard and Dietschy[22] accounts for several features of lipid absorption: (1) that absorption of short and medium chain fatty acids is independent of the presence of bile in the intestine; (2) that there is a moderate degree of malabsorption of long chain fatty acids in the absence of bile; and (3) that strongly nonpolar compounds, such as cholesterol, fat-soluble vitamins, and hydrocarbons, are essentially unabsorbed under these conditions.

The view of the fat assimilation process as developed to this point has simplified the problem by dealing with only 2 of the intraluminal phases. The micelles and the molecular dispersed phase, as previously discussed, are generated from the oil phase by lipolysis. Several more product phases of differing physical structures most probably exist in the intestinal content during the active digestion period. This is supported by the relatively low bile salt concentration, except for the initial phase of digestion when the gallbladder empties to put the bile acid pool in circulation.[26] The fat absorption process is rather specific. Most characteristic is the dependence of absorption of less polar molecules on the simultaneous absorption of triglyceride split products and bile salts. The effect of the TG split products is to solubilize the nonpolar fat into the mixed micelle and thereby to favor transport into the unstirred water layer. Other factors of importance are the aqueous solubility and the partition between the aqueous phase/villus membrane. It is well known that the products of lipolysis (monoglycerides and fatty acids) favor the solubility of nonpolar lipids into the mixed micelle.[27] The specificity in fat uptake thus depends on several factors in a kinetic system that transports lipids from the oil phase of the dietary fat to the cell sap of the enterocytes. The transport through the villus membrane is considered to be by passive diffusion.

Additional factors must be considered to explain the specificity in absorption of the sterols. *Cholesterol* absorption has been shown to be dependent on bile salts in vivo. This cannot be explained only as an effect of the nonpolarity of cholesterol; it is possible that the bile salts have a specific effect on the permeability of the cell membrane. Bile salts cannot be replaced by other types of detergent in vivo, even if they can solubilize cholesterol into a micellar form and promote the absorption of other lipids, such as monoglyceride and fatty acid.[28] Furthermore, there is a marked specificity in sterol absorption that is yet not explained, and small differences in the chemical structure of the sterol side chain have a profound effect. Sitosterol, which differs from cholesterol by an additional ethyl group in the 24-position, is absorbed with an efficiency of only 10% of that of cholesterol.[29] In vitro experiments with isolated intestinal preparations have yielded different results; cholesterol is taken up from non–bile salt micellar solutions,[30] and there is no difference between cholesterol and sitosterol uptake from bile salt solution.[31] Care obviously must be taken about applying data drawn from in vitro studies to the in vivo situation.

In a rare familial state of unknown etiology, plant sterols (chiefly β-sitosterol) are absorbed almost as efficiently as cholesterol. This leads to *β-sitosterolemia* and *xanthomatosis*.[32] In patients with this disorder, the normal mechanism responsible for selectivity in absorption of dietary sterols seems to have been lost.

The digestion and absorption of *phospholipids* (PL) have attracted some recent interest. The daily intake of PL (chiefly phosphatidylcholine) of about 2 g is small relative to the amount contained in bile. Both are digested by phospholipase A_2 of pancreatic juice as a prerequisite to absorption as lysophospholipid and fatty acid. The biliary PLs are important for the cosolubilization of cholesterol in bile and have been shown to have an important role in the overall fat absorption process.[33] Intraluminal PL is important in the translocation of dietary TG fat to the chyle.[34] Whether this is a specific effect of the lysophospholipid absorbed or is due to the availability of choline is not definitely known. High doses of dietary PL have been shown to decrease cholesterol absorption in vivo as well as in vitro.[35] A similar effect is obtained in the absence of phospholipase A_2, indicating that intact PL in the luminal contents tends to hold cholesterol back, possibly by affecting the intraluminal partition and in this way reducing its monomer activity.

Cellular Phase

The foregoing consideration of the fat absorptive process indicates that the products of lipolysis, *monoglyceride and fatty acids*, are the main lipids entering the cytoplasm on the interior side of the villus membrane. In contrast to what has been learned about transport up to the outer side of the villus membrane, almost nothing is known about transport beyond this point.

Microscopically, fat is first seen inside the lumen of the endoplasmic reticulum. A fatty acid binding protein with a molecular weight of 12,000 has been isolated from the enterocyte cytosol and its role in the transport of fatty acid from the membrane to the endoplasmic reticulum has been stressed by Ockner and Manning.[36] The importance of this protein is not yet clear and there is no information about how other fats, such as monoglycerides and sterols, are transported in the cell sap. The common end point is the presence of fat droplets inside the bulbous expansions of the smooth endoplasmic reticulum, where the long chain fatty acids are re-esterified to form TG.[37]

For resynthesis of fatty acid and monoglycerides into TG, 2 different pathways have been recognized: (1) the monoacylglycerol pathway catalyzed by the triacylglycerol synthetase localized in the interior membrane of the smooth endoplasmic reticulum, and (2) the phosphatidic acid or glycerophosphate pathway confined to the rough endoplasmic reticulum. It has been shown that the total cellular PL pool increases during fat absorption as a part of an expansion of the membrane system. The interpretation advanced is that this represents an increase in membrane lipid synthesis in addition to the formation of chylomicron surfactant.[38] The triacylglycerol synthetase of the enterocyte microsomal fraction has been isolated as a complex whose activity is dependent on phosphatidylcholine.[39] The absorbed lysophospholipids that originate in dietary and biliary PL are to a large extent resynthesized to PL and appear in the chylomicrons. An excess of PL over that needed for chylomicron formation is completely hydrolyzed and converted to TG.

Dietary or biliary cholesterol is found in the lipid droplets of the smooth endoplasmic reticulum membranes, mainly as free cholesterol.[37] The cholesterol in the chylomicron is largely esterified and 2 different mechanisms have been suggested to account for this synthesis. One hypothesis holds that the sterol ester hydrolase of the pancreatic juice is absorbed intact into the mucosal cell and affects cholesterol ester synthesis, energy being derived from the phase transitions involved.[40] The other postulate is that cholesterol synthesis occurs from the microsomal acyl-CoA-cholesterol acyltransferase system isolated from the enterocyte. However, experimental results do not support any rate-limiting effect of pancreatic or intestinal cholesterol ester hydrolase on intracellular cholesterol esterification during absorption.[41]

Delivery

The dietary long chain fatty acids leave the mucosal cell and the small intestine mainly in the TG form contained in the bulk of the chylomicrons. These lipoprotein particles with a diameter about 1 μ also contain fractions of nonpolar lipids, the sterols, the fat-soluble vitamins, hydrocarbons, and other hydrophobic molecules. In addition, they contain PL and some protein. As already discussed, TG is synthesized by the endoplasmic reticulum of the enterocyte and given off to its lumen as fat droplets. The latter are further completed during transport through the Golgi system and are finally fed out into the lateral intracellular spaces. Information as to the mechanism of the assembly, intracellular transport, and secretion of the chylomicrons is based on the integration of ultrastructural and chemical experimental results. The ultrastructural work indicates that nascent chylomicrons accumulate within Golgi vesicles and that secretion occurs by exocystosis.[42] The secretory vesicle membranes are seen to fuse with the lateral plasmalemma and the chylomicrons are discharged into the intracellular space, pass through the basement membrane, and gain access to the lymphatics through gaps between endothelial cells. The endoplasmic reticulum can be considered to represent a complex continuous intracellular system of tubular structures; alongside them, the absorbed lipids are transported while they undergo an orderly sequence of assembly that terminates in the secretion of complete chylomicrons. PL and cholesterol/cholesterol esters are probably added early to the triglyceride droplets.

Apo-B and apo-A are probably found preformed in the tubular system and added before the nascent chylomicrons enter the Golgi apparatus. In the human disease *abetalipoproteinemia,* lipid droplets accumulate in the vesicles of the smooth endoplasmic reticulum and do not enter the Golgi system. The exact reason for this is not clear; either the apoproteins are deficient or the Golgi membrane formation is defective. Most probably, apoprotein-lipid assembly occurs within the endoplasmic reticulum. Available evidence indicates that the Golgi system is the site of terminal glycosylation and that the secretion of lipoproteins by the Golgi apparatus is dependent on the addition of specific carbohydrates. This concept is further supported by the finding that fat fed to rats treated with galactosamine accumulates as large lipid droplets in the intercellular spaces.[43] The importance of the microtubular apparatus for the movement of the secretory vesicles to the plasmalemma is indicated by the finding that colchicine (a chemical known to interfere with the microtubular system) has inhibitory effects on chylomicron release.[44]

The chylomicron secreted by the enterocyte is, in effect, a lipoprotein particle with a core of triglyceride containing some cholesterol ester and other nonpolar lipids dissolved and covered on the surface by the amphiphilic PL, cholesterol, and apoprotein. The apoprotein species of the newly synthesized chylomicron are difficult to define, as the lymph draining the intestine contains all major apolipoprotein derived by filtration from plasma. However, apo-B, apo A-I, and apo A-IV seem to be synthesized by the intestine, apo A-IV being the one most inducible during fat absorption.[45]

Short and medium chain fatty acids (chain

length C4 to C12) are present in dietary fat, mostly in mixed TG. These fatty acids are preferentially split by lingual lipase, pancreatic lipase, and possibly the bile salt–stimulated lipase of milk and pancreas.[46] They are water soluble and partition into the aqueous phase of intestinal content. Their absorption rate is high.

The metabolism of the *medium chain fatty acids* (MCTs) (fatty acid chain length C8 to C12) has attracted special interest in medicine, as these acids are *absorbed independent of pancreatic lipase and bile.* The MCTs undergo hydrolysis by pancreatic lipase in the lumen more effectively than do long chain triglyceride. They may also be absorbed without previous complete hydrolysis. The assimilation of MCT-derived fatty acids or monoglyceride may not need bile to overcome the resistance of the unstirred water layer; they therefore can be expected to be absorbed as well in the absence of bile. After being absorbed, most of the MCTs are partitioned into the venous blood and leave the intestine as free ionized fatty acids partly bound to albumin. The MCTs occur only to a limited extent in the chylomicron as components of TG and then almost only in the form of the C12 fatty acid. MCT fat assimilation, hence, is largely independent of bile, pancreatic function, and factors that impair protein synthesis or obstruct lymphatic transport from the intestine. Their further metabolism also differs from long chain fatty acids. Only to a very limited extent (C12) are they incorporated into adipose tissue or other lipid stores. In general, they are rapidly metabolized to carbon dioxide and water in the liver.

Summary

Dietary fat is composed mainly of nonpolar, long chain triacylglycerols, is virtually water insoluble, and exists in physical form as an emulsion stabilized with rather nonspecific covers of phospholipid and protein. In this form, fat is not available for assimilation by the intestinal tract. Through lipolytic processes catalyzed by enzymes secreted into the content of the gastrointestinal tract, dietary fat is converted to more polar products that can more favorably interact with water. Bile disperses the products of lipid digestion and provides a vehicle to overcome the diffusion barrier covering the villus surface.

Absorbed lipids are resynthesized into fat, again mainly TG, and appear as fat droplets inside the canalicular system of the endoplasmic reticulum that traverses the enterocyte. Inside this tubular system, the end product of assimilation—the chylomicron—is assembled by ordered chemical processes. The chylomicron, in turn, is delivered by exocytosis to the lymphatic system in the form of a lipoprotein with a TG core covered with phospholipids and some specific apoproteins.

Dietary fat and the chylomicron may seem analogous, both chemically and physically. The difference between them is that chylomicron fat is distributed in a rather homogeneous particle size with a cover specifically built to be transported in the blood and be acted upon by lipoprotein lipase of the capillary endothelium after the uptake of apo C-II from plasma.

Acknowledgment: I am grateful to Dr. Mats Lindström for constructive discussions and the drawing of the figures.

References

1. Patton JS. Gastrointestinal lipid digestion. *In:* Johnson LR, ed. Physiology of the Gastrointestinal Tract, Vol. 2. New York: Raven Press, 1981: 1123–46.
2. Thomson ABR, Dietshy JM. Intestinal lipid absorption: Major extracellular and intracellular events. *In:* Johnson LR, ed. Physiology of the Gastrointestinal Tract, Vol. 2. New York: Raven Press, 1981: 1147–220.
3. Hamosh M, Scanlon JW, Ganot D, Likel M, Scanlon KB, Hamosh P. Fat digestion in the newborn. Characterization of lipase in gastric aspirates of premature and term infants. J Clin Invest 1981; 67:838–46.
4. Patton JS, Rigler MW, Liao TH, Hamosh P, Hamosh M. Hydrolysis of triacylglycerol emulsions by lingual lipase—A microscopic study. Biochim Biophys Acta 1982; 212:400–7.
5. Hamilton JA, Small DM. Solubilization and localization of triolein in phosphatidylcholine bilayers: A 13C NMR study. Proc Natl Acad Sci USA 1981; 78:6878–82.
6. Borgström B, Erlanson C. Interaction of serum albumin and other proteins with porcine pancreatic lipase. Gastroenterology 1978; 75:382–6.
7. Borgström B, Erlanson-Albertsson C, Wieloch T. Pancreatic colipase: Chemistry and physiology. J Lipid Res 1979; 20:805–16.
8. Borgström B, Wieloch T, Erlanson-Albertsson C. Evidence for a pancreatic pro-colipase and its activation by trypsin. FEBS Lett 1979; 108:407–10.
9. Hildebrand H, Borgström B, Békássy A, Erlanson-Albertsson C, Helén I. Isolated co-lipase deficiency in two brothers. Gut 1982; 23:243–6.
10. Blackberg L, Hernell O. The bile-salt-stimulated lipase in human milk: Purification and characterization. Eur J Biochem 1981; 116:221–5.
11. Borgström B. Importance of phospholipids, pancreatic phospholipase A_2, and fatty acid for the digestion of dietary fat. Gastroenterology 1980; 78:954–62.
12. Lagerlöf H, Johansson C, Kerstin E. Human gastric and intestinal response to meals studied by a multiple indicator dilution method. Mt Sinai J Med 1976; 43:1–98.
13. Borgström B, Hildebrand H. Lipase and co-lipase activities of human small intestinal contents after a liquid test meal. Scand J Gastroenterol 1975; 10:585–91.

14. Borgström B, Dahlquist A, Lundh G, Sjövall J. Studies of intestinal digestion and absorption in the human. J Clin Invest 1957; 36:1521–36.
15. DiMagno EP, Go VLW, Summerskil WHJ. Relations between pancreatic enzyme outputs and malabsorption in severe pancreatic insufficiency. N Engl J Med 1973; 288:813–5.
16. DiMagno EP, Malagelada JR, Go VLW, Moertel CG. Fate of orally ingested enzymes in pancreatic insufficiency. N Engl J Med 1977; 296:1318–22.
17. Ihse I, Lilja P, Lundquist I. Intestinal concentrations of pancreatic enzymes following pancreatic replacement therapy. Scand J Gastroenterol 1980; 15:137–44.
18. Patton JS, Carey MC. Watching fat digestion. Science 1979; 204:145–8.
19. Lindström M, Ljusberg-Wahren H, Larsson K. Aqueous lipid phases of relevance to intestinal fat digestion and absorption. Lipids 1981; 16:749–54.
20. Carey MC. The enterohepatic circulation. *In:* Arias I, Popper H. Schacter D, Shafritz A, eds. The Liver: Biology and Pathology. New York: Raven Press, 1982:429–65.
21. Westergaard H, Dietschy JM. Delineation of the dimensions and permeability characteristics of the major diffusion barriers to passive mucosal uptake in the rabbit intestine. J Clin Invest 1974; 54:718–32.
22. Westergaard H, Dietschy JM. The mechanism whereby bile acid micelles increase the rate of fatty acid and cholesterol uptake into the intestinal mucosa cell. J Clin Invest 1976; 58:97–108.
23. Smithson KW, Miller DB, Jacobs, LR, Gray GM. Intestinal diffusion barrier: Unstirrred water layer or membrane surface mucous coat. Science 1981; 214:1241–4.
24. Borgström B, Lundh G, Hofmann AF. The site of absorption of conjugated bile salts in man. Gastroenterology 1963; 45:229–38.
25. Lack L, Weiner IM. Intestinal absorption of bile salts and some biological implications. Fed Proc 1963; 22:1334–8.
26. Mansbach CM, Cohen RS, Leff PB. Isolation and properties of the mixed lipid micelles present in intestinal content during fat digestion in man. J Clin Invest 1975; 56:781–91.
27. Neiderhiser DH, Roth HP. Effect of phospholipase on cholesterol solubilization by lecithin in bile salt solution. Gastroenterology 1970; 58:26–31.
28. Watt SM, Simmonds WJ. The specificity of bile salts in the intestinal absorption of micellar cholesterol in the rat. Clin Exp Pharmacol Physiol 1976; 3:305–22.
29. Hassan AS, Rampone AJ. Intestinal absorption and lymphatic transport of cholesterol and β-sitosterol in the rat. J Lipid Res 1979; 20:646–53.
30. Feldman EB, Cheng CY. Mucosal uptake in vitro of cholesterol from bile salt and surfactant solutions. Am J Clin Nutr 1975; 28:692–98.
31. Sylvén C. Influence of blood supply on lipid uptake from micellar solutions by the rat small intestine. Biochim Biophys Acta 1970; 203:365–75.
32. Miettinen TA. Phytosterolaemia, xanthomathosis and premature atherosclerotic arterial disease: A case with high plant sterol absorption, impaired sterol elimination and low cholesterol synthesis. Eur J Clin Invest 1980; 10:27–35.
33. O'Doherty PJA, Kakis G, Kuksis A. Role of luminal lecithin in intestinal fat absorption. Lipids 1973; 8:249–55.
34. Tso P, Balint JA, Simmonds WJ. Role of biliary lecithin in lymphatic transport of fat. Gastroenterology 1976; 13:1362–7.
35. Beil FU, Grunda SM. Studies on plasma lipoproteins during absorption of exogenous lecithin in man. J Lipid Res 1980; 21:525–36.
36. Ockner RK, Manning JA. Fatty acid binding protein in small intestine. Identification, isolation and evidence for its role in cellular fatty acid transport. J Clin Invest 1974; 54:326–38.
37. Sjöstrand FS, Borgström B. The lipid component of the smooth-surface membrane-bounded vesicles of the columnar cells of the rat intestinal epithelium during fat absorption. J Ultrastruct Res 1967; 20:140–60.
38. Shaikh NA, Kuksis A. Expansion of phospholipid pool size of rat intestinal villus cells during fat absorption. Can J Biochem 1982; 60:444–51.
39. Manganaro F, Kuksis A. Modulation of acylglycerol synthetase activities of rat intestinal mucosa by homogenization and sonication. Can J Biochem 1981; 59:736–42.
40. Gallo LL, Newbill T, Hyun J, Vahouny GN, Treadwell CR. Role of pancreatic cholesterol esterase in the uptake and esterification of cholesterol by isolated intestinal cells. Proc Soc Exp Biol Med 1977; 156:277–81.
41. Watt SM, Simmonds WJ. The effect of pancreatic diversion on lymphatic absorption and esterification of cholesterol in the rat. J Lipid Res 1981; 22:157–65.
42. Sabesin SM, Frase S. Electron microscopic studies of the assembly intracellular transport and secretion of chylomicrons by rat intestine. J Lipid Res 1977; 18:496–511.
43. Sabesin SM. Ultrastructural aspects of the intracellular assembly, transport and exocytosis of chylomicrons by rat intestinal absorptive cells. *In:* Rommel K, Goebell H, eds. Lipid Absorption: Biochemical and Clinical Aspects. Lancaster, England: MTP Press Ltd, 1976:113–50.
44. Glickman RM. Chylomicron formation by the intestine. *In:* Rommel K, Goebell H, eds. Lipid Absorption: Biochemical and Clinical Aspects. Lancaster, England: MTP Press Ltd, 1976, 99–112.
45. Krause BR, Sloop CH, Castle CK, Roheim PS. Mesenteric lymph apolipoproteins in control and ethinyl estradiol-treated rate: A model for studying apolipoproteins of intestinal origin. J Lipid Res 1981; 22:610–9.
46. Staggers JE, Fernando-Warnakulasuriya JP, Wells MA. Studies in fat digestion, absorption and transport in the suckling rat. II. Triacylglycerols: Molecular species, stereospecific analysis and specificity of hydrolysis by lingual lipase. J Lipid Res 1981; 22:675–9.

Chapter 93

Carbohydrate Assimilation

Michael D. Levitt

Carbohydrates are the major dietary source of calories for most population groups in the world. The average American consumes about 1600 calories (400 g) per day of carbohydrate consisting of 55% starch, 35% sucrose, 5% lactose, and 3% fructose.[1] In addition to these readily absorbable carbohydrates, lesser quantities of a variety of poorly absorbed carbohydrates, such as cellulose, are also ingested.

With the exception of small amounts of the monosaccharide fructose, which is contained in fruits and honey, almost all ingested carbohydrate consists of 2 or more monosaccharides linked by glycosidic bonds. Since only the monosaccharide form can be absorbed with any degree of rapidity, digestion to monosaccharides is a prerequisite of normal carbohydrate absorption. The subsequent transport of monosaccharides across the small bowel mucosa then requires specific transport mechanisms. Thus, malabsorption of carbohydrate can result from defects in either digestion or mucosal transport.

The basic physiology and biochemistry of carbohydrate assimilation have been extensively studied and are well understood at the molecular level. In contrast, our ability to assess quantitatively the efficiency of absorption of carbohydrate in man is surprisingly primitive. Consequently, the *in vivo* efficiency of the carbohydrate digestive and absorption mechanisms remains to be defined precisely.

Carbohydrate Structure and Digestion

The structure of each of the major dietary carbohydrates and the enzymes involved in the digestion of these carbohydrates are shown in Figure 93–1.

Starch is a large polymer of glucose containing roughly 1000 to 10,000 glucose molecules per starch molecule. *Amylose,* which makes up about 20% of dietary starch, consists of long, straight chains of glucose molecules linked together in such a way that the first carbon (C-1) of one glucose is bound to the fourth carbon (C-4) of the next glucose in what is known as an α-1,4-glucosidic bond. The other 80% of ingested starch, *amylopectin,* has straight glucose chains connected by branches in a lattice-like pattern (Fig. 93–1). The branching bonds consist of α-1,6-linkages in which the C-6 of the glucose of one chain is linked to the C-1 of the first glucose of the branching chain.

The digestion of starch to its component glucose moieties involves the sequential actions of multiple enzymes. The pancreas and salivary glands secrete *α-amylase,* an endoamylase that can readily attack only internal α-1,4-bonds, i.e., when there are at least 2 glucose molecules on either side of the α-1,4-bond to be hydrolyzed. Hence, this enzyme cleaves amylose to maltose (glucose-glucose) and maltotriose (glucose-glucose-glucose) but liberates negligible free glucose. These 2 oligosaccharides are then hydrolyzed to glucose by either of 2 enzymes that are attached to the brush border, i.e., glucoamylase (formerly called maltase) and sucrase, both of which are effective maltases.[2]

The digestion of amylopectin is complicated by the presence of the α-1,6-branching linkages that are resistant to the action of α-amylase. Thus α-amylase splits amylopectin into smaller branched structures called *limit dextrins,* which contain both α-1,4-, and α-1,6-linkages. The glucose moieties of these limit dextrins are then sequentially removed from the non-reducing end of the limit dextrins by brush border enzymes, as shown in Figure 93–2.[3] The first 2 glucoses of the limit

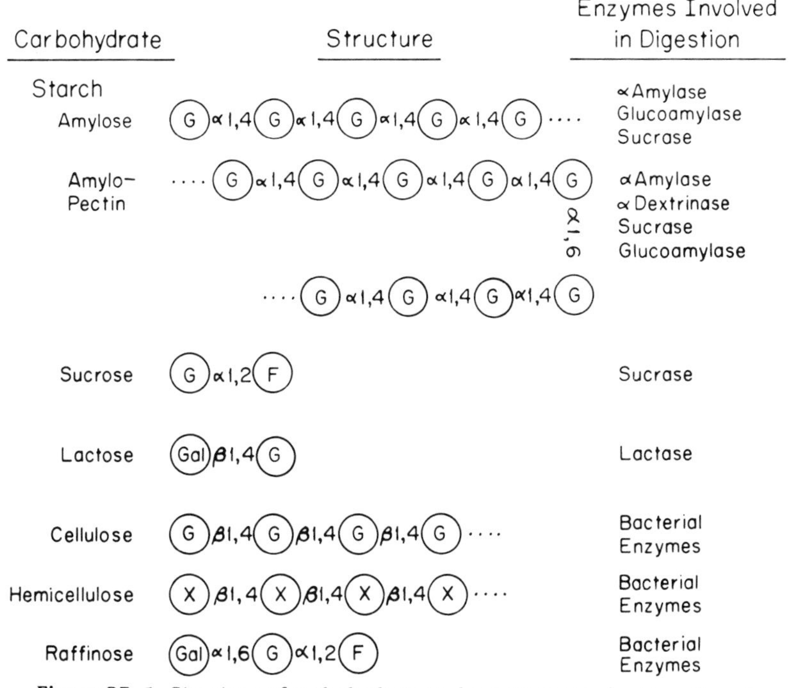

Figure 93–1. Structure of carbohydrate and enzymes required for digestion.

Figure 93–2. Sequence of cleavage of a model α-limit dextrin, 6^3 maltotriosylmaltotriose, by constitutive α-glucosidases of the brush border membrane. O = glucose limits, ∅ = reducing glucose unit; horizontal links denote α → 1,4 linkages and vertical links indicate α-1,6 linkages. The α-dextrin is hydrolyzed by sequential removal of a glucose unit from the non-reducing end of the molecule. With the exception of the removal of the α(1 → 6) linked glucose stub, which requires α-dextrinase, other cleavage steps are catalyzed by action of more than one enzyme. (From Gray GM. *In*: Johnson, LR, ed. Physiology of the Gastrointestinal Tract. New York: Raven Press, Copyright 1981. Reproduced with permission.)

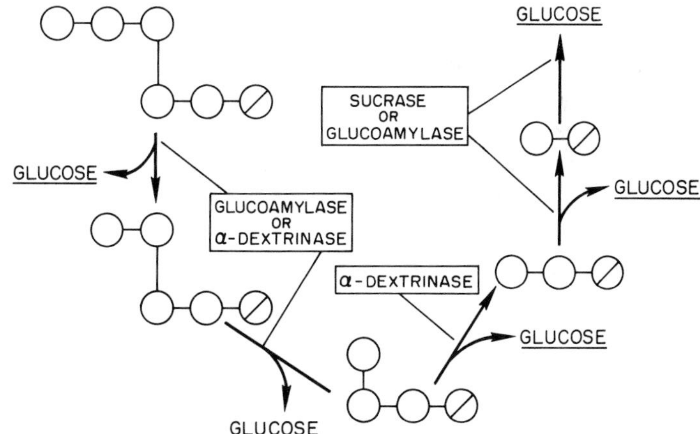

dextrins are removed by the action of either glucoamylase or α-dextrinase (formerly known as isomaltase). Alpha-dextrinase then hydrolyzes the α-1,6-linkage. Lastly, sucrase or glucoamylase hydrolyzes the remaining α-1,4-linkages of maltotriose.

Sucrose, a disaccharide composed of glucose linked to fructose, is hydrolyzed to its component monosaccharides by the brush border enzyme sucrase. *Lactose,* which consists of galactose linked to glucose, is split to its component monosaccharides by the brush border enzyme lactase.

A variety of carbohydrates contain bonds that cannot be cleaved by the pancreatic or brush border enzymes. For example, vegetables (particularly legumes) contain oligosaccharides, such as *raffinose* and *stachyose* (see Fig. 93–1). Since these oligosaccharides cannot be digested in the small bowel, they pass intact into the colon.

Fiber is another form of non-absorbable carbohydrate. By definition, fiber is a polymeric material found in plants that is not digested to a monomer form during passage through the human s' ɔmach and small bowel and hence cannot be absorbed in the small bowel. These polymers may be slowly attacked by bacterial enzyme systems in the colon and thus are not totally resistant to digestion in the gut. *Cellulose* is a glucose polymer in which the glucose molecules are linked by β-1,4-glycosidic bonds. Pancreatic and salivary amylase are stereospecific for α-1,4-linkages and have no activity against the β-1,4-bonds of cellulose. Other forms of fiber include *pectin,* a galacturonic acid polymer, and *lignin,* a non-carbohydrate consisting of polypropanes.

Intestinal Transport of Monosaccharides

The low permeability of the brush border membrane to water-soluble molecules of the size of the monosaccharides glucose, galactose, and fructose requires the intermediation of specific transport mechanisms for the rapid absorption of these compounds.

Glucose and galactose share a common active transport system that allows these sugars to be pumped from lumen to blood against a steep concentration gradient. Thus, the concentration of glucose in luminal contents can be reduced to negligible levels while blood glucose levels remain at 80 mg/dl.

The active transport mechanism for glucose and galactose has been extensively studied in the *in vivo* intestine and in a variety of *in vitro* preparations, including everted gut sacs, intestinal rings, isolated mucosa or epithelial cells, and brush border membranes. *In vitro* studies indicate that no active glucose transport occurs in the absence of luminal Na^+.[4,5] While such dependence on luminal Na^+ is less evident in *in vivo* studies, it seems likely that the low Na^+ concentration measured in bulk luminal contents in these studies does not adequately reflect the Na^+ concentration in the unstirred water layer adjacent to the brush border. *Pari passu* with the enhancement of glucose absorption by Na^+, glucose enhances the absorption of luminal Na^+. This enhancement of Na^+ absorption by glucose has been put to practical use in the treatment of cholera patients with oral solutions containing glucose and electrolytes.[6]

Presently available information on the mechanism of active glucose transport in the epithelial cell can be summarized as follows (Kimmich[7] has published an excellent and thorough review of intestinal absorption of sugar to which the interested reader is referred for detailed discussion of this subject): A carrier mechanism is present in the brush border membrane that binds glucose and Na^+, the affinity for glucose being markedly enhanced by the binding of Na^+ to the carrier. The mobility of this carrier is such that a shift from the luminal surface to the intracellular surface of the brush border is facilitated by attachment of Na^+ and glucose to the carrier. Loss of Na^+ and then glucose from the carrier favors the return of the free binding sites of the carrier back to the luminal surface.

Figure 93–3 schematically illustrates how such a carrier might function. A carrier protein molecule, which is capable of changing its configuration, fills a pore in the brush border membrane. The binding of both Na^+ and glucose to the carrier causes it to change its configuration in such a way that the Na^+ and glucose are now exposed to the interior of the cell. Because the Na^+ concentration of the cell interior is much lower than that of the lumen, the Na^+ tends to dissociate from the carrier. The loss of Na^+ reduces the affinity of the carrier for glucose, which also enters the cell interior. The loss of Na^+ and glucose causes the carrier to return to its

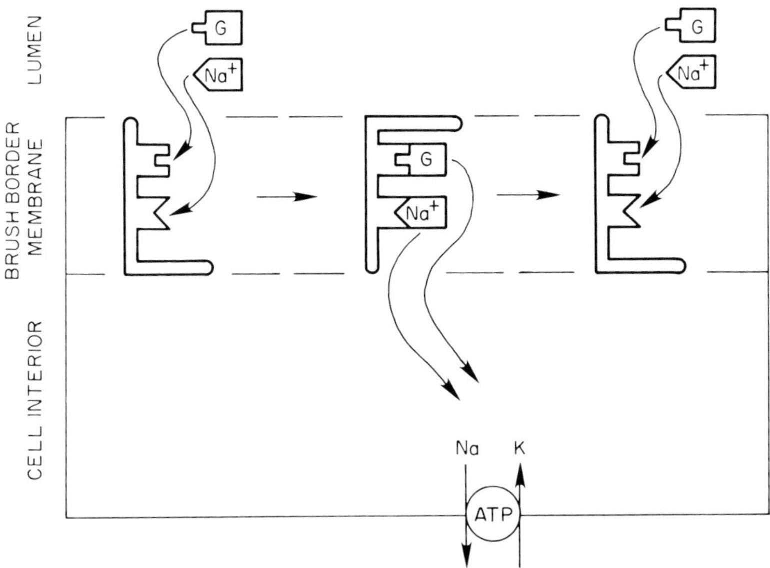

Figure 93–3. Schematic representation of how Na^+ and glucose might interact with carrier to yield active transport.

original configuration in which the binding sites for Na^+ and glucose are once again exposed to luminal contents.

The driving force for uphill glucose transport in this schema is 2-fold. *First,* there is the chemical gradient for Na^+ across the brush border, as the luminal Na^+ concentration is always a good deal higher than the concentration of intracellular Na^+. Intracellular Na^+ is maintained at low levels through the action of sodium-potassium adenosine triphosphatase (Na-K ATPase) pump on the basal surface of the epithelial cell, which continually pumps Na^+ out of the cell against a Na^+ gradient. This basally located Na^+ pump thus indirectly provides the energy for the active transport of glucose at the brush border. The *second* driving force for active glucose transport is provided by the electrical potential of the brush border membrane, the luminal surface of which is positive relative to the intracellular compartment. When Na^+ binds to the carrier, the carrier becomes positively charged, favoring translocation of the carrier-glucose-Na^+ complex to the interior surface of brush border membrane. Evidence that such an electrical gradient is involved in glucose transport is provided by *in vitro* studies in which the intracellular Na^+ concentration was manipulated to levels above that of the luminal solution.[8] If glucose absorption were driven solely by the chemical gradient for Na^+, glucose should be transported on the carrier back into the lumen as Na^+ moved from cell to lumen. Such reverse glucose transport was not observed, indicating that the carrier is influenced by factors other than just the chemical concentration gradient for Na^+. Presumably, the electrical potential of the membrane is this driving factor.

The role for an electrical force as well as a chemical Na^+ gradient in active glucose transport is supported by theoretical calculations indicating that the chemical gradient is insufficient to produce the observed rates of transport of glucose against steep concentration gradients.[9] Indeed, the enormous ability of the epithelial cell to concentrate glucose should theoretically require the binding by the carrier of 2 Na^+ molecules per glucose molecule, a prediction that is supported by actual measurements of the cotransport of these 2 molecules.[10]

While most attention has been directed toward the active glucose transport mechanism of the brush border, the subsequent movement of glucose out of the basal or lateral aspect of the cell also appears to involve a specific transport process. Although this basal-lateral exit pump is much less efficient than the brush border transport mechanism, the high intracellular glucose concentrations generated by the brush border pump allow it to work with sufficient efficiency that exit of glucose from the cell is not the rate-limiting step in absorption.

Fructose is absorbed by a facilitated diffusion mechanism that permits an absorption rate much faster than would otherwise be expected for a water-soluble molecule the size of fructose. While fructose cannot be absorbed against a concentration gradient, the blood levels of fructose are maintained at a very low level, allowing the efficient passive absorption of this sugar. Nevertheless, fructose is absorbed at an appreciably slower rate than is glucose, and hydrolysis of sucrose in the gut results in luminal concentrations of fructose that are appreciably higher than that of glucose.[11]

Carbohydrate Digestion and Absorption in Normal Subjects

The digestion of starch begins in the mouth with the action of salivary amylase. However, such digestion is thought to be minimal because of the rapid inactivation of salivary amylase by the acid pH of the stomach (amylase is inactive below pH 5 and irreversibly denatured at a pH below 3).

Carbohydrates are emptied from the normal stomach at a controlled rate. Although the digestion and absorption of carbohydrates in the small bowel are very efficient, extremely rapid gastric emptying can overload these processes, with resultant malabsorption of both starch and disaccharides.

In the duodenum, starch is rapidly broken down by pancreatic α-amylase to oligosaccharides. The quantity of amylase secreted by the pancreas is said to be many times greater than that necessary to bring about starch digestion[1]; and, normally, this digestion is thought not to be the rate-limiting step in starch absorption. The oligosaccharides resulting from the action of α-amylase, as well as sucrose or lactose, must diffuse through the unstirred water layer adjacent to the mucosa to reach the brush border, where they are digested to monosaccharides by the action of the brush border enzymes. Glucose and galactose are then actively absorbed and fructose is absorbed by facilitated diffusion.

The location of the disaccharidases on the brush border is useful in that the liberated monosaccharides are functionally "trapped" in high concentration in the unstirred layer relative to their concentration in bulk luminal contents. Thus, the absorption rate of monosaccharides is maximized, while luminal osmotic activity is minimized. The relation between the rate of digestion of disaccharides and the subsequent transport of their component monosaccharides is such that digestion is not the rate-limiting step in the assimilation of sucrose or maltose.[11] Nevertheless, only low concentrations of the component monosaccharides build up in bulk luminal contents. In contrast, the hydrolysis of lactose is frequently rate-limiting, even in subjects who possess what is considered to be "normal" lactase levels.[11]

Knowledge of the overall efficiency of the absorption process for carbohydrates in the normal small bowel has been limited by the lack of sensitive techniques for measuring malabsorption of a small fraction of an ingested carbohydrate load. Studies utilizing intubation of the terminal ileum or breath H_2 analysis to measure malabsorption (Chapters 27 and 101) suggest that carbohydrates that were commonly considered to be readily absorbable are not completely absorbed by the normal small bowel. Breath H_2 studies indicated that about 10% to 15% of the carbohydrate of 100 g of bread made from white, all-purpose wheat flour reached the colon of healthy subjects.[12] In contrast, gluten-free wheat flour was completely absorbed, suggesting that the linkage of protein to the starch in natural wheat flour retarded the absorptive process. Corn flour and potato flour were also malabsorbed but less so than wheat flour[13]; rice flour was the only natural flour to be completely absorbed. Terminal ileal aspiration showed that up to 8% of a 12.5-g dose of lactose was not absorbed by subjects with apparently "normal" lactase levels.[14] Lastly, ingestion of large doses of sucrose apparently leads to malabsorption of some of the fructose moiety.[15]

Vegetables contain a variety of indigestible, and therefore non-absorbable, carbohydrates. An appreciable fraction of the carbohydrate of legumes is not absorbed in the small bowel. While it has been assumed that this malabsorbed carbohydrate largely represents indigestible oligosaccharides, such as raffinose and stachyose,[16] the possibility remains that a high concentration of α-amylase inhibitors in legumes inhibits the digestion of otherwise digestible starches. Cellulose, hemicellulose, pectin, and other forms of fiber provide a variable load of non-absorbable carbohydrate, depending on the composition of the diet (roughly 17 g/day of fiber in the average American diet).

The total amount of dietary carbohydrate that reaches the colon has not been directly measured in man. However, the caloric requirement for the metabolism and turnover of the colonic bacteria has led to the theoretical estimate that as much as 70 g of carbohydrate is delivered to the colon bacteria each day.[17] While a small fraction of this carbohydrate may be endogenous in origin (mucous glycoproteins), the great bulk is apparently derived from dietary sources. Since fiber provides only about 17 g of non-absorbable carbohydrate, the remainder of the caloric requirements of the colonic flora presumably is supplied largely by malabsorption of carbohydrates formerly assumed to be completely absorbed.

Disease States Leading to Carbohydrate Malabsorption

Disease states can lead to excessive carbohydrate malabsorption through interference with either the normal digestive and/or the transport processes.

While little or no digestion of carbohydrate occurs in the stomach, this organ plays a role in the normal assimilation of carbohydrate by limiting the rate at which ingested carbohydrates are delivered to the small intestine. A high percentage of partially gastrectomized subjects incompletely absorbed 100 g of glucose, in contrast to the nearly complete absorption of this load by healthy controls.[18] Postgastrectomy subjects with chronic diarrhea also incompletely absorbed smaller doses of carbohydrates (25 g of sucrose or 25 g of starch), whereas their counterparts without diarrhea completely absorbed this load. This malabsorption did not appear to result from abnormal digestive or absorptive function *per se*, but rather from rapid gastric emptying. The latter, in turn, caused very rapid small bowel transit. In some of these subjects, ileal aspiration after large carbohydrate loads showed a small bowel transit time of less than 5 minutes. While the digestive and absorption processes are extremely efficient, a 5-minute exposure time in the small bowel is insufficient for complete carbohydrate assimilation. Such rapid transit with subsequent carbohydrate malabsorption may be readily simulated in normal subjects by rapid infusion of carbohydrates into the duodenum.[18]

It has been claimed that patients with pancreatic insufficiency do not have starch malabsorption because salivary amylase, residual pancreatic amylase, and brush border glucoamylase can bring about complete digestion of the starch.[1] However, studies utilizing breath H_2 as an indicator of carbohydrate malabsorption showed that patients with end-stage alcoholic pancreatitis do not completely absorb rice flour, in contrast to the complete absorption of this flour by controls.[19]

Lactose, sucrose, and small glucose polymers resulting from amylase digestion of starch must diffuse through an unstirred water layer adjacent to the brush border enzyme. While the existence of such a water layer is certain,[20] its thickness *in vivo* has not been adequately measured in either health or disease. It is not clear, therefore, if conditions that might be associated with poor luminal mixing, such as atonic gut or villous atrophy (which would result in decreased villous stirring), could increase this layer and lead to malabsorption. It is known that malabsorption occurs in conditions associated with a dilated, atonic gut, such as scleroderma or partial gut obstruction. However, this malabsorption has been attributed to bacterial overgrowth rather than poor luminal mixing.

Defective hydrolysis of disaccharides due to a deficiency of brush border enzymes is a common cause of carbohydrate malabsorption (Chapter 104). This condition can be secondary to processes producing anatomic injury to the mucosa, such as celiac or tropical sprue and gastroenteritis, or as an isolated primary defect in enzyme synthesis with an otherwise normal-appearing mucosa. In the secondary form, all the disaccharidases are reduced, while in the primary form, only a single enzyme is decreased.

Following digestion to monosaccharides, glucose and galactose require active transport for rapid absorption. A variety of diseases that injure the small bowel mucosa may reduce the efficiency of these transport processes and cause carbohydrate malabsorption. Although not extensively studied, the same disease states that injure the mucosa and lead to secondary disaccharidase deficiency (celiac sprue, tropical sprue, and gastroenteritis) result in defective monosaccharide transport. Thus, malabsorption occurring in these conditions may be due to defects in either digestion and/or transport.

A rare form of *glucose-galactose malabsorption* exists in which there is a congenital defect in the active transport process for these monosaccharides. Fructose absorption is normal, and patients can be maintained in good health by the dietary substitution of fructose and glycerol for glucose and galactose.

A final cause of carbohydrate malabsorption is a short small bowel resulting from the surgical removal of gut secondary to extensive Crohn's disease, mesenteric infarction, or as treatment for morbid obesity (Chapter 108). In this situation, the digestion and absorptive functions of the remaining gut are normal, but transit through the short gut is too rapid to permit the normal assimilation of carbohydrates.

Fate of Carbohydrates in the Colon

Since monosaccharides are not transported across the colonic mucosa, carbohydrates, *per se*, cannot be absorbed from the large bowel. However, these carbohydrates are rapidly fermented by the colonic bacteria, yielding products that can be absorbed by the colon. The rate at which such bacterial reactions occur depends upon the form of the carbohydrate. Soluble carbohydrates (non-fiber) are rapidly attacked by bacteria with conversion to monosaccharides, followed by fermentation reactions. Fiber is more slowly degraded.

The major end-products of these bacterial fermentation reactions in the colon are various volatile fatty acids (formic, acetic, propionic, and butyric), alcohols, and gases (CO_2 and H_2). The colonic mucosa is extremely permeable to alcohols, and organic acids are both rapidly absorbed and metabolized by the colon.[21] The benefit of this bacterial fermentation to the host is 2-fold. *First*, the bulk of the caloric value present in carbohydrate remains in the fermentative products. Thus, the absorption and subsequent oxidation of the organic acids by the host salvage most of the calories of the malabsorbed carbohydrate. Some animals with a very large cecum, such as porcupines, obtain a good share of their caloric intake through the absorption of organic acids produced from bacterial fermentation in the cecum.[22] Studies in jejuno-ileal bypass patients showed that up to 20 g of malabsorbed sucrose could be salvaged by the human colon.[23] It is possible that colonic compensation plays a role in the ability of such patients to maintain above normal weight despite the malabsorption induced by the shortened gut.

A *second* beneficial feature of the colonic salvage of carbohydrates is the resulting reduction in luminal osmoles. Fecal water is roughly isotonic and therefore every 300 mOsm of solvent will yield 1000 ml of fecal water. As little as 10 g of unabsorbed glucose (55 mOsm) in the colon would "hold" almost 200 ml of water and produce diarrhea. Consequently, colonic salvage of unabsorbed carbohydrate prevents the chronic diarrhea that would otherwise ensue from the low levels of carbohydrate that continually escape absorption in the small bowel.

The quantity of carbohydrate that can be salvaged by the human colon is limited; if sufficient carbohydrate is unabsorbed, diarrhea ensues. Illustrative is the observation that when increasing doses of lactulose (a non-absorbable disaccharide) were fed to normal subjects, diarrhea was always associated with the presence of the intact sugar in the feces, but not with an excess of organic acids.[24] This observation suggests that the rate-limiting step in carbohydrate salvage by the colon is bacterial conversion to organic acids rather than the colonic absorption of the organic acids.

The quantity of carbohydrate that may be salvaged in the colon probably varies according to a number of factors, including the type of carbohydrate malabsorbed, the rate at which the carbohydrate is delivered to the colon, the fermentative capacity of the colonic bacteria, and the ability of the colon to absorb bacterial fermentation products. For example, starch, with its low osmotic activity, would cause less fluid to enter the colon than an equal quantity of glucose. This lower fluid volume would provide less of a stimulus for evacuation, and the colon might have a more prolonged period during which to salvage the carbohydrate. Lactose taken with a meal seems to be better tolerated by lactase-deficient subjects than the same dose of lactose taken as a tolerance test (diluted in water). Presumably, the slower gastric emptying of lactose taken with a meal results in the delivery of the lactose to the colon over a longer period than is the case with the tolerance test, in which the lactose is delivered to the colon in a fairly compact bolus. Lastly, there appear to be individual differences in the susceptibility of subjects to diarrhea following ingestion of similar doses of non-absorbable carbohydrates, such as lactulose. This suggests individual differences in colonic bacterial fermentation or the absorptive function of the colon.

When either lactose or an equal mass of glucose plus galactose was ingested by lactase-deficient subjects in a blinded fashion, it was found that there was no appreciable difference in the symptoms (gas, bloating, diarrhea) after an 18-g dose taken with breakfast[25] (Chapter 104). When the dose was increased to 50 g, almost all subjects had symptoms with lactose ingestion. Assuming a 50% absorption of lactose by lactase-deficient subjects,[14] virtually every normal colon can handle about 9 g of lactose ingested with a meal, while a 25-g load exceeds the colonic salvage ability of most subjects.

During the fermentation of carbohydrate to organic acids, gases such as H_2 and CO_2 are liberated by the colonic bacteria. Other bacteria consume these gases and the quantity excreted represents the balance between these 2 processes. In general, the passage of large quantities of rectal gas suggests that excessive carbohydrate is reaching the colon. For instance, the flatulence following the ingestion of baked beans is thought to result from the large quantities of non-absorbable oligosaccharides (raffinose and stachyose) present in legumes.[16]

Fiber is, by definition, an indigestible sugar polymer, and virtually all ingested fiber reaches the colon. *Bran*, the most commonly ingested form of fiber, consists of varying concentrations of cellulose and hemicellulose. The colonic bacteria are capable of slowly degrading fiber, thereby releasing sugars that are then fermented to absorbable products. However, a large fraction of the bran remains intact in the colon and this bran hydrates, producing an increased water content and bulk of feces. In patients with constipation and prolonged colonic transit times, this increased fecal bulk shortens the transit time and yields increased laxation. It also has been claimed that in patients with rapid colonic transit times and diarrhea, fiber may slow transit with an improvement in the diarrhea.

Clinical Diagnosis of Carbohydrate Malabsorption

As just discussed, some carbohydrate routinely escapes absorption in the small bowel of normal subjects and diarrhea is prevented by subsequent colonic salvage. Diarrhea occurs only when carbohydrate malabsorption is in excess of this salvage capacity. Such excess carbohydrate malabsorption should be considered in any patient with diarrhea. The likelihood that the diarrhea is attributable, at least in part, to carbohydrate, is enhanced if large quantities of gas are passed along with the diarrhea. Carbohydrate-induced diarrhea should clear with fasting or elimination of the malabsorbed carbohydrate from the diet. To be stressed in this regard is that diarrhea should be attributed to the malabsorption of a specific carbohydrate only if the patient is consuming appreciable quantities (at least 15 g/day) of that carbohydrate. A particularly common mistake in clinical practice is to attribute diarrhea to lactase deficiency when, in fact, the patient is ingesting little or no lactose.

A variety of clinical tests of differing specificity, sensitivity, and availability are used to verify malabsorption of carbohydrate. These tests are described in Chapters 27 and 104 and are discussed as they apply in Chapters 104 to 108. Because of their pertinence to any consideration of carbohydrate assimilation, they are summarized here as well.

Challenge tests consist of feeding large doses (at least 50 g) of a carbohydrate and determining if diarrhea occurs. The value of such testing is limited by difficulty in controlling all the associated variables. For example, in patients with chronic diarrhea, it is difficult to be certain if a loose bowel movement after the test carbohydrate actually resulted from malabsorption of that carbohydrate.

A degree of objectivity and specificity is added to the challenge test if blood sugar concentrations are measured following ingestion of a test carbohydrate in what is commonly called a *tolerance test*. In these tests large doses (at least 50 g) of a carbohydrate are ingested and blood samples are obtained at 0, 15, 30, 60, and 90 minutes for glucose or reducing sugar measurements. Normal digestion and absorption of the test carbohydrate lead to an increase of at least 20 mg/dl in blood glucose concentration at one of the time periods. Although commonly used in clinical practice to document disaccharide malabsorption, this type of test has several drawbacks: (1) the test requires ingestion of large doses of disaccharides, which may produce severe diarrhea in some patients; (2) the results of the tests are influenced by factors other than carbohydrate digestion and absorption, such as gastric emptying and intermediary glucose metabolism; and (3) tolerance tests reflect the quantity of carbohydrate absorbed rather than the fraction not absorbed. Tests that reflect the quantity of substance absorbed are insensitive to malabsorption of a small fraction of a carbohydrate load. For example, the test cannot detect malabsorption of 10 g of a 100-g load of carbohydrate, since the 90 g absorbed yields a normal rise in blood sugar. However, malabsorption of 10 g of carbohydrate causes diarrhea and gas. The lack at present of quantitative data concerning the malabsorption of carbohydrate stems from the unavailability of a simple test that can quantify malabsorption, analogous to the quantitative fecal fat determination used in the study of fat absorption.

Breath H_2 analysis reflects the quantity of a carbohydrate load that is not absorbed.[26] This test is based on the observations that (1) nearly all H_2 produced in man results from the metabolism of the colonic flora; (2) H_2 production is markedly enhanced when exogenous carbohydrate is delivered to the colonic flora; and (3) a rather constant fraction of the colonic H_2 is absorbed into the blood and excreted in the breath.[27] Thus, an increase in breath H_2 concentration after ingestion of a carbohydrate load signifies malabsorption of the carbohydrate, and the quantity of H_2 excreted is roughly proportional to the quantity of carbohydrate malabsorbed. While a small percentage of patients may not produce H_2 despite apparent carbohydrate malabsorption, H_2 measurements generally have good sensitivity and specificity.[28]

Another simple test that reflects the quantity of carbohydrates not absorbed is measurement of the *pH* or reducing sugar content *of the feces*. Although used in pediatrics, this test has not been employed commonly as an indicator of carbohydrate malabsorption in adults. It is not clear to what extent its lack of use in adults results from ability of the adult colon to maintain a normal pH and eliminate reducing sugars despite appreciable carbohydrate malabsorption.

Research techniques employing intestinal intubation have been used to assess carbohydrate malabsorption quantitatively.[29] Double lumen tube techniques utilize constant perfusion of a length of gut (usually 15 to 30 cm) with a solution containing a test sugar and a non-absorbable marker, such as polyethylene glycol (PEG). Analysis of the infusate and fluid aspirated at the distal end of the segment for carbohydrate and PEG concentration makes it possible to quantitate the carbohydrate absorption in the perfused segment. Data from such perfusion studies have provided much of the existing knowledge concerning the rate of carbohydrate digestion and absorption of gut segments in health and disease. Such studies are too complex, however, to be applied clinically. In addition, such techniques do not measure the ability of the total gut to absorb an ingested carbohydrate load. Rather, they provide a measure of the ability of a gut segment to absorb carbohydrate delivered at a constant rate.

The only available means of quantitating the ability of the entire gut to absorb ingested carbohydrates is by intubation of the terminal ileum. A meal containing carbohydrate and PEG is ingested and the terminal ileum is either simply aspirated or constantly perfused and aspirated by means of a double lumen tube. Analysis of the aspirate allows for direct calculation of the quantity of an ingested carbohydrate that was not absorbed during passage through the small intestine.

References

1. McMichael HB. Disorders of carbohydrate digestion and absorption. Clin Endocrinol Metab 1976; 5:627–49.
2. Gray GM. Carbohydrate absorption and malabsorption. *In*: Johnson LR, ed. Physiology of the Gastrointestinal Tract. New York: Raven Press, 1981: 1063–72.
3. Gray GM, Lally BC, Conklin KA. Action of intestinal sucrase-isomaltase and its free monomers on an α-limit dextrin. J Biol Chem 1979; 254:6038–43.
4. Crane RK. Intestinal absorption of sugars. Physiol Rev 1960; 40:789–825.
5. Goldner AM, Schultz SG, Curran PF. Sodium and sugar fluxes across the mucosal border of rabbit ileum. J Gen Physiol 1969; 53:362–83.
6. Hirschhorn N, Kinzie JL, Schar DB, et al. Decrease in net stool output in cholera during intestinal perfusion with glucose-containing solutions. N Engl J Med 1968; 279:176.
7. Kimmich GA. Intestinal absorption of sugar. *In*: Johnson LR, ed. Physiology of the Gastrointestinal Tract. New York: Raven Press, 1981: 1035–61.
8. Kimmich GA. Sodium-dependent accumulation of sugars by isolated intestinal cells. Evidence for a mechanism not dependent on the Na^+-gradient. *In*: Heinz E, ed. Na^+-Linked Transport of Organic Solutes. Berlin: Springer-Verlag, 1972: 116–29.
9. Schafer JA, Heinz E. The effect of reversal of Na^+ and K^+ electrochemical gradients on the active transport of amino acids in Ehrlich ascites tumor cells. Biochim Biophys Acta 1971; 249:15–33.
10. Kimmich GA, Randles J. Evidence for an intestinal Na^+:

sugar transport coupling stoichiometry of 2.0. Biochim Biophys Acta 1980; 596:439–44.
11. Gray GM, Santiago NA. Disaccharide absorption in normal and diseased human intestine. Gastroenterology 1966; 51:489–98.
12. Anderson IH, Levine AS, Levitt MD. Incomplete absorption of the carbohydrate in all-purpose wheat flour. N Engl J Med 1981; 304:891–2.
13. Levine AS, Levitt MD. Malabsorption of starch moiety of oats, corn and potatoes. Gastroenterology 1981; 80:1209.
14. Bond JH, Levitt MD. Quantitative measurement of lactose absorption. Gastroenterology 1976; 70:1058–62.
15. Ravich WJ, Bayless TM, Thomas M. Fructose: Incomplete intestinal absorption in humans. Gastroenterology 1983; 84:26–9.
16. Steggerda FR. Gastrointestinal gas following food consumption. Ann NY Acad Sci 1968; 150:57–66.
17. Smith CJ, Bryant MP. Introduction to metabolic activities of intestinal bacteria. Am J Clin Nutr 1979; 32:149–57.
18. Bond JH, Levitt MD. Use of pulmonary hydrogen (H_2) measurements to quantitate carbohydrate malabsorption: study of partially gastrectomized patients. J Clin Invest 1972; 51:1219–25.
19. Mackie RD, Levine AS, Levitt MD. Malabsorption of starch in pancreatic insufficiency. Gastroenterology 1981; 80:1220.
20. Dietschy JM, Salee VL, Wilson FA. Unstirred water layers and absorption across the intestinal mucosa. Gastroenterology 1971; 61:932–4.
21. Progress report. Short chain fatty acids in the human colon. Gut 1981; 22:763–79.
22. Johnson JL, McBee RH. The porcupine cecal fermentation. J Nutr 1967; 91:540–6.
23. Bond JH, Currier B, Buchwald H, Levitt MD. Colonic conservation of malabsorbed carbohydrate. Gastroenterology 1980; 78:444-7.
24. Saunders DR, Wiggins HS. Conservation of mannitol, lactulose, and raffinose by the human colon. Am J Physiol 1981; 241:G397–402.
25. Newcomer AD, McGill DB, Thomas PJ, Hofmann AF. Tolerance to lactose among lactase-deficient American Indians. Gastroenterology 1978; 74:44–6.
26. Levitt MD, Donaldson RM. Use of respirator hydrogen (H_2) excretion to detect carbohydrate malabsorption. J Lab Clin Med 1970; 75:937–45.
27. Levitt MD. Production and excretion of hydrogen gas in man. N Engl J Med 1969; 281:122.
28. Newcomer AD, McGill DB, Thomas PJ, Hofmann AF. Prospective comparison of indirect methods for detecting lactose deficiency. N Engl J Med 1975; 293:1232–5.
29. Fordtran JS, Ingelfinger FJ. Absorption of water, electrolytes, and sugars from human gut. *In*: Code CF, ed. Handbook of Physiology: A Critical, Comprehensive Presentation of Physiological Knowledge and Concepts. Section 6. Alimentary Canal. Volume III. Intestinal Absorption. Washington DC: American Physiological Society, 1968: 1457–90.

Chapter 94

Protein Assimilation

Siamak A. Adibi

All animal species require a large-scale supply of amino acids daily to maintain body proteins and in situations of growth and injury to synthesize new ones. Proteins are the carriers of amino acids in nature. A critical function of the gastrointestinal tract is the hydrolysis of these proteins to free amino acids for delivery to the portal circulation. This function is completed in 3 phases. The first phase is accomplished in the gut lumen, the second phase on the brush-border membrane of intestinal mucosa, and the third and final phase within the cytoplasm of intestinal epithelium.

Physiology of Digestion and Absorption

Gut Lumen Phase. Proteins are digested in the gut lumen phase by gastric and pancreatic enzymes. Although gastric secretion contains several different classes of proteolytic enzymes, the major group consists of the pepsins (Chapter 62). Pepsins are secreted as pepsinogens, but in the presence of acid are autocatalytically activated by cleavage of a small peptide from pepsinogen. Proteolysis in the stomach requires an acidic pH below 5. Therefore, gastric enzymes, upon entering the duodenum where the pH is usually above 5, no longer have any proteolytic action. The digestion of protein in the duodenum and elsewhere in the intestine is the function of pancreatic enzymes (Chapter 207). Pancreatic secretion contains several proteolytic enzymes, including *trypsin, chymotrypsin, elastase,* and *carboxypeptidase.* These enzymes, like the pepsins, are secreted in inactive forms. Conversion of trypsinogen to trypsin requires *enterokinase,* which is an enzyme secreted by the intestinal mucosa. Trypsin in turn is responsible for conversion of chymotrypsinogen to chymotrypsin and proelastase to elastase and procarboxypeptidase to carboxypeptidase. The products of action of these enzymes are free amino acids and oligopeptides. Oligopeptides are not hydrolyzed in the gut lumen, inasmuch as they are not suitable substrates for pancreatic proteolytic enzymes.

Protein digestion *in vivo* has been studied by monitoring the concentration of bovine serum albumin in the gut lumen after ingestion by healthy subjects of a nutritionally balanced test meal containing 50 g of this protein.[1, 2] The results showed that complete digestion of bovine serum albumin requires the entire length of the small intestine and a period longer than 4 hours. Although most digestion (approximately 60%) occurs in the proximal small intestine, a significant fraction of ingested protein reaches the ileum. However, very little bovine serum albumin escapes digestion by the time it reaches the terminal ileum, since the total amount of protein passing into the colon without digestion during the 4-hour postprandial period was about 500 mg.

Free amino acids and oligopeptides accumulate in the gut lumen of individuals ingesting the bovine serum albumin test meal. The oligopeptides are mostly dipeptides, tripeptides, and tetrapeptides. Sharp increases occur in the concentrations of amino acids in peptide form, in both the jejunum and the ileum (Fig. 94–1). These increases are more pronounced in the jejunum than in the ileum. In contrast to increases in amino acid concentrations in peptide forms, increases in concentrations of amino acids in free form are quite modest and similar in both the jejunum and the ileum (Fig. 94–1). The fact

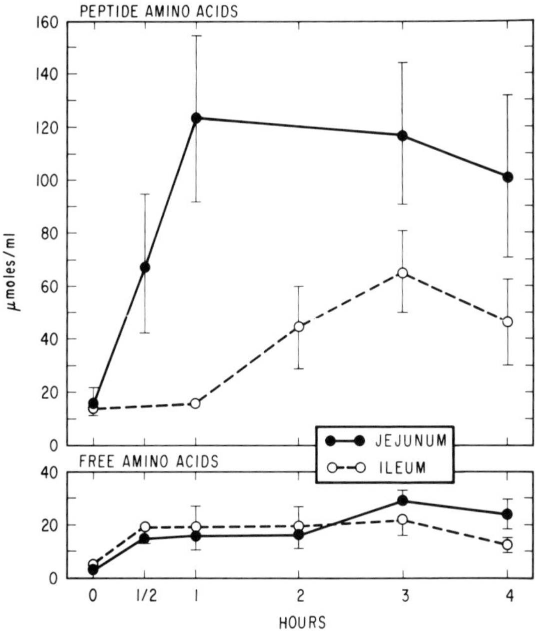

Figure 94–1. Concentrations (mean ± SEM) of peptide amino acids and free amino acids in the intestinal aspirates of 4 normal human volunteers obtained before and after a test meal. The test meal contained 50 g of bovine serum albumin, 120 g of carbohydrate, and 50 g of fat. The concentration of amino acid in peptide form is the difference in the concentration of the same amino acid in the protein-free filtrate of an intestinal aspirate, before and after acid hydrolysis. The following amino acids were included in both peptide and free amino acid fractions: aspartic acid, threonine, serine, asparagine, glutamine, glutamic acid, glycine, alanine, valine, methionine, isoleucine, leucine, tyrosine, proline, phenylalanine, lysine, histidine, and arginine. (Redrawn from Adibi and Mercer.[1])

that protein in the test meal was the source of the observed increases in amino acid and peptide concentrations in the gut lumen was established by failure to find any increase in these concentrations when the same meal was ingested but without the protein.[1]

Brush-Border Membrane Phase. The function of the brush-border membrane of the intestinal epithelium after a protein meal is to clear the mixture of amino acids and oligopeptides, mostly the latter, from the gut lumen. Clearance of these products of protein digestion from the gut lumen takes place through 3 separate mechanisms. The amino acids are taken up by amino acid carrier systems, dipeptides and tripeptides are taken up by the peptide carrier system, and oligopeptides with greater than 3 amino acid residues are hydrolyzed to absorbable products by the peptide hydrolase enzymes.

Amino Acid Carrier Systems. Although several amino acid carrier systems have been described, there is firm evidence for the existence of only 2 such systems. One system is largely responsible for the transport of *neutral amino acids,* such as leucine and methionine, and the other is responsible for transport of *basic amino acids,* such as lysine and arginine (this is further discussed later in considering disorders of amino acid transport). These transport systems have not yet been isolated to a degree sufficient to allow analysis of their chemical composition. Nevertheless, a good deal of information is available about their functional characteristics, including energy and sodium requirements and varied affinities for different amino acids.

Transport of both neutral and basic amino acids is *active,* meaning that by expenditure of energy, transport occurs against a higher concentration gradient within the enterocytes. Under favorable conditions of energy metabolism, when preparations of small intestine are incubated with an amino acid, intracellular concentration usually exceeds extracellular concentration. This phenomenon ordinarily does not occur *in vivo,* since amino acids, upon entry into the absorbing epithelial cells, are transferred to the portal circulation.

In vitro studies have shown that the intestinal transport of amino acids is markedly influenced by the concentration of sodium on the mucosal side of the intestine.[3] However, when amino acid solutions devoid of sodium are perfused into the jejunum of human volunteers, the rate of amino acid absorption is as great as when sodium is added.[4] Despite the absence of sodium in the perfusion solution, the body maintains an intraluminal concentration averaging about 55 mEq/liter. This concentration is much lower than the concentration of sodium (140 to 150 mEq/liter) required for an optimal rate of amino acid transport *in vitro.* The explanation for this difference is not yet entirely clear. It has been suggested that the concentration of sodium in the microenvironment of the brush-border membrane could be much higher than the intraluminal concentration and could account for the absence of the effect of exogenous sodium on amino acid absorption *in vivo.* Another explanation could be that, inasmuch as there is no accumulation of amino acids within the enterocytes *in vivo,* sodium is not needed to provide the driving force for the movement of amino acids across the brush-border membrane.

When the jejunum of healthy human volunteers is perfused with test solutions containing equimolar concentrations of 18 common dietary amino acids, a highly reproducible and consistent pattern of absorption is obtained (Fig. 94–2). Methionine and branched-chain amino acids (leucine, isoleucine, and valine) display the highest rates of absorption, and glutamic acid and aspartic acid show the lowest rates.[5] Several factors appear to account for this pattern: *First,* amino acids with a longer side chain have a higher affinity for the absorption sites and, consequently, have a higher rate of absorption. *Second,* amino acids with either positive charges (e.g., arginine and lysine) or negative charges (e.g., glutamic acid and aspartic acid) in their side chains do not have as strong an affinity as neutral amino acids for the absorption sites. Consequently, they are absorbed more slowly. *Third,* amino acids with high affinities competitively inhibit absorption of amino acids with low affinities.[6] The affinities of individual amino acids for the absorption sites have been assessed by determining the rates of amino acid absorption over a range of concentrations perfused into human intestine.[7] From the Lineweaver-Burk plots of absorption kinetics, the K_m values (concentration that produces one-half of the maximum absorption rate) for individual amino acids have been calculated. The apparent K_m value is regarded as an index of affinity for absorption sites—the lower the K_m value, the higher the affinity. For example, the molecular structure of leucine and valine is identical except for one less methyl group (CH_3^+) in the valine side chain, but the K_m value is twice that of leucine (Fig. 94–3).

Finally, segmental perfusion studies in the intestine of healthy human volunteers have shown that the capacity of amino acid transport is far greater in the jejunum than in the ileum.[7] The functional behavior of the carrier system in both segments, however, appears similar.[7] For example, amino acids with more lipophilic side chains are preferred in both segments.

Peptide Carrier System. For a long time it was widely believed that free amino acid absorption was the only mechanism for assimilation of the amino acid constituents of dietary protein. This notion became untenable in view of a series of studies that showed large-scale absorption of dipeptides and tripeptides in the intestine of man and experimental animals.[8, 9] The uptake of these oligopeptides is accomplished by a common carrier mechanism that is capable of uphill transport. Available evidence indicates the existence of only one peptide carrier system, since neutral, basic, and acidic dipeptides compete for the same system for transport.[10] Apparently, peptide uptake, unlike amino acid uptake, is indifferent to the net charge on the amino acid side chain. Nevertheless, the peptide carrier system is substrate-specific, considering that it does not transport amino acids or peptides with greater than 3 amino acid residues.

There are quantitative and qualitative differences in intestinal absorption of amino acids from solutions of dipeptides and tripeptides, as compared with solutions containing the amino acid residues of these peptides in free form.[11–13] For example, when jejunal ab-

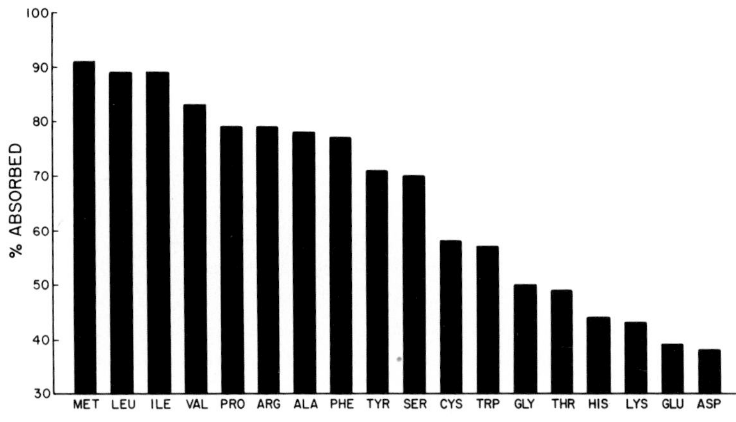

Figure 94–2. Mean absorption of amino acids from test solutions containing 18 common dietary amino acids, each at a concentration of 8 mM, infused into the jejunum of 3 human subjects. (Redrawn from Adibi et al.[5])

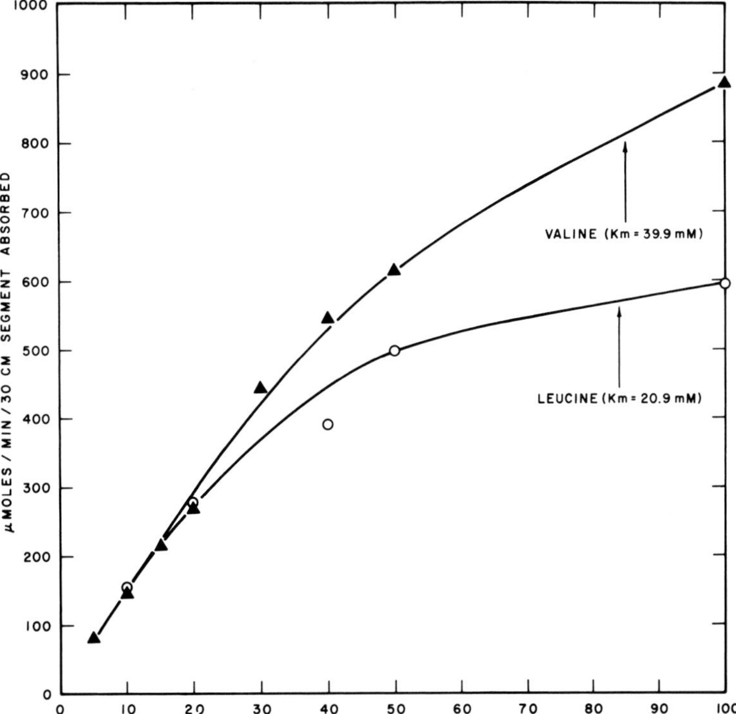

Figure 94–3. Mean absorption rates of leucine and valine from test solutions containing either leucine or valine infused into the jejunum of 5 of 9 human subjects. (Redrawn from Adibi.[7])

sorption rates of glycine and leucine from solutions containing these amino acids (e.g., glycylleucine) are compared with absorption of the same amino acids from solutions containing free glycine and free leucine at equimolar concentrations, 2 important differences are observed (Fig. 94–4). *First,* both glycine and leucine absorption rates are significantly greater from the dipeptide solution than from the corresponding free amino acid solution. *Second,* the difference between absorption of glycine and leucine, which occurs as a result of inhibition of leucine absorption by glycine, is much smaller from the dipeptide than from the corresponding amino acid solution. These differences in absorption can be explained by the fact that the peptide carrier system is more efficient than the carrier system for neutral amino acids.[14] Furthermore, a lack of hydrolysis prior to absorption largely prevents the neutral amino acid carrier system from exerting its preference for leucine over glycine.

Peptide Hydrolases. There is very little peptide hydrolase activity in the gut lumen, whereas the intestinal mucosa is a rich source of these enzymes. Several peptide hydrolases have been isolated from the brush-border membrane of the intestinal mucosa.[10] Among

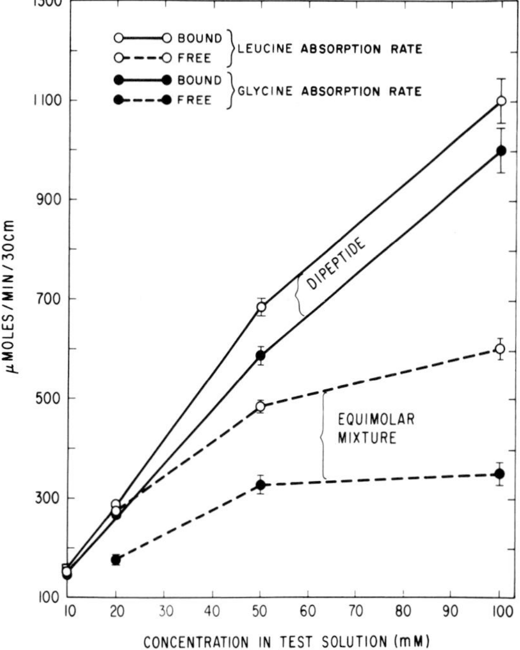

Figure 94–4. The jejunal absorption rates of glycine and leucine (mean ± SEM) from test solutions containing either glycyl-L-leucine or an equimolar mixture of free glycine and free leucine in equivalent amounts. The studies were performed in 5 normal volunteers. (Redrawn from Adibi.[11])

these enzymes, the amino-oligopeptidases appear to be the predominant enzymes. Amino-oligopeptidases sequentially remove an amino acid from the N-terminal end of oligopeptides. Although the substrates for the brush-border peptide hydrolases are peptides with 2 to 8 amino acid residues, the hydrolytic activity against these peptides varies markedly.[10] The activities, expressed as a per cent of total cellular activity, are 5% to 12% for dipeptides, 10% to 60% for tripeptides, 90% for tetrapeptides, and 98% for higher peptides. These data show a remarkable coordination between hydrolytic and transport systems for assimilation of peptides. The hydrolase activity is small against peptides that can be transported intact, but high against peptides that cannot be transported. Therefore, the chief function of the brush-border membrane enzymes appears to be hydrolysis of unabsorbable peptides to absorbable products (tripeptides, dipeptides, and amino acids). Nevertheless, these brush-border enzymes may hydrolyze some dipeptides and, particularly, some tripeptides. As far as dipeptides are concerned, this hydrolysis does not appear critical for their assimilation.[11] On the other hand, the brush-border peptide hydrolases appear to play an important role in intestinal assimilation of certain tripeptides that are poorly water-soluble, such as trileucine.[12]

Studies in human intestine have shown that the capacity for dipeptide absorption and hydrolysis is different in the jejunum and the ileum. While the capacity for dipeptide absorption is greater in the jejunum, the capacity for hydrolysis is greater in the ileum.[11] The physiologic implication of the greater capacity for dipeptide hydrolysis in distal small intestine is not yet clear.

Mucosal Cytoplasmic Phase. Several peptide hydrolases have been isolated from the cytoplasm of absorbing epithelial cells of the small intestine.[10] These enzymes are entirely different from the ones found in the brush-border membrane. The substrates for the cytoplasmic enzymes are peptides with 2 to 4 amino acid residues.[10] The activities expressed as the per cent of the total cellular activity are 80% to 95% for dipeptides, 30% to 60% for tripeptides, trace to 10% for tetrapeptides, and none for higher peptides.

The order of activities of the cytoplasmic enzymes is the reverse of the activities of brush-border peptide hydrolases. Hence, the cytoplasmic enzymes appear very specialized for completing the hydrolysis of absorbed peptides. In fact, because of substantial hydrolase activity against dipeptides and tripeptides, hardly any of the absorbed peptides accumulate in mucosal cells or reach the portal circulation in intact form. Certain peptides, however, may reach the portal vein in intact form.[10] Except for proline-containing peptides, peptides reaching the systemic circulation are efficiently hydrolyzed by extraintestinal tissues in the body.[15]

Amino acids produced as a result of intracellular hydrolysis of dipeptides and tripeptides within the intestinal mucosa, together with amino acids absorbed from the gut lumen, are transported to the portal circulation by means of a special mechanism located in the basolateral membrane.

Protein Malabsorption

Disorders of Digestion. There is a marked reduction in the formation of peptides from dietary protein infused directly into the gut lumen of patients with *pancreatic insufficiency*.[16] This reduction is considerably improved by the ingestion of pancreatic enzymes prior to introduction of protein into the gut lumen. The intraluminal digestion of protein is also reduced in diseases of the small intestine, such as *celiac-disease*[16] (Chapter 103). The mechanism of impairment of protein digestion in the intestine of patients with celiac disease is not entirely clear. It is possible that the intestinal mucosa may play a role in protein digestion, and this role may be reduced by intestinal disease. Indeed, studies in rats have shown that in the absence of luminal pancreatic enzyme activity brought about by pancreatic duct occlusion, 37% of ingested protein is still absorbed.[17] The mechanism responsible for protein digestion in these rats has not been fully investigated, but it does not appear to be due to pancreatic enzymes bound to the mucosal surface.

Selective disorders of protein digestion exist, including *congenital enterokinase deficiency*[18, 19] and *trypsinogen-trypsin deficiency*.[20] In the presence of these congenital deficiencies, protein malnutrition occurs in early childhood. Diagnosis is based on the demonstration of reduced trypsin activity with normal lipase and amylase activities. The distinction between isolated enterokinase and trypsinogen-trypsin deficiencies is made by the presence or absence of a rise in trypsin activity after addition of enterokinase to duodenal fluid.

The disorders of digestion contributing to protein malabsorption are not confined to whole protein. Encompassed as well is mucosal hydrolysis of peptides. In fact, it was once hypothesized that the mechanism of celiac disease was a deficiency of a mucosal peptidase involved in the hydrolysis of gluten.[21] This hypothesis was based on the following observations: (1) Celiac disease is effectively treated by elimination of gluten from the diet, and the disease relapses when gluten is reintroduced; (2) pre-digestion of gluten with an extract of hog intestinal mucosa prevents the toxic effect of gluten in patients with celiac disease; and (3) peptidase activity is reduced in the intestinal mucosa of patients with celiac disease. However, subsequent studies showed that the reduction in peptidase activity returns to near normal when the patient's diet is devoid of any gluten.[21] Therefore, reduction in peptidase activity does not appear to be an etiologic factor in the pathogenesis of this disease, but rather a reflection of the damaged mucosa.

Disorders of Absorption. Diffuse diseases of the intestinal mucosa, such as celiac disease, reduce both amino acid and peptide absorption.[22–24] This does not occur, however, if the damage to the intestinal mucosa is patchy, as in dermatitis herpetiformis.[23] The greater amino acid absorption from solutions containing peptides than free amino acids is even further magnified in the intestine of patients with celiac disease.[22] This appears to be due to a greater sensitivity of the amino acid carrier system to toxic effects. Some patients with celiac disease may actually have increased amino acid absorption in the distal intestine, if this segment escapes the deleterious effect of gluten.[25] The mechanism and nutritional significance of this increased absorption in the distal intestine remain uncertain.

Diseases affecting organs other than the small intestine also alter amino acid absorption in the intestine. For example, patients with pancreatic insufficiency and kidney failure seem to have reduced absorption of neutral amino acids.[26, 27] Peptide absorption in these patients does not appear to be significantly affected.[26, 27]

In addition to the generalized disorders of amino acid absorption, there are certain *selective disorders* of amino acid transport.[28] Among these, the ones that have been most extensively studied are *cystinuria and Hartnup's disease*. When jejunal biopsy specimens of cystinuric patients are incubated with amino acids *in vitro*, the samples are defective in the uptake of basic amino acids, but do actively accumulate the neutral ones. In contrast, the intestinal mucosa of patients with Hartnup's disease is defective in its uptake of neutral amino acids. The reason for the transport of cystine by the basic amino acid carrier system is not well understood, but impaired transport of this cystine may lead to renal damage in cystinuric patients. The transporting epithelial cells of both the intestine and the kidney share the same genetic defects of amino acid transport. In the case of the kidney, however, failure to reabsorb filtered cystine results in cystine precipitation in renal tubules and, consequently, damage to renal parenchyma. In all these patients, intestinal transport of dipeptides appears to be intact. Hence, there is no apparent evidence of protein malnutrition.[29]

A few reports have appeared of defective intestinal transport of individual free amino acids, such as methionine, tryptophan, and proline.[28] However, there is insufficient evidence to establish the existence of several different carrier systems for individual neutral amino acids in human intestine. Thus far, no genetic defect of peptide transport systems has been described; considering the physiologic importance of peptide transport in assimilation of dietary proteins, such a defect is probably incompatible with life.

Effect of Malnutrition on Protein Absorption

The small intestine and pancreas are metabolically active tissues with relatively high rates of protein synthesis. They are very sensitive, therefore, to the effects of malnutrition. Both experimental and clinical observations have shown hypoplasia and hypofunction of these tissues in malnutrition. Starvation and protein deprivation reduce the rate of amino acid absorption in the jejunum of human volunteers.[30] This reduction occurs without any apparent change in intestinal morphology. In patients with *protein-calorie malnutrition*, brought about as a result of jejunoileal bypass for treatment of obesity (Chapter 236), there is a reduction in the amino acid absorption rate in the functioning jejunum.[31] Dipeptide absorption, however, remains normal,[31] suggesting a greater resistance of the peptide carrier systems to the effects of malnutrition.

Therapeutic Implications

Patients who are not able to eat because of loss of appetite or disorders in the upper gastrointestinal tract may need enteral nutrition[32] (Chapter 234). An important consideration in enteral nutrition is the choice of the nitrogen source. The available choices are free amino acid mixtures and protein hydrolysates. Experience with free amino acid mixtures has not been generally favorable. They are hypertonic and may cause diarrhea. Furthermore, enteral nutrition with amino acids as the nitrogen source has shown poor nitrogen retention, since the ingested nitrogen appears to be converted to urea rather than to body proteins.[33] For a number of reasons, dipeptides and tripeptides are superior to free amino acids as substrates for enteral nutrition. They are more efficiently absorbed,[11–14] and their substitution for amino acids in enteral solutions reduces or eliminates the hypertonicity problem. Because of these considerations, many current enteral preparations utilize protein hydrolysates as the nitrogen source.

A protein hydrolysate is a mixture of peptides of unknown size and composition and free amino acids. The size and composition determine whether a peptide is a substrate for the peptide carrier system. For example, oligopeptides with greater than 3 amino acid residues are not transported by the peptide carrier system, and the rate of amino acid absorption from a solution containing these peptides may in fact be considerably smaller than from a corresponding amino acid mixture.[13] Another problem with protein hydrolysates is the possibility of inhibition of the activity of mucosal peptide hydrolases by the amino acids present in protein hydrolysates.[10] These problems could be resolved by using a crystalline mixture of dipeptides or tripeptides containing the appropriate amino acid composition.[34] However, such a mixture is not currently available commercially. In its absence, protein hydrolysates seem to be superior to crystalline amino acids as the nitrogen source for enteral nutrition.

References

1. Adibi SA, Mercer DW. Protein digestion in human intestine as reflected in luminal, mucosal, and plasma amino acid concentrations after meals. J Clin Invest 1973; 52:1586–94.
2. Chung YC, Kim YS, Shadchehr A, Garrido A, MacGregor IL, Sleisenger MH. Protein digestion and absorption in human small intestine. Gastroenterology 1979; 76:1415–21.
3. Rosenberg IH, Coleman AL, Rosenberg LE. The role of sodium ion in the transport of amino acids by the intestine. Biochim Biophys Acta 1965; 102:161–71.
4. Adibi SA. Leucine absorption rate and net movements of sodium and water in human jejunum. J Appl Physiol 1970; 28:753–7.
5. Adibi SA, Gray SJ, Menden E. The kinetics of amino acid absorption and alteration of plasma composition of free amino acids after intestinal perfusion of amino acid mixtures. Am J Clin Nutr 1967; 20:24–33.
6. Adibi SA, Gray SJ. Intestinal absorption of essential amino acids in man. Gastroenterology 1967; 52:837–45.
7. Adibi SA. The influence of molecular structure of neutral amino acids on their absorption kinetics in the jejunum and ileum of human intestine in vivo. Gastroenterology 1969; 56:903–13.
8. Adibi SA. Intestinal phase of protein assimilation in man. Am J Clin Nutr 1976; 29:205–15.
9. Matthews DM, Adibi SA. Peptide absorption. Gastroenterology 1976; 71:151–61.
10. Adibi SA, Kim YS. Peptide absorption and hydrolysis. *In:* Johnson LR, ed. Physiology of the Gastrointestinal Tract. New York: Raven Press, 1981: 1073–95.
11. Adibi SA. Intestinal transport of dipeptides in man: relative importance of hydrolysis and intact absorption. J Clin Invest 1971; 50:2266–75.
12. Adibi SA, Morse EL, Masilamani SS, Amin PM. Evidence for two different modes of tripeptide disappearance in human intestine: Uptake by peptide carrier systems and hydrolysis by peptide hydrolases. J Clin Invest 1975; 56:1355–63.
13. Adibi SA, Morse EL. The number of glycine residues which limits intact absorption of glycine oligopeptides in human jejunum. J Clin Invest 1977; 60:1008–16.
14. Adibi SA, Soleimanpour MR. Functional characterization of dipeptide transport system in human jejunum. J Clin Invest 1974; 53:1368–74.
15. Adibi SA, Morse, EL. Enrichment of glycine pool in plasma and tissues by glycine, di-, tri-, and tetraglycine. Am J Physiol 1982; 243:E413–7.
16. Cerda JJ, Brooks FP, Prockop DJ. Intraduodenal hydrolysis of gelatin as a measure of protein digestion in normal subjects and in patients with malabsorption syndromes. Gastroenterology 1968; 54:358–65.
17. Curtis KJ, Gaines HD, Kim YS. Protein digestion and absorption in rats with pancreatic duct occlusion. Gastroentrology 1978; 74:1271–6.
18. Lebenthal E, Antonowicz I, Shwachman H. Enterokinase and trypsin activities in pancreatic insufficiency and diseases of the small intestine. Gastroenterology 1976; 70:508–12.
19. Ghishan FK, Lee PC, Lebenthal E, Johnson P, Bradley CA, Greene HL. Isolated congenital enterokinase deficiency: recent findings and review of the literature. Gastroenterology 1983; 85:727–31.
20. Townes PL, Bryson MF, Miller G. Further observations on trypsinogen deficiency disease: Report of a second case. J Pediatr 1967; 71:220–4.
21. Adibi SA. Dipeptide absorption and hydrolysis in human small intestine. *In:* Matthews DM, Payne JW, eds. Peptide Transport in Protein Nutrition. New York: Elsevier, 1975: 147–66.
22. Adibi SA, Fogel MR, Agrawal RM. Comparison of free amino acid and dipeptide absorption in the jejunum of sprue patients. Gastroenterology 1974; 67:586–91.
23. Silk DBA, Kumar PJ, Perrett D, Clark ML, Dawson AM. Amino acid and peptide absorption in patients with coeliac disease and dermatitis herpetiformis. Gut 1974; 15:1–8.
24. Nutzenadel W, Fahr K, Lutz P. Absorption of free and peptide-linked glycine and phenylalanine in children with active celiac disease. Pediatr Res 1981; 15:309–12.
25. Schedl HP, Pierce CE, Rider A, Clifton JA, Nokes G. Absorption of L-methionine from the human small intestine. J Clin Invest 1968; 47:417–25.
26. Milla PJ, Kilby A, Rassam UB, Ersser R, Harries JT. Small intestinal absorption of amino acids and a dipeptide in pancreatic insufficiency. Gut 1983; 24:818–24.

27. Sterner G, Lindberg T, Denneberg T. Small intestinal absorption of glycine and glycyl-glycine in patients with chronic renal failure. Acta Med Scand 1983; 213:375–9.
28. Thier SO, Alpers DH. Disorders of intestinal transport of amino acids. Am J Dis Child 1969; 117:13–23.
29. Matthews DM. Intestinal absorption of peptides. Physiol Rev 1975; 55:537–608.
30. Adibi SA, Allen ER. Impaired jejunal absorption rates of essential amino acids induced by either dietary caloric or protein deprivation in man. Gastroenterology 1970; 59:404–13.
31. Fogel MR, Ravitch MM, Adibi SA. Absorptive and digestive function of the jejunum after jejunoileal bypass for treatment of human obesity. Gastroenterology 1976; 71:729–33.
32. Adibi SA. Recent advances in parenteral and enteral nutrition. *In*: Kern F Jr, Blum AL, eds. The Gastroenterology Annual I. New York: Elsevier, 1983: 253–67.
33. Smith JL, Arteaga C, Heymsfield SB. Increased ureagenesis and impaired nitrogen use during infusion of a synthetic amino acid formula. N Engl J Med 1982; 306:1013–8.
34. Steinhardt HJ, Adibi SA. Kinetics and characteristics of absorption of essential and non-essential amino acids from a mixture of twelve dipeptides in human intestine. Gastroenterology 1983; 84:1323.

Chapter 95

Water and Mineral Transport

Martin H. Kalser

Water Transport

Water transport in the normal gastrointestinal tract is highly efficient for conserving and recycling water for the organism. The overall efficiency is 90%; when 2000 ml of water is ingested per day, fecal water is only 200 ml. However, the efficiency is much greater when the endogenous secretion of 7 liters of water is added, to make a total 9000 ml that must be reabsorbed. Efficiency thus approaches 98% (Table 95–1).

Absorption of water is *passive* and secondary to the transport of solute and ions. The rate of net water absorption is dependent upon the membrane characteristics of the specific part of the intestinal tract involved (Chapter 91) (Table 95–2). The jejunum is most permeable to passive transfer of water and ions. It is thus a "leaky" membrane where both simultaneous inward and outward fluxes of water and solute take place rapidly. The latter occur by virtue of the paracellular pathway of rather large aqueous channel pores between mucosal cells and the low potential difference (PD). When a large hypertonic meal is ingested, isotonicity is rapidly reached.

In addition to absorption through the paracellular pathway of aqueous channels, water is absorbed with solute and ions through the transcellular route. There is a maximum rate of water absorption for the small intestine and colon; in the small intestine it is 12 liters/24 hours. When this is exceeded, the excess is delivered to the colon. Water absorption is most efficient in the colon, where 87% of the water entering through the ileocecal valve is absorbed. The maximum load that the colon can absorb, however, is about 5 liters delivered from the ileocecal valve. When this is exceeded, diarrhea results.

Water can be absorbed from the intestinal lumen when the osmolality of the luminal solution is greater than that of plasma. The "double membrane model" explains the passive movement of water from high osmolality of the lumen to isotonicity of plasma. The first membrane is a "tight" membrane separating the aqueous channel from the lumen; the second membrane is the capillary wall membrane, which separates the aqueous

Table 95–1. WATER INGESTION AND ABSORPTION

Intake (ml)	Net Absorption (ml)	Total Absorption (%)
Oral—2000	Jejunum—5500	61
Endogenous—7000	Ileum—2000	23
Salivary—1500	Colon—1300	14
Gastric—2500	*Total*—8800	98
Bile—500		
Pancreas—1500		
Intestinal—1000		

Table 95–2. MEMBRANE CHARACTERISTICS

Site	Type	PD	Resistance	Permeability
Jejunum	"Leaky"	Low	Lower	Permeable
Ileum	Moderate			
Colon	"Tight"	High	High	Impermeable

channel from the plasma. The capillary membrane is a "loose" membrane that is more permeable than the first membrane to ions such as sodium. Sodium is actively absorbed from the hypertonic luminal solution to the aqueous channel. This causes hyperosmolality in the aqueous channel together with the development of a hydrostatic pressure. This increased pressure forces water through the less permeable membrane of the capillary into the plasma, an osmotic "uphill" passive transport of water (Fig. 95–1).

Ion Transport

Membrane Characteristics (Fig. 95–2). There is close correlation between the various membrane characteristics at each level of the intestine and the type of transport that occurs in that area of the gut. Most proximally in the jejunum, the junctions at the intercellular spaces are "loose," the paracellular pathway affording the major pathway of net absorption. Thus *solvent drag*, passive absorption along an osmotic gradient, is greatest in this area. The transepithelial electrical *potential differences* (PD) are very low, as are the electrical differences. Consequently, the jejunum has a very high passive permeability to small ions and water, and large quantities of small solute molecules, ions, and water are absorbed in this region of the gut. Proceeding distally along the gut, the membrane becomes progressively "tighter," allowing less passive flow. The colon has the "tightest" membrane and the highest transmembrane PD. Active rather than passive transport is the dominant mechanism in the ileum and colon.

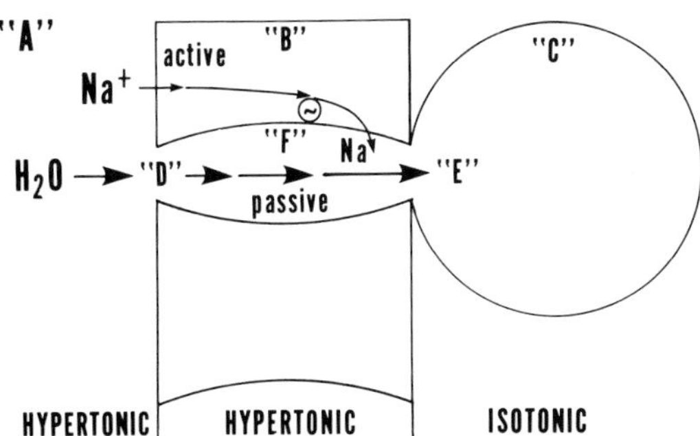

Figure 95–1. Schematic drawing demonstrating (1) "uphill" transport of water from a hypertonic luminal solution ("A"), (2) to an isotonic plasma in the capillary ("C"), (3) through a tight membrane ("D") of the paracellular aqueous channel ("F"), (4) through the more permeable basement membrane of the mucosal cell ("B") and the capillary membrane ("E"), (5) to the plasma in the capillary. The process is dependent upon the active transport of sodium ion from the lumen through the intestinal mucosal cell to the aqueous channel, resulting in channel hyperosmolality and increased hydrostatic pressure. This drives the water "uphill" from the hypertonic luminal solution to the plasma in the capillary.

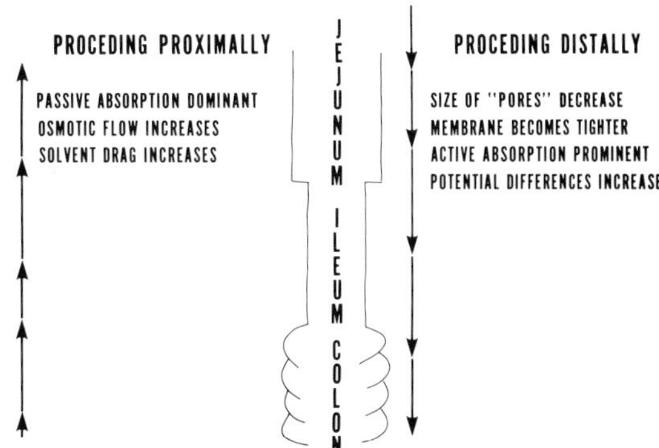

Figure 95–2. Schematic representation of the change in membrane characteristics in various parts of the small bowel and colon.

Sodium Absorption

Absorption of this ion is most efficient. The intestine functions to conserve all ingested and endogenously secreted sodium. In contrast to the 250 to 300 mEq of sodium ingested plus the 250 to 300 mEq secreted into the gut for a total of 500 to 600 mEq/24 hours, only 4 mEq is lost normally in the feces. This represents an efficiency of 98%. The concentration of sodium decreases from 135 mEq/liter in the jejunum to 125 mEq/liter in the ileum to 40 mEq/liter in the distal colon. Several mechanisms of net sodium absorption, passive and active, are involved. The majority of sodium is absorbed in the jejunum, but the greatest efficiency is in the colon, where almost total conservation of sodium is accomplished. Several mechanisms are involved in sodium absorption, varying with the locus in the gut.[1,2]

Glucose can stimulate sodium absorption by 2 mechanisms. With high luminal concentrations of glucose, sodium absorption is passive, secondary to the bulk flow of water. In this process, glucose goes from a high concentration in the lumen to a lower concentration in the capillaries. This is the *solvent drag* mechanism described in Chapter 91. It is a major mechanism in the jejunum, where the paracellular pathways are maximally utilized owing to the larger diameter of the intercellular junctions at the aqueous channels. The net result is to allow passive permeability to small molecules, small ions, and water. Solvent drag is minimal in the ileum and does not occur in the colon.

D-Hexoses as well as amino acids can also stimulate active sodium transport in the jejunum and ileum, but not in the colon. The active absorption of the glucose or amino

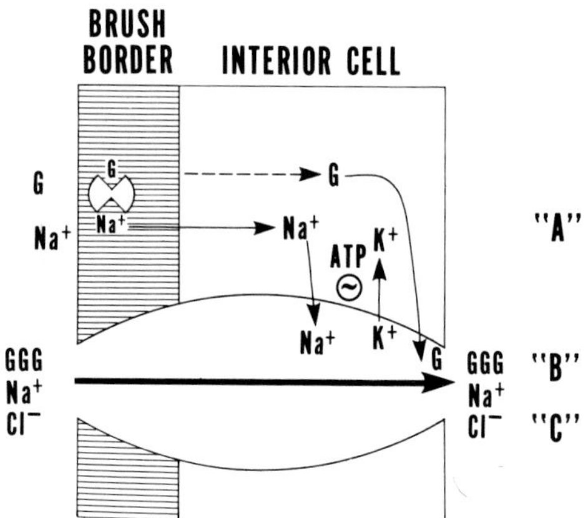

Figure 95–3. Schematic illustration of the effect of glucose on sodium transport. "A" represents the active absorption of glucose (G) and sodium (Na^+) by a common carrier through the brush border. This activates the "sodium pump" to extrude sodium from the cell through the sodium-potassium (K^+) ATPase energy system. Other solutes, such as D-amino acids, can stimulate sodium absorption by this mechanism in the small intestine but not in the colon. "B" represents the passive absorption of *solvent drag* with sodium being transported with bulk water flow as glucose is absorbed passively along a concentration gradient. This is the major route in the jejunum for glucose-stimulated sodium absorption. "C" represents passive chloride absorption.

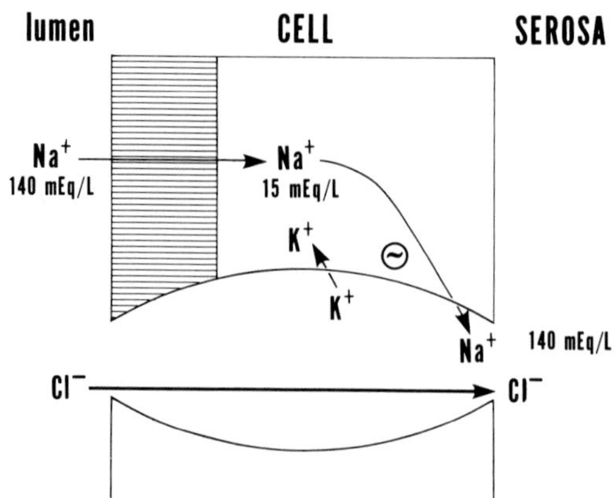

Figure 95–4. Schematic representation of non-coupled electrogenic active transport of sodium in a 2-step manner. The first step, entrance into the cell, is along an electrochemical gradient. The second, or extrusion, is the active step involving the ATPase sodium-potassium pump. Chloride is transported in the paracellular space passively secondary to PD created by sodium transport.

acid involves a common carrier with sodium through the brush border. The increased intercellular concentration of sodium stimulates the sodium pump for extrusion of sodium (Fig. 95–3).

There are 2 other major mechanisms of sodium absorption without coupling to glucose: (1) the electrogenic mechanism, and (2) the coupled sodium-hydrogen and chloride-bicarbonate mechanism. The electrogenic mechanism involves the sodium pump (described earlier) in the extrusion of sodium from the cell. The entrance of sodium into the cell is along an electrochemical gradient, which is not coupled to the active transport of solute as glucose or L-amino acid (Fig. 95–4).

Coupled Anion-Cation Exchange. Active sodium transport by the intestinal mucosa is closely linked to hydrogen transport (Fig. 95–5) coupled with chloride-bicarbonate exchange. The sodium-H^+ exchange is present in both the jejunum and ileum, but the chloride-bicarbonate exchange is predominantly in the ileal mucosa. This theory is compatible with observations in the human gut. Ion transport in the ileum does not generate a potential difference, and this exchange is non-electrogenic, since net ion movement is the result of interaction of H^+ and HCO^-_3. Also, carbonic anhydrase inhibitors retard sodium and chloride absorption in the ileum.

Site of Absorption. Considerable sodium net absorption occurs in the jejunum, primarily as a result of solvent drag. The jejunal

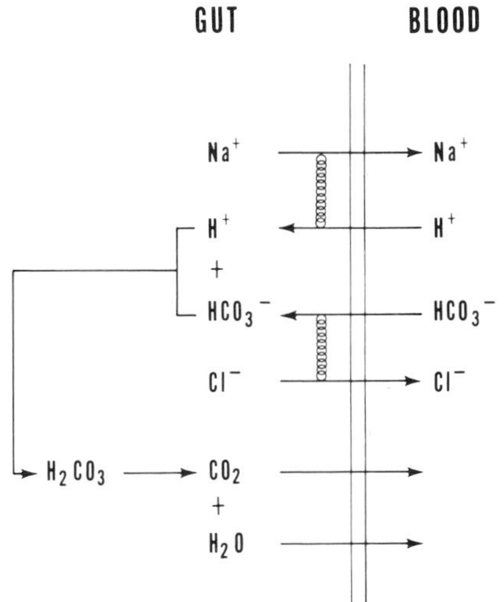

Figure 95–5. This is a schematic representation of the active sodium and chloride transport in the ileum and colon. There is an active double cation exchange carrier system, whereby sodium is absorbed simultaneously linked with hydrogen ion secretion. Normally there is a simultaneous and equal absorption of chloride linked to bicarbonate secretion. When both exchanges are operative at the same rate, hydrogen ion and bicarbonate react with one another in the lumen with formation of carbonic acid, which then breaks down to carbon dioxide and water. The carbon dioxide can diffuse across the ileal mucosa and the water is absorbed.

In chloridorrhea the chloride-bicarbonate exchange is non-functioning, while the sodium and hydrogen exchange is functioning normally. (See text for further explanation.)

mucosa is capable of absorption by other mechanisms, such as glucose- and amino acid–stimulated absorption and electrogenic and sodium-hydrogen exchange.

Sodium transport by ileal mucosa is entirely active and very efficient. The major mechanisms are electrogenic and sodium-hydrogen exchange.

The colon is the most efficient part of the gut for the final conservation of sodium. Of the 100 or so mEq of sodium entering the colon, only 5 mEq is lost in the feces. Thus, over 90% of the sodium entering the colon is absorbed. The efficiency of sodium absorption is evident in that active sodium net absorption persists until the sodium concentration falls to 15 to 25 mEq/liters. This active process is also against an electrical gradient. Glucose or amino acids do not stimulate sodium transport. The mechanisms of sodium absorption in the colon are electrogenic or by the sodium pump (Fig. 95–4) and the sodium-hydrogen coupled exchange (Fig. 95–5).

Aldosterone given 40 to 60 minutes pretreatment facilitates sodium absorption. The action occurs by enhancing sodium entrance into the cell.

Potassium Absorption

Of the 40 to 60 mEq of potassium ingested per day, 9 mEq is excreted in the feces. Potassium is absorbed primarily in the jejunum by passive transport. The concentration of potassium is a function of the PD. Intraluminal potassium concentration varies inversely with the PD across the mucosa. In the jejunum, where the PD is lowest, the concentration of potassium is lowest, while in the colon, which has the highest PD, the concentration of potassium is highest. Concentration in the ileum is intermediate. Thus, passive absorption of potassium occurs when the intraluminal concentration is greater than 6 mEq/liter in the jejunum or 12 mEq/liter in the ileum. In the colon, potassium is excreted by an active secretory process. This potassium excretion is stimulated by exogenous aldosterone or endogenous mineralocorticoid secretion.[3,4]

Anion Absorption

Chloride absorption in the jejunum is primarily passive secondary to the absorption of sodium, regardless of the mechanism of sodium transport. As mentioned, the jejunum is a "leaky" membrane, enabling rapid rates of chloride absorption with sodium (Figs. 95–4 and 95–5). The sodium absorption may be by the active transcellular mechanism or by solvent drag. In either mechanism, the sodium transport generates a PD that, in turn, creates the electrical gradient for chloride paracellular transport.

The ileum and colon absorb chloride by an active mechanism against a considerable concentration gradient. The colon can absorb chloride when the luminal concentration is as low as 25 mEq/liter. The major mechanism of chloride absorption is neutral chloride-bicarbonate exchange, which is believed to be coupled with sodium-hydrogen exchange (Fig. 95–5).[5]

The concentration of chloride in the jejunum is similar to that in plasma. Chloride concentration falls in the ileum (50 to 70 mEq/liter) and is as low as 25 mEq/liter in the colon. Chloride absorption is very complete in the colon. Of the 36 mEq delivered through the ileocecal valve per day, only 2 mEq is normally excreted in the feces.[3,4]

Bicarbonate is actively secreted into the ileum and colon. The concentration of bicarbonate increases from the jejunum to the colon. In the jejunum it is 6 mEq/liter, in the ileum 45 mEq/liter, and in the colon 75 mEq/liter. Bicarbonate concentration normally is greater in the feces than in plasma, accounting for the alkalinity of feces. The mechanism of bicarbonate secretion is the active chloride-bicarbonate exchange (Fig. 95–5).

Congenital Chloridorrhea

This is a syndrome of severe diarrhea occurring in infants and children with metabolic alkalosis, hypochloremia, hyponatremia, and hypokalemia. The diarrhea begins at birth or shortly thereafter and is associated with episodes of fever, vomiting, and dehydration. Laboratory studies show metabolic alkalosis and hypokalemia, as well as low serum sodium and chloride concentrations. This may be a fatal disease in infancy, but the exact mortality is not known. In one report,[6] 2 siblings died in infancy of the same apparent disorder, while another sibling survived. As patients grow older, the ability to adapt apparently increases and the symptoms become less severe.[6]

The pathophysiology involves the impairment of active chloride transport in the ileum and colon. The normal mechanism of active chloride absorption in the colon is an ion exchange of plasma bicarbonate secreted into the intestinal lumen simultaneously in exchange for absorption of chloride. This is coupled to sodium absorption and hydrogen secretion (Fig. 95–5). As noted previously, chloride absorption is very efficient in the ileum and colon and occurs with active transport against a large electrochemical gradient. In chloridorrhea, chloride continues to be absorbed passively along an electrochemical gradient. It was previously believed that there was a reversal of the bicarbonate and chloride exchange with active secretion of chloride from plasma. However, the defect appears not to be a reversal, but rather a non-functioning of the active chloride absorptive system. Sodium absorption is normal, with active transport against an electrochemical gradient. This involves the exchange of hydrogen from plasma. The hydrogen ion secreted into the gut lumen, however, is not completely neutralized by the bicarbonate, since the latter is not fully secreted into the ileum.

The net result of the failure to have active chloride absorption with bicarbonate exchange is acidification of ileal contents and increased chloride concentration (as high as 130 mEq/liter). Fluid accumulates in the ileum and colon. The stool is acid with a high chloride content; also, ammonium concentration is greater than the sum of the concentrations of potassium and sodium. Normally, the potassium concentration in stool is 90 mEq/liter and sodium is 40 mEq/liter, for a total of 130 mEq/liter. Chloride concentration normally is only 15 mEq/liter, but in this syndrome may be as high as 150 mEq/liter. The metabolic alkalosis results from loss of chloride ions. The hyponatremia and hypokalemia follow the excessive loss of fluid as a result of the diarrhea, which is of the osmotic type.

The diagnosis is established by the acid pH of the stool and the laboratory findings of metabolic alkalosis, hypokalemia, hypochloremia, and hyponatremia in an infant or child with severe diarrhea. The most definitive means of establishing the diagnosis is analysis of feces for chloride, potassium, and sodium concentration with demonstration of a markedly increased chloride concentration that exceeds the sum of the concentrations of sodium and potassium. Treatment in the form of a low chloride intake and very large doses of non-chloride potassium supplements has been successful. This decreases the diarrhea and, as the patient grows older, the situation tends to improve.[6]

Calcium Absorption

Calcium absorption involves a sophisticated system of active gut transport within the mucosal cells and synthesis of a carrier protein. The rate of absorption is controlled by a specific hormone, a metabolite of vitamin D, which is elaborated by the kidney.

Absorption is also influenced by parathyroid hormone and glucocorticosteroids. Other factors that affect transport are age, pregnancy, and dietary calcium intake. Malabsorption syndromes, the various types of sprue, biliary cirrhosis, chronic renal failure, and certain drugs are associated with impaired calcium absorption.

Assimilation. An adult subject in a steady state will ingest about 1 g of calcium/day, half of which is from milk or milk products, or 15 mg/kg of body weight. In addition, about 200 to 300 mg (3 to 4 mg/kg) is secreted into the gut from the various digestive juices, with the major fraction being bile (100 mg/day). The endogenous pool mixes with the ingested calcium to form the total pool available for absorption. Of this, 8 mg/kg is absorbed, representing a true absorption of 40% of the total calcium. At low calcium intakes, fecal calcium (representing primarily endogenous calcium) may exceed dietary calcium. Net absorption of dietary calcium increases to a maximum of 30% of ingested calcium on a daily intake of 45 mg/kg.[7] In perfused human intestine, the rate of absorption increases in a linear fashion from concentration gradients of 0.6 to 4.0 mM, indicating that with high concentrations, part of the calcium may be absorbed by diffusion.[6]

Digestion. Digestion of calcium in foodstuffs involves ionization of the bound calcium. Ionization of the calcium compounds, e.g., as calcium caseinate of milk, is probably an essential preliminary step to intestinal transport. Many calcium compounds, such as carbonates and phosphates, are insoluble, and their solution is also essential. Solubilization of precipitates and ionization of bound calcium require an acid pH. In the acid pH of the stomach, calcium is converted to calcium chloride.

Site of Absorption. The preferential site of calcium absorption is the duodenum or proximal jejunum, with the rate in the former being 3 times as rapid as in the latter. This has been demonstrated both by *in vivo* isolated loop perfusion studies and by *in vitro* everted gut sac techniques. Similarly, active transport against a concentration gradient is most operative in the duodenum and upper jejunum; little, if any, active transport occurs in the ileum. An adaptive increase in calcium transport to low calcium intake is most marked in the duodenum and much less so in the ileum.[8] However, following resection of the jejunum or bypassing of the duodenum, calcium transport proceeds normally, and calcium deficiency does not occur unless there is impaired absorption of vitamin D. Thus, calcium absorption can occur in the ileum to maintain calcium homeostasis.

Mucosal Transport. Calcium transport from mucosa to serosa is an active process. *In vitro* gut sac studies demonstrate that calcium transport fulfills the criteria of active transport, being transported against an electrical and a chemical gradient.

There is a bidirectional flux of calcium from lumen to blood and blood to lumen, but the latter movement occurs at a greatly decreased rate compared with the former. The unilateral lumen to serosa flux is 5- to 10-fold greater than the opposite flux from serosa to mucosa. This process is impaired in vitamin D–depleted animals.

Transport from lumen to serosa involves 3 steps. The first, which is the rate-limiting step, is the transport of calcium across the brush border of the cell. In the second step, calcium is transported across the cell by a specific protein, calcium-binding protein (CaBP). The third and final step is the extrusion of calcium from the cell. The compound 1,25-dihydroxy-vitamin D is essential for all 3 steps.[9] In the second step (transport of calcium across the cell), vitamin D controls the synthesis and concentration of the calcium-binding protein. In the third step (extrusion of calcium from the cell), the energy-requiring pump is vitamin D dependent.

Control of Absorption. Absorption of calcium is controlled by vitamin D metabolites and, to a lesser degree, by parathyroid hormone. Active absorption of calcium is severely inhibited in the absence of activated vitamin D. As noted, vitamin D is needed in all 3 steps of calcium transport, including brush border uptake, transport across the mucosal cell, and active extrusion from the cell (Fig. 95–6). Parathyroid hormone to a lesser degree is involved directly in the intestinal mucosal transport of calcium; it also

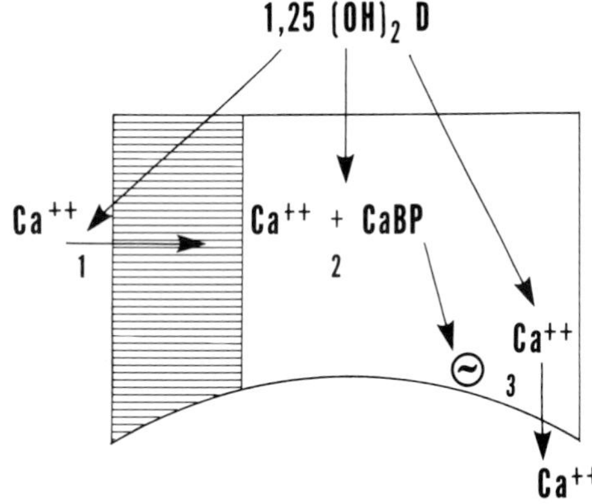

Figure 95–6. Schematic representation of the action of 1,25-dihydroxy-vitamin D (1,25-$(OH)_2D$) on the transport of calcium by the intestinal mucosal cell. It enhances the uptake at the brush border (1) as well as transport across the interior of the cell. The latter is accomplished by enhancing formation of calcium-binding protein (CaBP), which acts as a carrier (2). Vitamin D also augments the energy system for extrusion of the calcium from the cell (3).

indirectly controls calcium absorption by its control of vitamin D hydroxylation in the renal cortex.

Vitamin D Metabolism (Fig. 95–7). Vitamin D exists in 2 forms: vitamin D_2 (ergocalciferol) and vitamin D_3 (cholecalciferol). The former is a synthetic substance that is added to food products and is the major dietary source of vitamin D in the United States. While vitamin D_3 is found in certain foods, such as fish and eggs, it is produced in the skin by ultraviolet light. Both vitamin D_2 and vitamin D_3 are metabolized to the dihydroxy form, and both are commonly referred to as vitamin D.[9]

Both forms of vitamin D are affected by intestinal fat absorption (Chapter 92) inasmuch as ingested vitamin D (D_2 and D_3) is fat soluble and is absorbed with the fat. Both forms undergo an enterohepatic circulation during which they are secreted into the bile and then into the duodenum. Thus, interruption of normal fat assimilation can lead to deficiencies of both ingested and endogenous vitamin D.

Vitamin D is converted to an active calcium-regulating hormone by the kidney after being partially hydroxylated by the liver. Hydroxylation to 25-hydroxy-vitamin D (25-OH-D) (calcifediol) occurs in the hepatic cell microsomes. There is a feedback control of synthesis of this compound that is dependent on its concentration in hepatocytes and not on serum calcium levels. When the liver cell concentration of this form of vitamin D decreases, synthesis is increased. This monohydroxylate vitamin D is further hydroxylated by the renal cortex to an active hormone that regulates intestinal calcium absorption. The monohydroxyl form (25-OH-D) has

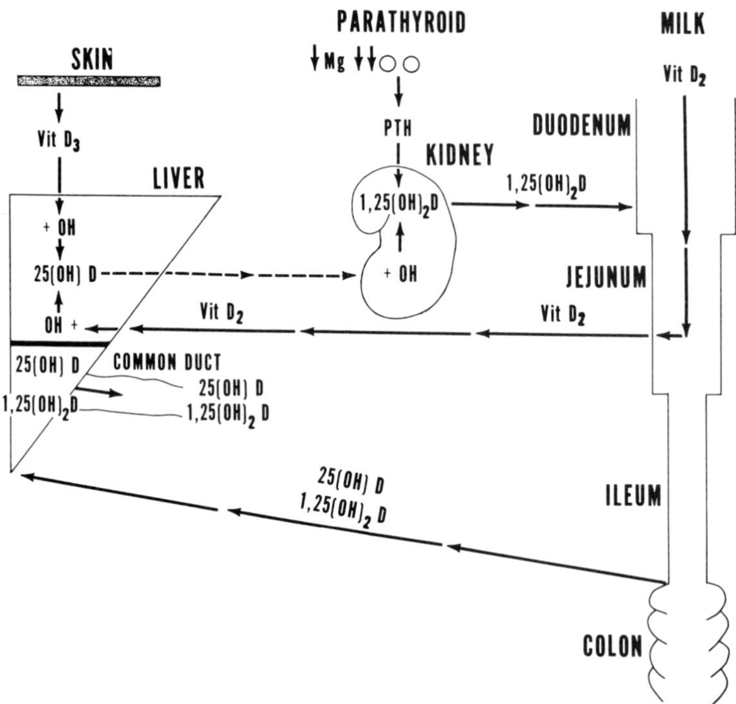

Figure 95–7. Schematic representation of vitamin D metabolism. Endogenous vitamin D_3 is formed by ultraviolet light in the skin, while exogenous vitamin D_2 (added to milk and other foods) is absorbed in the jejunum. Both vitamin D_2 and D_3 are hydroxylated in the liver to 25-monohydroxide vitamin D (25-(OH) D). They then are transported to the kidney where they are hydroxylated to 1,25-dihydroxy vitamin D (1,25-(OH)$_2$D). This is under the influence of parathyroid hormone (PTH). Very depressed levels of serum magnesium will inhibit release of PTH. The 1,25-(OH)$_2$D controls calcium absorption in its 3 steps (Fig. 95–6). The lower part of the figure demonstrates the enterohepatic circulation of 25-(OH) D and 1,25-(OH)$_2$D. Both are secreted with bile into the common bile duct and thence to the duodenum. They are then reabsorbed in the distal ileum and transported back to the liver to begin the cycle again. Interruption of the enterohepatic circulation from cholestasis or severely decreased ileal function can lower serum levels of 1,25-(OH)$_2$D and 25-(OH) D and impair calcium absorption.

about 1% of the physiologic activity of the dihydroxy vitamin D formed in the kidney.

The renal cortical cells hydroxylate the monohydroxyl form to the active form, 1,25-dihydroxy-vitamin D [1,25-$(OH)_2D$]. The renal cortex can also hydroxylate the monohydroxylate to 24,25-dihydroxy-vitamin D [24,25-$(OH)_2D$], a relatively inactive form of vitamin D.[10,11]

Control of Renal Hormone. Synthesis and secretion by the kidneys of the active hormone 1,25-$(OH)_2D$ in effect primarily control calcium absorption and are directly related to serum calcium levels. The level of serum calcium acts through its influence on parathyroid hormone (PTH) secretion. The latter, in turn, influences serum phosphorus levels by means of its control of renal tubular reabsorption of phosphate. A decrease in serum calcium levels below 10 mg/dl stimulates PTH secretion, and this increases the synthesis and release of 1,25-$(OH)_2D$. Intestinal absorption of calcium is thereby increased. High serum levels of calcium decrease PTH release, and this shuts off the synthesis and release of 1,25-$(OH)_2D$.

Thus, control of calcium absorption by the intestine is through a feedback mechanism influenced by serum calcium levels. When these are low, the secretion of the active renal hormone is increased, and when the serum calcium levels are elevated, the secretion of this hormone is depressed. This mechanism is dependent on a normal parathyroid gland, normal renal function, and normal absorption of vitamin D.

Calcium-Binding Protein. The renal hormone directly enhances calcium absorption by augmenting synthesis of the protein carrier for calcium transport (CaBP) in the mucosal cell.[8] The renal hormone associates with a receptor in the chromatin of the nucleolus, which is the DNA-containing portion of the mucosal cell. This activates the biochemical expression of genetic information, with DNA-directed synthesis of messenger RNA followed by translation into the functional protein CaBP. The appearance and relative amount of CaBP in the intestinal mucosal cell closely correlate with the rate of calcium transport. In animals, it is present in the highest concentration in duodenal mucosa, which has the most rapid rate of active calcium transport. The concentration of this protein is increased with vitamin D administration.

Phosphorus. The relative rates of synthesis of the active and inactive forms of renal hormone are influenced by phosphorus. Low serum phosphorus levels increase the secretion of the active form, 1,25-$(OH)_2D$. This effect of phosphorus has been reported to be independent of serum calcium levels. When the concentration of inorganic phosphorus in the renal cortex is less than 4 mg/g of tissue, there is increased synthesis of the active form, and when the concentration of phosphorus in the tissue rises above this level, the synthesis of the active form is turned off. It has been postulated that PTH at least partially exerts its effect through renal phosphate reabsorption.[10] With increased secretion of PTH, renal tubular reabsorption of phosphate is inhibited. This causes a fall in the concentration of inorganic phosphorus in the renal cells, which, in turn, causes the increased synthesis of the active form.[10]

Parathyroid Hormone. The parathyroid gland, through secretion of PTH, plays an important role in calcium absorption. The mechanism involves enhancement of secretion of the active renal hormone 1,25-$(OH)_2D$. Complete ablation of the parathyroid gland results in decreased synthesis of 1,25-$(OH)_2D$ and decreased mucosal transfer of calcium, as demonstrated by the everted gut sac technique. This is reversed by the administration of parathyroid extract. Primary hyperparathyroidism is associated with increased retention of isotopic calcium, which probably reflects an increased rate of absorption.

Glucocorticoid Steroids. A definite antagonism between vitamin D and glucocorticosteroids has been well established, but there are conflicting theories as to the mechanism. The intestinal mucosa of cortisone-treated animals exhibits decreased calcium transport. This effect may be noted in both the uptake of calcium at the mucosal surface and the transfer of calcium to the serosal surface. Two theories have been advanced: (1) cortisone has an independent effect in inhibiting calcium transport by the intestinal mucosa, and (2) cortisone acts by alteration of vitamin D metabolism.[10] It appears more likely that the effect of corticosteroids is on the inhibition of the intestinal calcium transport system.[12]

Adaptation. An increased rate of active transport of calcium occurs experimentally in pregnancy and with a low calcium diet. Both *in vivo* animal balance studies and *in vitro* everted gut sac techniques demonstrate that calcium absorption and transport are greater in animals that have a low calcium diet as opposed to a normal calcium intake.[7] This is associated with an increased concentration of CaBP. As noted previously, low serum calcium levels increase 1,25-dihydroxy-vitamin D synthesis by the kidney, and this, in turn, may increase the rate of synthesis of CaBP.

Similarly, the mucosa of young rats transports calcium at a greater rate than does that of older rats. During the last week of pregnancy, rats also have a more rapid transport rate as compared with non-pregnant controls. While active calcium transport is essentially limited to the duodenum and most proximal small bowel during regular calcium intake, transport in a subject on a low calcium diet, while remaining maximal in the proximal gut, can also be demonstrated throughout the rest of the small bowel.[8]

Calcium Malabsorption

Malabsorption of calcium can occur from many causes, including direct impairment of intestinal mucosal transport of calcium, intestinal intraluminal events, disturbances of vitamin D metabolism, deficiency of PTH, and very severe magnesium deficiency. Several of the factors that have a negative impact on calcium absorption may also affect vitamin D absorption. As an example, diminished concentration of conjugated bile salts in the jejunum will result in impaired micelle formation and steatorrhea (Chapter 92). Vitamin D is fat soluble, and micelle formation is necessary for its assimilation. Therefore, impaired absorption of this vitamin will result from bile salt insufficiency. In addition, the unabsorbed free fatty acids will form insoluble calcium soaps that will be excreted in the feces. Consequently, less calcium ions will be available for absorption.

Vitamin D Malabsorption. Impaired absorption of vitamin D is most severe in advanced cholestasis and celiac sprue and may lead to hypocalcemia. Vitamin D malabsorption also occurs in pancreatic disease, but calcium absorption does not appear to be affected. Absorption was measured by the use of tritium-labeled vitamin D given orally and determination of radioactivity by a 6-day fecal collection. Normal absorption was 62% to 91%. In patients with celiac sprue there was a high correlation between fecal fat and vitamin D malabsorption and hypocalcemia.[13]

Patients with steatorrhea secondary to exocrine pancreatic deficiency have normal serum calcium levels even though vitamin D absorption is impaired.[13] Presumably the normal jejunal mucosa in pancreatic steatorrhea enables the active absorption of calcium to continue.

Serum Vitamin D Levels. The vitamin D serum level, determined by measurement of serum 25-hydroxy-vitamin D (25-OHD), is a sensitive indicator of overt vitamin D deficiency.[9] The normal level is 15 to 28 ng/ml.[14] The serum concentration of the more active form, 1,25-dehydroxy-vitamin D [1,25-$(OH)_2D$], is much lower.

Decreased Serum Vitamin D Levels. Inadequate intake of exogenous vitamin D_2, which is added to milk, as well as lack of adequate exposure to ultraviolet sunlight, may result in lower serum values of vitamin D. Many patients with a lactose deficiency avoid milk, and this may become a contributing factor.

Almost any cause of impaired fat assimilation may result in vitamin D deficiency, including intestinal mucosal disease, pancreatic insufficiency, gastric resection, or conjugated bile salt deficiency. The last occurs with cholestatic liver disease, as well as with ileal disease and resection. Ileal malfunction, in addition, interrupts the enterohepatic circulation of vitamin D, thereby accentuating its malabsorption.

Direct impairment of calcium absorption can occur secondary to duodenal or jejunal mucosal disease and drugs that directly affect calcium transport.

CELIAC DISEASE (Chapter 105). Celiac disease, in which mucosal function is compromised, results in direct impairment of intestinal mucosal transport of calcium. Calcium is lost for absorption by combining with unabsorbed fatty acids in the form of insoluble soaps. Increased oxalate acts in a manner similar to that of free fatty acids to produce unabsorbable, insoluble calcium oxalate salts. Increased ingestion of inorganic phosphates similarly limits calcium absorption.[15]

ANTICONVULSANT MEDICATIONS. These drugs can act by one or both of 2 mechanisms: (1) by direct inhibition of intestinal transport of calcium; this occurs with phenytoin but does not have any effect on vitamin

D metabolism; and (2) by affecting vitamin D metabolism with formation in the liver of polar, inactive compounds other than 25-(OH) D. The effect of these medications on calcium absorption varies with the drug, the dosage, and individual susceptibility.[12]

RENAL INSUFFICIENCY. Chronic renal failure may be associated with osteodystrophy resulting from failure to synthesize the active renal hormone 1,-25-$(OH)_2D$ from the precursor 25-(OH) D, with resulting impaired absorption of calcium and parathyroid hyperplasia. Impaired formation of this hormone by the kidney may occur before the renal mass is greatly reduced as a result of a rise in renal cell inorganic phosphorus. The phosphorus may then shut off hydroxylation of the active compound.[9] Production of 25-(OH) D by the liver and absorption of vitamin D are normal in renal failure. The administration of small amounts of 1,25-$(OH)_2D$ to patients with advanced renal disease resulted in elevation of the serum calcium and phosphorus concentrations, with markedly improved intestinal absorption of calcium and decrease in fecal calcium of up to 72%.[16] Failure to elaborate the active renal hormone impairs intestinal transport of calcium.

CHRONIC CHOLESTASIS (Chapter 148). Cholestasis, as occurs with biliary atresia or hypoplasia in infants and primary biliary cirrhosis in adults, is associated with calcium malabsorption, steatorrhea, and vitamin D deficiency. Serum vitamin D levels are low.[17] Factors contributing to low levels of vitamin D include (1) steatorrhea secondary to lack of an adequate concentration of conjugated bile salts to form micelles, and (2) interruption of the enterohepatic vitamin D circulation. Some patients with these syndromes are given cholestyramine for the pruritus associated with high levels of retained serum bile acids. This substance can bind vitamin D. However, serum 25-(OH) D levels are low, even in patients not receiving cholestyramine.[17] Although these patients have osteomalacia due to vitamin D deficiency, the major bone lesion is osteoporosis.[18] Treatment with 25-(OH) D does not appear to improve the basic bone disease.

CROHN'S DISEASE. When this disorder involves the ileum, it may be associated with calcium and vitamin D malabsorption with osteomalacia.[14] Since the ileum is the intestinal region most affected in Crohn's disease, direct calcium transport in the duodenum and jejunum remains normal. The serum levels of 25-(OH) D are frequently low. Contributing to these depressed serum values is loss of ileal function, which impairs both the reabsorption of conjugated bile salts and their enterohepatic circulation. If the bile salt pool is sufficiently diminished, steatorrhea may result from lack of formation of a micellar phase. Exogenous vitamin D absorption will also be impaired. Since vitamin D and its active metabolites undergo an enterohepatic circulation, there is excess fecal loss when this mechanism is interrupted by ileal dysfunction. Medications that these patients may receive can also have a negative influence on calcium and vitamin D absorption. Glucocorticoid steroids inhibit direct intestinal transport of calcium. Cholestyramine is sometimes given to patients who have a bile salt–induced diarrhea following short ileal resections. While it is effective in controlling the diarrhea, binding of vitamin D by cholestyramine results in excess fecal loss of this vitamin. A lactose-free or milk-free diet is sometimes recommended for these patients because of intestinal lactase deficiency. However, milk is a source of added exogenous vitamin D and lack of milk can accentuate vitamin D deficiency.

FAMILIAL HYPOPHOSPHATEMIA. This is a group of diseases characterized by hypophosphatemia, normal serum calcium levels, and skeletal abnormalities appearing shortly after birth. The disorders are characterized as being "hereditary vitamin D–resistant rickets." The *first type,* an autosomal recessive disease, is a primary disorder of vitamin D metabolism with secondary hyperparathyroidism. The basic genetic defect is an apparent deficient activity of renal hydroxylase with impaired synthesis of 1,25-$(OH)_2D$ from the precursor 25-(OH) D. It is therefore a primary abnormality in intestinal absorption of calcium that occurs shortly after birth and is associated with secondary hyperparathyroidism and consequent hypophosphatemia. The treatment is vitamin D in extremely high doses throughout childhood and adulthood or 1,25-$(OH)_2D$ in physiologic doses of 1 μg/day.[19]

The *second type,* inherited primarily in an X-linked fashion, is simple hypophosphatemia. There is impaired absorption of phosphates by the intestinal mucosa and a primary and selective disorder of calcium-sensitive phosphate transport in the renal tubules that is not dependent on PTH responsiveness. The primary defect may be impairment of transepithelial absorption of phosphate. Treatment is careful use of phosphate salts in combination with large doses of vitamin D to prevent hypocalcemia and raise the serum phosphate levels to the normal range. With increased doses of vitamin D, there is an increase in absorption of calcium and a return to the normal rate of growth in patients of both sexes.

The *third type,* and probably the largest pathogenetic source of hypophosphatemia, is that group of diseases characterized by disorders of renal tubular reabsorption, the so-called *Fanconi syndrome.* Treatment involves phosphate replacement and high doses of vitamin D (up to 100 times normal intake).[19]

Magnesium Absorption

Magnesium absorption is related to intake. In normal man, about 0.4 to 0.5 g is ingested per day. The highest concentrations are found in meat, cheese, and spinach. About one-third of the ingested magnesium is absorbed.[8] Absorption occurs throughout the small bowel. The rate of transport is greatest in the proximal jejunum and progressively decreases distally. The mechanism of transport is passive diffusion throughout. Isolated gut sac techniques using radioactive Mg disclose kinetics compatible with passive diffusion. There is no competition for transport between magnesium and calcium.[20]

Hypomagnesemia

Clinical Syndrome. The major clinical features of hypomagnesemia are intertwined with those of hypocalcemia when both are present. With primary hypomagnesemia, however, the major manifestations are neurologic and consist of irregular muscular twitching, particularly twitching and tetany that are intractable and do not respond to calcium infusion. The major clue is convulsions, which can be severe, repeated, and intractable and are unresponsive to the usual anticonvulsive measures. Mental depression and depressed consciousness are also clinical manifestations.

Etiology. The major gastrointestinal causes of hypomagnesemia are steatorrhea with generalized malabsorption, alcoholism, and primary hypomagnesemia. The last is a specific syndrome described in infants and, in some instances, in adolescents. There is no evidence of generalized malabsorption. Rather, these patients have an apparent primary hypomagnesemia due to an isolated defect of intestinal absorption of magnesium.[21]

Hypomagnesemia may also be a consequence of a generalized malabsorption syndrome occurring with intestinal transport defects of intestinal mucosal disease. These vary from celiac sprue to the short bowel syndrome. Hypomagnesemia is usually a manifestation of the more severe cases. There are also apparent cases of hypomagnesemia resulting from protracted diarrhea, particularly in infants and young children, and hypomagnesemia can be caused by excessive renal loss of magnesium.

Laboratory Data. In primary hypomagnesemia, both serum calcium and serum magnesium concentrations are low, but serum phosphorus concentration and alkaline phosphatase activity may be normal. The serum magnesium level is normally 1.5 to 2.0 mEq/liter; in symptomatic hypomagnesemia, it is usually less than 1.0 mEq/liter. In hypomagnesemia associated with hypocalcemia due to vitamin D deficiency, as occurs in steatorrhea, both the calcium and phosphorus levels are low and the alkaline phosphatase activity is high, the biochemical picture of osteomalacia.

Mechanism of Hypocalcemia. The hypocalcemia found in association with severe hypomagnesemia is the result of deficient secretion of PTH. The reaction of the end-organ bone and kidney to PTH is increased in the presence of mild hypomagnesemia. However, in the presence of severe hypomagnesemia with low serum calcium concentrations, the PTH serum levels fall. When PTH is not released, the serum calcium level falls.[22]

Treatment. The treatment of hypomagnesemia consists of oral or parenteral magnesium. For short-term maintenance, magnesium can be given IM in the form of 2 ml of 50% magnesium sulfate with lidocaine (Xylocaine). Magnesium gluconate tablets (0.5 g) may be administered orally, 2 to 3 before meals 3 times a day. In patients with hypomagnesemia from any cause, serum calcium and magnesium levels should be monitored closely.

Iron Assimilation

Assimilation of iron is unique because the amount assimilated from dietary sources is dependent upon body needs. This stands in contrast to other minerals, with which there is no feedback control of absorption. Transfer of iron from the intestinal lumen to the plasma is increased in the presence of iron deficiency, whereas in iron overload transfer is decreased (Chapter 166). Factors in iron assimilation include the amount and form of dietary iron and mucosal cellular function.

Dietary. The average intake of iron is 10 to 20 mg/24 hours. With a carnivorous diet this is mainly in the form of myoglobin and hemoglobin. About 10% is absorbed in a steady state, while menstruating women absorb a greater amount, and iron-deficient patients absorb several-fold greater amounts. After acute blood loss, increased absorption of iron does not occur until 3 to 4 days later. Ferrous ion is more readily absorbed than the ferric form.

Intraluminal Actions

Elemental Iron. Iron in the ionic state is released from digested food by the action of hydrochloric acid and proteolytic enzymes in the stomach. Ferric ion is reduced to the ferrous state by ascorbic acid in the diet. In the presence of a low pH, the ferrous ion mixes with a mucopolysaccharide of about 200,000 daltons. After the mixing of the ferrous ion with this large molecular ion-binding protein, an iron complex is formed that remains stable as the pH is increased to neutrality. Within the duodenum, the ferrous ion is displaced from this soluble macrocomplex and is bound to smaller molecules (ligands) (molecular weight, 2000 daltons) forming smaller complexes. The binding substances include ascorbic acid and citric acid, as well as hexoses and certain amino acids, particularly cysteine. These smaller soluble complexes are probably formed close to the brush border, where the hexoses and amino acids are released by the action of brush border enzymes.[23]

Ferric iron polymerizes to form large colloidal gel complexes as the iron passes into the small bowel, where the pH is higher than in the stomach. Finally, this form of iron precipitates as ferric hydroxide.

Dietary factors influence ionic iron absorption. Citric and ascorbic acids, sugars, and amino acids facilitate the process, while phytate and phosphates inhibit it. Iron in wine is poorly absorbed. The amount of ionizable iron released from food is materially decreased in gastric atrophy.

Heme Iron. The metal-containing porphyrin, which supplies the major dietary source of iron in a meat-eating population, is split from myoglobin and hemoglobin in the stomach. As the heme passes from the stomach into the duodenum, the products of protein digestion by pancreatic enzymes become important. These small peptides prevent polymerization of heme to large complexes that cannot be absorbed. Heme is apparently absorbed into the cell as such without release of ionic iron until it is within the cell.

Cellular Actions (Fig. 95–8). There are 3 phases to iron transport through the mucosal cell: (1) uptake, (2) transport within the cell, and (3) release from the cell. Both heme and ionic iron are taken up by the cells. This is an active process with the most rapid rate of absorption occurring in the duodenum. Human duodenal mucosal transport studies suggest that *iron uptake is the rate-limiting step* in iron absorption.[24] When the rate of iron uptake is decreased, there is increased absorption of cobalt, nickel, zinc, manganese, and cadmium, suggesting a common carrier for iron and these elements. Iron uptake takes place in 2 phases: a very rapid uptake, 15 to 40 minutes after administration of iron, and a slower, more prolonged phase. Iron is believed to be transferred to specific receptors on the enterocyte.

The transfer within the cell is a separate process, believed to be carrier mediated. Heme is broken down intracellularly to iron and the remainder of the porphyrin molecule. The pathway of iron is then dependent upon whether the control mechanism for iron enhances or blocks iron absorption. When iron is to be absorbed, it is carried to the serosal surface, released, and combined with transferrin to be carried in the plasma. The release of iron from the mucosal cell is a separate step and is not rate limiting. When body iron stores are such that iron is not absorbed in significant quantities, it is shunted to intracellular ferritin, where it remains until the mucosal cell is shed into the lumen (Chapter 166). The iron is then excreted in the feces.

Site of Absorption. The major site of iron

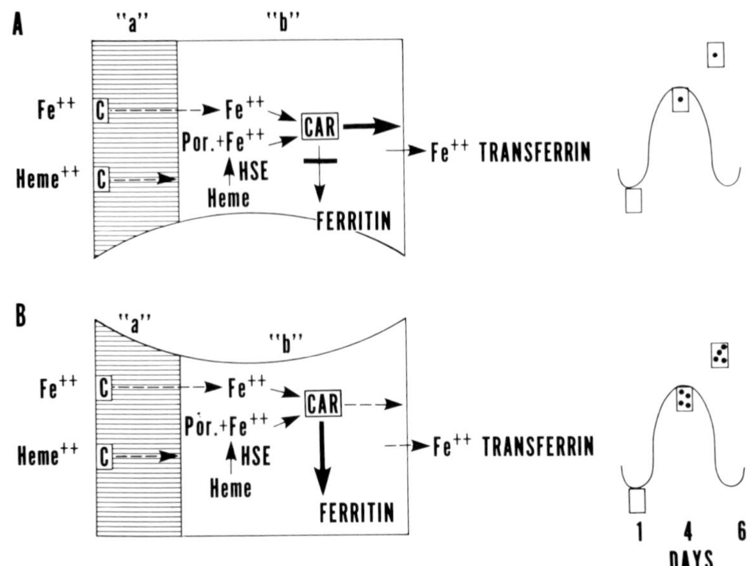

Figure 95–8. Schematic representation of iron absorption. "A" represents absorption after blood loss and iron deficiency states. Both ionic iron and heme iron are carried across the brush border with a carrier "C." The heme iron is broken down by heme-splitting enzymes (HSE) within the cell to non-iron–containing porphyrin and ferrous iron. The major part of the ferrous iron is carried by a carrier (CAR) and extruded from the cell to combine with transferrin in the plasma and then is transported within the blood. There is very little iron that combines with ferritin to remain in the cell (horizontal line to ferritin). The right side of the drawing represents a mucosal cell formed at day 1 at the base of the villus crypt. When this cell reaches the tip of the villus (day 4), it contains very little of the absorbed iron combined with ferritin (single dot). This cell is then sloughed off the villus and the iron and ferritin are lost in the feces.

"B" represents iron absorption when iron reserves are adequate or iron overload is present. Iron absorption is the same as in "A" except that almost all of this iron is bound *intracellularly* to ferritin *(thick arrow)* and very little iron is extruded from the cell to combine with transferrin in the plasma *(thin broken arrow)*. The mucosal cell at the right side contains significant intracellular iron bound to ferritin when it reaches the tip of the villus *(several dark dots)*. The cell containing this absorbed iron is then sloughed off and the absorbed iron, under this circumstance, is lost in the feces.

absorption, both in the ionic form and in heme, is in the duodenum and the most proximal jejunum.[25] Uptake and serosal transfer of ionic and heme iron are greatest in the duodenum and least in the ileum. Another factor is that as the iron proceeds distally in the gut, the physical state of the iron becomes more resistant to uptake by mucosal cells. This is because of the formation of insoluble macromolecules and the absence of sugar and small peptides as binding substances for iron at the brush border. However, because of the prolonged contact with the ileal mucosa, some absorption of iron takes place in this locus.

Control of Absorption. As noted earlier, in iron-deficient states absorption of iron is increased, whereas in iron overload absorption is decreased. The exact controlling factors, however, are not well established. Following acute blood loss, there is a lag of several days before an increase in iron absorption appears.[26] The major factors controlling the amount of iron reaching the plasma are the total body stores of iron and the rate of erythropoiesis. Other factors that have been postulated to influence total iron absorption are mucosal cell iron concentration when the mucosal cell is formed at the base of the crypt, local hypoxia, and plasma transferrin saturation.[27] It is also known that in iron overload ferritin is increased within the mucosal cell. Iron uptake, which is the rate-limiting step in iron absorption, is probably one mechanism of control.[28]

To summarize, iron absorption is an inef-

Table 95–3. ION TRANSPORT

Ion	Locus Absorption	Mechanism	Control	Remarks
		A. Cation		
Sodium	Jejunum	Passive (major) Active (minor)	None	Glucose absorption
	Ileum	Active	None	H^+ exchange
	Colon	Active	Aldosterone	H^+ exchange
Potassium	Jejunum	Passive	None	Luminal conc. >8 mEq/liter
	Colon	Secreted	None	
Iron	Duodenum	Active	Feedback	Body stores
Calcium	Duodenum	Active	Feedback	Serum calcium Vitamin D
Magnesium	Small bowel	Passive	None	
		B. Anion		
Chloride	Jejunum	Passive	None	With Na^+
	Ileum	Active	None	$Cl^- - HCO_3^-$ exchange
Phosphate	Small bowel	Passive Active	?	Vitamin D needed
Bicarbonate	Small bowel	Active	None	Dependent on H^+ secretion

ficient complex process compared with sodium absorption. Only 10% of the ingested iron is absorbed as compared with 99% of sodium. Iron, whether in the ionic state or in heme, must first be released from foodstuffs by an action of acid and pepsin in the stomach. The ferric iron is not absorbed. The ferrous iron combines with a macromolecular mucopolysaccharide secreted by the stomach that renders the ferrous iron reactive. Iron from this macromolecular complex is then released in the duodenum but must combine with small binding substances, such as hexoses and amino acids, before traversing the brush border. Heme, the major source of dietary iron in a carnivorous population, enters the mucosal cell directly as such. Within the cell the iron is liberated from heme by a specific intracellular enzyme system, with the iron entering the cellular space. Part of the intracellular iron is readily transferred by a carrier to the serosal surface and released and combined with transferrin in plasma. Part of the iron may be kept in the cell in the form of ferritin and may be lost when the mucosal cell is shed. A mechanism for control of iron absorption exists in that with iron deficiency states an increased amount of iron is absorbed, whereas in iron overload less iron is absorbed. The mechanism may be shunting of intracellular iron to cell storage as ferritin or a decreased rate of carrier-mediated cellular transfer and serosal release. The major factors controlling the amount of iron reaching the plasma are the total body stores of iron and the rate of erythropoiesis.

Summary

(Table 95–3)

Calcium and iron are absorbed by an active process with a control mechanism for the amount absorbed. The most rapid rate of absorption is in the duodenum. Sodium is absorbed most efficiently from the jejunum to the colon. In the jejunum, the mechanism is primarily passive (solvent drag), but in the ileum and colon it is active in order to conserve sodium so that over 90% of ingested and internally secreted sodium is absorbed. Potassium and magnesium absorption is passive in the jejunum and ileum. Potassium is secreted in the colon. Chloride is absorbed passively in the jejunum and actively in the ileum.

References

1. Fordtran JS. Stimulation of active and passive sodium absorption by sugars in the human jejunum. J Clin Invest 1975; 55:531–9.
2. Fordtran JS, Lochlear TW. Ionic constituents and osmolality of gastric and small intestinal fluids after eating. Am J Dig Dis 1966; 11:503–11.
3. Schultz SG. Ion transport by mammalian large intestine. *In:* Johnson LR, Ed. Physiology of the Gastrointestinal Tract. New York: Rowen Press, 1981: 991–1002.
4. Turnberg LA. Potassium transport in the human small bowel. Gut 1971; 12:811–9.
5. Turnberg LA, Bieberdorf FA, Mordowski SG, et al. Interrelations of chloride, bicarbonate, sodium and hydrogen transport in human ileum. J Clin Invest 1970; 49:557–65.
6. Turnberg LA. Abnormalities in intestinal electrolyte transport in congenital chloroidorrhea. Gut 1971; 12:544–50.
7. Nordin BEC. Measurement and meaning of calcium absorption. Gastroenterology 1968; 54:294–303.
8. Kimberg DV. Effects of vitamin D and steroid hormones on intestinal calcium transport. N Engl J Med 1969; 280:1396–1401.

9. Kaplan MM. Metabolic bone disease associated with gastrointestinal diseases. Viewpoints Dig Dis 1983; 15:9–12.
10. Deluca HF. The kidney as an endocrine organ. Production of 1,25-dihydroxy vitamin D. N Engl J Med 1973; 389:359–63.
11. DeLuca HF. Recent advances in metabolism of vitamin D. Ann Rev Physiol. 1981; 43:199–209.
12. Hahn TJ. Drug induced disorders of vitamin D and mineral metabolism. Clin Endocrine Metab 1980; 9:107–25.
13. Thompson GR, Lewis B, Booth GG. Absorption of vitamin D_3-H^3 in control subjects and patients with malabsorption. J Clin Invest 1966; 45:94–101.
14. Driscoll RH Jr, Meredith SC, Sitrin M, Rosenberg IH. Vitamin D deficiency and bone disease in patients with Crohn's disease. Gastroenterology 1982; 83:1252–8.
15. Alpers DH. Nutrition, vitamins and minerals. American Gastroenterologic Association Unit XIII-B. Timonium, Md: Milner-Fenwick, 1980.
16. Brickman AS, Colburn JW, Norman AW. Action of 1,25-dihydroxy-cholecalciferol, a potent kidney produced metabolite of vitamin D_3 in uremic man. N Engl J Med 1972; 287:891–6.
17. Herlong HF, Recher RR, Maddrey WC. Bone disease in primary biliary cirrhosis: histologic features and response to 25-hydroxy vitamin D. Gastroenterology 1982; 83:103–8.
18. Armand SD. 25-Hydroxy vitamin D_3 treatment of bone disease in primary biliary cirrhosis. Gastroenterology 1982; 83:137–9.
19. Scrivnar CR. Familial hypophosphatemia. The dilemma of treatment. N Engl J Med 1973; 289:531–2.
20. Aldor TM, Moore EQ. Magnesium absorption by everted sacs of rat intestine and colon. Gastroenterology 1970; 59:745–52.
21. Paunier L, Ingeborg CR, Kooh SY. Primary hypomagnesemia with secondary hypocalcemia in an infant. Pediatrics 1968; 41:385–92.
22. Fuh SM, Tasjian AA, Matsuo N. Pathogenesis of hypocalcemia in primary hypomagnesemia. J Clin Invest 1973; 52:153–64.
23. Jacobs A. Iron absorption. *In*: Dawson A, ed. Intestinal Absorption and Its Derangements. J Clin Pathol (London) 1971: 55–9.
24. Wheby MS, Suttle GE, Ford KT III. Intestinal absorption of hemoglobin iron. Gastroenterology 1970; 58:647–54.
25. Cox TM, Peters T. The kinetics of iron uptake in vivo by human duodenal mucosa; Studies in normal subjects. J Physiol 1979; 289:469–78.
26. Powel LW, Halliday JW. Iron absorption and overload. Clin Gastroenterol 1981; 10:707–35.
27. Conrad ME, Weintraub IR, Crosby WH. The role of the intestine in iron kinetics. J Clin Invest 1964; 43:963–72.
28. Powel LW, Halliday JW. Iron metabolism, iron absorption and iron storage disorders. Viewpoints Dig Dis 1982; 14:13–6.

Chapter 96

Absorption of Cobalamin (Vitamin B_{12}), Folate, and Other Water-Soluble Vitamins

Martin H. Kalser

Cobalamin (Vitamin B_{12})

Cobalamin is a specific compound with biologic activity in humans that has been attributed to vitamin B_{12}. Castle was the first to demonstrate that the treatment of pernicious anemia involved both an extrinsic factor, present in liver, and an intrinsic factor, normal gastric juice. The feeding of both of these factors to patients with pernicious anemia induced a remission of the disease.[1, 2] Modern chemical methods have since demonstrated that the extrinsic factor is vitamin B_{12} or, in its pure form, cobalamin, while the intrinsic factor has been shown to be a glycoprotein. Cobalamin is a cobalt-containing compound with a corrin ring. Originally it was believed to contain cyanide and was called cyanocobalamin, but the cyanide was subsequently recognized as an artifact of chemical processing.[2]

Cobalamin is unusual in that it cannot be synthesized by any mammalian tissue; it must be synthesized by bacteria or protozoa and then is absorbed and stored in body tissues. The microorganisms also produce inactive analogs classified as cobanamides. Cobalamin is present in liver and muscles. In humans, animal protein serves as the dietary source of cobalamin, which is ingested combined with protein.

The important factors in cobalamin absorption include the amount of vitamin ingested and the normal gastric secretion of acid, intrinsic factor, and perhaps pepsin. The integrity of the distal ileal mucosa is also an essential factor for cobalamin assimilation. The role of pancreatic and biliary secretions in clinical deficiencies of this vitamin is not established, although they do affect cobalamin assimilation.

In ruminant mammals the bacteria in the gut synthesize vitamin B_{12} for absorption and storage in the various body tissues. Humans can obtain this vitamin only by ingestion of animal products in which the vitamin B_{12} is combined with protein. Liver and kidney are the richest sources, but other meats, milk, fish, and eggs all contain substantial amounts. Grains, fruits, and vegetables do not contain cobalamin, so that vegetarians can eventually develop cobalamin insufficiency.[2, 3] The average western diet includes about 10 to 20 μg/day, which is about 10 times the minimal daily requirement for adults.[2] Between 30% and 60% of the normal dietary intake is absorbed, but when larger doses of 100 μg are given, only 1% may be absorbed.[2]

Cobalamin-Binding Proteins. Three proteins transport cobalamin (Table 96–1). R-protein and intrinsic factor transport cobalamin within the gastrointestinal tract, and transcobalamin carries it to the target organs by way of the blood. R-proteins and intrinsic factor are glycoproteins; transcobalamin II is

Table 96–1. COBALAMIN BINDERS

Carrier	Source	Structure	Specific for IF	Function
Intrinsic factor (IF)	Stomach parietal cells	Glycoprotein	Yes	Combines with cobalamin; necessary for ileal receptor uptake
R-proteins				
Salivary	Salivary glands	Glycoprotein	No	In stomach combines with cobalamin for transport to duodenum
Bile-liver	Liver	Glycoprotein	No	Hepatic storage; enterohepatic circulation
Gastric	Probably salivary glands	Glycoprotein	No	As salivary proteins
Other tissues	Multiple sites	Glycoprotein	No	Storage
Transcobalamin				
I*	Plasma	Glycoprotein	No	Slow release of cobalamin; probably plasma storage
II	Plasma	Polypeptide	Yes	Major form of cobalamin transport to specific tissue receptors; rapid turnover
III*	Granulocytes	Glycoprotein	No	Storage?

*Transcobalamin I and II are actually R-proteins.

a polypeptide. All of these proteins bind cobalamin tightly at a single binding site.[4] Intrinsic factor is the most specific cobalamin-binding protein, binding only colabamin; R-proteins bind a wide variety of cobalamin-like molecules (cobanamides) with the same range of affinity; and transcobalamin is intermediate in specificity, binding a few cobanamides in addition to cobalamin.

Intrinsic Factor. Intrinsic factor (IF) is a glycoprotein with a molecular weight of 44,000 in humans. Its secretion by the human stomach is stimulated by histamine, pentagastrin, and cholinergic drugs and is inhibited by cimetidine. With pentagastrin stimulation, there is a disparity between the secretion of hydrogen ion and that of IF. Intrinsic factor is secreted more rapidly and reaches a peak before acid secretion begins peaking. After peaking, IF output falls to basal levels rapidly. By the time acid secretion is maximal, IF output has fallen to control levels.

The secretory pattern of IF is also distinctively different from that of pepsinogen. Intracellularly, IF is present on the perinuclear envelope, the rough endoplasmic reticulum, the Golgi apparatus, and the tubulovesicular membrane system of the parietal cell.[2] IF is synthesized *de novo* within the parietal cell. It is not known whether the agents that stimulate the secretion of IF also stimulate its synthesis. IF is secreted in amounts greater than are needed to bind the average daily intake of cobalamin; in fact, in 1 hour the human stomach secretes enough IF to bind all the cobalamin present in the daily diet. IF secretion is thus independent of HCl or pepsinogen secretion.[2]

IF binds almost instantaneously with cobalamin, and the binding has extremely high affinity. The site on the IF molecule that binds cobalamin is different from the site that attaches to the mucosal cell of the ileum.[2] An acid pH inhibits the combining of IF with cobalamin, while an alkaline pH facilitates it.[6]

R-Protein Binders. R-binders are an immunologically distinct class of proteins that bind not only cobalamin but also its analogs, non-cobalamin coronoids, which have alterations in the coronoid end or the nucleotide portion of the molecule. Each R-protein molecule has 2 binding sites. The R-proteins are glycoproteins present in many of the body secretions, including serum, bile, saliva, and gastric and pancreatic juices. Gastric R-binder binds 10 to 50 μg of coronoids/day; bile R-binders, 2 to 6 μg/day; and pancreatic R-binders much less. Most of the gastric R-protein is from swallowed saliva. Deficiency of R-protein does not result in any clinical abnormality that can be attributed to impaired assimilation of cobalamin.[2]

Transcobalamin. There are 3 transcobalamin proteins. Transcobalamins I and III are actually R-proteins that are present in the blood. Transcobalamin I, which carries 90% of endogenous cobalamin, represents a storage form of the endogenous (hepatic?) vitamin, which is delivered slowly to the tissues. It is not known whether cobalamin bound to transcobalamin I ever interacts with that bound to transcobalamin II.

Transcobalamin II is synthesized primarily in the liver and to a lesser extent in the kidneys, intestine, and monocytes. There is a very small amount of transcobalamin II in plasma (about 25 μg/liter). Absorbed cobalamin binds rapidly and virtually exclusively to the unsaturated apotranscobalamin II. Turnover is rapid, with a half-life of about 90 minutes. Cobalamin bound to transcobalamin II is rapidly taken up by tissues throughout the body, and the transport protein is degraded to small fragments for excretion, probably by the kidneys.

Uptake of cobalamin by cells takes place in 2 phases. The first is rapid, requires divalent cations, but does not consume energy; cobalamin is presumably taken up by cell surface receptors, which are specific for transcobalamin II. The second phase requires several hours and probably represents transfer of cobalamin from the surface to the interior of the cell.[2, 5] The transcobalamin-II–cobalamin complex is internalized by endocytosis, and the cobalamin is liberated when the transcobalamin is degraded within the lysosomes.[2]

Transcobalamin II is essential for the absorption and distribution of cobalamin. Its congenital absence results in a clinical deficiency particularly evident in the nervous system (see below). Because transcobalamin II is the major transporter of cobalamin to almost all body cells, it is likely that every cell within the body contains receptors for it. These receptors can bind the transcobalamin-II–cobalamin complex as well as transcobalamin II alone, but they cannot bind R-proteins or IF, either free or complexed with cobalamin.

Transcobalamin III is present in granulocytes, and the free form found in serum is probably released from granulocytes after blood is collected; it has a short life of about 5 minutes.[2] Transcobalamin III delivers cobalamin rapidly and exclusively to liver cells. It also binds the analogs of cobalamin, preventing their dissemination in tissues. These analogs are initially of microorganism origin and enter the body during certain infections.[6]

Phases of Absorption. Absorption of cobalamin takes place in a sequential manner. Beginning in the stomach there is release of cobalamin from dietary protein and enzymes. This is followed, again in the stomach, by binding of cobalamin to R-proteins, which are primarily of salivary origin. Within the duodenum there is breakdown and digestion of the R-proteins with release of cobalamin, followed by combining of cobalamin in the alkaline environment of the duodenum with the intrinsic factor secreted by the stomach.

IF–cobalamin complex traverses the jejunum intact and attaches to specific receptors of the ileal mucosal cells. Cobalamin is absorbed by those cells and passes into the portal blood for transport to the liver, where most of it is stored. A small amount enters the bile and undergoes enterohepatic circulation (Fig. 96–1).

Stomach. Within the stomach, 3 events occur: (1) break-up of the cobalamin–protein and cobalamin–enzyme complexes, which are ingested; (2) secretion of IF; and (3) combining of R-proteins from saliva with free cobalamin molecules.

The exact mechanism of the breakdown of the ingested cobalamin complexes is unknown. The acid milieu is apparently of more importance than pepsin secretion.[2] The break-up occurs rapidly and is not a rate-limiting step in cobalamin absorption. The breakdown of the ingested complex is of some importance since, in humans, failure to absorb cobalamin from the ingested protein–cobalamin complex has been demonstrated in association with normal absorption of crystalline cobalamin. The patients described have achlorhydria with increased serum gastrin levels and serum anti-IF antibodies; their stomach secretion does contain IF. No clinical evidence of cobalamin deficiency is associated with this defect, although it has been postulated that such patients will later develop clinical pernicious anemia.[3, 8]

In an acid pH, cobalamin combines almost 100% with R-proteins and virtually not at all with IF.[9] However, if the gastric contents are made alkaline by addition to ingested bicarbonate, IF can compete with R-protein for binding of cobalamin.[6] Gastric R-protein is almost entirely derived from swallowed saliva and represents a salivary secretion.[4] Absence of R-protein does not lead to clinical cobalamin malabsorption or deficiency.

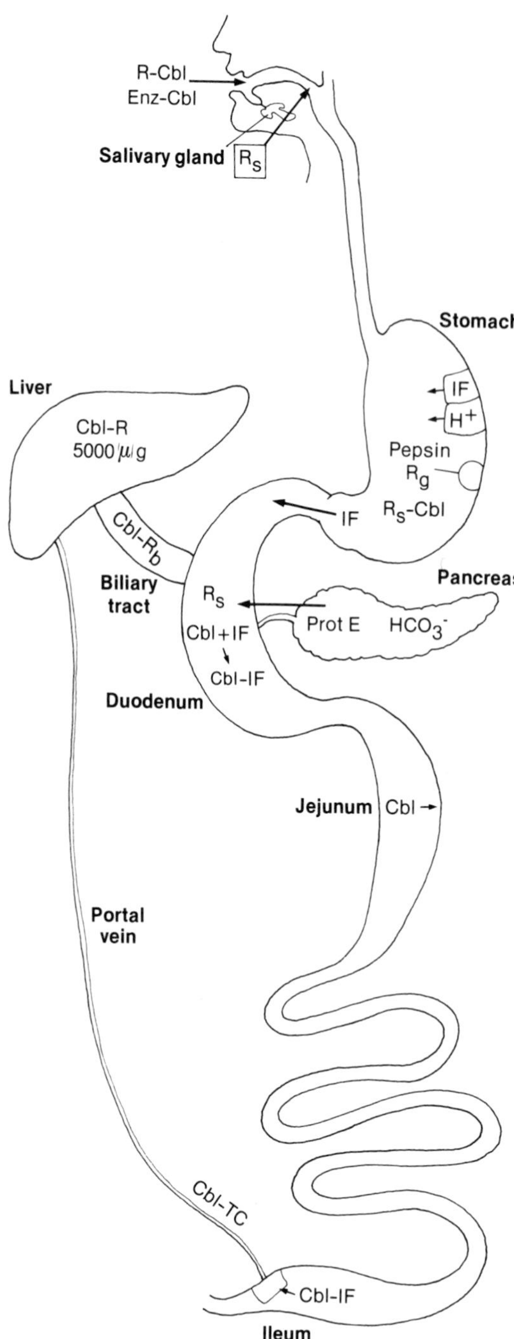

Figure 96–1. Absorption of cobalamin. R-Cbl = R-protein–cobalamin compound; Enz-Cbl = enzyme–cobalamin complex; R_s = R-binder protein (salivary gland); IF = intrinsic factor; H^+ = HCl; R_g = R-protein from stomach; Prot E = proteolytic enzyme; HCO_3^- = bicarbonate; Cbl-IF = cobalamin–intrinsic factor complex; Cbl = cobalamin; Cbl-TC = cobalamin–transcobalamin complex; Cbl-R_b = cobalamin-bile–R-protein complex. (See text for explanation.)

Thus, in the normal state the products leaving the stomach are (1) a complex of R-protein with ingested cobalamin and (2) secreted free IF.

Pancreas. Pancreatic secretions of bicarbonate and proteolytic enzymes also play a role in the assimilation of cobalamin. Although this role is not clearly established, certain facts are known. Absorption of crystalline cobalamin is impaired in patients with pancreatic insufficiency,[10, 11] yet the demonstration of a macrocytic anemia in such patients is rare. There are isolated reports[12] of megaloblastic anemia in these patients, but many patients with pancreatic insufficiency are chronic alcoholics; folate levels have not been noted in these reports. There is no correlation between cobalamin malabsorption and trypsin or chymotrypsin concentration in duodenal aspirates of patients with pancreatic insufficiency and cobalamin malabsorption.[4] A new specific pancreatic proteolytic enzyme has been reported to be necessary for cobalamin absorption, but this finding has not been confirmed.[13]

Trypsin and cobanamide inhibit the ability of R-proteins to compete with IF for cobalamin,[14] a finding that has been interpreted as indicating that trypsin degrades R-protein, making the cobalamin available for IF complex formation.

Transfer of cobalamin from R-protein to IF depends upon pH. At pH 2, cobalamin binds to R-protein 50 times more readily than to IF, but at pH 8, in the presence of trypsin, cobalamin binds to IF 150 times more readily than to R-protein. Thus, the transfer of cobalamin from R-protein to IF is rapid when pH changes.[6] Cobalamin–IF affinity in the absence of trypsin is also pH-dependent, being 3 times greater at pH 8 than at pH 2.[4] Bicarbonate has been shown to reverse the cobalamin malabsorption seen in patients with pancreatic insufficiency.[10]

Liver and Bile. The liver is the respository of a large reserve of cobalamin: 5 mg on average, or 1000 to 2000 times the normal daily dietary intake. These large hepatic stores account for the delay of several years in the clinical appearance of deficiency after cobalamin malabsorption begins, such as following ileal resection (Chapter 108).

Enterohepatic circulation of cobalamin occurs in the same way as circulation of bile salts (Chapter 97). Cobalamin (Cbl) is secreted from the liver combined with bile R-protein. In the normal state the Cbl-bile–R-protein complex is degraded in the duodenum, where the cobalamin combines with IF. The Cbl–IF complex that includes the cobalamin derived from bile is then recycled in the same manner as ingested cobalamin, being actively absorbed in the ileum and transported by way of the portal vein to the liver. A small fraction of the cobalamin in bile is not absorbed in the ileum and is lost in the feces. Approximately 2 to 9 μg of cobalamin is secreted into the bile per day.[4] Bile R-protein is extremely sensitive to degradation by pancreatic proteolytic enzymes, even with enzyme concentrations that are in the range seen with pancreatic insufficiency.[4]

Bile acids may also directly influence cobalamin absorption. Malabsorption of cobalamin was noted in some patients with common bile duct T-tube drainage; the malabsorption reversed when the T-tube was removed.[4] It has been postulated that bile acids play a role in facilitating uptake at the ileal receptors by dissociating the Cbl–IF complex within the ileal mucosal cell brush border.[4]

Duodenum. Events with the duodenum are the sum of the actions of the pancreatic enzymes, bicarbonate secretion, and the Cbl–protein complex in the bile. The Cbl–R-protein complex entering from the stomach dissociates because of degradation of the protein binder by pancreatic enzymes, releasing cobalamin to combine with IF; this association is enhanced by the alkaline pH of the duodenum resulting from bicarbonate secretion. The Cbl-IF complex is a dimer, with the IF molecule shrinking slightly as it combines with the nucleotide portion of the vitamin. The complex is somewhat protected from digestion by proteolytic enzymes.[1]

Small Intestine. Both active and passive absorption of cobalamin occur within the small intestine. Active absorption is by far the more important; passive absorption occurs only with pharmacologic doses given orally.

Active absorption takes place in the distal third of the ileum, where specific receptors are located. In humans the overall capacity to absorb cobalamin is limited, only 1 to 2 μg being absorbed from any given dose, even when there is excess IF.[2] The number of receptors for the Cbl–IF complex on the surface of an ileal mucosal cell is small compared with other receptors; there are probably no more than 300 to 400/cell, or 1/microvillus.[2] The limited number of receptors most probably accounts for the limited absorptive capacity of the ileum for cobalamin. The receptors are distributed in a patchy fashion that varies considerably from individual to individual. In general, resection of 100 cm or less of the ileum does not result in vitamin B_{12} malabsorption. The ileal receptors are most likely specific for the IF part of the Cbl–IF complex, so that the IF molecule is interposed between the receptor and the cobalamin molecule. The receptor sites are highly specific: purified receptor shows specific binding in humans to the CBl–IF complex but not to free cobalamin, free IF, or Cbl–R-protein complexes.[15]

The ileal receptor has been isolated and is an integral protein of about 200,000 molecular weight with 83% of its protein mass facing outside the lipid bilayer of the microvillus. It is thus similar to other receptors in the small bowel.[16] Attachment of the complex is rapid and does not require energy but does require the presence of calcium ions and a pH greater than 5.6.[2] It is believed that calcium forms specific "bridges," which maintain the appropriate configuration of the ileal receptors. The bridges may actually link the Cbl–IF complex to the receptor.

What happens after the Cbl–IF complex attaches to the ileal receptor until cobalamin appears in the portal blood is not clear. It is known that this is a relatively slow process (several hours) and one that is believed to require energy. Cobalamin appears at the serosal surface of the cell in a free form, not combined with IF. The unknown factor responsible for the separation of IF from cobalamin within the ileal cell has been termed "releasing factor." Whether transcobalamin II plays a role in the transport of cobalamin within the ileal cell or in its release from the cell is also not known. Following its release from the mucosal cell, cobalamin combines with transcobalamin II in the portal vein plasma and then combines with R-proteins to be stored in the liver. Part of it undergoes enterohepatic circulation, as previously described.

Passive absorption of cobalamin takes place throughout the small intestine. Only about 1% of cobalamin not bound to IF is absorbed passively. The passive absorption process is thus inefficient, but it reaches a rapid peak. The mechanism becomes apparent only with pharmacologic doses of cobalamin, which must be taken daily to maintain the process. Passive absorption is inefficient because cobalamin is a large molecule with a radius that far exceeds that of the aqueous pores of the jejunum (Chapter 91). Moreover, cobalamin contains hydrophilic groups, making it highly soluble in water and virtually insoluble in the lipid layer of biologic membranes. Thus, passive absorption of cobalamin does not play a significant role in normal or abnormal cobalamin absorptive states.[2]

Tissue Use of Cobalamin. Cobalamin is essential to the formation of 2 important coenzymes, methylcobalamin and adenosylcobalamin. Conversion of methylmalonate to succinate requires adenosylcobalamin, and formation of methionine from homocysteine requires methylcobalamin. Patients who are deficient in cobalamin or who suffer from a disorder of cobalamin metabolism demonstrate methylmalonate and homocysteine in the urine. Thus, the vitamin is crucial for tissue viability.[2]

Malabsorption. Cobalamin malabsorption can be caused by inborn defects of assimilation or by acquired diseases or surgical procedures.

Adult pernicious anemia is the classic clinical syndrome of cobalamin malabsorption. Progressive gastritis with atrophy of the glandular structure leads to a loss of parietal cells. When IF secretion is less than 1% of normal, cobalamin assimilation becomes impaired. The disease chiefly affects persons beyond middle age, although there is a juvenile form occurring in the second decade of life. It is inherited as an autosomal dominant trait and apparently requires an environmental factor for its expression.[1]

Juvenile pernicious anemia probably represents an early onset of the adult form of the disorder. The age of onset is between 10 and 18 years. There is lack of IF secretion from the gastric mucosa, histamine-fast achlorhydria, and gastric mucosal atrophy. Antibodies to gastric parietal cells and IF are detected in the serum. There often is associated hypofunction of endocrine glands, including hypoparathyroidism, hypothyroidism, and adrenocortical hormone insufficiency. Diagnosis is established by demonstrating impaired vitamin B_{12} absorption, achlorhydria, and antibodies to IF in the serum. Treatment is with parenteral vitamin B_{12}.[17]

In isolated reports, the basic defect in cobalamin assimilation is not associated with the secretion of IF or with the absorption or transport of the vitamin. Rather there is a defect in the liberation of cobalamin in the stomach from the ingested protein–cobalamin or enzyme–cobalamin complex with a failure to liberate cobalamin. It has been postulated that this may be an early phase of pernicious anemia.[8]

Congenital Defects. It has been estimated that the body stores of cobalamin at birth are 25 g. Based on known adult requirements, it has also been estimated that infants would need 0.04 g or less daily, but because of their rapid growth, infants would be sustained by their hepatic stores of cobalamin for only about 600 days. Hence, development of cobalamin deficiency within the first 2 years of life suggests a congenital defect in cobalamin assimilation.[17] There could be defective IF secretion (qualitative or quantitative) by the parietal cells of the stomach, defective ileal transport, or failure to elaborate transcobalamin II (Table 96–2).

Acquired defects in cobalamin assimilation are also listed in Table 96–2. These include (1) defects associated with gastrectomy and consequent failure of secretion of IF (Chapter 72); (2) bacterial overgrowth, in which certain bacteria metabolize ingested vitamin B_{12} in the jejunum and hence the cobalamin does not reach the ileal absorptive sites (Chapter 107); (3) certain parasitic infections; and (4) the consequences of disease or of surgical removal of the ileum (Chapter 108). Pancreatic insufficiency can also lead to impaired cobalamin assimilation but rarely or never to clinical manifestations of disease due to this deficiency. Zollinger-Ellison syndrome also interferes with cobalamin assimilation by disturbing the pH in the small intestine.

Isolated deficient IF secretion is a disease with onset of symptoms of anemia before the age of 2½ years and as early as 6 or 7 months.[17] It is not genetically related to adult pernicious anemia. There is a selective quantitative lack of IF secretion with preservation of normal acid secretion and normal gastric mucosal histology. Antibodies to IF are not present in the serum. The diagnosis is established by demonstrating a megaloblastic anemia, absence of IF from the gastric juice, and

Table 96–2. COBALAMIN MALABSORPTION

Type	Age at Onset	Mechanism	Clinical Manifestations	References
Early onset				
Intrinsic factor (IF) absence	6 mo	Isolated lack of IF in gastric juice	Megaloblastic anemia	17
Inert IF	13 yr	IF present but no uptake of Cbl-IF by ileal receptors	Anemia, anorexia, sore tongue	18
Familial vitamin B_{12} deficiency	< 10 yr	Ileal mucosal cell defect in transport of cobalamin	Familial; proteinuria, delayed development, parental consanguinity	19
Transcobalamin II deficiency	6 wk	Lack of serum transcobalamin II → lack of transport post absorption	Megaloblastic anemia, thrombocytopenia, mental retardation	7
Pernicious anemia				
Juvenile	10–20 yr	IF absence	Achlorhydria, gastric atrophy, antibodies to IF, endocrine abnormalities	17
Adult	Adult	IF absence	Megaloblastic anemia, neurologic deficiency	1
Acquired				
Gastrectomy	Adult	IF deficiency	See Chapter 72	
Pancreatic insufficiency	Adult	Bicarbonate and trypsin deficiency interfering with R-protein degradation	See Chapter 217	10, 11
Bacterial overgrowth	Varies	Bacterial uptake in jejunum	See Chapter 107	
Ileotomy	Postoperative	No ileal receptors	See Chapter 106	
Vegetarian (absolute)	Adult	No intake	Anemia	2
Drug-induced				
Biguanide	With medication	IF decreased	Transient or permanent deficiency	21
Cimetidine	With medication	IF decreased	Usually none	20

impaired cobalamin absorption, which is corrected by the administration of exogenous IF. Patients respond well to supplemental parenteral vitamin B_{12} injections.

Another congenital syndrome leading to cobalamin malabsorption involves the secretion of a biologically inert IF.[18] In the original description of this syndrome, the onset of the megaloblastic anemia was at age 13. Free cobalamin given orally was not absorbed unless given with normal quantities of human gastric juice from a normal volunteer. The patient's gastric juice did not correct the cobalamin malabsorption of a totally gastrectomized volunteer, nor did it promote cobalamin uptake by homogenates of guinea pig intestinal mucosa. The gastric juice was acid and contained normal quantities of immunologically identifiable IF. The gastric biopsy was normal. Small bowel transport function, as determined by D-xylose and fat absorption, were normal. Serum concentration of transcobalamin II was normal. There was normal affinity of the patient's IF for cobalamin. The primary abnormality therefore lay in the incapacity of the patient's IF to attach to the ileal mucosa and thus facilitate vitamin B_{12} absorption. The parents of the patient were first cousins, and the consanguinity suggested that the abnormality was due to a double dose of a gene that codes for the synthesis of a biologically inert IF. It was suggested that each parent was heterozygous for the abnormal gene, which was codominant with the normal one. The presenting symptoms were those of the anemia, with anorexia, fatigue, and a sore red tongue. Serum folate levels were normal. In this syndrome, treatment is also with parenteral vitamin B_{12}.

Ileal mucosal transport defect is a familial syndrome with selected vitamin B_{12} malabsorption associated with proteinuria. The onset of the symptoms of anemia are usually within the first decade of life, with weakness, easy bruising, oral ulcers, and delayed development being found. Neurologic signs of decreased vibratory sensation may be present. There is a report of 3 siblings having this disease.[19] Complete studies indicated that there was adequate secretion of IF and gastric acid. Intestinal absorption of fat and D-xylose was not impaired. Mucosal biopsies from the terminal ileum examined by light and electron microscopy were normal. *In vitro* uptake of free and IF-bound vitamin B_{12} by isolated ileal mucosal cells was normal. This would indicate that ileal surface receptors for the cobalamin–IF complex were normal. Addition of IF to ingested cobalamin did not enhance absorption. There were no IF antibodies in the serum. The fundamental abnormality in this familial syndrome appears to be localized to the absorptive process within the intestinal mucosal cell. There is presumably a defect in the transport of cobalamin after it is attached to the ileal brush border receptors. These patients respond well to vitamin B_{12} given parenterally.

An inherited deficiency of synthesis of transcobalamin II causes a severe megaloblastic anemia with megaloblastic changes in the bone marrow; this disorder has been reported at 6 weeks of age.[7] There is associated thrombocytopenia and mental retardation. The neurologic changes persist despite therapy. Proteinuria is not present. Diagnosis was established by demonstrating that the serum did take up vitamin B_{12} and that *in vitro* bone marrow cells did not take up this vitamin, so that there was markedly decreased vitamin B_{12} binding capacity. All endogenous vitamin B_{12} was bound to transcobalamin I, and there was an absence of transcobalamin II by gel filtration.

Drug Effects. Cimetidine given in doses of 1000 mg/day reduces absorption of protein-bound cobalamin, whereas a single daily dose of 400 mg given at night has no effect, even when therapy continues long-term. The higher dose of cimetidine does not inhibit absorption of free cobalamin, although it does decrease IF secretion by one third. It is believed that the clinical effect of cimetidine is on the HCl and proteolytic enzymes that are needed to split cobalamin from protein and enzymes within the stomach. It is doubtful that even long-term cimetidine therapy at higher dosages would lead to clinically evident cobalamin deficiency.[20]

Biguanide therapy can cause cobalamin malabsorption, observed in 36% of patients given metaformin and 11% of those given phenformin. In 50% of patients, vitamin B_{12} absorption returned to normal when the therapy was discontinued. IF added to oral cobalamin did not correct the malabsorption in some cases, suggesting that some factor other than depression of IF secretion was involved. In other patients, addition of IF to oral cobalamin did correct the malabsorption. Cobalamin malabsorption that persisted after biguanide therapy was discontinued was corrected with the addition of IF. Several of these patients had achlorhydria. It is postulated that some patients may be left with permanent depression of IF secretion.[21]

Folate (Folic Acid, Folatin)

Folates are water-soluble vitamins that are not synthesized by mammals but are essential for synthesis of deoxyribonucleic acid. A folate derivative is also required for the formation of methionine from homocysteine, to which it donates a methyl group. Folates are present in various foods, and enzymatic digestion is needed for their absorption by jejunal mucosal cells. Movement across the mucosal cell is primarily by active transport, although passive absorption occurs with pharmacologic doses. Folates are stored in the liver, where the total body reserve is 5 to 10 mg. With severe malabsorption, this reserve can be depleted in weeks to months, and markedly diminished intake of folates or absent dietary folates will also give rise to clinical symptoms within this time period. Folate deficiency also occurs with jejunal mucosal disease, as in celiac disease or tropical sprue; with alcoholism; and following administration of certain drugs, including oral contraceptives, phenytoin, and sulfasalazine. Folate deficiency in itself can induce histologic changes in the jejunal mucosa (Fig. 96–2). A syndrome of a specific isolated defect in folate assimilation has been reported.

Folates are synthesized by bacteria and plants, not by animal tissue. Thus, folates must be ingested from dietary sources on a fairly continuous basis.

Dietary Sources. Folic acid, folates, and folacins are generic terms describing a family of heterocyclic compounds possessing the

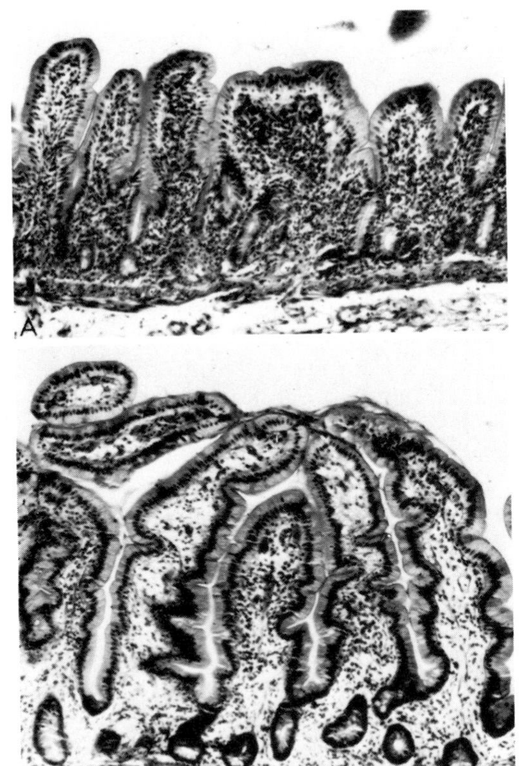

Figure 96–2. Low magnification light micrographs of 2 peroral jejunal biopsy specimens from a folate-deficient patient with severe marrow megaloblastosis, before and after folate replacement. Before treatment *(A)*, the villi are short and the mucosal thickness is reduced. The cellularity within the lamina propria is increased. After folate *(B)*, the villi, total mucosal thickness, and the cellularity of the lamina propria are normal. (Hematoxylin and eosin stain: original magnification, × 50, × 2). (From Hermos JA, et al. Ann Intern Med 1972; 76:957. Reproduced with permission.)

general properties of water-soluble vitamins and consisting of 3 essential and sequential components: pteridine, *p*-aminobenzoic acid, and one or more L-glutamic acid units (Fig. 96–3). The L-glutamic acid residues, beyond the first, are attached through γ-peptide bonds. The monoglutamate form (pteroylglutamate) is the compound commercially available for treatment of patients with folate deficiency, but most of the folate in the diet consists of polyglutamates.

The average daily intake of folate in the United States is about 1000 μg, about 10% to 20% of which is in the monoglutamate form and is totally available for absorption. The better sources of folate include yeast, liver, bananas, and some leafy vegetables. Orange juice, soybeans, egg yolk, and wheat germ are other sources. The proportion of monoglutamate varies, being high in cow's milk and low in orange juice. Both monoglutamate and polyglutamate folates are primarily ingested in a reduced and usually methylated form. Folates in food are vulnerable to destruction by cooking, and folates are sensitive to light, to aerobic conditions, and to extremes of pH, all of which result in breakdown of the folate molecule.[1]

Assimilation. The site of maximum absorption of folate is the jejunum. Folate assimilation is impaired when there is jejunal disease, such as celiac disase or tropical sprue,[21, 22] and is further impaired by the fact that folate deficiency itself can cause structural changes in the jejunal mucosa.

Assimilation involves 3 steps: (1) digestion, with breakdown of polyglutamate folates into the monoglutamate form; (2) uptake by the mucosal cells; and (3) release from the cell into the portal blood. Folate is then stored in the liver, and some of it undergoes enterohepatic circulation. The rate-limiting step in folate assimilation is uptake into the intestinal mucosal cells.[22]

Digestion. Most dietary folate is in the form of polyglutamates, and the availability of folate to the tissues depends on the digestion of the polyglutamates with release of folate in the monoglutamate form. The process involves splitting of the additional glutamic acid units by pteroylpolyglutamate hydrolases. Collectively, these enzymes are referred as "conjugases" because of their ability to hydrolyze conjugated folate. The terminal glutamate is cleaved off by splitting the γ-glutamyl bond.[22] Humans have 2 pteroylpolyglutamate hydrolases, one localized in the brush border and the other in the mitochondrial-lysosomal fraction of the mucosal cell. Perfusion studies have demonstrated that hydrolysis is present in the lumen. This strongly suggests that hydrolysis takes place in or near the mucosal border of the epithelial cell, which would be an indication that the brush border hydrolases are the more important ones[21] (Fig. 96–4). Gastric and pancreatic proteases do not have the ability to deconjugate folate because of the unique γ-glutamyl bonds of the polyglutamates.

Mucosal Transport. Transport across mucosal cells takes place preferentially in the

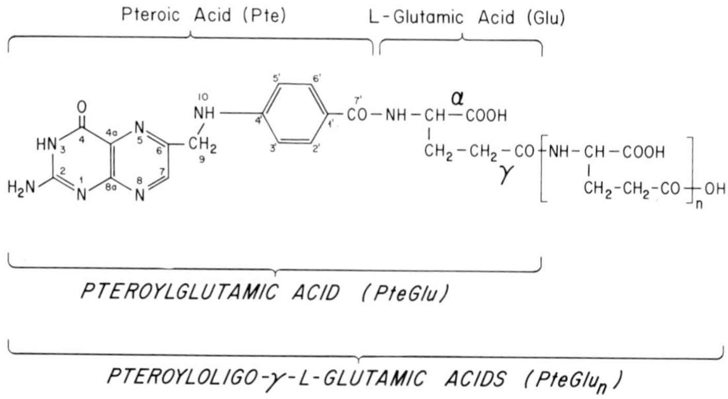

Pteroic Acid (Pte) L-Glutamic Acid (Glu)

PTEROYLGLUTAMIC ACID (PteGlu)

PTEROYLOLIGO-γ-L-GLUTAMIC ACIDS ($PteGlu_n$)

Figure 96–3. Structural formula of pteroyloligo-γ-L-glutamic acids ($PteGlu_n$). (From Godwin HA et al. J Biol Chem 1972; 247:2266. Reproduced with permission.)

proximal jejunum, but the mucosal cells of the entire small intestine contain the necessary conjugases. If the proximal intestine is bypassed or resected, the distal ileum is able to assume a significant proportion of folate assimilation.[22]

Monoglutamate folates are actively transported against a concentration gradient in a process that requires energy and sodium and is inhibited by lack of oxygen and cyanide. Maximal transport occurs at or near pH 6, and transport decreases by half at pH 5 or 7.[21] The structurally specific transport system is shared by reduced and unreduced or formyl-substituted monoglutamyl folates and by methotrexate. The specific process is coded genetically, since its congenital absence has been demonstrated to lead to megaloblastic anemia.[21] Although a specific folate-binding protein has been observed in the membrane of intestinal mucosal cells, it has not been found to be involved in the folate transport system.

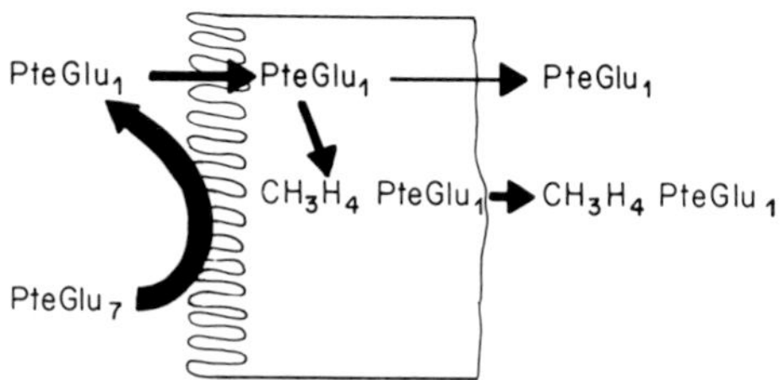

Figure 96–4. Proposed schema of digestion and absorption of polyglutamyl folate by the intestine. Hydrolysis of pteroylheptaglutamate ($PteGlu_7$) to pteroylmonoglutamate ($PteGlu_1$) by intestinal enzymes is rapid, and the overall rate of transport into the mesenteric circulation is controlled by the movement of the monoglutamyl folate. Under appropriate conditions a substantial portion of monoglutamate is reduced and methylated in the intestinal cell and appears in the circulation as 5-methyltetrahydrofolate ($CH_3H_4PteGlu_1$). (From Rosenberg IH. N Engl J Med 1975; 293:1303. Reproduced with permission.)

Within the cell, the monoglutamate is reduced and then methylated.[23] It is the methyltetrahydrofolate that appears in the blood to be transported within the portal bloodstream. Release of folate from the mucosal cell to the blood has been assumed to be by simple diffusion. However, in tumor cells there is a specific release mechanism for folate.[22]

Passive absorption has been demonstrated to occur by simple diffusion when there is a high folate concentration in the lumen. This mechanism predominates when pharmacologic doses of folic acid are ingested.

Liver and Bile. The total body stores of folate are estimated to be 5 to 10 mg and are primarily in the liver. There is an enterohepatic circulation of about 100 μg/day, which enters the intestine from the bile and is handled in the same way as ingested folate. In jejunal malabsorption syndromes, clinically evident deficiencies can occur relatively more rapidly because of malabsorption not only of ingested folate but also of folate present in bile.[22]

Pancreas. Pancreatic insufficiency paradoxically enhances absorption of folate because folate is best absorbed at pH 6. In the absence of bicarbonate secretion from the pancreas, the pH in the duodenum tends to be lower than when pancreatic secretion of bicarbonate is present.[22]

Delivery to Tissues. Normal folate levels in tissues during periods of dietary deprivation are maintained by release of stores from the liver into the bile. Thus, the folate enterohepatic cycle plays its principal role in maintaining adequate delivery to tissues when intake of folate is low. Methyltetrahydrofo-

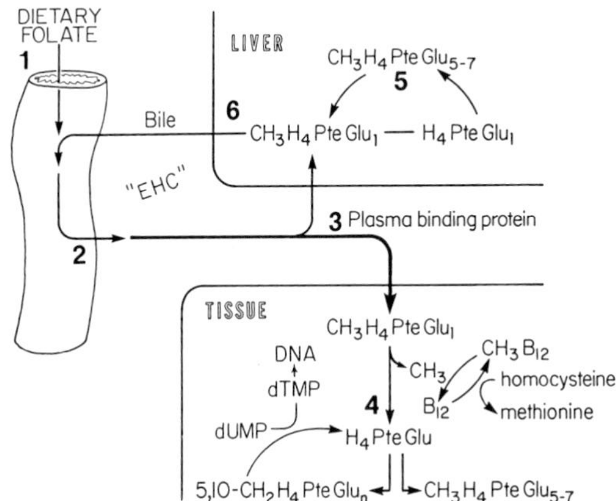

Figure 96–5. Important elements in normal folate homeostasis include (1) the level of folate in the diet, (2) intestinal absorption, (3) transport to liver and other tissues, (4) the intracellular metabolic steps involved in methionine and DNA synthesis, (5) liver uptake and incorporation into an intracellular folate polyglutamate ($CH_3H_4PteGlu_{5-7}$) pool, and (6) the transport of methyltetrahydrofolate monoglutamate ($CH_3H_4PteGlu_1$) into bile for reabsorption and supply to tissues (the folate enterohepatic cycle, FEHC). (From Hillman RS, Steinberg SE. Reproduced with permission from the Annual Review of Medicine, Vol 33, © 1982 by Annual Reviews Inc.)

late monoglutamate stored in hepatocytes is transported by way of the bile to the small intestine for reabsorption and distribution, probably involving a plasma-binding protein[25] (Fig. 96–5).

Ethanol. Alcohol has multiple effects on folate assimilation and utilization. There are both chronic effects from long-term ingestion of ethanol and acute effects of several hours' duration following the ingestion of a single large amount of ethanol. The effects of chronic alcohol ingestion include decreased folate intake, impaired small intestinal mucosal absorption, increase in serum folate–binding protein (although it is not usually known whether this increase leads to increased sequestration of folate in the serum), and finally an effect on the hepatocyte itself, leading to impaired storage. The acute effects primarily involve the enterohepatic circulation of folate[25] (Fig. 96–6).

Folate deficiency in alcoholics is primarily due to decreased protein (and therefore folate) intake and is seen in poorly nourished rather than well-nourished alcoholics. There may be secondary jejunal malabsorption, as discussed earlier. With prolonged alcoholism, uptake of folate by the liver may be abnormal.

Ethanol given in a sufficient amount to achieve a blood level of 150 to 200 mg/dl diminishes serum folate concentration to deficient levels within 48 to 72 hours. The bile folate level also falls, despite adequate liver stores. The acute ingestion of alcohol has no apparent effect on the uptake of folate by the liver, but does increase synthesis of folate polyglutamates, which is accompanied by reduction in the amount of methyltetrahydrofolate in the bile. The monoglutamate accumulates instead in the hepatocyte. The total effect is a marked decrease in the amount of folate in the enterohepatic circulation, so that there is less available for absorption in the jejunum. The acute effect is entirely reversible when the normal supply of folate is restored and alcohol is cleared from the system. The megaloblastic erythropoiesis is relieved as well as soon as alcohol ingestion is interrupted.[25]

Malabsorption. Malabsorption of folate occurs in chronic diseases of the jejunum: celiac disease (Chapter 105), tropical sprue (Chapter 106), and Whipple's disease (Chapter 109). Resection of the jejunum, leaving an intact ileum, does not lead to folate malabsorption. There are also specific disorders of folate assimilation.

Congenital Malabsorption. An inborn and isolated defect in folate absorption becomes

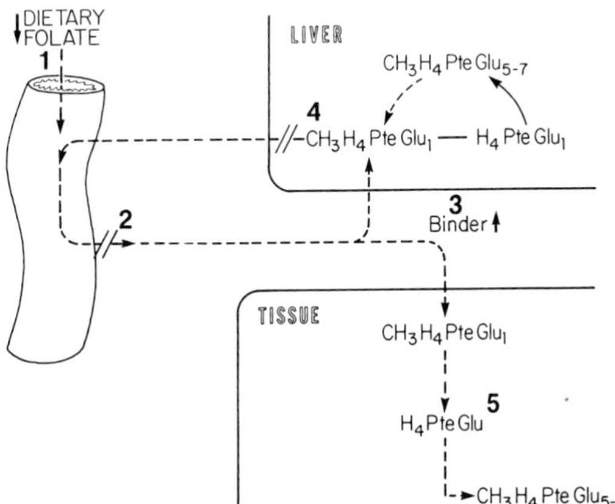

Figure 96–6. The toxic effect of alcohol involves several aspects of normal folate transport and metabolism, including (1) the intake of folate in the diet, (2) intestinal absorption, (3) the level of binder protein in the plasma, (4) the transport of methyltetrahydrofolate from the liver into bile, and (4/5) the formation of intracellular folate polyglutamate. (From Hillman RS, Steinberg SE. Reproduced with permission from the Annual Review of Medicine, Vol 33, © 1982 by Annual Reviews Inc.)

clinically evident by the onset of megaloblastic anemia at the age of 2 or 3 months. Other parameters of intestinal absorption are normal. The syndrome is characterized by relapsing megaloblastic anemia, mental retardation, convulsions, and a neurologic movement disorder.[1, 22, 26] The abnormality of absorption involves all folate forms and is not a deficiency in intestinal mucosal cell conjugases, since the monoglutamate is not absorbed either. Levels of folate in cerebrospinal fluid are low, and while serum levels can be returned to normal with pharmacologic doses of folate given orally or parenterally, cerebrospinal fluid levels remain low. Thus, it has been postulated that there are 2 transport defects, one in the intestinal mucosal cell and one in the central nervous system.[26]

Drug Effects. Sulfasalazine (salicylazosulfapyridine), a drug widely used in the treatment of inflammatory bowel disease, causes a low serum folate level and macrocytosis in some patients. The impaired assimilation of folate is caused by the whole sulfasalazine molecule and not by its components; sulfasalazine is broken down by bacteria in the colon and remains intact in the jejunum unless there is bacterial overgrowth. Jejunal perfusion studies as well as studies on isolated jejunal segments suggest that sulfasalazine has 2 effects: inhibition of jejunal conjugases and interference with binding at the mucosal cell surface. The latter effect occurs despite the fact that there is little similarity between the molecular structures of folate and sulfasalazine. The same studies suggest that clinical folate deficiency may be prevented by increasing dietary folate, by taking sulfasalazine between meals, or by taking supplemental folic acid.[27, 28]

Patients taking the aniconvulsant drug phenytoin (Dilantin) may develop folate deficiency with megaloblastic anemia. The drug probably limits folate transport by interfering either with mucosal cell uptake or with transport across the cell. It does not have an effect on conjugase activity at the brush boorder.[22]

Oral contraceptives have been reported to lower serum folate levels in some instances.[23] The mechanism of action is not known.

Methotrexate is a folate analog that acts as an antimetabolite, principally by competitive inhibition of folic acid reductase. Methotrexate interferes with DNA synthesis and thus with cellular replication. Because of their similar structure, there is competition for mucosal cell uptake by methotrexate and folate.[22]

Other Water-Soluble Vitamins

Relatively little investigative work has been devoted to the gastrointestinal assimilation of other water-soluble vitamins. The initial impression was that they were absorbed by passive transport, but it has been shown that in some instances active transport is involved.[29]

Thiamine (Vitamin B_1). Thiamine is absorbed by 2 mechanisms, one active and the other passive. At physiologic concentrations, transport is active, and it is transported by an active mechanism against a concentration gradient. Pharmacologic doses are transported passively along a concentration gradient. Active absorption is greatest in the duodenum and then decreases progressively through the rest of the small intestine. Saturation transport kinetics have been demonstrated, and structural analogs inhibit thiamine transport in a competitive manner. The results of these studies are compatible with a thiamine-binding protein acting as a carrier for absorption. It has been suggested that the cellular mechanism for active transport is located at a point beyond the brush border. Phosphorylation of thiamine does occur in the gut wall but is separate from thiamine transport. It is postulated that phosphorylation acts to concentrate thiamine in the cell. The exit across the basolateral membrane is considered from bacterial studies to be an energy-dependent process, modulated at least in part by the sodium pump mechanism present at that membrane. Stimulation of the sodium pump increases thiamine transport, while inhibition decreases it.

Vitamin B_6. This vitamin is actually a group of vitamins with similar biologic activity, including pyridoxine, its free analog pyridoxal, and pyridoxamine, together with their phosphorylated compounds. Pyridoxine, the most common form ingested, is derived from plants. Most vitamin preparations are marketed in this form and it is the one also used in the fortification of foods. The phosphorylated forms of pyridoxal and pyridoxamine are the principal forms found in animal tissues.

Limited experimental work has been reported on vitamin B_6 assimilation. It appears that the free forms, including pyridoxine, as well as the phosphorylated forms, are absorbed by passive diffusion. The process is non-saturable and not energy-dependent. Within the lumen, hydrolysis is accomplished by alkaline phosphatase. A small percentage of the phosphorylated vitamin may be absorbed as an intact molecule. It is unknown whether there is binding of the active vitamin to any other substances. Within the cell, part of the free vitamin is phosphorylated by the cytoplasmic enzyme pyridoxal kinase. Since the principal form appearing on the serosal side is the free, non-phosphorylated form of the vitamin, the phosphorylated vitamin formed within the cytoplasm in turn appears to undergo a phosphatase-mediated hydrolysis.[31]

Ascorbic Acid (Vitamin C). Among mammals, primates are unique in having a dietary requirement for L-ascorbic acid. This requirement is associated with a specific mechanism for the absorption of this vitamin, and species that do not have the dietary requirement also do not have the specific absorptive mechanism. The mechanism is sodium-dependent and saturable, consistent with active absorption.

The sodium gradient hypothesis is a transport model that best accommodates the available information on ascorbic acid absorption. According to the hypothesis adapted for this vitamin, ascorbic acid and sodium bind to a protein carrier located in the brush border membrane. It is likely that there is a one-to-one co-transport of ascorbic acid and sodium. Both the sodium and the vitamin are translocated into the cell, at which time they dissociate from the carrier. The sodium is then transported out of the cells by the sodium pump mechanism involving the Na^+,K^+-ATPase at the basolateral membrane. While the sodium is being extruded from the cell, ascorbic acid remains within the cell, reaching a concentration that exceeds that on the serosal surface. Presumably then, ascorbic acid exits the cell in a passive manner along a concentration gradient. A secondary active transport mechanism is involved because accumulation of ascorbic acid against an electrochemical gradient is dependent upon sodium transport across the brush border but only indirectly dependent on the cellular metabolic energy to operate the sodium pump.

Absorption of ascorbic acid fulfills the criteria for active transport, being a saturable process requiring energy and operating against an electrochemical gradient. It is also sodium-dependent and requires a brush border carrier. The rate-limiting step is the uptake into the brush border, while the exit from the cell apparently is a passive mechanism. A feedback mechanism based on the circulating level of ascorbic acid in the body has been postulated. Guinea pigs placed on a high ascorbic acid diet showed a significant reduction in uptake of ascorbic acid after 2 to 4 weeks. The clinical implication is that individuals taking huge doses of ascorbic acid may eventually limit their capacity to absorb the vitamin, which would render them susceptible to a rebound phenomenon of low ascorbic acid absorption and ascorbic acid insufficiency if their vitamin C intake suddenly fell. The result could be a clinical syndrome of rebound scurvy.[32]

Niacin. Availability of niacin from dietary sources is dependent upon the digestion of the pyridine nucleotides. This involves a series of enzymes to hydrolyze the phosphate bonds. Transport across the intestinal mucosa appears to be by a passive mechanism, but the details are not known.

Pantothenate. The sources of pantothenate in the diet are coenzyme A and phosphopantothenate. Digestion involves progressive dephosphorylation. Finally, the sulfhydryl group is removed by the enzyme pantothenase. The absorption of the liberated pantothenate is by simple diffusion. The crucial factor is whether there is sufficient pantothenase, which determines the rate of vitamin absorption from coenzyme A.

References

1. Castle WB, Godwin HA. Assimilation of vitamin B_{12} and folic acid. *In*: Bockus HL, ed. Gastroenterology. 3rd Ed. Vol. II. Philadelphia: WB Saunders, 1976: 95–108.
2. Donaldson RM Jr. Intrinsic factor and transport of cobalamin. *In*: Johnson LR, ed. Physiology of the Gastrointestinal Tract. New York: Raven Press, 181: 641–58.
3. Carmel R. Subtle cobalamin malabsorption in a vegan patient. Arch Intern Med 1982; 142:2206–7.
4. Herzlich B, Herbert V. The role of the pancreas in cobalamin (vitamin B_{12}) absorption. Am J Gastroenterol 1984; 79:489–93.
5. Allen RH. Intestinal absorption and plasma transport of cobalamin (vitamin B_{12}). Fed Proc 1984; 43:2424–5.
6. Allen RH, Seetharam B, Podell ER, Alpers DH. Effect of proteolytic enzymes on the binding of cobalamin to R-protein and intrinsic factor. J Clin Invest 1978; 61:47–54.
7. Burrow JF, Mollen DL, Sladden RA, Sourai N, Greory M. Inherited deficiency of transcobalamin II causing megaloblastic anemia. Br J Haematol 1977; 35:676–7.
8. King CE, Toskes PP. Evolution of protein bound cobalamin malabsorption. Arch Intern Med 1983; 143:2219.
9. Mercoulis G, Parnenter Y, Nicolos J, Jimenez M, Gerrard P. Cobalamin malabsorption due to non-degradation of R-proteins in the human intestine. J Clin Invest 1980; 66:430–40.

10. Veeger W, Abels J, Hellemans N. Effect of sodium bicarbonate and pancreatin on the absorption of vitamin B_{12} and fat in pancreatic insufficiency. N Engl J Med 1962; 267:1341–4.
11. Toskes PP, Hansell J, Cerda J, Deren JJ. Vitamin B_{12} malabsorption in chronic pancreatic insufficiency. N Engl J Med 1971; 289:627–32.
12. LeBauer E, Smith K, Greenberger NJ. Pancreatic insufficiency and vitamin B_{12} malabsorption. Arch Intern Med 1968; 122:423–5.
13. Toskes PP, Deren JJ, Conrad ME. Trypsin-like nature of the pancreatic factor that corrects vitamin B_{12} malabsorption associated with pancreatic dysfunction. J Clin Invest 1973; 52-1660–4.
14. Allen RH, Seetharam B, Allan NC, Podell ER, Alpers DH. Correction of cobalamin malabsorption in pancreatic insufficiency with a cobalamin analogue that binds with high affinity to R protein but not intrinsic factor. J Clin Invest 1978; 61:1628–34.
15. Seetharam B, Alpers DH, Allen RH. Isolation and characterization of the ideal receptor for intrinsic factor cobalamin. J Biol Chem 1981; 256:3785–90.
16. Seetharam B, Bagur SS, Alpers DH. Interaction of receptor for intrinsic factor cobalamin with synthetic and brush border lipids. J Biol Chem 1982; 257:183–9.
17. McIntyre OR, Sullivan LW, Jeffries GH, Silver RH. Pernicious anemia in childhood. N Engl J Med 1965; 272:981–6.
18. Katz M, Lee SK, Cooper BA. Vitamin B_{12} malabsorption due to biologically inert intrinsic factor. N Engl J Med 1972; 287:425–9.
19. MacKenzie JL, Donaldson RM Jr, Trier JS, Mathon VI. Ileal mucosa in familial selective vitamin B_{12} malabsorption. N Engl J Med 1972; 286:1021–5.
20. Streeter AM, Goulston KJ, Fracp FA, Bathor FA, Helmer RS. Cimetidine and malabsorption of cobalamin. Dig Dis Sci 1982; 27:13–7.
21. Adams JF, Clark JS, Ireland JT, Kesson CM, Watson WS. Malabsorption of vitamin B_{12} and intrinsic factor secretion during biguanide therapy. Diabetologia 1983; 24:16–18.
22. Rosenberg IH. Intestinal absorption of folates. *In*: Johnson LR, ed. Physiology of the Gastrointestinal Tract. New York: Raven Press, 1981: 1221–30.
23. Rosenberg IH. Folate absorption and malabsorption. N Engl J Med 1975; 293:1303–8.
24. Rosenberg IH. Digestion and absorption of dietary folate. Fed Proc 1984; 43:2248–9.
25. Hillman RS, Steinberg SE. The effects of alcohol on folate metabolism. Ann Rev Med 1982; 33:345–54.
26. Pomez M, Colman N, Herbert V, Schwartz E, Cohen AR. Therapy of congenital folate malabsorption. J Pediatr 1981; 98:76–9.
27. Reisenauer AM, Halsted CH. Human jejunal brush border conjugase. Biochem Biophys Acta 1981; 659:62–9.
28. Halsted CH, Gandhi G, Tomura T. Sulfasalazine inhibits the absorption of folates in ulcerative colitis. N Engl J Med 1981; 305:1513–7.
29. Rose RC. Transport and metabolism of water soluble vitamins in intestine. Am J Physiol 1981; 240:G97–101.
30. Hoyumpa AM Jr. Intestinal absorption of thiamine. Fed Proc 1984; 43:2423–4.
31. Middleton HM III. Intestinal absorption of vitamin B_6. Fed Proc 1984; 43:2426–7.
32. Rose AC. Ascorbic acid transport and metabolism in intestine and kidney. Fed Proc 1984; 43:2425–6.
33. Henderson LM. Digestion and absorption of NAD and CoA. Fed Proc 1984; 43:2427–8.

Chapter 97

Bile Acid and Cholesterol Homeostasis

Charles M. Mansbach, II • Scott M. Grundy

Since experiments by Schoenheimer in 1924 first suggested that bile acids were the operational component for the intestinal absorption of cholesterol, numerous investigations have identified biochemical and physiologic interrelationships between these materials. The synthesis of bile acids from cholesterol was demonstrated by Bloch et al. in 1943[1]; in 1952 Siperstein et al.[2] and Bergstrom[3] identified this pathway as a major excretory route for cholesterol. Subsequently, clinical investigators concentrated their initial research efforts on either bile acid metabolism or cholesterol metabolism. Eventually they had to come to grips with factors mutually responsible for control of both materials.[4] Clinical investigators with interests predominantly in the field of atherosclerosis have concentrated on the metabolism of cholesterol and other lipids in the peripheral blood, whereas gastroenterologists have been concerned chiefly with absorption of bile acids and the importance of these materials to the absorption of cholesterol and other lipids. Our purpose will be to examine these relationships as they exist in normal human physiology and in the context of gastrointestinal disorders known to alter bile acid–cholesterol homeostasis.

Bile Acid Metabolism

In normal man the bile acid pool is essentially confined to the enterohepatic space (Fig. 97–1). Plasma concentrations of bile acids are negligible[5] and amounts excreted in urine are low (<5 mg/day).[6] On the other hand, gross calculations based on estimates of renal plasma flow of bile acids (1 to 2 μg/ml of plasma and a renal plasma flow of 350 ml/minute) suggest an appreciable (500

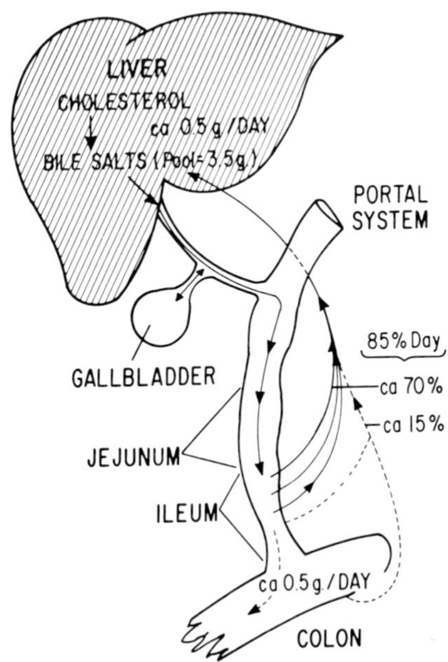

Figure 97–1. Schematic representation of the enterohepatic circulation of bile acids. The solid lines entering the portal system represent conjugated bile acid absorbed via ileal transport. The broken lines represent unconjugated bile acids resulting from bacterial action.[40]

to 1000 mg/day) potential loss of the bile acid pool by this route. Such degradation is prevented in normal man by a renal conservation mechanism. Two factors probably operate to minimize the urinary excretion of bile acids. The first is extensive binding of these substances to plasma proteins (mainly albumin but also to HDL lipoprotein),[7,8] which limits glomerular filtration. The second factor is tubular reabsorption, first detected in patients with hepatic disease and shown to involve both di- and trihydroxy bile acids.[5] Subsequent work in dogs characterized the reabsorptive process as a proximal tubular secretory flux that is specifically (carrier) mediated, possibly by the organic anion secretory system of the kidney.[9,10] However, the potential exists for bile acid excretion to be increased in urine during periods of hepatic excretory failure. Studies in rats have shown that the tubular fractional reabsorption of both taurocholate and taurochenodeoxycholate is decreased by conjugated bilirubin, enhancing their urinary excretion.[11] This, combined with the enhanced sulfation of bile acids under these conditions, leads to a large increase in the renal pathway of bile acid excretion (200 mg or more/24 hours).[7,12,13]

After an overnight fast the bile acid pool is confined chiefly to the gallbladder and biliary tree. This distribution reflects a highly specialized and efficient system or systems for intestinal absorption and hepatic uptake and secretion of bile acids. The physiologic importance of these transport systems to the economy of the bile acid pool is made evident by a brief consideration of the function and reutilization of these materials.

Bile acids are released into the upper intestine at the ampulla of Vater in response to a meal. Contraction of the gallbladder is mediated by the hormone cholecystokinin-pancreozymin (CCK-PZ). The components of the meal that promote gallbladder contraction are peptides, essential amino acids, and hydrolyzed lipid.[14] Whole proteins and nonessential amino acids are ineffective.[15] The release of bile acids is, furthermore, under the control of a feedback regulatory loop in which bile acids in the upper intestine inhibit their further release from the gallbladder.[16]

Bile acids are crucial for the solubilization of cholesterol in the gallbladder and biliary tree[17] (Chapter 179) and for the solubilization and absorption of cholesterol[18,19] and lipid-soluble vitamins[20,21] in the intestinal lumen. Bile acids greatly facilitate digestion and absorption of fat[22] (Chapter 92). Since bile acids contain both hydrophilic and hydrophobic functional groups, they provide characteristic detergent and emulsifying properties. Several physical factors determine the effectiveness of bile acids as detergents.[23] The pH of the surrounding milieu and the pKa (dissociation constants) of bile acids are important in this process, since they will determine the proportion of uncharged molecules in solution. For example, unconjugated bile acids, such as cholic acid, are less effective detergents, inasmuch as they possess sufficiently high pKa's to be un-ionized at physiologic pH, whereas taurine and glycine conjugates of these bile acids (pKa 1.9 to 4.8) are much more readily dissociated. Furthermore, in order to maintain cholesterol in micellar solution in the gallbladder a critical concentration of conjugated bile acids must be maintained; similarly, optimal absorption of dietary fats depends on adequate micellar solubilization of lipolytic products. Since these requirements for bile acids far exceed amounts present in the total body pool plus the liver's capacity to synthesize bile acids (discussed later), it is apparent that specialized absorptive mechanisms must be available for recycling and reutilization of bile acids. The magnitude of this recycling process may be appreciated from certain simple calculations. First, it has been estimated that the *total conjugated bile acid pool* in normal man[24,25] averages 3.5 g by isotope dilution methods.[26] Second, measurements of the concentration of bile acids in the intestinal lumen of normal man during the 3 to 4 hours of the digestion and absorption of a test meal indicate that the total bile acid pool must be absorbed and resecreted into the intestine at least twice with every meal[27]; this means that approximately 21 g of conjugated bile acids (6 times the bile acid pool) is emptied into the small intestine during a 3-meal day. In contrast, the daily fecal loss is only 250 to 400 mg/day.[28–30] In the steady state this excretory loss must be matched by *de novo* synthesis of bile acids from cholesterol.[31]

Although the broad outline of the enterohepatic circuit of bile acids is present in the near-term fetus, bile acid composition and synthetic rates are significantly different as compared with adults. In dogs,[32] monkeys,[33] and humans,[34] the bile acid pool size is reduced, as is the bile acid synthetic rate compared with adult levels. Additionally, the bile acid pool composition differs from adults in that the percentage of the pool represented by cholate is increased in newborn monkeys[33] and newborn humans,[35] taurine rather than glycine conjugates predominate,[33] and secondary bile acids are present in reduced amounts.[33–35] Ileal active transport of taurocholate is also reduced in fetal dogs[36] and neonatal rats[37] as compared with adults, but is at adult levels by 5 weeks in dogs[36] and at 26 days (weaning 21 days) in rats.[37] The sum of these effects on bile acid metabolism is that bile acid concentrations in the postprandial duodenum are considerably lower in near-term human fetuses than in adults.[34]

Intestinal Absorption of Conjugated and Unconjugated Bile Acids

Animal Models. The remarkable efficiency in recirculation and reutilization of bile acids prompted considerable search for a specialized absorptive system. The specific mechanisms responsible for bile acid absorption, as demonstrated by *in vitro* and *in vivo* experiments in a variety of species of animals, have been the subject of several reviews.[38–42] These investigations have clearly demonstrated uptake of bile acids against an electrochemical gradient *(active transport)* in the ileum of all species studied, but not in other portions of the small intestine or colon. Current data concerning the ileal receptor site for bile acids indicate a requirement for Na^+ that enhances the binding of bile acid to its receptor.[43] The data further suggest that the receptor has 2 recognition components for bile acids.[44] One recognizes the steroid moiety. The other is suggested to be a cationic site on the membrane that has a coulombic interaction with the negatively charged bile salt. This transport system is operative for all naturally occurring bile acids, conjugated and unconjugated. As with other intestinal transport systems, bile acid transport requires sodium ions and is inhibited by ouabain, an inhibitor of sodium, potassium, and adenosine triphosphatase. *In vitro* and *in vivo* animal experiments of bile acid transport by Lack and Weiner[45] and Heaton and Lack[46] have demonstrated mutual inhibition between the several types of bile acids; dihydroxy bile acids are better inhibitors than trihydroxy compounds. This could mean that the apparent affinity of dihydroxy compounds for the ileal transport system is greater than that of trihydroxy bile acids.

Dietschy et al.[47] have considered the process of *passive intestinal absorption* of bile acids. Their *in vitro* studies in isolated rat intestine invoked nonionic diffusion as the major mechanism involved in passive absorption of bile acids. From these and other studies[41] in several species of animals, it is apparent that passive diffusion takes place throughout the small bowel and colon. In the ileum this would proceed in parallel with active transport. Taurocholate and other similar compounds, because of their low solubility and low pKa (strong tendency to ionize), do not participate in this passive process. Cholic acid and other unconjugated bile acids possess sufficient lipid solubility and a sufficiently high pKa to undergo nonionic diffusion. Glycine-conjugated bile acids possess pKa's that are intermediate between these groups. Studies designed to assess the extent of passive diffusion from the proximal small intestine have been complicated by species variations as well as by possible artifacts inherent in the experimental design.[40,41] For example, when taurocholate (the bile acid least likely to be absorbed passively) was dissolved in buffered saline solution and placed in tied-off segments of the proximal small bowel, very little taurocholate was recovered from a common bile duct fistula in rabbits and guinea pigs. In contrast, a considerable portion was returned to the liver from similar segments in dogs. Playoust et al.[48] sampled common bile duct bile in 3 groups of dogs in which the bile acid pool was labeled with ^{14}C-taurocholate. In dogs lacking an ileum, digestion of one fat-containing meal resulted in 97% loss of the taurocholate pool, but the recovery of radioactive taurocholate was the same in dogs with resection of the jejunum as in those without any resected bowel. These observations suggest that *loss of the proximal small intestine has no effect on the enterohepatic circulation of taurocholate.*

Normal Humans. From the foregoing considerations it is apparent that assessment of the quantitative importance of each level of the gastrointestinal tract to bile acid absorption, and thus the maintenance of the enterohepatic bile acid circulation, requires an experimental model that enables measurement of the enterohepatic return of specific conjugated and unconjugated bile acids during normal digestion-absorption. Optimally, the degree of deconjugation of bile acids should also be known at each level, as well as the physicochemical characteristics of the luminal milieu.

Current data suggest that at least 70% and possibly up to 82% of the bile acid pool is reabsorbed each day as conjugated bile acid through the specialized transport system located in the distal 100 to 150 cm of ileum, just proximal to the ileocecal valve (Fig. 97–1). Furthermore, 3% to 15% of the bile acid pool is reabsorbed daily as unconjugated bile acid. These data are supported by studies in which conjugated bile acids were separately labeled in the amino acid and steroid moiety. When the glycine portion was labeled (the predominant bile acid conjugant in man), it was found to have a faster turnover time than the steroid moiety.[49,50] The taurine and cholyl moieties of taurocholate, however, were found to have essentially the same turnover rate.[51] The precise sites of reabsorption of unconjugated bile acids have not been identified clearly. From physicochemical considerations noted earlier, it is clear that unconjugated bile acids, when formed within the intestinal lumen, may be absorbed by a passive process throughout the entire small intestine; they are also subject to absorption by the specialized transport system in the distal small intestine. Thus, the site and extent of intestinal absorption by passive processes depend upon the activity of microorganisms capable of deconjugating bile acids. Such microorganisms are known to reside chiefly in the colon and, to a far lesser extent, in the terminal ileum of normal man.[52,53] Passive colonic absorption of deconjugated bile acids may represent a further means for the conservation of bile acids.[54]

A pool of secondary bile acids, predominantly glycine and taurine conjugates of deoxycholic acid, was found in the earliest qualitative studies of intestinal bile acid content in normal man.[55, 56] This finding confirmed the well-recognized luminal bacterial metabolism of bile acids demonstrated in various animal species.[57 60] Investigations have shown that hydrolysis of conjugated bile acids occurs regularly during enterohepatic circulation in normal man.[61] Bacterial metabolic alterations of sodium taurocholate-24-^{14}C and sodium glycocholate-24-^{14}C are apparent following their IV administration to normal subjects (Fig. 97–2). In these studies, samples of cholecystokinin-stimulated gallbladder bile were obtained from the duo-

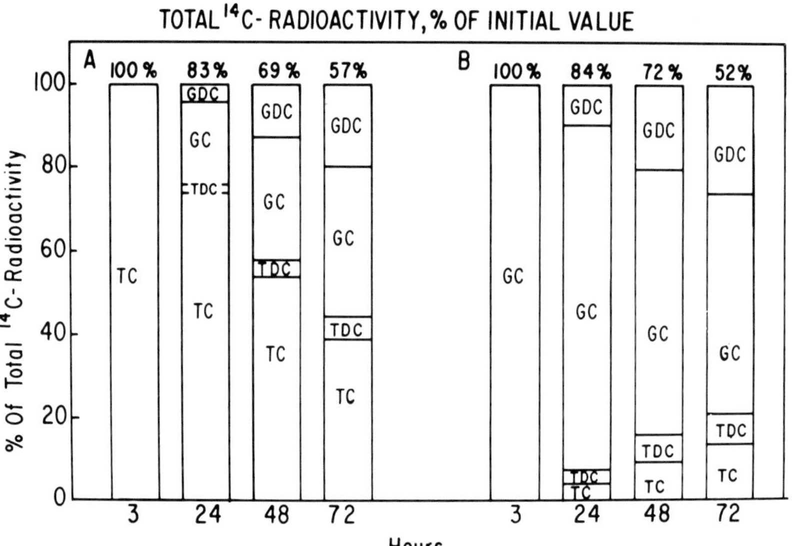

Figure 97–2. Composition of ^{14}C-radioactivity in duodenal fluid obtained at designated time periods after IV injection of sodium taurocholate-24-^{14}C (A) and sodium glycocholate 24-^{14}C (B); average values in 4 normal subjects. Data are expressed in terms of percentage of ^{14}C-radioactivity contributed by each bile acid fraction to the total recoverable ^{14}C-radioactivity. Total recoverable ^{14}C-radioactivity expressed as a percentage of the initial 3-hour value is shown at the top of each column. GDC = glycodeoxycholate; GC = glycocholate; TDC = taurodeoxycholate; TC = taurocholate.[133] (Adapted from Garbutt JT, Wilkins RM, Lark L, et al.[89])

denum at the designated time intervals, and individual bile acids were fractionated. Following taurocholate-^{14}C administration, the percentage of glycocholate-^{14}C recovered increased progressively with time, whereas the administration of glycocholate-^{14}C was associated with a progressive increase in the percentage of taurocholate-^{14}C recovered. This sequence could arise only as a result of bacterial hydrolysis followed by reabsorption of the unconjugated ^{14}C-cholate and subsequent hepatic conjugation with glycine and taurine. Furthermore, it is apparent (Fig. 97–2) that ^{14}C radioactivity accumulates progressively in glycine and taurine conjugates of deoxycholate following IV administration of either taurocholate-24-^{14}C or glycocholate-24-^{14}C to normal humans. Indeed, by 72 hours, 25% to 30% of the residual total ^{14}C radioactivity in duodenal fluid was present in conjugates of this secondary bile acid. These observations are consistent with well-recognized metabolic pathways for trihydroxy bile acid metabolism.[62,63] The presence of organisms in the intestinal flora of normal man that are capable of both hydrolysis and 7-α-dehydroxylation[64-66] adds further physiologic significance to such data. Deoxycholate-^{14}C formed in the more distal region of the small intestine or colon may be absorbed by passive diffusion, returning to the liver and being conjugated there with glycine or taurine.

From the foregoing, it may be assumed that conjugated bile acids are absorbed intact mainly by the ileal transport system in normal man. However, a significant but quantitatively unknown portion of the glycine-conjugated dihydroxy bile acid pool is absorbed passively in the jejunum.[67] Thus, measurement of the rate of disappearance of taurocholate-24-^{14}C (the conjugated bile acid least likely to be absorbed intact by any route other than ileal transport) should provide a fairly accurate assessment of the daily return of conjugated trihydroxy bile acid by ileal transport. Such measurements (Fig. 97–3) indicate a daily loss of approximately 30%. The estimate of daily reabsorption of bile acids by ileal transport, amounting to approximately 70% (see Fig. 97–1), seems reasonable from these observations. Studies using unconjugated ^{14}C-chenodeoxycholic acid have suggested a more efficient absorption of this bile acid.[68] If this were due to more effective ileal transport of glycine and taurine conjugates of chenodeoxycholic acid, then the estimate of 70% reabsorption by the ileal route would be minimal for total conjugated bile acids.

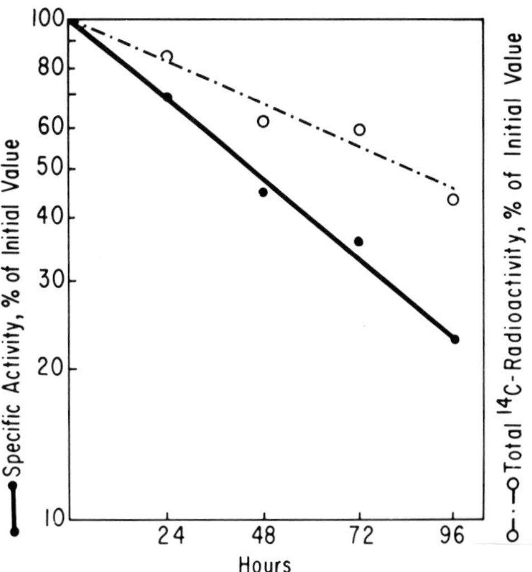

Figure 97–3. The rate of disappearance of sodium taurocholate-24-^{14}C from the enterohepatic circulation; average values in 4 normal medical students. The solid line is derived from the decline of specific activity, counts/minute/μg of sodium taurocholate. The broken line represents the decline in total ^{14}C-radioactivity, normalized for volume change. The differences between the ordinates of the lines represent the return of bacterially modified bile acid absorbed as conjugated ^{14}C-cholic acid and ^{14}C-deoxycholic acid, which then recirculates enterohepatically in the conjugated form.[40]

The daily absorption of bacterially modified bile acid (unconjugated ^{14}C-cholic acid and ^{14}C-deoxycholic acid) following the administration of taurocholate-24-^{14}C may be estimated from differences between the percentages of the decline in specific activity of this conjugated bile acid and the decline in total ^{14}C radioactivity normalized for volume change (Fig. 97–3). These amount to approximately 15% per day. Absorption of unconjugated bile acid following bacterial metabolism would be expected to occur primarily in the colon and to a lesser extent in the terminal ileum. In the cleansed human colon, chenodeoxycholate is absorbed 9 times more rapidly and deoxycholate 6 times more rapidly than cholate.[54] Despite the lack of more precise kinetic information, it is clear that this system also contributes importantly to the maintenance of the enterohepatic circulation of bile acids (approximately 15% per day [see Fig. 97–1]).

These data should be considered in light of our previous discussion of the overall

Table 97–1. BILE ACID KINETICS IN HEALTHY HUMANS*

Type of Bile Acid	Pool Size (mg)	Fractional Turnover Rate (days^{-1})	Daily Synthesis (mg)
Cholic	1195	0.261	299
Deoxycholic	720	0.258	171
Chenodeoxycholate	1011	0.210	177
Lithocholic	74	1.0	106

*From Matern S, Gerock W. Physiol Biochem Pharmacol 1979; 85:125–204. Reproduced with permission.

efficiency of these absorptive systems. The figure of 85% reabsorption (see Fig. 97–1) refers to the fraction of the total bile acid pool that returns in 24 hours. Since the pool, which averages about 3 g, recirculates at least 6 times per day, the absorption for each cycle is greater than 95%. The combined data from several laboratories with regard to bile acid pool size, fractional turnover rate, and daily synthesis rates are shown in Table 97–1.

The metabolism and absorption of glycine and taurine conjugates of chenodeoxycholic acid during enterohepatic circulation are only partially understood. Bacterial metabolic conversions of these conjugated bile acids have not been measured in normal man and may not be identical with the metabolism of cholate conjugates shown in Figure 97–2. Lithocholic acid, produced by bacterial 7-α-dehydroxylation of chenodeoxycholate, is a relatively insoluble monohydroxy bile acid; it appears to be firmly bound to intestinal bacteria during its passage through the colon. Indeed, lithocholate is present in relatively minimal quantities in gallbladder bile obtained from the duodenum of normal subjects.[68,69] Palmer[70] has demonstrated that lithocholic acid and its conjugates can undergo sulfation during enterohepatic circulation. These 3-α-sulfate esters may account for approximately 50% of the total lithocholic acid compounds in human bile. Such sulfation may further curtail intestinal absorption[71] and enhance fecal elimination rates of these potentially toxic bile acids, which have been implicated in a number of experimental pathologic processes: cirrhosis of the liver, bile ductular hyperplasia, and gallstone formation in animals[36,72-77,80,81] and fever following IM injection in man.[78,79] Furthermore, the position and extent of sulfation of bile acids greatly affect their absorption. Sulfation at the 3α, 7α, 3α–7α positions is progressively more poorly transported.[80] Indeed, bile acid sulfation may be an adaptive mechanism for eliminating bile acids from the organism in the setting of biliary obstruction, where the extent to which bile acids are sulfated is increased.[81]

Patients with Ileal Disorders. Interruption of the enterohepatic circulation of bile acids has been demonstrated in subjects with surgically created ileal dysfunction caused by ileal resection. Similar losses of bile acids have also been observed in subjects who have an anatomically intact intestinal tract but who have diffuse disease of the ileum due to regional enteritis (Crohn's disease), amyloid infiltration, or radiation damage. Although the precise degree of ileal disease necessary to produce these losses is not known, present data suggest that *functional loss of the distal one half to one third of the small intestine markedly reduces the absorption of bile acids* (Chapter 108).

The methods used to assess bile acid absorption in these patients include: (1) sequential measurements of the specific activity of bile acids in duodenal contents after the IV or oral administration of isotopically labeled conjugated or unconjugated bile acids,[24,25,82-84] (2) measurements of fecal excretion of radioactivity after the oral or IV administration of cholate-24-^{14}C,[85, 86] and (3) assay of the concentration of bile acids in luminal fluid during the digestion and absorption of a test meal[82-84, 87, 88, 90] (Fig. 97–3). For example, studies utilizing sequential measurements of specific activity of sodium taurocholate-^{14}C or sodium glycocholate-^{14}C have shown virtually complete disappearance of radioactivity in the bile acid administered 24 hours after IV injection.[24,66,89] In fact, even after one meal and an overnight fast, 90% to 95% of glycocholate and glycochenodeoxycholate is lost to the bile acid pool.[97] The specific activity at the 24-hour sampling time, expressed as a percentage of the initial 3-hour value in patients with ileal disease, has been compared with that in normal subjects (Fig. 97–4).[89] It is evident from these studies that the presence of significant ileal disease results in

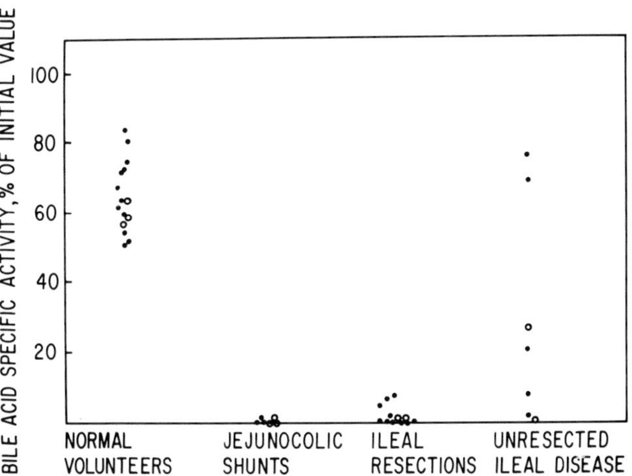

Figure 97–4. Disappearance of ^{14}C-labeled taurocholate (closed circle) or glycocholate (open circle) from the enterohepatic circulation 24 hours after IV injection in normal volunteer subjects and patients with ileal disorders. The specific activity (cpm/μg) in the corresponding chromatographically separated fractions of duodenal content is expressed as a percentage of the initial value obtained 3 hours after injection of the label, which is considered 100%.[89]

an inability to maintain conjugated trihydroxy bile acids in the enterohepatic circulation. Patients with unresected ileal disease show the widest spectrum of values, ranging from normal (2 patients with less than 20 cm of terminal ileum involved by regional enteritis) to nearly complete absence of radioactivity 24 hours after administration. Analyses of the fecal excretion of bile acids in similar subjects[91] have shown daily excretion ranging from 1.9 to 4 g, the latter amount being equal to the estimated total bile acid pool size in normal subjects. These methods estimate the net loss over a 24-hour period, which may entail at least 6 enterohepatic cycles of bile acids (the loss during one cycle is presently unknown). Serial determinations of the intraluminal concentration of bile acids during the ingestion of several meals in subjects with ileal resection have demonstrated markedly reduced values.[84] Actually, this has been observed as early as 1 hour after the feeding of a single meal.[92] In their entirety, *these studies point up the importance of the ileal transport site in man in maintaining enterohepatic circulation of conjugated bile acids.*

Since bacterial modification enables transport of bile acids by passive processes throughout the length of the intestinal tract, the recirculation of unconjugated bile acid may represent an important compensatory mechanism in patients who have lost ileal function. The colonic flora is regularly exposed to larger quantities of bile acid in this situation. Furthermore, the absence of an ileocecal valve or the presence of partially obstructed segments of remaining small intestine, which many of these subjects exhibit, may result in the development of a small intestinal flora capable of metabolizing bile acids. Measurements of the total ^{14}C radioactivity remaining 24 hours after the injection of sodium taurocholate-^{14}C have shown obvious differences between the values obtained in subjects with ileal disorders and those in normal man (Fig. 97–5). The total ^{14}C radioactivity remaining in the enterohepatic circulation in patients with ileal disorders is markedly reduced. These patients were arbitrarily separated into 2 groups based on the clinical and roentgenologic assessment of the presence or absence of small intestinal stasis. Although there was a slight increase in the 24-hour residual radioactivity present in the group with small intestinal stasis, neither group maintained normal amounts of radioactive bile acids throughout the study period. These observations suggest a lessened capacity for recirculation of both the parent compound and its metabolic products in patients with ileal disorders.[89]

There is a wide variation in values obtained from subjects with unresected regional enteritis, which may result from differences in the extent of functional damage to the ileal transport site, as well as the location and enzymatic capacity of the bacterial flora. Analysis of the chemical composition of the total ^{14}C radioactivity remaining 24 hours after injection of taurocholate-^{14}C (Fig. 97–6) further supports the role of reabsorption of bacterially modified bile acids as a compensatory contribution to the total bile acid pool in patients with ileal disorders. In patients with ileal disease, virtually all of the recovered ^{14}C radioactivity represents bacterial metabolic

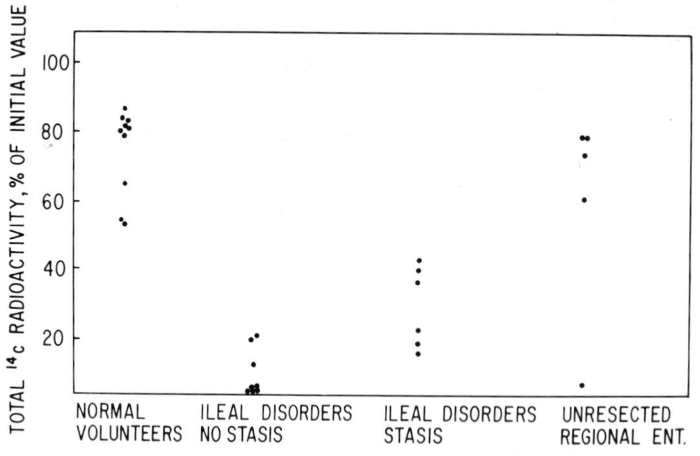

Figure 97–5. Disappearance of total ^{14}C-radioactivity, normalized for volume change, from the enterohepatic circulation 24 hours after IV injection of taurocholate-^{14}C in normal volunteer subjects and patients with ileal disorders. The total ^{14}C-radioactivity in duodenal contents is expressed as a percentage of the initial 3-hour value, which is considered 100%. The presence of intestinal stasis was determined by clinical and roentgenologic assessment.[89]

products. The major modification in subjects with rapid intestinal transit of barium and the absence of small intestinal stasis is deconjugation, resulting in the presence of glycocholate-^{14}C in the duodenal contents 24 hours after taurocholate-^{14}C injection. Subjects with partial small intestinal obstruction appear to modify the injected taurocholate-^{14}C more extensively. Residual radioactivity is composed predominantly of conjugates of deoxycholate-^{14}C, implying a metabolic sequence involving both deconjugation and 7-α-dehydroxylation of the injected trihydroxy bile acid.[89] These findings support the hypothesis that stagnant segments of bowel are more likely to support the growth of bacteria and increase the modification of bile acids.[52, 93] It seems clear that reabsorption of unconjugated bile acids is important to the overall economy of patients with ileal disorders, yet varies widely in individual patients; i.e., those with stasis and increased luminal metabolism of bile acids tend to have a greater contribution to their enterohepatic circulation via passive absorption of unconjugated bile acids.

Cholestyramine Administration. Oral administration of cholestyramine, an anionic exchange resin, results in an increased loss of fecal bile acids.[94-96] This material has been shown to bind bile acids *in vitro*[97] and in the lumen of the gut.[94-96] The effects of such bile acid sequestration on bile acid metabolism have been studied in normal,[98] obese,[99] and hypercholesterolemic patients,[94-96] and in patients after cholecystectomy with T-tube drainage of the common bile duct.[100] Although the dosage used in these studies has varied considerably (between 10 and 24 g), it is clear that cholestyramine administration not only causes a loss of bile acids from the enterohepatic circulation, but also considerably alters the composition of the bile acid pool. For example, cholestyramine given to normal subjects (16 g/day) results in a marked reduction in the relative proportions of ^{14}C-

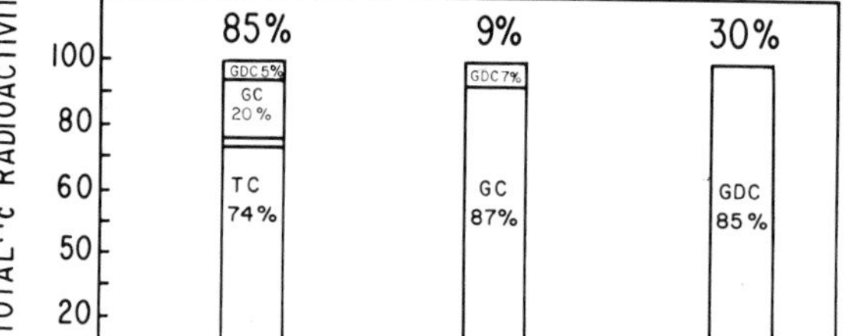

Figure 97–6. Composition of ^{14}C-radioactivity in duodenal contents obtained 24 hours after the intravenous injection of taurocholate-^{14}C. Data are expressed in terms of percentage of the ^{14}C contributed by each bile acid fraction to the total recoverable ^{14}C-radioactivity. The total residual ^{14}C-radioactivity at 24 hours expressed as a percentage of the initial value obtained at 3 hours is shown at the top of the bars. GDC = glycodeoxycholate; GC = glycocholate; TDC = taurodeoxycholate; TC = taurocholate.[273]

labeled metabolic products of cholate and in chenodeoxycholate remaining in the enterohepatic circulation.[98] After 6 weeks of cholestyramine administration, cholic acid averaged 85% of the total bile acids, with chenodeoxycholic and deoxycholic acid averaging 15% and less than 1% of the total, respectively. In comparison, cholate averaged 43%, chenodeoxycholate 38%, and deoxycholic acid 19% of the total bile acid pool before cholestyramine administration.[98] Furthermore, these observations demonstrate enhanced synthesis of bile acids during cholestyramine administration, in that measurements of the total bile acid pool provide values that are identical with those obtained prior to cholestyramine administration.[98] Thus, the normal bile acid pool is maintained, despite a 2- to 3-fold increase in fecal bile acid excretion.[94]

Bile Acid Synthesis and Conjugation

Animal Models. Extensive *in vivo* and *in vitro* studies, principally in the dog, rat, and mouse, have established that bile acids are derived from cholesterol[1-3] (Fig. 97–7). This conversion appears to occur *only in the liver,*[96] and bile acids thus formed are designated *primary bile acids.* The chemical structure of primary bile acids in mammals and a variety of nonmammalian vertebrates and the biologic significance of these variations have been studied extensively by Haslewood.[60] Cholic and chenodeoxycholic acids are the major primary bile acids in most mammalian species (Fig. 97–7). Investigations of the metabolic pathways in the synthesis of primary bile acids have principally involved the parenteral administration of labeled sterols (potentially intermediate in the pathway of bile acid synthesis) to rats with a bile fistula and the identification of metabolites in subcellular liver fractions of rats following *in vitro* incubations with labeled precursors.[101,102] Almost all results have supported the suggestion by Bergstrom[103] that modifications of the sterol nucleus preceded degradation of the side chain.

Considerable evidence has implicated the 7-α-hydroxylation of cholesterol as the initial rate-controlling step in the biosynthesis of cholic acid and chenodeoxycholic acid.[104-106] It is now evident that in rat liver the cholesterol 7-α-hydroxylase, which catalyzes this reaction, is located in the endoplasmic reticulum.[107-109] In rats, this enzyme undergoes a diurnal cycle with maximal levels from 6 PM to 12 PM and minimal levels between 6 AM and 12 AM.[110] This parallels the early evening feeding habits of rats and can be reversed on changing the rats' feeding schedule. Additionally, the peak to trough levels of enzyme activity have enabled the calculation of the T½ of the enzyme (2 hours). In man, 7-α-hydroxylase activity has been shown to vary with serum cholesterol.[111] Physicochemical requirements of this enzyme system have been reviewed.[112] It has also been suggested that this enzyme system is cytochrome P_{450}–dependent,[113] in keeping with the report that phenobarbital administration (in pharmacologic amounts) augments bile acid synthesis in monkeys.[114] In the rat, cholesterol-7-α-hydroxylase is very sensitive to modification of the enterohepatic circulation of bile acids. Thus, the activity of this enzyme system in liver microsomes rises in about 18 hours after creation of a bile fistula and achieves a plateau within about 3 days, a time course virtually indistinguishable from the change in bile acid synthesis.[104, 115, 116] Furthermore, this rise in enzyme activity

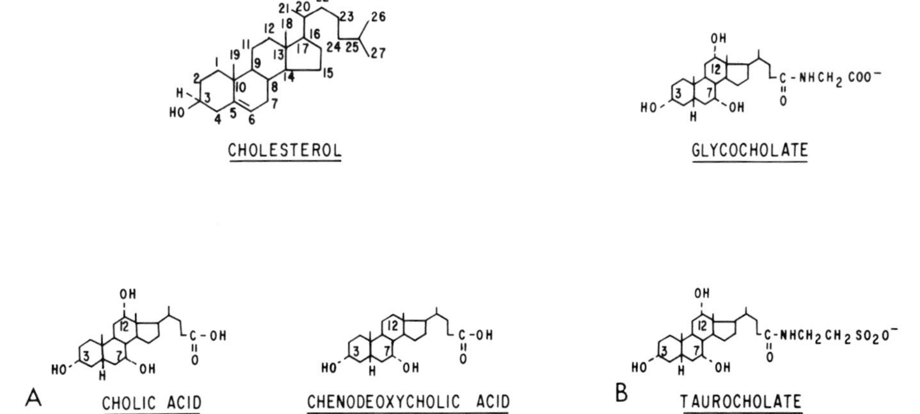

Figure 97–7. Chemical structure of cholesterol and major primary bile acids in man *(A)*. Chemical structure of glycine and taurine conjugates of cholic acid *(B)*.

has been shown to be the result of de novo enzyme synthesis. Reinfusion of bile acids into the distal end of the common bile duct in the rat with a bile fistula results in inhibition of the compensatory bile acid synthesis.[117] In monkeys, after complete interruption of bile acid enterohepatic circulation by ileectomy, a maximum 10-fold increase in the rate of bile acid synthesis has been reported.[118]

Prior to their secretion in bile, bile acids are conjugated with glycine and taurine (Fig. 97–7). Bile acid conjugation occurs in a 2-step process. Studies in rats[119] have shown that the first step in which the bile acid is activated by choloyl-CoA synthetase to its CoA derivative occurs in microsomes. The second step, mediated by the enzyme, bile acid–CoA: amino acid *N* acyltransferase, conjugates the activated bile acid with either glycine or taurine. This enzyme is present in the cytosolic fraction of hepatocytes. It appears that a single enzyme conjugates the bile acids. The proportion of bile acids conjugated with either glycine or taurine is determined by the K_m of the enzyme and substrate availablity.[120] For example, in the rat, whose bile acids are predominantly conjugated with taurine, the K_m for taurine is only 0.8 mM, whereas the K_m for glycine is 31 mM. Variations in the relative conjugation of bile acids with glycine and taurine are well recognized within mammalian species.[121] Hamsters and monkeys show a relative glycine preponderance similar to man. A further increase in the relative conjugation of bile acids with glycine has been demonstrated in the hamster following creation of a bile fistula.

Normal Humans and Patients with Interruption of Bile Acid Enterohepatic Circulation. The mechanisms of bile acid synthesis in man are only partially understood. Studies of subcellular fractions obtained from liver biopsy specimens in patients during cholecystectomy have concluded that 7-α-hydroxycholesterol is a precursor of both cholate and chenodeoxycholate.[122] The synthesis of chenodeoxycholic acid and, to a lesser extent, cholic acid from 26-hydroxycholesterol has been identified in patients with T-tube drainage following cholecystectomy.[123] This pathway, which is also operative in the rat and hamster, requires an initial oxygenase attack on the side-chain in liver mitochondria and has been considered less important quantitatively than bile acid synthesis by way of the 7-α-hydroxylase system.[119] However, the relative role of these systems in pathophysiologic states is presently unknown.

Estimation of bile acid synthesis has been obtained from isotope dilution techniques[24-26,68,69,82,98] and by measurement of fecal bile acids[28,30,94] in the metabolic steady state. The results of these and other studies indicate that normal humans usually synthesize from 250 to 500 mg of bile acids daily. Although it has been clearly demonstrated that cholesterol is the substrate for bile acid synthesis,[124-127] studies measuring fecal bile acid excretion have not demonstrated an increased production of bile acid after cholesterol feeding in normal man.[128,129] This failure to enhance bile acid synthesis may be partially due to the relatively small amounts of cholesterol that can be absorbed by man, as well as the likelihood that this amount is sufficient to inhibit hepatic cholesterol synthesis. An alternative is failure to accelerate bile acid synthesis from substrate delivered by this route. In contrast, interruption of the bile acid enterohepatic circulation in subjects given cholestyramine or in patients with ileal disorders results in a marked enhancement of bile acid synthesis. This would indicate that the conversion of cholesterol to bile acids is controlled by a negative feedback mechanism involving bile acids.[105]

Values for pool sizes of bile acids determined by isotope dilution methods in normal humans have been similar before and during 6 weeks of cholestyramine administration (12 g/day).[98] Since fecal excretion of bile acids is enhanced severalfold during cholestyramine administration,[94] the finding of normal pool sizes indicates a concomitant increase in bile acid synthesis. A compensatory increase in cholesterol synthesis also occurs in this situation. In the case of ileal disorders, estimates obtained from isotope dilution studies and measurements of fecal excretion suggest enhanced (3- to 15-fold) rates of bile acid synthesis.[24,25,82,91,130] Incomplete loss of bile acids from the enterohepatic circulation results in a lesser synthetic response than does more complete interruption. Nevertheless, marked variations apparently occur in patient response to maximal interruption. Such observations indicate a need for more precise identification of individual factors controlling bile acid synthesis, such as minor alterations in hepatic function and cholesterol absorption and synthesis.

Both primary and secondary bile acids are secreted into the canaliculus in the conjugated form. Virtually all bile acids are partitioned between glycine and taurine conjugates.[15,131,132] Glycine-conjugated bile acids predominate in normal adults; the relative conjugation of bile acids with glycine and taurine (G:T ratio) averages approximately 3:1.[55,82,88,133] Furthermore, the G:T ratio of each of the 3 major bile acids (cholic, chenodeoxycholic, and deoxycholic) is essentially identical.[55,82] Oral administration of a taurine load to normal adults enhances relative conjugation of bile acids with taurine (within 3 days), resulting in G:T ratios less than unity; large increases in glycine intake, in contrast, do not change this proportion.[134] Cystine loading will also lower the G:T ratio in normal adults, but to a lesser degree than taurine feeding. Taurine is derived chiefly from meats and seafood, and there is little effect on taurine blood levels following ingestion of these foods.[135] All the factors determining the availability of taurine for bile acid conjugation are not understood, whereas endogenous and exogenous glycine is ubiquitous. While there is no direct evidence from measurements of the biosynthesis of primary bile acids, it might be speculated that these synthetic pathways may be influenced by the relative availability of taurine to the conjugating system.[61,120]

The relative availability of taurine to the conjugating system may be depleted in 2 pathophysiologic situations: enhanced bile acid synthesis and/or enhanced deconjugation of bile acids during their enterohepatic circulation, as in bacterial overgrowth. In both circumstances, the requirements for bile acid conjugation are increased and a relatively greater conjugation with glycine may be readily demonstrated. Indeed, G:T ratios average 9:1 in normal subjects within 5 days after the administration of cholestyramine, a situation in which enhanced synthesis predominates.[98] Elevated G:T ratios are unchanged during a 6 week period of cholestyramine administration, returning promptly (within 5 days) to normal values following discontinuation of this agent. In patients with ileal disorders, the G:T ratio averages 15:1.[25,82,88,133] Bile acid synthesis may be greatly enhanced in these patients, but also varying degrees of bacterial overgrowth may be present concomitantly and the patients may also be nutritionally depleted. The administration of taurine to such patients will promptly (within 3 days) reverse the G:T ratio toward normal and, in fact, result in some instances in ratios of less than 1.[128]

Clinical Sequelae Related to Loss of Bile Acid Enterohepatic Circulation. The sequelae that may be related to loss of the bile acid–transporting capacity of the ileum can be separated into 2 major categories: (1) those arising as a direct result of excessive bile acid entering the colonic lumen, and (2) those arising through inability to maintain adequate bile acid concentrations in the biliary tree and intestinal lumen. Such sequelae are schematically represented in Figure 97–8.

The intactness of the enterohepatic circulation of bile acids can be tested by 3 methods:

1. Measuring the proportion of the bile acid pool conjugated with glycine as com-

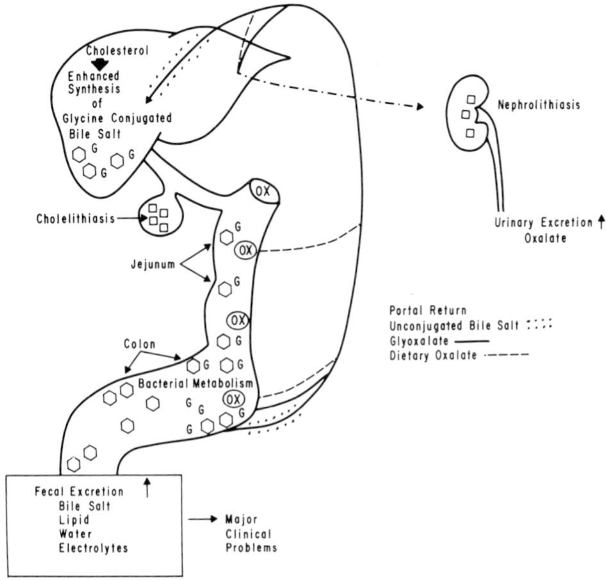

Figure 97–8. Clinical sequelae associated with interruption of the enterohepataic circulation of bile acid through loss of ileal function. Enhanced synthesis and reconjugation of reabsorbed bacterial metabolic products result in the development of a predominantly glycine-conjugated bile acid pool. Loss of the capacity to recirculate conjugated bile acid is associated with cholelithiasis and steatorrhea. Bacterial metabolism of the increased quantities of glycine-conjugated bile acid reaching the colon may contribute to the urgent effects of dihydroxy bile acid at this site, resulting in watery diarrhea, as well as produce glyoxalate, which after further hepatic metabolism contributes to hyperoxaluria and nephrolithiasis.[273] The major source of urinary oxalate in these patients with hyperoxaluria appears to be from a markedly enhanced absorption of dietary oxalate.[154]

pared with taurine. As stated earlier, glycine conjugates become more predominant when bile acid loss is excessive.

2. Administering (^{14}C-glycine) glycocholate by mouth and observing the output of (^{14}C) CO_2 in the breath.[136,137] In cases of an interrupted enterohepatic circulation, intestinal bacterial overgrowth, or cholangitis,[138] the amount of $^{14}CO_2$ appearing in the breath will be excessive (Chapter 27).

3. Observing the retention of radiolabeled bile acids within the enterohepatic space, as detailed earlier.

Excessive Bile Acid Entering the Colonic Lumen. Hofmann[139] has coined the term "cholerheic enteropathy" to describe the syndrome of watery diarrhea associated with the loss of bile acids into the colonic lumen when ileal reabsorption is insufficient. Inhibition of colonic salt and water absorption has been demonstrated *in vitro* and *in vivo* and has been attributed to dihydroxy bile acids.[140] The trihydroxy bile acid cholate apparently does not produce this effect. Both enhanced synthesis of chenodeoxycholate and increased bacterial conversion of cholate to deoxycholate may be expected to contribute to the amount of dihydroxy bile acid present in the colonic lumen. Therapeutic efforts have been directed primarily at intraluminal binding of these substances with nonabsorbable inert materials. Although a bile acid–binding capacity is demonstrable with various vegetables,[141] neomycin, lignin, and methylcellulose, cholestyramine has proved to be the most useful agent. This sequestrant has been shown to be very effective in reducing fecal volume, particularly in patients with ileal disorders who manifest only mild steatorrhea.[142] The mechanism of action has been presumed to be related to the binding of dihydroxy bile acid to the resin, but it may also be related to enhanced cholate synthesis, which appears to be the preferred pathway during cholestyramine administration.[98] Administration of cholestyramine to some patients with ileal disorders may worsen the diarrhea as a result of increased production of hydroxy fatty acids; these fatty acids are apparently produced in increased amounts following malabsorption of fat. Thus, this sequela requires precise identification of its mechanism prior to initiating effective therapy.[94,142]

Excessive Oxalate Absorption. An effect of the steatorrhea often manifested by these patients, which is abetted by the increased bile acid perfusion of the colon, is increased frequency of renal stones that often contain oxalate[139, 143-145] (Chapter 108). In an extreme case, acute renal failure due to oxalate precipitation in the kidney has been reported.[146] Normal man excretes 40 mg of oxalate or less into the urine each day, even on a high oxalate diet.[147] The urinary oxalate is derived 30% from absorbed oxalate, 30% from oxidation of ascorbate, and 40% from oxidation of glyoxalate.[148] In patients with steatorrhea of any cause and an intact colon, the quantity of urinary oxalate increases in direct proportion to the amount of steatorrhea.[149] However, hyperoxaluria is not usually seen unless fecal fat excretion exceeds 15 g/day.[149-151] Steatorrhea from a variety of causes has been associated with hyperoxaluria,[147,149] but the hyperoxaluria following ileal resection or disease has been the most closely studied[150,152-155] and is the most closely associated with the development of nephrolithiasis.[156] It is clear that the excessive oxalate excretion comes from enhanced absorption of dietary oxalate[150,154] and that it is primarily the colon that is responsible in both rats[164] and humans.[150,158,159] The increased absorption of oxalate is likely due to its increased solubility in fecal water in patients with steatorrhea. Normally, oxalate is precipitated from solution by Ca^{2+} and thus made unavailable for absorption. In patients with steatorrhea, excessive fatty acids are present to which the Ca^{2+} preferentially binds,[151] leaving oxalate in solution. Currently, oxalate is thought to be absorbed passively,[160,161] although preliminary evidence using Ca^{2+} in the incubating medium of *in vitro* studies suggests that an active component also exists.

Prevention of stone formation in patients with demonstrated hyperoxaluria is directed toward reducing urinary oxalate.[158] This may be accomplished by lowering the oxalate content of the diet.[162] However, an incomplete knowledge of the oxalate content of a variety of foodstuffs makes dietary manipulation of oxalate excretion unreliable as the sole means of treatment.[163] Calcium supplementation of the diet (up to 3 g/day) with careful monitoring of urinary calcium excretion also reduces urinary oxalate,[164,165] as does reducing dietary fat intake.[159] Finally, cholestyramine (often given to bind bile acids in the treatment of cholerheic enteropathy) also binds oxalate[145] and is effective in reducing urinary oxalate excretion.[145]

Inability to Maintain Adequate Bile Acid

Concentrations in the Biliary Tree and Intestinal Lumen. Patients with ileal disorders appear to have an increased prevalence of gallstone formation.[166,167] The reader is referred to Chapter 179 for basic information relative to this problem.

The presence of steatorrhea in patients with ileal disorders is well recognized. In the absence of efficient recirculation of conjugated bile acids, these patients must depend upon enhanced hepatic synthesis of these substances to obtain an effective concentration necessary for the solubilization of dietary fat. Several studies of intraluminal bile acid concentration during ingestion of a test meal have distinctly demonstrated decreased bile acid concentration in these patients.[83,84,87,92,142,168] Additional investigations in patients with this syndrome and minimal steatorrhea have shown no alteration in the stoichiometry of the association of the products of fat digestion with the bile acid mixed micelle, which would promote lipid absorption.[168] Hence, the steatorrhea seen in these patients is likely to be due to reduced efficiency of lipid absorption secondary to the low intraluminal bile acid concentration associated with a reduced length of intestine. Although oral supplements of bile acid will decrease the degree of steatorrhea, they also tend to increase the quantity of bile acid entering the colon and therefore may increase the watery diarrhea.

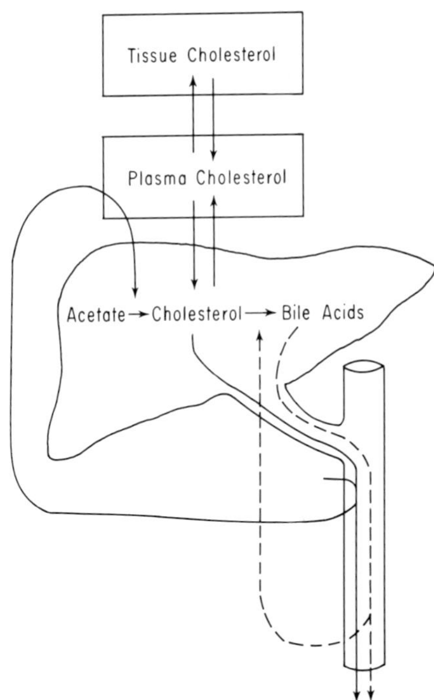

Figure 97–9. Schematic representation of cholesterol metabolism in man. Cholesterol is synthesized in the liver from acetate and partially converted into bile acids. Both cholesterol and bile acids are secreted into bile. Cholesterol is partially reabsorbed in the upper intestine and returns to the liver via the lymphatic circulation. In the liver, cholesterol inhibits its own formation from acetate. Hepatic cholesterol is the source of most of the plasma cholesterol. Bile acids are reabsorbed in the ileum, and they return to the liver by the portal circulation; in the liver, bile acids inhibit their own synthesis from cholesterol.

Cholesterol Metabolism

The major pathways of cholesterol metabolism in man are shown in Figure 97–9. The intestine regulates the input of cholesterol into the body by controlling the amount absorbed. The liver is a key organ regulating the overall economy of cholesterol. It is one of the major sites of cholesterol synthesis, and it controls the fate of cholesterol, i.e., its conversion into bile acids, its secretion into bile, and its input into plasma with lipoproteins. The plasma lipoproteins deliver cholesterol to peripheral tissues and thereby influence the synthesis of cholesterol in these tissues. Cholesterol in peripheral tissues must be returned to the liver (reverse cholesterol transport) for its final catabolism (conversion to bile acids or secretion into bile). In the following section, the basic pathways of cholesterol metabolism will be examined. Also to be discussed are the mechanisms of transport of cholesterol in lipoproteins and abnormalities in lipoprotein metabolism.

Cholesterol Absorption. Cholesterol enters the intestinal tract from 2 sources: the diet and the bile. A minor contribution may be secretion by the intestinal mucosa. The average intake of cholesterol in the United States is 450 to 500 mg/day; hepatic secretion of cholesterol into bile ranges from 750 to 1250 mg/day.[169] Biliary cholesterol is entirely unesterified, but a portion of dietary cholesterol can be esterified with fatty acids. Any esters are hydrolyzed rapidly in the intestinal lumen by pancreatic cholesterol esterase.[170]

Mechanisms for cholesterol absorption are shown schematically in Figure 97–10. Before absorption, cholesterol must be solubilized by mixed micelles containing conjugated bile acids and hydrolytic products of triglycerides and lecithin—fatty acids, monoglycerides, and lysolecithin.[22,171] Free (unesterified) cholesterol is dissolved in the hydrophobic cen-

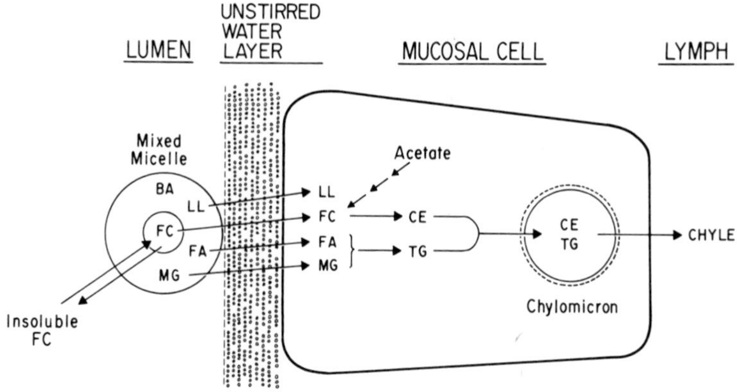

Figure 97–10. Mechanisms of cholesterol absorption. Intestinal free unesterified cholesterol (FC) is solubilized in the intestinal lumen by mixed micelles containing bile acids (BA), lysolecithin (LL), fatty acids (FA), and monoglycerides (MG). FC passes through an unstirred layer of water, along with other micellar constituents, and is taken up by the intestinal mucosa. BA are not absorbed. Small amounts of FC are also synthesized by mucosal cells. FC is converted into cholesterol ester (CE), and FA and MG are resynthesized into triglycerides (TG). CE and TG are incorporated into chylomicrons, which are secreted into bile.

ter of the micelle (Chapter 92). Bile acids are crucial detergents of the micelle, being required for cholesterol absorption; when bile acids are diverted from the intestine, as in total biliary obstruction, no cholesterol is absorbed. Since cholesterol must be in a soluble state before it can be absorbed, its absorption is limited by amounts that can be solubilized into micelles. Absorption of cholesterol is never complete because luminal cholesterol cannot be dissolved completely. Amounts absorbed depend on the intraluminal availability of bile acids, fatty acids, and monoglycerides, all of which expand mixed micelles and enhance absorption.[172,173] Absorption of cholesterol is greater in the upper intestine, where micelles are relatively large; it is less in the lower intestine, probably because of disruption of micelles by absorption of their fatty components.[174]

In addition to dissolving cholesterol, micelles promote cholesterol absorption by facilitating transport across the unstirred layer of water adjacent to the surface of the luminal cell.[175,176] The transport occurs by simple diffusion. Movement through the unstirred layer, and not penetration of the microvillus membrane, appears to be the rate-limiting step for cholesterol absorption. The micelle as a whole does not penetrate to cell membrane. Passage of cholesterol through the structured lipid of the membrane occurs by monomolecular passive diffusion. Whether micelles specifically facilitate cholesterol uptake into the mucosal cell has not been determined, but the requirement of bile acids for cholesterol absorption suggests such a role.

Reduction of cholesterol absorption results from any process that interferes with formation of mixed micelles in the upper intestine. Decreased biliary secretion of bile acids is one such cause; it can result from biliary obstruction or enhanced losses in ileal disease. Products of triglyceride digestion, fatty acids and monoglycerides, promote cholesterol absorption; their decreased availability, by low-fat diets or pancreatic insufficiency, reduces absorption. A large phase of neutral lipids in the intestinal lumen can compete with micelles for cholesterol, thereby decreasing mucosal uptake. Examples are incomplete hydrolysis of triglycerides, excess intestinal phospholipids,[177] and the plasma cholesterol–lowering agent sucrose polyester.[178] Cholesterol absorption likewise can be reduced by displacing cholesterol from micelles with sitosterol[179] or by neomycin.[180]

Hyperabsorption of sterols apparently can occur under certain circumstances. In the rare disease *hyperbetasitosterolemia* the normal barrier against sitosterol absorption is removed.[181] The result is excessive influx of sitosterol into plasma and tissues, xanthomatosis, and probably premature atherosclerosis. The intestine apparently absorbs excess cholesterol as well. The cause of this disorder is unknown. Hyperabsorption of cholesterol theoretically could produce hypercholesterolemia, but if such a metabolic defect exists, it likely is rare. *Familial hypercholesterolemia is not associated with excess cholesterol absorption.*[182] Still, absorption of cholesterol is not "saturated" by endogenous cholesterol; increasing dietary cholesterol can raise total plasma cholesterol levels.[183] The rate of cholesterol absorption seemingly is proportional to intake up to about 1000 mg/day[184]; above this value, absorption is essentially "saturated."

Intestinal Excretion. About half the cholesterol entering the intestine is not absorbed and passes into the large intestine. In the colon, cholesterol is attacked by anaerobic microorganisms[185] and partially transformed into 2 other neutral steroids (Figure 97–11); 5β-reduction of the double bond of cholesterol yields coprostanol, while oxidation of the latter produces coprostanone. Similar changes occur with the plant sterols. In some people these steroids can be degraded further to poorly characterized nonsteroidal products. Colonic neutral steroids are essentially unabsorbed.

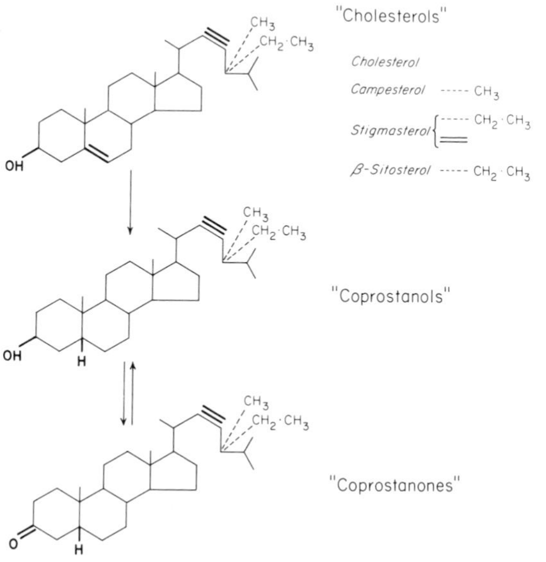

Figure 97–11. Fecal neutral sterols. The major fecal sterols excreted in human feces include cholesterol and the structurally related plant sterols (compesterol, stigmasterol, and β-sitosterol). These sterols are converted by intestinal bacteria into coprostanol (and its related plant sterols) and coprostanone (and its related plant sterols).

The neutral steroids have been implicated in cancer of the colon[186-188] (Chapter 139). Increased colonic cholesterol, or its transformation products, may follow diets rich in fats and cholesterol. High rates of colon cancer have been reported for populations consuming high-fat, high-cholesterol diets. These claims are consistent with a carcinogenic role for fecal steroids. Unfortunately, little is known about mechanisms of colon carcinogenicity. Whether increased or decreased conversion of cholesterol to secondary neutral steroids contributes to colonic carcinoma remains conjectural. Indeed, one study claimed that a familial absence of bacterial products of cholesterol is associated with a higher of rate of colon cancer.[188]

Intestinal Metabolism. After uptake of cholesterol by the intestinal mucosa, most is esterified by the enzyme acyl-CoA cholesterol acyltransferase (ACAT). In addition to luminal uptake, mucosal cells have the capacity to synthesize cholesterol.[189-192] In certain experimental animals, such as the rat and baboon, the intestine seemingly produces an appreciable fraction of the body's synthesis of cholesterol.[189,190,193] The human intestine can synthesize cholesterol,[94,190] but its contribution to total body synthesis is unknown. Cholesterol production by the intestine may be regulated by bile acids.[192] In the presence of bile acids, mucosal synthesis is inhibited; with bile diversion, it is enhanced.[27] Newly absorbed cholesterol is esterified and incorporated into chylomicrons. Most of chylomicron-cholesterol is transported to the liver. The metabolism of chylomicrons is described in more detail in the subsequent section on Lipoprotein Metabolism.

Hepatic Metabolism. Cholesterol in the liver comes from 3 sources: (1) newly absorbed cholesterol (delivered by chylomicrons), (2) cholesterol from peripheral tissues (delivered by plasma lipoproteins), and (3) cholesterol synthesized within the liver cell. The liver is probably the major site of cholesterol made in the body. Amounts produced by the human liver are unknown, but studies in primates suggest that at least half of whole body synthesis occurs in this organ.[190] In persons of normal weight, total body synthesis ranges from 9 to 13 mg/kg/day or for a normal 70-kg man, about 650 to 900 mg/day.[169] If data from nonhuman primates can be extrapolated to man, the human liver

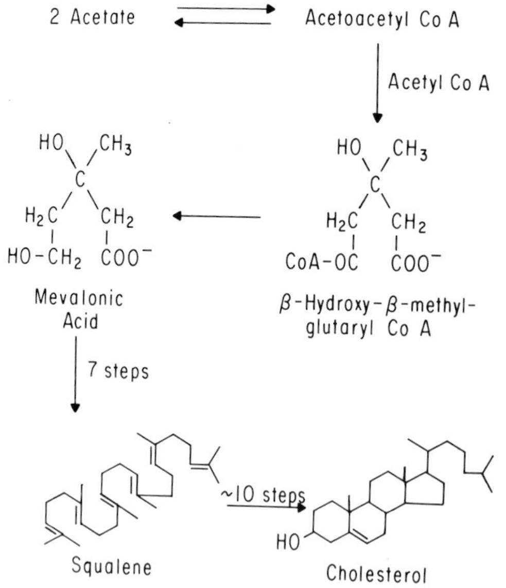

Figure 97–12. Essential steps in biosynthesis of cholesterol. Through condensation of 3 molecules of acetyl CoA, β-hydroxy-β-methyl-glutaryl CoA is produced. The conversion of the latter product into mevalonic acid appears to be the rate-controlling step in cholesterol synthesis. Further condensation reactions lead to the hydrocarbon squalene, and after ring closure and several other steps, cholesterol is produced.

would make approximately 325 to 450 mg of cholesterol per day. The precursor for sterol synthesis is acetyl coenzyme A (CoA) and at least 21 steps are included in the synthetic pathway for cholesterol.[194,195] The key steps in cholesterol synthesis are outlined in Figure 97–12. Initial steps in cholesterol synthesis include the sequential formation of acetoacetyl CoA, β-hydroxyl-β-methyl glutarate (HMG CoA), and mevalonic acid. The conversion of HMG CoA to mevalonic acid appears to be the rate-determining reaction of cholesterol formation. Through a series of condensation reactions, mevalonic acid is transformed into the long-chain hydrocarbon squalene, which in another sequence of reactions is cyclized and transformed into cholesterol.[194]

Cholesterol exerts a feedback inhibition on its own synthesis in the liver.[196-199] The site of feedback inhibition is primarily at the conversion of HMG CoA to mevalonic acid, which is mediated by an enzyme, HMG CoA reductase. The mechanisms by which this inhibition are mediated have not been determined fully. Both allosteric inhibition of the enzyme and reduction of enzyme synthesis are probably involved. Also, the specific agent responsible for feedback inhibition is disputed; while it is thought generally that cholesterol itself is the major inhibitory factor, oxygenated products of cholesterol (for example, 25-hydroxy-cholesterol and 7-keto-cholesterol have also been found to actively inhibit HMG CoA reductase.[200-203] Whether these latter products are important physiologically remains to be determined.

Although cholesterol derived from chylomicron remnants clearly inhibits hepatic synthesis, the feedback potential for cholesterol from other sources has been a matter of dispute. Newly synthesized cholesterol almost certainly is locally active in feedback regulation; cholesterol delivered by other plasma lipoproteins may also be inhibitory. High levels of plasma cholesterol *per se* are not necessarily associated with a marked reduction in cholesterol synthesis; in familial hypercholesterolemia, for example, total body synthesis of cholesterol is not suppressed.[204-207] It is conceivable that chylomicron cholesterol is more potent than cholesterol from other lipoproteins in feedback regulation. Earlier studies suggested that cholesterol in different lipoprotein species may vary in potency for feedback inhibition,[208] but these studies are difficult to interpret.

Rates of hepatic cholesterogenesis depend on several factors besides feedback regulation by cholesterol itself. One factor may be bile acids. The role of bile acids in regulating synthesis of hepatic cholesterol is controversial and probably is complex. Bile acids may influence cholesterol synthesis in at least 3 ways: (1) Since bile acids affect cholesterol absorption, they indirectly affect cholesterol synthesis by influencing the amount of cholesterol returning to the liver in chylomicrons.[199,209,210] (2) Bile acids suppress their own synthesis from cholesterol.[4,211] This inhibition should increase concentrations of cholesterol in the hepatocyte and the latter, in turn, should feed back on cholesterol synthesis. (3) Bile acids may directly interfere with some step in the biosynthesis of cholesterol,[4,211] although this mechanism is doubted by some investigators. In any case, bile acids probably affect cholesterol synthesis by more than a single mechanism.

Finally, synthesis of cholesterol in the liver depends on food intake. Production rates during feeding exceed those during fasting; this may reflect availability of dietary substrate.[214-216] Chronically high intakes of calories, when associated with obesity, also cause overproduction of cholesterol.[217-220] Restriction of calories in obese patients reduces cholesterol synthesis.[217] Whether the saturation of dietary fatty acids, independent of total fat intake, influences cholesterol synthesis is unresolved. Polyunsaturated fatty acids can increase cholesterol synthesis in some patients[221]; this effect, however, is not universal.

Hepatic cholesterol can have 3 fates: (1) a portion can be converted to bile acids, (2) another portion can be secreted into bile as cholesterol itself, and (3) still another portion can enter plasma with lipoproteins. Transformation of cholesterol to bile acids occurs only in the liver. Normally, about 30% to 50% of the daily production of cholesterol is converted into bile acids. The first step in this conversion—the formation of 7-α-hydroxycholesterol—is the rate-limiting step. A second fate of hepatic cholesterol is direct secretion into bile. In the steady state, when extrahepatic pools of cholesterol are constant, biliary cholesterol is equivalent to newly synthesized cholesterol plus that recycled from the intestine. In adults of normal weight, daily secretion rates of biliary cholesterol range from 800 to 1200 mg.[169] Finally, the remaining hepatic cholesterol is incorporated into lipoproteins. The amount secreted with lipoproteins probably is about 1000 mg/day.

Biliary Secretion. The detailed mechanisms whereby cholesterol enters the bile are in dispute. In general terms, cholesterol in bile is solubilized by mixed micelles containing bile acids and lecithin. The ways in which mixed micelles form are not well understood. Studies in several animal species have shown that biliary secretion of lecithin is closely linked to outputs of bile acids[222-227]; this connection can be attributed entirely to the ability of bile acids to form micelles and not to their enhancement of bile flow. Other studies in experimental animals and in man indicate that cholesterol secretion, in turn, is linked to outputs of lecithin. These relationships can pehaps be explained best by assuming that bile acids are secreted into bile canaliculi and thereafter leach cholesterol and lecithin out of canalicular membranes. If this mechanism does pertain, the composition of lipids in bile should depend on several factors, including availability of bile acids, types of bile acids present, and the composition of the canalicular membranes. When adequate amounts of bile acids are available, they take up membranous lecithin in relatively constant ratios. Lecithin/bile acid ratios are similar for all species. Amounts of cholesterol in bile micelles, however, are not the same for all species.[222-227] Presumably, the ratio of cholesterol to lecithin in canalicular membranes varies according to species. The ratio is particularly high in man. Consequently, humans produce biliary micelles containing more cholesterol than do most other species.

Supersaturated Bile. Since humans often have large amounts of cholesterol in the micelles of bile, the danger of cholesterol crystallization is high. If amounts of cholesterol exceed the solubilizing capacity of bile acids and lecithin, the bile becomes overloaded with cholesterol; in this situation the chances for gallstone formation increase[228,229] (Chapter 179). Bile containing more cholesterol than can be solubilized readily by available bile acids and lecithin is called supersaturated or "lithogenic" bile. Supersaturated bile can arise in at least 3 ways. First, there may be a deficiency of bile acids in the enterohepatic circuit (EHC).[230-232] Second, biliary secretion of cholesterol can be excessive.[217,230,233] And third, secretion of cholesterol in the fasting state may be disproportionately high relative to outputs of the solubilizing lipids.[227] Any of these factors, or combinations of them, can increase the risk for cholesterol gallstones. Each is considered in detail in Chapter 179. Only the essentials are summarized here.

BILE ACID DEFICIENCY. A reduction in pool size of bile acids has been found in many patients with cholesterol stones, for which defective regulation of bile acid synthesis appears most likely.[230] Normally, losses of bile acids by fecal excretion are readily replaced by newly synthesized bile acids. This is accomplished by efficient feedback regulation. Some patients, however, have a sluggish response; a fall in the bile acid pool in these patients does not evoke sufficient new synthesis to re-expand the pool to normal levels. These patients thus have chronically low pools of bile acids, which may predispose them to supersaturated bile and gallstone disease.

INCREASED SECRETION OF CHOLESTEROL. Another cause of supersaturated bile is excessive secretion of biliary cholesterol,[217,230,233] the major cause for which is increased whole body synthesis. The most common cause of overproduction of cholesterol is a high caloric intake associated with obesity.[218-220] The long-recognized association between obesity and gallstones may be explained by a high total body synthesis of cholesterol.[217] All cases of increased biliary cholesterol, however, are not due to obesity. Certain genetic forms of hypertriglyceridemia without obesity may be associated with increased synthesis and thus enhanced biliary secretion of cholesterol.[234-236] Pregnancy may be another cause of excess biliary cholesterol.

INFLUENCE OF FASTING ON BILIARY LIPID COMPOSITION. In several animal species (e.g., dogs, rats, and monkeys) biliary cholesterol outputs are linked tightly to those of lecithin over a wide range of bile acid secretion rates.[222-224] A tight coupling of cholesterol and lecithin, however, does not always exist in man (Fig. 97–13); when outputs of bile acids decline during fasting, owing to storage of bile acids in the gallbladder, bile saturation can increase strikingly. The result is a diurnal variation in biliary lipid composition, with bile being more saturated during fasting than in the feeding state.[237]

The diurnal variation in the biliary lipid composition of humans is greater than in other species. This is most likely explained by variation in the composition of the canalicular membrane during the day and night. The controlling factor may be synthesis of biliary lecithin. During the day, when food is being ingested, the flux of bile acids through the liver is high; at this time the production of lecithin seemingly is at a maximum, and the cholesterol/lecithin ratio likewise is lowest. During prolonged fasting the stimulus for lecithin synthesis is reduced; consequently, the formation of lecithin declines. The amount of cholesterol entering the canalicular membrane, in contrast, may not be so tightly dependent on caloric intake and bile acid flux. For example, it may not be tied closely to the diurnal variation in cholesterol synthesis. The plasma cholesterol may be a continuous source of hepatic cholesterol, even during the night. As a result, biliary cholesterol outputs do not decline markedly during fasting. This causes a rise in the ratio of cholesterol to lecithin with fasting. Saturation of bile, in turn, increases.[227]

The degree of increase in bile saturation during fasting is variable. Some people develop more supersaturated bile than others. This variability depends on several factors. Patients with low pools of bile acids have unusually great reductions in secretion of bile acids with fasting.[227] The increase in saturation during fasting consequently is accentuated in these people. Obese patients, on the other hand, have increased availability of cholesterol; they too have a marked increase in saturation during the night. Types of bile acids in the EHC may also affect the composition of bile. Cholic acid seemingly mobilizes cholesterol from the liver better than does chenodeoxycholic acid.[238] Saturation of bile, therefore, is greater when cholic acid predominates in bile. Other factors must also affect the composition of bile during fasting. These have not been elucidated, however, but they could be important in the pathogenesis of cholesterol gallstones.

Secretion of biliary cholesterol in humans thus appears more complex than in many animals. This complexity is probably due to the necessity to dispose of relatively more cholesterol. In contrast to certain animals such as the dog and rat, humans do not have the same ability to transform cholesterol into bile acids; while dogs and rats convert about two thirds of each day's production of cholesterol into bile acids, man converts only about one third. Humans hence are forced to excrete most of

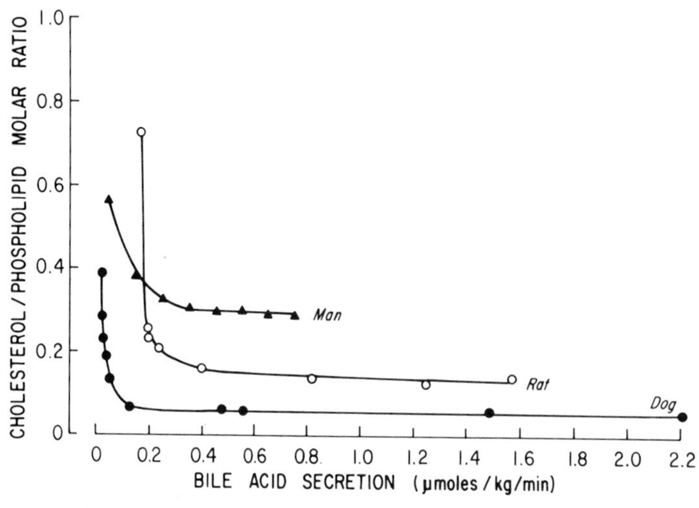

Figure 97–13. Cholesterol:phospholipid molar ratios at various rates of bile acid output in different species. In dogs, there is a tight coupling of cholesterol to lecithin over a wide range of bile acid outputs. Only at very low outputs does uncoupling occur. Rats show a similar pattern except that uncoupling occurs at higher outputs. In man, the cholesterol:phospholipid ratio is still higher and uncoupling occurs at even higher secretion rates of bile acids.

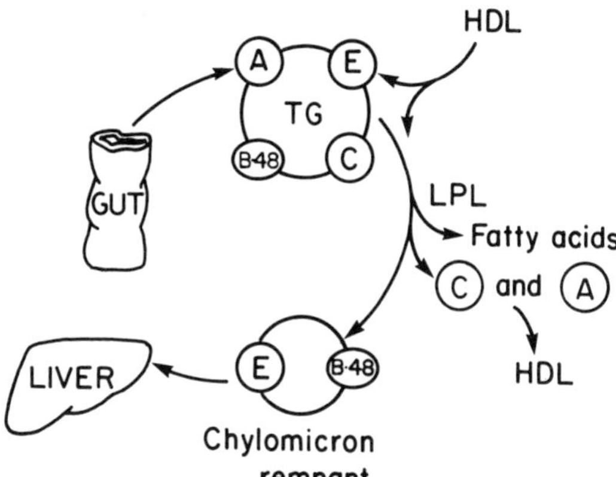

Figure 97–14. Metabolism of chylomicrons. Chylomicrons contain mainly triglycerides (TG) in their lipid core. They contain several apolipoprotein species in their surface coat. Apo A-1 is secreted by the intestine, as is apo B-48. The apo Es and apo Cs appear to be derived from HDL. Chylomicrons interact with lipoprotein lipase (LPD) to release fatty acids. The apo Cs and As are also released and return to HDL. The result is a chylomicron remnant that contains newly absorbed cholesterol ester (and small amounts of TG) along with apo B-48 and the apo Es. The chylomicron remnant is removed from the circulation by the liver.

their excess body cholesterol as cholesterol itself rather than as bile acids. This "species defect" in transformation of cholesterol into bile acids leads to an overloading of the efficient lecithin-dependent secretion of cholesterol. Most people can cope with the usual loads of newly synthesized and dietary cholesterol, but their mechanisms for solubilizing cholesterol are of marginal effectiveness; any slight deviation, because of either increased cholesterol synthesis or reduction of bile acid pools, leads to supersaturation and frequently to cholesterol gallstones.

Lipoprotein Metabolism

Since lipids are insoluble in aqueous solutions, they cannot circulate freely in plasma; instead, they are complexed with specialized proteins called apoproteins. The resulting lipid-apoprotein complexes are designated *lipoproteins.* The lipoproteins are composed of a central core of neutral lipids (cholesterol esters and triglycerides) and a membranous coating of unesterified cholesterol, phospholipids, and apoproteins. The lipoproteins, or their precursors, are produced in both the liver and the gut. In the following discussion the metabolism of the major lipoproteins will be considered.

Chylomicrons. Fatty acids and monoglycerides taken up by the intestinal mucosa are resynthesized into triglycerides. Mucosal triglycerides, along with any absorbed cholesterol, are incorporated into large lipoproteins called *chylomicrons.* The major "structural" apoprotein of chylomicrons is a form of apolipoprotein B designated B-48.[239] Most soluble apoproteins, apo As, Cs, and Es, have also been identified with chylomicrons. The metabolism of chylomicrons is outlined in Figure 97–14. These particles are secreted into intestinal lymph, enter the blood stream through the thoracic duct, and pass in peripheral capillary beds. At the surface of capillary endothelial cells, they come into contact with an enzyme, lipoprotein lipase, which hydrolyzes triglycerides to fatty acids and glycerol. During lipolysis, soluble apoproteins and surface components of chylomicrons are released into the circulation, where they are taken up by other lipoproteins. When lipolysis is almost complete, a cholesterol-rich residual lipoprotein, called a chylomicron "remnant," is released back into the circulation and is cleared rapidly by the liver.

Very Low Density Lipoproteins (VLDL). Like the gut, the liver secretes triglyceride-rich lipoproteins called VLDL. The metabolism of VLDL is outlined in Figure 97–15. VLDL resemble chylomicrons except that

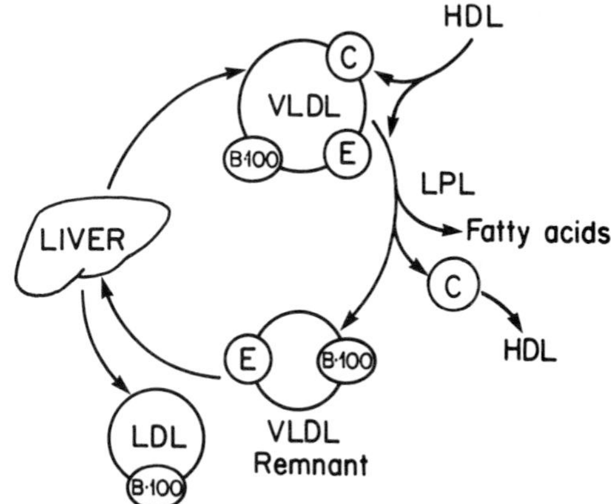

Figure 97–15. Metabolism of VLDL. Triglyceride-rich VLDLs are secreted by the liver. They contain apo B-100. The apo Es may be secreted with VLDL, but more apo E may be derived from HDL. The apo Cs also come from HDL. VLDL-triglycerides undergo lipolysis by lipoprotein lipase (LPL) with formation of a VLDL remnant. The remnants apparently attach to apo E receptors on liver cells. A portion is removed by the liver. The remainder lose their apo E and triglyceride, but return to the circulation as LDL. The almost exclusive apoprotein of LDL is apo B-100.

they are smaller. Also, VLDL contain another form of apolipoprotein B, apo B-100.[239] Since this is the major form of apoprotein B in fasting plasma, it will be designated simply as "apo B." The other apoproteins on circulating VLDL—apo Cs and apo Es—are soluble in plasma and seem to be derived in part from high density lipoproteins (HDL). As VLDL circulate, triglycerides undergo lipolysis. The soluble apoproteins are released into plasma, but apo B stays with the lipoprotein.

Partially catabolized VLDL are called VLDL remnants. They can have 2 fates. Under certain circumstances they are removed by the liver, similar to chylomicron remnants. In the usual course of events, however, most VLDL remnants are transformed to low density lipoproteins (LDL).

Low Density Lipoproteins (LDL). Pathways of formation and removal of LDL are presented in Figure 97–16. The LDL are the major cholesterol-carrying lipoproteins in man. Their core contains mainly cholesterol ester and little triglyceride; their surface coat has only one apoprotein, apo B (B-100). It appears from current evidence that some LDL may be secreted "directly" by the liver, a phenomenon most likely explained by hepatic secretion of very small VLDL (nascent LDL) that are rapidly converted to LDL.

The means of removal of LDL from plasma have been subject to intense investigation.

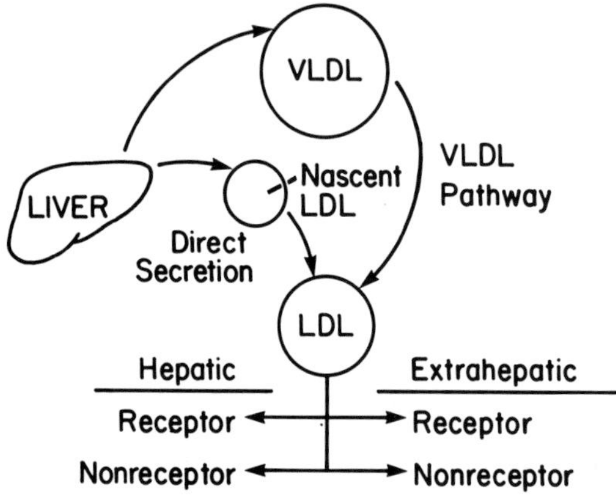

Figure 97–16. Metabolism of LDL. LDL is derived from 2 sources. VLDLs are converted to LDL through the steps shown in Figure 97–15. Another source is "direct" secretion of LDL by the liver; this pathway most likely involves a precursor lipoprotein, nascent LDL. The removal of LDL from plasma occurs by way of either the liver or the extrahepatic tissues. In either, uptake can be through receptor or nonreceptor pathways.

The basic mechanisms have been worked out using tissue cultures. One pathway is a high-affinity, receptor-mediated uptake of LDL by cells.[240] The rate of uptake of LDL by this pathway is a function of the number of binding sites on cells; binding to the LDL receptor is followed by internalization and digestion in lysosomes. The cholesterol esters of LDL are hydrolyzed and released into the cytoplasm; some cholesterol is used for cell membranes. When unesterified cholesterol exceeds the need for cell membranes, the excess cholesterol inhibits the cell's own synthesis of cholesterol; cholesterol is also stored in the cell as inert cholesterol ester. If the cell accumulates more cholesterol than it needs, synthesis of LDL receptors is reduced, thereby decreasing uptake of LDL.

Circulating LDL can be cleared by other means as well. One mechanism is by phagocytosis. This pathway has been called the "scavenger" pathway because it may consist in part of phagocytic cells of the reticuloendothelial system.[240] Nonreceptor removal of LDL may become important when the receptor pathway is saturated by high concentrations of LDL. Several types of nonreceptor pathways actually may participate in LDL catabolism, some of which may not be part of the reticuloendothelial system. Sites of LDL removal in man are not known, but studies in experimental animals indicate that the liver may remove from 40% to 60% of the total. The remainder is taken up by a variety of other tissues.

High Density Lipoproteins (HDL). Cholesterol entering peripheral cells during catabolism of LDL cannot be degraded. Mechanisms must therefore be provided for its return to the liver, where it can be excreted. Although pathways of this "reverse cholesterol transport" have not been defined fully, an attractive concept is that another lipoprotein, HDL, plays an important role. Current concepts of HDL metabolism are presented in Figure 97–17. Formation of HDL is a multistep process that begins in the liver, and, to a lesser extent, in the intestine and is completed in the plasma. Both the liver and the gut apparently produce a particle called "nascent" HDL.[241,242] This particle is disc-shaped and composed mainly of apoproteins (A-I, A-II, and E) and phospholipids. It has an affinity for unesterified cholesterol, which is removed from either cell membranes or other lipoproteins. Cholesterol transferred to

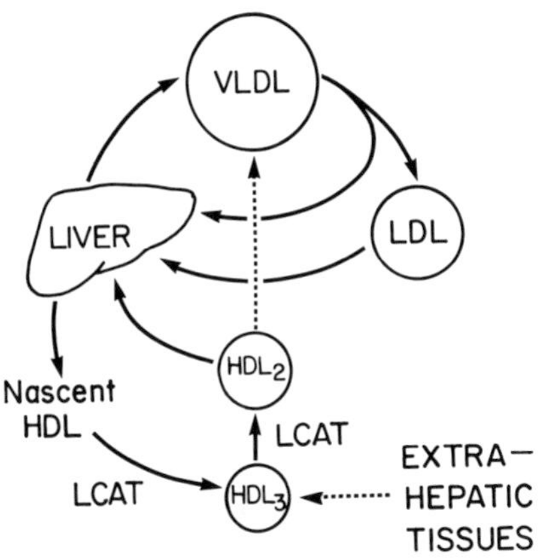

Figure 97–17. Pathways of HDL metabolism. The precursor for circulating HDL appears to be nascent HDL; this lipoprotein is produced mainly in the liver and, to a lesser extent, by the intestine. Nascent HDL takes up unesterified cholesterol from extrahepatic tissues (and from other lipoproteins). Esterification of cholesterol through action of the enzyme LCAT leads to the formation of the small particle HDL_3. Further uptake of cholesterol produces the larger HDL_2. Cholesterol in HDL_2 may return to the liver by several pathways: HDL_2 may be taken up directly by the liver; alternatively, HDL-cholesterol is transferred to VLDL, where it can return to the liver by way of VLDL remnants (or LDL).

HDL undergoes esterification with a fatty acid through a reaction catalyzed by lecithin-cholesterol acyltransferase (LCAT)[243]; the enzyme is so named because it transfers an acyl group (fatty acid) from lecithin to cholesterol. LCAT is activated by apo A-I. As cholesterol ester is formed, it moves into the core of HDL and thereby imparts a spherical shape to the lipoprotein. The product of this sequence is thought to be a small form of HDL (HDL_3).

HDL_3 interacts with other lipoproteins. For example, in the catabolism of triglyceride-rich lipoproteins (chylomicrons and VLDL), surface components (unesterified cholesterol, phospholipids, and C and E apoproteins) are transferred to the surface coat of HDL.[244] HDL can also transfer some of its cholesterol ester to VLDL in exchange for triglycerides.[245] In these multiple reactions, HDL_3 appears to be converted to a larger particle, HDL_2. The fate of HDL is poorly understood; whether it is removed intact from the circulation has not been determined. It can, however, return its cholesterol back to the liver by first transferring it to VLDL; the latter can transport cholesterol to the liver by the mechanisms outlined earlier.

Hyperlipoproteinemia

An increase in plasma lipoproteins can result from metabolic abnormalities of genetic origin, from dietary excess, or from secondary disease. The following discussion reviews the causes (as they are understood), the clinical manifestations, and the appropriate therapy for the different categories of hyperlipoproteinemia (HLP).

Genetic Hyperlipoproteinemias

Primary Type 1 HLP. This phenotype is characterized by a marked increase in circulating chylomicrons. Most cases are caused by *familial deficiency of lipoprotein lipase.*[246] In this disorder, plasma triglyceride levels usually are in the range of 2000 to 5000 mg/dl. Because of an absence of lipoprotein lipase, chylomicrons cannot be cleared from plasma. The defect is present from birth and usually becomes clinically apparent in infancy or early childhood. Clinical manifestations are eruptive skin xanthomas, lipemia retinalis, and acute pancreatitis. Premature atherosclerosis is not a feature of this disease. Plasma concentrations of LDL and HDL are reduced, often markedly. Levels of VLDL are either normal or mildly increased. The major danger of this condition is pancreatitis, which is the result of severely elevated chylomicrons. The only effective therapy is removal of most of the fat from the diet; best results are obtained when the diet contains less than 15% of total calories as fat.

Primary Type 2 HLP. An elevation of LDL is the feature of this type of HLP. The most striking increases of LDL are found in *familial hypercholesterolemia.*[246] Patients with this disorder have marked hypercholesterolemia, tendon xanthomas, and premature atherosclerosis. Clinical atherosclerotic disease often occurs in the second or third decades of life. The disease manifests autosomal dominant inheritance. Heterozygotes are relatively common, about 1/500 people, but homozygotes are rare, about 1/1 million people. Total plasma cholesterol in heterozygotes ranges from 350 to 500 mg/dl; the excess cholesterol is mainly in LDL. VLDL are normal or sometimes slightly increased, while HDL concentrations are often low.

The primary defect in familial hypercholesterolemia is a deficiency of LDL receptors on the surface of cells.[247] Clearance of LDL consequently is reduced. For unexplained reasons, the production of LDL can also be increased, accentuating the hypercholesterolemia. Currently, the best treatment is a combination of cholesterol-lowering drugs. Bile acid sequestrants are the first choice. The second drug can be nicotinic acid,[247] neomycin,[248] or probucol.[249] An alternative to bile acid sequestrants for interrupting the EHC of bile acids is the ileal exclusion operation.[250]

The most common cause of primary type 2 HLP is *polygenic hypercholesterolemia.* This term encompasses a group of related disorders in which concentrations of LDL are increased.[251,252] The disorder constitutes approximately 85% of all cases of primary hypercholesterolemia. Decreased clearance of LDL may be the major defect, although overproduction of LDL also may contribute.[253] Epidemiologic data indicate that the risk for coronary heart disease (CHD) in patients with polygenic hypercholesterolemia is increased 2 to 4 times over that of people with cholesterol concentrations in the low-normal range.[254] Patients with polygenic hypercholesterolemia should be treated first with a diet low in saturated fats and cholesterol.[255] Those who do not respond adequately can then be treated with bile acid sequestrants or, alternatively, with nicotinic acid, neomycin, or probucol.

Some patients with the type 2 phenotype will have *familial combined hyperlipidemia.*[251,252] These patients show increases in either LDL alone (type 2a HLP) or in both LDL and VLDL (type 2b HLP). To confirm the diagnosis, multiple lipoprotein phenotypes must be found in the same family. Type 2a patients with familial combined hyperlipidemia can be treated as are those with polygenic hypercholesterolemia. In those with type 2b, nicotinic acid should be a particularly good drug because it lowers both VLDL and LDL.[256] This drug also reduces the overproduction of lipoproteins, which seems to be the underlying defect of this disorder.

Primary Type 3 HLP. The primary form of the type 3 phenotype is *familial dysbetalipoproteinemia.*[257] This pattern is caused in part by poor catabolism of VLDL. Accumulation of VLDL remnants, called beta-VLDL, results. Chylomicron remnants can also be elevated. The genetic abnormality in most cases is a deficiency in one of the isoforms of apoprotein E, namely, apo E-3. This apoprotein seemingly is required for normal conversion of VLDL remnants to LDL and for the rapid removal of chylomicron remnants from the circulation. Actually, deficiency of apo E-3 is relatively common, being present in about 1% of the population.[257] Clinical hyperlipidemia, however, is much rarer, occurring in about 0.01%. The development of hyperlipidemia seemingly requires overproduction of VLDL, as well as deficiency of apo E-3.[258] Increased production of VLDL can be due to a primary disorder, such as familial combined hyperlipidemia, or to secondary overproduction, as occurs in obesity and diabetes mellitus. Atherosclerotic disease, especially peripheral vascular disease, almost certainly is accelerated in type 3 HLP. Without VLDL overproduction and hyperlipidemia, a mild increase in remnants of VLDL and chylomicrons has not been shown to impart greater risk for atherosclerotic disease.[246] The treatment of type 3 HLP is aimed at decreasing production and promoting clearance of the abnormal lipoproteins. Fibric acid derivatives will enhance clearance of remnants. Decreased synthesis of VLDL can be obtained by nicotinic acid in patients with primary overproduction, by insulin in diabetics, and by weight reduction in obese patients.

Primary Type 4 HLP. This form of hyperlipidemia is associated with an increase only of VLDL. Several different genetic diseases can cause this pattern. Most are not well classified because their metabolic defects have not been determined.

One important disorder responsible for the type 4 phenotype is *familial combined hyperlipidemia.*[251,252] It is characterized by multiple lipoprotein phenotypes in the same family. Some family members have increased VLDL; others have elevated LDL; still others have increases in both lipoproteins. This disorder usually does not become manifest until adulthood. Xanthomas rarely occur, but patients are at increased risk for CHD regardless of their lipoprotein phenotype. Familial combined hyperlipidemia may be the major cause of atherosclerosis in as many as 10% of cases of premature CHD. The primary metabolic defect appears to be overproduction of apo B.[256] The result is increased input of lipoproteins; newly secreted lipoproteins may enter VLDL or LDL, or both. Patients who have a simultaneous overproduction of apo B and triglycerides will have increased VLDL and elevated triglycerides. Their hypertriglyceridemia is sometimes made worse by a simultaneous defect in clearance of lipoproteins.[236]

When this occurs, the type 5 phenotype can result. When synthesis of triglycerides is low, lipoproteins can enter LDL directly. The result can be hypercholesterolemia, as will be discussed subsequently.

Other families have *pure hypertriglyceridemia* (pure type 4 HLP) in affected members. At least 3 different metabolic defects may be responsible for this familial pattern: (1) Some families appear to have overproduction of both VLDL–apo B and VLDL-triglycerides (VLDL-TG).[259] These families probably share the same basic metabolic defect as do families with familial combined hyperlipidemia, except that none of the family members with pure hypertriglyceridemia has elevated LDL. The hypertriglyceridemia probably is associated with the increased risk for CHD. (2) Another familial form of pure type 4 HLP may be overproduction of VLDL-TG without increased synthesis of VLDL–apo B.[260] (3) Yet another group may have a primary defect in clearance of VLDL-TG.[236] Whether the latter 2 abnormalities impart increased risk for CHD has not been determined; limited data suggest that they do not.[261]

The best approach to treatment of primary type 4 HLP is a matter of dispute. If the hypertriglyceridemia is due in part to other diseases or dietary factors, these should be treated first. For type 4 patients with documented familial combined hyperlipidemia, nicotinic acid is probably the best available drug.[256] This agent specifically interferes with the overproduction of VLDL. If familial combined hyperlipidemia cannot be proved, a decision about therapy must depend on an overall assessment of the patient's risk for coronary disease. Factors favoring the decision to use drugs are: (1) severe hyperlipidemia, (2) a history of premature CHD in the patient or first degree relatives, and (3) a history of hypercholesterolemia in other family members. Again, the preferred drug is nicotinic acid, but if this cannot be tolerated, a fibric acid derivative can be employed. The combination of nicotinic acid and a fibric acid derivative can be useful in some patients with marked hypertriglyceridemia.

Primary Type 5 HLP. The type 5 phenotype indicates an increase in both chylomicrons and VLDL. Several poorly defined defects in clearance of triglyceride-rich lipoproteins may contribute to this pattern. Abnormalities in availability or function of lipoprotein lipase are likely present in most cases. The degree of chylomicronemia can vary, possibly related to the nature of the metabolic defect. An aggravating factor in many patients is a simultaneous overproduction of VLDL. Type 5 patients with severe chylomicronemia are prone to eruptive skin xanthomas and pancreatitis. An increased risk for atherosclerotic disease has not been proved, although peripheral vascular disease seems common. Chylomicronemia in some patients can be cleared with a fibric acid derivative,[262] and a trial with this drug is warranted. Many patients, however, do not respond to drug therapy and must be treated by restriction of fat in the diet. Reduction of fat intakes to as low as 10% to 15% of total calories may be required to prevent development of pancreatitis.

Another cause of primary type 5 HLP is *familial deficiency of apoprotein C-II.*[263] This is a rare disorder in which apo C-II, the apoprotein required for activation of lipoprotein lipase, is genetically absent. Elevated chylomicrons and VLDL are the result; they can be cleared rapidly by IV injection of apo C-II. This, however, is not a practical therapy, and the only available choice is decreased dietary intake of fat.

Secondary Hyperlipoproteinemias

Secondary Hypercholesterolemia. Diseases of several systems produce hypercholesterolemia. The hypercholesterolemia of hypothyroidism results from delayed clearance of LDL. The nephrotic syndrome causes overproduction of both VLDL and LDL; some patients demonstrate increases predominantly in LDL. Elevated plasma levels of LDL can occur in several other states (acute intermittent porphyria, anorexia nervosa, and Cushing's syndrome), but the pathogenesis of the hypercholesterolemia in these conditions has not been determined. Patients with dysglobulinemias of various types can produce autoantibodies that uniquely interact with LDL and cause its retention in plasma. In obstructive liver disease, hypercholesterolemia is the result of accumulation of excess unesterified cholesterol in plasma associated with an abnormal lipoprotein, lipoprotein X.

Secondary Hypertriglyceridemias. These can result from diabetes mellitus, the nephrotic syndrome, rarely dysproteinemia, and sometimes estrogen therapy. Both diabetes mellitus and the nephrotic syndrome cause overproduction of VLDL.[264] Diabetes may also impart decreased clearance of triglyceride-rich lipoproteins and is present in about 80% of patients with type 5 HLP.[262] Hyperlipidemia induced by diabetes and the nephrotic syndrome probably causes increased atherosclerotic disease.

Diet-Induced Hyperlipidemias

Diet-Induced Hypercholesterolemia. Several dietary factors can raise plasma LDL: saturated fatty acids, cholesterol, and sometimes excess intake of total calories. The diet-induced rise in LDL may be sufficient to enhance risk of CHD.[254] Without associated genetic factors, however, diet alone rarely induces marked hypercholesterolemia. Still, dietary excesses can accentuate polygenic hypercholesterolemia. Indeed, the interaction between genetic factors and diet may be responsible for many cases of hypercholesterolemia in American adults.

Diet-Induced Hypertriglyceridemia. Usual intakes of fat normally cause only mild postprandial chylomicronemia. In contrast, these produce striking hypertriglyceridemia in patients who have a clearance defect for chylomicrons (types 1 and 5 HLP). Dietary fats may also cause a mild but transitory increase in hepatic synthesis of VLDL. Saturated fats raise plasma VLDL somewhat more than do polyunsaturates[221] and perhaps stimulate more synthesis of VLDL. Much greater stimuli for VLDL synthesis are carbohydrates,[265] alcohol, and high intakes of total calories.[266] In normal individuals, overproduction of VLDL due to excess carbohydrates and alcohol causes only mild rises in plasma triglycerides—usually not to abnormal levels. The same is true for obesity.[266] Most patients with so-called "carbohydrate-induced" and "alcohol-induced" hyperlipidemia have a coexisting defect in clearance of VLDL or chylomicrons. Obesity likewise does not cause marked hypertriglyceridemia without a concomitant clearance defect for plasma triglycerides.

Drug Treatment of Hyperlipidemia

Bile Acid Sequestrants. Two nonabsorbable resins are available for bile acid binding, *cholestyramine* and *colestipol.* Both have quaternary amine groups that interact with the acidic moiety of bile acids. When given by mouth, they remove bile acids from the enterohepatic circulation. The result is decreased return of bile acids to the liver, loss of feedback inhibition on bile acid synthesis, and increased conversion of cholesterol to bile acids. Cholesterol concentrations in the liver cell decline, causing increased production of LDL receptors. The liver thereby extracts more LDL from the blood stream[267] and LDL concentrations fall. For reasons not understood, the liver can secrete more VLDL in some patients during resin therapy,[268] and plasma triglycerides may rise. The daily dose of cholestyramine usually is 16 g; for colestipol it is 20 g. Lower doses may be almost as effective in some patients. The major side effect of bile acid sequestrants is constipation.

Nicotinic Acid. This drug lowers both VLDL and LDL. It inhibits the secretion of lipoproteins from the liver,[269] which accounts for its action in reducing both VLDL and LDL. It also retards the mobilization of free fatty acids from adipose tissue and this may partially explain its inhibition of VLDL synthesis. The drug may also interfere directly with hepatic formation or secretion of lipoproteins. Side effects of nicotinic acid are flushing of the skin, pruritus, skin rashes, abdominal distress when taken between meals, occasional hepatic dysfunction, and worsening of glucose tolerance in diabetics. The dose required for maximum lipid lowering is in the range of 3 to 6 g/day. The drug should be started in low doses and increased gradually as tolerated by the patient. The flushing phenomenon often can be mitigated by low dose aspirin.

Fibric Acid Derivatives. Drugs of this type currently available in the United States are *clofibrate* and *gemfibrozil.* Their major action is to lower VLDL levels. Clofibrate accelerates VLDL clearance by activating lipoprotein lipase.[256] Gemfibrozil has the same effect, but it also inhibits secretion of VLDL; this combined action possibly makes gemfibrozil the better drug for lowering plasma triglycerides in some patients. Various other fibric acid derivatives are being tested in the United States or are being used in other countries. The actions of these related drugs are similar but not identical. For example, some have a greater potential for lowering LDL than others. In general, however, none reduces concentrations of LDL as well as does nicotinic acid. Indeed, the fibric acids actually raise LDL in some patients. The drugs generally are safe, but side effects can occur, including abdominal discomfort, myalgia with a high serum creatine phosphokinase, and cholesterol gallstones. The last results from induction of supersaturated bile secondary to increased biliary cholesterol and decreased bile acid secretion.[270]

Neomycin. This antibiotic lowers LDL when given in doses of 2 g/day. The primary action of neomycin at this dose is to inhibit the absorption of cholesterol,[271] probably by disrupting intestinal micelles carrying cholesterol and thereby making cholesterol unavailable for absorption. At higher doses, neomycin can interfere with absorption of bile acids. The major side effect is gastrointestinal distress, which may be secondary to changes in the large bowel flora. Only trace amounts of neomycin are absorbed, and hearing impairment has not been documented. The possibility of hearing loss, however, must be kept in mind and checked for periodically.

Plant Sterols. The plant sterols are closely related in structure to cholesterol and when given by mouth compete with cholesterol for its absorption. Intestinal absorption of both dietary and biliary cholesterol is inhibited.[272] Decreased absorption of cholesterol lowers plasma LDL. The major plant sterol is *sitosterol.* The most effective dose of sitosterol for lowering plasma cholesterol is uncertain. The optimum dose may be as low as 3 g/day, but most investigations have been done with doses of 10 to 18 g/day. The plant sterols apparently are free of significant side effects. However, this is not true in a rare inherited disorder in which sitosterol is particularly efficiently absorbed, leading to elevated plasma levels of sitosterol, xanthomatosis, and possibly premature atherosclerosis.[171]

Probucol. The major action of probucol is to decrease LDL concentrations. It has little, if any, effect on the metabolism of cholesterol or bile acids. The drug promotes clearance of LDL from the circulation. It has no effect on VLDL levels, but HDL concentrations fall, together with LDL. Whether the latter change is detrimental is unknown. The dose of probucol is 500 mg twice daily. Few side effects have been reported.

References

1. Bloch K, Berg BN, Rittenberg D. The biological conversion of cholesterol to cholic acid. J Biol Chem 1943; 149:511–7.
2. Siperstein MD, Jayko ME, Chaikoff IL. Nature of the metabolic products of C^{14}-cholesterol excreted in bile and feces. Proc Soc Exp Biol Med 1952; 81:720–4.
3. Bergstrom S. The formation of bile acids from cholesterol in the rat. K Fysiografiska Sallskapets Forhandlingar (Lund) 1952; 22:91–6.
4. Dietschy JM, Wilson JD. Regulation of cholesterol metabolism. N Engl J Med 1970; 282:1128–38.
5. Rudman D, Kendall FE. Bile acid content of human serum. I. Serum bile acids in patients with hepatic disease. J Clin Invest 1957; 36:530–7.
6. Back PT. Identification and quantitative determination of urinary bile acids excreted in cholestasis. Clin Chim Acta 1973; 44:199–207.
7. Rudman D, Kendall FE. Bile acid content of human serum. II. The binding of cholanic acids by human plasma proteins. J Clin Invest 1957; 36:538–42.
8. Kramer W, Buscher P, Gerok W, Kurg G. Bile salt binding to serum components. Eur J Biochem 1979; 102:1–9.
9. Weiner IM, Glasser E, Lack L. Renal excretion of bile acids: Taurocholic, glycocholic, and cholic acids. Am J Physiol 1964; 207:1439–55.
10. Zins JR, Weiner IM. Bidirectional transport of taurocholate by the proximal tubule of the dog. Am J Physiol 1968; 215:840–5.
11. Barnes S, Gollan JL, Billing BH. The role of tubular reabsorption in the renal excretion of bile acids. Biochem J 1977; 166:65–73.
12. Summerfield JA, Billing BH, Schacleton CHL. Identification of bile acids in the serum and urine of cholestasis. Evidence for 6 α-hydroxylation of bile acids in man. Biochem J 1976; 154:507–16.
13. Thomassen PA. Urinary bile acids during development of recurrent cholestasis of pregnancy. Eur J Clin Invest 1979; 9:417–23.
14. Go VLW, Hofmann AF, Summerskill WHJ. Pancreozymin bioassay in man based on pancreatic enzyme secretion: Potency of specific amino acids and other digestive products. J Clin Invest 1970; 49:1558–64.
15. Meyer JH, Kelly GA. Canine pancreatic responses to intestinally perfused proteins and protein digests. Am J Physiol 1976; 231:682–91.
16. Malagelada JR, Go VLW, DiMagno EP, Summerskill WHJ. Interactions between intraluminal bile acids and digestive products on pancreatic and gallbladder function. J Clin Invest 1973; 52:2160–5.
17. Admirand WH, Small DM. The physico-chemical basis of cholesterol gallstone formation in man. J Clin Invest 1968; 47:1043–52.
18. Simmonds WJ, Hofmann AF, Theodor E. Absorption of cholesterol from a micellar solution: Intestinal perfusion studies in man. J Clin Invest 1967; 46:874–90.
19. Siperstein MD, Chaikoff IL, Reinhardt WO. C^{14} cholesterol. V. Obligatory function of bile in intestinal absorption of cholesterol. J Biol Chem 1952; 198:111–4.
20. Deuel HJ. The Lipids, Their Chemistry and Biochemistry. Vol 2. New York: Interscience Publishers, 1955:282.
21. Forsgren L. Studies on the intestinal absorption of labeled fat soluble vitamins (A, D, E and K) via the thoracic duct lymph in the absence of bile in man. Acta Chir Scand 1969; 399(Suppl):1–29.
22. Hofmann AF, Borgstrom B. The intraluminal phase of fat digestion in man. The lipid content of the micellar and oil phases of intestinal content obtained during fat digestion and absorption. J Clin Invest 1964; 43:247–57.
23. Hofmann AF, Small DM. Detergent properties of bile salts. Correlation with physiological function. Ann Rev Med 1967; 18:333–76.
24. Austad WI, Lack L, Tyor MP. Importance of bile acids and of an intact distal small intestine for fat absorption. Gastroenterology 1967; 52:638–46.
25. Heaton KW, Austad WI, Lack L, Tyor MP. Enterohepatic circulation of C^{14}-labeled bile salts in disorders of the distal small bowel. Gastroenterology 1968; 55:5–16.
26. Lindstedt S. The turnover of cholic acid in man. Acta Physiol Scand 1957; 40:1–9.
27. Borgstrom B, Dahlquist A, Lundh G, Sjovall J. Studies of intestinal digestion and absorption in the human. J Clin Invest 1957; 36:1521–36.
28. Connor WE, Witiak DT, Stone DB, Armstrong ML. Cholesterol balance and fecal neutral steroid and bile acid excretion in normal man fed dietary fats of different fatty acid composition. J Clin Invest 1969; 48:1363–75.

29. Grundy SM, Ahrens EH Jr. Measurements of cholesterol turnover, synthesis and absorption in man, carried out by isotope kinetic and sterol balance methods. J Lipid Res 1969; 10:91–107.
30. Moore RB, Anderson JT, Taylor HL, Keys A, Frantz ID Jr. Effect of dietary fat on the fecal excretion of cholesterol and its degradation products in man. J Clin Invest 1968; 47:1517–34.
31. Bergstrom S. Metabolism of bile acids. Fed Proc 1962; 21(Suppl 11):28–32.
32. Smallwood RA, Lester R, Piasecki GJ, Klein PD, Greco R, Jackson BT. Fetal bile salt metabolism. II. Hepatic excretion of endogenous bile salt and of a taurocholate load. J Clin Invest 1972; 51:1388–97.
33. Little, JM, Smallwood RA, Lester R, Piasecki GJ, Jackson BT. Bile salt metabolism in the primate fetus. Gastroenterology 1975; 69:1315–20.
34. Watkins JB, Szczepanik P, Gould JB, Klein P, Lester R. Bile salt metabolism in the human premature infant. Gastroenterology 1975; 69:706–13.
35. Watkins JB, Ingall D, Szczepanik P, Klein P, Lester R. Pool size and synthesis of bile salts in the newborn. N Engl J Med 1973; 288:431–4.
36. Lester R, Smallwood RA, Little JM. Fetal bile salt metabolism—intestinal absorption of bile salt. J Clin Invest 1977; 59:1009–16.
37. Little JM, Lester R. Ontogenesis of intestinal bile salt metabolism absorption in the neonatal rat. Am J Physiol 1980; 239:G319–23.
38. Dietschy JM. Mechanisms for the intestinal absorption of bile acids. J Lipid Res 1968; 9:297–309.
39. Dowling RH. The enterohepatic circulation. Gastroenterology 1972; 62:122–40.
40. Tyor MP, Garbutt JT, Lack L. Metabolism and transport of bile salts in the intestine. Am J Med 1971; 51:614–26.
41. Weiner IM, Lack L. Bile salt absorption: Enterohepatic circulation. *In*: Code CF, ed. Handbook of Physiology. Section 6, Alimentary Canal. Washington, DC: American Physiological Society, 1968:1439–55.
42. Matern S, Gerok W. Pathophysiology of the enterohepatic circulation of bile acids. Physiol Biochem Pharmacol 1979; 85:125–204.
43. Gallagher K, Mauskopf J, Walker JT, Lack L. Ionic requirements for the acute ileal bile salt transport system. J Lipid Res 1976; 17:572–7.
44. Bundy R, Mauskopf J, Walker JT, Lack L. Interaction of unchanged bile salt derivatives with the ileal bile salt transport system. J Lipid Res 1977; 18:389–95.
45. Lack L, Weiner LM. In vitro absorption of bile salts by small intestine of rats and guinea pigs. Am J Physiol 1961; 200:313–7.
46. Heaton KW, Lack L. Ileal bile salt transport: Mutual inhibition in an in vivo system. Am J Physiol, 1968; 214:585–90.
47. Dietschy JM, Soloman HS, Siperstein MD. Bile acid metabolism. I. Studies on the mechanism of intestinal transport. J Clin Invest 1966; 45:832–46.
48. Playoust MR, Lack L, Weiner IM. Effect of intestinal resection on bile salt absorption in dogs. Am J Physiol 1965; 208:363–9.
49. Hepner GW, Hofmann, AF, Thomas PJ. Metabolism of steroid and amino acid moieties of conjugated bile acids in man. I. J Clin Invest 1972; 51:1898–1905.
50. Hepner GW, Hofmann, AF, Thomas PJ. Metabolism of steroid and amino acid moieties of conjugated bile acids in man. II. J Clin Invest 1972; 51:1889–97.
51. Hepner GW, Sturman JA, Hofmann AF, Thomas PJ. Metabolism of steroid and amino acid moieties of conjugated bile acids in man. III. J Clin Invest 1973; 52:433–40.
52. Gorbach SL, Tabaqchali S. Bacteria, bile and the small bowel. Gut 1969; 10:963–72.
53. Kalser MH, Cohen R, Arteaga I, Yawn E, Mayoral L, Hoffert WR, Frazier D. Normal viral and bacterial flora of the normal human small and large intestine. N Engl J Med 1966; 274:500–5.
54. Mekhjian HS, Phillips SF, Hofmann AF. Colonic absorption of unconjugated bile acids. Dig Dis Sci 1979; 24:545–50.
55. Sjovall J. Bile acids in man under normal and pathological conditions. Bile acids and steroids 73. Clin Chim Acta 1960; 5:33–41.
56. Sobotka H. Physiological Chemistry of the Bile. Baltimore: William & Wilkins, 1937.
57. Wooten IDP, Wiggins HS. Studies in the bile acids. II. The non-ketotic acids of human bile. Biochem J 1953; 55:292–4.
58. Bergstrom S, Norman A. Metabolic products of cholesterol in bile and feces of rats. Steroids and bile acids. Proc Soc Exp Biol Med 1953; 83:71–4.
59. Gustafsson B, Bergstrom S, Lindstedt S, Norman A. Turnover and nature of fecal bile acids in germ free and infected rats fed cholic acid-24-^{14}C. Bile acids and steroids 41. Proc Soc Exp Biol Med 1957; 94:467–71.
60. Haslewood, GAD. The biological significance of chemical differences in bile salts. Biol Rev 1964; 39:537–74.
61. Garbutt JT, Lack L, Tyor MP: Physiological basis of alterations in the relative conjugation of bile acids with glycine and taurine. Am J Clin Nutr 1971; 24:218–28.
62. Norman A, Grubb A. Hydrolysis of conjugated bile acids by clostridia and enterococci. Acta Pathol Microbiol Scand 1955; 36:537–47.
63. Norman A, Shorb MS. In vitro formation of deoxycholic and lithocholic acid by human intestinal microorganisms. Proc Soc Exp Biol Med 1962; 110:552–5.
64. Aries V, Crowther JS, Drasar BS, Hill MJA. Degradation of bile salts by human intestinal bacteria. Gut 1969; 10:575–6.
65. Gustaffson BE, Midtvedt T, Norman A. Isolated fecal microorganisms capable of 7-α-dehydroxylating bile acids. J Exp Med 1966; 123:413–32.
66. Hill MJ, Drasar BS. Degradation of bile salts by human intestinal bacteria. Gut 1968; 9:22–7.
67. Krag E, Phillips SF. Active and passive bile acid absorption in man. J Clin Invest 1974; 53:1686–94.
68. Vlahcevic ZR, Miller JR, Farrar JT, Swell L. Kinetics and pool size of primary bile acids in man. Gastroenterology 1971; 61:85–90.
69. Vlahcevic ZR, Bell CC Jr, Buhac I, Farrar JT, Swell L. Diminished bile acid pool size in patients with gallstones. Gastroenterology 1970; 59:165–73.
70. Palmer RH. The formation of bile acid sulfates: A new pathway of bile acid metabolism in humans. Proc Nat Acad Sci 1967; 58:1047–50.
71. Low-Beer TS, Tyor MP, Lack L. Effects of sulfation of taurolithocholic and glycolithocholic acids on their intestinal transport. Gastroenterology 1969; 56:721–6.
72. Holsti T. Cirrhosis of the liver induced in rabbits by gastric instillation of 3-monohydroxycholanic acid. Nature (London) 1960; 186:250.
73. Hunt RD. Proliferation of bile ductules (the ductular cell reaction) induced by lithocholic acid. Fed Proc 1965; 24:431 (Abstract).
74. Hunt RD, Leville GA, Sauberlich HE. Dietary bile acid and lipid metabolism. III. Effects of lithocholic acid in mammalian species. Proc Exp Biol Med 1964; 115:277–80.
75. Palmer RH, Hruban Z. Production of bile duct hyperplasia and gallstones by lithocholic acid. J Clin Invest 1966; 45:1255–67.
76. Stolk A. Induction of hepatic cirrhosis in iguana by 3-monohydroxycholanic acid treatment. Exper 1960; 16:507–8.
77. Zaki FG, Carey JB Jr, Hoffbauer FW, Nwokolo C. Biliary reaction and choledocholithiasis induced in the rat by lithocholic acid. J Lab Clin Med 1967; 69:737–48.
78. Palmer RH, Glickman PB, Kappas A. Pyrogenic and inflammatory properties of certain bile acids in man. J Clin Invest 1962; 41:1573–7.
79. Palmer RH, Kappas A. Fever producing action of steroids. Med Clin N Am 1963; 47:101–12.
80. DeWitt EH, Lack L. Effects of sulfation patterns on intestinal transport of bile salt sulfate esters. Am J Physiol 1980; 238:G34–9.
81. Stiehl A. Bile salt sulphates in cholestasis. Eur J Clin Invest 1974; 4:59–63.
82. Abaurre R, Gordon SG, Mann JG, Kern F Jr. Fasting bile salt pool size and composition after ileal resection. Gastroenterology 1969; 57:679–88.

83. Hardison WG, Rosenberg IH. Bile salt deficiency in the steatorrhea following resection of the ileum and proximal colon. N Engl J Med 1967; 277:337–42.
84. Van Deest BW, Fordtran JS, Morawski SG, Wilson JD. Bile salt and micellar fat concentration in proximal small bowel contents of ileectomy patients. J Clin Invest 1968; 47:1314–24.
85. Meihoff WE, Kern F Jr. Bile salt malabsorption in regional ileitis. Ileal resection and mannitol-induced diarrhea. J Clin Invest 1968; 47:261–7.
86. Stanley M, Nemchausky B. Fecal C^{14}-bile acid excretion in normal subjects and patients with steroid wasting syndromes secondary to ileal dysfunction. J Lab Clin Med 1967; 70:627–39.
87. Krone CL, Theodor E, Sleisenger MH, Jeffries G. Studies on the pathogenesis of malabsorption. Medicine (Baltimore) 1968; 47:89–106.
88. McLeod GM, Wiggins HS. Bile salts and small intestinal contents after ileal resection and in other malabsorption syndromes. Lancet 1968; 1:873–6.
89. Garbutt JT, Wilkins RM, Lack L, Tyor MP. Bacterial modification of taurocholate during enterohepatic recirculation in normal man and patients with small intestinal disease. Gastroenterology 1970; 59:553–66.
90. Low-Beer TS, Wilkins RM, Lack L, Tyor MP. Effect of one meal on enterohepatic circulation of bile salts. Gastroenterology 1974; 67:490–7.
91. Woodbury JF, Kern F Jr. Fecal excretion of bile acids: A new technique for studying bile acid kinetics in patients with ileal resection. J Clin Invest 1971; 50:2531–40.
92. Mansbach CM, Garbutt JT, Tyor MP. Bile salt and lipid metabolism in patients with ileal disease with and without steatorrhea. Am J Dig Dis 1972; 12:1089–99.
93. Drasar BS, Shiner M, McLeod GM. Studies on the intestinal flora. I. The bacterial flora of the gastrointestinal tract in healthy and achlorhydric persons. Gastroenterology 1969; 56:71–9.
94. Grundy SM, Ahrens EH Jr, Salen G. Interruption of the enterohepatic circulation of bile acids in man: Comparative effect of cholestyramine and ileal exclusion on cholesterol metabolism. J Lab Clin Med 1971; 78:94–121.
95. Moore RB, Crane CA, Frantz ID Jr. Effect of cholestyramine on the fecal excretion of intravenously administered cholesterol-4-^{14}C and its degradation products in a hypercholesterolemic patient. J Clin Invest 1968; 47:1664–71.
96. Moutafis CD, Myant NB. The metabolism of cholesterol in 2 hypercholesterolemic patients treated with cholestyramine. Clin Sci 1969; 37:433–54.
97. Johns WH, Bates TR. Quantification of the binding tendencies of cholestyramine. I. Effect of structure and added electrolytes on the binding of unconjugated and conjugated bile salt anions. J Pharm Sci 1969; 58:179–83.
98. Garbutt JT, Kenney TJ. Effect of cholestyramine on bile acid metabolism in normal man. J Clin Invest 1972; 51: 2781–9.
99. Wood PD, Schioda R, Estrich DL, Splitter S. Effect of cholestyramine on composition of duodenal bile in obese human subjects. Metabolism 1972; 21:107–16.
100. Van der Linden W, Nakayama F. Change of bile composition in man after administration of cholestyramine (a gallstone dissolving agent in hamsters). Acta Chir Scand 1969; 135:433–8.
101. Danielsson H, Tchen TT. Steroid metabolism. *In:* Greenberg DM, ed. Metabolic Pathways. 3rd Ed. Vol. 2. New York: Academic Press, 1969:117–68.
102. Elliott WH, Hyde PM. Metabolic pathways of bile acid synthesis. Am J Med 1971; 51:568–79.
103. Bergstrom S. Formation and metabolism of bile acids. Bile acids and steroids 20. Recent Chem Prog 1955; 16:63–83.
104. Danielsson H, Einarsson K, Johansson G. Effect of biliary drainage on individual reaction in the conversion of cholesterol to taurocholic acid. Eur J Biochem 1967; 2:44–9.
105. Shefer S, Hauser S, Berkersky I, Mosbach EH. Feedback regulation of bile acid biosynthesis in the rat. J Lipid Res 1969; 10:646–55.
106. Shefer S, Hauser S, Berkersky I, Mosbach EH. Biochemical site of regulation of bile acid biosynthesis in the rat. J Lipid Res 1970; 11:404–11.
107. Anfinsen CB, Horning MG. Enzymatic degradation of the cholesterol side chain in cell free preparations. J Am Chem Soc 1953; 75:1511–12.
108. Danielsson H. On the oxidation of cholesterol in liver mitochondrial preparations. Acta Chim Scand 1960; 14:846–60.
109. Mendelsohn D, Staple E. The in vitro catabolism of cholesterol: Formation of 3-alpha, 7-alpha, 12-alpha-trihydroxycoprostane from cholesterol in rat liver. Biochemistry 1963; 2:577–9.
110. Gielen J, van Cantfort J, Robaye B, Renson J. Rat-liver cholesterol 7-α-hydroxylase. Eur J Biochem 1975; 55:41–8.
111. Nicolau G, Shefer S, Salen G, Mosbach EH. Determination of hepatic cholesterol 7-α-hydroxylase activity in man. J Lipid Res 1974; 15:146–51.
112. Boyd GS, Percy-Robb IW. Enzymatic regulation of bile acid synthesis. Am J Med 1971; 51:580–7.
113. Boyd GS, Brownie AC, Jefcoate CR, Simpson ER. Cholesterol hydroxylation in the adrenal cortex and liver. Biochem J 1971; 125:1P–2P.
114. Reddinger RN, Small DM. The effect of phenobarbital on bile salt metabolism and cholesterol secretion in the primate. J Clin Invest 1971; 50:76 (Abstract).
115. Boyd GS, Mitton JR, Simpson ER, Sulimovici SI. The hydroxylation of cholesterol by various mammalian tissues. Proceedings of the Seventh International Congress in Biochemistry. Ed V-2. 1967; 461–2.
116. Boyd GS, Scholan NA, Mitton JR. Factors influencing cholesterol 7-alpha-hydroxylase activity in the rat liver. *In:* Holmes WL, Carlson LA, Paoeletti R, eds. Proceedings of the Third International Symposium on Drugs Affecting Lipid Metabolism, Milan. New York: Plenum Press, 1969: 443–56.
117. Bergstrom S, Danielsson H. On the regulation of bile acid formation in the rat liver. Acta Physiol Scand 1958; 43:1–7.
118. Dowling RH, Mack E, Small DM. Effects of controlled interruption of the enterohepatic circulation of bile salts by biliary division and by ileal resection on bile salt secretion, synthesis and pool size in the Rhesus monkey. J Clin Invest 1970; 49:232–42.
119. Killenbeg PG. Measurement and subcellular distribution of choloyl-CoA synthetase and bile acid-CoA: Amino acid N-acyltransferase activities in rat liver. J Lipid Res 1978; 19:24–31.
120. Killenberg PG, Jordan JT. Purification and characterization of bile acid-CoA: Amino acid N-acyltransferase from rat liver. J Biol Chem 1978; 253:1005–10.
121. Bremer J. Species differences in the conjugation of free bile acids with taurine and glycine. Biochem J 1956; 63:507–13.
122. Bjorkhem I, Danielsson H, Einarsson K, Johansson G. Formation of bile acids in man: Conversion of cholesterol into 5-beta-cholestane-3 alpha, 7 alpha, 12 alpha-triol. J Clin Invest 1968; 47:1573–82.
123. Anderson KE, Kok E, Javitt NB. Bile acid synthesis in man: Metabolism of 7-α-hydroxycholesterol-^{14}C and 26-hydroxycholesterol-^{3}H. J Clin Invest 1972, 51:112–7.
124. Carey JB Jr. Conversion of cholesterol to trihydroxycoprostanic acid and cholic acid in man. J Clin Invest 1964; 43:1443–8.
125. Hanson RF. The formation and metabolism of 3-alpha, 7-alpha-dihydroxy 5-beta-cholestan-26-oic acid in man. J Clin Invest 1971; 50:2051–5.
126. Rabinowitz JL, Herman RH, Weinstein D, Staple E. Isolation of 3-alpha, 7-alpha-dihydroxycoprostane derived from cholesterol in human bile. Arch Biochem Biophys 1966; 114:233–4.
127. Salen G, Ahrens EH Jr, Grundy SM. Metabolism of β-sitosterol in man. J Clin Invest 1970; 49:952–7.
128. Helstrom K. On the bile acid and neutral fecal steroid excretion in man and rabbits following cholesterol feeding: Bile acids and steroids 150. Acta Physiol Scand 1965; 63:21–35.
129. Wilson JD, Lindsey CA Jr. Studies on the influence of dietary cholesterol on cholesterol metabolism in the isotopic steady state in man. J Clin Invest 1965; 44:1805–14.
130. Hofmann AF, Poley JR. Cholestyramine treatment of diarrhea associated with ileal resection. N Engl J Med 1969; 281:397–402.

131. Bergstrom S, Danielsson H, Samuelsson B. Formation and metabolism of bile acids. *In*: Bloch K ed. Lipid Metabolism. New York: John Wiley and Sons, 1960: 291–336.
132. Ekdahl P, Sjovall J. On the conjugation and formation of bile acids in the human liver. I. On the excretion of bile acids by patients with postoperative choledochostomy drainage. Bile acids and steroids 61. Acta Chir Scand 1957; 114:439–52.
133. Garbutt JT, Heaton KW, Lack L, Tyor MP. Increased ratio of glycine to taurine conjugated bile salts in patients with ileal disorders. Gastroenterology 1969; 56:711–20.
134. Sjovall J. Dietary glycine and taurine on bile acid conjugation in man. Bile acids and steroids 75. Proc Soc Biol Med 1959; 100:676–8.
135. Jacobsen JG, Smith LH. Biochemistry and physiology of taurine and taurine derivatives. Physiol Rev 1968; 48:424–511.
136. Sherr, HP, Yasuhito S, Newman A, Banwell John, Wagner H, Hendrix T. Detection of bacterial deconjugation of bile salts by breath-analysis technic. N Engl J Med 1971; 285:656–61.
137. Fromm H, Hofmann AF. Breath test for altered bile acid metabolism. Lancet 1971; 2:621–5.
138. James OF, Agnew JE, Bouchier IA. Assessment of the ^{14}C glycocholic acid breath test. Br Med J 1973; 3:191–5.
139. Hofmann AF. The syndrome of ileal disease and the broken enterohepatic circulation: Cholerheic enteropathy. Gastroenterology 1967; 52:752–7.
140. Mekhjian HS, Phillips SF, Hofmann AF. Colonic secretion of water and electrolytes induced by bile acids. Perfusion studies in man. J Clin Invest 1971; 50:1569–77.
141. Birkner HJ, Kern F Jr. In vitro absorption of bile salts to food residues, salicylazosulfapyridine, and hemicellulose. Gastroenterology 1974; 67:237–44.
142. Hofmann AF, Poley JR. Role of bile acid malabsorption in pathogenesis of diarrhea and steatorrhea in patients with ileal resection. I. Response to cholestyramine or replacement of dietary long chain triglycerides by medium chain triglycerides. Gastroenterology 1972; 62:918–34.
143. Dowling RH, Rose GA, Sutor VJ. Hyperoxaluria and renal calculin in ileal disease. Lancet 1971; 1:1103–6.
144. Hofmann AF, Thomas PJ, Smith LH, McCall JT. Secondary hyperoxaluria in patients with ileal resection and oxalate nephrolithiasis. Gastroenterology 1970; 58:960 (Abstract).
145. Smith LH, Fromm H, Hofmann AF. Acquired hyperoxaluria-nephrolithiasis, and intestinal disease. Description of a syndrome. N Engl J Med 1972; 286:1371–5.
146. Mandell I, Krauss E, Millan JC. Oxalate induced acute renal failure in Crohn's disease. Am J Med 1980; 69:628–32.
147. Anderson H, Gillberg R. Urinary oxalate on a high-oxalate diet as a clinical test of malabsorption. Lancet 1977; 2:677–8.
148. Yendt ER, Cohanim M, Peters L. Reduction of urinary oxalate excretion in primary hyperoxaluria by diet. Trans Am Clin Climat Assoc 1979; 91:191–201.
149. McDonald GB, Earnest DL, Admirand WH. Hyperoxaluria correlates with fat malabsorption in patients with sprue. Gut 1977; 18:561–6.
150. Earnest DL, Johnson G, Williams HE, Admirand WH. Hyperoxaluria in patients with ileal resection: An abnormality in dietary oxalate absorption. Gastroenterology 1974; 66:1114–22.
151. Earnest DL, Williams HE, Admirand WH. A physiochemical basis for the treatment of enteric hyperoxaluria. Trans Assoc Am Phys 1975; 88:224–34.
152. Anderson H, Jagenburg R. Fat-reduced diet in the treatment of hyperoxaluria in patients with ileopathy. Gut 1974; 15:360–2.
153. Barilla DE, Notz C, Kennedy D, Pak CY. Renal oxalate excretion following oral oxalate loads in patients with ileal disease and with renal and absorption hypercalciurias. Am J Med 1978; 64:579–85.
154. Chadwick VS, Modha, K, Dowling RH. Mechanism for hyperoxaluria in patients with ileal dysfunction. N Engl J Med 1973; 289:172–6.
155. Rudman D, Dedonis JL, Fountain M, Chandler J, Gerron G, Fleming GA, Kutner M. Hypocitraturia in patients with gastrointestinal malabsorption. N Engl J Med 1980; 303: 657–61.
156. Dharmsathaphorn K, Freeman D, Binder H, Dobbins J. Increased risk of nephrolithiasis in patients with steatorrhea. Dig Dis Sci 1982; 27:401–5.
157. Saunders DR, Sillerz J, McDonald GB. Regional differences in oxalate absorption by rat intestine. Gut 1975; 16:543–54.
158. Bambach CP, Robertson WG, Peacock M, Hill GL. Effect of intestinal surgery on the risk of urinary stone formation. Gut 1981; 22:257–63.
159. Fairclough PD, Feist TG, Chadwick VS, Clark ML. Effect of sodium chenodeoxycholate on oxalate absorption from the excluded human colon—A mechanism for enteric hyperoxaluria. Gut 1977; 18:240–4.
160. Binder H. Intestinal oxalate absorption. Gastroenterology 1974; 67:441–6.
161. Schwartz SE, Stauffer JQ, Burgess LW, Cheney M. Oxalate uptake by everted sacs of rat colon. Biochim Biophys Acta 1980; 596:404–13.
162. Finch AM, Kasidas GP, Rose GA. Urine composition in normal subjects after oral injection of oxalate rich foods. Clin Sci 1981; 60:411–8.
163. Earnest DL. Enteric hyperoxaluria. Adv Intern Med 1979; 24:407–27.
164. Hylander E, Jarnum S, Neilsen K. Calcium treatment of enteric hyperoxaluria after jejuno-ileal bypass for morbid obesity. Scand J Gastroenterol 1980; 15:349–52.
165. Stauffer JP. Hyperoxaluria and intestinal disease. The role of steatorrhea and dietary calcium in regulating intestinal oxalate absorption. Am J Dig Dis 1977; 22:921–8.
166. Cohen S, Kaplan M, Gottlieb L, Patterson J. Liver disease and gallstone disease in regional enteritis. Gastroenterology 1971; 60:237–45.
167. Heaton KW, Read AE. Gallstones in patients with disorders of the terminal ileum and disturbed bile salt metabolism. Br Med J 1969; 3:494–6.
168. Mansbach CM II, Newton D, Stevens RD. Fat digestion in patients with acid malabsorption but minimal steatorrhea. Dig Dis Sci 1980; 25:353–62.
169. Grundy SM, Metzger AL. A physiological method for estimation of hepatic secretion of biliary lipids in man. Gastroenterology 1972; 62:1200–17.
170. Treadwell CR, Vahouney GV. Cholesterol absorption. *In*: Code CF, ed. Handbook of Physiology, Vol 3, Section 6. Alimentary Canal. Washington DC: American Physiological Society, 1968: 1407.
171. Hofmann AF, Borgstrom BJ. Physico-chemical state of lipids in intestinal content during their digestion and absorption. Fed Proc 1962; 21:43–50.
172. Pihl A. The effect of dietary fat on the intestinal cholesterol and on the cholesterol metabolism in the liver of rats. Acta Physiol Scand 1955; 34:183–96.
173. Swell L, Flick DF, Field H Jr, et al. Role of fat and fatty acid in absorption of dietary cholesterol. Am J Physiol 1955; 180:124–8.
174. Simmonds WJ, Hofmann AF, Theodor E. Absorption of cholesterol from a micellar solution: Intestinal perfusion studies in man. J Clin Invest 1967; 46:874–90.
175. Westergaard H, Dietschy JM. The mechanism whereby bile micelles increase the rate of fatty acid and cholesterol uptake into the intestinal mucosal cell. J Clin Invest 1976; 58:97–108.
176. Simmonds WJ. Uptake of fatty acid and monoglyceride. *In*: Rommel K, Goebell H, Bohmer R, eds. Lipid Absorption: Biochemical and Clinical Aspects. Lancaster, England: MTP Press Ltd, 1976: 51–64.
177. Biel FU, Grundy SM. Studies on plasma lipoproteins during absorption of exogenous lecithin in man. J Lipid Res 1980; 21:525–36.
178. Crouse JR, Grundy SM. Effects of sucrose polyester on cholesterol metabolism in man. Metabolism 1979; 28:994–1000.
179. Grundy SM, Ahrens EH Jr, Davignon J. The interaction of cholesterol absorption and cholesterol synthesis in man. J Lipid Res 1965; 10:304–15.
180. Sedaghat A, Samuels P, Crouse J, Ahrens EH Jr. Effects of neomycin on absorption, synthesis, and/or flux of cholesterol in man. J Clin Invest 1975; 55:12–21.
181. Bhattacharyya AK, Connor WE. Beta-sitosterolemia and xanthomatosis: A newly described lipid storage disease in two sisters. J Clin Invest 1974; 53:1033–43.

182. Connor WE, Lin D. The intestinal absorption of dietary cholesterol by hypercholesterolemic (Type II) and normocholesterolemic humans. J Clin Invest 1970; 53:1062–70.
183. Mattson FH. Effect of dietary cholesterol on serum cholesterol in man. J Clin Nutr 1972; 25:589–94.
184. Quintao E, Grundy SM, Ahrens EH Jr. The effects of dietary cholesterol on regulation of total body cholesterol in man. J Lipid Res 1971; 12:233–47.
185. Miettinen TA, Ahrens EH Jr, Grundy SM. Quantitative isolation and gas-liquid chromatographic analysis of total dietary and fecal neutral steroids. J Lipid Res 1965; 6:411–24.
186. Mower HF, Ray RM, Shoff R, Stemmerman GN, Nomura A, Glober GA, Kamiyama S, Shimada A, Yamakawa H. Fecal bile acids in two Japanese populations with different colon cancer risks. Cancer Res 1979; 39:328.
187. Reddy BS, Hedges AR, Laakso K, Wynder EL. Metabolic epidemiology of large bowel cancer: Fecal bulk and constituents of high-risk North American and low-risk Finnish population. Cancer 1978; 42:2832.
188. Lipkin M, Reddy BB, Weisburger J, Schetcher L. Nondegradation of fecal cholesterol in subjects at high risk for cancer of the large intestine. J Clin Invest 1982; 67:304–7.
189. Dietschy JM, Siperstein MD. Effect of cholesterol feeding and fasting on sterol synthesis in seventeen tissues of the rat. J Lipid Res 1967; 8:97–104.
190. Dietschy JM, Weis HJ. Cholesterol synthesis by the gastrointestinal tract. Am J Clin Nutr 1971; 24:70–6.
191. Dietschy JM, Gamel WG. Cholesterol synthesis in the intestine of man: Regional differences and control mechanisms. J Clin Invest 1971; 50:872–80.
192. Dietschy JM. The role of bile salts in controlling the rate of intestinal cholesterogenesis. J Clin Invest 1968; 47:286–300.
193. Dietschy JM, Wilson JD. Cholesterol synthesis in the squirrel monkey. Relative rates of synthesis in various tissues and mechanisms of control. J Clin Invest 1968; 47:166–74.
194. Bloch K. The biological synthesis of cholesterol. Science 1965; 150:19–28.
195. Frantz ID Jr, Schoefer GJ Jr. Sterol biosynthesis. Ann Rev Biochem 1967; 36:691–726.
196. Gould RG. Lipid metabolism and atherosclerosis. Am J Med 1951; 11:209–27.
197. Tompkins GM, Sheppard H, Chaikoff IL. Cholesterol synthesis by liver. III. Its regulation by ingested cholesterol. J Biol Chem 1953; 201:137–41.
198. Gould RG, Taylor CB, Hagermann JS, et al. Cholesterol metabolism. I. Effect of dietary cholesterol on the synthesis of cholesterol in dog tissue in vitro. J Biol Chem 1953; 201:519–28.
199. Siperstein MD, Guest MJ. Studies on the site of the feedback control of cholesterol synthesis. J Clin Invest 1960; 39:642–52.
200. Kandutsch AA, Chen HW. Inhibition of sterol synthesis in cultured mouse cells by 7α-hydroxycholesterol, 7β-hydroxycholesterol and 7-ketocholesterol. J Biol Chem 1973; 248:8408–17.
201. Kandutsch AA. Consequences of blocked sterol synthesis in cultured cells—DNA synthesis and membrane composition. J Biol Chem 1977; 252:409–15.
202. Brown MS, Dana SE, Goldstein JL. Regulation of 3-hydroxy-3-methy-glutaryl coenzyme A reductase activity in cultured human fibroblasts: Comparison of cells from a normal subject and from a patient with homozygous familial hypercholesterolemia. J Biol Chem 1974; 249:789–96.
203. Brown MS, Faust JR, Goldstein JL. Role of the low density lipoprotein receptor in regulating the content of free and esterified cholesterol in human fibroblasts. J Clin Invest 1975; 55:783–93.
204. Bilheimer DW, Goldstein JL, Grundy SM, Brown MS. Reduction in cholesterol and low density lipoprotein synthesis after portacaval shunt surgery in a patient with homozygous familial hypercholesterolemia. J Clin Invest 1975; 56:1420–30.
205. Grundy SM, Ahrens EH Jr, Salen G. Interruption of the enterohepatic circulation of bile acids in man: Comparative effects of cholestyramine and ileal exclusion on cholesterol metabolism. J Lab Clin Med 1971; 78:94–121.
206. Miettinen TA. Mechanisms of hyperlipidemias in different clinical conditions. Adv Cardiol 1973; 8:85–99.
207. Bilheimer DW, Stone NJ, Grundy SM. Metabolic studies in familial hypercholesterolemia: Evidence for a gene-dosage effect in vivo. J Clin Invest 1979; 64:524–33.
208. Nervi FO, Dietschy JM. Inhibition of hepatic cholesterogenesis by different lipoproteins. Circulation 1974; 50(Suppl III):46.
209. Frantz ID Jr, Schneider HS, Hinkelman BT. Suppression of hepatic cholesterol synthesis in the rat by cholesterol feeding. J Biol Chem 1954; 206:465–9.
210. Bhattacharyya EPM, Siperstein MD. Feedback control of cholesterol synthesis in man. J Clin Invest 1963; 42:1613–8.
211. Bergstrom S, Danielsson H. On the regulation of bile acid formation in the rat liver. Acta Physiol Scand 1958; 43:1–7.
212. Fimograri GN, Rodwell VN. Cholesterol biosynthesis: Mevalonate synthesis inhibited by bile salts. Science 1965; 147:1038.
213. Back P, Hamprecht B, Lynen F. Regulation of cholesterol biosynthesis in rat liver: Diurnal changes of activity and influence of bile acids. Arch Biochem Biophys 1969; 133:11–21.
214. Shefer S, Hauser S, Bekersky I, et al. Biochemical site of regulation of bile acid biosynthesis in the rat. J Lipid Res 1970; 11:404–11.
215. Edward PA, Muroya H, Gould RG. In vivo demonstration of the circadian rhythm of cholesterol biosynthesis in the liver and intestine of the rat. J Lipid Res 1972; 13: 396–401.
216. Dietschy JM, Brown MS. Effect of alterations of the specific activity of the intracellular acetyl CoA pool on apparent rates of hepatic cholesterogenesis. J Lipid Res 1974; 15:508–16.
217. Bennion LJ, Grundy SM. Effects of obesity and caloric intake on biliary lipid metabolism in man. J Clin Invest 1975; 56:996–1011.
218. Nestel PJ, Whyte HM, Goodman DS. Distribution and turnover of cholesterol in humans. J Clin Invest 1969; 48:982–91.
219. Miettinen TA. Cholesterol production in obesity. Circulation 1971; 44:842–50.
220. Nestel PJ, Schreibman PH, Ahrens EH Jr. Cholesterol metabolism in human obesity. J Clin Invest 1973; 52:2389–97.
221. Grundy SM. Effects of polyunsaturated fats on lipid metabolism in patients with hypertriglyceridemia. J Clin Invest 1975; 55:269–82.
222. Wheeler HO, King KK. Biliary excretion of lecithin and cholesterol in the dog. J Clin Invest 1972; 51:1337–50.
223. Hardison WG, Apter JT. Micellar theory of biliary cholesterol excretion. Am J Physiol 1972; 222:61–7.
224. Dowling RH, Mack E, Small DM. Biliary lipid secretion and bile composition after acute and chronic interruption of the enterohepatic circulation in the Rhesus monkey. IV. Primate biliary physiology. J Clin Invest 1971; 50:1917–26.
225. Thureborn E. Human bile composition changes due to altered enterohepatic circulation. Acta Clin Scand 1962; 303(Suppl):1.
226. Nilsson S, Scherstern T. Importance of bile acids for phospholipid secretion into human bile. Gastroenterology 1962; 57:525–32.
227. Mok HYI, Von Bergman K, Grundy SM. Effects of interruption of enterohepatic circulation on biliary lipid secretion in man. Am J Dig Dis 1978; 23:1067–75.
228. Admirand WH, Small DM. The physiochemical basis of cholesterol gallstone formation in man. J Clin Invest 1968; 47:1043–52.
229. Holzbach RT, Marsh M, Olszewski M, et al. Cholesterol solubility in bile—evidence that supersaturated bile is frequent in healthy man. J Clin Invest 1973; 52:1467–79.
230. Grundy SM, Metzger AL, Adler R. Mechanism of lithogenic bile formation in American Indian women with cholesterol gallstones. J Clin Invest 1972; 51:3026–43.
231. Vlahcevic ZR, Bell CC Jr, Buhac I, et al. Diminished bile acid pool size in patients with gallstones. Gastroenterology 1970; 59:165–73.
232. Swell LC, Bell CC Jr, Vlahcevic ZR. Relationship of bile acid pool size to biliary lipid excretion and the formation of lithogenic bile in man. Gastroenterology 1971; 61:716–22.
233. Grundy SM, Duane WC, Adler RD, Aron JM, Metzger AL.

Biliary lipid outputs in young women with cholesterol gallstones. Metabolism 1974; 23:67–73.
234. Sodhi HS, Kudchokar BJ. Synthesis of cholesterol in hypercholesterolemia and its relationship to plasma triglycerides. Clin Exp Metab 1973; 22:895–912.
235. Einarsson K, Hellstrom K, Kallner M. Bile acid kinetics in relation to sex, serum lipids, body weights, and gallbladder disease in patients with various types of hyperlipoproteinemia. J Clin Invest 1974; 54:1301–11.
236. Beil U, Grundy SM, Crouse JR, Zech L. Triglyceride and cholesterol metabolism in primary hypertriglyceridemia. Arteriosclerosis 1982; 2:44–57.
237. Metzger AL, Adler R, Heymsfield S, Grundy SM. Diurnal variation in biliary lipid composition: Possible role in cholesterol gallstone formation. N Engl J Med 1973; 288:333–6.
238. Einarsson KA, Grundy SM. Effects of feeding cholic acid and chenodeoxycholic acid on cholesterol absorption and hepatic secretion of biliary lipids in man. J Lipid Res 1980; 21:23–34.
239. Malloy MJ, Kane JP. Hypolipidemia. Med Clin N Am 1982; 66:469–84.
240. Goldstein JL, Brown MS. The LDL receptor defect in familial hypercholesterolemia. Implications for pathogenesis and therapy. Med Clin North Am 1982; 66:335–62.
241. Hamilton RL, Williams MC, Fielding CJ, Havel RJ. Discoidal bilayer structures of nascent high density lipoproteins from perfused rat liver. J Clin Invest 1976; 58:667–80.
242. Green PHR, Tall AR, Glickman RM. Rat intestine secretes discoid high density lipoprotein. J Clin Invest 1978; 65:528–35.
243. Glomset JA, Nicholes AV, Norum KR, King W, Forte T. Plasma lipoproteins in familial lecithin:cholesterol acyltransferase: Further studies of very low and low density lipoprotein abnormalities. J Clin Invest 1973; 52:1078–92.
244. Tall AR, Small DM. Plasma high-density lipoproteins. N Engl J Med 1978; 299:1232–6.
245. Myers LH, Phillips NR, Havel RJ. Mathematical evaluation of methods for estimation of the concentration of the major lipid components of human serum lipoproteins. J Lab Clin Med 1976; 88:491.
246. Frederickson DS, Goldstein JL, Brown MS. The familial hyperlipoproteinemias. *In:* Stanbury JB, Wyngaardern JB, Frederickson DS, eds. The Metabolic Basis of Inherited Disease. 4th Ed. New York: McGraw-Hill, 1978.
247. Kane JP, Tun P, Malloy MJ, et al. Synergism in drug treatment of familial hypercholesterolemia. *In:* Goto AM Jr, Smith LC, Allen B, eds. Atherosclerosis V. New York: Springer-Verlag, 1980: 78.
248. Miettinen TA. Effects of neomycin alone and in combination with cholestyramine on serum cholesterol and fecal steroids in hypercholesterolemic subjects. J Clin Invest 1979; 64:1485.
249. Miettinen TA, Toivonen I. Treatment of severe and mild hypercholesterolemia with probucol and neomycin. Postgrad Med J 1975; 51(Suppl 8):71.
250. Buchwald H, Moore RB, Barco RL. Ten years' clinical experience with partial ileal bypass in management of hyperlipidemias. Ann Surg 180:384–92.
251. Goldstein JL, Hazzard WR, Schrott HG, Bierman EL, Motulsky AG. Hyperlipidemia in coronary heart disease. I. Lipid levels in 500 survivors of myocardial infarction. J Clin Invest 1973; 52:1533–43.
252. Goldstein JL, Schrott HG, Hazzard WR, Bierman EL, Motulsky AG. Hyperlipidemia in coronary heart disease. II. Genetic analysis of lipid levels in 176 families and delineation of a new inherited disorder, combined hyperlipidemia. J Clin Invest 1973; 52:1544–68.
253. Kesaniemi YA, Grundy SM. Significance of low density lipoprotein production in the regulation of plasma cholesterol level in man. J Clin Invest 1982; 70:13–22.
254. The Pooling Project Research Group. Relationship of blood pressure, serum cholesterol, smoking habit, relative weight and ECG abnormalities to incidence of major coronary events: Final report of the pooling project research group. J Chron Dis 1978; 31:201–306.
255. Grundy SM, Bilheimer D, Blackburn H, et al. Rationale of the Diet-Heart Statement of the American Heart Association. Circulation 1982; 65:839A–54A.
256. Grundy SM. Hypertriglyceridemia: Mechanisms, clinical significance, and treatment. Med Clin North Am 1982; 66:519–35.
257. Havel RJ. Familial dysbetalipoproteinemia. New aspects of pathogenesis and diagnosis. Med Clin North Am 1982; 66:319–30.
258. Berman M, Hall M III, Levy RI, Eisenberg S, Bilheimer DW, Phair RD, Goebel RH. Metabolism of apo B and apo C lipoproteins in man: Kinetic studies in normal and hyperlipoproteinemic subjects. J Lipid Res 1978; 19:37.
259. Kissebah AH, Alfarsi S, Peters PW. Integrated regulation of very low density lipoprotein triglyceride and apolipoprotein-B kinetics in man: Normolipemic subjects, familial hypertriglyceridemia, and familial combined hyperlipidemia. Metabolism 1981; 30:856–68.
260. Chait A, Albers JJ, Brunzell JD. Very low density lipoprotein overproduction in genetic forms of hypertriglyceridaemia. Eur J Clin Invest 1980; 10:17–22.
261. Brunzell JD, Schrott HG, Motulsky AG, Bierman EL. Myocardial infarction in familial forms of hypertriglyceridemia. Metabolism 1976; 25:313–20.
262. Brunzell JD, Bierman EL. Chylomicroenemia syndrome. Interaction of genetic and acquired hypertriglyceridemia. Med Clin N Am 1982; 66:455–68.
263. Breckenridge WC, Little JA, Steiner G, Chow A, Poapst M. Hypertriglyceridemia associated with deficiency of apolipoprotein C-II. N Engl J Med 1978; 298:1265.
264. Abrams JJ, Ginsberg H, Grundy SM. Metabolism of cholesterol and plasma triglycerides in nonketotic diabetes mellitus. Diabetes 1982; 31:903–10.
265. Melish J, Le NA, Ginsberg H, et al. Dissociation of apoprotein B and triglyceride production in very-low-density lipoproteins. Am J Physiol 1980; 239:E354.
266. Grundy SM, Mok, HYI, Zech L, et al. Transport of very low density lipoprotein triglycerides in varying degrees of obesity and hypertriglyceridemia. J Clin Invest 1979; 63:1274–83.
267. Shepherd J, Packard CJ, Bicker S, et al. Cholestyramine promotes receptor mediated low density lipoprotein catabolism. N Engl J Med 1980; 302:1219.
268. Beil U, Grundy SM, Crouse JR, Zech L. Triglyceride and cholesterol metabolism in primary hypertriglyceridemia. Arteriosclerosis 1982; 2:44–57.
269. Grundy SM, Mok HYI, Zech L, Berman M. Influence of nicotinic acid on metabolism of cholesterol and triglycerides in man. J Lipid Res 1981; 22:24.
270. Grundy SM, Mok HYI. Colestipol, clofibrate, and phytosterols in combined therapy of hyperlipidemia. J Lab Clin Med 1977; 89:354.
271. Sedaghat A, Samuel P, Crouse JR, et al. Effects of neomycin on absorption, synthesis and/or flux of cholesterol in man. J Clin Invest 1975; 55:12.
272. Grundy SM, Ahrens EH Jr, Davignon J. The interaction of cholesterol absorption and cholesterol synthesis in man. J Lipid Res 1969; 10:304.
273. Garbutt JT, Lack L, Tyor MP. The enterohepatic circulation of bile salts in gastrointestinal diseases. Am J Med 1971; 51:627–36.

Chapter 98

Intestinal Drug Absorption

Arvey I. Rogers • F. Scott Corbett

General Considerations

Oral preparations account for more than 80% of all drugs prescribed. It is essential, therefore, to understand the multiple factors that influence their intestinal absorption, a step second in importance only to drug ingestion and gastric emptying as a determinant of ultimate therapeutic effectiveness. The major intent of this chapter is to present clinically relevant information concerning drugs and gastrointestinal physiology relating to *intestinal* absorption of drugs. Sublingual and rectal absorption will not be considered, although either route may be a convenient means of drug administration when there is vomiting or altered consciousness.

Many drugs and dosage formulations have been and continue to be developed because of the need to (1) overcome disadvantages of specific medications (e.g., mucosal irritation or ulceration, drug destruction by acid or enzymes, precipitation or insolubility in gastro-intestinal secretions, formation of non-absorbable complexes with other drugs or foods, variable absorption rates influenced by gastric emptying, mixing completeness, and intestinal motility); (2) improve compliance (improve taste and ease of swallowing, reduce side effects, reduce frequency of dosing); and (3) provide sustained pharmacologic action in order to maintain overnight therapeutic effectiveness, eliminate drug peaks with their related side effects, and decrease the frequency of patient dosing errors. Preparations designed to overcome disadvantages and improve compliance include enteric-coated tablets and capsules; suspensions, powders, and emulsions; incorporated chelating agents; and a variety of flavored and unflavored preparations such as elixirs, syrups, solutions, tinctures, and fluid extracts. Tablets within tablets, slowly disintegrating tablets, pellets in capsules, slowly dissolving salts in solid and liquid suspension, and drugs embedded in ion exchange or inert plastic matrices are still other structurings designed to provide sustained pharmacologic action.[1,2]

A number of assumptions are necessarily made by the individual prescribing a medication: (1) the medication will control or cure the illness dictating its use, (2) the medication is what it is claimed to be and is biologically available, (3) the dosage frequency and relationship of drug administration to meals are correct, (4) the patient will take the medication as prescribed, (5) the patient will tolerate the medication, (6) several administered drugs do not interact so as to impair each other's absorption or extraintestinal metabolism, and (7) the drug does not alter gut function and/or structure, thereby modifying its absorption.

An implicit assumption underlying medical therapy by the oral route is that the medication prescribed is absorbed normally from the intestinal tract, a clear requisite for the expected pharmacologic action on the selected target organ. Intestinal absorption of drugs is influenced to a great extent by many of the same basic factors that affect the digestion and absorption of nutrients, water, and electrolytes. The indeterminant local and systemic effects on gut structure and function by many illnesses limit our understanding of drug absorption. Nevertheless, by combining proved observations and theoretical considerations, it is possible to construct a concept of the principles of drug absorption, to make certain rational assumptions given a set of observations, and to apply both the concept and the assumptions regarding intestinal drug absorption to provide good patient care.

Figure 98–1 diagrams the role of the intestine in the overall process of drug absorption

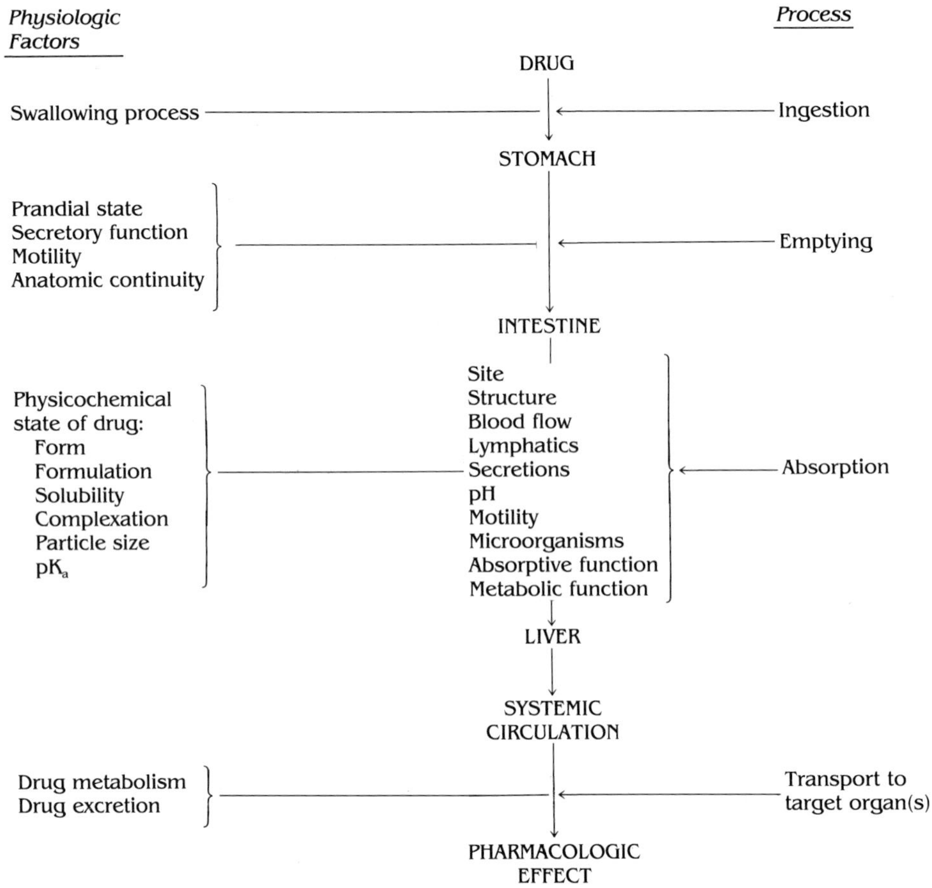

Figure 98–1. Physiology of drug absorption.

and pharmacologic effectiveness. Levine[3] appropriately focused only on the drug and the absorbing intestinal unit when he considered intestinal drug absorption. He emphasized (1) the physicochemical properties of the drug, (2) the non-absorptive physiologic functions of the gastrointestinal tract, (3) the structure of the absorbing surface, and (4) the metabolic activity and functions of the absorbing cell.

The effective total absorption of many drugs may be decreased by the liver through a phenomenon known as the "first pass effect." As this effect is perceived, drugs may be metabolized extensively by the liver as they pass initially with the blood through this structure before reaching the systemic circulation and the target organ. The intestine contains various cytochrome systems that are qualitatively similar but are only one-tenth to one-twentieth as effective as the liver in "first pass" metabolism. In addition, certain factors (i.e., barbiturates, glutethimide, cigarette smoking) may induce gut-associated drug-metabolizing enzyme systems, sometimes making adjustments in dosage necessary to ensure effectiveness.[4]

Physicochemical Properties of Drugs

As illustrated in Figure 98–1, there are at least 6 characteristics ascribed to the physicochemical state of the drug being presented to the intestinal surface for absorption. These are form, formulation, solubility, complexation, particle size, and pK_a. Each factor influences the rate and degree of drug absorption to some degree. These, in turn, determine overall absorptive efficiency and pharmacologic effectiveness.

Solid preparations must first dissolve before absorption can take place, and tablets must disintegrate even before the drug they contain can undergo dissolution. Varying rates and completeness of dissolution are likely to result in differing absorption rates among the various brands of tablets and capsules. This fact has significant clinical implications and may result in reported discrepancies among investigators.[5] Some important generic drugs whose brand name preparations have been shown to be absorbed with differing efficiency are chloramphenicol, digoxin, griseofulvin, nitrofurantoin, phenytoin, prednisone, spironolactone, sulfonamides, tetracyclines, tolbutamide, warfarin, and certain slow-release capsules and tablets or enteric-coated preparations.[4] While some brand name preparations have nearly identical bioavailability characteristics, it is nonetheless a sound principle to maintain a patient on a specific brand name drug once stabilization has been achieved. The unpredictable absorptive and metabolic characteristics among preparations mitigates against making frequent brand name changes. However, a slight difference in absorptive efficiency of various formulations is of less significance if the drug involved has a long half-life and is being utilized for long-term therapy.

The absorbing surface of the intestine is a lipoidal membrane with aqueous "pores" through which drugs and other foreign substances are absorbed by varying mechanisms, e.g., simple diffusion, filtration through pores, and specialized active transport processes (Chapter 91). Most drugs are absorbed by *passive diffusion* of unionized molecules, with the maximal absorptive site being the proximal small intestine.[6] The dissociation constant of a drug and the degree to which its non-ionic forms are lipid soluble (lipid/water partition coefficient) are major determinants of its absorption. Most drugs are weak acids or bases and are present in solution as both ionized and unionized species. Drugs that are poorly ionized, have a high lipid/water absorption coefficient for the non-ionic form, and have a small radius (4 Å; molecular weight 100 to 200) undergo rapid absorption. Ionized groups on drugs, usually COO^- or NR_2H^+, interact strongly with water dipoles and penetrate lipid membranes poorly or not at all.

Concentration and pH gradients across membranes also influence absorption rates. The pH gradients are of theoretical importance in determining whether a weak electrolyte is absorbed or secreted. At acidic pH, weak acids (warfarin, sulfonylureas, and anti-inflammatory drugs) are more un-ionized and better absorbed; thus, the stomach acts as the initial site of absorption for these agents.[4] At basic pH, weak bases are more un-ionized and better absorbed. Alkaline pH favors ionization of weak acids, while acid pH favors ionization of weak bases. During transport through the small intestine, where pH approaches neutrality, weakly acidic drugs are more ionized; however, drug absorption is even more rapid, owing to the much larger surface area to which the drug is exposed. Weakly basic drugs (i.e., antihistamines, antidepressants, narcotic analgesics, beta-blockers, and ephedrines) are highly ionized in the acid environment of the stomach, where absorption is poor, but exist in an unionized form in the intestine, from which absorption is rapid. Under normal circumstances, pH extremes in man do not exist throughout the intestine. Were this to occur, however, there are data suggesting that a cell surface–associated microenvironment of pH 5.3 may be the final determinant accounting for efficient absorption of weak acids from an alkaline milieu.[7,8] In general, drugs will be adequately absorbed if the pK_a of a weak acid is greater than 2 and that of a weak base less than 10.

Certain drugs, such as propantheline, neostigmine, and prolidoxime containing quaternary ammonium groups, remain completely ionized throughout the gastrointestinal tract. Theoretically, therefore, they should be poorly and erratically absorbed. Their anionic salts are well absorbed, however, and there is a phosphatidopeptide fraction isolated from intestinal tissue that further enhances their absorption. These observations suggest that certain cationic substances may be absorbed through combination with endogenous anionic membrane-associated carriers. Binding with intestinal mucus–associated polysaccharide interferes with absorption of these compounds and others. When inactive cationic compounds are administered concurrently, more active drug is absorbed. The inefficient absorption of tetracycline is attributed in part to the formation of chelates with polyvalent ions, such as calcium and magnesium, and with proteins. The removal of calcium by the co-administration of tripalmitin enhances tetracycline absorption. The same effect has been shown for combinations of EDTA and tetracyclines, since EDTA chelation of calcium ion ensures that tetracycline calcium-protein chelation will not occur.[9]

Non-Absorbing Gut Properties

Motility, digestion and secretion, blood flow and lymphatic circulation, and microorganisms are among the important anatomic, physiologic, and biologic factors that may modify drug absorption independent of the physicochemical properties of the drug.

Motility. Gastric emptying and small intestinal transit time may influence the predictable rate and efficiency of drug absorption. Fasting, liquid meals, and meals of large volume or carbohydrate content accelerate gastric emptying, whereas fatty foods, solids, and hypertonic meals delay it. Delayed gastric emptying allows more time for tablet dissolution, increases gastric blood flow, and enhances the absorption through gastric mucosa of a weakly acidic drug (if its non-ionic form is soluble). Emptying rates and hence absorption rates are unpredictable and unreliable. Certain drugs may undergo inactivation when exposed for prolonged periods to an acid-peptic environment. Rapid gastric emptying, e.g., physiologic or surgically induced, shortens optimal dissolution time required for solid preparations, but generally does not result in impaired intestinal absorption unless associated accelerated intestinal transit time appreciably reduces intestinal mucosal surface contact time. Intestinal transit time prolonged by diseases, e.g., scleroderma, amyloidosis, hypothyroidism, intestinal pseudo-obstruction, or strictures, may impair drug absorption if bacterial overgrowth supervenes and bacterial metabolism alters drugs or luminal environmental characteristics.

Of further interest are observations linking effects of drugs modifying gastric emptying on the absorption of other drugs administered concomitantly. Nimmo[6] demonstrated that metoclopramide enhanced the absorption of paracetamol (acetaminophen) and tetracycline, presumably by enhancing gastric emptying. Metoclopramide has similarly been shown to enhance the absorption of ampicillin.[10]

Nimmo[6] additionally demonstrated that propantheline delayed gastric emptying and slowed the absorption of paracetamol in 6 convalescent hospitalized patients without gastrointestinal disease. Previous studies had demonstrated a similar effect of propantheline on the absorption of digoxin and riboflavin.[11,12] Amphetamines, desipramine, and phenobarbital have been reported to impair the absorption of anticonvulsants, phenylbutazone, and griseofulvin, respectively.[13–15] Alteration in gastrointestinal motility is hypothesized as the basis for these observations. Aluminum hydroxide has been demonstrated to relax gastric smooth muscle, impair contractile response to acetylcholine, and delay gastric emptying in man.[16] Thus, slowing of gastric emptying by aluminum-containing antacids has been linked to reduced rates of diazepam absorption and overall reduced isoniazid (INH) absorption in man when antacids are administered concomitantly with these drugs.[17,18]

Digestion and Secretion. Certain drugs will be susceptible to acid or enzymatic hydrolysis in the stomach, effects that can be reduced or eliminated by coating the tablets or by administering concomitant bicarbonate or H_2-receptor blockers. This is especially true regarding pancreatic enzyme administration.[19] Diseases or drugs enhancing gastrointestinal secretion (infectious diarrheas; diseases associated with gastrin, prostaglandin, or vasoactive intestinal polypeptide [VIP] excess; sprue; lactase deficiency states; certain diuretics; cathartics) may result in significant drug dilution in the intestinal lumen leading to impaired absorption because of reduced drug concentration per unit of absorbing surface area.[3,20]

An aspect of drug absorption that has just begun to receive attention concerns drug diffusion from plasma to the gut lumen, i.e., drug excretion or secretion. This process is driven by the concentration gradient of membrane-permeable drug species, generally non-ionized, non–protein bound molecules. The rate of diffusion from plasma into the lumen is limited by the relatively low concentrations of drugs in plasma and tissue fluids because of local blood flow, metabolism, and renal excretion. This fact usually favors the diffusion of drugs from the lumen to plasma.[21] The addition of activated charcoal, however, adsorbs drugs in the lumen, thereby effectively reducing diffusible drug to zero. This process optimizes the drug concentration gradient in the direction favoring diffusion of drug from plasma into the lumen.[21]

The effect of adding activated charcoal to the gut lumen not only limits absorption of various drugs but results in enhancement of the gastrointestinal secretion or excretion of drugs that have been administered IV.[22] This effect continues for several hours after a drug has been administered. These properties of activated charcoal make it especially important in the management of drug overdose, since the preparation may be administered by nasogastric tube to the unconscious patient. In effect, this use of activated charcoal provides a technique for gastrointestinal dialysis.[21] Drugs whose absorption has been effectively controlled by activated charcoal include aspirin, acetaminophen, phenobarbital, digoxin, phenytoin, nortriptyline, and phenylpropanolamine.[21,23] Concomitant adsorption of N-acetylcysteine (Mucomyst) limits the use of activated charcoal in acetaminophen overdose.

Blood Flow and Lymphatics. Little of practical import is known concerning the role of intestinal blood flow and lymphatic circulation in the absorption of drugs. Extremes of reduced arterial flow, passive venous congestion, or lymphatic obstruction that compromise small intestinal structure and function generally would be expected to impair drug absorption. Low cardiac output states associated with congestive heart failure, mesenteric vascular insufficiency complicating atherosclerosis of mesenteric vessels, and mucosal atrophy consequent to prolonged arterial ischemia are examples of clinical disorders that may be associated with altered drug absorption. There are few specific studies, however, that can be presented to confirm or refute this speculation. It is not known what factors enhance drug absorption in man under normal circumstances of arterial and lymphatic circulation. Alcohol administration in rats appears to increase gastric mucosal blood flow, perhaps thereby augmenting barbiturate absorption from the stomach; a similar effect was not observed for intestinal absorption. The absorption of *p*-aminosalicylate and tetracycline, which are absorbed poorly by way of the lymphatics, was increased in rats when concurrently administered tripalmitin enhanced lymphatic flow.[3] Though similar studies are lacking in man, it seems reasonable to assume that the oral administration of most drugs given in close relationship to meals will enhance absorption for the same reasons that nutrients, water, and electrolytes are absorbed.

Microorganisms. The role of resident microorganisms in the metabolism and absorption of drugs by the human intestine is receiving increasing attention. They may either enhance or reduce bioavailability of therapeutically administered drugs. For example, salicylazosulfapyridine (sulfasalazine, Azulfidine) becomes active therapeutically only when colonic flora split the azo linkage existing between the sulfapyridine and salicylate moieties constituting the parent compound.[24] The delivery of topically active 5-aminosalicylate to the inflamed colon is required for any significant therapeutic benefit to be realized. Concomitant administration of antibacterial agents may therefore impair therapeutic effectiveness of sulfasalazine. Other compounds are being developed that do not depend upon prior bacterial cleavage or binding with a sulfonamide to ensure delivery of 5-aminosalicylate to the target organ.

Microbial metabolism of digoxin may account for partial therapeutic refractoriness and the need for a higher drug dosage in some patients.[25] The reduced metabolites of digoxin are excreted in the urine and stool of such patients. Stool flora can institute the reduction reaction *in vitro*. The addition of antibiotics to the *in vitro* preparation will inhibit this action, as will the oral administration of tetracycline or erythromycin. The antibiotic effect is made evident by the disappearance of reduced metabolites in the urine or stool. These observations have implications other than those already discussed. It is possible that gut flora normally exert some degree of regulation of digoxin absorption through microorganism metabolism in some, and possibly all, patients. If such a patient receives antibiotics for an intercurrent infection, microorganism regulation of digoxin absorption could undergo disruption, resulting in unimpaired digoxin absorption and possible digitalis intoxication. How frequently this mechanism accounts for digitalis intoxication is not known.

Intestinal flora may likewise alter the metabolism of estrogens. This is seen in the failure of oral contraceptives in women taking ampicillin, chloramphenicol, rifampin, or sulfamethoxypyridazine.[26] Breakthrough bleeding has also been noted to be more frequent during concurrent antibiotic therapy.[27]

Drug toxicology may be related to intestinal flora. Two trace metabolites of L-dopa, m-tyramine and m-hydroxyphenylacetic acid (MHPA), are produced by intestinal flora and excreted in urine.[28,29] An increase in the urinary excretion of MHPA occurs when L-dopa is administered to patients with parkinsonism in a preparation retarding absorption. It is felt that prolonged contact time with intestinal flora results in increased metabolism of L-dopa and unacceptable increase in gastrointestinal intolerance.

Microbial beta-glucuronidases may deconjugate compounds that normally undergo glucuronidation in the liver and are excreted in the feces by way of the biliary tract. Deconjugation enhances intestinal absorption, establishing thereby an enterohepatic circulation for a particular drug, such as diethylstilbestrol and possibly morphine and indomethacin. Antibiotic administration may interrupt the enterohepatic circulation of these compounds and alter drug pharmacokinetics.[30]

Intestinal Absorbing Unit

Structure of Surface. Sallee et al.[31] observed that there is an unstirred layer on the surface of the small intestinal mucosa. This would suggest that earlier *in vitro* studies of drug absorption utilizing isolated everted intestinal sacs may require confirmation by current *in vitro* methods that consider the effects of this layer on absorption dynamics. The functional characteristics of the absorbing surface membrane, discussed earlier, assume a lipoidal membrane with aqueous pores without considering the unstirred layer. Future studies may force modification of existing concepts.

Obviously, factors that grossly or microscopically modify the structure of the absorbing surface can be expected to alter absorption of drugs as well as nutrients, water, and electrolytes. These factors include spontaneously occurring intestinal malabsorption syndromes, irradiation, neomycin, alcohol, colchicine, p-aminosalicylate, and chemotherapeutic agents.[32] Reversible modification of surface structure and/or function may be induced by certain anionic or non-ionic surfactants that enhance drug absorption. The widening of intercellular channels by chelating agents has been observed to enhance drug absorption. Siber et al.[33] also demonstrated a dose-related increase (2- to 20-fold) in the absorption of large molecules (molecular weight 11,000) from the small intestine of patients receiving 5-fluorouracil therapy for metastatic colon carcinoma.

Function of Absorbing Cell. The absorption, metabolism, and biotransformation of certain drugs by the intestine depend upon intact gut-associated enzyme systems. The so-called presystemic elimination of drugs involves the intestine and the liver, the contribution of each being dependent upon the rate of diffusion through and the metabolism by the intestinal mucosa. Limited drug bioavailability appears to be a result of rapid metabolism, which begins in the intestinal mucosa and ends in the liver.[34] Drug induction of gut-associated drug-metabolizing enzymes is an exceptional occurrence; however, data suggesting that certain chemicals in our environment may induce these enzyme systems are being increasingly advanced.[35] Most notable are observations to the effect that cigarette smoke reduces blood levels of orally administered phenacetin in humans without altering the metabolic rate in the liver. These observations point to the effect of smoking on intestinal mucosa.[35] In rats, smoke inhalation increases paracetamol oxidation by intestinal mucosa 100%.[36] In humans, tobacco smoke appears to produce small increases in the metabolism of theophylline, antipyrine, nicotine, imipramine, and pentazocine but does not appear to alter the presystemic elimination of meperidine, phenytoin, nortriptyline, and warfarin. Of additional interest is that certain vegetables and combustion products associated with meat spoilage or charcoal-broiled meat may induce intestinal enzyme systems.

Lastly, factors that inhibit enzymes active in the Krebs cycle may impair drug transport, which is partially energy dependent. Furthermore, when water and electrolyte transport is impaired, the absorption of drugs dependent on pore filtration processes, ion transport, and carrier-mediated transport processes may be impaired.

Factors Altering Drug Absorption

It was earlier pointed out in this chapter that for drug absorption to proceed normally, the drug must first arrive at a normal absorbing surface in a form suitable for absorption; it must remain there long enough in a form and in a concentration that enhance absorption; and it must be absorbed by a normal epithelial cell without being metabolized by that cell. All factors known to impair drug absorption or modify its prehepatic, presystemic bioavailability can be related to a defect in one or several of these absorption requisites (Table 98–1). A more detailed but clinically relevant analysis of factors altering drug

Table 98–1. DRUG ABSORPTION FACTORS

- I. The Drug
  - A. Solid or enteric-coated form
  - B. Insolubility
  - C. Complexes with drugs or food
  - D. Excessive ionization
  - E. Low lipid/water partition coefficient
  - F. Large particle size
- II. The Stomach
  - A. Delayed gastric emptying
    1. Intrinsic motility defect
    2. Postprandial state
    3. Pyloric outlet obstruction
    4. pH extremes
    5. Drug interaction
  - B. Rapid gastric emptying (unregulated postoperatively, fasting)
- III. The Intestine
  - A. Lumen
    1. Enzymatic digestion
    2. Dilution by intestinal secretions
    3. Complexities with food or ions
    4. Obstruction
  - B. Mucous membrane
    1. Surface mucopolysaccharide
    2. Disease, drug, irradiation damage
    3. Biotransformation phenomena
  - C. Epithelial cell
    1. Impaired Na^+ ion transport
    2. Inhibited Krebs cycle
    3. Competition for absorptive pathways
    4. Disease, drug, irradiation damage
    5. Biotransformation phenomena

absorption considers the drug; the gut; the interaction of the drug with the gut, other drugs, and nutrients; and the influence of the disease on gut structure and function and drug absorption. The prescribing health professional must be aware of all these factors if he is to make rational drug choices, properly select combinations of drugs, choose among the several available forms of preparation of the drug, determine the dosing schedule, and correctly interpret the reason(s) for treatment failure as they relate to inability to achieve therapeutic blood levels of an orally administered drug.

Effect of Diet and Drugs. Food or food components can reduce, slow, or increase drug absorption, depending upon the type of food, the physical state of the drug, the influence of the meal on gut motility, and the physical or chemical interactions between the drug and the food. In general, food slows the absorption of drugs by lengthening gastric emptying time and reducing immediate access to the absorbing surface. Slower absorption should not be equated with reduced therapeutic efficacy, however, since total absorption is more important in this regard. A delay in gastric emptying may favor disintegration and dissolution of a solid preparation, thereby enhancing absorption. Furthermore, the incremental gastric emptying of a drug may favor its intestinal absorption when absorptive sites are quickly saturated. This effect has been demonstrated for riboflavin and may be invoked to explain improved postprandial absorption of hydrochlorothiazide. L-dopa and methyldopa, related structurally to amino acids, are not absorbed well when administered with protein meals because of competition for carriers among the different amino acids. Fiber sources, such as wheat bran and pectin, retard drug absorption, notably that of acetaminophen. Earlier concerns about retarded digoxin absorption in patients on high fiber diets proved to be clinically insignificant. Fiber-induced shortening of intestinal transit time may reduce drug exposure time to intestinal bacteria, which must metabolize the drug to make it effective therapeutically.[37]

Certain antibiotics are less well absorbed in the presence of food and should therefore be prescribed 1 hour before or 3 hours following a meal. These include oral penicillins (except amoxicillin), erythromycin, lincomycin, rifampin, isoniazid, and the tetracyclines. Complexes formed between the tetracyclines and divalent and trivalent cations are usually insoluble, non-absorbable chelates; the antibiotic is inefficiently absorbed when taken within 2 hours of ingesting foods or beverages containing calcium (milk, cottage cheese and other cheeses, yogurt, and ice cream) or iron (iron-fortified cereals or

Table 98–2. INFLUENCE OF FOOD ON DRUG ABSORPTION*

Food Impairs Absorption of	Food Enhances Absorption of
Most antibiotics	Propranolol
Aspirin	Hydralazine
Propantheline	Hydrochlorothiazide
L-Dopa	Propoxyphene
Methyldopa	Griseofulvin
Rifampin	Nitrofurantoin
Isoniazid	Spironolactone
Phenobarbital	
Methotrexate	
Acetaminophen	
Digoxin	
Furosemide	
Potassium ions	

*Modified from Roe DA.[37]

meat). The addition of EDTA to the antibiotic formulation offsets chelate formulation and may have therapeutic significance under certain circumstances.[9]

Table 98–2 lists drugs and the effect of meals on their absorption.

Table 98–3 provides a partial listing of drugs and their effects on the absorption of other drugs.

Effect of Diseases. It is virtually impossible to provide a useful listing of all the diseases that have been shown to influence drug absorption. To determine whether alterations in drug absorption are likely in a specific clinical setting, it is necessary only to be familiar with the requisites for normal absorption and to know whether a specific disease modifies them. Table 98–4 presents a partial listing of diseases and relates them to the drug absorption requisite that is impaired.

Epilogue

Current understanding of drug absorption by the human gastrointestinal tract is based primarily on *in vitro* studies that have been challenged because the methods used did not consider the role of the unstirred layer on small intestinal surface mucosal epithelium. Presently held concepts may well have to undergo substantial revision in the future. The prevailing view at present is that most orally ingested drugs are weak acids and bases that are absorbed from the proximal small intestine by simple diffusion, the effi-

Table 98–3. DRUGS THAT MAY IMPAIR DRUG ABSORPTION*

Drugs or Drug Category	May Affect Absorption of	Drugs or Drug Category	May Affect Absorption of
I. Antacids		VI. Miscellaneous	
A. Al^{+++} or Mg^{++}-containing, standard doses	1. Tetracycline 2. Diazepam, chlordiazepoxide 3. Cimetidine	A. Cholestyramine	1. Acetylsalicylic acid 2. Chlorothiazide 3. Warfarin 4. Digitalis 5. Hydrochlorothiazide 6. Iron 7. Phenobarbital 8. Phenylbutazone 9. Potentially diffuse malabsorption of drugs dependent on bile salts 10. Quinidine 11. Thyroxine
B. Large doses	4. Nalidixic acid 5. Nitrofurantoin 6. Penicillin G 7. Sulfonamides 8. Isoniazid		
II. Antibiotics			
A. Neomycin	1. Diffuse impairment		
B. Tetracycline, puromycin, actinomycin D	2. Diffuse impairment 3. Iron		
C. Wide variety	4. Metabolism of sulfasalazine	B. Sulfasalazine	1. Folic acid
III. Antimetabolites		C. Kaolin and pectin	1. Lincomycin 2. Promazine
A. Colchicine	1. Folic acid 2. Vitamin B_{12}	D. Cathartics (Mg^{++})	1. Potential decrease secondary to dilution in gut lumen
B. Alkylating and alkaloid agents	3. Diffuse; large molecules	E. Anticholinergics; narcotics	1. Potential decrease secondary to delayed gastric emptying
IV. Anticonvulsants			
A. Phenytoin	1. Folic acid		
B. Barbiturates	2. Warfarin 3. Folic acid 4. Griseofulvin	F. Metoclopramide	1. A variety of drugs secondary to more rapid gastric emptying (tetracycline, ampicillin, paracetamol)
V. Oral contraceptives	1. Folic acid		

*Based on data from references 6, 8, 16, 17, 24, 32, and 38 to 55.

Table 98–4. DISEASES AFFECTING DRUG ABSORPTION

Organ	Dysfunction	Disease(s)	Consequence(s)
Esophagus	Reduced emptying Regurgitation	Achalasia Scleroderma Peptic stricture	Unpredictable and unregulated gastric delivery, reduced absorption rate
Stomach and duodenum	Impaired emptying	Pyloroduodenal scarring Gastroparesis due to drugs, disease, vagotomy	Unpredictable gastric emptying, delivery rates to the intestine, and intestinal absorption rate
	Rapid emptying	Gastric surgery	Reduced intestinal contact time, reduced absorption
Small intestine	Altered structure	Sprue, chemotherapy, radiation, ischemia, infection	Impaired absorption secondary to altered absorbing unit *or*
	Reduced length	Resection	Reduced surface area
	Slow transit (with bacterial overgrowth)	Scleroderma, hypometabolic states, pseudo-obstruction, amyloidosis, strictures, fistulas	Steatorrhea, drug metabolism by bacteria, epithelial cell damage—reduced absorption
	Dilution of luminal contents	Sprue, disaccharidase deficiency state, secretory diarrheal disorders	Reduced drug concentration at absorbing unit surface
Pancreas	Exocrine insufficiency	Chronic pancreatitis Duct obstruction, inflammation, neoplasm	Malabsorption of fat-soluble preparations
Liver and biliary tract	Bile salt lack	Liver failure Obstructive jaundice	Malabsorption of fat-soluble preparations

ciency of which is determined by drug pK_a and the lipid/water partition coefficient for its non-ionic component. Factors that (1) impair gastric emptying, (2) result in the drug's complexing with other drugs or food, (3) retard dissolution of solid or particulate tablets, (4) induce major directional shifts in intestinal pH, or (5) alter intestinal structure or function may reduce drug absorption, bioavailability, and therapeutic efficacy. The role of microorganisms as regulators of drug absorption and of foodstuffs and chemicals on enzyme induction within the intestinal epithelial cell is receiving increasing attention. An appreciation of the processes that regulate normal absorption will enable a rational approach to be made to the patient who fails to respond to medical therapy because of impaired drug absorption.

References

1. Goodman LS, Gilman A. The Pharmacologic Basis of Therapeutics. 6th Ed., New York: Macmillan, 1980.
2. Schanker LS. Intimate study of drug action, absorption, distribution, and excretion. *In:* DiPalma JR, ed. Drill's Pharmacology in Medicine. New York: McGraw-Hill, 1971: 21.
3. Levine RR. Factors affecting gastrointestinal absorption of drugs. Am J Dig Dis 1970; 15:171.
4. Graham GG, Kennedy M. Drug absorption and bioavailability. Med J Austral 1978; 2:143.
5. Kramer PA, Chpron MS, Benson J, Mercik SA. Tetracycline absorption in elderly patients with achlorhydria. Clin Pharmacol Ther 1978; 23:467.
6. Nimmo J: The influence of metoclopramide on drug absorption. Postgrad Med J 1973; July Suppl, p 25.
7. Hogben CAM, Tocco DJ, Brodie BB, Schanker LS. On the mechanism of intestinal absorption of drugs. J Pharmacol Exp Ther 1959; 125:275.
8. Martin EW: Hazards of Medication. Philadelphia: JB Lippincott, 1971.
9. Poiger H, Schlattar C. Compensation of dietary induced reduction of tetracycline absorption by simultaneous administration of EDTA. Eur J Clin Pharmacol 1978; 14:129.
10. Gothani G, Pentikainen P, Vapaatalo HI, Wackman R, Afbjorksten K. Absorption of antibiotics: Influence of

metoclopramide and atropine on serum levels of pirampicillin and tetracycline. Ann Clin Res: 1972; 4:228.
11. Manninen V, Apajalahti A, Melin J, Karesoja M. Altered absorption of digoxin in patients given propantheline and metaclopramide in paracetamol absorption. Br Med J 1973; 1:587.
12. Levy G, Gibaldi M, Procknal JA. Effect of an anticholinergic agent on riboflavin absorption in man. J Pharmacol Sci 1972; 61:798.
13. Frey WH, Kampmann E. Interaction of amphetamine with anticonvulsant drugs. Acta Pharmacol Toxicol 1966; 24:310.
14. Consola S et al. Griseofulvin-phenobarbital interactions in man. Eur J Pharmacol 1970; 10:239.
15. Riegelman S, Rowland M, Epstein WL. Griseofulvin-phenobarbital interaction in man. JAMA 1970; 213:426.
16. Hurwitz A, Robinson RG, Vats TS, Whittier FC, Herrin WF. Effects of antacids on gastric emptying. Gastroenterology 1976; 71:268.
17. Greenblatt DJ, Allen MD, MacLaughlin DS, Harmatz JS, Shader RI. Diazepam absorption: Effect of antacids and food. Clin Pharmacol Ther 1978; 24:600.
18. Hurwitz A, Schlozman DL. Effects of antacids on gastrointestinal absorption of isoniazid in rat and man. Am Rev Resp Dis 1974; 109:41.
19. Graham DY. Pancreatic enzyme replacement. The effect of antacids and cimetidine. Dig Dis Sci 1982; 27:485.
20. Levine RA. Cyclic AMP in digestive physiology. Am J Clin Nutr 1973; 26:876.
21. Levy G. Gastrointestinal clearance of drugs with activated charcoal. N Engl J Med 1982; 307:676.
22. Berg MJ, Berlinger WG, Goldberg MJ, Spector R, Johnson GE. Acceleration of the body clearance of phenobarbital by oral activated charcoal. N Engl J Med 1982; 307:642.
23. Dawling S, Crome P, Braithwaite R. Effect of delayed administration of activated charcoal on nortriptyline absorption. Eur J Clin Pharmacol 1978; 14:445.
24. Peppercorn MA, Goldman P. The role of intestinal bacteria in the metabolism of salicylazosulfapyridine. J Pharmacol Exp Ther 1972; 181:555.
25. Lindenbaum J, Rund DG, Butler VP, Jr, Tse-Eng D, Sha JR. Inactivation of digoxin by the gut flora: Reversal by antibiotic therapy. N Engl J Med 1981; 305:789.
26. Dossetar J. Drug interaction with oral contraceptives. Br Med J 1975; 4:467.
27. Reiner D. Rifampicin, "Pill" do not go well together. JAMA 1974; 227:608.
28. Sandler M, Goodwin BL, Ruthven CRJ, Calne DB. Therapeutic implication in Parkinsonism of m-tyramine formation from L-dopa in man. Nature 1971; 229:414.
29. Sandler M, Karoum F, Ruthven CRJ, Calne DB. M-hydroxylphenyl-acetic acid formation from L-dopa in man: Suppression by neomycin. Science 1969; 166:1417.
30. Walsh CT, Feierabend JF, Levine RR. The effect of lincomycin on the excretion of diethylstibestrol and its ureterotrophic action in rats. Life Sci 1975; 16:1689.
31. Sallee VL, Wilson FA, Dietschy JM. Determination of unidirectional uptake rates for lipids across the intestinal brush border. J Lipid Res 1972; 13:184.
32. Bartelink A. Drug-induced diseases of the gastrointestinal tract. *In:* Megler L, Peck HM, eds. Drug-induced Diseases. Vol. 4. Amsterdam: Excerpta Medica, 1972: 110.
33. Siber GR, Mayer RJ, Levin MJ. Increased gastrointestinal absorption of large molecules in patients after 5-fluorouracil therapy for metastatic colon carcinoma. Cancer Res 1980; 40:3430.
34. Remmer H. The role of the liver in drug metabolism. Am J Med 1970; 49:617.
35. Ullrich V, Kremers P. Multiple forms of cytochrome P450 in the microsomol monooxygenase system. Arch Toxicol 1977; 39:41.
36. Welch RM, Cavallito J, Loh A. Effect of exposure to cigarette smoke on the metabolism of benzo(a)pyrene and acetophenetidim by lung and intestine of rats. Toxicol Appl Pharmacol 1972; 23:749.
37. Roe DA. Interactions between drugs and nutrients. Med Clin North Am 1979; 63:985.
38. Caldwell JH, Greenberger NJ. Cholestyramine enhances digitalis excretion and protects against lethal intoxication. J Clin Invest 1970; 49:169.
39. Fenster LF, Weser E. Hepatic and gastrointestinal disorders. *In:* Melmon KL, Morrelli HF, eds. Clinical Pharmacology. New York: Macmillan, 1972: 109.
40. Franklin JL, Rosenberg IH. Impaired folic-acid absorption in inflammatory bowel disease: Effects of salicylazosulfapyridine (Azulfidine). Gastroenterology 1973; 64:517.
41. Gallo DG, Baily KR, Sheffner AJ. The interaction between cholestyramine and drugs. Proc Soc Exp Biol Med 1965; 120:60.
42. Halsted CH, Robles EA, Mezey E. Decreased jejunal uptake of labeled folic-acid (^{3}H-PGA) in alcoholic patients: Roles of alcohol and nutrition. N Engl J Med 1971; 285:701.
43. Halsted CH, Robles EA, Mezey E. Intestinal malabsorption in folate-deficient alcoholics. Gastroenterology 1973; 64:526.
44. Kabins SA. Interactions among antibiotics and other drugs. JAMA 1972; 219:206.
45. Krondl A. Present understanding of the interaction of drugs and food during absorption. Can Med Assoc J 1970; 103:360.
46. Morrelli HF, Melmon KL. The clinician's approach to drug interactions. Cal Med 1968; 109:380.
47. Morrelli HF, Melmon KL. Drug interactions. *In:* Melmon K L, Morrelli HF, eds. Clinical Pharmacology. New York: Macmillan, 1972: 585.
48. Prescott LF. Pharmacokinetic drug interactions. Lancet 1969; 2:1239.
49. Raisfeld IH. Clinical pharmacology of drug interactions. *In:* Annual Review of Medicine. Vol. 24. Palo Alto, Ca: Annual Reviews, 1973: 385.
50. Roe DA. Drug-induced vitamin deficiencies. Drug Ther 1973; 3:23.
51. Rosenberg IH. Drugs and folic-acid absorption. Gastroenterology 1972; 63:353.
52. Thomas FB, McCullough FS, Greenberger NJ. Effect of phenobarbital on the absorption of inorganic and hemoglobin iron in the rat. Gastroenterology 1972; 62:590.
53. Thomas FB, Salisbury D, Greenberger NJ. Inhibition of iron absorption by cholestyramine. Am J Dig Dis 1972; 17:263.
54. Ware AJ, Combes B. Influence of sodium taurocholate, cholestyramine, and Mylanta on intestinal absorption of glucocorticoids in the rat. Gastroenterology 1973; 64:1150.
55. Steinberg WM, Lewis JH, Katz DM. Antacids inhibit absorption of cimetidine. N Engl J Med 1982; 307:400.

Chapter 99

Intestinal Immunology

Stephen B. Hanauer • Sumner C. Kraft

Non-Immunologic Aspects of Host Enteric Defense

As the major organ system naturally engaged in antigen sampling, the digestive tract is uniquely endowed to absorb nutrients from the environment and yet exclude the systemic uptake of noxious elements. In the latter regard, both immunologic and non-immunologic processes serve to protect the gut and the body as a whole.[1] Table 99–1 lists a number of non-immunologic host enteric defense mechanisms.

Salivary secretions are important in preventing the proliferation of microorganisms in the mouth.[2] *Lysozyme* may be bacteriolytic,[1] whereas the coating of more distal mucosal surfaces by glycoproteins and glycolipids may inhibit the growth of intestinal bacteria[3] or interfere with their adherence to the mucosa.[4] For example, mucosal extracts have the capacity to block receptors on bacteria, thus retarding the association of bacteria with luminal surfaces.[5] Likewise, the local production and release of *mucins* may provide a selective barrier to the epithelial penetration of enterotoxins and other biologically active macromolecules.[6] Additionally, mucosal goblet cells may work in concert with intestinal mast cells and antigen-antibody complexes located in the bowel lumen to release mucus—a further demonstration of the synergy of specific and non-specific antigen handling by the gut.[7, 8]

Table 99–1. NON-IMMUNOLOGIC ENTERIC DEFENSE MECHANISMS

Salivary secretions
Mucus
Gastric acid
Bile salts
Epithelial cell turnover
Gut "closure"
Peristalsis
Intestinal microflora

Gastric acidity protects the small intestine from undue exposure to microorganisms[9, 10] and macromolecular antigens.[11] If bacteria do survive passage through the stomach, they encounter potentially inhibitory *bile salts.*[12, 13] However, neither the succus entericus nor pancreatic juices appear to exert a significant antibacterial effect *in vivo,* as evidenced by the bacterial overgrowth that occurs in patients with the blind loop syndrome[9] (Chapter 107).

An increase in the rate of *renewal of epithelial surfaces* may occur in the presence of bacterial, viral, and parasitic infections.[14] The luminal loss of epithelial cells, connective tissue stroma, and lymphocytes, in the presence of absorbed and exuded fluids, tends to dilute, dissolve, or wash away various antigens.[14, 15] Fetal intestinal epithelial cells lack a complete brush border and therefore are capable of the non-immunologic endocytosis of macromolecules, which are then transported to the lamina propria and general circulation. Shortly after birth, however, the intestinal epithelial cells of the infant undergo maturation and this non-specific capacity to engulf antigens and microorganisms diminishes—a process often referred to as "gut closure."[16]

Peristalsis tends to dislodge macromolecules, microbes, and parasites from the small intestinal surface and inhibits microbial proliferation,[1, 9] whereas bacterial overgrowth may occur in the presence of intestinal hypomotility and stagnation of luminal contents. The indigenous gut flora are further influenced by factors such as local sanitation, diet, and competitive relationships among organisms. Bacteria interact through alterations in oxidation-reduction potential, as well as by synthesizing inhibitory short-chain fatty acids or colicins that serve to control the local environment.[9] Additionally, antibiotic therapy can profoundly affect the microbial inhabitants of the gut and permit a normally suppressed species (e.g., *Clostridium difficile)* to proliferate and cause pathologic changes.

General Immunologic Principles
(Table 99–2)*

The lymphoid cells of the immune system are organized to react exquisitely to specific antigens. While the mechanisms of antigen recognition and processing require the integration of several additional cell types, including macrophages and other phagocytes, the effector lymphocytes classically are separated into the cell-mediated *(T-cell)* and humoral *(B-cell)* immune systems (Fig. 99–1). While both types of these lymphocytes originate from bone marrow–derived precursors, the T-cell lineage undergoes further differentiation after thymic processing.

Thymus-independent B cells are responsible for the ultimate synthesis of immunoglobulin. They apparently differentiate and mature in humans as a result of factors in the fetal bone marrow, liver, and spleen—possibly the equivalent of the bursa of Fabricius of avian species. The majority of the relatively short-lived and sedentary B cells inhabit distinct thymus-independent areas in peripheral lymphoid tissues, such as germinal centers in the lymph nodes and spleen; they

* See Table 99–2 for abbreviations used.

Table 99–2. SELECTED ABBREVIATIONS USED IN GENERAL IMMUNOLOGY

ADCC: antibody-dependent cell-mediated cytotoxicity

B cell/B lymphocyte: thymus-independent lymphocyte of humoral immune system

Con A: concanavalin A

DNA: deoxyribonucleic acid

E rosettes: lymphocytes (T cells) rosetted with sheep erythrocytes (in absence of antibody and complement)

Fab: antigen-binding fragment of immunoglobulin molecule produced by enzymatic digestion wtih papain

Fc: crystallizable fragment of immunoglobulin heavy chains obtained following enzymatic digestion with papain

GALT: gut-associated lymphoid tissue

HLA: histocompatibility locus antigen

IEL: intraepithelial lymphocyte

IgA: immunoglobulin A

IgA1/IgA2: subclasses of IgA

IgD: immunoglobulin D

IgE: immunoglobulin E

IgG: immunoglobulin G

IgM: immunoglobulin M

IPSID: immunoproliferative small intestinal disease

J chain: a plasma cell–produced glycoprotein component of polymeric immunoglobulin molecules that joins the heavy chains

K cell: null cell mediating ADCC

M cell: "membrane" cell that lacks microvilli and forms a thin bridge between adjacent columnar intestinal epithelial cells

MHC: major histocompatibility complex

MLN: mesenteric lymph node

NK cell: natural killer cell

OKT4: a monoclonal murine antibody that reacts most closely against the subset of human helper/inducer T cells

OKT8: a monoclonal murine antibody that reacts most closely against the subset of human suppressor/cytotoxic T cells

PHA: phytohemagglutinin

SC: secretory component

SCMC: spontaneous cell-mediated cytotoxicity

sIgA: secretory IgA

T cell/T lymphocyte: thymus-dependent lymphocyte of cell-mediated immune system

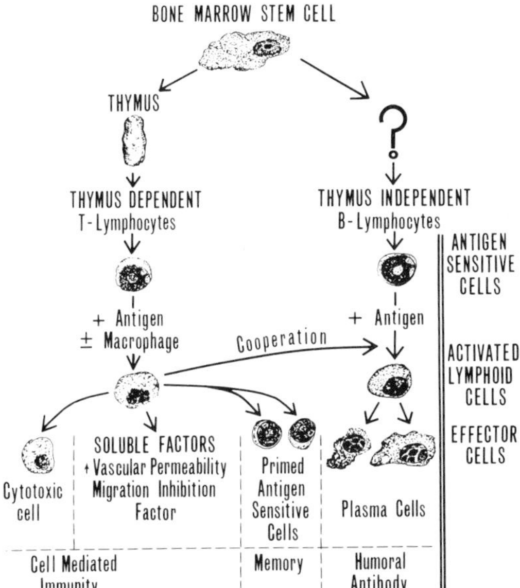

Figure 99–1. Schematic model for the derivation and function of the immunologic response. T lymphocytes mediate delayed type or cell-mediated immunity. B lymphocytes mediate humoral immunity.

constitute only about 15% of the circulating lymphocyte pool. As an individual B cell matures, the isotype of its surface immunoglobulin may undergo a transition directly from cell lines that bear IgM to separate cells bearing IgA, IgG, or IgE. Although some antigens (such as certain encapsulated bacterial polysaccharides and lipopolysaccharides) can directly stimulate the production of immunoglobulin by B cell–derived plasma cells, most antigens require the cooperation of *helper T cells* (see later) to elicit an optimal antibody response. In addition, *suppressor T cells* or monocytes/macrophages may interact with B cells to inhibit immunoglobulin and antibody production, functioning as important regulators of the expression of differentiated B-cell activity.

The longer-lived, recirculating thymus-dependent lymphocytes, or T cells, make up about 70% of lymphocytes in the blood and occupy the thymus-dependent areas of peripheral lymphoid tissues, such as the paracortex of lymph nodes and periarteriolar lymphoid sheaths of the spleen. Certain plant lectins, e.g., phytohemagglutinin and concanavalin A, are especially mitogenic for T cells and thus are useful functional markers of this lymphocyte population. However, human T cells are better identified by a propensity to form rosettes with sheep erythrocytes *(E rosettes).* T cells may be further differentiated into effector cells that are capable of mediating immunologic interactions with other T cells, B cells, or macrophages. This immunoregulation may occur by (1) helper or inducer function, suppression, amplification, or cytotoxicity; or (2) T-effector cells that produce soluble factors or lymphokines, such as transfer factor, macrophage chemotactic factor, macrophage inhibitory factor, lymphotoxin, or interferon. T-cell subsets often are classified according to these functional activities. They are classified as well by using a variety of monoclonal antibodies directed against stable cell-surface antigens that generally correspond to functional capabilities (e.g., mature, helper/inducer, or suppressor/cytotoxic T cells).

Functional heterogeneity is additionally exemplified by the cytotoxic capabilities of lymphocytes. Cytotoxic T cells, when stimulated, produce antigen-specific damage directed against cell-surface major histocompatibility complex (MHC)–coded transplantation antigens; this involves direct cell-cell interaction between the T cell and the target cell. Other cytotoxic lymphocytes carry receptors for the Fc region of immunoglobulins and participate in antibody-dependent cell-mediated cytotoxicity directed against target cells bearing antibody of the IgG or IgM isotypes. Since this "third population" of lymphocytes do not contain surface immunoglobulin and do not form E rosettes (in the absence of antibody and complement), they have been referred to as *null cells.* In contrast, so-called *natural killer* (NK) cells are capable of non-selective killing of nucleated target cells, termed spontaneous cell-mediated cytotoxicity. The importance of these various lymphocyte types in host-defense and host-tumor interactions is under intense investigation in many laboratories.

Antigen recognition and processing require the additional participation of non-lymphoid cells. Macrophages play a central role in the trapping of some antigens (especially those coated with antibody) that may find their way to the lymph node cortex, the walls of lymphatic sinusoids, or below specialized areas of the intestinal epithelium. Subsequently, T cells that share genetically identical portions of the MHC immune response region recognize and interact with soluble protein antigens derived from macrophages, requiring the physical binding of these 2 cell types. Such interactions lead to the induction of T-cell proliferation, macrophage-augmented phagocytosis and killing, and the secretion of additional mediators of the inflammatory response (e.g., complement components, lysozyme, proteases, hydrolases, prostaglandins, enzyme inhibitors). In concert with polymorphonuclear leukocytes, eosinophils, tissue mast cells, and biochemical mediators of inflammation (histamine, prostaglandins), lymphocytes and monocytes/macrophages direct the immune response throughout the body and are strategically arranged within the gut to react to the ubiquitous antigenic load.

Gut-Associated Lymphoid Tissue

While the non-immunologic mechanisms act to bar many foreign substances, the immunologic apparatus of the gut serves more specifically to defend the body against a virtually perpetual onslaught of antigens. Thus, the gut-associated lymphoid tissue (GALT) is a major division of the general immune system; indeed, approximately one-fourth of the intestinal mucosa is composed of lymphoid cells.[17] As indicated in Table 99–3, GALT may be categorized in terms of its non-aggregated and aggregated components, while subsets of lymphoid cells may

Table 99–3. GUT-ASSOCIATED LYMPHOID TISSUE (GALT)

Non-Aggregated
- Luminal leukocytes
- Intraepithelial lymphocytes, macrophages, and mast cells
- Lamina propria lymphoid cells
- Intestinal macrophages
- Tissue mast cells

Aggregated
- Peyer's patches
- Lymphoid follicles, microscopic
- Mesenteric lymph nodes

selectively migrate both within the gut wall and to remote non-enteric mucosal-associated sites.[18]

Non-Aggregated Lymphoid Tissue

Luminal Leukocytes. Prior to contact with the gastrointestinal epithelium, environmental substances may be exposed to lymphoid cells and other leukocytes within the gut lumen. Under experimental conditions, large numbers of lymphocytes have been observed on the luminal surface of Peyer's patches in mice infected with Giardia.[19] In normal rabbits, leukocytes on the luminal aspect of the epithelium appear to share an intimate relationship with intestinal microorganisms.[20] Functionally, these cells appear to be lymphocytes and macrophages that have migrated into the lumen from the mucosa, similar to luminal cells that have been described within bronchi.[21] The emigration of polymorphonuclear leukocytes into intestinal loops through antigen-induced, immune-mediated chemotaxis has been observed in guinea pigs,[22] and both neutrophils and lymphocytes have been reported to migrate across the gastric epithelium in increased numbers in human patients with gastric ulcers.[23] Certainly, neutrophils, lymphocytes, and eosinophils frequently are identifiable in the feces of humans with various infectious diarrheas and inflammatory bowel diseases.[24] Although the functional significance and ultimate fate of these luminal leukocytes remain uncertain, more than merely a passive cell-losing gastroenteropathy or an "intestinal sink" concept is suggested. There is no evidence of a back migration of luminal lymphoid cells across the intestinal epithelium.[25]

Intraepithelial Lymphocytes. The mucosal cells lining the gastrointestinal tract both contain and are interspersed with intraepithelial lymphocytes (IEL) and, under certain conditions, macrophages, mast cells, neutrophils, and eosinophils.[26, 27] Estimates of the prevalence of these cells in man range up to 20% of viable epithelial cells,[28] of which as few as 25% or as many as 75% are lymphocytes,[17, 27] depending on gut location, the presence or absence of disease, differences in methodology, and other variables.

The IEL population itself is far from homogeneous, being composed of varied cell sizes and sometimes containing granules on light and electron microscopy.[26, 29–34] Using immunohistochemical staining of tissue sections, the majority of IEL have reacted with T-cell antisera (90% of these T cells staining with the OKT8 monoclonal antibody that is most closely associated with the subset of suppressor/cytotoxic T cells).[35, 36] Mechanical and enzymatic tissue isolation techniques applied to human[27] and other bowel specimens,[26, 37–39] identify a more heterogeneous group of IEL, including T, B, and null cells. However, variations among techniques, species differences, and possible contamination with lymphoid cells of the lamina propria mandate caution in the interpretation of these data.[37, 40]

The T cell–enriched IEL population in guinea pigs proliferates *in vitro* in response to phytohemagglutinin and concanavalin A, includes antigen-specific responder T cells, and is capable of stimulation in mixed lymphocyte cultures; the B cell–enriched IEL population responds to lipopolysaccharide.[37, 38] Other studies in the guinea pig have demonstrated mitogen-induced cellular cytotoxicity using isolated IEL[41]; furthermore, both animal[41, 42] and human IEL[40] appear to have the capacity to participate in antibody-dependent and spontaneous cell-mediated cytotoxicity reactions.

Transfer studies in animals support the thymus-derived origin of the majority of IEL.[43, 44] Although the exact homing mechanism has yet to be defined, these IEL appear to enter the crypt epithelium by way of the blood stream,[43–48] and their distribution clearly is influenced by the nature of the luminal contents. In studies using lambs, for example, only 4 or fewer lymphocytes/100 epithelial cells were present throughout gestation; this number normally increased to 30 to 35 by 2 months after birth, whereas intestinal epithelium isolated from the flow of luminal contents contained far fewer IELs.[45] Similar sequelae of antigen deprivation have been reported in germ-free mice[46] and in studies of fetal mouse intestine grafted under the kidney capsule.[47]

The fate of IEL requires clarification. They cannot remain between epithelial cells for long without being shed into the lumen,[45] but this would not appear to be their usual disposition.[43,49] As discussed later, IEL may be primed by antigens and re-enter the lamina propria and circulation.[50] Their clinical importance has not been determined, although quantitative and qualitative differences among IEL have been reported in several diseases.[27, 34, 51]

Lamina Propria Lymphocytes. There are few lymphoid cells in the lamina propria of newborn or germ-free animals;[52] after birth, however, increasing numbers of these cells populate the lymphatic and vascular-rich connective tissues of the gut. This condition is referred to as "physiologic inflammation" and can be experimentally reproduced before birth by injecting antigens into the fetal intestine.[45] IgM-containing B cells and their progeny predominate initially, possibly stimulated by luminal lipopolysaccharide.[52]

The B-cell population of the intestinal lamina propria accounts for approximately 25% of the total lymphoid cell pool in normal adults.[27] Approximately 80% to 90% of the former contain IgA, compared with 2% to 5% in either the spleen or peripheral lymph nodes[53]; 60% to 70% of the small intestinal IgA cells are located within 200 μm of the lumen or base of the villi, providing 10^{10} IgA cells/meter of small bowel.[54] The rest of the lamina propria cells consist of T cells (50%) and null cells (25%); macrophages, mast cells, neutrophils, and eosinophils generally have been considered to make up less than 1% of the normal human lamina propria population.[27, 40]

The T-cell population of the lamina propria is composed of a greater proportion of helper/inducer cells[36] than is detectable among the IEL, although suppressor/cytotoxic cells are also present.[37, 40, 55] Most studies using isolated lamina propria lymphocytes demonstrate a capacity for both antibody-dependent and spontaneous cell-mediated cytotoxicity.[40, 42, 56, 57] Results, however, have differed, depending upon the methods used and the diseases studied.[58, 59]

Mucosal mast cells are morphologically and functionally heterogeneous in comparison with those located in other tissues.[60, 61] For example, they respond to different stimuli for histamine secretion, as well as to different pharmacologic modulators, and they require T cells for rapid proliferation in the presence of parasites.[62] While the human duodenal mucosa appears to contain approximately 20,000 mast cells/mm^3 and the distribution varies throughout the intestinal layers, improved methods for isolating these cells suggest that these numbers may be underestimates.[63] Clearly, the precise role of these multipotent cells in gastrointestinal diseases has yet to be determined.[62, 63] Likewise, studies suggest that mucosal eosinophils are recruited by lymphocytes in response to increased tissue utilization and also behave as modulators of immune responses involving IgE-mediated mast cell degranulation.[64]

Aggregated Lymphoid Tissue

Peyer's Patches. Large numbers of solitary lymphoid follicles are scattered throughout the intestinal lamina propria. They range in size from 0.6 to 3 mm in diameter and are present mainly above the muscularis mucosae but can be found in all layers of the bowel wall.[65] Both the solitary lymphoid follicles and Peyer's patches are more prominent in the ileum, where the latter consist of groupings of many lymphoid follicles aggregated into a mass, usually situated along the antimesenteric border. They can be recognized grossly as thickened and elongated oval nodules measuring up to 2 cm in diameter. Peyer's patches in man first appear at 24 weeks of gestation and tend to involute with age.[66]

Studies using isolated segments of fetal lamb ileum demonstrate histologically mature Peyer's patches at birth, prior to stimulation by luminal antigens.[45] Their architecture appears unaltered following antigenic contact. Follicles in isolated non-antigen-stimulated intestinal segments grow at the same rate as those in normal intestine after birth, but they begin to involute unless continuity with intact bowel is restored. Coinciding with the development of Peyer's patches according to these studies, the thoracic duct lymphocyte output increases by 4-fold over the first 3 weeks of life and there is a 40-fold increase in small lymphocytes that contain surface immunoglobulin. Such changes are nullified in fetal lambs in whom Peyer's patches have been removed, suggesting that Peyer's patches may be primary lymphoid organs during an *in utero* period of genetically predetermined growth; later, antigenic stimulation may amplify specific clonal proliferation.[45]

If this aggregated lymphoid tissue is found to be the mammalian equivalent of the avian central lymphoid organ (the bursa of Fabricius), this role would seem to be limited to uterine life. For example, the quantitative level of cellular proliferation in Peyer's patches in the mouse is insufficient for a central B-cell generating organ.[67] Furthermore, since Peyer's patches contain both functional T and B lymphocytes,[68] and in view of the previously noted responses of the fetal lamb intestine to antigen,[45] a continuing role as a central lymphoid organ seems unlikely; these lymphoid aggregates therefore must constitute part of the peripheral immune system.

The anatomy of Peyer's patches continues to be an area of fertile investigation, as more highly refined probes are used to identify lymphoid subpopulations. Morphologic studies of individual patches also make note of an overlying specialized follicle-associated epithelium that covers a dome region rich in lymphocytes, plasma cells, and macrophages.[69, 70] While the dome region and the interfollicular zone of Peyer's patches are predominantly T-cell areas,[20] the full development of both the T- and B-cell zones of Peyer's patches is thymus-dependent.[71] The germinal centers of the follicles consist mainly of B cells and plasma cells[70] accompanied by occasional helper T cells.[72, 73] Paracortical lymphocytes are either of the suppressor/cytotoxic T-cell subset[72, 73] or devoid of T-cell surface phenotypic markers.[70]

The domed surfaces of lymphoid follicles and Peyer's patches bulge into the intestinal lumen between villi; the tonsils and appendix also are covered with a similar epithelial coat.[19, 69, 74–77] The number of goblet cells is reduced; this creates a breach in the mucous layer and allows luminal particles to reach unique "M" (membrane) cells that lack microvilli and form thin bridges between the microvillus-covered columnar epithelial cells.[69, 75] The lack of a developed terminal web between M cells allows lymphoid cells migrating within the follicle and its specialized epithelium to cluster close to the intestinal lumen.[69] The internal vesicles of M cells are capable of transporting luminal moieties to the underlying macrophages and lymphocytes.[75, 78] The M cells arise from partially differentiated cuboidal epithelial cells that migrate from adjacent crypts, possibly promoted by chemotactic factors and an inhibition of goblet cell migration over Peyer's patches.[77] Microvascular connections between the dome epithelium and the capillaries supplying perifollicular crypts afford a potential pathway for chemical or cellular mediators to influence the migration of cuboidal M-cell precursors.[79] Radioactive labeling studies in mice have confirmed the motility and migration of lymphoblasts below M cells, providing an efficient mechanism for antigen sampling and transport.[77, 78] Evidence for the bidirectional transport of horseradish peroxidase, coupled with the presence of adjacent plasma cells, raises the possibility that M cells may be involved in transferring locally produced immunoglobulins into the intestinal lumen[75] (Fig. 99–2).

Although Peyer's patches are enriched with B-cell precursors that are destined to populate the intestinal lamina propria with IgA-producing cells,[80] these *in situ* B cells appear incapable of secreting antibody.[68, 81] Likewise, lymphoid cells from Peyer's patches seem incapable of mediating either

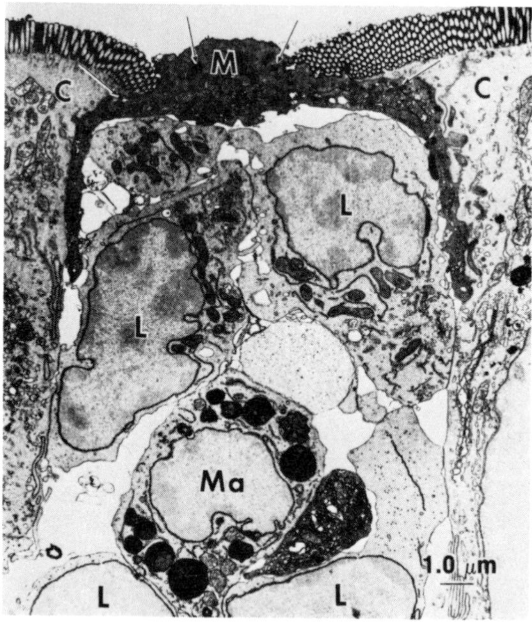

Figure 99–2. Mouse Peyer's patch "M" cell (M) surrounding several lymphocytes (L) and a macrophage (Ma). Arrows mark vesicles transporting horseradish peroxidase. Portions of 2 adjacent columnar epithelial cells (C) are shown. (From Owen RL, Nemanic P. Scanning Electron Microsc 1978; 2:367–78. Reproduced with permission.)

antibody-dependent or spontaneous cell-mediated cytotoxicity, suggesting an absence of K cells.[41] On the other hand, functional T cells have been isolated from Peyer's patches,[17, 68, 82, 83] including subpopulations capable of mediating graft-versus-host reactions.[84]

In summary, Peyer's patches play an active role in sampling luminal antigens, which then stimulate the maturation and release of the precursors of IgA-producing cells into the lymphatic circulation. Within the Peyer's patch, these antigen-sensitive precursors may clonally expand and migrate or may proliferate locally and generate additional secondary IgA precursors, without maturation to plasma cells.[85] The regulatory mechanisms of helper and suppressor T-cell interactions that are involved within the mucosal follicular microenvironment await further clarification.[17, 82, 85]

Mesenteric Lymph Nodes. Unlike Peyer's patches, the mesenteric lymph nodes (MLN) of fetal lambs respond vigorously to antigen that is introduced into the intestines. These fetal lymph nodes consist of a thin band of cortex with medullary cords that are populated by undifferentiated small lymphocytes; germinal centers are absent and lymphoid cells are scarce in the sinuses. With *in utero* antigenic challenge, germinal centers appear within the enlarging cortices, immunoblasts proliferate, sinuses become filled with lymphoid cells, and plasmacytes appear in the medullary cords. Following the same embryologic development as peripheral lymph nodes, the MLN become highly reactive after birth unless a germ-free environment is maintained.[45] The MLN are constantly exposed to antigenic materials that may then be filtered out by resident macrophages.[86]

In re-injection experiments, large radiolabeled MLN lymphocytes localize preferentially to the intestinal lamina propria or return to the MLN (and to a lesser extent to the lungs, mammary glands, and proestrial cervix) without a tendency to "home" back to peripheral lymph nodes.[18, 87] Although MLN lymphocytes are capable of repopulating the lamina propria, they do not appear to be essential for the selective migration to the gut of antibody-containing cells that had been generated by intestinal immunization.[88] The following section discusses cell migration in more detail.

Circulatory Patterns of Gut-Associated Lymphoid Tissue

Studies of the circulatory patterns of lymphoid cells have further defined the concept of gut-associated lymphoid tissue (GALT), emphasizing it to be a compartment of a more generalized mucosa-associated lymphoid system.

The continuous and dynamic process of populating the gut with lymphoid cells begins before birth,[89] as demonstrated by the recirculation of lymphocytes through Peyer's patches in fetal lambs.[90] In such an environment, free of extrinsic antigen, there is no evidence of a differential pattern of lymphocyte circulation.[91] In mature sheep, however (after cannulating efferent lymphatic vessels from peripheral lymph nodes, the thoracic duct, and MLN), injected radiolabeled small lymphocytes of intestinal origin are observed to migrate preferentially back to the intestine. Conversely, subcutaneously derived lymphocytes return to peripheral lymphoid tissues.[92–94] In earlier studies in rats, large lymphoblasts of thoracic duct origin were shown to "home" back to the lamina propria of the small intestine.[95,96] This selective migration back to the gut of lymphoblasts of intestinal origin has been widely confirmed.[43,97–99]

Many of the lymphoblasts isolated from the MLN,[43,97,100,101] Peyer's patches,[80] and the thoracic duct[95] either bear surface or cytoplasmic IgA or are committed precursors of IgA-producing cells. The IgA-secreting cells in the gut are maintained by the traffic of large lymphocytes entering the blood through the thoracic duct and migrating back to the lamina propria, where differentiation to plasma cells is completed.[87] Although less than 5% of thoracic duct lymphocytes are producers of IgA, as manifested by cytoplasmic IgA, the presence of surface IgA appears to be a better indicator of those immunoblasts that are destined for migration to the lamina propria.[87] Using isolated intestinal loops in rats sensitized to cholera toxin, the antitoxin-containing cells that migrate back to the intestine (1) are almost all of the IgA isotype, (2) do not migrate back to segments that do not contain Peyer's patches, (3) are derived from both large non-recirculating and small circulating lymphocytes, and (4) continue to persist.[88]

Studies of cell migration patterns in sheep

identify 2 separate populations of T lymphocytes, i.e., T cells from the thoracic duct with preferential circulation through the gut and T cells derived from subcutaneous lymph nodes that are destined for peripheral migration.[92] This dichotomy applies to T lymphoblasts in mice[43,48,102]; there is a similar homing back to both the lamina propria and the intraepithelial region of T lymphoblasts derived from MLN and the thoracic duct lymph.

Demonstration of preferential cell trafficking within gut, mammary gland, respiratory, and genitourinary epithelia has expanded the concept of a common mucosa-associated lymphoid system.[18] An early report of highly specific IgA-antibody titers in the milk, but not the serum, of sows perorally exposed to transmissible gastroenteritis virus suggested the migration of gut-sensitized cells to the mammary glands.[103] Rabbit studies also indicated high levels of colostral IgA antibodies (in the absence of specific serum antibodies) following oral exposure to dinitrophenolated pneumococci.[104] Links between the intestinal, urinary, and bronchial tracts have been established as well in rats experimentally infected or colonized with *E. coli.* In animals previously exposed to the same bacterial serotypes, the rapid secretory IgA response in the urine suggests an anamnestic response made possible by the initial homing of gut-primed cells to the urinary tract.[105] In humans, the ingestion of killed *Streptococcus mutans* produced strain-specific IgA antibodies in the saliva and tears, again in the absence of serum antibodies, adding further support to the concept of a generalized mucosal immune system.[106]

Transfer studies demonstrate homing of MLN lymphoblasts to the gut, lungs, mammary glands, and proestrial cervix, in preference to peripheral lymph nodes.[18,87,107] This provides a mechanism for the appearance at distal mucosal sites of antigen-sensitive cells capable of producing IgA. The lymphoid follicles of the lamina propria of the respiratory tract are morphologically similar to those of the gut, and lymphoid cells from the bronchial-associated lymphoid tissue have the capacity to repopulate GALT with IgA-producing cells.[21] Further documentation of specific cell traffic is provided by the spectrotypic analysis (isoelectric focusing) of IgA antibodies in the intestinal, mammary, and salivary secretions of enterically immunized rats; cells with identical clonotype potential seeded these widely separated secretory surfaces.[108]

The antigen-specific trafficking of lymphocytes is not limited to B cells, since analyses of colostral cellular activity demonstrate the transfer of T cell–mediated tuberculin sensitivity to breast-fed neonates.[109] The highest level of specific T-cell activity in colostrum occurs immediately after the onset of lactation; thus, these T cells may represent another subpopulation of gut-associated lymphocytes that had migrated to the breast during pregnancy.

The demonstration of a common mucosa-associated lymphoid system raises basic questions regarding the mechanisms of selective cell homing to these secretory sites. Some organ-specific trafficking to lymph nodes appears to be controlled by interactions between lymphocytes and the endothelial cells of high endothelial venules.[89,110,111] The latter are specialized vessels that direct the movement of lymphocytes from the blood into lymph nodes and Peyer's patches, as well as into areas of inflammation. For example, the preferential binding of peripheral lymph node lymphocytes and Peyer's patch lymphocytes to their respective high endothelial venules has been demonstrated.[112] Conversely, the homing characteristics of uncommitted B and T cells appear to be largely independent of the organ of origin; yet, B cells migrate preferentially to Peyer's patches and MLN, while T cells seem to migrate more to peripheral lymph nodes. This would suggest at least 2 complementary sets of lymphoendothelial receptors.[111]

There does *not* seem to be a specialized site within the lamina propria for newly arrived antibody-containing cells to accumulate.[113] In the isolated intestinal loop model, a uniform distribution of such cells occurs above and below the crypts. However, after entering the lamina propria of immunized loops, *specific* immunocytes accumulate around the crypt region, while *non-specific* antibody-containing cells disperse, die, or migrate.[113]

As already discussed, antigen may play a limited role as an attractor of sensitized lymphoid cells, e.g., the *in utero* homing of lymphocytes in fetal sheep prior to extrinsic antigen exposure.[94] The selective trafficking of lymphoid cells to gut mucosal tissues also has been demonstrated in cesarean-born neonatal rats and in sterile heterotropic transplants of syngeneic fetal gut in rats and mice.[114] The preservation of both the structural morphology of high endothelial venules and the separate B- and T-cell areas in these transplanted fetal tissues is felt to contribute to the homing process.[21]

Nevertheless, antigen certainly has a profound effect on the location, magnitude, and persistence of intestinal immune responses.[88] Studies of isolated intestinal loops in cholera toxoid–primed rats document the accumulation by way of cell division of antibody-producing cells in stimulated loops, while cells without specific antibody migrate through unstimulated loops but do not persist in these segments.[88,113] T-cell lymphoblasts similarly localize in the gut in response to exposure to parasites, even before the development of pathologic changes.[102]

The predominance of the IgA response at mucosal surfaces might suggest that secretory component (SC) could serve as an important target of homing; however, the experimental injection of anti-SC antibodies does not inhibit the subsequent accumulation of IgA precursor cells.[87] Another potential mechanism for the homing of lymphoid cells involves genetic coding for Ia antigens on epithelial cells, which could act as receptors for IgA-producing cells; this has been suggested by studies of the mammary gland.[115] Furthermore, the molecular determinants of lymphoid cell migration may be influenced by hormonal factors with respect to the genital organs, but apparently not the gut or respiratory mucosa.[21] Either bronchial or gastric immunization can trigger the remote-site stimulation of mammary and salivary immunoglobulin secretion,[116] but the homing of MLN cells to mammary and genital tissues can be greatly affected by manipulating endocrine hormones.[18,117,118] Changes in migratory patterns and responses to antigenic challenges can also be induced by nutritional factors, such as protein deprivation[119] or vitamin A deficiency,[120] that have the potential to alter the surface glycoprotein receptors of lymphocytes.

Obviously, intricate mechanisms govern lymphocyte migration and localization and the controlling factors remain poorly understood.

Secretory Immune System

Morphologic Considerations. As a result of the migration of B-cell precursors, the intestinal mucosa and submucosa become richly endowed with plasma cells, which appear in the neonatal human intestine at 3 weeks of age and are initially of the IgM isotype.[121] The mean number of these cells remains relatively constant from 1 to 6 months of age, but the proportion and number of IgA-containing cells continue to increase for up to 2 years. IgA-producing cells are derived from precursors that previously carried surface IgM, the commitment to ultimate isotype expression being determined during early stages of antigen-independent development.[122] Isotype restriction may depend upon the stage of maturation at which a B cell is "triggered." Although there usually is a progression of IgM to IgG to IgA, the IgG step does not appear to be necessary.[122]

Table 99–4. IMMUNOGLOBULIN-CONTAINING CELLS IN NORMAL ADULT HUMAN INTESTINAL MUCOSA*

	IgA Cells	IgM Cells	IgG Cells
Jejunum	81%	17%	2.6%
Ileum	83%	11%	5.0%
Large bowel	90%	6%	4.2%

*Adapted from Brandtzaeg P, Baklien K.[54]

After the neonatal period, the preponderant intestinal immunoglobulin-containing cells are of the IgA isotype, resulting in up to 10^{10} IgA cells/meter of small intestine.[54] As shown in Table 99–4, the relative ratios of IgA:IgM:IgG cells are fairly uniform throughout the length of the bowel, with IgA cells accounting for between 80% and 90% of the detectable immunocytes. The majority of these cells are distributed less than 200 μm from the lumen or base of the villi, with lesser numbers located nearer to the muscularis mucosae.[54]

Secretory IgA. As described by Tomasi et al.,[123] the IgA molecule in secretions differs from the majority of the serum IgA molecules. Human serum IgA generally is detectable in 3 forms: (1) IgA monomers; (2) polymeric IgA, usually composed of dimers of 2 monomeric subunits linked covalently by disulfide bonds and a J chain; and (3) small amounts of secretory IgA, consisting of the polymeric IgA molecule with SC attached. Ninety per cent of the serum IgA is monomeric, whereas the predominant form in external secretions is secretory IgA (sIgA). Differences between serum IgA and sIgA may derive from the site of production, since human tissue culture experiments demonstrate bone marrow IgA synthesis to be 90% monomeric, while plasma cells isolated from the lamina propria, as well as their circulating precursors, produce mostly polymeric IgA that contains cytoplasmic J chains.[124,125]

There also are differences in the distribution of IgA between the serum and intestinal mucosa; the former contains approximately 90% IgA1 and 10% IgA2, while the latter has about 40% IgA2[126] (which is apparently more resistant to luminal degradation[65]). Lower levels of circulating IgA2 may reflect its more rapid clearance by secretory surfaces.[127] Although the mucosal production of immunoglobulins can be readily approximated by counting isotype-producing cells, intestinal fluid immunoglobulins are more difficult to quantitate and their source is controversial. While levels of immunoglobulins may be fairly constant in the duodenal fluid of healthy children and young adults from ages 2 weeks to 19 years, with IgG>IgM>IgA,[128] most of the IgG is thought to be derived from the serum of these individuals. On the other hand, IgA and IgM have SC attached, pointing to their source as the lamina propria plasma cells or the hepatobiliary tree (see later). Further studies, perhaps concurrently quantitating luminal immunoglobulin and mucus production, are needed for clarification.[129]

The sIgA dimer is an 11S molecule that consists of 2 7S IgA monomers covalently linked at their heavy chains by the J (joining) peptide.[130] J-chain synthesis is initiated early during the local immune response within the mucosal plasma cells, where the peptide is incorporated into either the IgA dimers or the IgM pentamers.[54] The combination of the J chains and the locally produced IgA or IgM induces a configuration that is thought to permit the complexing of the polymers with SC.[131] These relationships are schematically shown in Figure 99–3. Nevertheless, the intestinal immunocytes that produce IgA are heterogeneous with regard to J-chain content, SC affinity, and the proportions of monomers to polymers.

Secretory component is a glycoprotein of approximately 83,000 daltons that is produced principally by crypt epithelial cells, making sIgA a lymphoepithelial product of diverse cell types. Initially, SC can be identified in the endoplasmic reticulum and Golgi apparatus[54,132]; it is later incorporated into the lower two-thirds of the lateral plasma membrane of the epithelial cell, where it may serve as a receptor for J chain–containing IgA or IgM.[133,134] For example, the binding of polymeric IgA to the luminal surface of intestinal epithelial cells (Fig. 99–4) occurs concomitantly with the appearance of SC on the

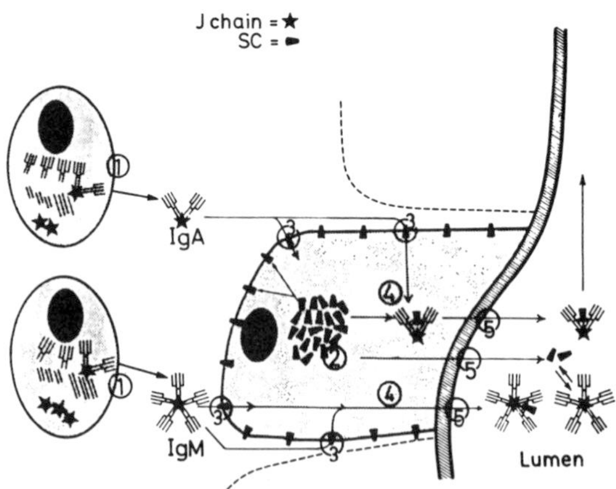

Figure 99–3. Schematic representation of gland-associated synthesis and transport of dimeric IgA pentameric IgM. (From Brandtzaeg P, Baklien K. Ciba Found Symp 1977; 46:77–108. Reproduced with permission.)

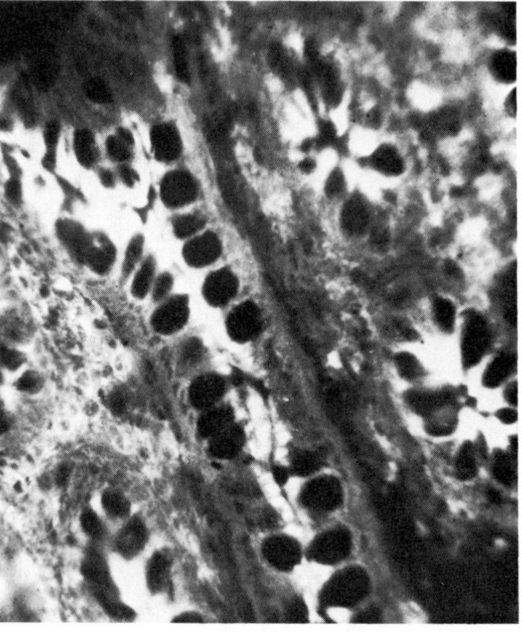

Figure 99–4. Longitudinal section of an adult human rectal gland *(center)* showing cytoplasmic IgA lining the apical portion of the ductular lumen. There is an absence of staining of the mucus portion of the goblet cells, nuclei, and basal cytoplasm. (From Gelzayd EA, et al. Science 1967; 157:930–1. Copyright 1967, American Association for the Advancement of Science. Reproduced with permission.)

epithelial membranes. This binding is blocked by adding sIgA that already contains SC, and the binding is inhibited in the presence of anti-SC antibodies but not monomeric IgA.[135]

Secretory component synthesis occurs independent of IgA synthesis; it begins in fetal life prior to the onset of IgA production and also occurs in patients with hypogammaglobulinemia. Individuals with IgA deficiency can produce SC and persons with SC deficiency can produce IgA[54,136]; however, a defect in the glandular transport of immunoglobulins has yet to be shown as a primary cause of disease.

The non-covalent complexing of polymeric IgA and SC stimulates pinocytosis by the epithelial cell. Within the pinocytotic vesicles, bonding is stabilized by disulfide exchanges and the secretory polymers are transported through the cell to be extruded into the gut lumen or along general glandular secretory pathways. IgA monomers produced by intestinal immunocytes either drain into the systemic circulation or are degraded in the intestinal lumen.[54,131,133]

The special structural properties imparted to sIgA by the combination of J chains and SC are felt to increase its resistance to proteolytic digestion within the enzyme-rich intestinal milieu.[137] Intraluminally, sIgA may distribute within the chyme and form complexes with mucinous components that coat the mucosal surface,[6,138] although the actual content of secretory immunoglobulins in mucin may be modest.[139]

The biologic functions of sIgA are diverse. The antigen-binding property of sIgA is enhanced by the 4 potential binding positions of the Fab segments of the dimeric immunoglobulin molecule. Antibacterial protective mechanisms include: (1) direct activity against lipopolysaccharide, pili, or fimbriae, resulting in immobilization, agglutination, or inhibition of adherence to the mucosal surface[105, 140]; (2) inhibition of bacterial division when associated with lactoferrin[105] or lysozyme and complement[65]; and (3) induction of an "antigenic drift," resulting in less virulent organisms secondary to genetic alterations of bacterial surface characteristics.[105] In combination with bacterial toxins or luminal enzymes, sIgA may induce antigenic inactivation or assist in proteolytic degradation.[140] By increasing the contact of bacteria with mucus, sIgA also may enhance immune exclusion.[141]

In addition, sIgA is known to combine with and neutralize viruses[142] and prevent uptake of viruses from the gut lumen.[140] Absorption of other macromolecular antigens may be impaired by the phenomenon of antigen-antibody complexing that interferes with adherence to epithelial surfaces and allows increased digestion by luminal enzymes.[138,143] An sIgA response to small quantities of antigen that escape exclusion and penetrate the mucosa could further limit absorption[144] and play a role in depressing the local inflammatory response by modulating IgG-mediated phagocytosis.[141] Antigen-antibody complexes also are known to enhance the release of goblet-cell mucus,[8] to act synergistically with other immunologic and physiologic protective mechanisms, and to inhibit reaginic-type hypersensitivity reactions at the surface of the intestinal epithelium.[7,65]

Compared with IgM or IgG, sIgA is not as effective a participant in inflammatory responses that are activated by the Fc portions of immunoglobulins. Although the alternate complement pathway may be activated by chemically aggregated IgA, sIgA-antigen complexes appear incapable of initiating activation of either the alternate or the classical complement system.[145] While sIgA does not opsonize bacteria in preparation for phagocytosis,[146] it can induce antibody-dependent cell-mediated antibacterial activity in the absence of complement.[147]

Regulation of Secretory IgA Production and Secretion. As described earlier, localization of the secretory immune response to the intestine requires the homing of IgA precursors or memory cells to the gut. The presence of luminal antigen and its subsequent processing by Peyer's patches are requisites for antibody-containing cells to persist and accumulate within intestinal segments.[88] The germinal centers of Peyer's patches are the sites of generation of the IgA-cell precursors and may play a role in the phenomenon of surface heavy-chain switching.[148] In the intestinal microenvironment, the potential to express isotypic and idiotypic antibody responses is stimulated by antigen-induced cell division and is associated with the loss of surface IgD.[149,150]

The role of T cells in regulating the intestinal IgA response has been studied more vigorously since the demonstration that both the clonal expansion of IgA memory cells[151] and the production of IgA antibody[152] require the presence of thymus-derived lymphocytes. Subsequently, T-cell subsets have been shown to have differing immunoregulatory activities in various tissues vis-à-vis either the enhancement or the suppression of isotypic antibody production.[153] More recently, the T-cell induction of immunoglobulin heavy-chain switching[154] and the presence of antigen-specific IgA helper T cells have been described.[155] Furthermore, murine T cells with Fc receptors for IgA are known to possess specific isotypic suppressor cell activity against IgA, without influencing IgG or IgM production[156]; the diminished mucosal IgA cells described in children with malnutrition may relate to a T-cell defect that secondarily influences the differentiation or localization of lymphocytes.[157] Although IgA precursors migrate to diverse sites, differentiation and proliferation may occur only in tissues with a "favorable" helper:suppressor T-cell ratio; the latter may be antigen-regulated.[158]

Finally, regulation of the secretion of immunoglobulins into intestinal fluids is partly dependent upon non-immunologic mechanisms. Since the intestinal secretion of IgA in rats can be stimulated by cholinergic agonists, the autonomic nervous system has been conceived as facilitating IgA transport into the lumen in coordination with the presence of swallowed antigens.[159] Also, concentrations of duodenal IgA and IgM in children selectively increase after the IV administration of secretin; this phenomenon appears to be associated with an enhanced local secretion of mucus.[160]

Hepatobiliary Aspects of the Secretory Immune System. The IgA produced in the lamina propria is not fully secreted into the gut lumen; a portion enters the portal, lymphatic, and systemic circulations. The role of the liver in the subsequent intestinal delivery of this circulating IgA was initially suggested by the observation of a 10-fold increase in the amount of IgA in rat bile as compared with serum[161]; the biliary IgA concentration increased significantly in the presence of common bile duct obstruction.[162] Subsequent experiments confirmed that the rodent hepatobiliary tract is capable of transporting dimeric IgA, in preference to IgM and monomeric IgA, after combining with SC.[163–166] This appears to involve a unique vesicular transport mechanism within hepatocytes that bypasses the Golgi apparatus.[167] While the transfer of circulating IgA dimers also occurs in humans,[165,166] the exact site of the hepatobiliary secretion of sIgA remains undetermined. There is evidence for both IgA and SC uptake in hepatocytes,[168] as well as in the epithelial cells of bile ducts.[169] The magnitude of the selective clearance of circulating dimeric IgA into bile in man does not seem to be as great as in the rat, suggesting that local synthesis accounts for the major portion of the sIgA appearing in human bile under physiologic conditions.[165]

In the presence of liver disease or biliary obstruction, changes may occur in the concentration of serum IgA. For example, infants with cholestatic jaundice associated with either extra- or intrahepatic biliary obstruction have shown marked increases in serum sIgA levels, the levels being much higher in those with intrahepatic disease.[170] On the other hand, the use of different methods of measurement demonstrated both the total amount of serum IgA and the proportion of polymeric IgA to be normal in 4 cases of total biliary obstruction.[171] Other studies have shown 2- to 4-fold elevations of serum IgA, mainly accounted for by increased proportions of polymeric IgA, in patients with alcoholic cirrhosis and other liver disorders.[172] Although these observations have not clarified the site of secretion of the biliary IgA, human T-tube drainage analyses suggest that at least 10% to 20% of intestinal IgA may be derived from sources within the biliary tree.[172]

Despite its uncertain source, several potential functions of biliary sIgA are apparent. The salvage of circulating polymeric IgA with return of secretory antibody to the intestinal lumen has been documented in rats.[173,174] Another important function would be the elimination of enterically derived antigens that enter the portal or systemic circulations. Thus, the sIgA in bile has been shown to agglutinate antigens *in vitro*,[174] and IgA antibodies are capable of mediating the clearance of specific antigens from blood to bile.[175,176] The formation of IgA-containing immune complexes with their subsequent biliary clearance is therefore a potential mechanism for eliminating undesirable circulating antigens and returning them to the intestine in an innocuous form without inciting the cascade of immune-mediated inflammatory reactions.[166] Although IgA-containing immune complexes have been identified as potential mediators of disease, disruption of the hepatobiliary transport of sIgA has yet to be implicated directly in the pathogenesis of any clinical disorder.[166]

In summary, IgA cells are delivered to secretory surfaces throughout the body, and sIgA appears in the corresponding secretions. Thus, the selective transport of IgA dimers, likely enhanced by the recognition of SC by epithelial receptors, appears to be a mechanism common to the epithelial cells of the intestines, liver, salivary glands, and mammary glands.[177,178]

Other Intestinal Immunoglobulins

IgM. IgM shares many of the secretory properties of IgA, in part related to the capacity to bind with SC.[54,171,179–181] As already noted, IgM-producing cells also are found within the lamina propria throughout the intestines. Although there tends to be a marked increase in the number of these IgM cells in individuals deficient in IgA,[182] suggesting at least a supportive role for IgM in defending the intestinal mucosa, the majority of the IgM in intestinal fluids appears to be partially digested by luminal enzymes.[139,183]

IgG. The absence of a J chain greatly limits the affinity of IgG for SC.[184] Therefore, the epithelial secretion of IgG is not known to occur, and its presence within the lumen of the gut is much more likely to be derived from the serum than from local production.[185] The content of IgG cells in the lamina propria is diminished compared with IgA and IgM cells,[54] except in the presence of inflammation.[186] An increase in the number of intestinal IgG cells also has been reported in patients with Hirschsprung's disease.[187]

IgE. While IgE is primarily a mucosal antibody and IgE cells can be found along the respiratory and gastrointestinal tracts,[55,188] the local synthesis of IgE does not significantly contribute to the immunoglobulin content of the secretions of the normal small bowel or colon; the major site of intestinal IgE production appears to be in the mesenteric lymph nodes. In rats infected with parasites, for example, IgE produced in the MLN is transported through the lymph and blood to the intestines, where it binds to the surface of subepithelial tissue mast cells.[189] In man, IgE may thus mediate allergic disorders of the intestines or provide a second line of defense against the absorption of food antigens[190]; in other animals, there is evidence that IgE becomes involved in host-parasite interactions[191] by enhancing cell mucus release[7] or by activating intestinal macrophages.[192]

Cellular Immune System

Distribution. The ingredients necessary to mount a cellular immune response are present within the intestinal lumen starting at birth. The initial exposure to external antigenic stimuli in the neonate occurs with the ingestion of colostrum, which contains a spectrum of functional T cells.[109,193] While these activated T cells represent a form of passive transfer of maternal cellular immunity,[109] the lymphocytes of the neonate subsequently migrate into the intestinal lumen in response to infectious agents and other exogenous antigens.[20]

The migratory pattern of T cells is similar to that of B-cell precursors.[102] In rodents, T-cell precursors migrate into the lamina propria in response to nematode infections and are essential for the expulsion of the worms during the enteric stages.[89,191] T-cell migration has also been studied following the intraperitoneal injection of allogeneic tumor cells into mice; cytotoxic T cells were observed in the lamina propria prior to localization within the Peyer's patches, MLN, or spleen.[194]

As discussed earlier, the heterogeneous intraepithelial lymphoid cell population includes an apparent abundance of the suppressor/cytotoxic T-cell phenotype. Likewise, the lamina propria is replete with T cells, null cells, macrophages, mast cells, and neutrophils. In this location, however, helper T cells seem to predominate,[36,195] as is true in the germinal centers of aggregated lymphoid follicles.[72] Thus, the gut is richly endowed with the components required to produce a variety of cell-mediated immunologic responses.[27,40]

T-Cell Regulatory Functions. The cellular immune system is engaged in a spectrum of immunoregulatory functions. Clearly, enhancement of the mucosal production of IgA, while suppressing IgG and IgM, involves intestinal T cells.[153–156,158] However, other local influences seem to provide additional protection.

Regulatory actions involving the epithelial cells themselves have been observed during experimental gastrointestinal infections and within small intestinal allografts; in these settings, crypt hyperplasia and villous atrophy usually occur in immunologically intact rats.[15] In contrast, T cell–depleted animals maintain normal villi in response to *Nippostrongylus brasiliensis*. In murine giardiasis, crypt mitoses are prevalent without villous enlargement.[15] Thus, increased epithelial cell turnover has been considered to be an additional mechanism available to protect the body against pathogens that persist by adhering to or penetrating the outer mucosal layer.[89]

In the setting of intestinal allograft transplantation in mice and dogs, the initial morphologic changes include not only a lymphocytic infiltrate, but also short or absent villi and elongated crypts.[15] The latter phenomena may relate to the effects of lymphokines as well as cellular products of secondarily activated monocytes, eosinophils, and neutrophils.[15,196] The intestinal mast cell may also play a key role by means of the production and release of serotonin, known to enhance jejunal crypt cell renewal. Additionally, vasoactive intestinal polypeptide (VIP), which is liberated following IgE-mediated reactions, can function to trigger epithelial cell fluid secretion—an "enteric tear" system.[190]

If these reactions fail to prevent mucosal penetration by food, microbes, or other antigens, still other regulatory phenomena may come into play. Local immunization stimulates a greater cell-mediated response than does parenteral inoculation, as measured indirectly by the production of migration inhibitory factor (MIF) by intestinal lymphocytes.[197] Non-specific immunity from activated macrophages also can protect against unrelated antigens and participate in the tissue response at mucosal surfaces that are subjected to constant antigenic stimulation.[15,197]

Tissue damage from absorbed antigens is further obviated by immunologic tolerance, a regulatory phenomenon that involves several cellular processes and is discussed in more detail in the section on the intestinal immune response.[198] The initial exposure to small amounts of antigen by the oral route is more likely to produce tolerance than is exposure to larger antigenic loads. Suppressor T cells are involved. They act in part by limiting DNA synthesis in the lymph nodes, spleen, lungs, and liver, a reaction that is antigen specific and may be inhibited by prior exposure to cyclophosphamide.[198,199]

Cytotoxicity. In addition to regulatory effects, the mucosal cellular immune system is well equipped to participate in cytotoxic reactions. Cytotoxic T cells that are induced by stimulation with foreign cell-surface antigens, or with host cell-surface antigens altered by chemicals or viruses, have been identified among the intestinal epithelial cells of the guinea pig.[37,41] Similar cells are present in the lamina propria of several species,[40,41,56,59] while precursor cytotoxic T cells exist in Peyer's patches.[68,200]

The cytotoxic effects of lymphocytes devoid of T-cell markers (and presumably of null or K cells) have been observed in assays for antibody-dependent cell-mediated cytotoxicity (ADCC) using either IEL[33] or lamina propria lymphocytes.[57–59] Other investigators, however, have failed to document ADCC using lamina propria or Peyer's patch lymphocytes in different assay systems.[83,201,202]

Natural killer (NK) cells include a separate functional class of non–T lymphocytes that also bear Fc receptors and are capable of antibody-independent or spontaneous cell-mediated cytotoxicity (SCMC).[203] This activity has been identified within the IEL population in guinea pigs.[41] Initial attempts at inducing SCMC using human lamina propria lymphocytes were unsuccessful[56,59]; subsequent animal studies suggested that this may relate to the heterogeneity and compartmentalization of subpopulations of NK cells. Large granular lymphocytes that appear to have T-cell markers and function as spontaneous killer cells have been isolated from the murine intestinal mucosa.[42] The emerging evidence therefore suggests that a full complement of cellular immune functions is available within the intestinal mucosa and its associated lymphoid tissues, providing the bowel with the capability of mediating the recognition, processing, and destruction of a wide variety of antigenic moieties.

Intestinal Immune Responses

Antigen Uptake. The combination of luminal processes, mechanical factors, and mucus,[7] intestinal antibodies,[121,144] and intraluminal lymphocytes[19,204] functions in concert as a mucosal barrier to contact with and penetrance by unwanted antigens. In neonates and infants, immunologically active components derived from colostrum and breast milk provide initial protection prior to the maturation of the mucosal barrier.[16] Colostrum contains both soluble factors (immunoglobulins, complement, lactoferrin, lysozyme, interferon) and cellular factors (macrophages, neutrophils, lymphocytes) that serve to protect against neonatal sepsis.[205,206] The highest concentrations of immunoglobulins and T-cell activity occur in colostrum immediately after the onset of lactation, with a rapid decline after the first week.[109] Although a small amount of the colostral IgA is absorbed during the first 24 to 36 hours of life,[109] the majority of the neonatal mucosal antibody available in humans is transmitted transplacentally in the form of IgG. In certain animal species, by comparison, the intestinal epithelial cells selectively transport maternal antibodies supplied in the breast milk.[16] In such animals, the uptake of labeled protein antigens into MLN is enhanced by immune complexes formed with breast milk.[207] Although maternally derived, passively acquired circulating antibody may not significantly suppress the immunologic response of young infants to ingested antigens,[208] breast milk in humans supplies transient cell-mediated immunologic protection for the relatively permeable infant gut.[109,209] Breast milk also has the capacity to facilitate the maturation of the infant's mucosal epithelial cells,[16] a process described as "*gut closure.*"[8,16,210]

Nevertheless, several studies indicate that macromolecules can cross the normal human mucosal barrier under physiologic conditions.[138,211,212] The small intestinal epithelium is permeable to macromolecular antigens that are engulfed by an endocytotic process. This process involves initial interactions with components of the microvillus membrane of intestinal absorptive cells, is most likely concentration dependent, and is increased during the first 3 months of extrauterine life, possibly representing a residual primitive absorptive mechanism.[8,16] The more frequent detection of food antigens in the circulation of premature infants during the first 3 months of life may therefore result from both increased uptake *and* immature lysosomal function impairing intracellular proteolysis.[16,213–216] After the first weeks of extrauterine life, the capacity to engulf antigens and microorganisms diminishes; this "closure" phenomenon may be due to the establishment of intestinal flora, an improved gastric barrier, the production of mucins, and the presence in colostrum of "mucosal growth factor."[16,217,218]

A separate mechanism for antigenic sampling within the intestinal epithelium involves the specialized intestinal M-cell system, providing antigens with direct access to the underlying lymphoid tissue. Using horseradish peroxidase as an experimental antigen, a concentration-dependent difference has been demonstrated between the absorptive capacity of M cells and that of conventional intestinal epithelial cells.[75] Lower levels of luminal antigen favor uptake by the M cells; at increased concentrations of the antigen, a more generalized uptake occurs by way of the microvilli of adjacent epithelial cells.

The route of antigen entry may be important in promoting local versus systemic immunity or immunologic responsiveness versus tolerance.[89,215] Antigen penetrating the mucosa through M cells gains ready access to the immune system. When enters by way of the endocytotic adsorptive process of the columnar epithelium, it is carried in phagosomes, partially digested by combining with lysosomes, and deposited in the intestinal space at the lateral cell border by means of exocytosis.[212] Once through the epithelial cells, antigen may be transported (1) by way of efferent lymphatics that drain from lymphoid follicles to mesenteric lymph nodes, (2) through villous lacteals that also drain into the mesenteric lymph node system en route to the thoracic duct, or (3) directly into mesenteric veins that drain into the portal venous system to the liver.[86,89] The relative importance of each of these routes of entry and transport needs further study; differences among antigens may depend upon concentration, molecular size, solubility, time course of exposure, surface properties, and whether they are self-replicating, as in the case of infectious agents.

Peyer's patches and the other intestinal mucosal lymphoid aggregates play a crucial role in the initial sampling of antigens. Although Peyer's patches are histologically mature at birth and are unaltered by luminal contact with antigen *in utero,* they will involute if isolated from the normal luminal stream. This would suggest that antigen may amplify the number of cells in specific clones after a period of genetically predetermined growth.[45,85] On the other hand, mesenteric lymph nodes dramatically enlarge after the intestinal flora becomes established and "gut closure" occurs.[219] Yet, the relative influence of MLN upon the immune response has not been evaluated, in comparison with numerous studies of the influence of Peyer's patches. The latter play a key role in the mucosal immune response, as measured by IgA synthesis,[220] specific antibody-containing cells,[88,221] and T-cell subsets.[200,222–224] The importance of the direct interaction of enteric antigens with Peyer's patch cells is supported by the *in situ* cell proliferation that follows antigenic stimulation, the presence of suppressor cells in Peyer's patches prior to their appearance in the spleen, and the differential response of Peyer's patches and the spleen to environmental antigens.[17,150,224] Transportation of antigen from the general circulation into Peyer's patches may prove to be an additional important aspect of the mucosal immune response.[225]

Sensitization. Beyond the neonatal period, and in the absence of a disrupted mucosal barrier, the introduction of most antigens into the gastrointestinal tract can produce a local intestinal response without apparent systemic immunity. This selective type of sensitizing or priming response involves the interaction of the humoral and cell-mediated immune systems, i.e., the local production of IgA reduces the subsequent absorption of antigen while suppressing the formation of circulating antibody.[226] The kinetics of the mucosal response varies with antigen dose, exposure time, the location of priming, and the properties of specific antigens.

In adult animals, non-replicating antigens often are ineffective at priming for a secretory immune response.[227] However, immunization with ferritin,[228] bovine serum albumin,[81,229,230] cholera toxin,[221,227] and other particulate and soluble bacterial antigens[106,231] is capable of inducing intestinal and, in some cases, systemic immune responses. In man, peroral immunization resulting in the mucosal production of specific IgA antibody has been demonstrated using bacteria[232,233] and viruses.[139,142,234] Measurement of the human mucosal immune response has been impeded by various problems associated with obtaining specimens and quantitating the degree of dilution or degradation of the secreted IgA. Since this often has been indirectly measured using salivary or mammary secretions, inferences regarding intestinal mucosal responses may not be reliable.[140]

Just as the antigen dose influences the amount absorbed and may relate to the ultimate immune response,[197] the time course and route of immunization may alter the balance between priming and suppression of the immune reaction to a particular antigen.[227,235,236] Thus, while both enteric and parenteral antigens may prime for a secondary intestinal plasma cell response, the route determines the eventual antibody isotype (enteric, mainly IgA; parenteral, mainly IgG). Such isotypic specificity may be directed by local populations of antigen-specific T lymphocytes[236] in possible combination with serum factors[237] that govern clonal expansion of the committed cells.[227]

Under certain circumstances, antigenic stimulation of the intestinal tract may affect the non-enteric immune system.[234,237–239] Again, a preponderance of the IgA isotype occurs, which may be directed by both splenic factors[26] and still to be determined hepatic influences.[166,240]

Tolerance. Tolerance, or the suppression of humoral or cellular immune responses, has long been recognized. Mucosal tolerance depends upon the properties of the specific antigenic stimulus as well as the dose,[198,199,241] duration and timing of exposure,[237,242] previous contact with the antigen,[243] and time at which the response is measured.[244] Tolerance may be mediated in part by a local and/or systemic IgA response acting to impede additional presentation of the antigen to the extraintestinal immune system. Unresponsiveness in such previously immunized hosts involves a direct effect of antibody with absorbed enteric antigen within gut lymphoid tissues.[245]

Suppression, in addition, depends upon the action of suppressor T lymphocytes[198,199,224,241] and circulating factors,[237] and is perhaps enhanced by the transport of antigen to the liver.[198,240] For example, protein feeding may interfere with carrier-dependent helper T-cell activity and antigen-stimulated T-cell proliferation.[198] This "regulatory option" may be dependent on the class of antigen and the subsequent suppressor effect may be due to: (1) deficient macrophage activity, causing enhanced suppressor induction; (2) the nature of the digestion of the protein, resulting in antigenic configurations that are not readily processed by macrophages; or (3) the transfer of antigens to the liver, where tolerance is further modulated.[198]

Other factors that will influence the development of suppression include both antigenic routing through the intestinal and systemic lymphoid tissues and the trafficking of lymphoid elements.[224,241] Therefore, future approaches to the use of immune modulation for immunizing patients against enteric pathogens, as well as therapeutic manipulations of inflammatory conditions of the intestinal tract, will require additional studies of the basic mechanisms involved in the immunologic apparatus of the gut and its interaction with systemic lymphoid organs.

Celiac Disease

Celiac disease (Chapter 105) has been considered the prototype of an immunogenetic disorder; e.g., when an antigenic determinant from gluten sensitizes a genetically susceptible individual, subtotal or total villous atrophy occurs above a lymphoplasmacytic infiltrate within the lamina propria. Such immunopathogenetic theories have been evolving for about 25 years and are based on both indirect and direct evidence.[246–248] Many of the morphologic features of celiac disease support an immune basis for the deleterious action of gluten in susceptible individuals. The early descriptions of the disorganized, irregular, flattened epithelial cells with damaged microvilli focused attention on the epithelium as a target of gluten-induced damage.[249] Although the accompanying lymphoid infiltration of the epithelium may be more apparent[34] than real[51,250] and may represent a crowding of lymphocytes into a reduced volume of epithelium, markedly increased immunoblastic activity within the epithelium appears to correlate with gluten sensitivity.[249] The evidence that these immunoblasts may influence epithelial cells and increase the proliferation of enterocytes has been reviewed,[196] and this article may be consulted for details.

Indirect evidence of the involvement of humoral immune phenomena in celiac disease includes increased numbers of IgA, IgM, and IgG cells in the jejunal mucosa of untreated patients as compared with treated patients or control subjects.[246] The negative correlation between the elapsed time from gluten challenge until clinical relapse and the increased number of jejunal IgG cells further implies a possible role for IgG in the pathogenesis of celiac disease.[251]

The serum concentration of IgA is increased in celiac disease, with some normalization occurring with treatment. Furthermore, IgA anti-gliadin antibodies may be a specific marker in active celiac disease; circulating anti-gliadin associated with IgG is additionally demonstrated in patients with other intestinal disorders.[252] Serum concentrations of IgG and IgM tend to be low in untreated patients, possibly due to intraluminal leakage inasmuch as normalization again occurs with treatment.[246] Dietary antibodies to milk, different food proteins, and reticulin and other tissue components have been identified in patients with celiac disease but are considered to be non-specific markers of mucosal damage.[246] Lowered serum complement levels are noted with active disease, concurrent with the mucosal deposition of complement components and the appearance of immune complexes in the sera of untreated patients. However, gluten-free diets reduce or eliminate these findings as the tissue abnormalities improve.[246] Additionally, mast cell degranulation may occur in response to gluten exposure and may participate in the inflammatory response.[253] These findings suggest that humoral-type immunologic reactions may participate in the tissue changes in celiac disease but that they most likely are secondary phenomena.

More evidence is accumulating for a cell-mediated immunologic reaction as a primary event in this disorder. While non-specific findings suggest a depression of peripheral blood T-cell numbers, skin test positivity, and phytohemagglutinin (PHA) responsiveness, the specific lymphocyte-mediated responses to gluten or gluten products are probably enhanced.[246] A combination of cell loss through the mucosa and the intestinal "trapping" of T cells produces an apparent lymphoreticular atrophy.[254] The intraepithelial lymphocytes in celiac disease appear to be gluten-sensitized immunoblasts[250] showing an increased mitotic index.[255] Lymphokine production in celiac disease can be demonstrated by exposing circulating mononuclear cells[246,256] and jejunal biopsy samples[247,257] to gluten fractions and measuring migration inhibition. In mucosal tissue culture studies in patients with treated celiac disease,[258] *in vitro* epithelial injury in response to gluten required exposure of the jejunal tissue to culture medium or cells from "exacerbation" tissue. Since this response could be inhibited by cortisol, the data further supported the concept of a cell-mediated immune event.

The recognition of genetic factors (Chapter 240) in celiac disease has provided much insight into host-environment interactions.

Thus, the predisposition to gluten sensitivity often is associated with the HLA-A1, B8 haplotype in linkage disequilibrium with DR3 at the major histocompatibility locus. The finding that the HLA-B8 antigen is more prevalent in numerous "autoimmune" disorders has led to studies in search of a generalized immune hyperresponsiveness in celiac disease. For instance, HLA B8–positive control leukocytes produce more migration inhibitory factor upon exposure to gluten fraction III than do non–HLA B8 leukocytes, although less than in untreated patients with celiac disease.[258] With the identification of HLA DR–like antigens in the epithelium of the human small intestine,[259] this potential receptor could explain both the genetic susceptibility and the necessity for environmental exposure to cause a cell-mediated host response. Such an interaction would alter the recognition site on the epithelial cell and incite the generation of immune products that would then damage the now "targeted" epithelial cell.[248,260] This could involve both soluble factors, such as immunoglobulins and lymphokines, and cellular factors, such as activated and/or cytotoxic lymphocytes.

Why some predisposed individuals with the proper environmental exposure do not demonstrate a pattern of tissue injury or seem to suddenly "turn-on" this untoward immune response in later life and why others fail to "turn-off" the response after gluten restriction remain unknown. New information is constantly being accumulated, e.g., preliminary reports that immunoglobulin heavy-chain allotype-linked genes may control the antibody response to wheat gliadin.[261]

IgA-Deficient Sprue

Selective IgA deficiency (Chapter 243) may be detected in about 1 in 400 to 700 individuals, of whom relatively few experience symptoms.[146,262] When malabsorption and diarrhea do occur, the morphologic findings on jejunal biopsy often are similar to celiac disease (Chapter 103), i.e., subtotal or total villous atrophy, except that IgA-containing plasma cells are absent from the lamina propria in patients with sprue.[182,262,263] The relationship of the IgA deficiency to the pathogenesis of any intestinal manifestation remains uncertain. Yet, selective IgA deficiency occurs more frequently in patients with celiac disease (1 in 40 patients) than in the general population, and the term "*IgA-deficient sprue*" has been coined.[262] Most of these patients respond favorably to gluten restriction alone[182] or to the additional withdrawal of milk products.[262] Although it is difficult to exclude a chance association between IgA deficiency and malabsorption, the likelihood that individuals with IgA deficiency have enhanced intestinal permeability is reflected by findings of increased serum antibody titers to food proteins and circulating immune complexes, suggesting sensitization to numerous dietary antigens.[62–64]

Nodular Lymphoid Hyperplasia

Lymphoid hyperplasia of the submucosa and mucosa of the gastrointestinal tract may be a variant of normal or may occur within a group of distinct clinicopathologic entities[265] (Chapter 112). Recent progress in air-contrast techniques permits the recognition of discrete follicles as small as 1 to 3 mm in diameter in up to one-third of adult human colons.[266] A similar nodular hyperplasia may also co-exist with defects in humoral immunity,[267] often with associated *Giardia lamblia* infection.[265] Malabsorption and other abnormalities frequently are present in such patients. The syndrome, therefore, has been referred to as "*nodular lymphoid hyperplasia of the intestines with dysgammaglobulinemia*" and is part of the spectrum of "*hypogammaglobulinemic lymphoid enteropathy*"[265] (Chapter 243). These nodules contain polyclonal IgM-bearing lymphocytes in hypogammaglobulinemic individuals[268] and IgA-deficient individuals.[269] In such persons, the hyperplasia appears to be an antigen-induced proliferation of B lymphocytes with a maturational arrest in the differentiation to mature plasma cells; this may conceivably relate to combinations of excessive T-cell suppression or to inadequate T-cell helper activity.[268]

In the absence of immunodeficiency, intestinal lymphoid hyperplasia may occur as a response to enteric infection as well as being recognized in normal children and young adults.[265,266] However, nodules greater than 7 mm in diameter, especially if ulcerated, would suggest an underlying inflammatory disease[266] and the possibility of an associated malignant lymphoma of the gastrointestinal tract.[262,265,270]

Alpha-Chain Disease

An aberrant monoclonal expansion of IgA-secreting B-cell derivatives forms the basis for a not uncommon form of malabsorption in developing countries, especially in the Middle East and Mediterranean basin, but also described sporadically in Asia and North America[271–275] (Chapter 112). Alpha-chain disease involves a proliferation of intestinal lymphoid and mesenteric lymph node cells that produce incomplete IgA molecules devoid of light chains and the rest of the Fab fragment.[274] The incomplete alpha heavy chains may be linked by J chains into polymers that are capable of recognizing SC.[271,272] These polymers produce variable serum electrophoretic patterns that include abnormal broad bands extending from the α_2- to the β_2-globulin region.[274,275] The observation that serum concentrations of IgG and IgM are usually low in spite of normal ratios of lambda and kappa light chains suggests some form of immune suppression.[271]

Malabsorption is a frequent clinical finding in alpha-chain disease. Although the disease usually is most prominent in the upper small intestine, the stomach may be involved in a cobblestone pattern,[272] rectal biopsies may show characteristic abnormalities,[276] and a respiratory form of the disease has been described.[271]

Histologic findings include a dense infiltration of lymphoid cells in the lamina propria that may extend through the muscularis mucosae and is associated with secondary villous atrophy.[277] Immunofluorescent staining will demonstrate the presence of alpha heavy chains without light chains in the lymphoid cell infiltrate.[271,273,275]

Information regarding the course of alpha-chain disease is limited, but the early stages may "respond" to antibiotics.[271,273] Progression from a benign phase to intestinal lymphoma is well recognized,[273,278–280] appears to be based on the expansion of a single clone of cells,[281] and has led the World Health Organization to consider this spectrum of disorders as *"immunoproliferative small intestinal disease"* (IPSID)[273,282] (Chapter 243).

The cause of alpha-chain disease remains unknown. The finding of an abnormal chromosomal pattern in a patient with alpha-chain disease suggests the need for further studies of genetic factors.[283] Defects in suppressor T cells also could account for the initial clonal expansion. While the cells that produce the abnormal alpha chain may be present in small numbers in normal individuals, the protein cannot be measured in normal serum.[271]

References

1. Walker WA. Host defense mechanisms in the gastrointestinal tract. Pediatrics 1976; 57:901–16.
2. Gibbons RJ, van Houte J. Bacterial adherence in oral microbial ecology. Annu Rev Microbiol 1975; 29:19–44.
3. Gorbach SL. Intestinal microflora. Gastroenterology 1971; 60:1110–29.
4. Springer GF. Importance of blood-group substances in interactions between man and microbes. Ann NY Acad Sci 1970; 169:134–52.
5. Freter R, O'Brien PCM, Halstead SA. Adhesion and chemotaxis as determinants of bacterial association with mucosal surfaces. Adv Exp Med Biol 1978; 107:429–37.
6. Edwards PAW. Is mucus a selective barrier for macromolecules? Br Med Bull 1978; 34:55–6.
7. Lake AM, Bloch KJ, Sinclair KJ, Walker WA. Anaphylactic release of intestinal goblet cell mucus. Immunology 1980; 39:173–8.
8. Walker WA. Antigen handling by the gut. Arch Dis Child 1978; 53:527–31.
9. Simon GL, Gorbach SL. Intestinal microflora. Med Clin North Am 1982; 66:557–74.
10. DuPont HL, Formal SB, Hornick RB, Snyder MJ, Libonati JP, Sheahan DG, LaBreck EH, Kalas JP. Pathogenesis of *Escherichia coli* diarrhea. N Engl J Med 1971; 285:1–9.
11. Kraft SC, Rothberg RM, Knauer CM, Svoboda AC Jr, Monroe LS, Farr RS. Gastric acid output and circulating anti-bovine serum albumin in adults. Clin Exp Immunol 1967; 2:321–30.
12. Dixon JMS. Fate of bacteria in small intestine. J Pathol 1968; 79:131–40.
13. Williams RC, Showalter R, Kern F Jr. In vivo effect of bile salts and cholestyramine on intestinal anaerobic bacteria. Gastroenterology 1975; 69:483–91.
14. Eastwood GL. Gastrointestinal epithelial renewal. Gastroenterology 1977; 72:962–75.
15. Ferguson A, MacDonald TT. Effects of local delayed hypersensitivity on the small intestine. Ciba Found Symp 1977; 46:305–19.
16. Walker WA. Gastrointestinal host defence: importance of gut closure in control of macromolecular transport. Ciba Found Symp 1979; 70:201–19.
17. Kagnoff MF. Immunology of the digestive system. *In*: Johnson LR, ed. Physiology of the Gastrointestinal Tract. New York: Raven Press, 1981: 1337–59.
18. Bienenstock J, Befus AD, McDermott M. Mucosal immunity. Monogr Allergy 1980; 16:1–18.
19. Owen RL, Nemanic PC, Stevens DP. Ultrastructural observations on giardiasis in a murine model. I. Intestinal distribution, attachment, and relationship to the immune system of *Giardia muris*. Gastroenterology 1979; 76:757–69.
20. Heatley RV, Bienenstock J. Luminal lymphoid cells in the rabbit intestine. Gastroenterology 1982; 82:268–75.
21. Bienenstock J, McDermott M, Befus AD, O'Neill M. A common mucosal immunologic system involving the bronchus, breast and bowel. Adv Exp Med Biol 1978; 107:53–9.
22. Bellamy JE, Nielsen NO. Immune-mediated emigration of neutrophils into the lumen of the small intestine. Infect Immun 1974; 9:615–9.
23. Steer HW. Ultrastructure of cell migration through the gastric epithelium and its relationship to bacteria. J Clin Pathol 1975; 28:639–46.
24. Harris JC, DuPont HL, Hornick RB. Fecal leukocytes in diarrheal illness. Ann Intern Med 1972; 76:697–703.
25. Laissue JA, Chanana AD, Cottier H, Cronkite EP, Joel DD. Fate of intraintestinal thymocytes labeled with

[125]iododeoxyuridine or tritiated thymidine. Proc Soc Exp Biol Med 1976; 152:262–5.
26. Arnaud-Battandier F. Immunologic characteristics of isolated gut mucosal lymphoid cells. *In:* Strober W, Hanson LA, Sell KW, eds. Recent Advances in Mucosal Immunity. New York: Raven Press, 1982: 289–99.
27. Bartnik W, ReMine SG, Chiba M, Thayer WR, Shorter RG. Isolation and characterization of colonic intraepithelial and lamina proprial lymphocytes. Gastroenterology 1980; 78:976–85.
28. Austin LL, Dobbins WO 3d. Intraepithelial leukocytes of the intestinal mucosa in normal man and in Whipple's disease: a light- and electron-microscopic study. Dig Dis Sci 1982; 27:311–20.
29. Marsh MN. Studies of intestinal lymphoid tissue. I. Electron microscopic evidence of 'blast transformation' in epithelial lymphocytes of mouse small intestinal mucosa. Gut 1975; 16:665–74.
30. Meader RD, Landers DF. Electron and light microscopic observations on relationships between lymphocytes and intestinal epithelium. Am J Anat 1967; 121:763–73.
31. Röpke C, Everett NB. Proliferative kinetics of large and small intraepithelial lymphocytes in the small intestine of the mouse. Am J Anat 1976; 145:395–408.
32. Toner PG, Ferguson A. Intraepithelial cells in the human intestinal mucosa. J Ultrastruct Res 1971; 34:329–44.
33. Ferguson A. Intraepithelial lymphocytes of the small intestine. Gut 1977; 18:921–37.
34. Ferguson A, Murray D. Quantitation of intraepithelial lymphocytes in human jejunum. Gut 1971; 12:988–94.
35. Selby WS, Janossy G, Jewell DP. Immunohistological characterisation of intraepithelial lymphocytes of the human gastrointestinal tract. Gut 1981; 22:169–76.
36. Janossy G, Tidman N, Selby WS, Thomas JA, Granger S, Kung PC, Goldstein G. Human T lymphocytes of inducer and suppressor type occupy different microenvironments. Nature 1980; 288:81–4.
37. Arnaud-Battandier F, Nelson DL. Immunologic characteristics of intestinal lymphoid cells of the guinea pig. Gastroenterology 1982; 82:248–53.
38. Arnaud-Battandier F, Lawrence EC, Blaese RM. Lymphoid populations of gut mucosa in chickens. Dig Dis Sci 1980; 25:252–9.
39. Collan Y. Characteristics of nonepithelial cells in the epithelium of normal rat ileum. Scand J Gastroenterol 1972; 7(Suppl 18):1–66.
40. Chiba M, Bartnik W, ReMine SG, Thayer WR, Shorter RG. Human colonic intraepithelial and lamina proprial lymphocytes: cytotoxicity *in vitro* and the potential effects of the isolation method on their functional properties. Gut 1981; 22:177–86.
41. Arnaud-Battandier F, Bundy BM, O'Neill M, Bienenstock J, Nelson DL. Cytotoxic activities of gut mucosal lymphoid cells in guinea pigs. J Immunol 1978; 121:1059–65.
42. Tagliabue A, Befus AD, Clark DA, Bienenstock J. Characteristics of natural killer cells in the murine intestinal epithelium and lamina propria. J Exp Med 1982; 155:1785–96.
43. Guy-Grand D, Griscelli C, Vassalli P. The gut-associated lymphoid system: nature and properties of the large dividing cells. Eur J Immunol 1974; 4:435–43.
44. Röpke C, Everett NB. Kinetics of intraepithelial lymphocytes in the small intestine of thymus-deprived mice and antigen-deprived mice. Anat Rec 1976; 185:101–8.
45. Reynolds J. Gut-associated lymphoid tissues in lambs before and after birth. Monogr Allergy 1980; 16:187–202.
46. Glaister JR. Factors affecting the lymphoid cells in the small intestinal epithelium of the mouse. Int Arch Allergy Appl Immunol 1973; 45:719–30.
47. Ferguson A, Parrott DMV. The effect of antigen deprivation on thymus-dependent and thymus-independent lymphocytes in the small intestine of the mouse. Clin Exp Immunol 1972; 12:477–88.
48. Guy-Grand D, Griscelli C, Vassalli P. The mouse gut T lymphocyte, a novel type of T cell. Nature, origin, and traffic in mice in normal and graft-versus-host conditions. J Exp Med 1978; 148:1661–77.
49. Pink IJ, Croft DN, Creamer B. Cell loss from small intestinal mucosa: a morphological study. Gut 1970; 11:217–22.
50. Marsh MN. Studies of intestinal lymphoid tissue. II. Aspects of proliferation and migration of epithelial lymphocytes in the small intestine of mice. Gut 1975; 16:674–82.
51. Marsh MN. Studies of intestinal lymphoid tissue. III. Quantitative analyses of epithelial lymphocytes in the small intestine of human control subjects and of patients with celiac sprue. Gastroenterology 1980; 79:481–92.
52. Porter P, Parry SH, Allen WD. Significance of immune mechanisms in relation to enteric infections of the gastrointestinal tract in animals. Ciba Found Symp 1977; 46:55–67.
53. Cebra JJ, Kamat R, Gearhart P, Robertson SM, Tseng J. The secretory IgA system of the gut. Ciba Found Symp 1977; 46:5–22.
54. Brandtzaeg P, Baklien K. Intestinal secretion of IgA and IgM: a hypothetical model. Ciba Found Symp 1977; 46:77–108.
55. Pucci-Favino A, Clancy R. Quantitative and functional aspects of T-cell populations in human gut mucosa. Ric Clin Lab 1979; 9:237–44.
56. Falchuk ZM, Barnhard E, Machado I. Human colonic mononuclear cells: studies of cytotoxic function. Gut 1981; 22:290–4.
57. Chiba M, Shorter RG, Thayer WR, Bartnik W, ReMine S. K-cell activity in lamina proprial lymphocytes from the human colon. Dig Dis Sci 1979; 24:817–22.
58. Fiocchi C, Battisto JR, Farmer RG. Gut mucosal lymphocytes in inflammatory bowel disease: isolation and preliminary functional characterization. Dig Dis Sci 1979; 24:705–17.
59. MacDermott RP, Franklin GO, Jenkins KM, Kodner IJ, Nash GS, Weinrieb IJ. Human intestinal mononuclear cells. I. Investigation of antibody-dependent, lectin-induced, and spontaneous cell-mediated cytotoxic capabilities. Gastroenterology 1980; 78:47–56.
60. Pearce FL, Befus AD, Gauldie J, Bienenstock J. Mucosal mast cells. II. Effects of anti-allergic compounds on histamine secretion by isolated intestinal mast cells. J Immunol 1982; 128:2481–6.
61. Lemanske RF Jr, Atkins FM, Metcalfe DD. Gastrointestinal mast cells in health and disease. J Pediatr 1983; 103:177–84, 343–51.
62. Mayrhofer G, Bazin H. Nature of the thymus dependency of mucosal mast cells. III. Mucosal mast cells in nude mice and nude rats, in B rats and in a child with the DiGeorge syndrome. Int Arch Allergy Appl Immunol 1981; 64:320–31.
63. Golder JP, Doe WF. Isolation and preliminary characterization of human intestinal macrophages. Gastroenterology 1983; 84:795–802.
64. Beeson PB. Role of the eosinophil. Ciba Found Symp 1977; 46:203–13.
65. Dobbins WO III. Gut immunophysiology: a gastroenterologist's view with emphasis on pathophysiology. Am J Physiol 1982; 242:G1–8.
66. Cornes JS. Number, size, and distribution of Peyer's patches in the human small intestine. I. The development of Peyer's patches. Gut 1965; 6:225–29.
67. Friedberg SH, Weissman IL. Lymphoid tissue architecture. II. Ontogeny of peripheral T and B cells in mice: evidence against Peyer's patches as the site of generation of B cells. J Immunol 1974; 113:1477–92.
68. Kagnoff MF, Campbell S. Functional characteristics of Peyer's patch lymphoid cells. I. Induction of humoral antibody and cell-mediated allograft reactions. J Exp Med 1974; 139:398–406.
69. Owen RL, Nemanic P. Antigen processing structures of the mammalian intestinal tract: an SEM study of lymphoepithelial organs. Scan Electron Microsc 1978; 2:367–78.
70. Sell S, Raffel C, Scott CB. Tissue localization of T and B lymphocytes in lagomorphs: anatomical evidence for a major role of the gastrointestinal associated lymphoid tissue in generation of lymphocytes in the adult. Dev Comp Immunol 1980; 4:355–66.
71. Guy-Grand D, Griscelli C, Vassalli P. Peyer's patches, gut IgA plasma cells and thymic function: study in nude mice bearing thymic grafts. J Immunol 1975; 115:361–4.
72. Poppema S, Bhan AK, Reinherz EL, McCluskey RT, Schlossman SF. Distribution of T cell subsets in human lymph nodes. J Exp Med 1981; 153:30–41.

73. Rouse RV, Ledbetter JA, Weissman IL. Mouse lymph node germinal centers contain a selected subset of T cells—the helper phenotype. J Immunol 1982; 128:2243–6.
74. Owen RL, Jones AL. Epithelial cell specialization within human Peyer's patches: an ultrastructural study of intestinal lymphoid follicles. Gastroenterology 1974; 66:189–203.
75. Owen RL. Sequential uptake of horseradish peroxidase by lymphoid follicle epithelium of Peyer's patches in the normal unobstructed mouse intestine: an ultrastructural study. Gastroenterology 1977; 72:440–51.
76. Curran RC, Jones EL. Immunoglobulin-containing cells in human tonsils demonstrated by immunohistochemistry. Clin Exp Immunol 1977; 28:103–15.
77. Bhalla DK, Owen RL. Cell renewal and migration in lymphoid follicles of Peyer's patches and cecum: an autoradiographic study in mice. Gastroenterology 1982; 82:232–42.
78. Wolf JL, Rubin DH, Finberg R, Kauffman RS, Sharpe AH, Trier JS, Fields BN. Intestinal M cells: a pathway for entry of reovirus into the host. Science 1981; 212:471–2.
79. Bhalla DK, Murakami T, Owen RL. Microcirculation of intestinal lymphoid follicles in rat Peyer's patches. Gastroenterology 1981; 81:481–91.
80. Craig SW, Cebra JJ. Peyer's patches: an enriched source of precursors for IgA-producing immunocytes in the rabbit. J Exp Med 1971; 134:188–200.
81. Bienenstock J, Dolezel J. Peyer's patches: lack of specific antibody-containing cells after oral and parenteral immunization. J Immunol 1971; 106:938–45.
82. MacDonald TT. Enhancement and suppression of the Peyer's patch immune response by systemic priming. Clin Exp Immunol 1982; 49:441–8.
83. Kagnoff MF, Campbell S. Antibody-dependent cell-mediated cytotoxicity; comparative ability of murine Peyer's patch and spleen cells to lyse polysaccharide-coated and uncoated erythrocytes. Gastroenterology 1976; 70:341–6.
84. MacDonald TT, Carter PB. Mouse Peyer's patches contain T cells capable of inducing the graft-versus-host reaction (GVHR). Transplantation 1978; 26:162–5.
85. Cebra JJ, Crandall CA, Gearhart PJ, Robertson SM, Tseng J, Watson PM. Cellular events concerned with the initiation, expression, and control of the mucosal immune response. *In:* Ogra PL, Dayton D, eds. Immunology of Breast Milk. New York: Raven Press, 1979: 1–18.
86. Hall J, Orlans E, Peppard J, Reynolds J. Lymphatic physiology and secretory immunity. Adv Exp Med Biol 1978; 107:29–34.
87. Husband AJ, Monié HJ, Gowans JL. The natural history of the cells producing IgA in the gut. Ciba Found Symp 1977; 46:29–42.
88. Husband AJ, Gowans JL. The origin and antigen-dependent distribution of IgA-containing cells in the intestine. J Exp Med 1978; 148:1146–60.
89. Ottaway CA, Rose ML, Parrott DMV. The gut as an immunological system. *In:* Crane RK, ed. International Review of Physiology, Gastrointestinal Physiology II. Vol. 19. Baltimore: University Park Press, 1979: 323–56.
90. Pearson LD, Simpson-Morgan MW, Morris B. Lymphopoiesis and lymphocyte recirculation in the sheep fetus. J Exp Med 1976; 143:167–86.
91. Cahill RNP, Poskitt DC, Hay JB, Heron I, Trnka Z. The migration of lymphocytes in the fetal lamb. Eur J Immunol 1979; 9:251–3.
92. Cahill RNP, Poskitt DC, Frost H, Trnka Z. Two distinct pools of recirculating T lymphocytes: migratory characteristics of nodal and intestinal T lymphocytes. J Exp Med 1977; 145:420–8.
93. Chin W, Hay JB. A comparison of lymphocyte migration through intestinal lymph nodes, subcutaneous lymph nodes, and chronic inflammatory sites of sheep. Gastroenterology 1980; 79:1231–42.
94. Hall JG. An essay on lymphocyte circulation and the gut. Monogr Allergy 1980; 16:100–11.
95. Gowans JL, Knight EJ. The route of re-circulation of lymphocytes in the rat. Proc R Soc Lond (Biol) 1964; 159:257–82.
96. Williams AF, Gowans JL. The presence of IgA on the surface of rat thoracic duct lymphocytes which contain internal IgA. J Exp Med 1975; 141:335–45.
97. Griscelli C, Vassalli P, McCluskey RT. The distribution of large dividing lymph node cells in syngeneic recipient rats after intravenous injection. J Exp Med 1969; 130:1427–51.
98. Hall JG, Smith ME. Homing of lymph-borne immunoblasts to the gut. Nature 1970; 226:262–3.
99. Rose ML, Parrott DMV, Bruce RG. Migration of lymphoblasts to the small intestine. II. Divergent migration of mesenteric and peripheral immunoblasts to sites of inflammation in the mouse. Cell Immunol 1976; 27:36–46.
100. McWilliams M, Phillips-Quagliata JM, Lamm ME. Characteristics of mesenteric lymph node cells homing to gut-associated lymphoid tissue in syngeneic mice. J Immunol 1975; 115:54–8.
101. McWilliams M, Phillips-Quagliata JM, Lamm ME. Mesenteric lymph node B lymphoblasts which home to the small intestine are precommitted to IgA synthesis. J Exp Med 1977; 145:866–75.
102. Parrott DMV, Rose ML. Migration pathways of T lymphocytes in the small intestine. Adv Exp Med Biol 1978; 107:67–74.
103. Bohl EH, Saif LJ, Gupta RKP, Frederick GT. Secretory antibodies in milk of swine against transmissible gastroenteritis virus. Adv Exp Med Biol 1974; 45:337–42.
104. Montgomery PC, Cohn J, Lally ET. The induction and characterization of secretory IgA antibodies. Adv Exp Med Biol 1974; 45:453–62.
105. Hanson LA, Ahlstedt S, Carlsson B, Kaijser B, Larsson P, Mattsby Baltzer I, Sohl Akerlund A, Svanborg Edén C, Svennerholm AM. Secretory IgA antibodies to enterobacterial virulence antigens: their induction and possible relevance. Adv Exp Med Biol 1978; 107:165–76.
106. Mestecky J, McGhee JR, Arnold RR, Michalek SM, Prince SJ, Babb JL. Selective induction of an immune response in human external secretions by ingestion of bacterial antigen. J Clin Invest 1978; 61:731–7.
107. McDermott MR, Bienenstock J. Evidence for a common mucosal immunologic system. I. Migration of B immunoblasts into intestinal, respiratory, and genital tissues. J Immunol 1979; 122:1892–8.
108. Montgomery PC, Lemaitre-Coelho IM, Vaerman JP. A common mucosal immune system. Antibody expression in secretions following gastrointestinal stimulation. Immunol Commun 1980; 9:705–13.
109. Ogra SS, Weintraub DI, Ogra PL. Immunologic aspects of human colostrum and milk: interaction with the intestinal immunity of the neonate. Adv Exp Med Biol 1978; 107:95–107.
110. Anderson ND, Anderson AO, Wyllie RG. Specialized structure and metabolic activities of high endothelial venules in rat lymphatic tissues. Immunology 1976; 31:455–73.
111. Stevens SK, Weissman IL, Butcher EC. Differences in the migration of B and T lymphocytes: organ-selective localization *in vivo* and the role of lymphocyte-endothelial cell recognition. J Immunol 1982; 128:844–51.
112. Butcher EC, Scollay RG, Weissman IL. Organ specificity of lymphocyte migration: mediation by highly selective lymphocyte interaction with organ-specific determinants on high endothelial venules. Eur J Immunol 1980; 10:556–61.
113. Husband AJ. Kinetics of extravasation and redistribution of IgA-specific antibody-containing cells in the intestine. J Immunol 1982; 128:1355–9.
114. Parrott DMV, Ferguson A. Selective migration of lymphocytes within the mouse small intestine. Immunology 1974; 26:571–88.
115. Hanson LA, Carlsson B, Cruz JR, Garcia B, Holmgren J, Khan SR, Lindblad BS, Svennerholm AM, Svennerholm B, Urrutia J. Immune response in the mammary gland. *In:* Ogra PL, Dayton D, eds. Immunology of Breast Milk. New York: Raven Press, 1979: 145–57.
116. Montgomery PC, Connelly KM, Cohn J, Skandera CA. Remote-site stimulation of secretory IgA antibodies following bronchial and gastric stimulation. Adv Exp Med Biol 1978; 107:113–22.
117. Lamm ME, Weisz-Carrington P, Roux ME, McWilliams M, Phillips-Quagliata JM. Development of the IgA system in the mammary gland. Adv Exp Med Biol 1978; 107:35–42.
118. Tomasi TB Jr, Larson L, Challacombe S, McNabb P. Mucosal immunity: the origin and migration patterns of cells in the secretory system. J Allergy Clin Immunol 1980; 65:12–9.

119. Barry WS, Pierce NF. Protein deprivation causes reversible impairment of mucosal immune response to cholera toxoid/toxin in rat gut. Nature 1979; 281:64–5.
120. McDermott MR, Mark DA, Befus AD, Baliga BS, Suskind RM, Bienenstock J. Impaired intestinal localization of mesenteric lymphoblasts associated with vitamin A deficiency and protein-calorie malnutrition. Immunology 1982; 45:1–5.
121. Perkkiö M, Savilahti E. Time of appearance of immunoglobulin-containing cells in the mucosa of the neonatal intestine. Pediatr Res 1980; 14:953–5.
122. Cooper MD, Kubagawa H, Vogler LB, Kearney JF, Lawton AR. Generation of clonal and isotype diversity. Adv Exp Med Biol 1978; 107:9–17.
123. Tomasi TB Jr, Tan EM, Solomon A, Prendergast RG. Characteristics of an immune system common to certain external secretions. J Exp Med 1965; 121:101–24.
124. Kutteh WH, Prince SJ, Mestecky J. Tissue origins of human polymeric and monomeric IgA. J Immunol 1982; 128:990–5.
125. Kutteh WH, Koopman WJ, Conley ME, Egan ML, Mestecky J. Production of predominantly polymeric IgA by human peripheral blood lymphocytes stimulated in vitro with mitogens. J Exp Med 1980; 152:1424–9.
126. André C, André F, Fargier MC. Distribution of IgA1 and IgA2 plasma cells in various normal human tissues and in the jejunum of plasma IgA-deficient patients. Clin Exp Immunol 1978; 33:327–31.
127. Mota G. Selective hydrolysis of human secretory IgA subclasses. Rev Roum Biochim 1977; 14:39–42.
128. Lebenthal E, Clark BA, Kim O. Immunoglobulin concentrations in duodenal fluid of infants and children. Am J Dis Child 1980; 134:834–7.
129. Spohn M, McColl I. Studies on human gastric mucosal immunoglobulin A. Biochim Biophys Acta 1979; 576:1–8.
130. Tomasi TB, Grey HM. Structure and function of immunoglobulin A. Prog Allergy 1972; 16:81–213.
131. Brandtzaeg P, Savilahti E. Further evidence for a role of secretory component (SC) and J chain in the glandular transport of IgA. Adv Exp Med Biol 1978; 107:219–26.
132. Jos J, Labbe F, Geny B, Griscelli C. Immunoelectronmicroscopic localization of immunoglobulin A and secretory component in jejunal mucosa from children with coeliac disease. Scand J Immunol 1979; 9:441–50.
133. Brandtzaeg P. Transport models for secretory IgA and secretory IgM. Clin Exp Immunol 1981; 44:221–32.
134. Brandtzaeg P. Polymeric IgA is complexed with secretory component (SC) on the surface of human intestinal epithelial cells. Scand J Immunol 1978; 8:39–52.
135. Crago SS, Prince SJ, Kulhavy R, Mestecky J. Molecular-cellular interactions in the secretory IgA system. Adv Exp Med Biol 1978; 107:209–17.
136. Strober W, Krakauer R, Klaeveman HL, Reynolds HY, Nelson DL. Secretory component deficiency. A disorder of the IgA immune system. N Engl J Med 1976; 294:351–6.
137. Brown WR, Newcomb RW, Ishizaka K. Proteolytic degradation of exocrine and serum immunoglobulins. J Clin Invest 1970; 49:1374–80.
138. Walker WA, Isselbacher KJ. Uptake and transport of macromolecules by the intestine. Possible role in clinical disorders. Gastroenterology 1974; 67:531–50.
139. Brown WR. Relationships between immunoglobulins and the intestinal epithelium. Gastroenterology 1978; 75:129–38.
140. World Health Organization. Intestinal immunity and vaccine development: a WHO memorandum. Bull WHO 1979; 57:719–34.
141. Magnusson K-E, Stjernström I. Mucosal barrier mechanisms. Interplay between secretory IgA (SIgA), IgG and mucins on the surface properties and association of salmonellae with intestine and granulocytes. Immunology 1982; 45:239–48.
142. Ogra PL, Karzon DT. Distribution of poliovirus antibody in serum, nasopharynx, and alimentary tract following segmental immunization of lower alimentary tract with poliovaccine. J Immunol 1969; 102:1423–30.
143. André C, Lambert R, Bazin H, Heremans JF. Interference of oral immunization with the intestinal absorption of heterologous albumin. Eur J Immunol 1974; 4:701–4.
144. Walker WA, Isselbacher KJ. Intestinal antibodies. N Engl J Med 1977; 297:767–73.
145. Colten HR, Bienenstock J. Lack of C3 activation through classical or alternate pathways by human secretory IgA anti-blood group A antibody. Adv Exp Med Biol 1974; 45:305–8.
146. Doe WF. An overview of intestinal immunity and malabsorption. Am J Med 1979; 67:1077–84.
147. Lowell GH, MacDermott RP, Summers PL, Reeder AA, Bertovich MJ, Formal SB. Antibody-dependent cell-mediated antibacterial activity: K lymphocytes, monocytes, and granulocytes are effective against Shigella. J Immunol 1980; 125:2778–84.
148. Butcher EC, Rouse RV, Coffman RL, Nottenburg CN, Hardy RR, Weissman IL. Surface phenotype of Peyer's patch germinal center cells: implications for the role of germinal centers in B cell differentiation. J Immunol 1982; 129:2698–707.
149. Parkhouse RME, Dresser DW. Effect of anti-IgD serum on immune responses. Adv Exp Med Biol 1978; 107:43–51.
150. Gearhart PJ, Cebra JJ. Differentiated B lymphocytes. Potential to express particular antibody variable and constant regions depends on site of lymphoid tissue and antigen load. J Exp Med 1979; 149:216–27.
151. Cebra JJ, Emmons R, Gearhart PJ, Robertson SM, Tseng J. Cellular parameters of the IgA response. Adv Exp Med Biol 1978; 107:19–28.
152. Lally ET, Zitron IM, Fiorini RC, Montgomery PC. Cellular aspects of the murine anti-hapten IgA response. Adv Exp Med Biol 1978; 107:143–50.
153. Elson CO, Heck JA, Strober W. T-cell regulation of murine IgA synthesis. J Exp Med 1979; 149:632–43.
154. Kawanishi H, Saltzman LE, Strober W. Characteristics and regulatory function of murine Con A-induced, cloned T cells obtained from Peyer's patches and spleen: mechanisms regulating isotype-specific immunoglobulin production by Peyer's patch B cells. J Immunol 1982; 129:475–83.
155. Kiyono H, McGhee JR, Mosteller LM, Eldridge JH, Koopman WJ, Kearney JF, Michalek SM. Murine Peyer's patch T cell clones. Characterization of antigen-specific helper T cells for immunoglobulin A responses. J Exp Med 1982; 156:1115–30.
156. Hoover RG, Lynch RG. Isotype-specific suppression of IgA: suppression of IgA responses in BALB/c mice by T_α cells. J Immunol 1983; 130:521–3.
157. Green F, Heyworth B. Immunoglobulin-containing cells in jejunal mucosa of children with protein-energy malnutrition and gastroenteritis. Arch Dis Child 1980; 55:380–3.
158. Elson CO, Heck JA, Strober W. T-cell regulation of IgA synthesis. *In*: Ogra PL, Dayton D, eds. Immunology of Breast Milk. New York: Raven Press, 1979: 37–47.
159. Wilson ID, Soltis RD, Olson RE, Erlandsen SL. Cholinergic stimulation of immunoglobulin A secretion in rat intestine. Gastroenterology 1982; 83:881–8.
160. Lebenthal E, Clark B. Immunoglobulin concentrations in the duodenal fluids of infants and children. II. The effect of pancreozymin and secretin. Am J Gastroenterol 1981; 75:436–9.
161. Lemaître-Coelho I, Jackson GDF, Vaerman J-P. Rat bile as a convenient source of secretory IgA and free secretory component. Eur J Immunol 1977; 7:588–90.
162. Lemaître-Coelho I, Jackson GDF, Vaerman J-P. High levels of secretory IgA and free secretory component in the serum of rats with bile duct obstruction. J Exp Med 1978; 147:934–9.
163. Orlans E, Peppard J, Reynolds J, Hall J. Rapid active transport of immunoglobulin A from blood to bile. J Exp Med 1978; 147:588–92.
164. Fisher MM, Nagy B, Bazin H, Underdown BJ. Biliary transport of IgA: role of secretory component. Proc Natl Acad Sci USA 1979; 76:2008–12.
165. Dooley JS, Potter BJ, Thomas HC, Sherlock S. A comparative study of the biliary secretion of human dimeric and monomeric IgA in the rat and in man. Hepatology 1982; 2:323–7.
166. Kleinman RE, Harmatz PR, Walker WA. The liver: an integral part of the enteric mucosal immune system. Hepatology 1982; 2:379–84.

167. Renston RH, Jones AL, Christiansen WD, Hradek GT. Evidence for a vesicular transport mechanism in hepatocytes for biliary secretion of immunoglobulin A. Science 1980; 208:1276–8.
168. Hsu S-M, Hsu P-L. Demonstration of IgA and secretory component in human hepatocytes. Gut 1980; 21:985–9.
169. Nagura H, Smith PD, Nakane PK, Brown WR. IgA in human bile and liver. J Immunol 1981; 126:587–95.
170. Goldblum RM, Powell GK, Van Sickle G. Secretory IgA in the serum of infants with obstructive jaundice. J Pediatr 1980; 97:33–6.
171. Delacroix DL, Jonard P, Dive C, Vaerman J-P. Serum IgM-bound secretory component (sIgM) in liver diseases: comparative molecular state of the secretory component in serum and bile. J Immunol 1982; 129:133–8.
172. Kutteh WH, Prince SJ, Phillips JO, Spenney JG, Mestecky J. Properties of immunoglobulin A in serum of individuals with liver diseases and in hepatic bile. Gastroenterology 1982; 82:184–93.
173. Hall J, Orlans E, Reynolds J, Dean C, Peppard J, Gyure L, Hobbs S. Occurrence of specific antibodies of the IgA class in the bile of rats. Int Arch Allergy Appl Immunol 1979; 59:75–84.
174. Vaerman JP, Lemaitre-Coelho IM, Jackson GDF. Role of the liver in the rat intestinal s-IgA system. Adv Exp Med Biol 1978; 107:233–9.
175. Socken DJ, Simms ES, Nagy BR, Fisher MM, Underdown BJ. Secretory component-dependent hepatic transport of IgA antibody-antigen complexes. J Immunol 1981; 127:316–9.
176. Kühn LC, Kraehenbuhl J-P. Role of secretory component, a secreted glycoprotein, in the specific uptake of IgA dimer by epithelial cells. J Biol Chem 1979; 254:11072–81.
177. Virella G, Montgomery PC, Lemaitre-Coelho IM. Transport of oligomeric IgA of systemic origin into external secretions. Adv Exp Med Biol 1978; 107:241–51.
178. Russell MW, Brown TA, Mestecky J. Role of serum IgA. Hepatobiliary transport of circulating antigen. J Exp Med 1981; 153:968–76.
179. Brandtzaeg P. Human secretory immunoglobulin M: an immunochemical and immunohistochemical study. Immunology 1975; 29:559–70.
180. Brown WR, Isobe K, Nakane PK, Pacini B. Studies on translocation of immunoglobulins across intestinal epithelium. IV. Evidence for binding of IgA and IgM to secretory component in intestinal epithelium. Gastroenterology 1977; 73:1333–9.
181. Brandtzaeg P. The secondary immune system of lactating human mammary glands compared with other exocrine organs. Ann NY Acad Sci 1983; 409:353–81.
182. Crabbé PA, Heremans JF. Selective IgA deficiency with steatorrhea: a new syndrome. Am J Med 1967; 42:319–26.
183. Richman LK, Brown WR. Immunochemical characterization of IgM in human intestinal fluids. J Immunol 1977; 119:1515–9.
184. Brandtzaeg P. Complex formation between secretory component and human immunoglobulins related to their content of J chain. Scand J Immunol 1976; 5:411–9.
185. Brown WR, Isobe Y, Nakane PK. Studies on translocation of immunoglobulins across intestinal epithelium. II. Immunoelectron-microscopic localization of immunoglobulins and secretory component in human intestinal mucosa. Gastroenterology 1976; 71:985–95.
186. Brandtzaeg P, Baklien K. Immunohistochemical studies of the formation and epithelial transport of immunoglobulins in normal and diseased human intestinal mucosa. Scand J Gastroenterol 1976; 11(Suppl 36):1–45.
187. Halpin TC Jr, Gregoire RP, Izant RJ Jr. Abnormal rectal immunoglobulin pattern in Hirschsprung's disease. Lancet 1978; 2:606–8.
188. Brown WR, Borthistle BK, Chen ST. Immunoglobulin E (IgE) and IgE-containing cells in human gastrointestinal fluids and tissues. Clin Exp Immunol 1975; 20:227–37.
189. Mayrhofer G. Sites of synthesis and localization of IgE in rats infested with *Nippostrongylus brasiliensis*. Ciba Found Symp 1977; 46:155–75.
190. Belut D, Moneret-Vautrin DA, Nicolas JP, Grilliat JP. IgE levels in intestinal juice. Dig Dis Sci 1980; 25:323–32.
191. Ogilvie BM, Love RJ. Co-operation between antibodies and cells in immunity to a nematode parasite. Transplant Rev 1974; 19:147–68.
192. Capron A, Dessaint JP, Joseph M, Rousseaux R, Capron M, Bazin H. Interaction between IgE complexes and macrophages in the rat: a new mechanism of macrophage activation. Eur J Immunol 1977; 7:315–22.
193. Parmely MJ, Williams SB. Selective expression of immunocompetence in human colostrum: preliminary evidence for the control of cytotoxic T lymphocytes including those specific for paternal alloantigens. *In:* Ogra PL, Dayton D, eds. Immunology of Breast Milk. New York: Raven Press, 1979: 173–83.
194. Davies MDJ, Parrott DMV. The early appearance of specific cytotoxic T cells in murine gut mucosa. Clin Exp Immunol 1980; 42:273–9.
195. Selby WS, Janossy G, Bofill M, Jewell DP. Lymphocyte subpopulations in the human small intestine. The findings in normal mucosa and the mucosa of patients with adult coeliac disease. Clin Exp Immunol 1983; 52:219–28.
196. Castro GA. Immunological regulation of epithelial function. Am J Physiol 1982; 243:G321–9.
197. Ganguly R, Waldman RH. Cell-mediated immunity on secretory surfaces. Adv Exp Med Biol 1978; 107:75–85.
198. Richman LK. Immunological unresponsiveness after enteric administration of protein antigens. *In:* Ogra PL, Dayton D, eds. Immunology of Breast Milk. New York: Raven Press, 1979: 49–62.
199. Asherson GL, Perra MACC, Thomas WR, Zembala M. Contact-sensitizing agents and the intestinal tract: the production of immunity and unresponsiveness by feeding contact-sensitizing agents and the role of suppressor cells. *In:* Ogra PL, Dayton D, eds. Immunology of Breast Milk. New York: Raven Press, 1979: 19–36.
200. Kagnoff MF. Effects of antigen-feeding on intestinal and systemic immune responses. I. Priming of precursor cytotoxic T cells by antigen feeding. J Immunol 1978; 120:395–9.
201. Bull DM, Bookman MA. Isolation and functional characterization of human intestinal mucosal lymphoid cells. J Clin Invest 1977; 59:966–74.
202. Clancy R, Pucci A. Absence of K cells in human gut mucosa. Gut 1978; 19:273–6.
203. Gupta S. Natural killer cells—immunologist's fancy? Gastroenterology 1980; 78:865–7.
204. Kraft SC. The intestinal immune response in giardiasis. Gastroenterology 1979; 76:877–9.
205. Ogra SS, Ogra PL. Components of immunologic reactivity in human colostrum and milk. *In:* Ogra PL, Dayton D, eds. Immunology of Breast Milk. New York: Raven Press, 1979: 185–95.
206. Ahlstedt S, Carlsson B, Fällström SP, Hanson LA, Holmgren J, Lidin-Janson G, Lindblad BS, Jodal U, Kaijser B, Sohl-Åkerlund A, Wadsworth C. Antibodies in human serum and milk induced by enterobacteria and food proteins. Ciba Found Symp 1977; 46:115–29.
207. Hunt JS, Kim Y, Halsey JF. Immune complexes facilitate uptake of antigen from the gut. Immunol Commun 1981; 10:21–6.
208. Rothberg RM, Rieger CHL, Kraft SC, Lustig JV. Development of humoral antibody following the ingestion of soluble protein antigen by passively immunized animals. Adv Exp Med Biol 1978; 107:123–32.
209. Galant SP. Biological and clinical significance of the gut as a barrier to penetration of macromolecules. (Phila) Clin Pediatr 1976; 15:731–4.
210. Walker WA. Cellular and immune changes in the gastrointestinal tract in malnutrition. Curr Concepts Nutr 1980; 9:197–218.
211. Walker WA. Antigen absorption from the small intestine and gastrointestinal disease. Pediatr Clin North Am 1975; 22:731–46.
212. Walker WA, Bloch KJ. Intestinal uptake of macromolecules: *in vitro* and *in vivo* studies. Ann NY Acad Sci 1983; 409:593–601.
213. Rothberg RM. Immunoglobulin and specific antibody synthesis during the first weeks of life of premature infants. J Pediatr 1969; 75:391–9.

214. Eastham EJ, Lichauco T, Grady MI, Walker WA. Antigenicity of infant formulas: role of immature intestine on protein permeability. J Pediatr 1978; 93:561–4.
215. Editorial. Antigen absorption by the gut. Lancet 1978; 2:715–7.
216. Udall JN, Pang K, Fritze L, Kleinman R, Walker WA. Development of gastrointestinal mucosal barrier. I. The effect of age on intestinal permeability to macromolecules. Pediatr Res 1981; 15:241–4.
217. Udall JN, Colony P, Fritze L, Pang K, Trier JS, Walker WA. Development of gastrointestinal mucosal barrier. II. The effect of natural *versus* artificial feeding on intestinal permeability to macromolecules. Pediatr Res 1981; 15:245–9.
218. Walker WA. Antigen penetration across the immature gut: effect of immunologic and maturational factors in colostrum. *In:* Ogra PL, Dayton D, eds. Immunology of Breast Milk. New York: Raven Press, 1979: 227–35.
219. Cottier H, Hess MW, Keller HU. Structural basis for lymphoid tissue functions: established and disputed sites of antigen-cell and cell-to-cell interactions *in vivo*. Monogr Allergy 1980; 16:50–71.
220. Keren DF, Holt PS, Collins HH, Gemski P, Formal SB. The role of Peyer's patches in the local immune response of rabbit ileum to live bacteria. J Immunol 1978; 120:1892–6.
221. Pierce NF. The role of antigen form and function in the primary and secondary intestinal immune response to cholera toxin and toxoid in rats. J Exp Med 1978; 148:195–206.
222. Kagnoff MF. Functional characteristics of Peyer's patch cells. III. Carrier priming of T cells by antigen feeding. J Exp Med 1975; 142:1425–35.
223. Kagnoff MF. Functional characteristics of intestinal Peyer's patch lymphoid cells. Ann NY Acad Sci 1976; 278:539–45.
224. Mattingly JA, Waksman BH. Immunologic suppression after oral administration of antigen. I. Specific suppressor cells formed in rat Peyer's patches after oral administration of sheep erythrocytes and their systemic migration. J Immunol 1978; 121:1878–83.
225. Myrvik QN, Ockers JR. Transport of horseradish peroxidase from the vascular compartment to bronchial-associated lymphoid tissue. J Reticuloendothel Soc 1982; 31:267–78.
226. Editorial. Gut reaction to antigen. Lancet 1979; 1:763.
227. Fuhrman JA, Cebra JJ. Special features of the priming process for a secretory IgA response. B cell priming with cholera toxin. J Exp Med 1981; 153:534–44.
228. Crabbé PA, Nash DR, Bazin H, Eyssen H, Heremans JF. Antibodies of the IgA type in intestinal plasma cells of germfree mice after oral or parenteral immunization with ferritin. J Exp Med 1969; 130:723–44.
229. Rothberg RM, Kraft SC, Farr RS, Kriebel GW Jr, Goldberg SS. Local immunologic responses to ingested protein. *In:* Dayton DH Jr, Small PA Jr, Chanock RM, Kaufman HE, Tomasi TB Jr, eds. The Secretory Immunologic System. Washington, DC: US Government Printing Office, 1971: 293–307.
230. Lim PL, Rowley D. The effect of antibody on the intestinal absorption of macromolecules and on intestinal permeability in adult mice. Int Arch Allergy Appl Immunol 1982; 68:41–6.
231. Ebersole JL, Molinari JA. The induction of salivary antibodies by topical sensitization with particulate and soluble bacterial immunogens. Immunology 1978; 34:969–79.
232. Girard JP, de Kalbermatten A. Antibody activity in human duodenal fluid. Eur J Clin Invest 1970; 1:188–95.
233. La Brooy JT, Davidson GP, Shearman DJC, Rowley D. The antibody response to bacterial gastroenteritis in serum and secretions. Clin Exp Immunol 1980; 41:290–6.
234. Ogra PL, Karzon DT, Righthand F, MacGillivray M. Immunoglobulin response in serum and secretions after immunization with live and inactivated poliovaccine and natural infection. N Engl J Med 1968; 279:893–900.
235. Pierce NF, Koster FT. Induction and dissemination of an intestinal immune response to cholera toxin/toxoid in rats. *In:* Ogra PL, Dayton D, eds. Immunology of Breast Milk. New York: Raven Press, 1979: 63–72.
236. Pierce SK, Cancro MP, Klinman NR. Individual antigen-specific T lymphocytes: helper function in enabling the expression of multiple antibody isotypes. J Exp Med 1978; 148:759–65.
237. Kagnoff MF. Effects of antigen-feeding on intestinal and systemic immune responses. IV. Similarity between the suppressor factor in mice after erythrocyte-lysate injection and erythrocyte feeding. Gastroenterology 1980; 79:54–61.
238. Heremans JF, Bazin H. Antibodies induced by local antigenic stimulation of mucosal surfaces. Ann NY Acad Sci 1971; 190:268–75.
239. Rothberg RM, Kraft SC, Michalek SM. Systemic immunity after local antigenic stimulation of the lymphoid tissue of the gastrointestinal tract. J Immunol 1973; 111:1906–13.
240. Rogoff TM, Lipsky PE. Role of the Kupffer cells in local and systemic immune responses. Gastroenterology 1981; 80:854–60.
241. Asherson GL, Zembala M, Perera MACC, Mayhew B, Thomas WR. Production of immunity and unresponsiveness in the mouse by feeding contact sensitizing agents and the role of suppressor cells in the Peyer's patches, mesenteric lymph nodes and other lymphoid tissues. Cell Immunol 1977; 33:145–55.
242. André C, Heremans JF, Vaerman JP, Cambiaso CL. A mechanism for the induction of immunological tolerance by antigen feeding: antigen-antibody complexes. J Exp Med 1975; 142:1509–19.
243. David MF. Prevention of homocytotropic antibody formation and anaphylactic sensitization by prefeeding antigen. J Allergy Clin Immunol 1977; 60:180–7.
244. Kagnoff MF. Immunological unresponsiveness after enteric antigen administration. *In:* Strober W, Hanson LA, Sell KW, eds. Recent Advances in Mucosal Immunity. New York: Raven Press, 1982: 95–111.
245. Pierce NF. Suppression of the intestinal immune response to cholera toxin by specific serum antibody. Infect Immun 1980; 30:62–8.
246. Asquith P, Haeney MR. Coeliac disease. *In:* Asquith P, ed. Immunology of the Gastrointestinal Tract. Edinburgh: Churchill Livingstone, 1979: 66–94.
247. Marsh MN. The small intestine: mechanisms of local immunity and gluten sensitivity. Clin Sci 1981; 61:497–503.
248. Falchuk ZM. Update on gluten-sensitive enteropathy. Am J Med 1979; 67:1085–96.
249. Marsh MN. Studies of intestinal lymphoid tissue. The cytology and electron microscopy of gluten-sensitive enteropathy, with particular reference to its immunopathology. Scand J Gastroenterol 1981; 16(Suppl 70):87–106.
250. Ferguson A. Celiac disease and gastrointestinal food allergy. *In:* Ferguson A, MacSween RNM, eds. Immunological Aspects of the Liver and Gastrointestinal Tract. Baltimore: University Park Press, 1976: 153–202.
251. Scott H, Ek J, Baklien K, Brandtzaeg P. Immunoglobulin-producing cells in jejunal mucosa of children with coeliac disease on a gluten-free diet and after gluten challenge. Scand J Gastroenterol 1980; 15:81–8.
252. Unsworth DJ, Kieffer M, Holborow EJ, Coombs RRA, Walker-Smith JA. IgA anti-gliadin antibodies in coeliac disease. Clin Exp Immunol 1981; 46:286–93.
253. Dollberg L, Gurevitz M, Freier S. Gastrointestinal mast cells in health, and in coeliac disease and other conditions. Arch Dis Child 1980; 55:702–5.
254. Ashkenazi A, Levin S, Idar D, Handzel ZT, Altman Y, Or A, Barzilai N. Cellular immunity in children with coeliac disease. Eur J Pediatr 1982; 138:250–3.
255. Marsh MN, Miller V. Raised epithelial lymphocyte mitotic index—a prospective marker of childhood celiac sprue. Gastroenterology 1983; 84:1241 (Abstract).
256. O'Farrelly C, Feighery C, Greally JF, Weir DG. Cellular response to alpha-gliadin in untreated coeliac disease. Gut 1982; 23:83–7.
257. Howdle PD, Bullen AW, Losowsky MS. Cell-mediated immunity to gluten within the small intestinal mucosa in coeliac disease. Gut 1982; 23:115–22.
258. Simpson FG, Bullen AW, Robertson DAF, Losowsky MS. HLA-B8 and cell-mediated immunity to gluten. Gut 1981; 22:633–6.
259. Scott H, Solheim BG, Brandtzaeg P, Thorsby E. HLA-DR-like antigens in the epithelium of the human small intestine. Scand J Immunol 1980; 12:77–82.

260. Neild GH. Coeliac disease: a graft-versus-host-like reaction localised to the small bowel wall? Lancet 1981; 1:811–2.
261. Weiss JB, Austin RK, Schanfield MS, Kagnoff MF. Celiac disease: immunoglobulin heavy chain allotype-linked genes control the immune response to wheat gliadin. Gastroenterology 1983; 84:1348 (Abstract).
262. Ross IN, Asquith P. Primary immune deficiency. *In:* Asquith P, ed. Immunology of the Gastrointestinal Tract. Edinburgh: Churchill Livingstone, 1979: 152–82.
263. Ammann AJ, Hong R. Selective IgA deficiency: presentation of 30 cases and a review of the literature. Medicine 1971; 50:223–36.
264. Cunningham-Rundles C, Brandeis WE, Pudifin DJ, Day NK, Good RA. Autoimmunity in selective IgA deficiency: relationship to anti-bovine protein antibodies, circulating immune complexes and clinical disease. Clin Exp Immunol 1981; 45:299–304.
265. Ranchod M, Lewin KJ, Dorfman RF. Lymphoid hyperplasia of the gastrointestinal tract. A study of 26 cases and review of the literature. Am J Surg Pathol 1978; 2:383–400.
266. Kenney PJ, Koehler RE, Shackelford GD. The clinical significance of large lymphoid follicles of the colon. Radiol 1982; 142:41–6.
267. Crooks DJM, Brown WR. The distribution of intestinal nodular hyperplasia in immunoglobulin deficiency. Clin Radiol 1980; 31:701–6.
268. Nagura H, Kohler PF, Brown WR. Immunocytochemical characterization of the lymphocytes in nodular lymphoid hyperplasia of the bowel. Lab Invest 1979; 40:66–73.
269. Jacobson KW, deShazo RD. Selective immunoglobulin A deficiency associated with nodular lymphoid hyperplasia. J Allergy Clin Immunol 1979; 64:516–21.
270. Matuchansky C, Morichau-Beauchant M, Touchard G, Lenormand Y, Bloch P, Tanzer J, Alcalay D, Babin P. Nodular lymphoid hyperplasia of the small bowel associated with primary jejunal malignant lymphoma. Evidence favoring a cytogenetic relationship. Gastroenterology 1980; 78:1587–92.
271. Doe WF. Alpha heavy chain disease and related small-intestinal lymphoma. *In:* Asquith P, ed. Immunology of the Gastrointestinal Tract. Edinburgh: Churchill Livingstone, 1979: 306–15.
272. Hibi T, Asakura H, Kobayashi K, Munakata Y, Kano S, Tsuchiya M, Teramoto T, Uematsu Y. Alpha heavy chain disease lacking secretory alpha chain, with cobblestone appearance of the small intestine and duodenal ulcer demonstrated by endoscopy. Gut 1982; 23:422–7.
273. Khojasteh A, Haghshenass M, Haghighi P. Immunoproliferative small intestinal disease: a "third-world lesion." N Engl J Med 1983; 308:1401–5.
274. Seligmann M. Immunochemical, clinical, and pathological features of alpha-chain disease. Arch Intern Med 1975; 135:78–82.
275. Doe WF, Danon F, Seligmann M. Immunodiagnosis of alpha chain disease. Clin Exp Immunol 1979; 36:189–97.
276. Rhodes JM, Jewell DP, Janossy G. Alpha-chain disease diagnosed by rectal biopsy. Br Med J 1980; 280:1043–4.
277. Nassar VH, Salem PA, Shahid MJ, Alami SY, Balikian JB, Salem AA, Nasrallah SM. "Mediterranean abdominal lymphoma" or immunoproliferative small intestinal disease. II: Pathological aspects. Cancer 1978; 41:1340–54.
278. Galian A, Lecestre M-J, Scotto J, Bognel C, Matuchansky C, Rambaud J-C. Pathological study of alpha-chain disease, with special emphasis on evolution. Cancer 1977; 39:2081–101.
279. Doe WF. Alpha chain disease. Clinicopathological features and relationship to so-called Mediterranean lymphoma. Br J Cancer 1975; 31(Suppl 2):350–5.
280. Lewin KJ, Kahn LB, Novis BH. Primary intestinal lymphoma of "Western" and "Mediterranean" type, alpha chain disease and massive plasma cell proliferation: a comparative study of 37 cases. Cancer 1976; 38:2511–28.
281. Ramot B, Levanon M, Hahn Y, Lahat N, Moroz C. The mutual clonal origin of the lymphocytoplasmocytic and lymphoma cell in alpha-heavy chain disease. Clin Exp Immunol 1977; 27:440–5.
282. World Health Organization Memorandum. Alpha chain disease and related small-intestinal lymphoma. Bull WHO 1976; 54:615–24.
283. Gafter U, Kessler E, Shabtay F, Shaked P, Djaldetti M. Abnormal chromosomal marker ($D_{14}q+$) in a patient with alpha heavy chain disease. J Clin Pathol 1980; 33:136–44.

Chapter 100

Ecology of the Gastrointestinal Tract

Gerald T. Keusch and Sherwood L. Gorbach (Bacteria) • Robert J. Pauley (Viruses) • Dexter H. Howard (Fungi and Actinomycetes)

Bacteria

Gerald T. Keusch • Sherwood L. Gorbach

"There are more animals living in the scum on the teeth in a man's mouth, than there are men in a whole kingdom, especially in those who don't ever clean their teeth, whereby such a stench comes from the mouth of many of 'em, that you can scarce bear to talk to them, which is called by many people "having a stinking breath," though in sooth tis most always a stinking mouth. For my part, I judge, from myself (howbeit I clean my mouth like I've already said) that all the people living in our United Netherlands are not as many as the living animals that I carry in my own mouth this very day."

In these words 300 years ago Antony van Leeuwenhoek reported the very first glimpse of the indigenous bacteria.[1] Indeed, the number of bacteria in a single gram of heavily colonized dental plaque or colonic content[2] exceeds the total world population of humans by 100-fold and presents a set of coexistence problems for this enormous population of microbes. They comprise more species than countries in the United Nations (over 400 known organisms in stool),[3] are of different color, size, and shape (as observed in a Gram-stained specimen), exhibit variable tolerance to the presence of oxygen (from indifference to extreme intolerance), have distinctive metabolic needs and functions, and demonstrate individual life styles expressed in choice of niche or habitat.[4] With so many different organisms living in such close contact (Fig. 100–1), it becomes obvious that to survive they must interact both physically and metabolically not only with one another but with the host as well. The microbial flora is a remarkable ecosystem; it is therefore necessary to discuss the microbial ecology of the gastrointestinal tract and not just the flora.[5]

Definitions and Methods

Methodology clearly limits our knowledge of intestinal microecology. Not very long ago, it was believed that stool, which can be considered a 25% to 30% aqueous suspension of bacteria, was composed mostly of dead organisms because only a small percentage of those observed visually could be grown microbiologically. A major revolution of the past few decades is the understanding that stool is a living ferment. Further, the vast majority of the viable organisms are anaerobic, i.e., they do not grow in the presence of oxygen. This realization has necessitated the development of anaerobic techniques to permit growth, taxonomic classification, and enumeration of the different *obligate anaerobes*. The degree of oxygen intolerance varies from organisms that can survive for hours in

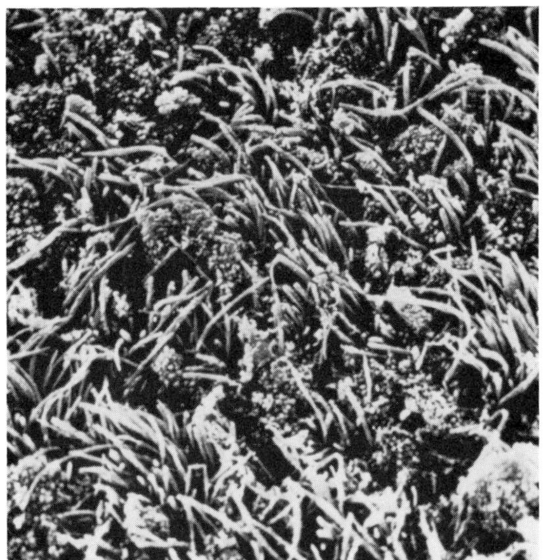

Figure 100–1. Scanning electron micrograph of the microbial flora of dental plaque. Note the density of the microorganisms and the diversity of their morphologic features.

the presence of oxygen but cannot multiply to extremely oxygen-sensitive strains that are killed almost immediately by molecular oxygen and must be collected, transported, and cultured under strict conditions that exclude oxygen. The mixture of organisms is so complex and the methodology is so demanding that a complete analysis of a single stool with present laboratory techniques requires about 1 year.[6, 7]

Most is known about the smallest portion of the flora, those organisms capable of growing in the presence of oxygen, called *aerobes,* or those capable of growing in either the presence or absence of air, classified as *facultative anaerobes.* The latter group includes coliforms, especially *Escherichia coli.* Even among the aerobes or facultative anaerobes, however, there are problems in the recovery of those species present in smaller numbers than the predominant organisms.

Sampling. Since it is easy to obtain specimens from the 2 ends of the intestinal tract, the mouth and the anus, our knowledge of the flora during life has been largely restricted to these sites. Special methods have been developed to overcome the relative inaccessibility of the intervening portions of the bowel.[5] The methods range from single or multiple lumen long tubes with weighted mercury bags to facilitate passage[8] to a telemetrically operated mini-sampling capsule[9] opened by electronic signal at some point during its fantastic voyage to sample the gut contents.

The multiple lumen long tube has been used to aspirate samples from several sites in the gut at the same time, e.g., on either side of the ileocecal valve.[8] To minimize contamination during passage, the openings of the tube have been sealed with agar plugs and filled with sterile deoxygenated water.[5] The tube could then be opened at the desired location by blowing out the plug, with sampling accomplished by aspiration.

Each method has disadvantages, including (1) contamination and possible changes in physiology caused by the presence of the tube (largely avoided by the unattached capsule method) and (2) the long delay between sample collection and recovery of the electronic capsule in the passed stool, which undoubtedly permits the growth of some organisms and may distort the relative proportions of others.

Some investigators have employed needle aspiration of intestinal contents during surgery to obtain samples of gut fluids from otherwise inaccessible sites.[10] However, patients undergoing bowel surgery would not have a typical or normal flora because of acquisition of hospital strains, preoperative antibiotic bowel preparation or enemas, preoperative starvation, anesthesia, or the underlying disease state.

Comparative analysis of the data obtained by these various methods suggests that intubation techniques are the easiest and are probably no less reliable than other methods.[4]

Anaerobic Microbiology. Various types of reduced media, jars, and chambers have been used to obtain anaerobic conditions for culture.[5, 11] A major innovation, the roll tube method, was introduced in 1950 by Hungate.[12] This technique permitted benchtop manipulation to obtain anaerobiosis by a stream of oxygen-free gas. By using a thin layer of agar prepared on a rolling culture tube pre-reduced prior to inoculation and streaking the inoculum in a spiral pathway along the constantly rotating tube in the apparatus, anaerobiosis was maintained and individual colonies could be obtained for quantitative studies. Though cumbersome, Hungate's method has been extensively and successfully used to define the complex microbiology of the rumen, but it has not been very useful for clinical microbiology.

Adaptation of an anaerobic chamber to the

benchtop in the form of the plastic glove box (Fig. 100–2) has served well for clinical purposes.[13] The use of pre-reduced, oxygen-free media with inorganic oxygen scavangers has improved the efficiency of the glove box in culturing highly anaerobic organisms, permitting microscopic analysis and manipulations such as antimicrobial sensitivity testing within it. Even so, this methodology is beyond the capability of laboratories in small community hospitals.

The introduction of the commercially produced Gas-Pak system, a simple jar in which an anaerobic environment can be readily generated, has solved this problem.[14] This method can be used for clinically important organisms, since they can tolerate exposure to air—at least for a few hours.[15] However, many anaerobic species in the normal flora cannot survive oxygenated conditions, and the Gas-Pak system is unsuitable as a research technique to evaluate the composition or function of the intestinal flora.

Isolation and Enumeration. As a general rule, the most numerous and least fastidious bacterial species in the flora are the least difficult to isolate.[5, 11, 13] It is necessary to suppress these components of the flora as well as provide for the special metabolic needs of the fastidious microbes to permit their growth. Selective media are used for this purpose, but there are inherent difficulties involved. Such media not only prevent the growth of unwanted species, but may also partially inhibit growth of the desired organism, leading to underestimation of their number.[16] Furthermore, unless the media are metabolically appropriate, fastidious microbes will not grow at all. It should be evident that selective media are only selective for those species that are known and are being sought. Bacteria present in low concentrations and not apparent on general nonselective media cannot be identified if the selective media do not favor their growth.[4]

Enumeration involves the counting of colonies arising from single organisms in diluted samples of the material being cultured. The assumption that one colony-forming unit (cfu) results from a single bacterium depends on the diligence with which the sample is dispersed. That the organisms recovered are representative of the whole sample under study depends upon the thoroughness with which the sample is mixed and the randomness of the collection procedure.

Identification of microorganisms proceeds by traditional analysis of size, shape, Gram stain characteristics, colonial morphology, growth characteristics, and metabolic reactivity. Recent additions are biochemical characterization of cell wall components, antigenic characteristics, studies of DNA homology with reference strains, and use of gas-liquid chromatography (GLC) to identify fermentation products such as short chain fatty acids.[17, 18] In fact, the individual GLC pattern of certain anaerobes can be so characteristic that it is directly useful for classifying and identifying isolates, at least to the genus level and sometimes to the species level as well (Fig. 100–3).[18]

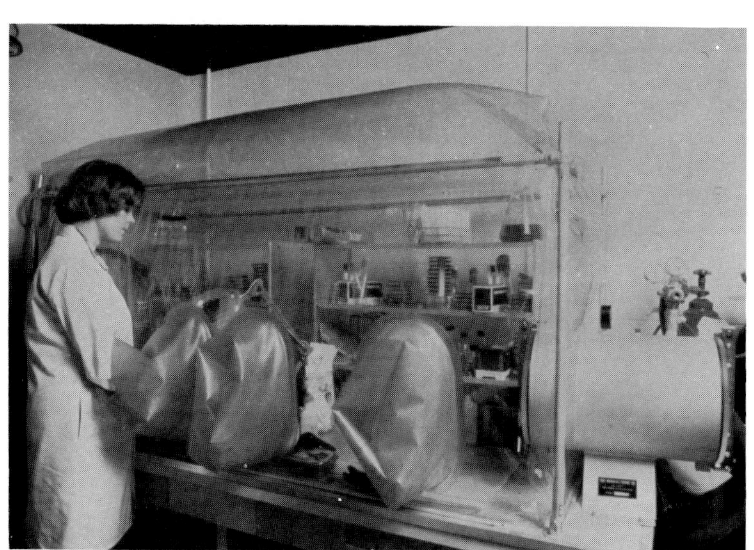

Figure 100–2. A plastic glovebox for anaerobic microbiology.

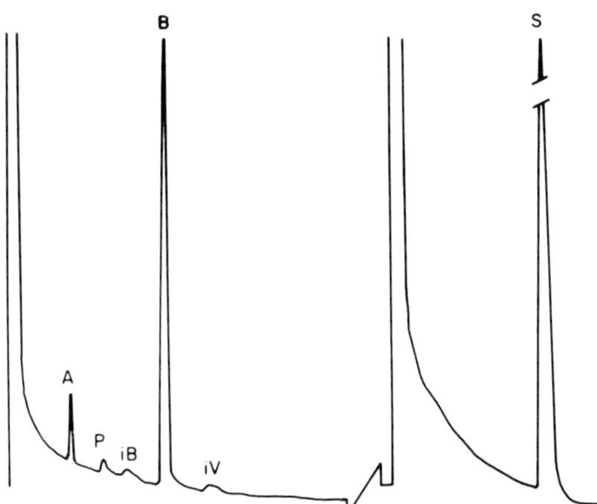

Figure 100–3. Gas liquid chromatography of the contents of a mixed aerobic-anaerobic rectal abscess. The peaks identified are: A = acetic acid; P = propionic acid; iB = isobutyric acid; B = butyric acid; iV = isovaleric acid; and S = succinic acid. The presence of large amounts of volatile acids, and especially succinic acid, is characteristic of infection with *Bacteroides fragilis.*

Composition of Normal Flora

The nature and numbers of microorganisms differ from one part of the intestinal tract to another (Table 100–1).[2, 4, 5, 8, 9, 11, 13, 19-21]

Mouth. In spite of the constant flow of air through the oral cavity, the mouth flora is predominantly anaerobic, existing mostly in the gingival crevices and in dental plaque.[22, 23] The predominant organisms include *Bacteroides (melaninogenicus, oralis), Fusobacterium, Veillonella, Lactobacillus, Peptostreptococcus,* and spirochetes among the anaerobes and *Neisseria* and *Streptococcus (mutans, salivarius, sanguis)* among the aerobes.

Stomach. Oral bacteria are washed with saliva into the stomach; however, the vast majority are destroyed by gastric acid.[22] Concentrations of bacteria are generally low, less than 10^3 cfu/ml and are primarily composed of relatively acid-resistant species, such as *Streptococcus, Staphylococcus, Lactobacillus,* fungi, and even smaller numbers of *Peptostreptococcus, Fusobacterium,* and *Bacteroides.*[8, 19-21] The gram-positive organisms predominate, and a striking feature is the absence of Enterobacteriaceae as well as *Bacteroides fragilis* and *Clostridium.*

The gastric flora can become more complex when the ability to achieve an acid pH is altered by buffering of ingested food or by hypochlorhydria due to intrinsic pathology or surgery.[22] The gastric flora also reflects organisms ingested with and protected within food (at least for a time after ingestion of a meal). Both the emptying time and the completeness of emptying can affect the isolation of different organisms.

Small Intestine. Sparsely populated in its proximal portions, the distal small intestine constitutes a zone of transition from the minimal flora of the stomach to the lush and diverse bacterial flora of the colon.[8, 19-21, 24] The bacteria ordinarily encountered in the duodenum, jejunum, and initial portions of the ileum are similar to those encountered in the stomach. As the ileocecal valve is approached, however, the number and variety of gram-negative bacteria begin to in-

Table 100–1. COMPOSITION OF THE INTESTINAL FLORA OF ADULT HUMANS*

	Bacterial Concentration (Log_{10}/ml or g)			
Bacterial Species	*Stomach*	*Jejunum*	*Ileum*	*Colon*
Total Viable count	$0–10^3$	$0–10^5$	$10^2–10^7$	$10^{10}–10^{12}$
Aerobes or facultative anaerobes				
Enterobacteria	$0–10^2$	$0–10^3$	$10^2–10^7$	$10^4–10^{10}$
Streptococci	$0–10^3$	$0–10^4$	$10^2–10^6$	$10^5–10^{10}$
Staphylococci	$0–10^2$	$0–10^3$	$10^2–10^5$	$10^4–10^9$
Lactobacilli	$0–10^3$	$0–10^4$	$10^2–10^5$	$10^6–10^{10}$
Fungi	$0–10^2$	$0–10^2$	$10^2–10^4$	$10^4–10^6$
Anaerobes				
Bacteroides	Rare	$0–10^3$	$10^3–10^7$	$10^{10}–10^{12}$
Bifidobacteria	Rare	$0–10^4$	$10^3–10^9$	$10^8–10^{12}$
Streptococci	Rare	$0–10^3$	$10^2–10^6$	$10^{10}–10^{12}$
Clostridia	Rare	Rare	$10^2–10^6$	$10^6–10^{11}$
Eubacteria	Rare	Rare	Rare	$10^9–10^{12}$

*The oral flora defies simple characterization, for its composition varies with the site (tongue, tooth, gingival crevice), the duration of time of undisturbed growth (e.g., without tooth brushing) prior to sampling, and the nature of the diet (carbohydrate content and *S. mutans*). (See Nolte WA, reference 23.)

crease.[4, 8, 19-21, 25, 26] Coliforms are found consistently, and the number of anaerobic organisms, both gram-positive and gram-negative (such as *Bifidobacterium, Clostridium, Bacteroides,* and *Fusobacterium*), rises sharply. The ability of the distal ileum to support this anaerobic flora is reflected in the redox potential of −150 mv, which is only slightly lower than the −200 mv of the cecum.[27]

Colon. A further dramatic increase in the flora occurs as soon as the ileocecal valve is crossed. Here, the number of bacteria present approaches the theoretical limits of packing cells of such size in space. Nearly one-third of the dry weight of the feces consists of bacteria.[28] The anaerobes outnumber the aerobes or facultative flora by 1000- to 10,000-fold. The predominant isolates are *Bacteroides, Bifidobacterium, Eubacterium,* and anaerobic cocci *(Peptostreptococcus),* with small numbers of *Staphylococcus, Lactobacillus,* group D streptococci, and the Enterobacteriaceae, among which *E. coli* strains predominate.[6-8, 10, 19-21, 24, 29-31]

Microbial interactions are significant in defining this indigenous microflora. The facultative flora help to maintain the reduced environment of the colon by using available oxygen diffusing across the mucosa. Metabolic products of one species also affect the growth of other species and may even have autoregulatory effects. Among the best known are colicins, antibiotic substances produced by strains of *E. coli.* Other organisms, including *Bacillus subtilis* and *Pseudomonas aeruginosa,* can make similar substances. Short chain fatty acids produced by anaerobic microorganisms (including acetic, propionic, and butyric) are inhibitory to the growth of many bacteria, particularly at the pH and Eh levels found in the colon.[32, 33]

Ecologic Considerations

The information just reviewed indicates that there is a distinctive longitudinal distribution of microorganisms in the intestinal tract. Experimental animal studies suggest that a cross-sectional distribution of populations exists as well, at least in mice.[34, 35] A number of studies demonstrate the presence of a unique population of bacteria associated with the epithelium that are quite different from those organisms colonizing the lumen. Electron microscopic studies show these organisms to be present in the mucous layer overlying the microvillous border (Fig. 100–4), especially in the crypts of the distal small bowel.[36] Although bacilli and cocci can be found in the mucus overlaying the proximal small bowel epithelium in humans, these organisms prove to be similar in nature to the flora present in the luminal fluids, even though they seem to be firmly adherent and are not removed by vigorous washing.[37, 38]

Many factors appear to influence the nature and site selectivity of the indigenous flora.

Colonization of the Newborn. A fecal flora is rapidly acquired after birth.[39-42] The nature of the early flora appears to depend on a number of factors, including the method of delivery, the gestational age of the newborn, and whether the infant is bottle or breast fed. For example, in one study virtually all bottle-fed, full-term, vaginally delivered infants had an anaerobic flora within the first week of life, including *Bacteroides fragilis* in nearly two-thirds.[40] In contrast, only 59% of abdominally delivered full-term infants harbored anaerobes by the end of the first week of life, and *B. fragilis* was found in only 9%. Breast feeding reduced the prevalence of *B. fragilis* and increased the prevalence of *Bifidobacterium bifidus. Veillonella* spp. were preferentially isolated from newborns delivered by cesarean section, whereas preterm infants were less likely to be colonized by any anaerobic organism. The aerobic coliform flora was rapidly acquired in the vaginally deliv-

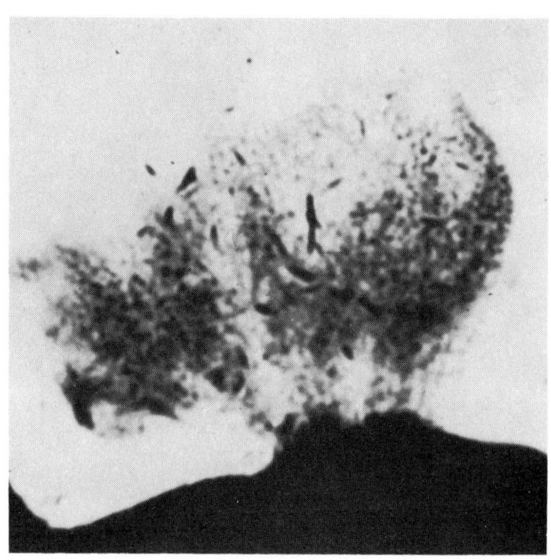

Figure 100–4. Colonizing bacteria present in the mucus over a goblet cell in the small intestinal epithelium.

ered babies; 70% were positive for this organism by 48 hours compared with only 29% of cesarean births. *E. coli* predominated in the former, while *Klebsiella* were dominant in the latter group. The presence of aerobes paralleled the appearance of anaerobes, and in most instances when anaerobes were found, more than one species was isolated. These data suggest that the colonic flora is rapidly acquired during vaginal delivery and more slowly when delivery is by cesarean section.

Serotyping *E. coli* strains from mother-infant pairs indicates that the infant acquires these organisms primarily from the mother rather than from the environment, although the dominant maternal serotype does not necessarily become dominant in the newborn.[43-45] The peroral route of inoculation is also indicated by studies of newborns with congenital small bowel obstructions.[46] In such infants a fecal-type flora is found immediately proximal to the obstructed region, while the distal bowel remains sterile.

In breast-fed infants, the *Bifidobacterium* population rises over the first week or 2 of life to become a stable and dominant component of the fecal flora until the weaning period.[39, 41, 42] *Clostridium* spp. may appear in such infants, but they do not persist.[47] In contrast, formula-fed infants have a more diverse flora, resembling that of weaned infants and adults.[39, 40, 42, 47, 48] The properties in breast milk that promote a dominant *Bifidobacterium* flora are not well understood but may involve both nutritional and immunologic factors.[16, 49-55]

There are some data on the establishment of the oral flora in the newborn period. Within the first week of life, a predominant gram-positive flora consisting of α-streptococci (especially *S. salivarius* and *mitis*) and lactobacilli is established.[56-58] *Streptococcus mutans,* however, does not colonize the newborn epithelium very well until dentition, since its ecologic niche appears to depend upon dental plaque.[59] Other components of the adult mouth flora, such as *Bacteroides melaninogenicus*, spirochetes, and some *Actinomycetes* appear to develop after puberty, although the reasons for this are not known.[60, 61]

Stability of the Microflora. The composition of the fecal flora appears to vary more from individual to individual than it does in particular subjects studied over time.[26, 29, 62] Even so, particular serotypes of *E. coli* can fluctuate over time in an individual subject. This is readily observed in hospitalized patients who rapidly acquire hospital-associated serotypes.[63] The ability of new strains to colonize may be a specific property of certain strains and not of others.[63-65] Whereas several investigations have found that stable artificial implantation of *E. coli* was generally difficult, this could be accomplished with ease using certain strains. The overall impression (and the remarkable observation) about the flora is that it is indeed quite consistent in individuals in spite of the continuous introduction of new species and strains.[4]

These observations are consistent with the definition of an indigenous or "autochthonous" flora in mice by Dubos et al.[34] In essence, adaptation of microbe and host is perceived to be so far advanced that no immune or other response is elicited by the autochthonous flora. The information available from human studies suggests that it is possible to distinguish between normal (long-term) colonizers of the intestinal tract and those organisms capable of transient residence only. The normal inhabitants appear to be ecologically regulated and to occupy specific and distinctive niches or habitats within the intestine.[4, 6, 8, 19-21, 24, 29, 31, 34, 37-39, 58, 65] Under normal conditions all niches are occupied and are resistant to displacement, except perhaps by pathogenic strains with particular virulence factors that contribute to this ecologic disturbance. Transient colonization by non-pathogenic strains requires a prior perturbation of the resident flora, e.g., the changes induced by antimicrobial therapy.[4, 19] Otherwise, the habitat defined by host physiology, microbial interactions and environmental pressures is remarkably resistant to change. Indeed, it appears to be the very complexity of the ecosystem that results in this stability, and the usual flora is again restored after perturbations induced by various exogenous factors.

Microbial Factors

Bacterial Colonization Determinants. It is now clear that specific determinants of the bacterial surface can mediate cell-to-cell adherence with certain types of mammalian cells.[66] These interactions have been postulated to be similar to the receptor-ligand interactions of soluble molecules or macromolecules, with several important distinctions.[67]

First, cell-to-cell contacts involve enormous

surface areas; therefore, it is appropriate to conceptualize the process as megavalency of binding sites. Even if each individual contact is a non-covalent and reversible binding, the sheer number of sites involved makes it unlikely that all will become free at the same time to permit the adherent cells to separate. In practice, the binding becomes irreversible.

Second, the large size of the interacting cells raises the question of surface charge in determining the cell-to-cell interaction. Both bacterial and mammalian cells have net negative charges due to the ionization of surface groups such as carboxyls on teichoic, glucuronic, or hyaluronic acids of prokaryotes or sialic acids of eukaryotes. The 2 surfaces are, therefore, mutually repulsive, but nonetheless come into close apposition, indicating that attracting forces must exist to overcome these charge effects. Charge may not be uniformly distributed over the surface, so that regions exist in which the weak interactions of focal ionic attractions, Van der Waals forces, hydrogen bonding, or hydrophobic interactions are sufficient to mediate attachment. Since the magnitude of each of these forces is affected by distance, temperature, and ionic strength of the fluid phase, the situation is indeed complex.

Third, the larger the size of the adhering cells, the more important are geometric considerations such as the radius of curvature of the surface profiles in attachment.[68] As the radius decreases, repulsive forces decrease more rapidly than attractive forces, resulting in increasing net attraction. As the distance between the cells narrows, displacement of water can take place from 2 apposing hydrophobic regions such as segments of peptides with many apolar amino acids, hydrogen atoms, or methyl or methoxy groups on carbohydrates or lipids, resulting in a favorable change in free energy and tight adherence.

With these considerations in mind, we could predict that bacterial adherence factors would be positioned on a long, thin appendage, with a small radius of curvature relative to the cell surface itself, with a lower net negative charge than the rest of the cell, and with a high concentration of hydrophobic segments.[67, 68] This is indeed what nature has chosen to do in many instances, employing finger-like projections or appendages of the bacterial surface called fimbriae (if uniform in structure) or fibrillae (if thinner and somewhat irregular in composition) (Fig. 100–5).

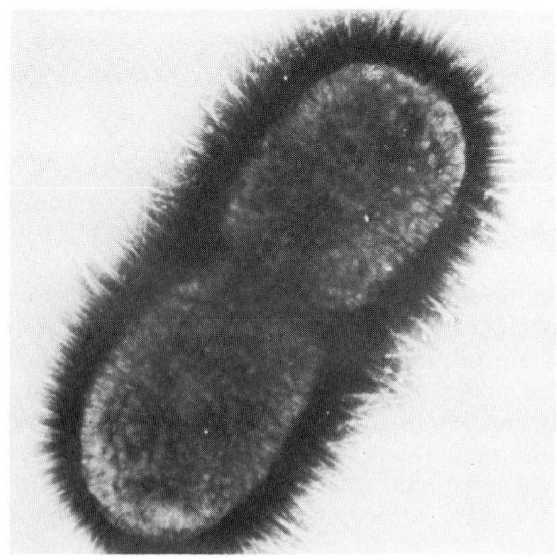

Figure 100–5. Colonization pili present on the surface of enterotoxigenic *E. coli* appear as a hair-like fuzzy layer over the surface of the organism.

These structures often contain a concentration of apolar amino acids, are quite hydrophobic, and contain specific recognition sites. In many instances, they are under genetic control of plasmids. These include CFA-I and II for human *E. coli* enteric pathogens, K-88 pili antigens for porcine strains, and K-99 pili antigens for strains pathogenic for calves and lambs. We are only beginning to understand the role of such colonization factors in pathogenic bacteria, and at present only know in conceptual terms their potential role in normal flora interactions.

Capsular adhesive factors may be of importance in other organisms.[66-68] Glycans and lipoteichoic acid are involved in adherence of *Streptococcus mutans* or *S. pyogenes* in the oral cavity, while K-1 polysaccharide may serve a similar role for *E. coli* lower in the intestinal tract. We can only speculate at this time about the mechanism used by the 400 or so other constituents of the intestinal biota.

Microbial Interactions. The association of 2 or more species of bacteria exerts important influences on their mutual existence and on the possibilities for enrichment of the flora. For example, strict anaerobes on mucosal surfaces, when exposed to oxygen directly or by diffusion across the epithelium, are invariably found in the presence of an aerobic or facultative flora, which helps to maintain a reduced environment by utilizing available oxygen.[20]

In some instances, one organism creates an ecologic niche for another otherwise poorly colonizing species. This interaction, termed interbacterial aggregation, has been shown for *S. salivarius* and *Veillonella* sp. in the mouth.[69] The former produces a glucosyltransferase utilized by the latter for adherence to the smooth surface of teeth.

IgA Protease. Because the predominant immunoglobulin in secretions is secretory IgA, a molecule capable of inhibiting the attachment of certain microorganisms to epithelial cell surfaces,[70-72] the discovery of specific IgA proteases of bacterial origin is of potential interest as a determinant of colonization.[73] The enzyme, as isolated and purified from several species of bacteria, has great specificity for the Ig-A1 immunoglobulin subtype of human, gorilla, or chimpanzee origin. Cleavage occurs in the hinge region in a peptide segment deleted from the IgA protease-resistant IgA-2 subtype and involves either a prolyl-threonyl or a prolyl-seryl peptide bond, depending on the bacterial species of origin of the enzyme. The result of the peptide bond hydrolysis is intact Fab_{α} and Fc_{α}, with a sharp reduction in antibody activity compared with the intact molecule.[73]

The hypothesis that this enzyme might account for some of the specificity of the intestinal flora is seriously challenged by the restricted number of organisms known to produce it and its absence in many of the most numerous constituents of the normal flora.[74] IgA protease is made by several distinctive pathogens, including *Neisseria gonorrhoeae* and *N. meningiditis, Streptococcus pneumoniae* and *S. sanguis* (one of the common viridans streptococci causing bacterial endocarditis), and *Hemophilus influenzae*. Although each of these organisms can colonize a mucosal surface without causing disease, only *S. sanguis* is considered a part of the indigenous microflora. It is, without doubt, the source of the IgA protease in dental plaque, but whether the enzyme contributes in any way to co-colonization with *S. mutans* is uncertain.

Even if the latter is possible, the role of the microbial protease-resistant IgA-2 as a regulator of bacterial adherence must still be addressed. The present evidence suggests, but does not prove, a role for IgA protease in the pathogenesis of certain infections, since the enzyme is found *in vivo* in local secretions over colonized mucosa, and its elaboration correlates with virulence in different species of the enzyme-producing genera of organisms. Even if this enzyme is a virulence factor in the positive strains, it cannot be an essential determinant, for other mucosal pathogens are clearly among the IgA protease-negative strains.

Host Factors. The *in vitro* doubling time of *E. coli* under optimal nutritional conditions is about 20 minutes. If this rate of multiplication occurred *in vivo,* a single organism would multiply to over 10^{14} in a little over 14 hours and would totally overwhelm the host. *In vivo* studies of microbial generation time in animals suggest a much slower doubling time, on the order of 6 to 24 hours.[75] This is undoubtedly a reflection of the simultaneous multiplication and clearance of organisms and not simply the effects of a limited supply of nutrients, for bacterial populations in the gut increase dramatically shortly after death of the host, indicating the nutritional adequacy of the environment.[4]

Intestinal Motility. One important host mechanism limiting the proliferation of organisms in the small bowel is gut motility. Peristaltic movement tends to roll up bacteria within intestinal mucus and to propel them in a caudad direction.[76] Its importance in maintaining the proximal small bowel relatively bacteria-free is amply demonstrated when motility is impaired.[20, 77] Surgical blind loops, strictures with partial obstruction, prior surgery, radiation therapy, or localized inflammatory processes such as Crohn's disease are associated with bacterial overgrowth.[4, 20, 21, 27, 78, 79] Diverticulosis of the small bowel also results in exuberant microbial proliferation. When there is a single, large duodenal diverticulum, the rest of the bowel is normal and overgrowth is limited to the diverticulum itself and the bowel just distal to it.[78, 80] Not surprisingly, disorders of intestinal motility such as scleroderma, diabetic neuropathy, and idiopathic intestinal pseudo-obstruction also result in extensive small bowel colonization.[79, 81-84] In addition, bacterial overgrowth may occur in patients with cirrhosis, in malnourished hosts, in patients receiving abdominal x-irradiation, and in some elderly individuals, with no known systemic illness or anatomic abnormality.[79, 85-87]

With good microbiologic methods a complex flora containing 20 or so species of bacteria can be isolated from the small bowel in these patients.[21, 78, 88] The bacterial count is generally in the range of 10^7 to 10^9 cfu/ml, but may reach as high as 10^{11} cfu/ml in some patients. The physiologic consequences depend on the specific nature of the flora, in particular, the presence of anaerobes (see later discussion).

Gastric Acid. Acid production in the stomach acts as a defense mechanism against exogenous pathogenic microorganisms, as well as suppressing colonization of the proximal small bowel by both the oropharyngeal organisms and the fecal flora.[20, 22, 89, 90] Hypochlorhydria due to atrophic gastritis, prior gastric surgery, or the use of hydrogen-ion secretion blockers such as cimetidine increases the susceptibility of patients to enteric infections such as cholera or salmonellosis.[91, 92] In experimental human studies, administration of such pathogenic organisms along with sodium bicarbonate dramatically reduced the infectious inoculum by as much as 100,000-fold.[93] In the presence of hypochlorhydria, the concentration of organisms in the stomach and small bowel increases. The flora can include greater numbers of the usually sparse streptococci, lactobacilli, and fungi, as well as coliforms and gram-negative anaerobes.

Enteric Secretions. Although unconjugated bile acids are inhibitory to bacterial growth *in vitro,* there is no evidence of significant antibacterial activity *in vivo.*[94, 95] Indeed, bacterial overgrowth may be a cause of diarrhea by deconjugating bile salts in the intestinal lumen.[96] There is also no evidence of any inhibitory effects of pancreatic juice or succus entericus on bacterial proliferation.[4]

Epithelial Cell Membrane Structures. Preference for a colonization site of mucosal microorganisms may be determined by specific recognition between microbial and mammalian surface structures.[97] In many instances, these appear to be a recognition between sugar-binding proteins (lectins) and characteristic oligosaccharides on the interacting membranes. Site specificity could therefore be related to the presence of such receptors. Indeed, there are important differences, both qualitative and quantitative, in the glycolipids and glycoproteins of the epithelial membranes of the intestinal tract, including differences between cells in different regions of the gut, between cells in different parts of the crypt or villus within the same region of the gut, and between apical and basal-lateral membranes of the same cell.[98-100] Recognition molecules are not necessarily fixed in space within the membrane; their distribution and mobility can be altered, serving as a potential regulatory mechanism for their function. Membrane fluidity and cytoskeletal elements are important for topographic reorganization of receptors within the plane of the membrane. Fluidity, related at least in part to the ratio of cholesterol to phospholipid, increases from the duodenum to ileum.[101]

Both glycoplipid and glycopeptide components are present in these membranes. The glycoproteins can be broadly separated into "O-glycosidic" and "N-glycosidic," differing in the type of linkage between carbohydrate side chain and protein.[102] The former contains an alkali-labile O-glycosidic linkage between N-acetyl-D-galactosamine (GalNAc) and hydroxyamino acids and is abundant in mucin. The latter contains oligosaccharides that are attached to the membrane via alkali-resistant N-glycosidic linkages between N-acetyl-D-glucosamine (GlcNAc) and asparagine in the protein moiety. Six monosaccharides are commonly found in these glycoproteins, including GalNAc, GlcNAc, mannose (Man), galactose (Gal), fucose (Fuc), and sialic acid (NeuNAc). GalNAc is present in O-glycosidic types, and Man is present in N-glycosidic types, while the other sugars occur in either type. Many membrane glycoproteins contain both types of carbohydrate side chains. These variations, as well as the primary sequence and stereochemical disposition, permit an almost endless number of distinctive stereospecific structures capable of serving as unique recognition molecules. O-glycosidic molecules have in common the linkage of GalNAc to hydroxyamino acids, but differ tremendously in the length and composition of the sugar side chain. N-glycosidic molecules have in common a trisaccharide of Manβ1$\rightarrow$4 GlcNAcβ1$\rightarrow$4 GlcNAc linked to asparagine and may be divided further into high mannose, complex, hybrid, and polylactosamine varieties. These are distinguished by the addition to the core trisaccharide of 5 to 9 α-linked Man residues; a complex oligosaccharide made up of GlcNAc, Gal, Fuc, and NeuNAc; a combination of high Man and complex side chains; or repeating units of lactosamine (GlcNAcβ1$\rightarrow$3 Gal), respectively.

Evidence in animal models utilizing specifically colonizing *E. coli* strains indicates the involvement of glycoconjugates containing terminal GalNAc or GlcNAc in pig intestine in the binding of K-88–positive strains or GM_2-ganglioside in the case of bovine intestine and K-99–positive bacteria.[103, 104] Comparable data in the human gut are not yet available. Indeed, for most organisms that demonstrate site-selective colonization, the nature of the cell surface receptor is unknown.

Intestinal Immunity. The mucous membranes, being exposed to the enormous load of the microflora, must have mechanisms to prevent systemic invasion. Many of the organisms that appear to be innocuous when confined to their natural habitat provoke disease and even death when they penetrate the epithelium. Phagocytic cells must perform this defense function in part, for when a patient is rendered granulocytopenic by disease or drugs, systemic invasion by the enteric flora, most often facultative gram-negative bacilli, is common.

Antibody in secretions, particularly secretory IgA (S-IgA), may play a regulatory role in colonization by commensals.[105] Adherence of microbes to epithelial cells can be effectively inhibited by S-IgA antibody, at least *in vitro* and in *in vivo* experimental systems.[70-72] However, since a vast normal flora exists in regions literally bathed in secretory immunoglobulin, there must be special conditions that impede this mechanism. Perhaps this is one role of the IgA protease of some mucosal bacteria, as discussed previously.[73, 74] The problem is enigmatic at present.

The intestinal tract is highly organized as a specialized organ of the immune system.[106, 107] Antigen-sampling sites occur throughout the gut, intestine, including the tonsils, Peyer's patches, appendix, and isolated mucosal lymphoid nodules. Mucus secretion is often reduced in amount in these areas, permitting bacteria to closely approach specialized M cells. These cells overlie the follicular lymphocytes and function in the uptake and transport of antigen to macrophage antigen-presenting cells and lymphocytes in the lamina propria.[108] Antigen can also reach regional mesenteric lymph nodes, and responding lymphoid cells can later be found in thoracic duct lymph. Such cells can home back to the gut or to other organs of the mucosal immune system, including the breast and lung. Sensitized lymphocytes are found in the lamina propria and between enterocytes on the villi. Both B and T cells, the latter often containing granules and resembling mast cells, are thus poised and ready to respond to antigens presented at the luminal surface.[106] Therefore, it seems necessary to postulate the existence of regulatory turn-off signals from normal flora constituents, for otherwise both T and B cell immune mechanisms should be operative.

Diet. Diet has variable effects on the flora. Fecal microbial counts can differ tremendously among individuals consuming a similar diet.[26] This flora will remain stable in each subject during a period of up to 2 weeks of feeding of an elemental liquid diet. Even though stool weight and frequency of passage are significantly reduced, there are no differences in average counts of aerobes, anaerobes, or coliforms.[109, 110]

In other studies, volunteers were sequentially fed a control diet, a meatless diet, a high-beef diet, and a control diet again, each for a 1-month period.[111] Minimal changes were observed, the most striking of which were a slight increase in the number of anaerobes during the high-beef diet and a mild increase in coliforms during the meatless diet.

In contrast, diet can affect the oral flora, with a striking reduction in the number of *S. mutans* in the mouth brought about by restricted carbohydrate intake.[112] The explanation is that this organism must synthesize a high-molecular-weight extracellular glucan from dietary glucose as a prerequisite for colonization.[113] Elimination of sugar in the diet prevents colonization of tooth surfaces and reduces the incidence of dental caries due to *S. mutans.*

Such studies have been performed by classic microbiologic enumeration techniques and are subject to considerable error that can mask important changes. Recent studies have used metabolic criteria to detect diet-related changes, especially in the context of bacterial metabolism of potentially carcinogenic substances. This approach shows that diet can indeed significantly alter metabolic activities of the intestinal flora, and these will be discussed later.

Physiologic Effects of the Flora

Morphologic Considerations. The ability to raise animals in a germ-free state and to colonize them selectively with one or more known microorganisms has demonstrated that "normal" histology of the gut is determined by the presence of the bacterial flora.[114-116] Without the resident flora, the intestinal wall appears thinner, contains few inflammatory or lymphoid cells, has a noticeable absence of plasma cells, and has small, poorly developed Peyer's patches that contain few germinal centers. These differences are largely accounted for by a reduction in the lamina propria and its constituent cell types. Additionally, the villi are shorter, thinner, and more pointed at the tips; the crypts are more shallow; and the total surface area of the intestine is reduced in the germ-free animal compared with the conventional animal. Turnover of epithelial cells is slowed in the germ-free animal; the proportion of mature to immature cells is increased, and the former are more cuboidal in shape.

These features are altered rapidly when a flora is introduced.[115] The first change is infiltration of the lamina propria by macrophages, histiocytes, lymphocytes, and plasma cells, constituting a mild chronic inflammatory reaction that imparts the typical "normal" appearance to the mucosa. Another quite dramatic change is a reduction in the size of the cecum, which may be enlarged up to 10 times "normal" size in the germ-free state and may constitute almost one-third of the animal's total weight.[114] This change is most efficiently effected by introduction of either *Bacteroides* or *Clostridium* spp.[115, 117, 118] The differences in the size of the cecum may be related to its reduced ability to absorb water in the germ-free colon.[115] As a result, the cecum is dilated and filled with hypotonic fluid, which is low in chloride and bicarbonate. Although the reasons for this are unknown, the absence of a flora may result in an increase in osmotically active molecules and/or biologically active mediators of intestinal secretion in the gut.[117, 119]

Functional Characteristics. The germ-free state also results in a more alkaline intraluminal pH, a more positive oxidation-reduction potential or Eh (reflecting the absence of bacterial metabolism and oxygen consumption), and a decrease in gastric emptying, intestinal motility, and transit time.[114, 120] Carbohydrate absorption is enhanced, perhaps owing to a lack of competitive utilization by bacteria, resulting in more substrate available to the host.

The flora can synthesize important vitamins, but to the extent that these compounds may be absorbed, there is no indication that this replaces any dietary vitamin source.[19] If anything, dietary and flora sources are additive and complementary. In contrast, the presence of normal fecal flora in the upper small bowel can result in clinical vitamin B_{12} deficiency due to competitive microbial utilization.[27]

Metabolism of Sex Hormones. Estrogens are normally excreted in bile as conjugated glucuronides or sulfates and following deconjugation by the gut microflora are reabsorbed to enter into an enterohepatic circulation.[121] Virtually all of the small amount of estrogen excreted in feces is in the deconjugated form, attesting to the completeness of action of bacterial β-glucuronidase and sulfatase activities.[122] Elegant studies have followed the fate of labeled IV estriol.[123] Initial metabolism in the liver results in the production of estriol-3-sulfate-16-glucuronide, which is excreted into bile. This doubly conjugated compound is then reduced to free estriol by the flora and absorbed into the intestinal mucosal cell in which the hormone is glucuronidated at the 16 position. This metabolite is recirculated back to the liver and conjugated again with sulfate, subsequently reappearing in bile and completing the enterohepatic pathway.[124, 125] The mucosal cell also glucuronidates a portion of the estriol at the 3 position. This compound does not enter the enterohepatic circulation and is instead rapidly excreted in urine. The summation of these reactions is a transglucuronidation from the 16 to the 3 position, which requires enzymatic modifications by both the flora and the mucosal cells. Because the synthesis of estriol-3-glucuronide (E-3-G) occurs exclusively in colonic epithelium, its appearance in urine is an indicator of estrogen reabsorption in the large bowel.

One would predict that antibiotics should reduce E-3-G excretion in urine. This has been demonstrated by several investigators using absorbable antibiotics such as penicillin or ampicillin or non-absorbable drugs such as neomycin.[126–128] Reduction in urinary E-3-G excretion is accompanied by a reduction in total plasma conjugated estriol and estriol-16-glucuronide levels.[129] Ampicillin has been demonstrated to increase fecal excretion of conjugated estrogens by 60-fold, with only a small increase in excretion of unconjugated metabolites.[130] Over 90% of the reduction in urinary estriol levels in this situation is accounted for by the decrease in E-3-G.[131] These data are strong evidence of the role of the colonic flora in these reactions.

Other steroid hormones are also affected by antibiotic administration. During ampicillin therapy, glucuronide conjugation metabolites of progesterone transiently decrease in urine and subsequently return to normal.[129, 132] At that time, however, 5β-pregnane-3α,20α-diol sulfate is decreased by over 80%. In a study in beagle dogs, ampicillin also transiently increased the stool content of glucuronide conjugated androgen metabolites.[133]

Other transformations of sex hormones occur in stool as well.[121, 134] Reductive and oxidative reactions have been demonstrated *in vitro,* the type of reaction depending on the density of the bacterial inoculum. At high concentrations of bacteria (which simulate the *in vivo* environment), Eh is high and the reductive reactions predominate, whereas the reverse is true when low inocula of bacteria are used. Consistent with the latter observations, it has been possible to introduce double bonds into the steroid nucleus ring only when low concentrations of bacteria are added along with an oxidizing agent.[121]

Drug Metabolism. The intestinal flora can metabolize a variety of ingested compounds including therapeutically administered drugs. Indeed, this may be essential for the bioavailability of at least some agents.[135] At the same time, bacterial metabolism can alter drug activity and/or toxicity.[136] Systemic drug metabolism often results in conjugated or esterified hydrophilic derivatives that are more readily excreted; flora metabolism often produces better absorbed lipophilic derivatives by hydrolysis or reduction of glycosidic bonds or by deconjugations, dehydroxylations, or decarboxylations. When these reactions occur sequentially, an enterohepatic circulation can ensue (to be discussed). However, because of the complexity of the microbial ecosystem, the natural environment in which drug metabolism occurs may be difficult to simulate *in vitro.*[136] While experimental studies reveal that a variety of reactions can be performed by the gut flora (Table 100–2), there is no proof that metabolic transformations demonstrated in culture are carried out *in vivo,* even when it is shown that the relevant organism is indeed present in substantial numbers and conditions are stringently controlled.

Probably the 2 most important factors involved in determining whether a compound is metabolized by intestinal bacteria are the distribution of relevant microorganisms within the gut and the route of administration and absorption of the drug.[136] Poorly absorbed compounds may reach the colon in high concentration, where they are exposed to a metabolically active flora. The time course of biotransformations is largely dependent on intestinal transit time and the density of the metabolically capable flora. These reactions are probably best studied in animals, since there is no *a priori* reason to believe that the same events do not occur in humans.[136]

Table 100–2. METABOLIC CONVERSIONS BY THE ENTERIC FLORA

Reaction Type	Chemical Group Involved
Hydrolysis	Glycosides, glucuronides, sulfate esters, sulfamates
Dehydroxylation	C-hydroxyl, N-hydroxyl
Decarboxylation	Carboxyl
Dealkylation	O-alkyl, N-alkyl
Dehalogenation	Halogens
Deamination	Amines
Reduction	Double bonds, nitro groups, azo groups, aldehydes, ketones, alcohols, N-oxides, nitrates

One well characterized human situation involves the drug salicylazosulfapyridine (sulfasalazine, Azulfidine), which consists of a sulfonamide, sulfapyridine, joined by an azo bond at the N-4 position to the amino nitrogen of 5-aminosalicylate.[137] When given by mouth, the bulk of the drug reaches the cecum in unchanged form. There, the azo linkage is split by the flora to produce the 2 individual component drugs.[136] Sulfapyridine is promptly absorbed, glucuronidated in the liver, and excreted in the urine. The salicylate is in part excreted unchanged in feces and in part absorbed, acetylated, and eliminated in the urine. Only a tiny fraction of the parent drug appears in the urine, since it must be metabolized to be absorbed. The efficacy of this drug in ulcerative colitis may be a consequence of its ability to deliver the therapeutically active molecule 5-aminosalicylate topically to the colon.[137]

The synthetic disaccharide 4-β-D-galactopyranosyl-D-fructose (lactulose) is used in treating hepatic encephalopathy. Lactulose is not hydrolyzed by small intestinal β-galactosidase (lactase) and passes unchanged to the colon, where it is split by bacterial action and metabolized to lactic and acetic acids.[138] The result is a fermentative diarrhea, an acid stool, and protonation of ammonia and amines that serves to inhibit their absorption. The last action is believed to be the key to the therapeutic efficacy of the drug. The same mechanisms account for the suppression of chronic shigellosis by lactulose, since decreased pH, increased Eh, and short-chain acids are inhibitory to the growth of this pathogen in the bowel.[139]

More recently, Lindenbaum et al.[140] reported that microbial metabolism of digoxin results in formation of inactive reduced metabolites such as dihydrodigoxin or dihydrodigoxigenin, altering the therapeutic effects of the drug. In about 10% of patients, such reduction products constitute a significant portion of the urinary metabolites. This proportion is increased still further when poorly absorbed formulations of digoxin are given. It was found that the stool flora from subjects excreting the reduction products could perform this reaction *in vitro,* whereas the flora from the non-reducers could not. When tetracycline or erythromycin was administered to the former group, the reduced metabolites disappeared from the urine and stool. Addition of an antibiotic *in vitro* to stool cultures from patients producing reduced products abrogated the *in vitro* conversion of digoxin as well.

The implications of the digoxin data are that a proportion of patients receiving the drug are partially refractory to this agent and require a higher dose because of bacterial metabolism. This introduces the potential for drug-drug interaction if such patients receive antibiotics for an intercurrent infection, for this might precipitate digitalis toxicity by eliminating the drug-inactivating flora. The incidence of toxicity due to this mechanism is unknown at the present time, and its relevance to other drug interactions is a matter of conjecture.

The role of the intestinal flora in the metabolism of estrogens has already been discussed. In view of these pathways, it is not surprising that failure of oral contraception has been reported during periods of antibiotic therapy. This association has been reported in women taking ampicillin, chloramphenicol, rifampin, or sulfamethoxypyridazine.[141, 142] In other reports, breakthrough bleeding has been noted to be more frequent when concurrent antibiotic therapy is being used, again suggesting an effect of the flora on steroid hormone metabolism.

The flora may contribute to the toxicology of drugs by other mechanisms. For example, sodium and calcium cyclamate (the salts of cyclohexylsulfamic acid) were widely used as non-nutritive artificial sweeteners. These compounds are poorly absorbed and have a long elimination time from the body, with about 50% being excreted unchanged in feces and another 30% in urine.[136] After a single dose, trace amounts (less than 0.002% of the administered dose) are converted to the carcinogen cyclohexylamine and excreted in urine; this metabolite causes bladder carcinoma in rodents. When cyclamate is given to humans on a daily basis, the urinary levels of cyclohexylamine increase dramatically, up to several thousand–fold. This conversion does not occur when cyclamate is given parenterally, but can be accomplished *in vitro* by incubating the drug with the fecal flora, especially after priming by oral administration of cyclamate for a few days.[143] Because of these alarming findings, cyclamates were removed from the market in 1969.

Two of the trace metabolites of L-dopa that appear in the urine, m-tyramine and m-hydroxyphenylacetic acid (MHPA), are produced by the intestinal flora.[144-146] These metabolites disappear from the urine when neomycin is administered to patients, and they are not found in germ-free rats given L-dopa.[147] When L-dopa is administered to Parkinson's disease patients in a formulation that retards absorption, the prolonged contact with intestinal bacteria markedly increases the concentration of MHPA in urine, which is associated with an unacceptable increase in gastrointestinal intolerance.

The enterohepatic circulation of some drugs is determined by metabolic conversions by the intestinal flora. The liver tends to oxidize compounds in preparation for excretion, while the flora tends to reduce compounds and increase absorption. Sequential oxidation and reduction of a drug could produce an enterohepatic circulation. As an example, diethylstilbestrol (DES) is glucuronidated in the liver and excreted in bile.[148] Unless the compound is deconjugated, it is excreted in stool. The deconjugation is accomplished by microbial β-glucuronidase. Thus, antibiotic therapy can inhibit the absorption of conjugated DES, effectively interrupting the enterohepatic circulation.[149] Other possible examples in which pharmacokinetics (and possibly toxicity) might be affected by bacterial metabolism of glucuronidated drugs include morphine and indomethacin.[136]

Pathophysiologic Effects of the Flora

Intestinal Flora and Cancer. A role for the intestinal flora in carcinogenesis has been suggested as a possible explanation for epidemiologic differences in incidence of certain tumors between distinctive populations.[150] Colon cancer, for example, is more frequent in Western populations than in Orientals. The factors are thought to be environmental rather than genetic, since the frequency increases in Orientals living in the West and consuming Western diets.[151, 152] The epidemiologic key is currently believed to be contained in the high-fat intake of the typical Western diet,[153] perhaps mediated through effects on the gut flora.[154]

Investigations of populations with high and low risk for colon cancer, however, do not find significant differences in the composition of the flora. Specifically, there is no evidence for the existence of a "high-risk" colon cancer microbiota.[6, 30, 155] However, when the colonic contents are examined by metabolic rather than by microbiologic criteria, differences begin to emerge.[4] The underlying assumption of such an approach is that potential carcinogens ("procarcinogens") are ingested with the diet, either as natural constituents or as food additives or pollutants, and that chemical modification is needed to activate or "unmask" their carcinogenic potential.[156] Most of these studies employ animal models and report that the colonic flora produces enzymes capable of converting certain procarcinogens to carcinogens. These enzyme activities include β-glucosidase, β-glucuronidase, nitroreductase, azoreductase, 7α-dehydroxylase, and cholesterol dehydrogenase.[157, 158]

One example in the animal studies is the experimental colon cancer induced by cycasin, the β-glucoside of methylazoxymethanol.[4, 136] Inclusion of cycasin in the diet of rats results in a high incidence of colon cancer in conventional animals but not in germ-free animals, whereas the deconjugated aglycone, methylazoxymethanol, is equally active in either type of rat. In adult animals, cycasin is carcinogenic only after oral administration, whereas in newborns with high levels of tissue β-glucosidase, it is carcinogenic by any route, including subcutaneous or intraperitoneal administration. Adult animals have low tissue levels of β-glucosidase, and they are susceptible to this chemical carcinogen only when the microbial flora can play a rôle.

A number of suspected or demonstrated carcinogens are nitrosoamines or N-hydroxy compounds. These may be formed as intermediaries in the metabolism of aromatic nitro compounds to aromatic amines by bacterial nitroreductase. The reduction of azo food dyes by bacterial azoreductase also yields substituted phenyl and naphthylamines, which can be carcinogenic as well.[4, 136, 157, 158]

These examples demonstrate the potential of the flora as a "biochemical entity" in the formation of carcinogens in the colon. Consistent with this view and in contrast to the relative stability of the composition of the flora in response to dietary changes, the metabolic activity appears to be much more responsive to diet,[4, 157] perhaps because many bacterial enzymes are substrate-induced. If the substrate happens to be a procarcinogen and the induced enzyme can convert it to a carcinogen, the potential for induction of tumors increases tremendously.

Recent studies have examined fecal bile acids as candidate carcinogens because of their structural resemblance to various polycyclic aromatic hydrocarbons of known carcinogenic potential.[154, 159] In this regard it is pertinent that high levels of animal fat in the diet augment bile flow and synthesis of conjugated bile acids, in turn inducing bacterial 7α-dehydroxylase in the stool, which is involved in conversion of primary to secondary bile acids.[160] Indeed, the concentration of secondary bile acids in stool correlates with the intake of a beef-containing Western-style diet, and the flora of such individuals contains more organisms capable of 7α-dehydroxylation.[154] Compared with vegetarians, the stool of meat eaters has an increased content of deoxycholic and lithocholic acids and of coprostanol and coprostanone, but not of cholic acid or cholesterol.[154, 161] The data suggest that the colonic flora of the meat eater is the more metabolically active. It has also been reported that activities of 7α-dehydroxylase and cholesterol dehydrogenase are elevated in patients with colon cancer.[159] The evidence is circumstantial, but the data are consistent with the hypothesis that the intestinal flora plays a role in carcinogenesis.

Diet appears to regulate bacterial β-glucuronidase, an enzyme capable of "retoxifying" compounds that have been glucuronidated in the liver. β-glucuronidase levels increase in the feces of meat eaters, and the enzyme can activate the procarcinogens N-hydroxy-N-2-fluorenylacetamide and DES-glucuronide in the bowel by hydrolysis of the glucuronide bond.[162] Experimental studies in the rat confirm the influence of diet on fecal β-glucuronidase, azoreductase, and nitroreductase. The incidence of dimethylhydrazine-induced colon cancer in rats was correlated with the inclusion of beef or beef fat in the diet.[157, 163, 164] This carcinogen is metabolized in the liver to methylazoxymethanol-β-glucuronide, which like cycasin is deconjugated to the active carcinogen by the intestinal flora.[4] The increase in the relevant enzymatic activity in the high-beef group was accompanied by a 3-fold increase in the incidence of tumors produced by dimethylhydrazine.[162–164]

Studies in humans showed higher levels of fecal β-glucuronidase, nitroreductase, azoreductase, and 7α-dehydroxylase in omnivores compared with strict vegetarians. When red meat was eliminated or fiber was added to the omnivore diet, a significant decrease in 7α-dehydroxylase activity was observed.[162]

For many decades, lactobacilli have received attention and notoriety as potential health-promoting components of the normal flora. No less a figure than Metchnikoff believed in the importance of yogurt cultures containing *Lactobacillus bulgaricus* in the longevity of Bulgarian peasants.[165] While there are few data to support such contentions, the idea remains a topic of conversation and continued speculation, even though *L. bulgaricus* is unable to colonize the human.[166] For example, a study on patients with colon cancer in Scandinavia found an association between low cancer risk and high intake of dairy products and increased fecal lactobacilli counts.[167] Experimental animal studies also show that when *L. acidophilus* is fed to rats consuming a high-beef diet, the levels of potentially important "procarcinogen enzymes" that ordinarily increase in the meat-fed animals, including β-glucuronidase, azoreductase, and nitroreductase, all fall significantly in the group receiving the bacterial inoculum.[168] If the hypotheses just described are true, a lactobacillus flora might indeed protect against tumor formation. Consistent with this idea, a significant delay has been demonstrated in the latency period for tumor formation in rats given dimethylhydrazine along with lactobacillus feedings.[168]

Bacterial Overgrowth Syndromes. Bacterial overgrowth in the proximal small bowel is facilitated by situations that subvert normal bacterial control mechanisms, such as disordered gut motility (scleroderma, diabetes), reduced gastric acid secretion (pernicious anemia), surgically effected alterations (gastrectomy), and localized inflammatory or obstructive processes of the gut (Crohn's disease, strictures). These underlying problems permit the growth of a normal fecal flora in a region of the intestinal tract ordinarily colonized by a sparse resident flora at most. Discussion of these syndromes is found in Chapter 107.

Tropical Sprue. This malabsorption syndrome, found in tropical areas and associated with bacterial overgrowth in the proximal small bowel, is fully reviewed in Chapter 106.

Antibiotic-Associated Colitis. Another instance of ecologic shifts of the flora resulting in pathologic changes is pseudomembranous colitis associated with antimicrobial therapy. This subject is specifically treated in Chapter 141.

Infant Botulism. Botulism usually is caused by ingested preformed neurotoxin that interrupts normal release of acetylcholine at the neurosmuscular junction. Although frequently found in soil, the causative organism, *Clostridium botulinum,* does not multiply well in humans, except rarely in contaminated wounds, which are a source for some cases of botulism. In general, proliferation of the organism and production of 1 of 7 antigenically distinct but pharmacologically similar toxins occur *ex vivo* in contaminated foods (see Chapters 118 and 119 for additional data). The major exception occurs in young infants, whose large bowel may be colonized by *C. botulinum,* resulting in toxin production, absorption, and a fatal neurologic disease called *infant botulism.*[169]

The syndrome occurs primarily in infants between 1 and 6 months of age, a time when there is apparently something conducive to the colonization of the bowel by the *Clostridium.* The organism is not present in younger or older infants. Changes in the gut flora have been proposed as determinants of susceptibility of infants of this age to infection.[170]

A similar "window of vulnerability" has been experimentally reproduced in mice, which are susceptible to oral challenge with *C. botulinum* only during the second week of life.[171] This corresponds to the period after initial colonization of the proiximal gut with lactobacilli and anaerobic streptococci in the first week of life. During the susceptible period, *E. coli* and enterococci first colonize the colon. At the start of the third week of life, when the animals are resistant to oral challenge with *C. botulinum,* the anaerobic flora, including *Bacteroides, Fusobacterium, Eubacterium,* and other clostridia, becomes established and dominant. The mechanism for the resistance to implantation before and after the second week of life is not known, and the evidence that the microecology of the flora is responsible is only indirectly supported by the available evidence.

References

1. van Leeuwenhoek A. Letter 39, 17 September, 1683. *In:* Dobell C, ed. Antony van Leeuwenhoek and his "Little Animals", Being Some Account of the Father of Protozoology and Bacteriology and His Multifarious Discoveries in These Disciplines. New York: Harcourt, Brace, 1932: 243.
2. Hardie JM, Bowden GH. The normal microbial flora of the mouth. *In:* Skinner FA, Carr JG, eds. The Normal Microbial Flora of Man. New York: Academic Press, 1974:47–83.
3. Moore WEC, Holdeman LV. Discussion of current bacteriologic investigations of the relationships between intestinal flora, diet, and colon cancer. Cancer Res 1975; 35:3418–20.
4. Simon GL, Gorbach SL. The intestinal flora in health and disease: A review. Gastroenterology 1984; 86:174–193.
5. Clarke RTJ. Methods for studying gut microbes. *In:* Clarke RTJ, Bauchop T, eds. Microbial Ecology of the Gut. New York: Academic Press, 1977:1–33.
6. Moore WEC, Cato EP, Holdeman LV. Some current concepts in intestinal bacteriology. Am J Clin Nutr 1978; 31:533–42.
7. Moore WEC, Holdeman LV. Special problems associated with the isolation and identification of bacteria in fecal flora studies. Am J Clin Nutr 1974; 27:1450–5.
8. Gorbach SL, Plaut AG, Nahas L, Weinstein L. Studies of intestinal microflora. II. Microorganisms of the small intestine and their relations to oral and fecal flora. Gastroenterology 1967; 53:856–67.
9. Hiryzmann M, Reuter G. Klinische erfahwgen mit einer neuen, atomatisch gesteureten Kapsel zur gewinnung von darminhalt und bakteriologische untersuchungen des inhalts hoherer darmabschnitte. Klin Prax 1963; 35:1408–12.
10. Bentley DW, Nichols RL, Condon RE, Gorbach SL. The microflora of the human ileum and intraabdominal colon: Results of direct needle aspiration at surgery and evaluation of the technique. J Lab Clin Med 1972; 79:421–9.
11. Drasar BS. Cultivation of anaerobic intestinal bacteria. J Pathol Bacteriol 1967; 94:417–27.
12. Hungate RE. The anaerobic mesophilic cellulolytic bacteria. Bacteriol Rev 1959; 14:1–49.
13. Arank A, Syed SA, Kenney EB, Freter R. Isolation of anaerobic bacteria from human gingiva and mouse cecum by means of a simplified glove box procedure. Appl Microbiol 1969; 17:568–76.
14. Brewer JH, Allgeier DL. Safe self-contained carbon dioxide-hydrogen anaerobic system. Appl Microbiol 1966, 14:985–8.
15. Loesche WJ. Oxygen sensitivity of various anaerobic bacteria. Appl Microbiol 1969; 18:723–7.
16. Finegold SM, Miller AB, Posnick DJ. Further studies on selective media for Bacteroides and other anaerobes. Ernaehrungsforschung 1965; 10:517–28.
17. Cummins CS, Johnson JL. Taxonomy of the clostridia: Cell wall composition and DNA homologies in *Clostridium butyricum* and other butyric acid-producing clostridia. J Gen Microbiol 1971; 67:33–46.
18. Gorbach SL, Mayhew JW, Bartlett JG, Thadepalli H, Onderdonk AB. Rapid diagnosis of anaerobic infections by direct gas-liquid chromatography of clinical specimens. J Clin Invest 1976; 57:478–84.
19. Donaldson RM Jr. Normal bacterial populations of the intestine and their relation to intestinal function. N Engl J Med 1964; 270:938–45, 994–1001, 1050–6.
20. Drasar BS, Hill MJ. Human Intestinal Flora. New York: Academic Press, 1974.
21. Gorbach SL. Intestinal microflora. Gastroenterology 1971; 60:1110–29.
22. Drasar BS, Shiner M, McLeod GM. Studies on the intestinal flora. I. The bacterial flora of the gastrointestinal tract in healthy and achlorhydric persons. Gastroenterology 1969; 56:71–9.
23. Nolte WA. Oral Microbiology. St. Louis: CV Mosby, 1982.
24. Kalser MH, Cohen R, Arteaga I, Yawn E, Mayoral L, Hoffert WR, Frazer D. Normal viral and bacterial flora of the human small and large intestine. N Engl J Med 1966; 274:500–5.
25. Cregan J, Hayward NJ. The bacterial content of the healthy small intestine. Br Med J 1953; 1:1356–9.
26. Gorbach SL, Nahas L, Lerner PI, Weinstein L. Studies of intestinal microflora. I. Effects of diet, age and periodic sampling on numbers of fecal microorganisms in man. Gastroenterology 1967; 53:845–55.
27. Donaldson RM Jr. The relation of enteric bacterial populations to gastrointestinal function and disease. *In:* Sleisenger M, Fordtran JS, eds. Gastrointestinal Disease, 2nd ed. Philadelphia: WB Saunders, 1978:79–92.
28. MacNeal WJ, Latzer LL, Kear JE. The fecal bacteria of healthy men. I. Introduction and direct quantitative observations. J Infect Dis 1909; 6:123–69.
29. Holdeman WV, Good IJ, Moore WEC. Human fecal flora: Variation in bacterial composition within individuals and a possible effect of emotional stress. Appl Environ Microbiol 1976; 31:359–75.
30. Moore WEC, Holdeman LV. Human fecal flora: The normal flora of 20 Japanese-Hawaiians. Appl Microbiol 1974; 27:961–79.
31. Moore WEC, Cato EP, Holdeman LV. Anaerobic bacteria of the gastrointestinal flora and their occurrence in clinical infections. J Infect Dis 1969; 119:641–9.
32. Byrne BM, Dankert J. Volatile fatty acids and aerobic flora in the gastrointestinal tract of mice under various conditions. Infect Immun 1979; 23:559–63.
33. Wolin MJ. Metabolic interactions among intestinal microorganisms. Am J Clin Nutr 1974; 27:1320–8.
34. Dubos R, Schaedler RW, Costello R, Hoet P. Indigenous, normal and autochthonous flora of the gastrointestinal tract. J Exp Med 1965; 122:67–77.
35. Savage DC. Microbial ecology of the gastrointestinal tract. Ann Rev Microbiol 1977; 31:107–33.
36. Savage DC, Blumershine RVH. Surface-surface association in microbial communities populating epithelial habitats in the murine gastrointestinal ecosystem: Scanning electron microscopy. Infect Immun 1974; 10:240–50.
37. Nelson DP, Mata LJ. Bacterial flora associated with the human gastrointestinal mucosa. Gastroenterology 1970; 58:56–61.
38. Plaut AG, Gorbach SL, Nahas L, Weinstein L. Studies of intestinal microflora and fluids. Gastroenterology 1967; 53:868–73.
39. Haenel H. Human normal and abnormal gastrointestinal flora. Am J Clin Nutr 1970; 23:1433–9.
40. Long SS, Swenson RM. Development of anaerobic fecal flora in healthy newborn infants. J Pediatr 1977; 91:298–301.

41. Mata LJ, Urrutia JJ. Intestinal colonization of breast-fed children in a rural area of low socioeconomic level. Ann NY Acad Sci 1971; 176:93–108.
42. Mitsuoka T, Kaneuchi C. Ecology of the bifidobacteria. Am J Clin Nutr 1977; 30:1799–1810.
43. Bettelheim KA, Breadon A, Faiers M, O'Farrell SM, Shooter RA. The origin of O serotypes of *Escherichia coli* in babies after normal delivery. J Hyg 1974; 72:67–70.
44. Bettelheim KA, Teoh-Chan CH, Chandler ME, O'Farrell SM, Layla R, Shaw EJ, Shooter RA. Further studies of *Escherichia coli* in babies after normal delivery. J Hyg 1974; 73:277–85.
45. Gareau FE, Mackel D, Boring J III, Payne FJ, Hammett FL. The acquisition of fecal flora by infants from their mother during birth. J Pediatr 1959; 54:313–18.
46. Bishop RF, Anderson CM. The bacterial flora of the stomach and small intestine in children with intestinal obstruction. Arch Dis Child 1960; 35:487–91.
47. Smith HW, Crabb WE. The faecal bacterial flora of animals and man: Its development in the young. J Pathol Bacteriol 1961; 82:53–66.
48. Olsen E. Studies on Intestinal Flora of Infants. Copenhagen: Ejnar Munksgaard, 1949.
49. Ford JE, Law BA, Marshall VME. Influence of the heat treatment of human milk on some of its protective constituents. J Pediatr 1977; 90:29–35.
50. Goldman AS, Smith CW. Host resistance factors in human milk. J Pediatr 1973; 82:1082–90.
51. Gyllenberg H, Roine P. The value of colony counts in evaluating the abundance of *"Lactobacillus" bifidus* in infant faeces. Acta Pathol Microbiol Scand 1953; 41:144–150.
52. Gyorgy P. Hitherto unrecognized biochemical difference between human milk and cow's milk. Pediatrics 1953; 11:98–107.
53. Kabara JJ. Lipids as host resistance factors of human milk. Nutr Res 1980; 38:65–73.
54. Ogra PL, Dayton DH, eds. Immunology of Breast Milk. New York: Raven Press, 1979.
55. Raptopoulou-Gigi M, Marwick K, McClelland DBL. Antimicrobial proteins in sterilized human milk. Br Med J 1977; 1:12–14.
56. Carlson J, Grahnen H, Jonsson G, Wikner S. Early establishment of *Streptococcus salivarius* in the mouths of infants. J Dent Res 1970; 49:415–8.
57. McAllister TA, Gwan J, Black A, Turner MJ, Kerr MM, Hutchison JH. The natural history of bacterial colonization of the newborn in a maternity hospital. Scott Med J 1974; 19:119–24.
58. McCarthy C, Snyder ML, Parker RB. The indigenous oral flora of man. I. The newborn to one year old infant. Arch Oral Biol 1965; 10:61–70.
59. Zinner DD, Jablon JM. Cariogenic streptococci in infants. Arch Oral Biol 1969; 14:1429–31.
60. de Araujo WC, Macdonal JB. The gingival crevice microbiota in five preschool children. Arch Oral Biol 1964; 9:227–8.
61. Ellen RP. Establishment and distribution of *Actinomyces viscosus* and *Actinomyces naeslundii* in the human oral cavity. Infect Immun 1976; 14:1119–24.
62. Zubrzycki L, Spaulding EH. Studies on the stability of the normal fecal flora. J Bacteriol 1962; 83:968–74.
63. Cooke EM, Ewins SP, Shooter R. The changing fecal population of *E. coli* in hospital medical patients. Br Med J 1969; 4:593–5.
64. Formal SB, Hornick RB. Invasive *Escherichia coli.* J Infect Dis 1978; 137:641–4.
65. Sears HI, Brownlee I. Further observations on the persistence of individual strains of *E. coli* in the intestinal tract of man. J Bacteriol 1952; 63:47–57.
66. Beachey E. Bacterial Adherence. Receptors and Recognition, Series B. Vol 6. London: Chapman and Hall, 1980.
67. Keusch GT. The role of bacterial adherence in infection. *In:* Majno G, Cotran RS, Kaufman N, eds. Current Topics in Inflammation and Infection. Baltimore: Williams and Wilkins, 1982:94–113.
68. Jones GW. The attachment of bacteria to the surfaces of animal cells. *In:* Reissig JL, ed. Microbial Interactions. Receptors and Recognition, Series B. Vol 3. London: Chapman and Hall, 1977: 139–76.
69. Wittenberger CL, Beaman AJ, Lee LN, McCabe RM, Donkersloot JA. Possible role of *Streptococcus salivarius* glucosyltransferase in adherence of *Veillonella* to smooth surfaces. *In:* Schlessinger D, ed. Microbiology—1977. Washington, DC: American Society for Microbiology, 1977: 417–21.
70. Brandtzaeg P, Fjellanger I, Gjbruldsen ST. Adsorption of immunoglobulin A onto oral bacteria *in vivo.* J Bacteriol 1968; 96:242–9.
71. Gibbons RJ. Bacterial adherence to mucosal surfaces and its inhibition by secretory antibodies. *In:* Meslecky J, Lawton AR, eds. The Immunoglobulin A System. New York: Plenum Press, 1974: 315–25.
72. Sirisinha S. Reactions of human salivary immunoglobulins with indigenous bacteria. Arch Oral Biol 1970; 15:551–4.
73. Plaut AG, Microbial IgG proteases. N Engl J Med 1978; 298:1459–63.
74. Kornfeld SJ, Plaut AG. Secretory immunity and bacterial IgA proteases. Rev Infect Dis 1981; 3:521–34.
75. Gibbons RJ, Kapsimalis B. Estimates of the overall role of growth in the gastrointestinal microflora of hamsters, guinea pigs, and mice. J Bacteriol 1967; 93:510–12.
76. Dixon JMS. The fate of bacteria in the small intestine. J Pathol Bacteriol 1960; 79:131–40.
77. Gorbach SL. Population control in the small bowel. Gut 1967; 8:530–2.
78. Drasar BS, Shiner M. Studies of the intestinal flora. II. Bacterial flora of the small intestine in patients with gastrointestinal disorders. Gut 1979; 10:812–9.
79. Gracey M. The contaminated small bowel syndrome: Pathogenesis, diagnosis, and treatment. Am J Clin Nutr 1979; 32:234–43.
80. Goldstein F, Cozzolino HJ, Wirts CW. Diarrhea and steatorrhea due to a large solitary duodenal diverticulum. Report of a case. Am J Dig Dis 1963; 8:937–43.
81. Ament ME, Shimoda SS, Saunders DR, Rubin CE. Pathogenesis of steatorrhea in three cases of small intestinal stasis syndrome. Gastroenterology 1971; 67:728–47.
82. Goldstein F, Wirts CW, Knowlessar OD. Diabetic diarrhea and steatorrhea: Microbiologic and clinical observations. Ann Intern Med 1970; 72:215–8.
83. Kahn LJ, Jeffries GH, Sleisenger MH. Malabsorption in intestinal scleroderma: Correction by antibiotics. N Engl J Med 1966; 274:1339–44.
84. Maldonado JE, Gregg JA, Green PS, Brown AL. Chronic idopathic intestinal pseudoobstruction. Am J Med 1970; 49:203–12.
85. Gorbach SL, Lal D, Levitan R. Intestinal microflora in Laennec's cirrhosis. J Clin Invest 1970; 49:36a.
86. Gracey M, Suharjono S, Stone DE. Microbial contamination of the gut: Another feature of malnutrition. Am J Clin Nutr 1973; 26:1170–4.
87. Roberts SH, James O, Jarvis EH. Bacterial overgrowth syndrome without "blind loop": A cause for malnutrition in the elderly. Lancet 1977; 2:1193–5.
88. Goldstein F, Mandle RJ, Schaedler RW. The blind-loop syndrome and its variants. Am J Gastroenterol 1973; 60:255–64.
89. Broido PW, Gorbach SL, Nyhus LM. Microflora of the gastrointestinal tract and the surgical malabsorption syndromes. Surg Gynecol Obstet 1972; 135:449–60.
90. Gray JDA, Shiner M. Influence of gastric pH on gastric and jejunal flora. Gut 1967; 8:574–81.
91. Gitelson S. Gastrectomy, achlorhydria and cholera. Isr J Med Sci 1971; 7:663–7.
92. Waddel WR, Kunz LJ. Association of salmonella enteritis with operation on the stomach. N Engl J Med 1956; 255:555–9.
93. Hornick RB, Music SI, Wenzel R, Cash R, Libonati JP, Snyder MJ, Woodward TE. The broad street pump revisited: Response of volunteers to ingested cholera vibrios. Bull NY Acad Med 1971; 47:1181–91.
94. Floch MH, Binder HJ, Filburn B, Gershengoren W. The effect of bile acids on intestinal microflora. Am J Clin Nutr 1972; 25:1418–26.

95. Lykkegaard Nielson M, Justesen T, Lenz K, Vagn Nielsen O, Lindkaer Jensen S. Bacterial flora of the small intestine and bile acid metabolism in patients with hepatico-jejunostomy roux-en-y. Scand J Gastroenterol 1977; 12:977–82.
96. Gorbach SL, Tabaqchali S. Bacteria, bile and the small bowel. Gut 1969; 10:963–72.
97. Keusch GT. Specific membrane receptors: Pathogenetic and therapeutic implications in infectious diseases. Rev Infect Dis 1979; 1:517–29.
98. Bonhours JF, Glickman RM. Rat intestinal glycolipids. II. Distribution and biosynthesis of glycolipids and ceramide in villus and crypt cells. Biochim Biophys Acta 1976; 441:123–33.
99. Herscovics A, Bugge B, Quaroni A, Kirsch K. Characterization of glycopeptides labelled from D-(2-^{3}H) mannose and L-(6-^{3}H) fucose in intestinal epithelial cell membranes during differentiation. Biochem J 1980; 192:145–53.
100. Kim YS, Perdomo A, Ochoa P, Issacs RA. Regional and cellular localization of glycosyltransferases in rat small intestine. Changes in enzymes with differentiation of intestinal epithelial cells. Biochim Biophys Acta 1975; 391:39–50.
101. Trier JS, Madara JL. Functional morphology of the mucosa of the small intestine. *In:* Johnson LR, ed. Physiology of the Gastrointestinal Tract, Vol 2. New York: Raven Press, 1981:925–61.
102. Kornfeld R, Kornfeld S. Structure of glycoproteins and their oligosaccharide units. *In:* Lennarz WL, ed. The Biochemistry of Glycoproteins and Proteoglycans. New York: Plenum Press, 1980:1–34.
103. Anderson MJ, Whitehead JS, Kim YS. Interaction of *Escherichia coli* K88 antigen with porcine intestinal brush border membrane. Infect Immun 1980; 29:897–901.
104. Faris A, Lindahl M, Wadstrom T. Gm_2-like glycoconjugate as possible erythrocyte receptor for the CFA/1 and K99 haemagglutinins of enterotoxigenic *Escherichia coli.* FEMS Micro Letters 1980; 7:265–9.
105. McNabb PC, Tomasi TB. Host defense mechanism at mucosal surfaces. Ann Rev Microbiol 1981; 35: 477–96.
106. Bienenstock J, Befus AD, McDermott M. Mucosal immunity. Monogr Allergy 1980; 16:1–18.
107. Ottaway CA, Rose ML, Parrott DM. The gut as an immunological system. Int Rev Physiol 1979; 19:323–56.
108. Owen RL, Nemanic P. Antigenic processing structures of the mammalian intestinal tract: A SEM study of lymphoreticular organs. Scan Electron Microsc 1978; 11:367–78.
109. Attebery HR, Sutter VL, Finegold SM. Effect of a partially chemically defined diet on normal human fecal flora. Am J Clin Nutr 1972; 25:1391–8.
110. Bounous G, Devroede GJ. Effects of an elemental diet on human fecal flora. Gastroenterology 1974; 66:210–14.
111. Hentges DJ. Fecal flora of volunteers on controlled diets. Am J Clin Nutr 1978; 31:S123–4.
112. de Stoppelaar JD, van Houte J, Backer-Dirks O. The effect of carbohydrate restriction on the presence of *Streptococcus mutans, Streptococcus sanguis* and iodophilic polysaccharide-producing bacteria in human dental plaque. Caries Res 1970; 4:114–23.
113. Gibbons RJ, van Houte J. Bacterial adherence in oral microbial ecology. Ann Rev Microbiol 1975; 29:19–44.
114. Abrams GD. Microbial effects on mucosal structure and function. Am J Clin Nutr 1977; 30:1880–6.
115. Kenworthy R. Observations on the reaction of the intestinal mucosa to bacterial challenge. J Clin Pathol 1971; 24:138–45.
116. Thompson GR, Trexler PC. Gastrointestinal structure and function in germ-free or gnotobiotic animals. Gut 1971; 12:230–5.
117. Coates ME, Fuller R. The gnotobiotic animal in the study of gut microbiology. *In:* Clarke RTJ, Bauchop T, eds. Microbial Ecology of the Gut. New York: Academic Press, 1977: 311–46.
118. Skelly BJ, Trexter PC, Tanami J. Effect of a clostridium species upon cecal size of gnotobiotic mice. Proc Soc Exp Biol Med 1962; 110:455–8.
119. Gracey M. Intestinal absorption in the "contaminated small-bowel syndrome." Gut 1971; 12:403–10.
120. Gordon HA. Is the germ-free animal normal? A review of its anomalies. *In:* Coates ME, ed. The Germ Free Animal in Research. New York: Academic Press, 1968:127–50.
121. Lombardi P, Goldin B, Boutin E, Gorbach SL. Metabolism of androgens and estrogens by human fecal microorganisms. J Steroid Biochem 1978; 9:795–801.
122. Adlercreutz H, Martin F. Oestrogen in human pregnancy feces. Acta Endocrinol 1976; 83:410–19.
123. Sandberg AA, Slaunwhite WR Jr. Studies on phenolic steroids in human subjects. VII. Metabolic fate of estriol and its glucuronide. J Clin Invest 1965; 44:694–702.
124. Inoue N, Sandberg AA, Graham JB, Slaunwhite WR Jr. Studies on phenolic steroids in human subjects. IX. Role of the intestine in the conjugation of estriol. J Clin Invest 1969; 48:390–6.
125. Levitz M, Katz J. Enterohepatic metabolism of estriol-3-sulfate-16-glucuronidate in women. J Clin Endocrinol Metab 1968; 28:862–8.
126. Pulkkinen MO, Willman K. Maternal oestrogen levels during penicillin treatment. Br Med J 1971; 4:48.
127. Pulkkinen MO, Willman K. Reduction of maternal estrogen excretion by neomycin. Am J Obstet Gynecol 1973; 115:1153.
128. Willman K, Pulkkinen MO. Reduced maternal plasma and urinary estriol during ampicillin treatment. Am J Obstet Gynecol 1971; 109:893–6.
129. Adlercreutz H, Martin F, Lehtinen T, Tikkanen MJ, Pulkkinen MO. Effect of ampicilin administration on plasma conjugated and unconjugated estrogen and progesterone levels in pregnancy. Am J Obstet Gynecol 1971; 128:266–71.
130. Adlercreutz H, Martin F, Pulkkinen M, Dencker H, Rimer U, Sjoberg NO, Tikkanen MJ. Intestinal metabolism of estrogens. J Clin Endocrinol Metab 1976; 43:497–505.
131. Tikkanen MJ, Pulkkinen MO, Adlercreutz H. Effect of ampicillin treatment on the urinary excretion of estriol conjugation in pregnancy. J Steroid Biochem 1973; 4:439–40.
132. Martin F, Peltonen J, Laatikainen T, Tikkanen M, Pulkkinen M. Excretion of unconjugated and conjugated progesterone metabolites in pregnancy urine during ampicillin administration. Clin Chim Acta 1974; 55:71–80.
133. Martin F, Bhargava AS, Adlercreutz H. Androgen metabolism in the beagle: Endogenous C_{19} O_2 metabolites in bile and faeces and the effect of ampicillin administration. J Steroid Biochem 1977; 8:753–60.
134. Eriksson H, Gustafsson J-A. Excretion of steroid hormones in adults: Steroids in faeces from adults. Eur J Biochem 1971; 18:146–50.
135. Boxenbaum HG, Bekersky I, Jack ML, Kaplan SA. Influence of gut microflora on bioavailability. Drug Metab Rev 1979; 9:259–79.
136. Goldman P. Biochemical pharmacology of the intestinal flora. Ann Rev Pharmacol Toxicol 1978; 18:523–39.
137. Goldman P, Peppercorn MA. Salicylazosulfapyridine in clinical practice. Gastroenterology 1973; 65:166–9.
138. Elkington SG, Floch MH, Conn HD. Lactulose in the treatment of chronic portal-systemic encephalopathy. A double blind clinical trial. N Engl J Med 1969; 281:408–412.
139. Levine MM, Hornick RB. Lactulose therapy in shigella carrier state and acute dysentery. Antimicrob Agents Chemother 1975; 8:581–4.
140. Lindenbaum J, Rund DG, Butler VP Jr, Tse-Eng D, Saha JR. Inactivation of digoxin by the gut flora: Reversal by antibiotic therapy. N Engl J Med 1981; 305:789–94.
141. Dossetar J. Drug interaction with oral contraceptives. Br Med J 1975; 4:467–8.
142. Reimer D. Rifampicin, "Pill" do not go well together. JAMA 1974; 227:608.
143. Drasar BS, Renwick AG, Williams RT. The conversion of cyclamate into cyclohexylamine by gut bacteria. Biochem J 1971; 123:26–7P.
144. Sandler M, Goodwin BL, Ruthven CRJ, Calne DB. Therapeutic implications in Parkinsonism of m-tyramine formation from L-dopa in man. Nature 1971; 229:414–6.
145. Sandler M, Goodwin BL, Ruthven CRJ, Hunter KR, Stern GM. Variation of levodopa metabolism with gastrointestinal absorption site. Lancet 1974; 1:238–40.

146. Sandler M, Karoum F, Ruthven CRJ, Calne DB. M-hydroxyphenyl-acetic acid formation from L-dopa in man: Suppression by neomycin. Science 1969; 166:1417–8.
147. Goldin BR, Peppercorn MA, Goldman P. Contribution of host and intestinal microflora in the metabolism of L-dopa by the rat. J Pharmacol Exp Ther 1978; 186:160–6.
148. Adamson RH, Bridges JW, Evans ME, Williams RT. The role of gut bacteria in the aromatization of the quinic acid in different species. Biochem J 1969; 112:17–8.
149. Walsh CT, Feierabend JF, Levine RR. The effect of lincomycin on the excretion of diethylstilbestrol and its ureterotrophic action in rats. Life Sci 1975; 16:1689–92.
150. Wynder EL, Reddy BS. Metabolic epidemiology of colorectal cancer. Cancer 1974; 34:801–6.
151. Haenszel W, Berg JW, Segi M, Kurihara M, Locke FB. Large-bowel cancer in Hawaiian Japanese. J Natl Cancer Inst 1973; 51:1765–9.
152. Wynder EL, Kajitani T, Ishikawa S, Dodo H, Takano A. Environmental factors of cancer of the colon and rectum. Cancer 1969; 23:1210–20.
153. Armstrong B, Doll R. Environmental factors and cancer incidence and mortality in different countries, with special reference to dietary practices. Int J Cancer 1975; 15:617–31.
154. Hill MJ, Drasar BS, Aries V, Crowther JS, Hawksworth G, Williams REO. Bacteria and etiology of cancer of large bowel. Lancet 1971; 1:95–100.
155. Finegold SM, Sutter VL. Fecal flora in different populations, with special reference to diet. Am J Clin Nutr 1978; 31:S116–22.
156. Weisburger JH. Colon carcinogens: their metabolism and mode of action. Cancer 1971; 28:60–70.
157. Goldin BR, Gorbach SL. The relationship between diet and rat fecal bacterial enzymes implicated in colon cancer. J Natl Cancer Inst 1976; 57:371–5.
158. Scheline RR. Metabolism of foreign compounds by gastrointestinal microorganisms. Pharmacol Rev 1973; 25:251–3.
159. Mastromarino A, Reddy BS, Wynder EL. Metabolic epidemiology of colon cancer: Enzymic activity of fecal flora. Am J Clin Nutr 1976; 29:1455–60.
160. Hill MJ. The role of colon anaerobes in the metabolism of bile acids and steroids, and its relation to colon cancer. Cancer 1975; 36:2387–400.
161. Reddy BS, Wynder EL. Large-bowel carcinogenesis: Fecal constituents of populations with diverse incidence rates of colon cancer. J Natl Cancer Inst 1973; 50:1437–42.
162. Goldin BR, Swenson L, Dwyer J, Sexton M, Gorbach SL. Effect of diet and *Lactobacillus acidophilus* supplements on human fecal bacterial enzymes. J Natl Cancer Inst 1980; 64:255–61.
163. Goldin BR, Dwyer J, Gorbach SL, Gordon W, Swenson L. Influence of diet and age on fecal bacterial enzymes. Am J Clin Nutr 1978; 31:S136–40.
164. Goldin BR, Gorbach SL. The effect of *Lactobacillus acidophilus* dietary supplements on 1,2-dimethylhydrazinedihydrochloride-induced intestinal cancer in rats. J Natl Cancer Inst 1980; 64:263–5.
165. Metchnikoff E. The Prolongation of Life. New York: Putnam, 1908.
166. Rettger LF, Levy MN, Weinstein L, Weiss JE. *Lactobacillus acidophilus* and Its Therapeutic Applications. New Haven: Yale University Press, 1935.
167. Report from the International Agency for Research on Cancer Intestinal Microecology Group. Dietary fiber transit-time, fecal bacteria, steroids and colon cancer in two Scandinavian populations. Lancet 1977; 2:207–11.
168. Goldin BR, Gorbach SL. Alterations in fecal microflora enzymes related to diet, age, *Lactobacillus* supplements, and dimethylhydrazine. Cancer 1977; 40:2421–6.
169. Arnon SS, Chin J. The clinical spectrum of infant botulism. Rev Infect Dis 1979; 1:614–21.
170. Hentges DJ. The intestinal flora and infant botulism. Rev Infect Dis 1979; 1:668–71.
171. Sugiyama H, Mills DC. Intraintestinal toxin in infant mice challenged intragastrically with *Clostridium botulinum* spores. Infect Immun 1978; 21:59–63.

Viruses

Robert J. Pauley

Virus studies of the human alimentary tract flora in both normal and pathologic states have increased rapidly with the development of modern tissue culture methods. The most medically and economically significant gastrointestinal tract viruses, however, have been difficult to adapt to tissue culture techniques until only recently. Consequently, studies with these viruses were initially limited to detection by the laborious method of electron microscopy. Development of enzyme-linked immunosorbent assays has substantially advanced understanding of one important class of the human gastrointestinal viruses, the human rotavirus.

History

Recovery of the poliovirus in 1908 by Landsteiner and Popper[1] from monkeys inoculated with central nervous system tissue of a boy dying of poliomyelitis was a benchmark in virology. Another milestone in the identification of viral enteritis agents was achieved in 1969 when an outbreak of typical winter vomiting disease in Norwalk, Ohio, resulted in the identification of the Norwalk virus.[2] The isolated virus was shown to produce identical clinical symptoms in adult volunteers.[3] Still another high point was reached in 1973 when Australian scientists discovered the human rotavirus in duodenal tissue obtained by biopsy from acutely ill infants and young children with diarrhea.[4]

Classification

Numerous studies have led to the conclusion that there are 2 groups of human enteric viruses: (1) The *enteroviruses,* such as the polioviruses, coxsackieviruses, and echoviruses, which are not important causes of acute gastroenteritis,[5, 6] but are transient inhabitants of the gastrointestinal tract; and (2) the *acute gastroenteritis viruses,* i.e., the Norwalk-like viruses and the rotaviruses, which are important causes of acute gastroenteritis.[5–9] This section is concerned with the advances made in understanding the biologic, pathogenetic, and epidemiologic properties of these viruses. More in-depth reviews of the acute infectious non-bacterial gastroenteritis viruses are available and may be consulted for additional details.[5–9]

Enteroviruses

In 1957, several viruses isolated from the lower intestinal tract in humans were officially designated "enteroviruses." These viruses shared certain common properties, but were generally regarded as transient inhabitants. The enteroviruses, which are basically picornaviruses (for small RNA-containing virus), are worldwide in distribution and are subdivided into the polioviruses, the coxsackieviruses (group A and B), and the echoviruses (for enteric cytopathogenic human orphan). The viruses share these properties: a small icosahedral virus particle (22 to 30 nm), a single-stranded RNA genome, resistance to ether and acid pH, and heat sensitivity.

Human enteroviruses are only transient inhabitants of the gastrointestinal tract or producers of infection. Their survival depends upon successful implantation within susceptible cells. Apparently, a seasonal incidence occurs in healthy subjects, with an increase in positive isolations during the summer and autumn months. Worldwide epidemics erupt during the warm months in temperate climates, but sporadic disease is also seen throughout the year.[10]

Enteroviruses are demonstrable in fecal collections from healthy children (most frequently before the age of 4), and variations occur annually in both percentage and type of enterovirus isolated in any one geographic location.[11, 12] Thus, monthly surveys conducted in 150 children in southern Louisiana disclosed a peak isolation rate of 29.5% that occurred in July.[12]

The major means of enteroviral dissemination is probably the fecal-oral pathway; nonhuman viral reservoirs have not been reported.[13] The epithelial surfaces of the oropharynx and small intestine, particularly the ileum, are considered to be the loci of implantation and multiplication of many enteroviruses in man.[10, 13] Whether this is true for all enteroviruses is unknown, as replication of some viruses can occur outside the gastrointestinal tract. Once infection occurs, the fecal viral concentration is high (usually greater than 10,000 infectious particles/g).[13] Intestinal involvement may be by direct invasion of the gut or may reflect part of an advanced phase of a generalized viral disease. Evidence of intestinal tissue injury may or may not be present and is variably associated with viral replication.[14] The majority of viral infections of the human intestinal tract cause no demonstrable evidence of viral-induced tissue injury.

The polioviruses have been the most extensively studied and are felt to be an accurate reflection of the fate of any of the enteroviruses entering the human mouth. There is also evidence that some viruses continue to multiply in regional lymph nodes and are then disseminated by means of humoral or lymphatic pathways.[14] During this period, large quantities of virus are usually easily detected in the feces.

Goffe[14] has stressed the role played by the intestine vis-à-vis viral entry. First, the intestine serves as the site of viral replication. Evidence for this exists in necropsy material from which viruses have been recovered from washed intestinal walls and by the fact that polioviruses released at the intestinal level (by means of oral administration in a gelatin capsule) cause infection; there is some evidence that viruses may gain entry to the gut directly from the blood stream. Second, the intestine acts as a barrier to invasion. Last, the gut is capable of immune response (Chapter 99).

The naturally occurring poliovirus or the Sabin vaccine will produce an excellent immune response, presumably because of its ability to stimulate the production of both tissue and serum antibodies. Because the intestinal tract is resistant to repeated infection by a virus, the oral vaccine is preferred for this purpose. Patients who have antibody are more difficult to infect than those with no evidence of previous infection by the particular virus.[14] Another significant method of body defense is that of viral interference. During active infection by an enterovirus, there may be partial or complete resistance to infection by a second virus. Type-specific humoral antibodies develop during the infective period, reflecting the immune response of the gut. Within 2 weeks of colonization of the gastrointestinal tract, neutralizing antibodies appear and may last for years. Complement-fixing and hemagglutination-inhibitor antibodies appear shortly thereafter, but there is much variation for the different viruses.[13] When the enterovirus reaches its secondary or target organ, the role of the humoral antibody lessens, while factors such as sequestration of the virus in macrophages, the role of interferon, and cellular resistance become more important.[13] Development and availability of type-specific antisera have not only facilitated identification of enteroviruses but have also provided a basis for serologic classification. Enteroviruses are neutralized by human gamma globulin and by individual human sera.[15]

Many clinical syndromes are produced by the enteroviruses, including involvement of the skin, mucous membranes, central nervous system, heart, skeletal muscle, and various visceral organs. Members of the poliovirus family, although previously implicated in gastrointestinal disease, are no longer considered causative agents of diarrhea or gastrointestinal diseases.[7]

Viral Enteritis

Two epidemiologically distinct forms of viral gastroenteritis are common. One form is involved with family and community-wide outbreaks of gastroenteritis and tends to be benign and self-limited. The symptoms of illness usually last 24 to 48 hours and include diarrhea, vomiting, nausea, low-grade fever, abdominal cramps, headache, anorexia, malaise, and myalgia. The clinical features of the illness frequently vary from one patient to another, with vomiting or diarrhea also varying in prominence and frequency. Serious sequelae have not been described, and generally treatment is unnecessary. Among the descriptive labels used to denote this illness are *winter vomiting disease,* because the illness occurs most frequently from September to March, and *acute infectious* or *epidemic non-bacterial gastroenteritis.* The agents associated with this form of viral gastroenteritis are the *Norwalk-like viruses,* and these viruses may cause about one-third of the epidemics of viral gastroenteritis that occur in the United States.[16]

The second epidemiologically distinct form of viral gastroenteritis occurs predominantly in infants and young children and is usually sporadic, although it may reach epidemic proportions. The illness frequently produces severe diarrhea, that commonly lasts 5 to 8 days, with symptoms of fever and vomiting. Serious sequelae may occur as a result of severe dehydration, but may be prevented by fluid replacement. The agents associated with this form of viral gastroenteritis are the human *rotaviruses,* which are members of the reovirus family. It has been estimated that this second form of viral gastroenteritis is responsible for up to one-half of the worldwide cases of infantile diarrhea that require hospitalization[6] and that rotavirus is a major cause of worldwide morbidity and infant mortality in developing nations.[17] Table 100–3 summarizes the important properties of the 2 viral agents for which there is clear evidence of involvement in gastroenteritis.

Norwalk-like Viruses. These viruses are characterized as small particles (about 27 nm) that are resistant to ether, acid, and heating (Table 100–3). Three viruses in this group have been studied: (1) the Norwalk agent, recovered in 1969 from an outbreak of gastrointestinal disease in Norwalk, Ohio; (2) the Hawaii agent; and (3) the Montgomery County (Maryland) agent, for all of which the Norwalk virus is the prototype. A large number of Norwalk-like agents have been described[7] that share virus morphologic features, are derived from epidemics or family outbreaks of gastroenteritis, and have been isolated worldwide.

Advances in understanding of the Norwalk-like viruses have been impeded by inability to reproduce the virus in tissue cul-

Table 100–3. DOCUMENTED HUMAN VIRAL GASTROENTERITIS AGENTS

Characteristics	Norwalk-like Virus	Rotaviruses
Physical properties		
Size (nm)	27	60–70
Capsid		Double-shelled capsid
Nucleic acid	Presumed DNA and single-stranded linear	Double-stranded RNA, 11 segments/genome
Ether-stable	Yes	Yes
Heat-stable	Yes	Yes
Acid-stable	Yes	Yes
Density in CsCl	1.36 to 1.41 g/cm^3	1.35 to 1.37 g/cm^3
Biologic properties		
Growth in tissue culture	No	Yes (but poorly)
Animal infections and disease	±	+ (piglets, calves)
Antigens	?	Type-specific and type-common
Serotype	3 (at least)	3 (at least)
Virion characteristics		Virion RNA-dependent, RNA polymerase Virion hemagglutinin
Etiologic relationship to human enteritis	Established	Established
Methods to identify virus and diagnostic tests	Immune electron microscopy, volunteer studies	Electron microscopy Counterimmunoelectrophoresis Radioimmunoassay ELISA Animal inoculation Cell culture antigen production Serologic assays RNA electrophoresis
Clinical characteristics		
Method of transmission	Fecal-oral Contaminated water and shellfish	Fecal-oral
Incubation period	1 to 2 days	1 to 3 days
Duration of illness	1 to 2 days, usually	5 to 8 days, usually
Age affected by illness	Older children and adults	Infants and young children
Epidemiology	Usually winter Family and community epidemics	Usually winter Occasionally epidemic
Pathology		
Site of human infection	Small bowel	Small bowel
Mechanisms of immunity	Essentially unknown	Local intestinal IgA, antibody may be important

ture. Hence, knowledge of these viruses has been limited largely to electron microscopic identification of the virus in infectious fecal filtrates.[18] Immune electron microscopy (IEM) allows for the visualization of antigen-antibody interactions using convalescent serum from a person with a recent virus infection; the interaction results in aggregation of the 27-nm virus particles. The Norwalk-like viruses are considered parvovirus-like (small-sized, high density, DNA-containing viruses).[18] However, one study indicates that Norwalk-like virus may be related to the RNA-containing caliciviruses.[6]

Norwalk virus, although not detectable by electron microscopy within mucosal cells, produces a histologic lesion of the human proximal small bowel mucosa that disappears within 2 weeks.[19] By contrast, the gastric mucosa and colonic mucosa are normal in individuals with Norwalk illness.[20, 21] In the absence of a reliable animal model for infection with a Norwalk-like virus, detailed understanding of the pathology of the disease is difficult to obtain.

Serologic studies, using a radioimmunoassay to detect antibodies to the Norwalk virus, have advanced our understanding of the epidemiology of these agents. These studies are limited, however, by the absence of hyperimmune animal serum reagents for diagnostic purposes, and they rely upon defined fecal and serum samples from experimentally infected humans. Current evidence, summarized by Blacklow and Cukor,[7] indicates that there are 3 distinct Norwalk-like virus serotypes determined by volunteer cross-challenge and IEM; however, more may be found. Based on the seroresponses to Norwalk virus or the serologically related Norwalk-like viruses in 70 viral gastroenteritis epidemics, 34% of the epidemics were due to Norwalk-like virus.[16] The occurrence of serum antibody in the United States has been documented during late adolescence and early adulthood, but not during childhood; about 66% of adults have serum antibody.[22, 23] These findings are consistent with the concept that the Norwalk-like viruses are not significant agents in severe infant gastroenteritis. The Norwalk-like viruses are transmitted in a fecal-oral mode,[18] with shed virus being present in stools of volunteers.

An unusual feature of the Norwalk illness, and of the immunity in terms of serum antibody to the virus, is that the presence of serum antibody to the Norwalk virus seems to have no protective role in the illness.[24] This conclusion is based on the observation that volunteers who become ill following inoculation were at higher risk of the illness after a second inoculation with the virus, even though they had elevated Norwalk-like virus serum antibody levels. Individuals who were clinically well following the first inoculation were unaffected by the second inoculation. Importantly, the same correlation occurs regarding local jejunal antibody to Norwalk virus.[22] Therefore, these observations are in contrast to the traditional concept that seroconversion has a protective effect on virus infection and clinical illness. A possibly similar phenomenon, termed antibody-mediated enhancement of virus infection, has been described for other viruses, including rabies[25] and dengue[26] viruses, indicating that repeated exposure to produce a serologic response to an agent may possibly be a promoting factor in some illnesses.

Rotaviruses. The rotaviruses are characterized as 60 to 70 nm in diameter, double-shelled virus particles that lack an ether-sensitive envelope (Table 100–3). The rotaviruses are also called *human reovirus–like (HRVL) virus.* They belong to the reovirus family, which includes the rota-, reo-, and orbiviruses. On electron microscopy, the outer capsid margin of the virus particle appears like a rim of a wheel surrounding radiating spokes from the inner hub-like core. This appearance accounts for the name *rota,* which means wheel. The rotaviruses have been identified in sporadic and epidemic outbreaks of enteritis in infants and young children that have occurred worldwide. The peak occurrence of rotavirus illness is during the winter months.

The rotavirus is produced in high quantities in stool specimens, allowing for the direct visualization of the virus by electron microscopy[17, 27] and permitting biochemical studies on it. Electrophoretic analysis of the virion RNA genome has demonstrated 11 unique-sized segments of double-stranded RNA; the reovirus and orbivirus contain only 10 segments.[28, 29] Comparison of the double-stranded RNA species from various isolates has permitted the characterization of a large number of electrophoreotypes of rotaviruses.[30] For example, at least 19 different electrophoreotypes were found in 5 years in 2 hospitals in the Netherlands.[31]

The human rotaviruses have proved difficult to adapt to growth in *in vitro* cell culture systems. In terms of virus identification, the virus will undergo an incomplete replication cycle when it is centrifuged onto a monolayer of cells. Although virus antigens were detected within the cell monolayer, infectious virus was not produced.[32] One rotavirus strain was successfully grown in human cells only after extensive passage through gnotobiotic piglets.[33] Several reports[34–36] have described the serial passage of human rotaviruses in cell cultures, using rhesus monkey cells (MA-104), by several culture manipulations.

The pathologic characteristics of the human rotaviruses are similar to the Norwalk-like viruses, with virus particles observed in intestinal epithelial cells of duodenal biopsy specimens.[37]

The acute rotaviral gastroenteritis in hospitalized young children occurs most commonly from 6 to 24 months of age. The illness is characterized by severe watery diarrhea with fever and vomiting at the onset and resulting isotonic dehydration. Recovery is usually complete following parenteral fluid replacement and restriction of oral fluids as the primary therapeutic measures. Although the initial diagnostic test for human rotaviruses was limited to electron microscopic detection of the virus in stool samples, several other tests have been developed, including radioimmunoassay, enzyme-linked immunosorbent assay (ELISA), immunoelectroosmophoresis, and fluorescent antibody techniques. In a comparative analysis of these methods,[38, 39] the ELISA rotavirus test proved a simple and reliable method for the diagnosis of human rotavirus infections. The level of sensitivity is as good as or better than electron microscopy or other methods. A latex agglutination test has been introduced that appears to be sensitive and reliable and may be more suitable for general use in a clinical laboratory setting.[40]

Serologic studies for the detection of rotavirus antibodies have utilized several methods, including immunofluorescence, radioimmunoassay, and ELISA. The common rotavirus antigens are located on the inner shell, whereas the type-specific antigens are located on the outer capsid layers. Although various sources have indicated as many as 4 different serotypes of human rotaviruses, current evidence supports at most 3 serotypes on the basis of virus neutralization and ELISA tests.[41–43] However, other serotypes may exist that have not as yet been conclusively demonstrated. It is not clear at this point what relationship exists between the human rotavirus RNA electrophoreotypes, which are numerous, and the viral serotypes, although it is unlikely that variation in each RNA species would necessarily alter the serotype of the virus. Perhaps the sensitivity and reliability of the technique in analyzing and differentiating between the virus genomes have surpassed the immunologic methods necessary for reliable serologic testing.

The role of the immune system in human rotavirus disease is not understood. Transmission of this virus is by the fecal-oral route and nosocomial infections are common. Observations to the effect that breast-fed infants have a lower occurrence rate of rotavirus disease, that serum antibodies are common in older children and adults, and that humans who have rotavirus antibodies can be infected would all seem to support the hypothesis that although serum antibodies may not be protective against infection, local immune factors, such as secretory IgA, may be important in protection against rotavirus infection.[8, 17, 44] In adult volunteer studies,[45] rotavirus IgA antibody levels from jejunal fluid appeared to correlate better with resistance to clinical illness than did serum IgG antibody. The presence of serum or intestinal antibody to one rotavirus serotype did not correlate with protection against challenge with a different serotype. Therefore, intestinal rotavirus antibody may have an important role in resistance to disease.

Other Enteric Agents

A number of other agents have been observed by electron microscopy of diarrheal feces, but evidence that these agents have an epidemiologic role as medically significant pathogens has not been presented.[8] Among these agents are a *calicivirus,* which may account for several well-defined outbreaks among infants and schoolchildren.[46] Because the morphologic appearance of the calicivirus and the Norwalk-like virus is similar, they have not been clearly distinguished from each other. A non-cultivatable, *non-cytopathic enteric adenovirus* has been visualized in diarrheal stools and in feces from asymptomatic individuals,[8] but as yet no conclusive evidence for a role of this adenovirus in acute enteric disease has been presented. *Coronavirus* has not been shown to be an etiologic agent of acute diarrheal gastroenteritis in man, but may cause gastroenteritis in several animal species.[5] *Astroviruses* have been observed in the feces of children with mild gastroenteritis,[47] but an etiologic relationship to human enteritis has not been established.[48]

References

1. Landsteiner K, Popper E. Mikroskopische Praparte von einem menschlichen und zwei Affenruckenmarken. Wien Klin Wochenschr 1908; 21:1830–5.
2. Adler J, Zickl R. Winter-vomiting disease. J Infect Dis 1969; 119:668–73.
3. Dolin R, Blacklow NR, DuPont H, Formal S, Buschow RF, Kasel JA, Chames RP, Hornick R, Chanock RM. Transmission of acute infectious nonbacterial gastroenteritis by cross-challenge in volunteers. J Infect Dis 1971; 123:307–12.
4. Bishop RF, Davidson GP, Holmes IH, Ruck BJ. Detection of a new virus by electron microscopy of faecal extracts from children with acute nonbacterial gastroenteritis. Lancet 1973; 2:1281–3.
5. Schreibner DS, Trier JS, Blacklow NR. Recent advances in viral gastroenteritis. Gastroenterology 1977; 73:174–83.
6. Steinhoff MC. Viruses and diarrhea—A review. Am J Dis Child 1978; 132:302–7.
7. Blacklow, NR, Cukor G. Viral gastroenteritis. N Engl J Med 1981; 304:397–406.
8. Blacklow NR, Schreiber DS, Trier JS. Viral enteritis. Semin Inf Dis 1978; 256–77.

9. Holmes IH. Viral gastroenteritis. Prog Med Virol 1979; 1–36.
10. Wenner HA. Enteroviruses: Notes on epidemiology, pathogenesis and means of identification. Med Time 1964; 92:625–37.
11. Farmer GW, Vincent MM, Fuccillo DA, Horta-Barbosa L, Ritman S, Sever JL, Gitnick GL. Viral investigations in ulcerative colitis and regional enteritis. Gastroenterology 1973; 65:8–18.
12. Gelfand HM, Fox JP, Leblane, DR. Enteric viral flora of population of normal children in Southern Louisiana. Am J Trop Med 1957; 6:521–31.
13. Wenner HA. The enteroviruses. Am J Clin Pathol 1972; 57:751–61.
14. Goffe AP. Intestinal immunity in poliomyelitis. *In*: Davis A, ed. The Small Intestine. Philadelphia: FA Davis, 1965: 65.
15. Syverton JI. Enteroviruses. Gastroenterology 1961; 40:331–7.
16. Greenberg HB, Valdesuso J, Yolken RH, Gangarosa E, Gary W, Wyatt RG, Konno T, Suzuki H, Chanock RM, Kapikian AZ. Role of Norwalk virus in outbreaks of nonbacterial gastroenteritis. J Infect Dis 1979; 139:564–8.
17. Kapikian AZ, Kim HW, Wyatt RG, Rodriguez W, Ross S, Cline W, Parrott R, Chanock R. Reoviruslike agent in stools: association with infantile diarrhea and development of serologic tests. Science 1974; 185:1049–53.
18. Dolin R, Blacklow NR, DuPont H, Buscho R, Wyatt R, Kasel J, Hornick R, Chanock R. Biological properties of Norwalk agent of acute infectious nonbacterial gastroenteritis. Proc Soc Exp Biol Med 1972; 140:578–83.
19. Schreiber DS, Blacklow NR, Trier JS. The mucosal lesion of the proximal small intestine in acute infectious nonbacterial gastroenteritis. N Engl J Med 1973; 288:1318–23.
20. Agus SG, Dolin R, Wyatt RG, Tousimis AJ, Northrup RS. Acute infectious nonbacterial gastroenteritis: intestinal histopathology: histologic and enzymatic alterations during illness produced by the Norwalk agent, in man. Ann Intern Med 1973; 79:18–25.
21. Widerlite L, Trier JS, Blacklow NR, Schreiber D. Structure of the gastric mucosa in acute infectious nonbacterial gastroenteritis. Gastroenterology 1975; 68:425–30.
22. Blacklow NR, Cukor G, Bedigian MK, Echeverria P, Greenberg HB, Schreiber DS, Trier JS. Immune response and prevalence of antibody to Norwalk enteritis virus as determined by radioimmunoassay. J Clin Microbiol 1979; 10:903–9.
23. Kapikian AZ, Greenberg HB, Cline WL, Kalica AR, Wyatt RG, James HD, Lloyd NL, Chanock RM, Ryder RW, Kim HW. Prevalence of antibody to the Norwalk agent by a newly developed immune adherence hemagglutination assay. J Med Virol 1978; 2:281–94.
24. Parrino TA, Schreiber DS, Trier JS, Kapikian AZ, Blacklow NR. Clinical immunity in acute gastroenteritis caused by Norwalk agent. N Engl J Med 1977; 297:86–9.
25. Prabhakar BS, Nathanson N. Acute rabies death mediated by antibody. Nature 1981; 290:590–1.
26. Halstead SB. In vivo enhancement of Dengue virus infection in Rhesus monkeys by passively transferred antibody. J Infect Dis 1979; 140:527–33.
27. Flewett TH, Bryden AS, Davies H, Woode G, Bridger J, Derrick J. Relation between viruses from acute gastroenteritis of children and newborn calves. Lancet 1974; 2:61–3.
28. Kalica AR, Sereno MM, Wyatt RG, Mebus C, Chanock R, Kapikian AZ. Comparison of human and animal rotavirus strains by gel electrophoresis of viral RNA. Virology 1978; 87:247–55.
29. Schnagl RD, Holmes IH. Characteristics of the genome of human infantile enteritis rotavirus. J Virol 1976; 19:267–70.
30. Espejo RT, Munoz O, Serafin F, Romero P. Shift in the prevalent rotavirus detected by ribonucleic acid segment differences. Infect Immunol 1980; 27:351–4.
31. Buitenwerf J, van Alphen MM, Schaap GJP. Characterization of rotaviral RNA isolated from children with gastroenteritis in two hospitals in Rotterdam. J Med Virol 1983; 12:71–8.
32. Bryden AS, Davies HA, Thouless ME, Flewett T. Diagnosis of rotavirus infection by cell culture. J Med Microbiol 1977; 10:121–5.
33. Wyatt RG, James WD, Bohl EH, Thiel KW, Saif LJ, Kalica AR, Greenberg HB, Kapikian AZ, Chanock RM. Human rotavirus type 2: cultivation in vitro. Science 1980; 207:189–91.
34. Birch CJ, Rodger SM, Marshall JA, Gust ID. Replication of human rotaviruses in cell culture. J Med Virol 1983; 11:241–50.
35. Sato K, Inaba Y, Shirozaki T, Fujii R, Massumoto M. Isolation of human rotaviruses in cell culture. Arch Virol 1981; 69:155–60.
36. Urasawa T, Urasawa S, Taniguichi T. Sequential passage of human rotaviruses in MA-104 cells. Microbiol Immunol (Tokyo) 1981; 25:1025–35.
37. Davidson GP, Barnes GL. Structural and functional abnormalities of the small intestine in infants and young children with rotavirus enteritis. Acta Paediatr Scand 1979; 68:181–6.
38. Grauballe PC, Vestergaard BF, Meyling A, Genner J. Optimized enzyme-linked immunoabsorbent assay for detection of human and bovine rotavirus in stools: comparison with electron microscopy, immunoelectro-osmophoresis and fluorescent antibody techniques. J Med Virol 1981; 7:29–40.
39. Yolken RH, Leister FJ. Evaluation of enzyme immunoassays for the detection of human rotaviruses. J Infect Dis 1981; 144:379–80.
40. Haikala OJ, Kokkonen JO, Leinonen MK, Nurmi T, Mantyjarvi R, Sarkkinen H. Rapid detection of rotavirus in stool by latex agglutination: comparison with radioimmunoassay and electron microscopy and clinical evaluation of the test. J Med Virol 1983; 11:91–7.
41. Suzuki H, Konno T, Numazaki Y, Kitaoka S, Tetsuo S, Aki I, Tazawa F, Nakagom T, Nakagomi G, Ishida N. Three different serotypes of human rotavirus determined using an interference test with Coxsackievirus B1. J Med Virol 1984; 13:41–44.
42. Tufvesson B. Detection of a human rotavirus strain different from types 1 and 2—A new subgroup? Epidemiology of subgroups in a Swedish and Ethiopian community. J Med Virol 1983; 12:111–7.
43. Yolken RH, Wyatt RG, Zissis GP, Brandt CD, Rodriguez WJ, Kim HW, Parrott RH, Urrutia JJ, Mata L. Epidemiology of human rotavirus types 1 and 2 as studied by enzyme-linked immunosorbent assay. N Engl J Med 1978; 299:1156–61.
44. Totterdell BM, Chrystie IL, Banatvala JE. Cord blood and breast milk antibodies in neonatal rotavirus infection. Br Med J 1980; 280:828–30.
45. Kapikian AZ, Wyatt RG, Greenberg HB, Kalica AR, Kim HW, Brandt CD, Rodriguez WJ, Parrott RH, Chanock RM. Approaches to immunization of infants and young children against gastroenteritis due to rotaviruses. Rev Infect Dis 1980; 2:459–69.
46. Chiba S, Sakuma Y, Kogasaka R, Akibara M, Terashima H, Horino K, Nakao T. Fecal shedding of virus in relation to the days of illness in infantile gastroenteritis due to calicivirus. J Infect Dis 1980; 142:247–9.
47. Kurtz JB, Lee TW, Pickering D. Astrovirus associated gastroenteritis in a children's ward. J Clin Pathol 1977; 30:948–52.
48. Kurtz JB, Lee TW, Craig JW, Reed SE. Astrovirus infection in volunteers. J Med Virol 1979; 3:221–30.

Fungi and Actinomycetes

Dexter H. Howard

Ecology is defined as the interrelationship of organisms with their environment. Knowledge regarding the interaction of fungi or of actinomycetes with the gastrointestinal environment is scanty.[1]

Several yeasts, notably *Candida* spp. and *Rhodotorula* spp., are commensals of the intestinal tract,[2] and some of the anaerobic actinomycetes in the family Actinomycetaceae occur in the large bowel.[3] Filamentous molds are not known to inhabit the bowel but may be isolated occasionally from feces, in which they probably occur as transients. Fungal propagules that are ingested with food or those that occur in water find the gastrointestinal tract of humans an unfavorable environment. Few species survive the combined inhibitory effects of the elevated temperature of the human body, the lowered oxidation reduction potential of the gastrointestinal tract, and the acidity of the stomach.

Infections of the gastrointestinal tract by fungi or actinomycetes are unusual.[4] *Candida* spp. and certain filamentous molds in the order Mucorales[1, 5] occasionally invade the gastrointestinal tract of immunocompromised individuals, and several of the fungi that cause primary pulmonary mycoses may disseminate to the various organs that constitute the gastrointestinal tract. In general, however, this is rarely observed. Abdominal actinomycosis is recorded in the literature but is quite uncommon today. Thus, the fungi and actinomycetes are not very important incitants of infectious diseases of the gastrointestinal tract.

This section considers those fungi and actinomycetes that constitute the normal microbiota of the gastrointestinal tract and those few pathogens that occasionally invade the organs comprising that system.

Commensals and Opportunists

Actinomycetes

The actinomycetes are filamentous *bacteria* that belong to the order Actinomycetales. These are true bacteria and are accordingly comprised of prokaryotic cells. Many members of this order grow by apical extension, form a mycelial type of colony, and reproduce by fragmentation or spore formation. These morphologic features led early microbiologists to include the actinomycetes with the fungi and even to treat them as intermediary forms between bacteria and fungi. Clearly, the 2 groups are unrelated taxonomically, but the tradition of considering them together in certain medical discussions is continued in this section.

The order Actinomycetales is comprised of 9 families of medical importance. However, only one of the families, Actinomycetaceae, contains members that are consistently associated with the gastrointestinal tract.[1, 3] The family Actinomycetaceae is comprised of anaerobic actinomycetes that are found on the mucous membranes of the mouth and in the gastrointestinal tract. In these locations the anaerobic actinomycetes are commensals that live in harmless association with their mammalian hosts. Under certain conditions, however, these commensal actinomycetes may opportunistically invade the tissues and precipitate infections that are collectively known as actinomycosis.

Actinomycosis is a chronic, suppurative, granulomatous infection in which abscesses are formed deep within the tissues; sinus tracts emerge from the tissue and often empty through the skin surface. Within the pus draining from the sinus tracts are granules comprised of branching filaments of one of several closely related actinomycetes. The disease is generally classified according to location as cervicofacial, thoracic, or abdominal. The last is the form that arises in the gastrointestinal tract and is the only one to be considered in this section.

Abdominal actinomycosis results from invasion of tissue by commensal actinomycetes through perforations in the intestinal wall.[1] The perforations may be produced by a variety of traumatic events.[1, 3] The major clinical features of abdominal actinomycosis were described by Cope[6] in his classic consideration of actinomycosis. Very little work has been done on the fundamental mechanism of the host-parasite interaction after tissue penetration by the bacterium, and no serologic procedures are routinely employed in the United States to facilitate diagnosis.[1]

The interconnecting sinus tracts that occur in the disease penetrate directly through the abdominal wall. Within the pus that emerges are granules, frequently referred to as sulfur granules because of their yellowish color. The granules are composed of the branching filaments of the incitant of the deep tissue abscesses (Fig. 100–6). The actinomycetes that cause abdominal actinomycosis are, in decreasing order of importance, *Actinomyces israelii, Arachnia propionica,* and *Actinomyces naeslundii.*[3] A single case of thoracic actinomycosis was attributed to *Bifidobacterium eriksonii.* Two additional species of actinomycetes, *Actinomyces viscosus* and *Actinomyces odontolyticus,* are found in the oral microbiota and are currently viewed as contributors to dental caries.[1, 3, 7] *Actinomyces bovis* causes a disease of cattle similar to that seen in humans, but the organism is not associated with humans, either as a commensal or as a pathogen.

The 3 agents of abdominal actinomycosis, *Actinomyces israelii, Actinomyces naeslundii,* and *Arachnia propionica,* are similar in their morphology and physiology.[7] On most laboratory media, they produce colonies composed of branching filaments that fragment into bacillary forms. They are gram-positive but not acid-fast, and their walls do not contain diaminopimelic acid, arabinose, or mycolic acid.[3, 7] Most of the species mentioned in this brief discussion are facultative anaerobes, but *Bifidobacterium eriksonii* is an obligate anaerobe. Other features of the biology of the various members of the Actinomycetaceae are comprehensively described in other textbooks, 2 of very recent date.[1, 3, 7]

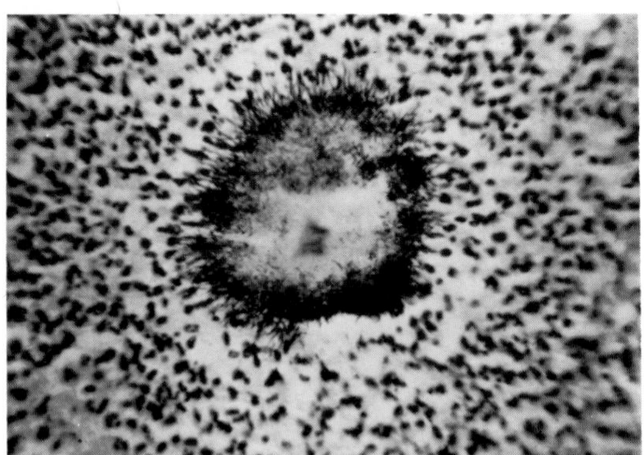

Figure 100–6. Gram stain of a sulfur granule in pus from a draining sinus tract of actinomycosis. The filaments are gram-positive (× 400). (From Rippon JW. Medical Mycology: The Pathogenic Fungi and the Pathogenic Actinomycetes. 2nd Ed. Philadelphia: WB Saunders, 1982. Reproduced with permission.)

None of the other families of actinomycetes has members that occur as commensals of humans. However, the exogenously acquired opportunists *Nocardia asteroides, N. brasiliensis,* and *N. caviae* (fam. Nocardiaceae) all produce primary pulmonary disease that may disseminate to almost any organ system, and, although rare, nocardial lesions of the liver and pancreas have been recorded.[4] These occurrences seem too uncommon to merit an elaborate consideration of the agents. Briefly, the 3 species mentioned are aerobes that produce heaped, waxy colonies composed of branching filaments that fragment into bacillary forms. The cells are gram-positive, partially acid-fast, and non–spore forming.[8]

Fungi

For the sake of convenience, the fungi will be considered under the separate headings of yeasts and molds. The yeasts are unicellular fungi that usually grow and reproduce asexually by a budding or fission process, while molds grow predominantly as filamentous elements called hyphae and reproduce by means of various types of spores and asexual propagules. The distinction, while arbitrary, is useful for purposes of discussion.

Yeasts. The term "yeast" is sometimes reserved for those forms that have a sexual phase of growth, e.g., *Saccharomyces* spp. Those yeasts lacking a sexual phase of growth (Fungi Imperfecti) are accordingly referred to as yeast-like fungi. In this brief treatment of the subject, the term yeast is used as defined in the preceding paragraph without further qualification.

The gastrointestinal tract is the location of several yeasts that live in commensal association with humans. There are, of course, a large number of transients, which are recovered from stools on occasion.[1, 9] The number of species that appear to be consistent residents of the bowel is rather restricted and encompasses *Candida* spp., *Rhodotorula* spp., *Torulopsis glabrata,* and *Trichosporon cutaneum.*[9] *Geotrichum candidum,* which can be isolated from this source, will also be considered under this heading; although it does not reproduce asexually by budding, it does produce ascospores in its sexual form of growth *(Endomyces candidum)* and is generally considered in discussions of commensal yeasts of the gastrointestinal tract. The number of reports on *Torulopsis glabrata* from the gastrointestinal tract is small; it is far more frequently encountered as a resident of the genitourinary tract. Other than occurrence, little is known of the factors involved in the commensal association of yeast with the other microbial members of the microbiota. However, some measure of control of numbers is operative because it is very well known that the use of broad-spectrum antibacterial antibiotics will consistently favor exaggerated growth of *Candida* spp. Experimental infections in animals have augmented these experiences in the human host. Work with germ-free chicks has shown that certain intestinal bacteria are inhibitory to *in vitro* growth and gut colonization by *Candida albicans.*[10] Extension of these studies has indicated that a competitive bacterial biota is more effective than an intact immune system (T cell) in preventing gastric candidiasis.[11, 12] The interesting fact that mice do not normally carry *C. albicans* as a commensal has led to the use of the infant mouse model in a detailed investigation of the host-parasite interaction in candidiasis.[13, 14]

Each of the yeasts known to occur as commensals of the bowel is also recognized as an opportunistic pathogen. Thus, the overall biology of these microorganisms will be discussed at this point.

Candida. No genus of fungus is better known for its opportunistic behavior than is *Candida.* The genus contains 7 species that are commensals of humans, *C. albicans, C. guilliermondii, C. krusei, C. parapsilosis, C. pseudotropicalis, C. stellatoidea,* and *C. tropicalis.*[1, 15] The principal characteristic that unites these species is the ability to produce pseudohyphae (i.e., chains of elongated yeast cells) on certain laboratory media. Of the 7 species that may occur as commensals, *C. albicans, C. parapsilosis, C. stellatoidea,* and *C. tropicalis* are most often encountered as pathogens in immunocompromised individuals.[2] Clinical disease may involve the esophagus, the bowel, or the perianal areas.[1, 2] The various clinical and other features when these sites are involved are considered in Chapters 57, 77, and 143.

Candida spp. are responsible for acute or subacute infections that may involve the skin, nails, and mucous membranes or may become systemic and involve any area of the body. The source of infection is generally endogenous from a commensal inhabitant of the gastrointestinal tract, but examples of contagion are known. Predisposing factors of recognized importance include maceration, physiologic changes, endocrinopathies, malnutrition, malignancies, antibacterial and immunosuppressive drugs, and genetic abnormalities of immunocompetency.[1, 2]

Identification of members of the genus *Candida* depends on morphologic and biochemical determinations.[2, 5] The fungus appears as blastoconidia (yeast cells) and filamentous elements in direct KOH mounts from scrapings, within stained biopsy material, or in tissue sections from necropsy specimens. In cultures on Sabouraud's glucose agar, *Candida* spp. grow as yeasty colonies composed predominantly of blastoconidia. Of the many species in the genus *Candida, C. albicans* is most commonly associated with human disease (*C. stellatoidea* is treated as a variety of *C. albicans* in this discussion; it will key out with *C. albicans* and is reported as such in most laboratories). Since other species may occur as inhabitants of the gastrointestinal tract, it is necessary to be able to distinguish these from *C. albicans.* The distinction is most commonly and easily made on the basis of the fact that *C. albicans* produces germ tubes (Fig. 100–7) under certain experimental conditions.[1, 5, 15] Confirmation of *C. albicans* may be obtained or identification of other species may be established by morphologic studies on corn meal agar with Tween-80 and assimilation of carbohydrates, for which commercial reagents are used.[15]

The host-parasite interactions have been subjected to extensive study, and some of the salient features have been reviewed.[2, 16] There is much work currently being directed toward developing ancillary serologic tests involving detection of either specific antibody or circulating antigen. No such test has achieved widespread use, however, at this time.

Other Yeasts. *Rhodotorula* spp. have on rare

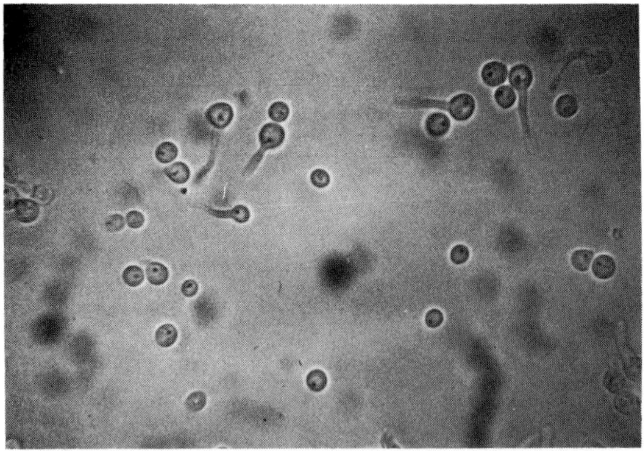

A

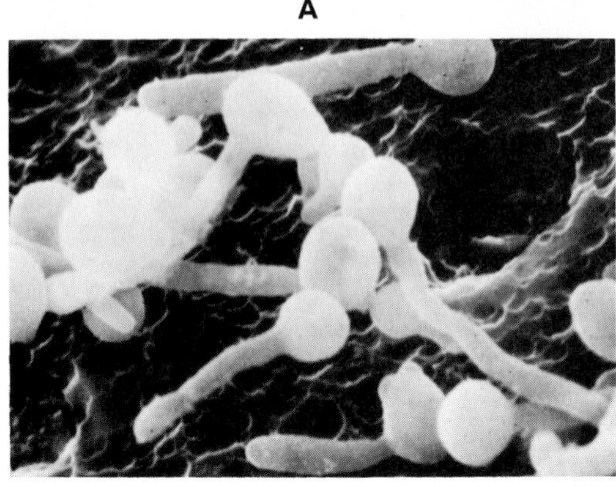

B

Figure 100–7. *A*, Germ tube formation by *Candida albicans*. The tubes develop after incubation of yeast cells in serum at 37°C (× 440). *B*, Scanning electron microscopic illustration of germ tubes. (From Rippon JW. Medical Mycology: The Pathogenic Fungi and the Pathogenic Actinomycetes. 2nd Ed. Philadelphia: WB Saunders, 1982. Reproduced with permission.)

occasions been isolated from patients in terminal stages of debilitating disease.[1] As the generic name indicates, the most outstanding characteristic of this yeast is the carotinoid pigment that it produces, which gives its colonies a pink coloration and has led to the colloquial name "pink yeast."

Trichosporon spp. are well-recognized although rare incitants of infection. These yeasts are identified in culture by the fact that they produce both arthroconidia and blastoconidia (yeast cells) as reproductive propagules.[1, 15]

Gastrointestinal involvement by *Geotrichum candidum* has been recorded a few times.[1] The commensal occurrence of *G. candidum* is well known[1, 2, 15] and makes establishment of an etiologic relationship to intestinal disease very difficult.[1] The fungus is seen in direct mounts as oblong to rectangular arthroconidia. The hyphae that form the white to creamy colonies that grow on culture break up into arthroconidia. Virtually nothing is known of host-parasite interactions.

There are a number of other yeast species that have been implicated in human disease on rare occasion. No doubt some of them reside for a time in the gastrointestinal tract and may precipitate infections endogenously from that location. Information of this sort is available from standard sources.[1–4]

Molds. As indicated in the introduction to this section, there are no filamentous molds that are recognized commensals of the gastrointestinal tract. Nevertheless, mold spores must be constantly ingested, and no doubt some survive for a period in the bowel. There is one very well-recognized opportunistic infection, i.e., mucormycosis, which arises from spores that have survived and are at least transient residents of the bowel. There is no evidence that such spores germinate under normal circumstances, but they do indeed survive and are poised to take opportunistic advantage of immunocompromised individuals.

Mucorales. The term "mucormycosis" is widely used for those mycoses caused by fungi belonging to the order Mucorales.[5, 17] In a conference on this topic published in

1980,[17] Edwards presented the clinical aspects of gastrointestinal mucormycosis as follows:

> Gastrointestinal mucormycosis is rare, even in patients with leukemia and lymphoma.[18] Generally, intrinsic abnormalities of the gastrointestinal tract, such as amebic colitis, typhoid, pellagra, and kwashiorkor[19, 20] have preceded infection. One patient, without an underlying systemic illness, developed mucormycotic ulcerations in the terminal ileum after therapy with antibiotics and steroids for anaerobic bacterial peritonitis.[19] Another patient developed gastric mucormycosis after nasogastric intubation.[20] The gastrointestinal organ most frequently involved is the stomach, with the large bowel next in frequency.[20, 21] Widespread dissemination from a primary gastrointestinal site may occur.[22] Infections of the ileum have also been reported.[20] Mucormycosis can extend from the gut lumen to the gallbladder, liver, pancreas, and spleen and may cause perforation or bowel obstruction.
>
> The Mucorales may either colonize (without invasion) or invade gastric ulcers.[23, 24] When they invade, the lesion extends and marked surrounding induration develops, with a black surface discoloration forming in the ulcer bed. Invasion was associated with a poor prognosis in contrast with an excellent prognosis when only colonization was present. Diagnosis depends on biopsy demonstration of tissue invasion. Stool and gastric cultures are of value.

The Mucorales is an order of the Zygomycetes, which contain the major opportunistic pathogens found in this class of fungi. The basic unit of asexual sporulation is a sporangiospore borne within a sporangium. This structure is not seen in the tissues, but rather non-septate hyphae with right angle branching are observed[4] (Fig. 100–8).

The Mucorales that are involved in opportunism are predominantly found within the family Mucoraceae. Three genera within this family are commonly isolated from patients with mucormycosis: *Mucor, Absidia,* and *Rhizopus.* All form sporangiospores within a sporangium. Ancillary morphologic structures can be used to distinguish among these 3 genera.[17] Work on host resistance factors, prospects for immunodiagnostic methods, and the status of current therapy were reviewed in the conference conducted by Lehrer et al.[17]

Aspergillus. Members of the genus *Aspergillus*[25] may be responsible for a wide spectrum of opportunistic disease, including infection or colonization of tissues or cavities. They may cause pulmonary infections of a localized or invasive type, or they may disseminate to involve almost any tissue of the body. They are also responsible for allergy and may cause a toxemia after ingestion of their by-products. Disseminated aspergillosis is a relatively rare disease of humans and involvement of the gastrointestinal tract is unusual.[1, 26] An excellent monographic treatment of the genus exists.[25]

Aspergillus fumigatus is the most common species involved in human aspergillosis, but several other species have been implicated from time to time.[1] *Aspergillus fumigatus* produces a moderately fast-growing, flat, velvety colony that is bluish-green in color and becomes brown upon aging. Typical *Aspergillus*-type sporulation[25] is observed with chains of conidia borne on one row of phialides pointing upward from the upper part of the vesicle. In the tissues of a host, the fungus generally shows only septate hyphae that branch at acute angles, but in some cases

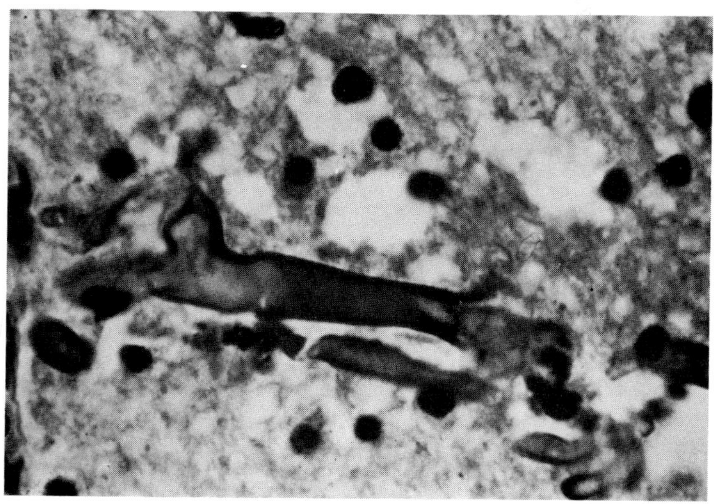

Figure 100–8. Broad, non-septate hyphae of one of the members of the Mucoraceae (periodic acid–Schiff and hematoxylin, × 800). (From Rippon JW. *In*: Freeman BA, ed. Burrows Textbook of Microbiology. 20th Ed. Philadelphia: WB Saunders, 1979. Reproduced with permission.)

of cavity colonization fully sporulating *Aspergillus* "heads" have been observed. Although a large number of species are known, only a few are encountered commonly. Host-parasite interactions have been reviewed by Schaffner et al.[27] and by Diamond et al.,[28] and several laboratories are currently engaged in developing immunologic tests for specific antigens in body fluids.

Pseudallescheria. This genus contains a single species, *P. boydii,* which may cause a spectrum of clinical diseases.[1] The types of opportunistic infections are very similar to those seen with *Aspergillus* spp.[1] Cases occurring in the gastrointestinal tract have not been reviewed, but one case of liver involvement has been recorded.[29]

The asexual conidia of this fungus are broadly clavate or ovoid and are borne singly and terminally on solitary conidiophores.[1] Practically nothing is known of host-parasite interactions, and no efforts are currently directed toward developing serodiagnostic methods.

Pathogens

None of the fungi described in this section occur naturally in the gastrointestinal tract. Each is acquired from an exogenous source. All of these fungi, except *Sporothrix schenckii,* are acquired primarily by inhalation and produce pulmonary infection from which site dissemination to other organ systems may occur. In rare instances, the gastrointestinal organs may be involved. *Sporothrix schenckii* is customarily acquired by inoculation, but some episodes of disseminated disease are known and it is thought that some of the cases were acquired by the pulmonary route.

Yeasts

Cryptococcus. In its most frequently recognized form, cryptococcosis is a chronic, wasting, frequently fatal disease characterized by a pronounced predilection for the central nervous system and caused by the yeast *Cryptococcus neoformans.* This organism could have been discussed in the preceding section on opportunists because almost two-thirds of the clinical cases occur in immunocompromised individuals. However, it appears that involvement of the central nervous system is a rare sequel to a far more common primary pulmonary form of disease, and there is a body of evidence suggesting widespread subclinical infection.[30] Thus, the overall behavior of *C. neoformans* is more akin to the pathogens discussed in this section than it is to the opportunists described previously.

The genus *Cryptococcus* contains a single species, *C. neoformans,* with 2 varieties, *neoformans* (A and D serotypes) and *gattii* (B and C serotypes), which produce disease in humans and animals.[31] The source of infection is exogenous and there is an interesting but not totally explained association of A and D serotypes of *C. neoformans* with pigeon dung.[1] The location of B and C serotypes in nature is not known.

Although cryptococcosis is acquired exogenously by inhalation, primary pulmonary disease is not often diagnosed. In the tissues of the host, the fungus appears as an encapsulated yeast cell. In cultures in the laboratory, the fungus produces somewhat mucoid yeast colonies consisting of encapsulated yeast cells. Confirmatory identification consists of the production of a brown-colored colony on *Guzotia* seed agar. The color is due to a melanin-like pigment formed by an active phenoloxidase produced by both varieties of *C. neoformans* from appropriate precursors found in the seed agar. *Cryptococcus neoformans* is the only species of *Cryptococcus,* and almost the only commonly encountered yeast, that produces this melanin-like pigment under these circumstances.[32] The phenoloxidase enzyme is related to virulence of the yeast.[33]

There are 4 antigenic types of *C. neoformans* based on capsular differences and labeled A, B, C, and D. Epidemiologic studies[34] have established that the B and C serotypes are more important incitants of infection in southern California than in other areas of the United States. Interestingly, the A and D serotypes, which are the most prevalent pathogens in all areas of the United States except southern California, are readily isolated from samples of pigeon dung. The B and C serotypes, however, have not been isolated from any environmental source. Other aspects of the worldwide distribution of serotypes have been published.[35]

A very useful serologic test is available for diagnosis of patients suspected of having cryptococcosis. The test involves a search for antigen in body fluids. Latex particles are coated with specific rabbit immune globulin against the antigenic types of *C. neoformans*. The particles are mixed with the patient's specimen, and agglutination indicates the presence of antigen. Aspects of the host-parasite interaction have been studied extensively,[5] but a thorough discussion is beyond the limits of this summary.

Molds

Blastomyces. Blastomycosis is a chronic disease caused by *Blastomyces dermatitidis*. It is characterized by the formation of suppurative and granulomatous lesions in any part of the body but with a marked predilection for lungs, skin, and bone. Involvement of organs of the gastrointestinal tract is infrequently seen.[1, 4]

Blastomycosis was once thought to be limited solely to the United States, with a majority of cases occurring along the Mississippi and Ohio River valleys. Scattered cases were then found in Canada, Mexico, Central America, and northern South America, and the disease is now known to be worldwide.[36]

Blastomyces dermatitidis is a dimorphic fungus. *In vivo* and in cultures at 37°C, it multiplies as blastoconidia (yeast cells). These cells are 8 to 15 μm in diameter, with a thick cell wall and a wide base at the juncture of the budding daughter cells. In nature and in cultures at room temperature, a mycelium is produced, which is made up of hyphae that bear round to ovoid conidia. These latter propagules are the infectious spores that are inhaled and that initiate infection. The ecologic location of *B. dermatitidis* is poorly understood.[36, 37] Aspects of the host-parasite interaction have been explored, and there is a substantial literature on serodiagnosis.[1, 5]

Coccidioides. Coccidioidomycosis is caused by *Coccidioides immitis*. The disease is probably the most infectious of the systemic mycoses; the majority of individuals who live in endemic areas for any length of time acquire the infection. Inhalation of infectious propagules may result in primary pulmonary disease, which is self-limited and benign, but a more progressive disease is seen in a small percentage of individuals. The progressive form is chronic, malignant, and disseminated to involve almost any organ system.[1] Wilson and Plunkett[38] stated in 1965 that the gastrointestinal tract is remarkably resistant to coccidioidal involvement, and this fact was reiterated in 1982 by Rippon[1] in his textbook.

The fungus is confined to the New World. No cases are acquired outside North, Central, or South America. In the United States, the fungus occurs only in the southwestern states.[36] Of course, infections can be acquired in the endemic areas and become manifest in non-endemic regions. Indeed, approximately 20% of cases occur outside areas endemic for the fungus.[39]

Coccidioides immitis is a well-adapted soil fungus whose ecology I have recently reviewed elsewhere.[37] The fungus is dimorphic. *In vivo* and *in vitro* at 37°C (under some cultural conditions), the organism consists of large spherules averaging 30 to 60 μm (up to 150 to 200 μm) in diameter that contain many small (2 to 5 μm) endospores. *In vitro* at room temperature the fungus grows as a mycelium consisting of hyphae that break up into arthroconidia (2.5 to 5 μ). These propagules are highly infectious. Aspects of the dimorphism of fungus, the host-parasite interaction, and serodiagnostic methods have received abundant study, and the vast literature has been summarized.[1, 5]

Histoplasma. Histoplasmosis, which is caused by *Histoplasma capsulatum*, presents a variety of clinical manifestations. Primary histoplasmosis is acquired by inhalation of infectious spores and is largely confined to the lungs. Progressive histoplasmosis is a rare sequel that is characterized by emaciation, leukopenia, and irregular fevers. In the latter form of the disease, liver involvement is common and intestinal ulcers have been observed.[1] In fact, intestinal ulcerations are a constant feature of the disease, as seen in bats.[1]

The fungus is worldwide in distribution with a notable intensity in the United States, where its highest frequency rate is in those states bordering on the Mississippi, Missouri, and Ohio River basins. A summary of the other features of the epidemiology and ecology of histoplasmosis is found in the review referred to earlier with respect to coccidioidomycosis.[37]

Histoplasma capsulatum is a dimorphic fungus. *In vivo* and *in vitro* at 37°C the fungus appears as ovoid, budding blastoconidia (yeast cells) measuring about 4 μm in diameter. In the tissue of an infected host, the blastoconidia are facultative intracellular parasites of the mononuclear phagocytes of the reticuloendothelial system (Fig. 100–9). *In vitro* at room temperature, *H. capsulatum* forms a mycelium consisting of hyphae that bear 2 types of conidia: characteristic tuberculate macroconidia (8 to 14 μm in diameter) and small, spherical microconidia (2 to 4 μm in diameter). The latter are the infectious elements inhaled from various natural locations.[1, 37] A vast literature exists on the dimorphism of the fungus, on host-parasite interactions, and on serodiagnostic methods.[1, 5]

Another variety of *H. capsulatum* is called *H. capsulatum* var. *duboisii*. This variety occurs predominantly in Africa and differs from var. *capsulatum* in the morphologic details of its parasitic form of growth. Disseminated forms of the disease do involve the gastrointestinal tract, but only a few studies on host-parasite interactions and serodiagnostic methods have been made.[1]

Paracoccidioides. Paracoccidioidomycosis is geographically limited to South and Central America.[36] The infection is a chronic granulomatous disease that begins as a primary pulmonary infection but may disseminate to form ulcerative granulomas of many organ systems. The gastrointestinal tract is occasionally involved.[1] The causative agent, *Paracoccidioides brasiliensis,* is presumably acquired by direct inhalation of infectious propagules, but the location of the fungus in nature is not known and exact information on geographic distribution is accordingly fragmentary.[36] Various features of the epidemiology of the disease are recorded.[1, 36]

Paracoccidioides brasiliensis is a dimorphic fungus. *In vivo* and *in vitro* at 37°C, it appears as single and multiple budding, thick-walled blastoconidia that are 10 to 60 μm in diameter. *In vitro* at room temperature the fungus grows as a mycelium consisting of hyphae that occasionally produce conidia. These propagules may be rare on some culture media, but must be produced more abundantly in nature since they are the only recognized infectious propagules.[1]

Various aspects of the dimorphism, the host-parasite interactions, and the serodiagnosis of *P. brasiliensis* have been studied.[1, 5]

Sporothrix. In its most commonly encoun-

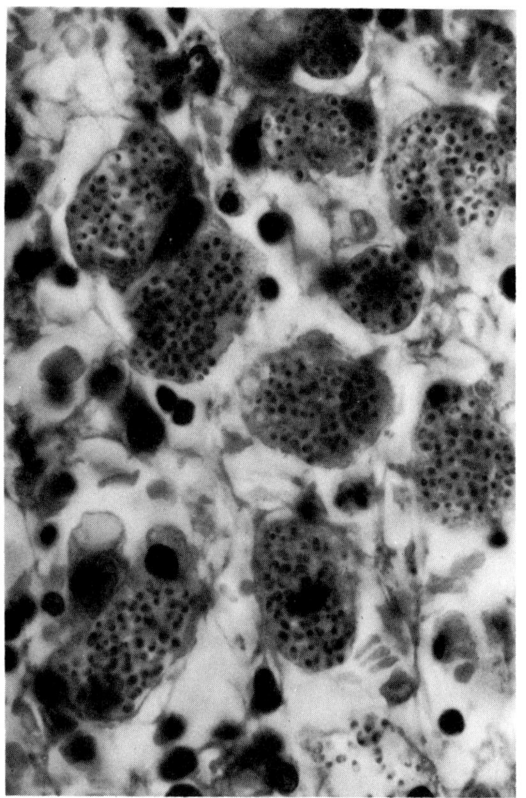

Figure 100–9. Yeast cells of *Histoplasma capsulatum* within histiocytes. The preparation is from a disseminated case of histoplasmosis (hematoxylin and eosin, × 400). (From Rippon JW. Medical Myocology: The Pathogenic Fungi and the Pathogenic Actinomycetes. 2nd Ed. Philadelphia: WB Saunders, 1982. Reproduced with permission.)

tered form, sporotrichosis is a chronic, suppurative, granulomatous disease caused by *Sporothrix schenckii*. The infection is acquired by direct implantation of fungal spores into subcutaneous tissues, where nodules develop. The nodules form abscesses that ulcerate and drain. A chain of secondary nodules that follow the course of the lymphatics may develop. The infection may also be acquired rarely by inhalation. Disseminated disease may arise by spread from primary cutaneous or pulmonary disease.[1] Although extremely rare, spread to organs of the gastrointestinal tract is known to occur.[1] Various features of the geographic distribution and epidemiology have been amply studied.[1, 36]

Sporothrix schenckii is a dimorphic pathogen. *In vivo* and *in vitro* at 37°C it grows as budding blastoconidia that are often bacilliform (1 to 3 × 3 to 10 μm). *In vitro* the fungus produces a mycelium consisting of hyphae that produce conidia (2 to 3 × 3 to 6 μm) in a petellate arrangement on delicate conidiophores. Aspects of this dimorphism have been studied in some detail;[5] features of the host-parasite interactions have received only scant attention and serodiagnostic methods are rarely used.[1]

Summary

The gastrointestinal tract is not a site favored by fungi or actinomycetes. The number of commensals is very small and confined to yeasts and anaerobic actinomycetes. Those commensals stimulated by immunocompromising events in the host are as likely to attack other organs systems as they are to cause profound disease of the gastrointestinal tract. Systemic fungal pathogens rarely produce disease of the bowel or accessory organs of the gastrointestinal tract. *Histoplasma capsulatum* and *Paracoccidiodes brasiliensis* do occasionally produce intestinal ulcerations.

References

1. Rippon JW. Medical Mycology: The Pathologenic Fungi and the Pathogenic Actinomycetes. Philadelphia: WB Saunders, 1982.
2. Odds FC. *Candida* and Candidosis. Baltimore: University Park Press, 1979.
3. Mitchell TG. Actinomycetes. *In* WK Joklik, HP Willett, DB Amos, eds. Zinsser Microbiology. 18th Ed. Norwalk, Conn: Appleton-Century-Crofts, 1984: 583–93.
4. Baker RD, ed. Human Infections with Fungi, Actinomycetes, and Algae. New York: Springer Verlag, 1971.
5. Howard DH, ed. Fungi Pathogenic for Humans and Animals. New York: Marcel Dekker, 1983.
6. Cope VZ. What Every Practitioner Ought to Know About Human Actinomycosis. London: Heinemann Medical Books, 1955.
7. Slack JM, Gerencser MA. *Actinomyces*, Filamentous Bacteria. Minneapolis: Burgess Publishing, 1975.
8. Goodfellow M, Minnikin DE. Nocardiform bacteria. Annu Rev Microbiol 1977; 31:159–80.
9. Mackenzie DWR. Yeasts from human sources. Sabouraudia 1961; 1:8–15.
10. Balish E, Phillips AW. Growth, morphogenesis and virulence of *Candida albicans* after oral inoculation in the germfree and conventional chick. J Bacteriol 1966; 91:1736–43.
11. Helstrom PB, Balish E. Effect of oral tetracycline, the microbial flora, and the athymic state on gastrointestinal colonization and infection of BALB/c mice with *Candida albicans*. Infect Immun 1979; 23:764–74.
12. Johnson WJ, Balish E. Macrophage function in germfree, athymic (nu/nu), and conventional-flora mice (nu/+) mice. J Reticuloendothel Soc 1980; 18:55–65.
13. Pope LM, Cole GT, Guentzel MN, Berry LJ. Systemic and gastrointestinal candidiasis in infant mice after intragastric challenge. Infect Immun 1979; 25:702–7.
14. Field LH, Pope LM, Cole GT, Guentzel MN, Berry, LJ. Persistence and spread of *Candida albicans* after intragastric inoculation of infant mice. Infect Immun 1981; 31:783–91.
15. McGinnis MR. Laboratory Handbook of Medical Mycology. New York: Academic Press, 1980.
16. Hector RF, Domer JE, Carrow EW. Immune responses to *Candida albicans* in genetically distinct mice. Infect Immun 1982; 38:1020–8.
17. Lehrer RI, Howard DH, Sypherd PS, Edwards JH, Segal GP, Winston DJ. Mucormycosis. Ann Intern Med 1980; 93:93–108.
18. Meyer RD, Rosen P, Armstrong D. Phycomycosis complicating leukemia and lymphoma. Ann Intern Med 1972; 77:871–9.
19. Calle S, Klatsky S. Intestinal phycomycosis (mucormycosis). Am J Clin Pathol 1966; 45:264–72.
20. Kahn LB. Gastric mucormycosis: report of a case with a review of the literature. S Afr Med J 1963; 37:1265–9.
21. Deal WB, Johnson JE. Gastric phycomycosis: report of a case and review of the literature. Gastroenterology 1969; 57:579–86.
22. Sartir AA, Alla MD, Mahgoub S, Musa AR. Systemic phycomycosis. Br Med J 1971; 1:440.
23. Lawson HH, Schmaman A. Gastric phycomycosis. Br J Surg 1974; 61:743–6.
24. Dannheimer IP, Fouche W, Nel C. Gastric mucormycosis in a diabetic patient. S Afr Med J 1974; 48:838–9.
25. Raper KB, Fennell DI. The Genus *Aspergillus*. Baltimore: Williams & Wilkins, 1965.
26. Ross DA, MacNaughton MC, Stewart WK. Fulminating disseminated aspergillosis complicating peritoneal dialysis in eclampsia. Arch Intern Med 1968; 121:183–8.
27. Schaffner A, Douglas H, Braude AI, Davis CE. Killing of *Aspergillus* spores depends on the anatomical source of the macrophage. Infect Immun 1983; 42:1109–15.
28. Diamond RD, Huber E, Haudenschild CC. Mechanism of destruction of *Aspergillus fumigatus* hyphae mediated by human monocytes. J Infect Dis 1983; 147:474–82.
29. Meadow M, Tripple M, Rippon J. Endophthalmitis caused by *Petriellidium boydii*. First report of a pediatric case. Am J Dis Child 1981; 135:378–80.
30. Schimpff SC, Bennett JE. Abnormalities in cell-mediated immunity in patients with *Cryptococcus neoformans* infection. J Allergy Clin Med 1975; 58:430–41.
31. Kwon-Chung KJ, Polacheck I, Bennett JE. Improved diagnostic medium for separation of *Cryptococcus neoformans* var. *neoformans* (serotypes A and D) and *Cyptococcus neoformans* var. *gattii* (serotypes B and C). J Clin Microbiol 1982; 15:535–7.

32. Polacheck I, Hearing VJ, Kwon-Chung KJ. Biochemical studies of phenoloxidase and utilization of catecholamines in *Cryptococcus neoformans.* J Bacteriol 1982; 150:1212–20.
33. Kwon-Chung KJ, Polacheck I, Popkin TJ. Melanin-lacking mutants of *Cryptococcus neoformans* and their virulence in mice. J Bacteriol 1982; 150:1414–21.
34. Bennett JE, Kwon-Chung KJ, Howard DH. Epidemiologic differences among serotypes of *Cryptococcus neoformans.* Am J Epidemiol 1977; 105:582–6.
35. Kwon-Chung KJ, Bennett JE. Epidemiologic differences between the two varieties of *Cryptococcus neoformans.* Am J Epidemiol 1984; 120:123–30.
36. Al-Doory Y. The Epidemiology of Human Mycotic Diseases. Springfield, Ill: Charles C Thomas, 1975.
37. Howard DH. The epidemiology and ecology of blastomycosis, coccidioidomycosis and histoplasmosis. Zbl Bakt Hyg 1984; A257:219–27.
38. Wilson JW, Plunkett OA. The Fungous Diseases of Man. Berkeley, Cal: University of California Press, 1965.
39. Drutz DJ, Huppert M. Coccidioidomycosis: factors affecting the host-parasite interaction. J Infect Dis 1983; 147:372–90.
40. Pappagianis D. Epidemiology of coccidioidomycosis. *In*: Stevens DA, ed. Coccidioidomycosis. New York: Plenum Medical, 1980: 63–85.

Chapter 101

Clinical Manifestations and Evaluation of Malabsorption

Martin H. Kalser

Malabsorption syndromes include a large heterogeneous group of disorders with the common characteristic of failure to assimilate one or more ingested foodstuffs normally. The defect is characterized by decreased or impaired function of almost any organ of the gut, including the liver, biliary tract, pancreas, and lymphatic system, as well as the intestine. There are important interrelationships such as, for example, the need of a normal ileum for fat assimilation even though the latter actually takes place in the jejunum. The clinical manifestations may vary from a severe symptom complex of weight loss, diarrhea, distention, and asthenia to symptoms of an isolated deficiency, such as occult anemia. The clinical approach is to identify the cause and the diseased organ, followed by appropriate therapy. Clinical suspicion originates in the history and physical examination. The routine hemogram and biochemical profile can give important clues by the presence of certain deficiencies in the blood, but more specialized tests of absorption are usually needed to help quantitate and identify the specific absorptive defect. Imaging techniques varying from barium meal studies to the more sophisticated procedures of ultrasonography and computed tomography, endoscopic procedures such as enteroscopy, and biopsy of the small bowel may be required to establish a definitive diagnosis.

Classification

The general classification of malabsorption syndromes is based on the site of defect of fat assimilation (Table 101–1). The *intraluminal phase* consists of 2 subphases: (1) the *lipolytic*, representing failure of pancreatic enzyme secretions to reach the duodenum in adequate concentration, and (2) the *micellar*, due to inadequate duodenal concentrations of conjugated bile salts. This phase can result from disease of the liver, biliary tract, or ileum or from jejunal bacterial overgrowth. Defects in the lipolytic phase are referred to as *maldigestion*, since the major defect is in the breakdown of large molecules. *Mucosal cell disease (mucosal phase)* results in several defects, including brush border enzyme deficiencies, uptake of various substances from the intestinal lumen, resynthesis of triglycerides, or formation of chylomicrons. Retroperitoneal lymphatic disease results in defect of delivery (*delivery phase*) of the fat containing chylomicrons to the lymph. A more complete classification is given in Table 101–2.

Table 101–1. DEFECTS OF FAT ASSIMILATION

Intraluminal defects
- Digestion
  - Pancreatic insufficiency (inflammation, malignancy, cystic fibrosis)
  - Acid pH (Zollinger-Ellison syndrome)
  - Inadequate mixing (postgastrectomy)
  - Excessive dilution
- Micelle formation
  - Decreased bile salt concentration
    - Liver disease
    - Biliary tract obstruction
    - Ileal dysfunction (resection or disease)
  - Deconjugation of bile salts
    - Bacterial overgrowth (blind loop syndrome)

Mucosal cell disease
- Primary (celiac and tropical sprue)
- Systemic disease
- Drug-induced
- Parasitic
- Malignancy
- Protein malnutrition
- Inflammatory disease

Delivery
- Lymphatic obstruction
- Chylomicron deficiency

Presentation

The classic presentation of malabsorption syndromes is of progressive weight loss, diarrhea, distention, weakness, and symptoms of specific deficiencies such as bleeding, tetany, or paresthesias. However, the full clinical syndrome in all of its manifestations may not be present.

Some degree of diarrhea and isolated deficiencies can be the presenting factors in malabsorption of intestinal etiology (Table 101–3). A macrocytic anemia developing during pregnancy may herald latent celiac disease. The anemia results from deficient folate absorption and hence insufficient folate to respond to the increased demands of the fetus. With duodenal and jejunal mucosal disease, microcytic anemia due to faulty iron absorption may be the only finding. Isolated impairment of vitamin B_{12} and macrocytic anemia without malabsorption of other substances also occur. Celiac disease may present as a bleeding diathesis (vitamin K malabsorption) or as bone pain without pathologic fractures (vitamin D and calcium malabsorption).

Evaluation

The objectives of the evaluation are to determine which organ is involved and the

Table 101–2. PHYSIOLOGIC AND DISEASE CLASSIFICATION OF MALABSORPTION SYNDROMES

- Maldigestion
  - Deficient pancreatic secretion
    - Chronic pancreatitis
    - Pancreatic malignancy
    - Cystic fibrosis
  - Physiochemical defect
    - Inadequate mixing (postgastrectomy)
      - Enzyme inactivation
      - Low pH (Zollinger-Ellison syndrome)
    - Congenital enterokinase deficiency
  - Brush border enzyme (small oligo molecule substrate)
    - Disaccharidase deficiencies
      - Lactase
      - Sucrase-isomaltase
      - Trehalase
- Malabsorption
  - Intraluminal defects
    - Bacterial overgrowth (blind loop syndrome)
    - Hepatocellular disease
    - Cholestasis, intra- or extrahepatic
    - Ileal dysfunction syndrome
      - Ileal resection > 3 ft
      - Diffuse ileal disease
  - Mucosal cell disease
    - Primary
      - Celiac sprue (gluten enteropathy)
      - Tropical sprue
    - Short bowel syndrome
      - Massive distal resection
      - Congenital
    - Endocrinopathies
      - Diabetes mellitus
      - Hypoparathyroidism
      - Thyrotoxicosis
      - Adrenocortical insufficiency
    - Drug-induced
      - Neomycin
      - Colchicine
    - Inflammatory
      - Acute bacterial enteritis
      - Crohn's disease
    - Malignancy
      - Lymphoma
        - Intestinal
        - Extraintestinal
      - Adenocarcinoma
      - Gut (esophagus, stomach)
      - Extraintestinal carcinoma
  - Dermatologic disease
    - Dermatitis herpetiformis
    - Psoriasis
    - Kohler-Dager syndrome
- Vascular
  - Radiation enteritis
  - Chronic mesenteric vascular insufficiency
- Systemic disorders
  - Dysgammaglobulinemia, heavy chain
  - Protein malnutrition
  - Amyloidosis
  - Mastocytosis
  - Collagen vascular (disseminated lupus erythematosus, scleroderma)
- Allergic
  - Milk allergy (infants)
  - Allergic protein-losing gastroenteropathy
- Unknown etiology
  - Whipple's disease
  - Collagenous sprue
  - Idiopathic steatorrhea
  - Pseudo-obstruction
  - Paneth cell deficiency
  - Congenital malrotation of intestine
- Lymphatic obstruction
  - Retroperitoneal malignancy
  - Congestive heart failure (severe right side)
  - Intestinal lymphangiectasia
- Genetic disorders (single enzyme)
  - Amino acid
    - Hartnup disease
    - Cysteinuria
    - Others
  - Mineral
    - Vitamin D–deficient rickets
    - Magnesium deficiency
    - Chloridorrhea
  - Vitamins
    - Selective vitamin B_{12} malabsorption
  - Fat
    - Abetalipoproteinemia
  - Carbohydrate
    - Glucose-galactose malabsorption

Table 101–3. PRESENTING SYMPTOMS IN MALABSORPTION SYNDROMES

Symptom	Laboratory Findings	Defect	Organ
Weight loss	Steatorrhea	Fat assimilation	Pancreas Small intestine Liver Biliary tract
Weakness	Anemia	Iron transport Folate transport Vitamin B_{12} absorption	Duodenum Jejunum Ileum
Diarrhea	Hypokalemia Hyponatremia	Water and electrolyte secretion	Jejunum Ileum
Bleeding	Abnormal prothrombin	Fat assimilation	Jejunum Ileum Liver Biliary tract
Tetany Osteomalacia	Hypocalcemia Hypophosphatemia High bone alkaline phosphatase	Vitamin D absorption Calcium absorption	Jejunum Ileum Liver Biliary tract
Edema	Hypoalbuminemia	Protein malabsorption Protein-losing enteropathy	Jejunum Ileum Retroperitoneum Lymph nodes

specific cause and then to institute appropriate therapy. The evaluation of malabsorption begins with the history and physical examination.

History and Physical Examination. There are several historical facts that provide a clue to the basis for malabsorption. A childhood history of diarrhea and failure to thrive is consistent with celiac disease (Chapter 105). A folate-deficient megaloblastic anemia developing during pregnancy suggests the same diagnosis. Celiac disease may first be manifest after surgery. Prolonged residence in tropical areas associated with longstanding diarrhea may suggest tropical sprue (Chapter 106). Diarrhea beginning with travel to certain endemic areas of the world suggests the possibility of giardiasis (Chapter 232). Symptoms of peptic ulcer associated with diarrhea and malabsorption are found in patients with the Zollinger-Ellison syndrome (Chapter 70). Previous gastric resection could mean that a bacterial overgrowth syndrome is present in the afferent loop (Chapter 107), while prior surgery on the small bowel for Crohn's disease alerts one to the possibility of short bowel syndrome (Chapter 108). The presence of early age onset of diabetes would be consistent with diabetic enteropathy.

Several skin disorders are sometimes associated with intestinal malabsorption. *Dermatitis herpetiformis* is seen with celiac disease (Chapter 105) and *scleroderma* may affect the entire gut, with small bowel stasis leading to jejunal bacterial overgrowth (Chapter 107). Peripheral neuropathy in a young man with a history of juvenile diabetes, diarrhea, and postural hypotension is consistent with diabetic enteropathy with an autonomic neuropathy. Lymphadenopathy may suggest retroperitoneal involvement, which could contribute to malabsorption. Positive Chvostek and Trousseau signs would indicate calcium malabsorption.

Hemogram and Biochemical Profile. The hemogram, including the red blood cell indices, can indicate whether a microcytic or macrocytic anemia is present. The anemia can be further classified by more specialized tests. A low prothrombin concentration in the absence of the hepatic dysfunction may indicate vitamin K malabsorption. In the biochemical profile, hypoalbuminemia may indicate protein loss through the gut or protein malabsorption. Hypocalcemia, with hypophosphatemia and elevated bone alkaline phosphatase, indicates biochemical osteomalacia, which in turn is highly suggestive of vitamin D and calcium malabsorption. Serum cholesterol is low in intestinal malabsorption as well as in liver disease and malnutrition in general. Hypokalemia may indicate increased fecal potassium loss from excess diarrhea.

Special Biochemical Tests. Once the diagnosis of intestinal malabsorption is suspected, special tests should be obtained (Chapter 27). A serum carotene level below 50 mg/dl is consistent with malabsorption. This should be interpreted as a screening rather than a specific test of intestinal dysfunction. The serum *magnesium* concentration must be followed in any patient with low calcium levels, since hypocalcemia may not respond to replacement therapy if low magnesium stores are not replaced.

The *oral 25-g* D-*xylose test* is a very useful and specific test for jejunal function, although it is also abnormal in some cases of bacterial overgrowth syndrome. Normal gastric emptying and renal function, as well as complete urinary collection, are necessary for a valid test. In most laboratories, the normal urinary 5-hour D-xylose content is greater than 4 or 4.5 g.

When anemia is found, *serum iron, iron binding capacity, folate,* and *vitamin* B_{12} levels should be obtained. Serum folate is a sensitive indicator of jejunal dysfunction since it is absorbed in the jejunum and body stores are limited. Iron absorption occurs primarily in the duodenum and may be impaired with duodenal-jejunal mucosal disease. Low serum vitamin B_{12} levels may be indicative of longstanding ileal disease, since this vitamin is absorbed in the distal ileum and body stores are conserved by the enterohepatic circulation and storage in the liver. Other causes of low serum vitamin B_{12} concentrations, such as pernicious anemia, must be ruled out.

Fecal fat should be determined in any type of malabsorption disorder. The various methods are discussed in Chapter 27. The microscopic examination, although qualitative, can be semi-quantitative when performed by experienced observers. The 72-hour fecal collection with determination of total fecal fatty acids and expressed as grams of neutral fat per day is probably the most accurate clinical method if properly done with adequate fat intake and complete stool collection.

Glucose and *lactose tolerance* tests have limited use in the evaluation of generalized intestinal malabsorption syndromes. A "flat" glucose tolerance curve with maximal elevation of blood glucose above fasting of 40 mg/dl is seen in jejunal mucosal disease but is non-specific. The lactose tolerance test may be of use in certain cases of disaccharidase malabsorption (Chapter 104).

Tests for Parasites. Examination for parasites such as giardia should be done when there is clinical suspicion (Chapter 232).

Imaging Procedures. Barium study of the small bowel is essential as part of the initial evaluation of any patient with suspected malabsorption. This can help localize the disease and possibly suggest a specific diagnosis, e.g., multiple jejunal diverticula, as a cause of bacterial overgrowth syndrome. The radiologic changes of malabsorption syndromes are discussed in Chapter 102. If lymphoma is suspected, abdominal ultrasonography or computed tomography is indicated.

Enteroscopy. This procedure makes possible gross visualization of abnormalities of the distal jejunum and establishment of the specific area of disease, from which biopsy samples can be obtained (Chapter 103). This has an advantage over peroral blind biopsy in that the areas of involvement in some mucosal disorders are patchy.

Small Bowel Biopsy. This is an essential procedure whenever the clinical work-up is suggestive of intestinal malabsorption due to involvement of jejunal mucosa in such entities as celiac disease, tropical sprue, or giardiasis. The capsule peroral biopsy instruments are the ones in common use and can provide a good specimen. The details of the technique are given in Chapter 47, while its role in malabsorption syndromes is discussed in Chapter 103.

Special Tests (Chapter 27). These tests may not be available in all institutions, but can be of help in proper diagnosis of specific entities.

The *Schilling test* is used in suspected vitamin B_{12} malabsorption. With the use of commercially available dual radioisotopes, the cause of vitamin B_{12} deficiencies can be readily elucidated. Briefly, one test preparation of vitamin B_{12}, labeled with a cobalt isotope, is bound to human gastric juice, while the other preparation is unbound vitamin B_{12}, labeled with another cobalt isotope. The urinary excretion of each isotope can be determined independently. In ileal dysfunction or bacterial overgrowth syndrome, excretion of both forms is low. In the latter disease, bowel sterilization can restore absorption to normal levels.

The *hydrogen breath test* is used in the diagnosis of suspected disaccharidase deficiency and bacterial overgrowth syndrome. The basis of the test is that bacteria ferment sugars into hydrogen and volatile fatty acids.

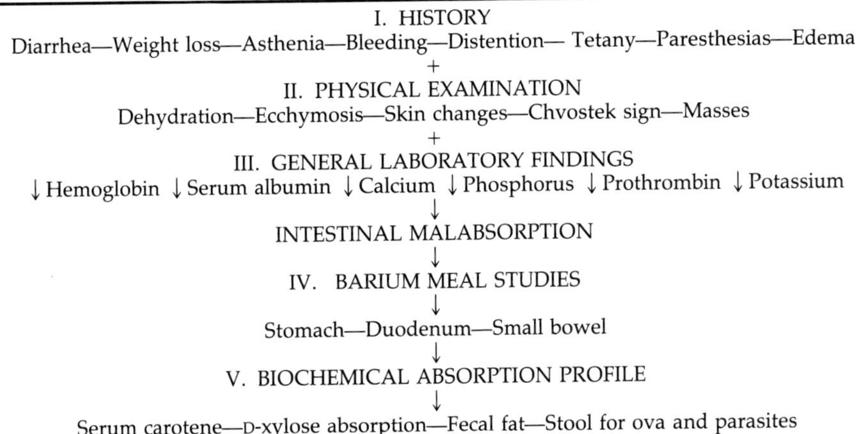

Figure 101–1. Approach to evaluation of malabsorption syndromes.

Expired hydrogen is measured after ingestion of a test sugar, such as lactose, in patients suspected of having lactase deficiency.

The *bile acid breath test* is used if there is suspected bile acid malabsorption due to ileal dysfunction or bacterial overgrowth syndrome. The basis of the test is that the amino acid (glycine) part of the conjugated bile salt molecule is labeled with ^{14}C glycine (cholyl-^{14}C glycine). Bacteria deconjugate and metabolize the glycine to $^{14}CO_2$, which is then expired. With ileal dysfunction, an excess of the conjugated bile salts reaches the colon, where colonic bacteria metabolize these salts. With bacterial overgrowth syndrome, the excess coliform bacteria in the jejunum deconjugate the bile salts.

The *^{14}C-D-xylose-radioactive breath test* has been introduced as a specific and sensitive test to diagnose bacterial overgrowth syndrome (Chapter 107). It is based on the fact that certain bacteria, when present in the jejunum in very high concentrations, metabolize D-xylose before it is absorbed.

Overview

A systematic approach (Fig. 101–1) is necessary to evaluate and establish the diagnosis in patients with possible malabsorption syndromes. A history of several symptoms, such as weight loss, diarrhea, weakness, fatigue, bleeding tendencies, bone pain, paresthesias, distention, or dependent edema, should arouse suspicion. Physical examination can be consistent with these symptoms. The general laboratory evaluation may disclose a microcytic or macrocytic anemia, decreased prothrombin concentration, hypoalbuminemia, hypokalemia, or hypocalcemia. Stool examination may disclose ova of *Giardia lamblia*. If pancreatic dysfunction appears to be the primary disease process, this should be pursued as outlined in Chapter 208. If suspicion remains of primary intestinal dysfunction, a barium meal study of the stomach, duodenum, jejunum, and ileum is carried out (Chapter 102). Specific tests of absorption can then be obtained. The latter include serum carotene concentration, 25-g D-xylose oral tolerance test, serum magnesium, serum folate, and vitamin B_{12} levels, and fecal fat determination. If the evaluation still suggests intestinal disease, jejunal biopsy must be obtained. This can be accomplished either by the peroral technique (Chapter 47) or by enteroscopy (Chapter 103). A more careful investigation for ova and parasites should also be done in such individuals (Chapter 232).

More highly specialized tests are available and have value in specific syndromes. The hydrogen breath test with an oral sugar load is of help in establishing the diagnosis of disaccharide deficiency. It is also used in suspected bacterial overgrowth syndromes. The radioactive conjugated bile salt absorption test (cholyl-^{14}C glycine) is used when there is suspected impairment of bile salt reabsorption with ileal dysfunction and also in the bacterial overgrowth syndrome. In addition to these tests, the ^{14}C-D-xylose breath test is specific for the diagnosis of bacterial overgrowth syndrome. The dual isotope Schilling test is used to determine more exactly the cause of vitamin B_{12} deficiency.

Finally, in difficult cases a therapeutic trial, such as a gluten-free diet for suspected celiac disease, may be the final pathway of establishing the definite diagnosis.

Chapter 102

Radiologic Features of Malabsorption Syndromes

Igor Laufer • Hans Herlinger

The radiologic examination of the small bowel in patients with known or suspected malabsorption can have 2 basic purposes: (1) the radiologic demonstration of a malabsorption pattern may be the first clue to the presence of a malabsorption state in patients with vague symptoms, such as abdominal pain, change in bowel habits, anemia, fatigue, or weight loss; and (2) in patients in whom the presence of a malabsorption state has been established by virtue of typical symptoms and biochemical findings, the role of the radiologic examination is to demonstrate or rule out an organic cause for the malabsorption and to detect any possible complications.

The "Malabsorption Pattern"[1,2]

Normally, the fine barium particles are kept in suspension by a combination of electrostatic surface charges and suspending agents. On radiographs, the small bowel will be seen as a more or less continuous barium column with a feathery mucosal pattern (Fig. 102–1). In most malabsorption states, there is an excess of fluid and mucus within the small bowel, resulting in the eventual clumping and flocculation of the barium particles. The typical radiographic features of the malabsorption pattern may be seen; these include *fragmentation* or *segmentation* of the barium column within dilated small bowel. The feathery mucosal pattern is lost because the flocculated barium can no longer depict the mucosal surface of the small bowel.[3] The "*moulage phenomenon*" refers to the featureless, toothpaste-like appearance of the barium suspension in loops of small bowel. This is an expression of the same flocculation process (Fig. 102–2) and is rarely seen with modern barium suspensions.

The degree and rapidity of flocculation depend on the amount of fluid and mucus within the small bowel; flocculation may be minimized by increasing the amount of barium entering the small bowel and by accelerating its transit. The *small bowel enema* (enteroclysis) is particularly valuable for this purpose. The infusion of the barium suspension directly into the small bowel results in transit that is sufficiently rapid to allow for

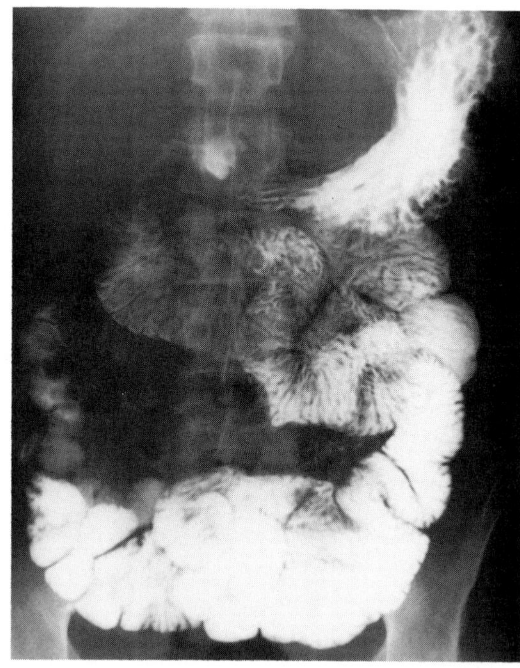

Figure 102–1. Normal small bowel. Note the feathery appearance of the mucosa of the small bowel as seen on a meal roentgenogram.

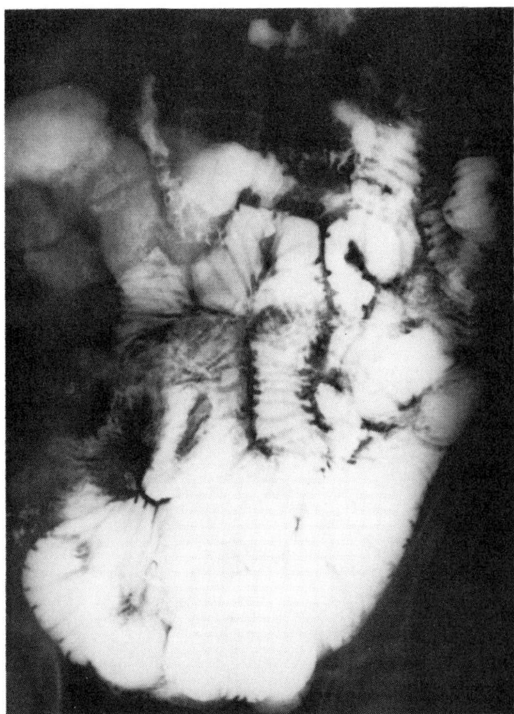

Figure 102–2. Malabsorption pattern. The small bowel is moderately dilated, with dilution and flocculation of the barium suspension in the proximal small bowel.

adequate imaging in most cases before significant flocculation occurs (Fig. 102–3).

The malabsorption pattern is most frequently seen in patients with celiac disease, although it may be found in other malabsorption states associated with hypersecretion, in Crohn's disease, in lymphoma, and occasionally in normal persons. It should be noted that the increased accumulation of normal fluid in the small bowel, as in patients with obstruction due to adhesions, usually does not result in flocculation of the barium suspension.

Barium Studies in Malabsorption

Certain basic guidelines must be observed in any type of barium study of the small bowel: (1) A sufficient quantity of a flocculation-resistant barium suspension of suitable density should enter the small bowel as rapidly as possible; (2) its passage through the small bowel should be accelerated; and (3) reliance must not be placed on survey films alone. Compression films taken during intermittent fluoroscopy are essential.

There are 2 general techniques that can be used to examine the small bowel:

1. *The small bowel meal* is a modification of the conventional small bowel follow-through study. A large quantity (500 to 600 ml) of a 50% w/v suspension of barium is ingested after the oral or IV administration of metoclopramide. The intent is to have a large bolus of barium pass quickly out of the stomach and through the small bowel. The upper gastrointestinal tract can be examined by single contrast during the administration of the barium. Intermittent fluoroscopy and compression spot films are required to study and record the filling and emptying of all small bowel loops. A drawback is that this method, however carefully applied, will prove to be inadequate in the more severe malabsorption states because of the frequent development of barium flocculation before imaging can be completed. In such patients, a small bowel enema (enteroclysis) is often required.

2. *Small bowel enema (enteroclysis).* In this study, a modified Bilbao-Dotter tube is passed beyond the ligament of Treitz into the proximal jejunum. A single-contrast study can be performed by the injection of barium through the tube until all loops of

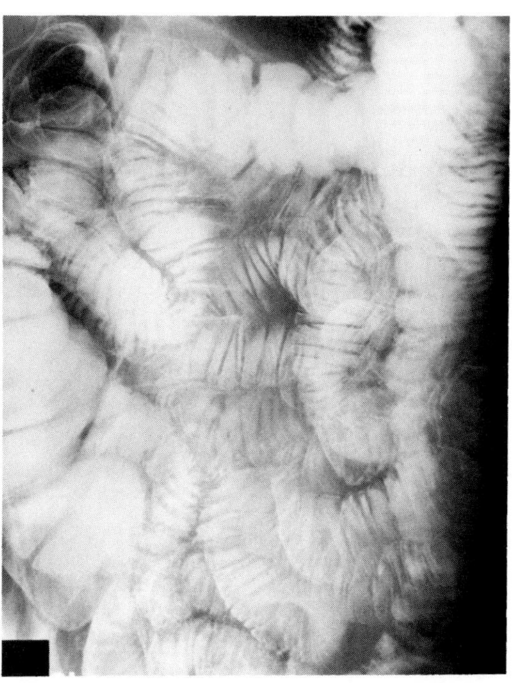

Figure 102–3. Small bowel enema in a patient with celiac disease. There is granularity and dilution of the barium suspension. However, because of the rapid transit, intestinal morphologic features can still be demonstrated.

small bowel are visualized.[4] Alternatively, a higher density barium can be injected and followed by a 0.5% solution of methylcellulose to obtain a double-contrast effect.[5] Both variations of this technique allow for the demonstration of anatomic detail throughout the small bowel before the abnormal intestinal contents destroy the imaging capacity of the barium suspension.

Radiographic Abnormalities in Malabsorption

Some of the common causes of malabsorption may produce either no detectable radiographic abnormality or only a minimal increase in intraluminal fluid. In other cases, the barium study may show a focal abnormality causing malabsorption, either by short circuiting the small bowel (as through an enteric fistula), or by bacterial overgrowth within blind loops (as in jejunal diverticulosis) (Fig. 102–4).

Diffuse disease of the small bowel may be more difficult to evaluate. However, the small bowel is capable of only a relatively limited number of responses to disease states. The major radiographic features are an increase of lumen diameter and abnormalities of the small bowel fold pattern.[6] The small bowel folds may be thick and straight or they may be unevenly thickened with nodulation. All of these abnormalities may be seen with or without evidence of fluid increase. These general characteristics will help to narrow the differential diagnosis. However, additional features such as distribution of disease, ulceration, bowel wall thickening, and abnormalities of peristalsis should be sought and may help to identify the underlying pathologic condition.

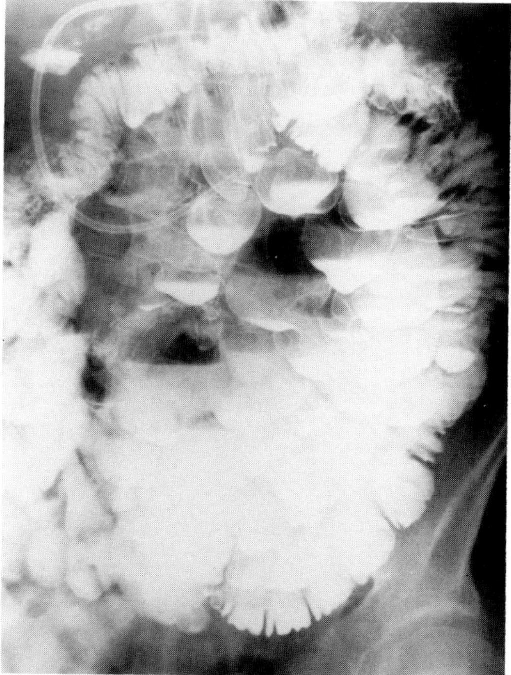

Figure 102–4. Jejunal diverticulosis. An upright film shows barium-fluid-air levels within multiple jejunal diverticula.

Table 102–1 lists, in abbreviated form, the differential diagnosis of the causes of malabsorption based on the predominant radiologic finding. The conditions are further subdivided into those that have an increase in intraluminal fluid and those that do not. In the following section, celiac disease is used as the model to illustrate the radiologic issues that arise in patients with malabsorption states. There are also short discussions of other malabsorptive states that have radiologic manifestations of interest.

Celiac Disease (Non-tropical Sprue, Gluten Enteropathy)

(Chapter 105)

The radiologic problems in the diagnosis of malabsorption can be illustrated with one of the most common causes of malabsorption, celiac disease. In severe cases, the small bowel meal shows only the non-specific signs of a malabsorption syndrome, such as dilatation, dilution, and segmentation (see Fig. 102–2). This pattern, as noted, is essentially a reflection of the excess fluid and mucus within the lumen of the small bowel causing disintegration of the barium column. Under these circumstances, accurate imaging of small bowel morphologic features is not possible. By using the small bowel enema technique, rapid transit of barium through the small bowel is achieved, allowing for adequate morphologic imaging before disintegration of the barium column. In uncomplicated cases of celiac disease, the small bowel enema may be normal or may show only minimal dilatation, dilution, and granularity of the barium (see Fig. 102–3).

In most patients with celiac disease, a normal circular fold pattern will be present throughout the small bowel. The effects of intraluminal fluid on flocculation of the bar-

Table 102–1. RADIOLOGIC FEATURES OF DISORDERS ASSOCIATED WITH MALABSORPTION

Radiologic Feature	No Fluid Increase	Fluid Increase
Normal	Maldigestion—bile salt or pancreatic enzyme deficiency Alactasia	Celiac disease Tropical sprue Dermatitis herpetiformis
Dilatation	Gastric surgery Scleroderma Dermatomyositis Pseudo-obstruction	Celiac disease
Folds—thickened, straight	Amyloidosis Radiation Macroglobulinemia Eosinophilic gastroenteritis	Zollinger-Ellison syndrome Abetalipoproteinemia
Folds—unevenly thickened, nodulation	Lymphoid hyperplasia Lymphoma Crohn's disease Whipple's disease Mastocytosis	Lymphangiectasia Giardiasis
Other structural lesions	Fistula Resection	Stricture Diverticulosis Blind loop

ium suspension may give a misleading impression of fold thickening. However, in the presence of hypoalbuminemia there may be thickening of the small bowel folds due to edema throughout the small intestine. Dilation of the lumen, most pronounced in the jejunum, is a frequent finding and correlates well with the severity of the disease process.[7] Jejunal dilatation has also been shown to occur in hypoalbuminemic states of other causes.[8] Intussusceptions are frequently seen during fluoroscopy in patients with celiac disease. They are usually transient and do not cause obstruction.[9] After successful treatment with a gluten-free diet, symptoms abate and the radiologic abnormalities return to normal.

The radiologic presentation of *tropical sprue*, of the rare enteropathy associated with *dermatitis herpetiformis*, and of *hypogammaglobulinemic sprue* or *collagenous sprue* can be indistinguishable from that of celiac disease.[10]

Another important role of radiology in patients with celiac disease is the demonstration of complications of the disease. Complications may be heralded by the loss of response to gluten withdrawal or by the development of abdominal pain, weight loss, or fever. The mucosal changes indicating these complications can often be missed during small bowel meal examination because of the presence of flocculation so that a more detailed examination of the small bowel, i.e., an intubation study, is often necessary.

It is now well recognized that there is an increased frequency of malignancy of the small bowel and esophagus in patients with celiac disease.[11,12] The small bowel malignancy may be either a lymphoma or a carcinoma. *Lymphoma* engrafted on celiac disease tends to be more widely spread throughout the small bowel than is true of primary lymphoma.[13] There may be a variety of radiologic manifestations, including nodular thickening of folds (Fig. 102–5), intraluminal nodules of varying sizes, infiltration of the bowel wall, and mesenteric masses. *Carcinoma* may present as either a polypoid mass or an annular stricture with destruction of the mucosa. *Ulcerative jejunoileitis* is a poorly understood condition that may be associated with celiac disease.[14] It may present as widespread inflammation throughout the small bowel resembling Crohn's disease. Other patients have focal ulceration that may go on to perforation or to stricture formation. The duodenum can also be involved.

Diseases Characterized Primarily by Dilatation

A variety of diseases presenting with malabsorption have as their prime radiologic

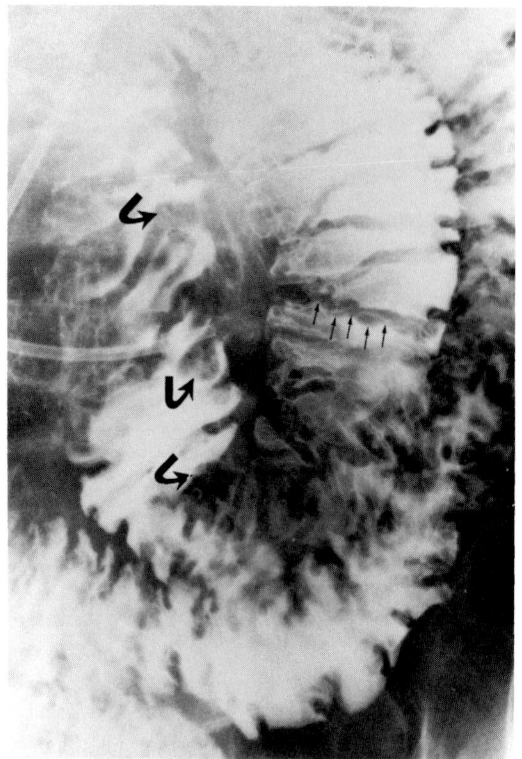

Figure 102–5. Lymphoma complicating celiac disease. A small bowel enema shows nodules *(curved arrows)* and nodular folds *(straight arrows)* as manifestations of lymphoma complicating celiac disease.

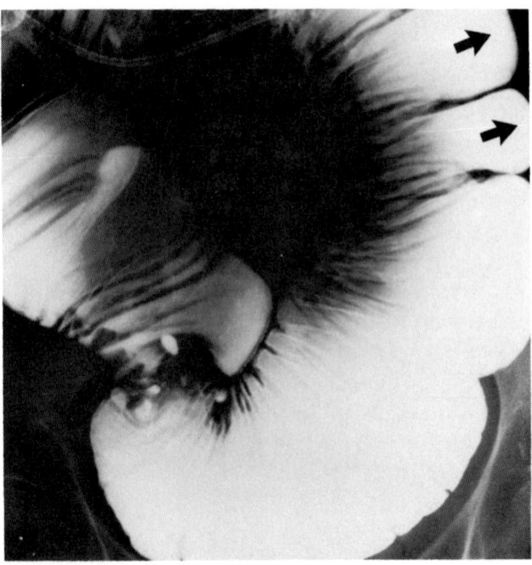

Figure 102–6. Systemic sclerosis. The small bowel is dilated with crowding of folds of normal width. This is the so-called "hide-bound" appearance of the small bowel. There are also wide-necked diverticula *(arrows)* characteristic of systemic sclerosis.

feature either focal or diffuse dilatation of the small bowel.

Scleroderma or *systemic sclerosis* has been reported to affect the small bowel in 57% of patients.[15] Half of these patients have mild steatorrhea. Fibrosis of the muscular layers of the bowel results in a hypotonic, dilated small bowel. The duodenum and upper jejunum are most often affected and hypersecretion is not a feature. The combination of luminal dilatation and tightly packed, thin, circular folds results in an appearance that has been called the *"hide-bound bowel"* (Fig. 102–6); this appearance is quite characteristic of scleroderma.[16] Wide-mouthed diverticula may be seen in the small bowel and in the colon as a result of asymmetric fibrosis in the bowel wall.[17] Occasionally, pneumatosis intestinalis may develop and may produce an asymptomatic pneumoperitoneum.[18]

Chronic intestinal pseudo-obstruction (Chapter 123) is a condition in which clinical symptoms suggest the presence of a bowel obstruction but no obstruction exists. It may be secondary to systemic diseases, such as systemic sclerosis, amyloidosis, or hypokalemia. There is also an idiopathic form in which no primary cause is found. Although the entire gastrointestinal tract may be affected, small bowel involvement usually predominates. Virtually all patients have esophageal involvement with aperistalsis and failure of relaxation of the lower esophageal sphincter.[19] Radiology is crucial in establishing the diagnosis since diagnostic laparotomy, with its potential for the formation of adhesions requiring repetitive surgery, should be avoided.[19] Barium studies show esophageal aperistalsis and dilated, fluid-filled small bowel that is either atonic or exhibits ineffective, non-propulsive contractions. The barium will ultimately be seen to enter the colon with no abrupt point of transition from dilated small bowel to bowel of normal caliber. Chronic stasis in the small bowel leads to bacterial overgrowth, malabsorption, and steatorrhea. It may take many days for the flocculated barium to be cleared from the intestinal tract.

Diseases Characterized by Fold Thickening

Folds in the small bowel may be thickened because of accumulation of fluid, blood, inflammatory exudate, tumor, or other infiltrate within the mucosa or submucosa of the bowel. Radiologically, the thickened folds may be straight and uniform or they may be uneven and nodular.

Uniform thickening of the small bowel folds results in a configuration that has been termed "stacked-coin" or "picket fence" because of its appearance.[6] This configuration is characteristically seen in patients with intramural *hemorrhage* or *ischemia* resulting in edema and hemorrhage in the bowel wall. However, these are generally acute events that do not result in chronic malabsorption with steatorrhea. Occasionally, milder forms of ischemia may produce epigastric pain and a mild degree of malabsorption. Barium studies in this situation may show no abnormality.[20]

Amyloid deposition in the small bowel frequently produces diarrhea, but malabsorption is uncommon. Barium studies show general and regular thickening of the folds and decreased peristaltic activity.[21] If amyloid is deposited into the muscularis propria, dilatation results. There is no fluid increase and therefore no flocculation. Rarely, amyloid deposits may coalesce to form multiple tumor-like masses.

Malabsorption with *steatorrhea* is an uncommon presentation in *Waldenström's macroglobulinemia*.[22] Barium studies have been reported to show diffuse fold thickening with punctate filling defects. The latter are caused by enlarged villi that contain amorphous material, believed to be macroglobulin.

Barium studies should be requested in patients with *Whipple's disease* only if the symptoms indicate small bowel involvement (Chapter 109). This need not be an early feature of this multisystem disease. Barium studies have been reported as normal in 13% of patients.[23] Most of the small bowel examinations showed coarse and irregular folds in the duodenum and jejunum, occasionally extending into the ileum (Fig. 102–7). Dilatation of the jejunum and increase in fluid do occur but are of moderate degree.[24] Occasionally, a pebble-like appearance of the mucosal surface has been found,[25] believed to be caused by enlarged villi. In a few patients, films of the abdomen may also show abnormality in the sacroiliac joints.

Intestinal lymphangiectasia is a protein-losing enteropathy due to congenital malformation of intestinal lymphatics or secondary to an infective process or malignancy (Chapter 110). A jejunal biopsy will show dilated lymphatics and distended villi. Small bowel examinations may merely demonstrate diffuse, non-specific fold thickening and hypersecretion.[26] Only if early flocculation can be avoided will it be possible to visualize a pattern of fine nodules superimposed on the enlarged folds, presumably representing the bleb-like engorgement of villi.

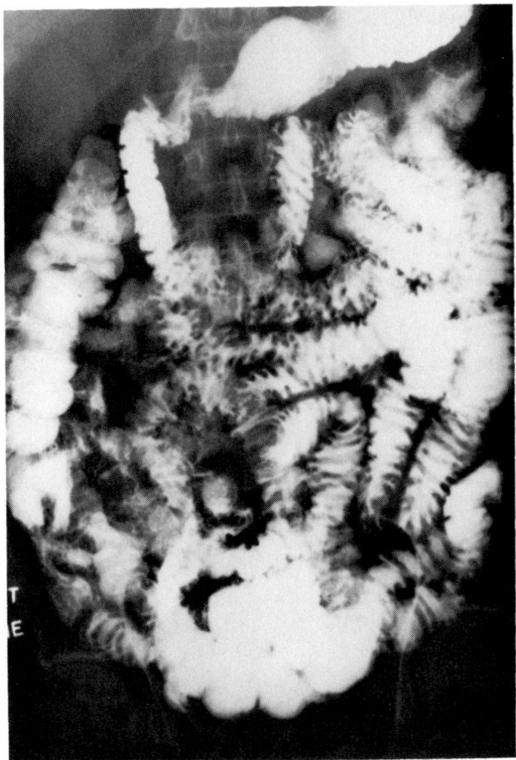

Figure 102–7. Whipple's disease. There is irregular thickening of mucosal folds throughout the small bowel, but particularly prominent distally. (Courtesy of Dr. Charles Mulhern, Jeanes Hospital, Philadelphia.)

Eosinophilic gastroenteritis is a condition with eosinophilic infiltration predominantly of the mucosa and is often associated with malabsorption[27] (Chapter 82). There is usually a pronounced eosinophilia in the peripheral blood. Gastric mucosal thickening is mostly confined to the antrum. The small intestine shows hypersecretion and segments with thickened folds and irritability. The jejunum tends to be more extensively affected than the ileum. Occasionally, there has been extension into the mucosa of the right side of the colon. Treatment with steroids usually results in clinical cure and resolution of the radiographic abnormalities.

One-third of patients with small bowel *Crohn's disease* may have demonstrable malabsorption, especially if the jejunum is involved.[28] The mechanism can be multifactorial but is mostly related to the duration of the disease process and to the extent of any bowel resection.[28] Hypersecretion and moderate flocculation of barium are frequently found in patients with more widespread, active disease.

Diarrhea is a frequent feature in patients with the *Zollinger-Ellison syndrome.* Low pH values in the jejunum lead to inactivation of pancreatic lipase and thus the steatorrhea. Barium studies show hyper-rugosity in the stomach and duodenum, often with multiple ulcers. The second portion of the duodenum tends to be dilated.[29] Jejunal folds are thickened and increased luminal fluid is present. There may be hyperperistalsis and flocculation may occur.

Mastocytosis is an uncommon systemic disease that involves the skin (urticaria pigmentosa) and is frequently associated with hepatosplenomegaly, sclerotic bone lesions, and peptic ulcers. A few patients also have steatorrhea and an intolerance to alcohol. Barium studies show thickened folds, mostly in the jejunum, and mucosal nodules, measuring about 5 mm in diameter.[29] Biopsy specimens demonstrate a cellular infiltrate of the mucosa, composed of a variable proportion of mast cells. The nodules may represent urticarial lesions of the small bowel mucosa.

Abetalipoproteinemia is a rare hereditary disease characterized by steatorrhea, neuromuscular and retinal abnormalities, acanthocytosis, and a total or near-total absence of serum betalipoprotein. It is manifested in the first or second decade of life and tends to be mistaken for celiac disease until either a lack of response to gluten withdrawal or its very different radiologic appearance points away from this diagnosis. Barium studies show thickened folds in the duodenum and jejunum, less so in the ileum. Mild hypersecretion, slight dilatation, and minimal flocculation have been described.[30] The distribution of the thickened folds resembles those found in giardiasis, Whipple's disease, and the Zollinger-Ellison syndrome.

Lymphoid hyperplasia and *giardiasis* are closely related disorders. Prominent lymph follicles are a normal feature in the terminal ileum. They are most pronounced in children and young adults, but may also be seen in older persons.[31] The term *"lymphoid nodular hyperplasia"* refers to the finding of innumerable small nodules measuring 1 to 3 mm in diameter throughout the small intestine (Fig. 102–8). The nodular hyperplasia is usually a response to a common variable immunodeficiency state.[32] Patients may have other gastrointestinal disorders, including malabsorption.

Infection with *Giardia lamblia* may develop in patients with lymphoid nodular hyperplasia or in otherwise normal hosts. Giardiasis results in fold thickening in the duodenum and jejunum, increased secretions, irritability of small bowel loops, and accelerated transit.[33] Occasionally, there is no radiographic abnormality.

Malabsorption Associated with Structural Abnormalities

The *short bowel syndrome* (Chapter 108) may follow resection of the small intestine. The distal ileum and the duodenum and proximal jejunum are of specific importance to the absorptive function of the small intestine. Provided they are spared, the loss of well

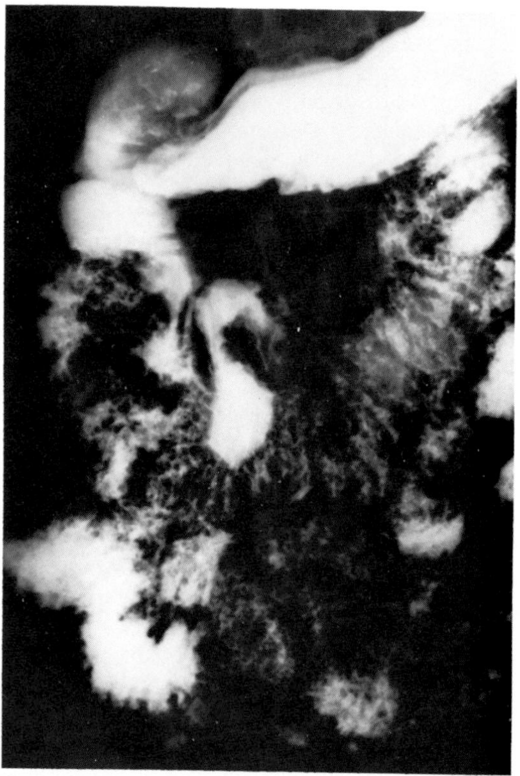

Figure 102–8. Lymphoid hyperplasia in a patient with hypogammaglobulinemia. The proximal small bowel has a finely nodular appearance due to lymphoid hyperplasia.

over half of the small bowel can be tolerated. In the event of their resection, significant malabsorption can occur even if the total loss of small bowel length amounts to less than 25%.[34] Resection of such magnitude may be required in cases of small bowel infarction, strangulation, or Crohn's disease.

Barium radiology can provide an estimate of the length of the residual small bowel and can demonstrate or rule out further active disease. The shortened bowel shows luminal dilatation and a greater number of folds of normal thickness, both expressions of an intensified absorptive function. Following resection of the distal ileum, there is a 3-fold increase in frequency of gallstones[35] and a tendency to form calcium oxalate renal calculi, both potentially visible on radiographs.

Radiology plays an important role in depicting the variety of possible structural alterations that can lead to *small bowel stasis*. Stasis causes bacterial overgrowth, malabsorption, and megaloblastic anemia. Patients who present with such an anemia, along with diarrhea and steatorrhea, need to be investigated for a cause of small bowel stasis, and this should include a barium meal study.

Jejunal diverticulosis is found mostly in older patients. The prevalence of jejunal diverticula at necropsy has been reported to be 4.6%.[36] It is not clear what size or number of diverticula are required before they may be regarded as the cause for malabsorption. It is also possible that even multiple jejunal diverticula may be missed during a follow-through type of barium examination if they are obscured by overlying loops. A tube study will show them reliably, especially if erect or decubitus views are included[37] (see Fig. 102–4).

Blind loops are still another cause of stagnation of small bowel contents. Most blind loops are postsurgical phenomena. No more than 1.5 cm of proximal intestine should be allowed to extend beyond a side-to-side anastomosis, whether enteroenteric or enterocolic.[38] If more bowel is retained, it can gradually enlarge, dilate, and eventually become a site of significant bacterial overgrowth leading to malabsorption.

Any pathologic process causing the normally rapid transit of small bowel contents to slow or stagnate will eventually lead to bacterial overgrowth and malabsorption. *Strictures* (most often due to Crohn's disease) or any impairment of motility (as in scleroderma) may present in this way. Stagnation, however, may then be only one of several factors responsible for malabsorption.

If wide enough to short circuit small bowel contents appreciably, the presence of *fistulas* can lead to malabsorption by a combination of mechanisms. Sufficient lengths of gut can be excluded to produce the equivalent of a short bowel syndrome; stagnation in bypassed gut will lead to bacterial overgrowth; in the case of an enterocolic fistula, continuous bacterial contamination may take place from the colon. Fistulas can be due to surgery (as in bypass operations), penetrating trauma, inflammatory disease (such as Crohn's disease or diverticulitis), or malignancy. Barium meal radiology is required to illustrate the pathologic anatomic features, information that is especially important before any attempt at surgical correction can be made.

References

1. Frazer AC, French JM, Thompson MD. Radiographic studies showing the induction of the segmentation pattern in the small intestine in normal human subjects. Br J Radiol 1949; 22:123.
2. Golden R. Radiologic Examination of the Small Intestine. Philadelphia: JB Lippincott, 1945.
3. Miller RE, Skucas J. Radiographic Contrast Agents. Baltimore: University Park Press, 1977.
4. Miller RE, Sellink JL. Enteroclysis: the small bowel enema—how to succeed and how to fail. Gastrointest Radiol 1979; 4:269.
5. Herlinger H. Small bowel. *In*: Laufer I, ed. Double Contrast Gastrointestinal Radiology with Endoscopic Correlation. Philadelphia: WB Saunders, 1979.
6. Goldberg HI, Shaft DJ. Abnormalities in small bowel contour and caliber; a working classification. Radiol Clin North Am 1976; 14:461.
7. Laws JW, Booth CC, Shawdon H, et al. Correlation of radiological and histological findings in idiopathic steatorrhoea. Br Med J 1963; 1:1311.
8. Farthing MJG, McLean AM, Bartram CI, Baker LRI, Kumar PJ. Radiologic features of the jejunum in hypoalbuminemia. AJR 1981; 136:883.
9. Cohen MD, Lintott DJ. Transient small bowel intussusception in adult coeliac disease. Clin Radiol 1978; 29:529.
10. Reeder MM, Palmer PES. Infections and infestations. *In*: Margulis AR, Burhenne HJ, eds. Alimentary Tract Radiology. 3rd Ed. St. Louis: CV Mosby, 1983.
11. Collins SM, Hamilton JD, Lewis TD, Laufer I: Small bowel malabsorption and gastrointestinal malignancy. Radiology 1978; 126:603.
12. Selby WS, Gallagher MD. Malignancy in a 19-year experience of adult celiac disease. Dig Dis Sci 1979; 24:684.
13. Trier JS. Complications of celiac sprue and potentially related diseases with similar intestinal histopathology. Gastroenterology 1978; 75:314.
14. Moritz M, Moran JM, Patterson JF. Chronic ulcerative jejunitis. Gastroenterology 1971; 60:96.
15. Bluestone R, MacMahon M, Dawson JM. Systemic sclerosis and small bowel involvement. Gut 1969; 10:185.
16. Horowitz AL, Meyers MA. The "hide-bound" small bowel of scleroderma: characteristic mucosal fold pattern. AJR 1973; 119:332.

17. Morson BC, Dawson IMP. Gastrointestinal Pathology. 2nd Ed. Oxford: Blackwell, 1979.
18. Meyers MA, Ghahremani GG, Clements JL, Goodman K. Pneumatosis intestinalis. Gastrointest Radiol 1977; 2:91.
19. Schuffler MD, Deitch EA. Chronic idiopathic intestinal pseudo-obstruction. A surgical approach. Ann Surg 1980; 192:752.
20. Goldberg HI, Brook Jeffrey R. Overview. *In*: Margulis AR, Burhenne HJ, eds. Alimentary Tract Radiology. 3rd Ed. St. Louis: CV Mosby, 1983.
21. Seliger G, Krassner RL, Beranbaum ER, Miller F. The spectrum of roentgen appearance in amyloidosis of the small and large bowel: Radiologic-pathologic correlation. Radiology 1971; 100:63.
22. Bedine MS, Yardley JH, Elliott HL, Banwell G, Hendrix TR. Intestinal involvement in Waldenström's macroglobulinemia. Gastroenterology 1973; 65:308.
23. Maizel H, Ruffin JM, Dobbins WO. Whipple's disease: A review of 19 patients from one hospital and review of the literature since 1950. Medicine 1970; 49:175.
24. Philips RL, Carlson HC. The roentgenographic and clinical findings in Whipple's disease. A review of 8 patients. AJR 1975; 123:268.
25. Marshak RH, Lindner AE, Maklansky D. Malabsorption. *In*: Margulis AR, Burhenne HJ, eds. Alimentary Tract Radiology. 3rd Ed. St. Louis: CV Mosby, 1983.
26. Shimkin PM, Waldmann TA, Krugman RL. Intestinal lymphangiectasia. AJR 1970; 110:827.
27. Marshak RH, Lindner AE, Maklansky D, Gelb A. Eosinophilic gastroenteritis. JAMA 1981; 245:1677.
28. Losowsky MS, Walker BE, Kelleher J. Malabsorption in Clinical Practice. London: Churchill Livingston, 1974.
29. Marshak RH, Lindner AE. Radiology of the Small Intestine. 2nd Ed. Philadelphia: WB Saunders, 1976.
30. Weinstein MA, Pearson KD, Agus SG. Abetalipoproteinemia. Radiology 1973; 108:269.
31. Robinson MJ, Padron S, Rywlin AM. Enterocolitis lymphofollicularis. Arch Pathol 1973; 96:311.
32. Thomas HC, Jewell DP. Clinical Gastrointestinal Immunology. Oxford: Blackwell, 1979.
33. Hartong WA, Gourley WK, Arvanitakis C. Giardiasis: Clinical spectrum and functional-structural abnormalities of the small intestinal mucosa. Gastroenterology 1979; 77:61.
34. Trier JS: The short bowel syndrome. *In*: Sleisenger MH, Fordtran JS, eds. Gastrointestinal Disease. 3rd Ed. Philadelphia: WB Saunders, 1983.
35. Hill GL, Mair WSJ, Goligher JC. Gallstones after ileostomy and ileal resection. Gut 1975; 16:932.
36. Noer T. Non-Meckelian diverticula of the small bowel. The incidence in an autopsy material. Acta Clin Scand 1960; 120:175.
37. Spiro HM. Clinical Gastroenterology. 2nd Ed. New York: Macmillan, 1970.
38. Maingot R. Abdominal Operations. 7th Ed. Chapter 129. New York: Appleton-Century-Crofts, 1980.

Chapter 103

Structural Changes in the Malabsorption Syndromes

Margot Shiner • Jamie S. Barkin

Morphologic Features

Margot Shiner

Identification and differentiation of disorders producing malabsorption rest principally on histologic examination of small intestinal tissue. Such tissue may be obtained by small bowel biopsy, which consists of peroral intubation of the small intestine with an instrument containing a cutting device enabling mucosal specimens to be sampled. Details of this biopsy technique are given in Chapter 47 and are further discussed from the standpoint of application in Chapter 105. Nevertheless, the procedure is reviewed briefly here as well because it is so essential to the evaluation of structural changes that occur in the gut in instances of the malabsorption syndrome.

Small Bowel Biopsy

Instruments. The technique for duodenal biopsy was independently developed by Royer et al.[1] and Shiner.[2] Numerous modifications have since been described.[3–8] Perhaps the most popular instruments in use today are the Crosby-Kugler capsule and the multipurpose instrument,[3] a small flexible version of the Wood gastric tube. Various modifications of the Crosby-Kugler capsule have also made it suitable for use in children of all ages.[9–13] A small intestinal biopsy capsule utilizing hydrostatic and suction principles was described by Baker and Hughes,[14] Ross and Moore,[15] and Flick et al.[16] This enables multiple biopsies to be retrieved without actually withdrawing the tube from the intestine. Various modifications of this system are also in use.[17–19] If, in children or adults, multiple biopsies are required for other than just diagnostic purposes, the instruments of choice are those employing pull-wire methods[2,3] or hydraulic principles.[14–16]

Technique. Various aids to speed the biopsy capsule into the small intestine have been described,[20] but the one essential is the placing of the capsule or biopsy head under fluoroscopic control. If screening facilities are not available, x-ray films may be taken.

Prior sedation of the patient may be necessary. Sedation is of great advantage in small children (under 3 years of age) and may be beneficial in older children and anxious adults. In children, trimeprazine tartrate (Vallegran, Temaril) may be given as a syrup, 1.5 to 2.5 mg/lb of body weight; for adults, diazepam (Valium), 5 to 20 mg by mouth or 10 mg IV, may be necessary. Before intubation, an oral surface anesthetic, such as 1% tetracaine (amethocaine) or lidocaine given as a spray, can be very useful but is not essential.

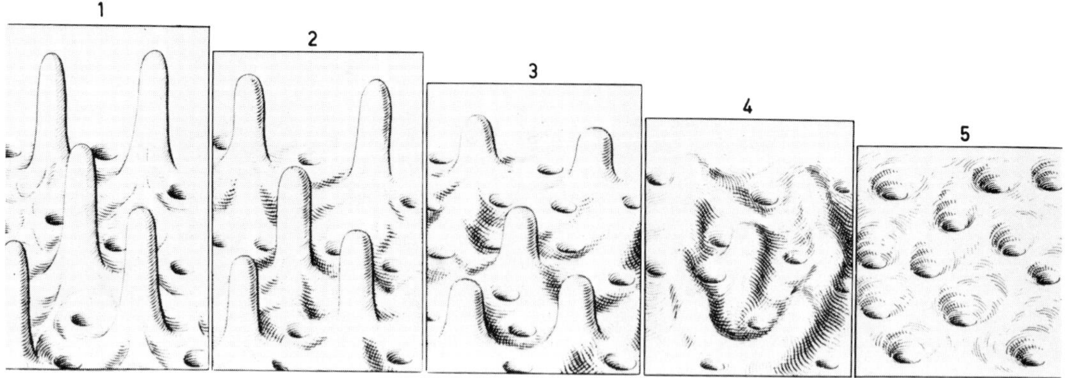

Figure 103–1. Schematic drawing of the surface of the jejunal mucosa as seen with the dissecting microscope showing the normal appearance (1) and the varying degrees of abnormalities (2 to 5). (Courtesy of Dr. J. V. Martins Campos.)

Following intubation, the position of the biopsy head should be checked fluoroscopically to ensure that enough of the tubing has been swallowed for the headpiece to reach the small intestine. Biopsy is usually taken at the ligament of Treitz (duodenojejunal flexure) or at any point beyond it.

Once obtained, the mucosal biopsies should be speedily retrieved from the biopsy capsule. Direct handling of the specimen should be avoided; it should be picked up with a needle placed on the undersurface (muscularis mucosae) or with fine forceps. Examination of the biopsy specimens with a dissecting microscope (magnification × 15 to 25) before histologic sectioning is of considerable diagnostic importance. For this, the specimens are submerged in either normal saline solutions or in a fixative such as formol saline. A surface view of the biopsy is thus obtained (Fig. 103–1), and the appearances correlate fairly closely with the corresponding histologic and pathologic sections (Figs. 103–2 to 103–4). Thus, the absence of villi

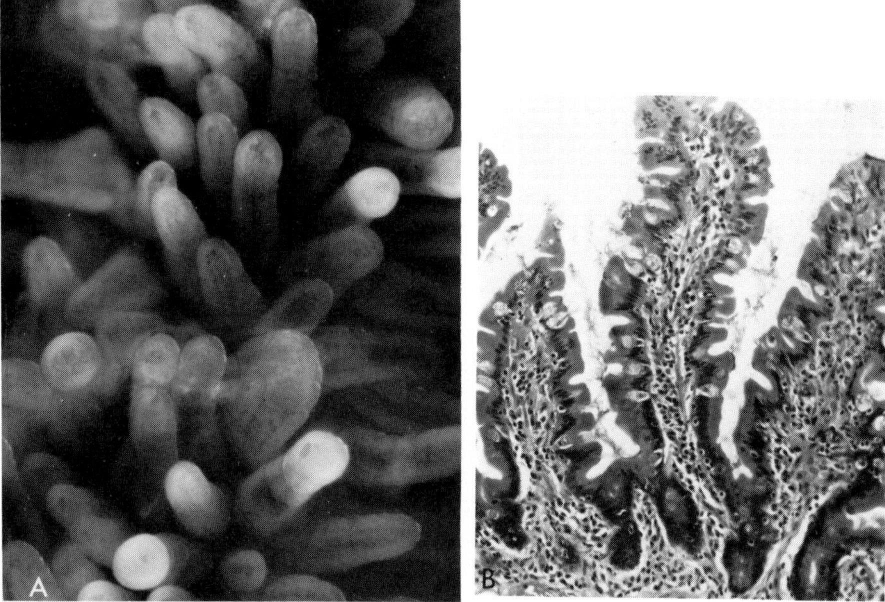

Figure 103–2. *A,* Finger-shaped and occasionally tongue-shaped villi as seen in the normal jejunal mucosa on dissecting microscopy. (Courtesy of W. Brackenbury and Dr. J. S. Stewart.) *B,* The same mucosa on histologic sectioning. Normal appearance.

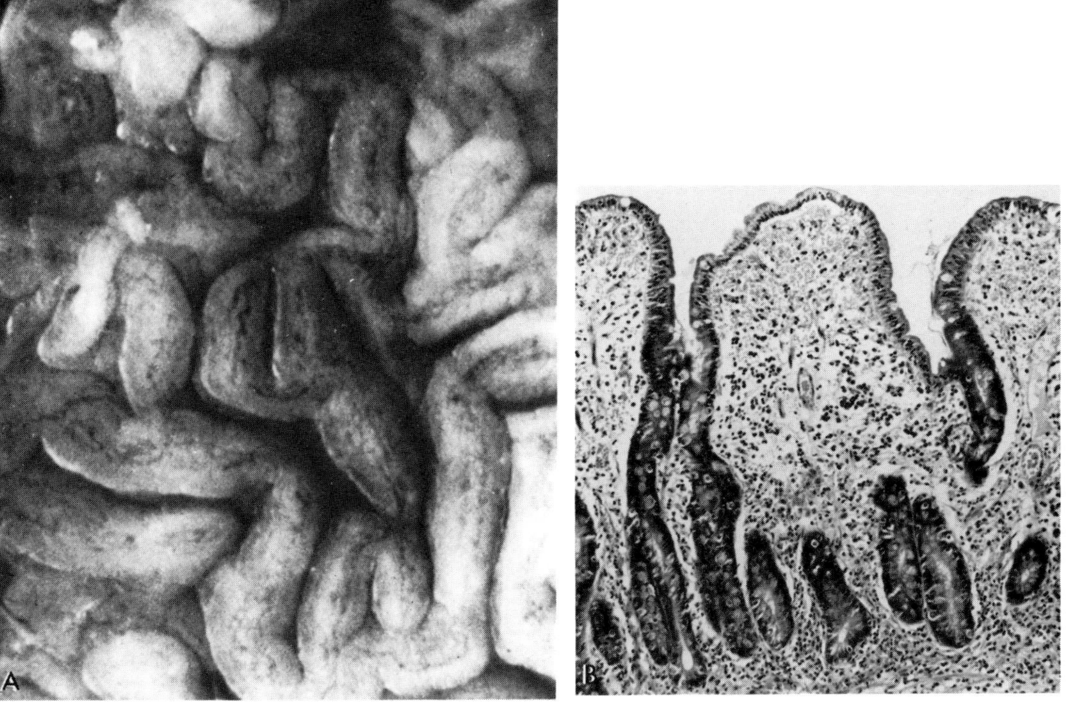

Figure 103–3. Surface view of the jejunal mucosa showing convolutions as seen with the dissecting microscope. (Courtesy of W. Brackenbury and Dr. J. S. Stewart.) *B,* The corresponding histologic appearance of the jejunal mucosa with partial villous atrophy.

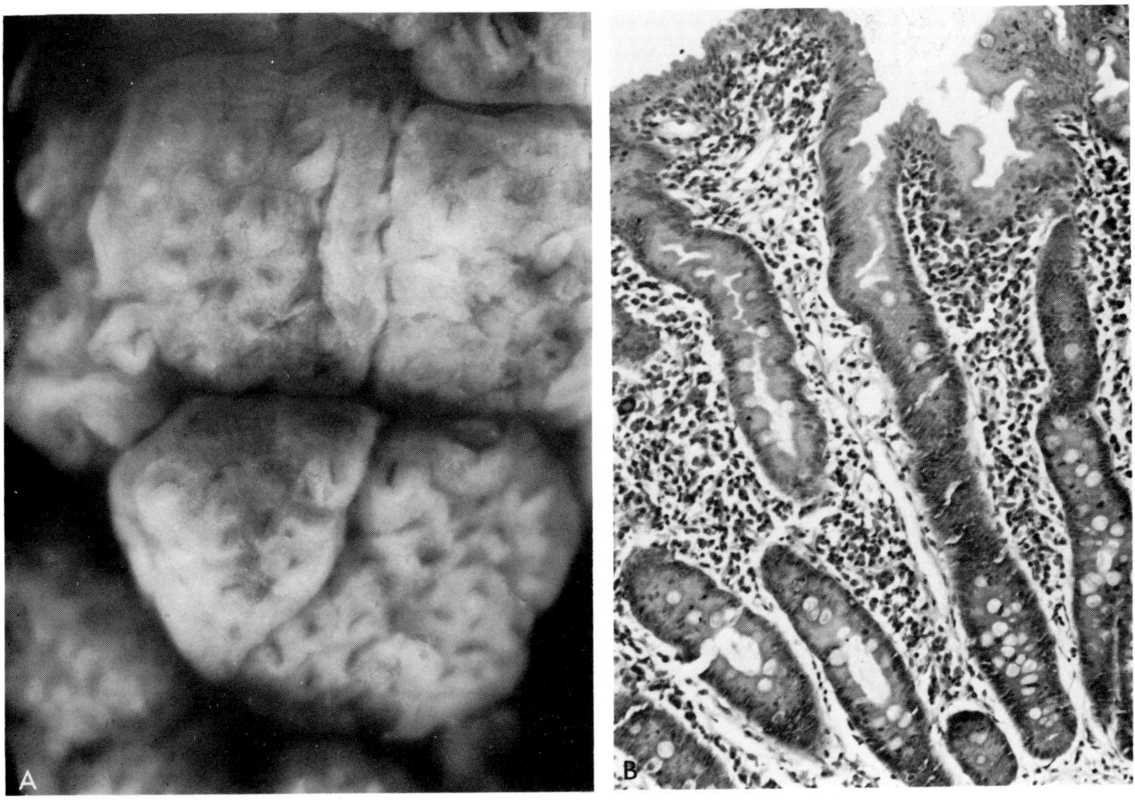

Figure 103–4. *A,* Surface view of the jejunal mucosa showing a mosaic appearance as seen with the dissecting microscope. (Courtesy of W. Brackenbury and Dr. J. S. Stewart.) *B,* The corresponding histologic section of the jejunal mucosa showing subtotal villous atrophy.

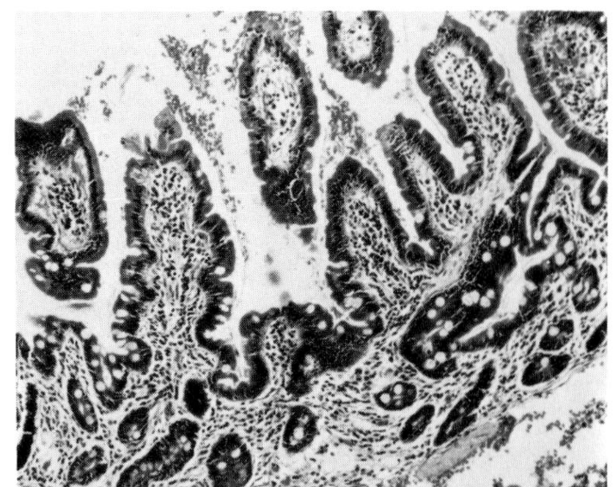

Figure 103–5. Example of improper orientation of a normal jejunal biopsy (compare with Figure 103–2). The villi and crypts are cut obliquely, and this gives the appearance of shortening of the villi and an increase in mucosal thickness.

gives a mosaic pattern to the biopsy surface and suggests the possibility of celiac disease (Chapter 105).

Because the excessive fragility of the mucosa is increased in pathologic states, some operators prefer to place the specimens in fixative for histologic preparations without prior orientation. Others[21] advocate straightening out the biopsy on copy paper before immersion into fixative. Correct orientation is of great importance (Figs. 103–5 to 103–7). A representative histologic section should contain villi and crypts of Lieberkühn cut in a vertical plane, the full thickness of the mucosa, including the muscularis mucosae; and an intact surface epithelium. Excessive fragmentation, particularly of the villi and their lining epithelium, is usually not seen in single non-retrieved biopsies. With multiple biopsies, repeated suction will cause a certain amount of fragmentation. The hydraulically operated tubes are liable to cause the greatest amount of fragmentation of the tissues because they are carried upward by a jet of fluid injected under considerable pressure.

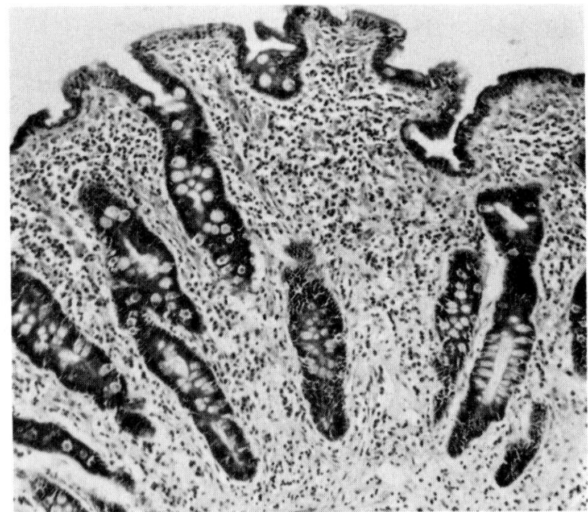

Figure 103–6. Correct orientation of jejunal mucosa showing subtotal villous atrophy.

The rate of failure to obtain adequate biopsy specimens should be below 25%, but may vary between 2% and 35%,[22,23] regardless of the instrument chosen.

Indications. Small intestinal biopsy is essential for the diagnosis of a number of diseases affecting the small bowel mucosa and causing malabsorption and is valuable in the exclusion of others. Follow-up biopsy is of importance in celiac disease after a period on a gluten-free diet to see if villous regeneration occurs in cow's milk protein intolerance and in alpha-chain disease. In Whipple's disease, it is imperative to check progress after antibiotic treatment by repeat biopsy to ensure the disappearance of the large foamy macrophages. Appropriate restriction of dietary fats should lessen fat retention within the absorbing villous epithelium in abetalipoproteinemia, and this should be verified by biopsy.

Indications for peroral biopsy in clinical research are numerous. Mucosal biopsies are employed for tissue and organ culture[24]; for incubation studies for biochemical and physiochemical investigations; and for scanning and electron microscopy, histochemistry, immunocytochemistry, and autoradiography. The fact that viable tissue from the small bowel can be retrieved safely and speedily makes the technique uniquely suitable for physiologic and pathologic studies of this portion of the gut.

Contraindications. Precautionary care with regard to coagulation defects and other contraindications to small bowel biopsy are discussed in Chapter 47. Several authors advise caution with biopsies performed in infants and underweight or malnourished children,[25,26] but I and others[23,27,28] find that the procedure is safe in experienced hands.

Complications. Complications vary from 0.14%[29] to 4.1%[30,31] and consist principally of hemorrhage and perforation.[23,32,33]

Structural Changes

The jejunal mucosa, the usual site for obtaining biopsies, should be uniformly and diffusely involved for biopsy to be diagnostic.

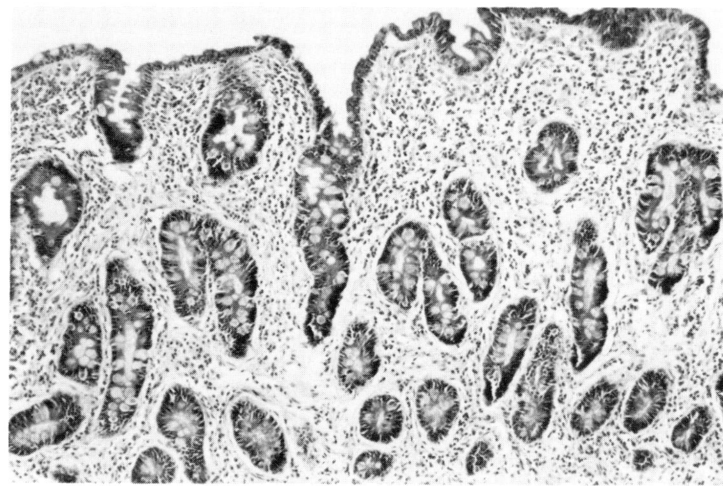

Figure 103–7. Incorrect orientation of part of the same biopsy as shown in Figure 103–6.

This situation obtains in instances of (1) total or subtotal villous atrophy (SVA) (Fig. 103–4) with glandular hypertrophy, (2) infiltration of the mucosa with macrophages showing positive staining with periodic acid–Schiff (PAS) (Fig. 103–8), and (3) retention of fat in the villous epithelium (Fig. 103–9).

The most common disorders exhibiting total or subtotal villous atrophy are non-tropical sprue (idiopathic steatorrhea, celiac sprue, adult celiac disease)[34] and celiac disease of childhood.[11] Total or subtotal villous atrophy may also be found in small bowel lymphoma[36] and carcinoma,[37] hypo- and agammaglobulinemia,[38,39] tropical sprue,[40] protein-calorie malnutrition,[41] dermatitis herpetiformis, food allergy, alpha-chain disease[35] (Fig. 103–10), systemic mastocytosis, idiopathic lymphangiectasia[42] (Fig. 103–11), and acute gastroenteritis.[43] With respect to hypo- and agammaglobulinemia associated with malabsorption, it should be noted that the absence of plasma cells within the small bowel mucosa would indicate that local antibody is not available.

The second form of diffuse involvement featuring PAS-staining macrophages is characteristic of Whipple's disease (Fig. 103–8).[44] The third form of diffuse involvement by fat is found in a rare disease starting in infancy and known as abetalipoproteinemia[45] (Fig. 103–9).

In non-tropical sprue, or celiac disease, small bowel biopsy is probably the single most important diagnostic investigation (Chapter 105) (Fig. 103–12). It is important, however, to repeat the biopsy after 6 to 12 months of treatment with a gluten-free diet, when patients with the gluten-sensitive type of sprue will usually show regeneration of the villous architecture[31,46] (Figs. 103–13 and 103–14).

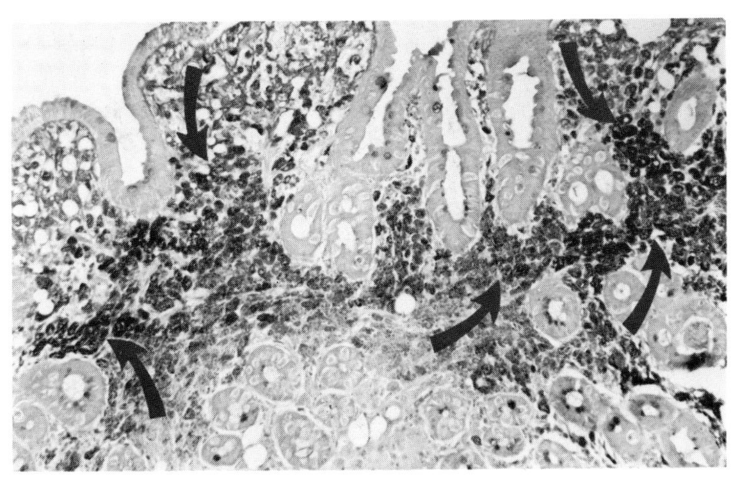

Figure 103–8. Jejunal biopsy from patient with untreated Whipple's disease. The section is stained with period acid–Schiff stain. The darkly staining cells are macrophages containing mucopolysaccharide material.

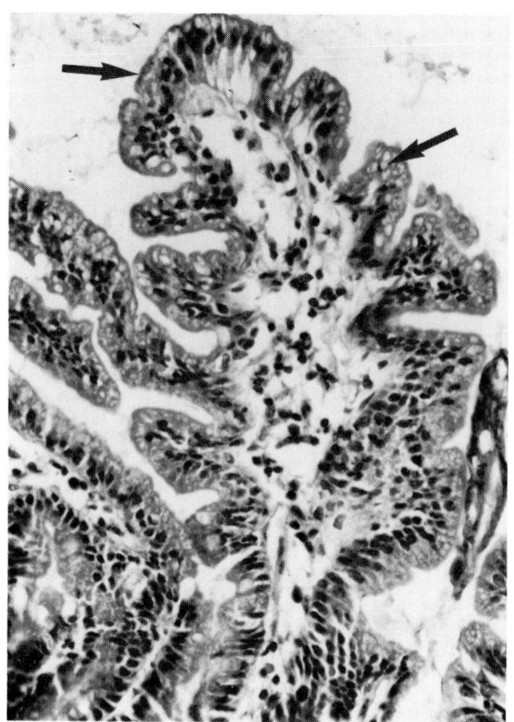

Figure 103–9. Jejunal biopsy from a patient with abetalipoproteinemia showing fat-laden epithelial cells *(arrows)* covering a villus.

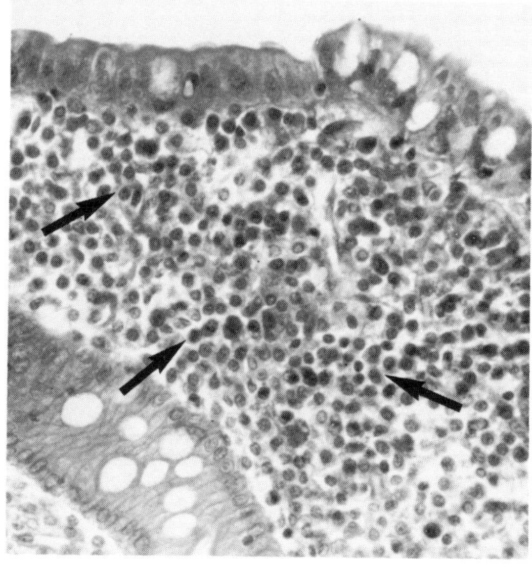

Figure 103–10. Jejunal biopsy from a patient with alpha-chain disease. Note the intense infiltration of the lamina propria with uniform mononuclear cells *(arrows)* confirmed as plasma cells by electron microscopy.

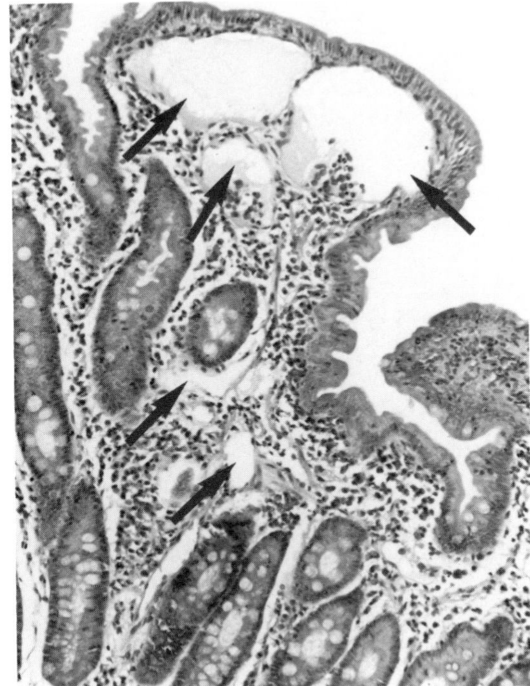

Figure 103–11. Jejunal biopsy from a patient with idiopathic lymphangiectasia. The mucosa shows subtotal villous atrophy with patchy but marked lymphatic dilatation in the lamina propria *(arrows)*.

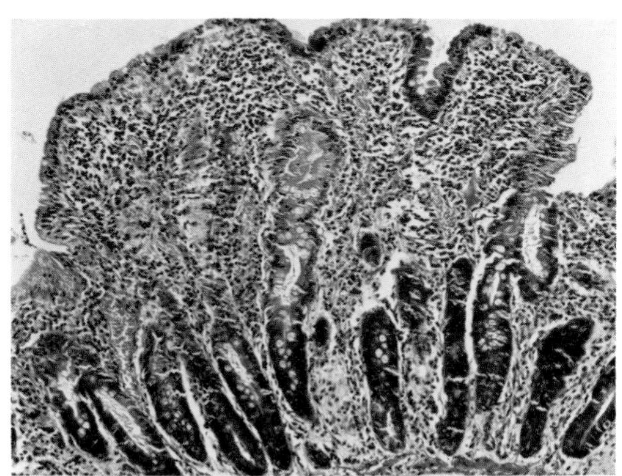

Figure 103–12. Jejunal biopsy from a child with celiac disease before treatment. Subtotal villous atrophy. Villi are virtually absent, the crypts are hypertrophied, and a dense infiltration with chronic inflammatory cells is seen.

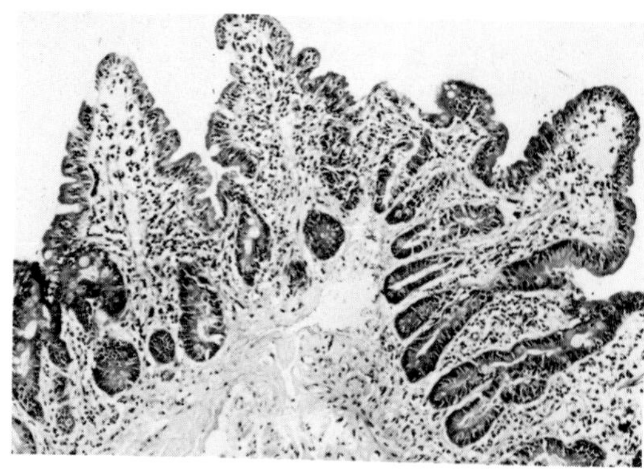
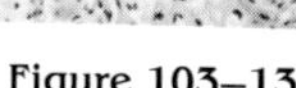

Figure 103–13

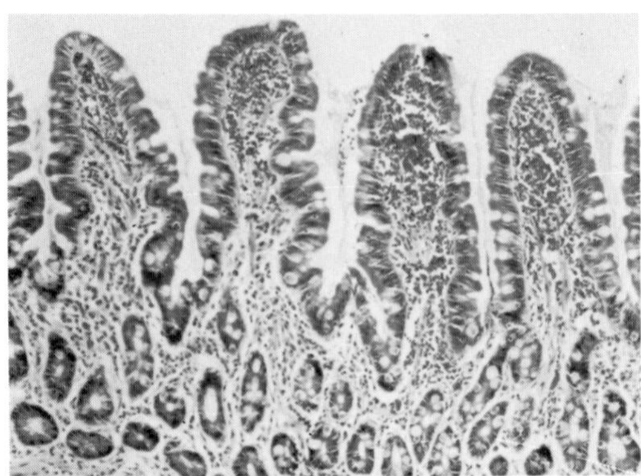

Figure 103–14

Figure 103–13. Same patient as in Figure 103–12, 5 months after start of gluten-free diet. Partial villous atrophy. The villi are short and broad, and the crypts are less elongated. Note the great reduction in inflammatory cells.

Figure 103–14. Same patient as in Figure 103–12, 12 months after start of gluten-free diet. The villi, though shorter than normal, are taller and more slender than in Figure 103–13. The crypts still show some hypertrophy. Inflammatory cell infiltration is less marked.

Many small bowel diseases affect the mucosa patchily. Peroral biopsy in these disorders may or may not be of specific diagnostic value, even when multiple specimens are taken. The following disorders are in this category: Crohn's disease,[47] amyloidosis,[21] parasitic infections[48–50] (Figs. 103–15 and 103–16), lymphomas[51] (Fig. 103–17), eosinophilic enteritis,[52] cow's milk protein intolerance, and gastroenteritis.[53,54]

Partial villous atrophy (PVA) is a real enigma. This type of villous atrophy has been well defined by morphometric measurements.[34,46] In most temperate climates, it usually is associated with disease but is not diagnostic in itself. Thus, it is commonly

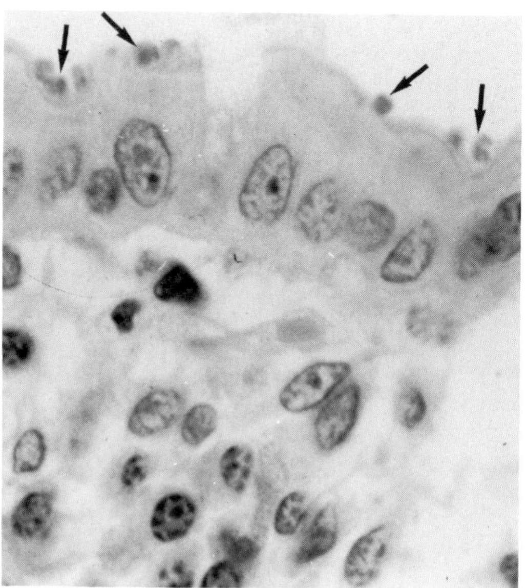

Figure 103–15. Jejunal biopsy from a patient with cryptosporidial infection. Small spherical bodies *(arrows)* are seen on the brush border of epithelial cells facing the bowel lumen (Epon embedding).

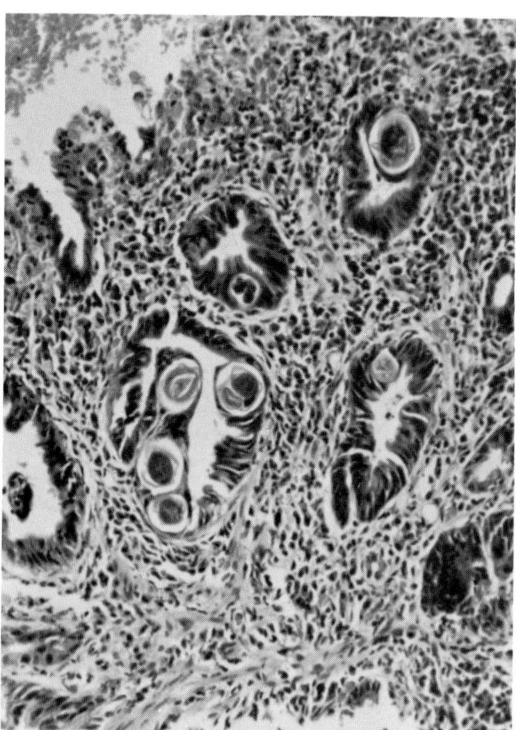

Figure 103–16. The jejunal mucosa in a patient with schistosomiasis. The ova appear to lie within the crypt lumen.

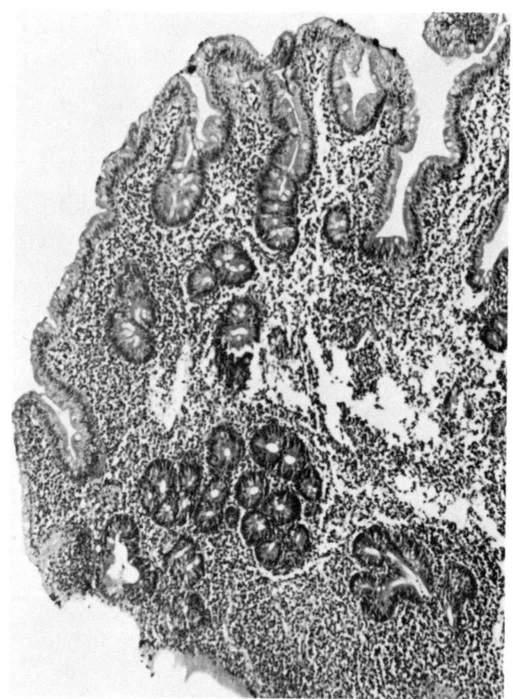

Figure 103–17. The jejunal biopsy in a patient with multiple lymphoma of the small intestine. The mucosa is densely infiltrated with lymphocytes of atypical appearance.

found in children and adults with non-specific diarrhea and diarrhea associated with parasitic infections[54] (Fig. 103–15), Crohn's disease,[47] ulcerative colitis[55] (Fig. 103–18), malabsorption associated with neomycin,[56] radiation damage affecting the small intestine,[57,58] and malnutrition[41] (Figs. 103–19). Rarely, severe villous atrophy may be seen in malnutrition in childhood (Fig. 103–20). In tropical countries, mild partial villous atrophy may be unassociated with any disease[62] (Fig. 103–21), or the villous changes may range from mild (Fig. 103–22) to very severe (Fig. 103–23) and may be indistinguishable from SVA. It is likely that the difference in appearances of the mucosal villi in normal subjects in Western regions and those in tropical climates is conditioned by luminal environmental factors, such as the frequent occurrence of parasites and other infections in tropical regions.

The small intestinal mucosa in dermatitis herpetiformis is associated with SVA in one-third to one-half of patients with this disorder.[59] Moreover, reports of healing of the skin lesions with use of a gluten-free diet have been published.[60] It is therefore important to test for malabsorption and small intestinal mucosal abnormalities in these patients.

In more advanced forms of non-tropical sprue, collagen deposition may be seen in the lamina propria of the villi beneath the villous epithelium.

Complementary Use of Scanning Electron Microscopy. The study of the surface appearances of the jejunal mucosa has been enhanced by the use of the scanning electron microscope (SEM), which combines high resolution with the 3-dimensional view of the dissection microscope. The surface gives a

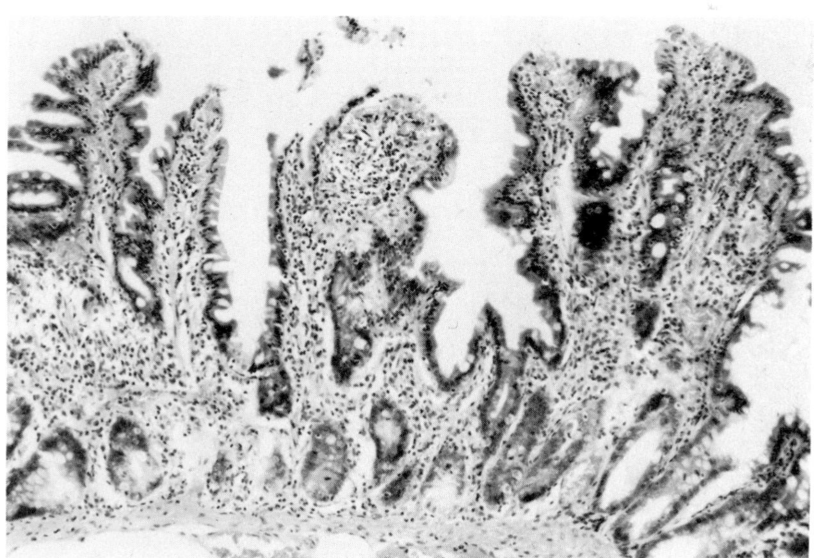

Figure 103–18. The jejunal mucosa in a patient with ulcerative colitis. The villi, though moderately tall, show fusion and distortion. The numbers of inflammatory cells in the lamina propria are increased. The crypts appears to be of normal length.

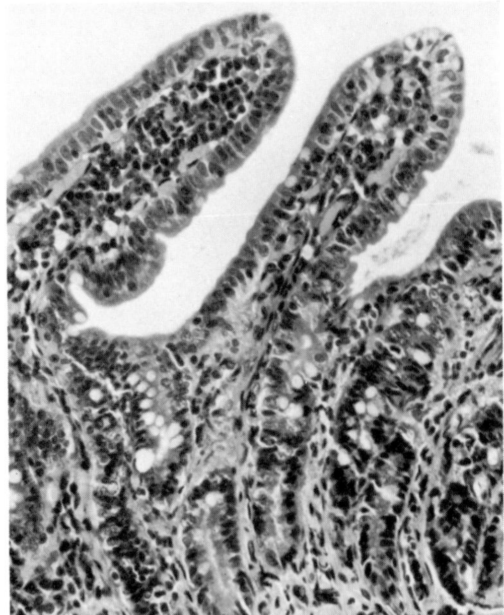

Figure 103–19. The jejunal mucosa in a patient with protein-calorie malnutrition showing partial villous atrophy with abnormal surface epithelium and increase in chronic inflammatory cells.

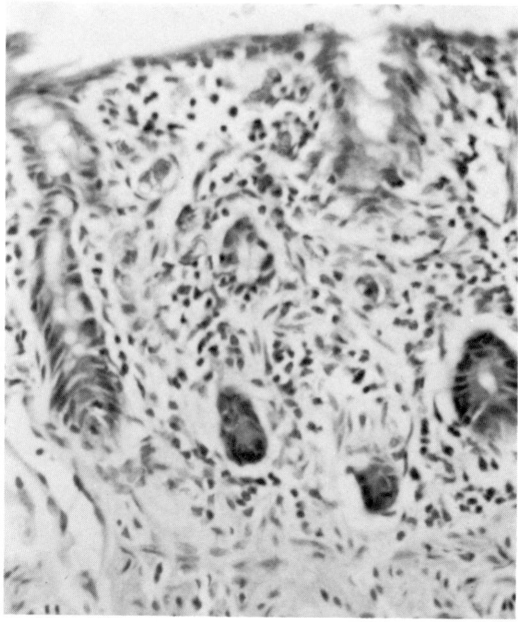

Figure 103–20. The jejunal biopsy in a child severely ill with protein-calorie malnutrition showing total villous atrophy. Note the similarity to the appearances in celiac disease (Fig. 103–112) except for the absence of crypt cell hypertrophy.

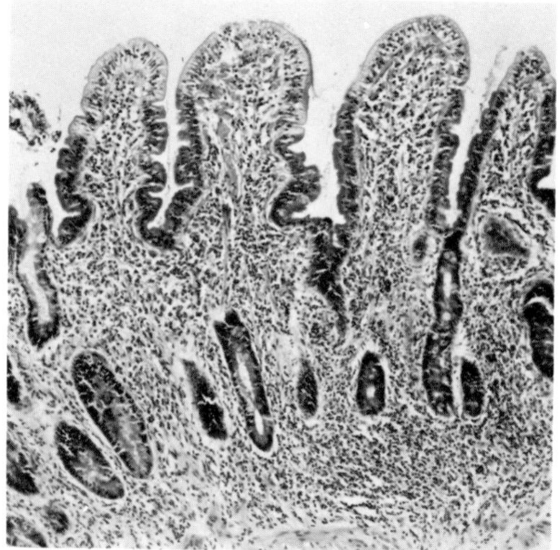

Figure 103–21. The jejunal mucosa from a patient without small bowel disease who was residing in a tropical country. The villi are shorter than normal, but the villous epithelium appears normal. No crypt cell hypertrophy. Extensive chronic inflammatory cell infiltration.

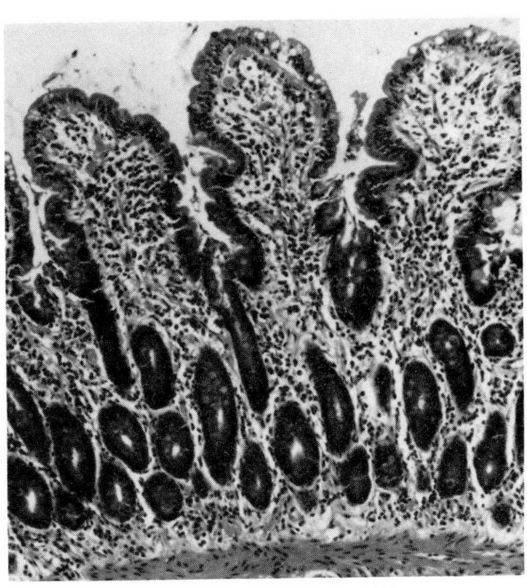

Figure 103–22. The jejunal mucosa from a patient with mild tropical sprue. Partial villous atrophy with crypt cell hyperplasia and moderate infiltration with chronic inflammatory cells. Compare with Figure 103–21.

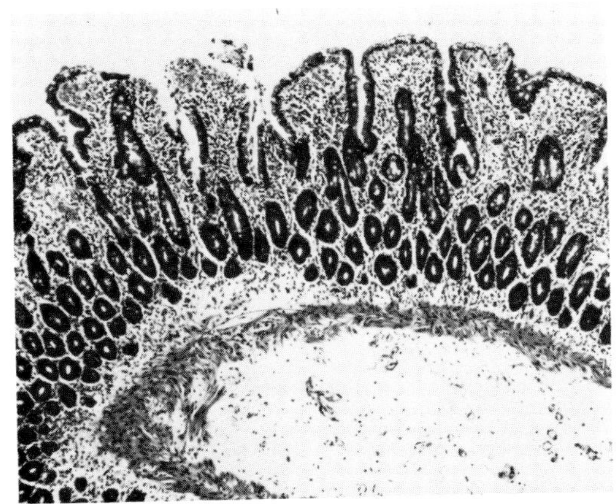

Figure 103–23. The jejunal biopsy from a patient with severe tropical sprue. The appearance is that of a severe partial villous atrophy with glandular hyperplasia.

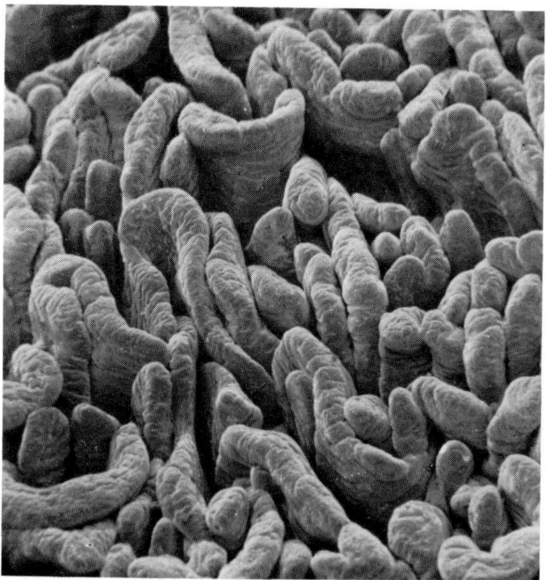

Figure 103–24

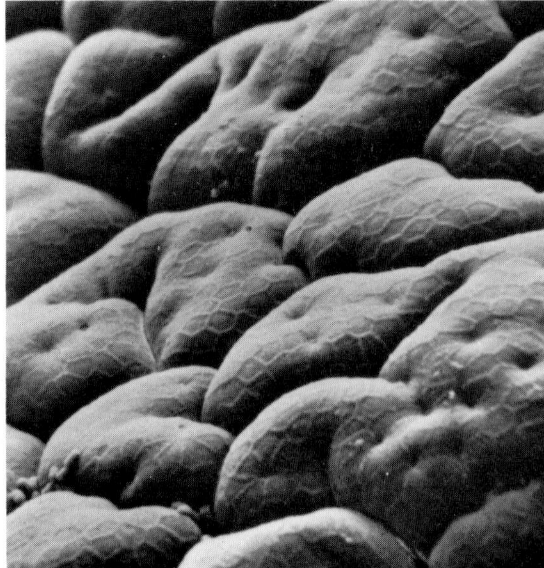

Figure 103–25

Figure 103–24. Human jejunal biopsy. This scanning electron micrograph shows a range of villous shapes, including some typical finger villi with a number of broader leaf forms. The image clarity and depth of focus are typical of this technique. Surface details can be made out on individual villi at a level of resolution not available to conventional dissection microscopic technique (× 80 approx.). (Courtesy of Drs. K. E. Carr and P. G. Toner.)

Figure 103–25. Human jejunal biopsy. At this slightly higher level of resolution, the scanning microscope shows part of the surface of a single villus. The coarse geographic pattern is caused by indentations of the villous surface. The fine polygonal pattern is accounted for by the apical cell boundaries of adjacent, closely packed columnar epithelial cells. The small pockmarks are the mouths of individual goblet cells (× 1000 approx.). (Courtesy of Drs. K. E. Carr and P. G. Toner.)

view as in a relief map of the overall pattern of the intestinal villi (Figs. 103–24 and 103–25). Furthermore, the relationship between the villi and the crypts can be studied in health and disease. The use of the SEM is at present limited to research, but can be helpful in the identification of parasites, such as *Giardia lamblia* (Fig. 103–26) and of bacterial adhesions to the surface of the villous epithelium (Fig. 103–27) in the case of diarrhea due to pathogenic bacteria.

Transmission electron microscopy can be useful in better defining the etiopathologic features of diseases associated with malabsorption. The fine structural changes of the absorbing epithelium in celiac disease consist of abnormalities in microvillous structure, an increase of intracytoplasmic lysosomes, abnormalities of mitochondria and ribosomes, and thickening of the basement membrane (basal lamina) (Figs. 103–28 to 103–31). In the lamina propria, the accumulation of fibrous tissue and collagen may further hinder absorption, and the infiltration of plasma cells would indicate intense immunologic reactions.[61] These can be more advantageously studied after gluten challenge in treated celiac patients.[61]

Various fine structural changes have been identified in relation to other intestinal diseases, such as bacterial invasion of the lamina propria and the presence of large phagocytic vacuoles in the macrophages in Whipple's disease (Fig. 103–32), flagellate protozoa in giardiasis (Fig. 103–33), coccidial parasites of cryptosporidiosis (Fig. 103–34), stasis in mucosal lymphatics and between epithelial cells in lymphangiectasia (Fig. 103–35), hyperplasia of mucosal mast cells in systemic mastocytosis (Fig. 103–36), or the fat-laden vacuoles within absorbing cells characteristic of abetalipoproteinemia (Fig. 103–37).

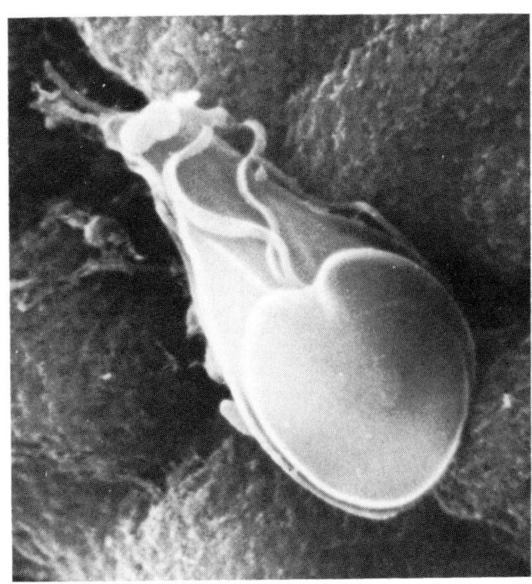

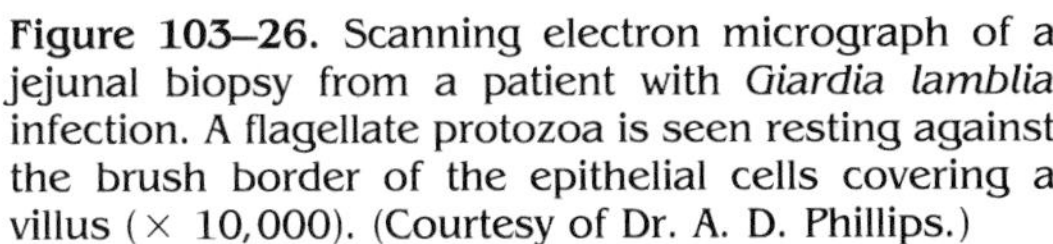

Figure 103–26. Scanning electron micrograph of a jejunal biopsy from a patient with *Giardia lamblia* infection. A flagellate protozoa is seen resting against the brush border of the epithelial cells covering a villus (× 10,000). (Courtesy of Dr. A. D. Phillips.)

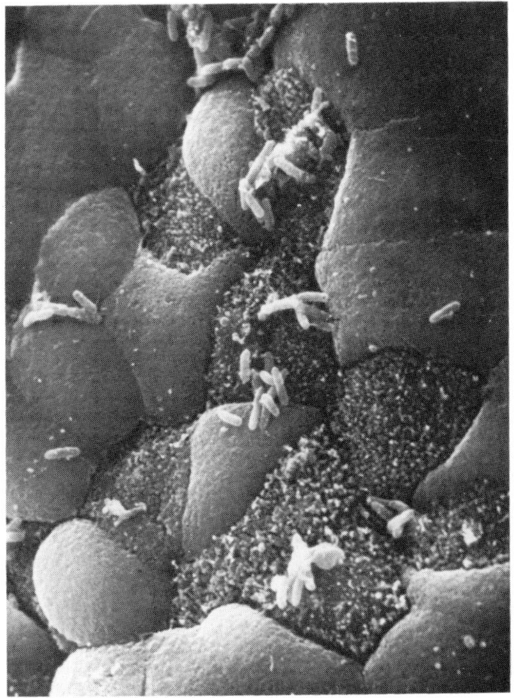

Figure 103–27. Scanning electron micrograph of a jejunal biopsy from a patient with severe diarrhea showing rod-shaped bacteria on the brush border of the epithelial cells (× 5000). (Courtesy of Dr. A. D. Phillips.)

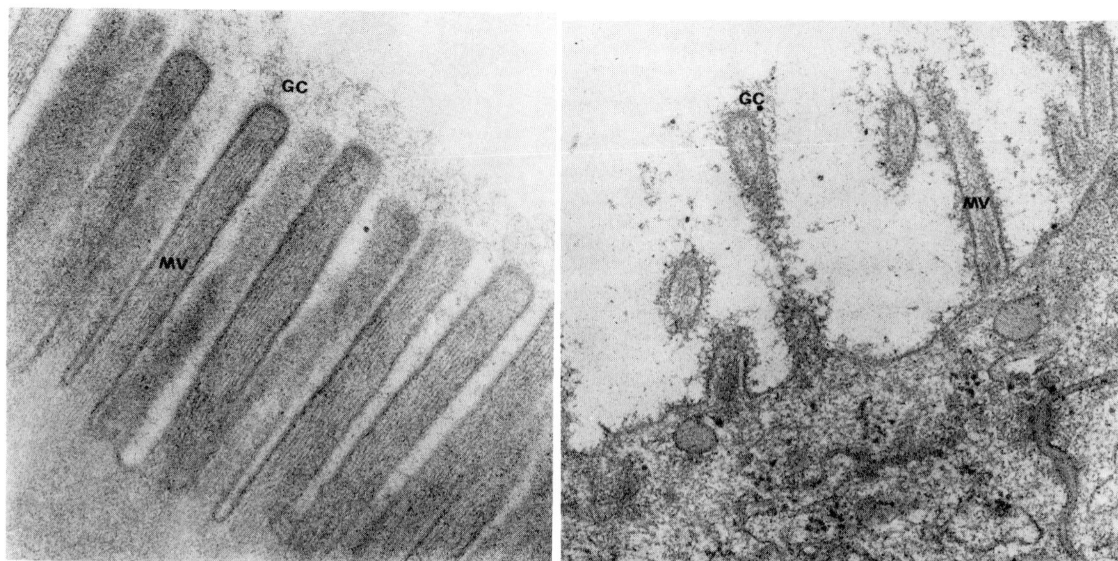

Figure 103–28

Figure 103–29

Figure 103–28. The microvilli of surface epithelia from a normal jejunal biopsy seen by transmission electron microscopy (× 80,000). MV = micovilli; GC = glycocalyx.

Figure 103–29. The microvilli of surface epithelia in subtotal villous atrophy seen by transmission electron microscopy. Specimen obtained from a patient with untreated adult celiac disease. The surface cells were grossly abnormal and the microvilli were short, scanty, and irregular (× 80,000). MV = microvilli; GC = glycocalyx.

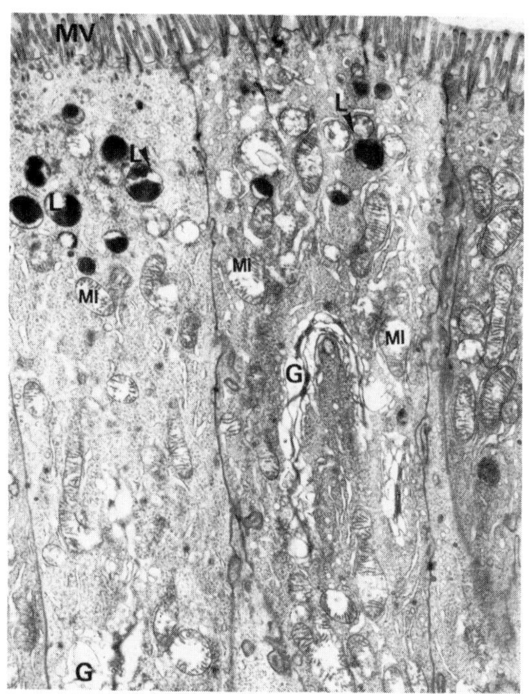

Figure 103–30. Transmission electron micrograph of epithelial cells from a jejunal biopsy in a patient with untreated celiac disease. Note the branching of the short microvilli (MV), the numerous lysosomes (L), the distention of the mitochondria (MI) with disruption of the cristae mitochondriales, and the dilatation of the Golgi vesicles (G) (× 21,000).

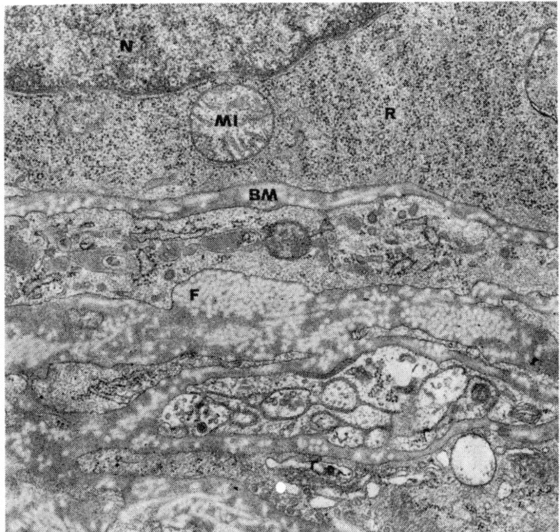

Figure 103–31. Transmission electron microscopy of the infranuclear region of the surface epithelium and its basement membrane (basement lamina). The latter shows thickening and increased density. The subepithelial connective tissue spaces also show thickening and the appearance of coarse electron-translucent fibrils, which may be collagen (× 30,000). N = nucleus; MI = mitochondria; R = ribosomes; BM = basement membrane; F = fibrils.

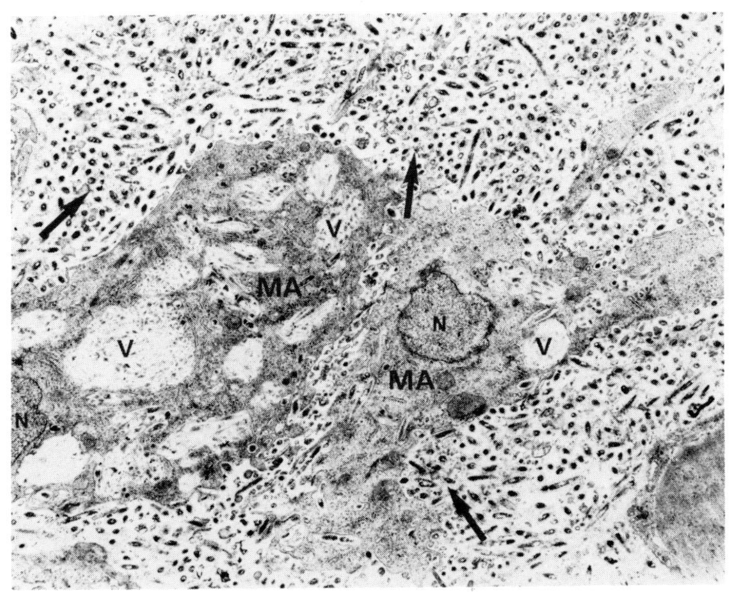

Figure 103–32. Transmission electron micrograph of the jejunal biopsy from a patient with untreated Whipple's disease. The lamina propria contains numerous rod-shaped and coccal forms of bacteria *(arrows)*. Two macrophages (MA) are seen containing large vacuoles (V) with bacterial bodies (× 8300). N = nuclei of macrophages. (Courtesy of Dr. F. Tavarela Veloso.)

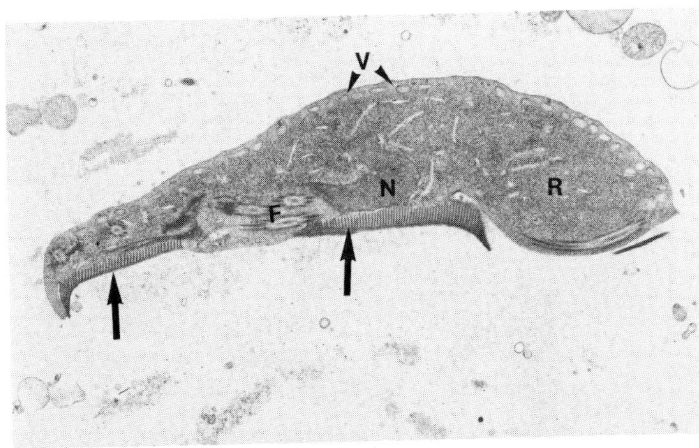

Figure 103–33. Ultrastructure of the protozoa *Giardia lamblia*. The body, wider at one end, contains a nucleus (N), a suction disc *(arrows)*, flagella (F) seen in cross section, numerous ribosomes (R), and a series of vacuoles (V) (× 33,000).

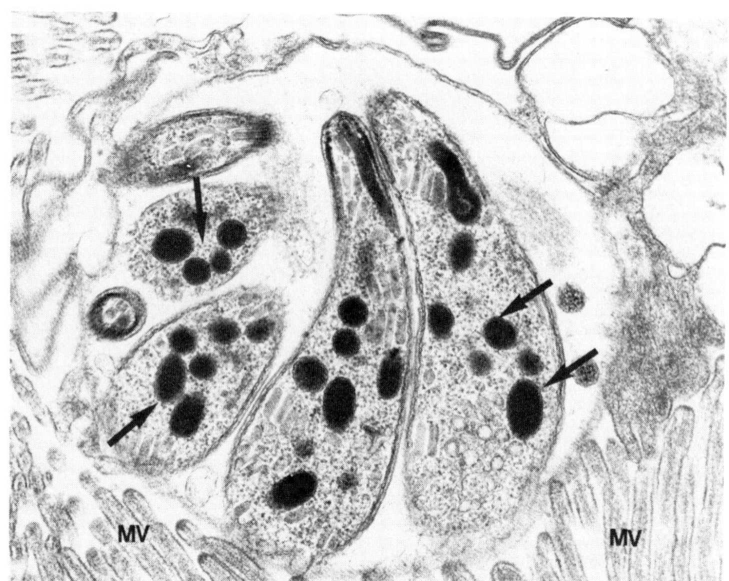

Figure 103–34. Ultrastructure of the spherical bodies shown in Figure 103–15, presumably cryptosporidia. A capsule surrounds several trophozoites that contain dense homogeneous bodies *(arrows)*, vacuoles, and rod-shaped structures. Note the close proximity to the intestinal microvilli (MV) (× 20,500). (Courtesy of Dr. R. Dourmashkin.)

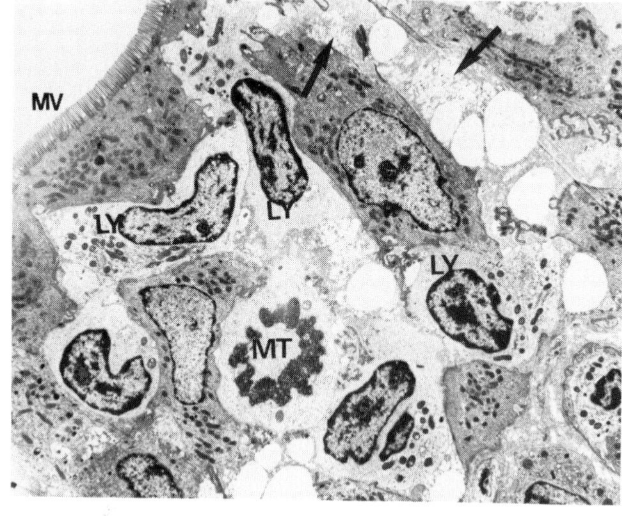

Figure 103–35. Ultrastructure of several epithelial cells in idiopathic lymphangiectasia (see Figure 103–14). These cells are held widely apart by large fluid spaces, probably caused by stasis in the mucosal lymphatics. Interepithelial lymphocytes (LY) and chylomicrons *(arrows)* are found in the spaces. A mitotic figure (MT) is seen, which may be a dividing lymphocyte (× 8800). MV = microvilli of epithelial cells.

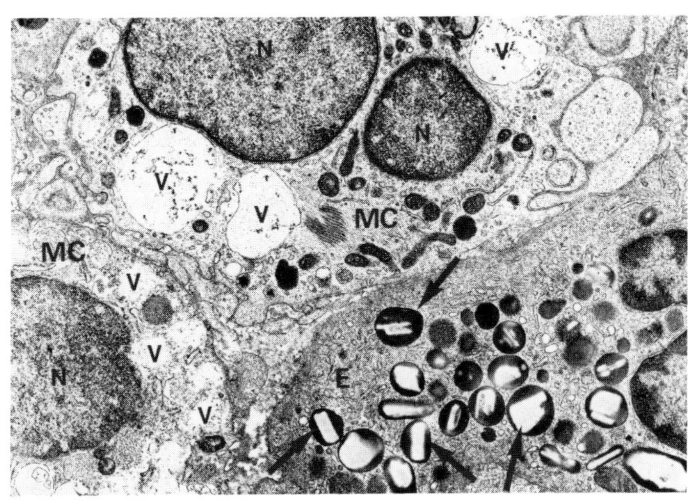

Figure 103–36. Ultrastructure of two mast cells (MC) and an eosinophil (E) in the lamina propria in systemic mastocytosis. Note that one of the mast cells contains 2 nuclei (N). The mast cell cytoplasm contains many vacuoles (V), which represent degranulated bodies. Eosinophils, recognized by their typical cytoplasmic granules *(arrows),* are numerous in the vicinity of the mast cells in this disease (× 16,000.)

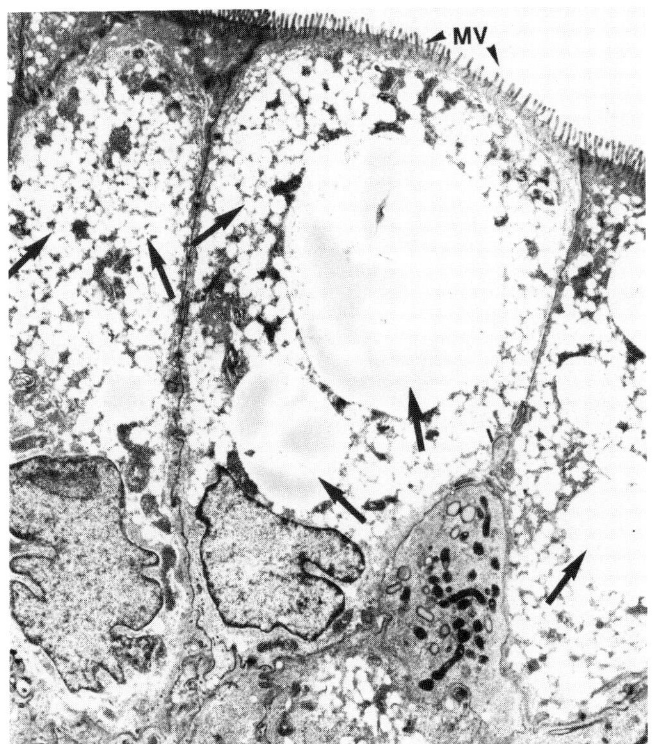

Figure 103–37. Ultrastructure of epithelial cells in abetalipoproteinemia (see Figure 103–9) showing numerous fat-containing vacuoles *(arrows)* within the cytoplasm. Note that the epithelial cells are tightly apposed laterally and that the fat appears to be trapped inside the cells. The microvilli (MV) are short and sparse (× 11,300).

References

1. Royer M, Croxatto O, Biempica L, et al. Biopsia duodenal por aspiracion bajo control radioscopico. La Prensa Medica Argentina 1955; 42:2515.
2. Shiner M. Duodenal biopsy. Lancet 1956; 1:17.
3. Brandborg LL, Rubin CE, Quinton WE. A multipurpose instrument for the suction biopsy of the esophagus, stomach, small bowel and colon. Gastroenterology 1959; 37:1.
4. Carey JB Jr. A simplified gastrointestinal biopsy capsule. Gastroenterology 1964; 46:550.
5. Crosby WH, Kugler HW. Intraluminal biopsy of the small intestine. The intestinal biopsy capsule. Am J Dig Dis 1957; 2:236.
6. Henning von N, Zeitler G, Neugebauer I. Ein Gerat zur Schleimhautbiopsie in tieferen Darmabschnitten. Dtsch Med Wochenschr 1959; 84:1961.
7. Ralston M, Wood IJ, Hughes A. Small-bowel biopsy with the suction biopsy tube. Aust Ann Med 1960; 9:103.
8. Roy Choudhury DC, Nicholson GI, Cooke WT. Simple capsule for multiple intestinal biopsy specimens. Lancet 1964; 2:185.
9. James WPT. Jejunal biopsy modified for paediatric use. Lancet 1968; 1:795.
10. McCarthy CF, Gough KR, Rodrigues M, et al. Peroral intestinal mucosal biopsy with a small Crosby capsule. Br Med J 1964; 1:1620.
11. Sakula J, Shiner M. Coeliac disease with atrophy of the small intestine mucosa. Lancet 1957; 2:876.
12. Schneider RE, Chang R. A paediatric tube and capsule for suction biopsy of the small intestinal mucosa designed for direct nasogastric intubation. Gut 1971; 12:399.
13. Sebus J, Fernandes J, Bult JA. A new twin hole capsule for peroral intestinal biopsy in children. Digestion 1968; 1:193.
14. Baker SJ, Hughes A. A multiple-retrieving small intestinal biopsy tube. Lancet 1960; 2:686.
15. Ross JR, Moore VA. Small intestinal biopsy capsule utilizing hydrostatic and suction principles. Gastroenterology 1961; 40:113.
16. Flick AL, Quinton WE, Rubin CE. A peroral hydraulic biopsy tube for multiple sampling at any level of the gastrointestinal tract. Gastroenterology 1961; 40:120.
17. Bolt RJ, French AB, Polland HM. A simplified multiple-retrieving small-bowel biopsy tube. Am J Dig Dis 1962; 7:773.
18. Lehmann KE. An instrument for multiple transoral biopsies of the gastrointestinal tract. Acta Med Scand 1961; 169:205.
19. Loder RM, Mueller VC, Trier JS, et al. An improved design for a hydraulic biopsy tube. Gastroenterology 1964; 46:418.
20. Evans N, Farrow LJ, Harding A, et al. New techniques for speeding small intestinal biopsy. Gut 1970; 11:88.
21. Rubin CE, Dobbins WO III. Peroral biopsy of the small intestine. Gastroenterology 1965; 49:676.
22. Crosby WH. Small intestinal studies: Methods for obtaining intraluminal contents and intestinal mucosa. Am J Dig Dis 1963; 8:2.
23. Shmerling DH. Peroral intestinal mucosal biopsies in infants and children. Helv Pediatr Acta, Suppl 22, 1970.
24. Trier JS, Bronwing TH. Epithelial-cell renewal in cultured duodenal biopsies in celiac sprue. N Engl J Med 1970; 283:1245.
25. Partin JC, Schubert WK. Precautionary note on the use of the intestinal biopsy capsule in infants and emaciated children. N Engl J Med 1966; 274:94.
26. Lillibridge C, Rubin CE. Unpublished observations. Quoted in Rubin CE, Dobbins WO III. Gastroenterology 1965; 49:676.
27. Jos J. La biopsie de la muqueuse intestinale chez l'enfant. Etude des syndromes de malabsorption. Paris: Imprimerie R Foulon et Cie, 1962.
28. McNeish AS. Jejunal biopsy in infants and underweight children. Arch Dis Child 1967; 42:623.
29. Sheehy TW. Intestinal biopsy. Lancet 1964; 1:959.
30. Hubble D. Diagnosis and management of coeliac disease in childhood. Br Med J 1963; 2:701.
31. Sheldon W, Tempany E. Small intestine peroral biopsy in coeliac children. Gut 1966; 7:481.
32. McDonald WG. Perforation and hemorrhage after gastrointestinal mucosal biopsy in a child. Gastroenterology 1966; 51:390.
33. Shackelton J, Haas L. Fatal peritonitis after jejunal biopsy with the Crosby capsule. Lancet 1962; 2:989.
34. Shiner M, Doniach I. Histopathological studies in steatorrhoea. Gastroenterology 1960; 38:419.
35. Doe WF, Henry K, Hobbs JR, et al. Five cases of alpha chain-disease. Gut 1972; 13:947.
36. Gough KR, Read AE, Naish JM. Intestinal reticulosis as a complication of idiopathic steatorrhoea. Gut 1962; 3:232.
37. Joske RA. Primary carcinoma of the jejunum with atrophic jejunitis and intestinal malabsorption. Gastroenterology 1960; 38:810.
38. Crabbe PA, Heremans JF. Normal and defective production of immunoglobulins in the intestinal tract. *In*: Shmerling DH, Berger H, Prader A: Modern Problems in Paediatrics, Vol 11. Basel: S Karger, 1968: 161.
39. Webster ADB, Slavin G, Shiner M, Platts-Mills TAE, Asherson GL. Coeliac disease with severe hypogammaglobulinaemia. Gut 1981; 22:153.
40. Swanson VL, Thomassen RW. Pathology of the jejunal mucosa in tropical sprue. Am J Pathol 1965; 46:511.
41. Shiner M, Redmond AOB, Hansen JDL. The jejunal mucosa in protein-energy malnutrition. A clinical, histological and ultrastructural study. Exp Mol Pathol 1973; 19:61.
42. Waldmann TA, Steinfled JL, Dutcher TF, et al. The role of the gastrointestinal system in "idiopathic hypoproteinemia." Gastroenterology 1961; 41:197.
43. Marsh MN. Studies of intestinal lymphoid tissue. The cytology and electron microscopy of gluten sensitive enteropathy with particular reference to the immunopathology. Scand J Gastroenterol 1981; 16(Suppl 70):87.
44. Dickinson CJ, Hartog M, Shiner M. A report of two cases of Whipple's disease diagnosed by peroral small intestinal biopsy. Gut 1960; 1:163.
45. Salt HB, Wolff OH, Lloyd JK et al. On having no beta-lipoprotein: A syndrome comprising a-beta-lipo-proteinaemia, acanthocytosis and steatorrhoea. Lancet 1960; 2:325.
46. Madanagopalan N, Shiner M, Rowe B. Measurements of the small intestinal mucosa obtained by peroral biopsy. Am J Med 1965; 38:42.
47. Shiner M, Drury RA. Abnormalities of the small intestinal mucosa in Crohn's disease (regional enteritis). Am J Dig Dis 1962; 7:744.
48. Brandborg LL, Goldberg SB, Breidenbach WC. Human coccidiosis—a possible cause of malabsorption: The life cycle in small bowel mucosal biopsies as a diagnostic feature. N Engl J Med 1970; 283:1306.
49. Hoskins LC, Winawer SJ, Gottlieb L, et al. Pathogenetic features of malabsorption accompanying intestinal giardiasis. Clin Res 1963; 11:184.
50. Sheehy TW, Meroney WH, Cox RS Jr, et al. Hookworm disease and malabsorption. Gastroenterology 1962; 42:148.
51. Eidelman S, Parkins RA, Rubin CE. Abdominal lymphoma presenting as malabsorption: A clinico-pathologic study of 9 cases in Israel and a review of the literature. Medicine 1966; 45:111.
52. Leinbach GE, Rubin CE. Eosinophilic gastroenteritis: A simple reaction to food allergy? Gastroenterology 1970; 59:874.
53. Shiner M. Ultrastructural features of allergic manifestations in the small intestine of children. Scand J Gastroenterol 1981; 16(Suppl 70):49.
54. Walker-Smith JA. Diseases of the Small Intestine in Childhood, 2nd ed. Tunbridge Wells, UK: Pitman Medical, 1979: 279.
55. Salem SN, Truelove SC, Richards WCD. Small intestinal and gastric changes in ulcerative colitis: A biopsy study. Br Med J 1964; 1:394.
56. Jacobson ED, Prior JT, Faloon WW. Malabsorptive syndrome induced by neomycin. Morphologic alterations in the jejunal mucosa. J Lab Clin Med 1960; 56:245.

57. Peterson HH, Clausen EG. Radiation injury to the small bowel with special consideration of surgical complications. Gastroenterology 1956; 31:47.
58. Whitehead R. Mucosal Biopsy of the Gastrointestinal Tract. Philadelphia: WB Saunders, 1973: 121.
59. Shuster S, Watson AJ, Marks J. Coeliac syndrome in dermatitis herpetiformis. Lancet 1968; 1:1101.
60. Fry L, McMinn RMH, Cowan JD, et al. Effect of gluten free diet on dermatological, intestinal and haematological manifestations of dermatitis herpetiformis. Lancet 1968; 1:557.
61. Shiner M. Ultrastructure of the Small Intestinal Mucosa: Normal and Disease-related Appearances. Berlin-Heidelberg, New York: Springer-Verlag, 1982.
62. Baker SJ, Ignatius M, Mathan VI, et al. Intestinal biopsy in tropical sprue. *In*: Intestinal Biopsy. Ciba Foundation Study Group No. 14, Boston: Little, Brown, 1962: 84.

Enteroscopic Findings

Jamie S. Barkin

Enteroscopy has not been widely used in the diagnosis of diseases of the small intestine because of the need for specialized endoscopes and techniques. Technologic improvements, however, have made enteroscopy suitable for regular use as a diagnostic procedure.

Instruments and Techniques

Standard endoscopes used for upper gastrointestinal tract examination can often be passed into the third part of the duodenum and occasionally even further when passage is made under fluoroscopic guidance. Passage into the jejunum may be facilitated by inserting a stiffening wire into the biopsy channel.[1] Another method of easing passage of the standard endoscope and achieving deeper entry into the gut is the use of a previously passed peroral pull-through guide. This method, however, has the drawback of requiring as long as 2 to 3 days for the guiding string to become securely placed.[1]

Special enteroscopes designed to procure passage into the small intestine have had only limited acceptance because of their floppy construction, relative unavailability, and difficulty in passage through the proximal gastrointestinal tract and then into the jejunum. The most frequently utilized special enteroscope (developed by the Olympus Corporation) has a 1-cm outside diameter, a 162-cm effective length, and bending angles in 4 directions.[2] A new prototype enteroscope resembling a small intestinal tube has been designed by Shinya and constructed and made available by the Olympus Corporation.[3] This instrument measures 250 cm in length and is 5 mm in diameter. It is propelled through the gut by intestinal peristaltic activity and usually must remain in place for 24 hours. Enteroscopy is possible during its withdrawal.

Intra-operative endoscopy of the small bowel may be accomplished with a standard long endoscope, such as is used for colonoscopy, when passage of the instrument is made by the endoscopist aided by the surgeon. The endoscopist passes the endoscope into the duodenum and the surgeon gently pleats the intestine over the instrument in a concertina-like fashion.[4] This procedure is particularly helpful to localize and determine the cause of bleeding.[5]

The standard colonoscope may also be used to enter into the small intestine and obtain small bowel biopsies.[6] We have found that entry into the small bowel is more readily achieved with the use of a pediatric colonoscope. Retrograde entry into the terminal portion of the ileum may also be effected with the standard colonoscope and biopsy obtained through this instrument.[7,7a]

Advantages of Enteroscopy

Endoscopic small intestinal biopsy has several potential advantages compared with standard capsule biopsy. The capsule must pass the antropyloric region of the stomach, which is frequently a time-consuming event and, in at least 3% of patients, fails to occur. In addition, radiologic confirmation is required to assure proper capsule biopsy location. This precludes its use in pregnant patients or in outpatient facilities where this equipment may not be available. Enteroscopy, by contrast, does not have these drawbacks and, further, allows visually directed biopsy of selected areas. The latter is especially advantageous in diseases that are patchy in distribution. Not only may multiple tissue samples be taken, but specimens of intestinal contents can be obtained as well.

Biopsy Material

In a study of the adequacy of tissue obtained at endoscopy by direct vision duodenal biopsy in 22 patients, Koren and Foroozan[8] found that at least one specimen was histologically adequate, and that 34 (76%) of 45 biopsies were of adequate size and orientation for histologic interpretation. Scott and Jenkins[9] obtained at least one satisfactory biopsy specimen in 87% of their patients.

Using a spiked forceps passed through a pediatric colonoscope, my associates and I were able to obtain at least one histologically adequate biopsy specimen from the jejunum in all 38 patients we have thus far examined (unpublished data). Our criteria for adequacy include the presence of at least 3 contiguous complete villous-crypt gland complexes oriented perpendicular to the muscularis mucosae and crush artifact that did not interfere with identification of tissues and/or cells. In addition, muscularis mucosae was present in at least one specimen from each patient and submucosa was also frequently present.

A feature pertinent to enteric biopsy in general is the observation reported by Scott and Losowsky[10] that small intestinal biopsies

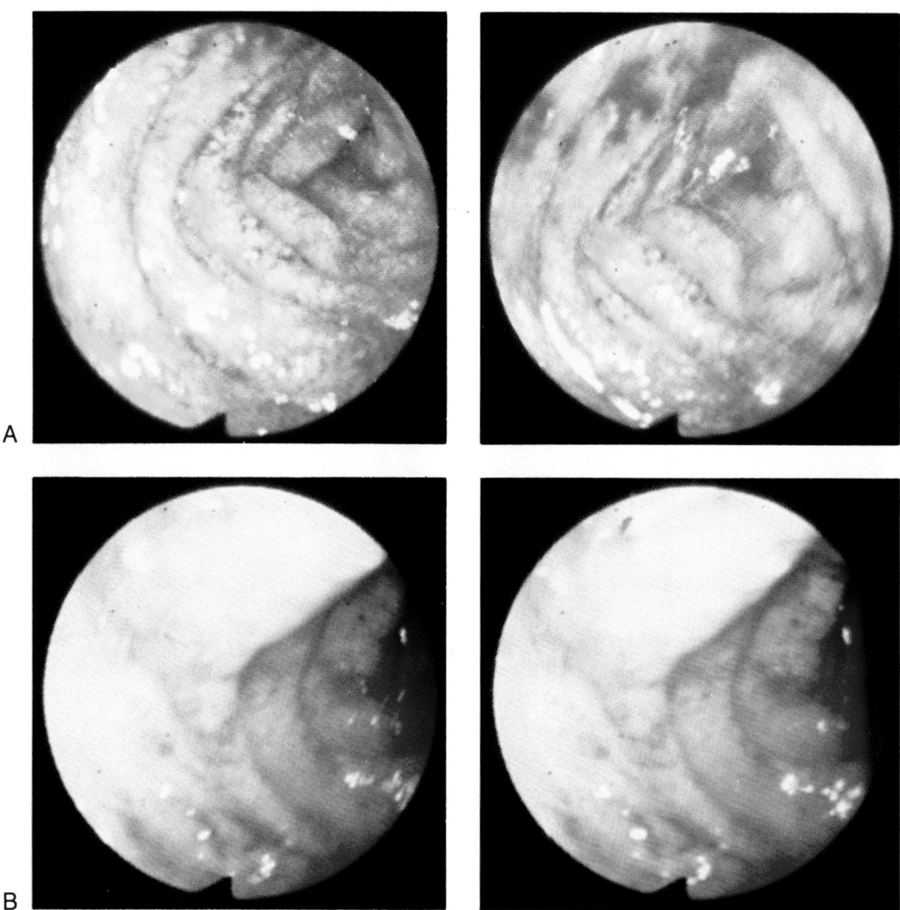

Figure 103–38. *A,* Enteroscopic appearance of Whipple's disease. There is yellow discoloration of thickened and blunted valvulae conniventes. The mucosa is granular. *B,* Enteroscopic appearance of intestinal lymphoma. The mucosa is nodular, friable, and distorted.

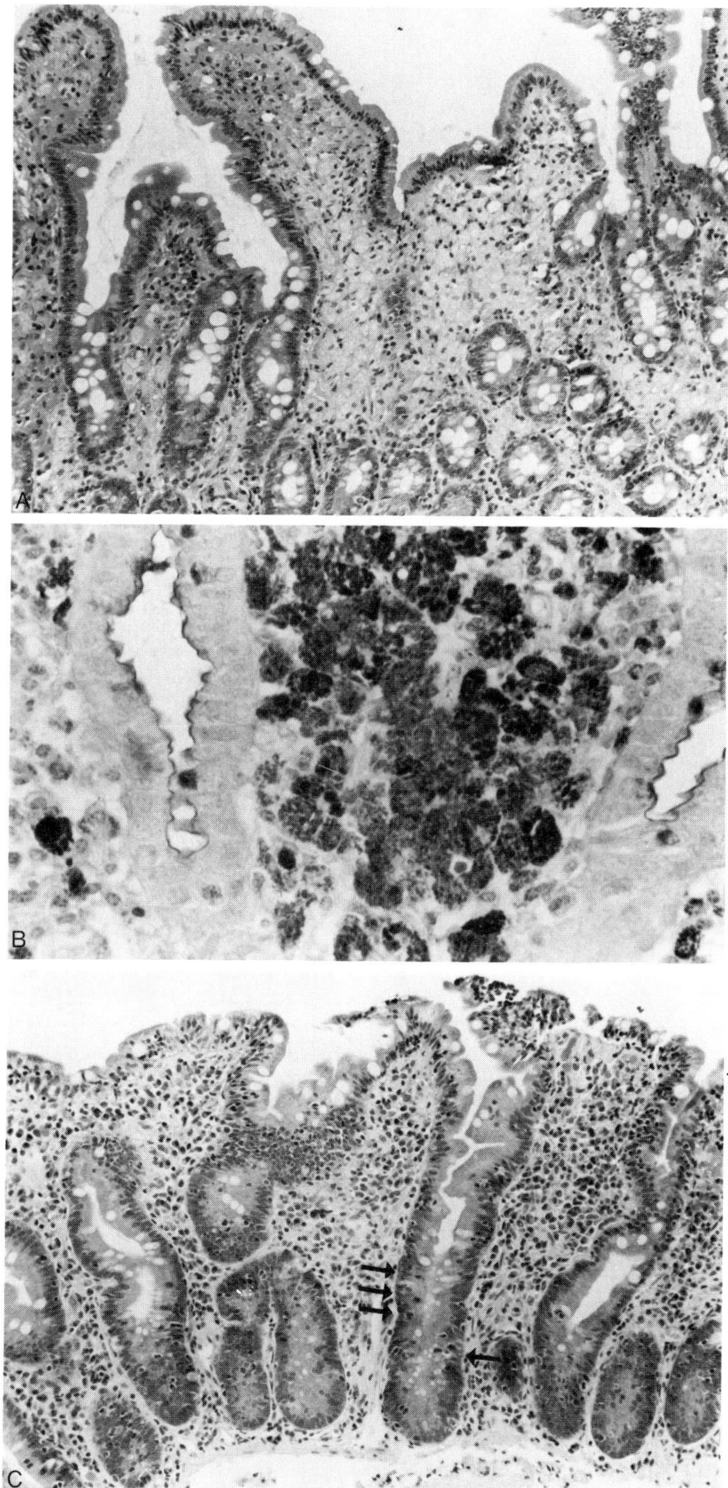

Figure 103–39. Microscopic sections of enteroscopic biopsies. *A* and *B*, *Whipple's disease. A*, The lamina propria is expanded focally by large, foamy histiocytes (hematoxylin and eosin, × 100). *B*, The histiocytes contain the characteristic diastase-resistant, periodic acid–Schiff (PAS) positive cytoplasmic granules (PAS, × 320). *C*, *Celiac sprue.* The luminal surface of the jejunal mucosa is flat. The lamina propria contains infiltrations of plasma cells and lymphocytes. Increased numbers of mitoses *(arrows)* are present in the crypts (hematoxylin and eosin, × 100). (Courtesy of Dr. Sharon Thomsen.)

taken from the distal end of the second part of the duodenum were comparable to those obtained from the duodenojejunal junction if "well oriented" histologic sections without massive infiltration of Brunner's glands were evaluated. Representative enteroscopic photographs and endoscopically obtained histologic specimens are shown in Figures 103–38 and 103–39.

Complications

Small bowel enteroscopy should have at least the same risks as standard upper gastrointestinal tract endoscopy and perhaps the potential for even greater risk. In the limited number of these examinations that have thus far been done, however, no adverse effects have been reported. As the procedure becomes more widely used and applied, the likelihood is that complications will occur and the actual risk will then become evident.

REFERENCES

1. Cotton PB, Williams C. Small intestinal endoscopy. *In*: Practical Gastrointestinal Endoscopy. 2nd Ed. Boston: Blackwell Scientific, 1982.
2. Ogoshi K, Hara Y, Ashizawa S. New technic for small intestinal fiberoscopy. Gastrointest Endosc 1973; 20:64–5.
3. Shinya H, McSherry C. Endoscopy of the small bowel. Surg Clin North Am 1982; 62:821–4.
4. Bowden TA, Hooks VH, Mansberger AR. Intraoperative gastrointestinal endoscopy. Ann Surg 1980; 191:680–7.
5. Greenberg GR, Phillips MJ, Tovee EB, Jeejeebhoy KN. Fiberoptic endoscopy during laparotomy in the diagnosis of small intestinal bleeding. Gastrointest Endosc 1976; 71:133–5.
6. Parker HW, Agayoff JD. Enteroscopy and small bowel biopsy utilizing a peroral colonoscope. Gastrointest Endosc 1983; 29:139–40.
7. Goldin E, Rachmilewitz D. Ileoscopic diagnosis of terminal ileitis. Gastrointest Endosc 1984; 30:11–4.

7a. Schuman BM. Ileoscopy—if forgotten it will be forsaken. Gastrointest Endosc. 1984; 30:213–4 (Editorial).

8. Koren E. Foroozan P. Endoscopic biopsies of normal duodenal mucosa. Gastrointest Endosc 1974; 21:51–4.
9. Scott BB, Jenkins D. Endoscopic small intestinal biopsy. Gastrointest Endosc 1981; 27:162–7.
10. Scott BB, Losowsky MS. Patchiness and duodenal jejunal variation of the mucosal abnormality in celiac disease and dermatitis herpetiformis. Gut 1976; 17:984–7.

Chapter 104

Disaccharide Malabsorption

James B. Hammond • Armand Littmann

Historical Background

Since at least the early part of the present century, pediatricians have recognized a relationship between the ingestion of dietary lactose and other carbohydrates and the development of diarrhea in infants.[1,2] However, the mechanism causing the diarrhea was not understood and the term "fermentative" was applied without substantiating evidence.[3] Also unappreciated were the clinical implications of earlier biochemical investigations such as the description in 1895 of intestinal lactase in the young of the dog and cow, which diminished with maturity,[4] and the characterization in 1907 of small intestinal lactase, sucrase, and maltase.[5,6]

Lactose intolerance associated with chronic diarrhea in an infant was first described by Durand in 1958.[7] The following year, Holzel and co-workers[8] presented evidence that lactose malabsorption was the cause of the diarrhea in their patients. Subsequent reports confirmed their observation and demonstrated that the malabsorption was due to a "deficiency of sugar-splitting enzymes."[9,10] Using tolerance tests, transitory disaccharide malabsorption during infantile diarrhea was demonstrated in 1962.[11]

In 1963, the first observations on lactose malabsorption in adults were reported. Intestinal lactase was demonstrated to be deficient, while the other disaccharidases were normal. Auricchio and co-workers[12] were the first to report enzyme assays on human mucosal specimens obtained at surgery. Soon afterward, the clinical syndrome of milk intolerance due to lactase deficiency in adults was described by Haemmerli et al.[13] in Zurich and by Dahlqvist et al.[14] in Chicago and Hines, Illinois. The latter study was based on previous investigations by Dahlqvist[15] utilizing an enzyme assay method adapted to small mucosal specimens obtained by peroral biopsy.[16].

The ethnic and geographic distribution of lactase deficiency was next defined, beginning with the report of Bayless and Rosensweig[17] in 1966 and leading to a genetic theory of origin proposed by Simoons in 1970.[18] More practical methods of diagnosis followed, most notable perhaps being the breath hydrogen test first described by Bond and Levitt in 1972.[19] Recently, food technology has impacted on treatment by the commercial production of a yeast lactase capable of converting the lactose of cow's milk to monosaccharides and thus making milk available in a well-tolerated form to lactose-intolerant individuals.[20]

Definition

Disaccharidase deficiency (DD) is defined as below normal activity of the intestinal mucosal disaccharidases. This general term implies that all of the disaccharidases are deficient. If the deficiency is restricted to 1 enzyme, such as lactase, or to 2 enzymes, such as sucrase and isomaltase, the specific terms are used—lactase deficiency or sucrase-isomaltase deficiency, respectively. Unless qualified, the term is non-committal regarding associated clinical symptoms. The diagnosis is established either directly by enzyme assay of mucosal biopsy specimens or indirectly by a method that quantitates a response to an orally administered disaccharide.

Disaccharide intolerance (DI) is defined as a characteristic symptom complex resulting from the ingestion of ordinary dietary quantities of disaccharides. Although the intolerance is due to disaccharidase deficiency in most patients, there are exceptions. The 2 terms are not equivalent. When symptoms are associated with the ingestion of only 1 or 2 disaccharides, the term is modified accordingly.

Disaccharide intolerance may be suspected clinically in a patient who consistently develops characteristic symptoms after ingesting foods with a high content of a certain disaccharide. However, until it is demonstrated that the symptoms are due to the disaccharide content of the food, the diagnosis should specify the food or foods that provoke symptoms (i.e., milk intolerance rather than lactose intolerance).

Functional Biochemistry

Role of Oligosaccharides and Disaccharides in Nutrition. Carbohydrates are the source of over half the total calories in the average adult diet in the United States. More than half the carbohydrate is in the form of starch, derived chiefly from cereals and potatoes, and over a third from sucrose, principally as cane sugar in prepared foods; a lesser amount is obtained from berries and other fruits.[21] Although lactose constitutes only 10% of the carbohydrates in average adult diets, other nutrients in milk and milk products are important; these include 75% of the calcium, 39% of the riboflavin, and 35% of the phosphorus provided by such diets.[22]

Dietary starches are almost entirely hydrolyzed in the duodenum by the α-amylase of pancreatic origin to the disaccharide maltose and the trisaccharide maltotriose; about 6% of α-amylase is constituted of α-limit dextrins, chiefly α-1-isomaltase. The activity of α-amylase is high, so that starch digestion is normally complete when the contents of a meal reach the distal duodenum. Even in disorders associated with pancreatic insufficiency, starch maldigestion is rare.[21]

Dietary carbohydrates are presented to the surface membrane of the jejunum in the form of isomaltose, maltotriose, and 3 major disaccharides—maltose, sucrose, and lactose.[22] Trehalose, a disaccharide contained in young mushrooms and in certain insects, is a minor component of modern Western diets.

Normal Digestion of Oligosaccharides and Disaccharides. The hydrolysis of oligosaccharides and disaccharides occurs at the mucosal surface,[23] where the disaccharidases are constituents of the plasma membranes of the microvilli of absorptive cells (Table 104–1).[24] Hydrolysis occurs rapidly, except for lactose, and is followed by absorption of the monosaccharide products. Lactose is hydrolyzed more slowly; its products are absorbed at approximately half the rate as an equivalent mixture of its monosaccharide components, glucose and galactose.[25] The hydrolytic step for lactose is therefore rate-limiting, in contrast to that for the other disaccharides.

The Oligosaccharidases and Disaccharidases. The activities of the disaccharidases are subject to 2 types of control mechanisms. One is product inhibition. As glucose, galactose, and fructose accumulate at the sites of hydrolysis, they inhibit the enzyme reactions. This constitutes a feedback mechanism modulating the rate of disaccharide hydrolysis and tending to adjust it to that of monosaccharide absorption.[26] A second mechanism is induction by substrate and product, a property limited to sucrase-isomaltase. The ingestion of relatively large amounts of sucrose, glucose, or fructose leads to an increase in the activity of this enzyme in the intestinal mucosa within 2 to 5 days; reduced consumption has an opposite effect.[27]

Table 104–1. INTESTINAL DISACCHARIDASES

Enzyme	Substrate	Dietary Source	Products	Properties
β-galactosidase, lactase*	Lactose	Milk, dairy products	Glucose and galactose	Hydrolytic step is rate-limiting; not inducible
α-Glucosidase-malto-oligosaccharidase†	—	Starch	Glucose	—
Glycoamylase, maltase, sucrase-α-dextrinase	Sucrose	Cane sugar, fruits	Glucose and fructose	Inducible
Sucrase-isomaltase complex	α-Dextrins (isomaltose)	Starch	Glucose	—
Trehalase	Trehalose	Mushrooms	Glucose	Enzyme activity very high

*Enzyme also has phlorizin hydrolase activity.
†Substrate specificity includes saccharides with 2 to 9 α-(1 → 4) linked glucose units.

The distribution of the disaccharidases along the small intestine is apparently optimal for absorption of hydrolytic products, being maximal in the jejunum and upper ileum, half-maximal in the duodenum, and absent in the terminal ileum.[28] Their relative activities in the mucosa are proportional to the usual dietary concentration of substrate. Maltase is most active. By comparison, sucrase is approximately one-half and lactase one-fourth as active. Under physiologic conditions, however, both maltose and sucrose digestion proceed at approximately equal rates.[25]

The disaccharidases are high-molecular-weight glycoproteins with pH optimums of about 6. Their turnover time in the brush border membrane is several hours, a small fraction of the 3-day life cycle of the absorptive cell. The rate of turnover is increased by intraluminal removal from the intestinal cell plasma membrane by pancreatic proteases, possibly augmented by bile acids and lysolecithin.[29,30] In pancreatic insufficiency with decreased activities of intraluminal proteases, mucosal disaccharidase activities are relatively high,[31] reflecting a decreased rate of degradation in relation to the rate of synthesis. This interpretation is corroborated by the observation that the therapeutic administration of pancreatic enzymes normalizes mucosal disaccharidases.[30]

During prenatal development of the disaccharidases, lactase presents a unique pattern. While sucrase and maltase activities reach levels near those of adults by the fourth to sixth month of fetal life, lactase does not appear until the last 8 weeks and reaches adult values near term.[32,33] Calculations based on lactase levels led to the prediction, subsequently confirmed, that full-term breast-fed infants would absorb lactose poorly and that absorption would be even more impaired in those born prematurely. The degree of lactose malabsorption in these infants does not appear to be deleterious. Indeed, it may be beneficial by creating conditions that promote the growth of lactose-fermenting non-pathogenic intestinal microflora.[34]

In the small bowel of the fully developed infant and young child, all disaccharidases are at levels of activity similar to those in adults. However, beginning as early as age 2 years in some racial groups (which is often the end of the period of breast-feeding) and as late as adolescence in others, the activities of lactase in the majority of the world's peoples drop sharply.[35] In most individuals of northern European ancestry and certain groups in Africa and India, lactase activity persists into adulthood (Table 104–2). These

Table 104–2. DIFFERENCES IN LACTOSE MALABSORPTION AMONG THE WORLD'S PEOPLES (ADULTS)*

I. Groups among whom malabsorption predominates (60% to 100% malabsorbers)
   A. Near East and Mediterranean: Arabs, Jews, Greek Cypriots, southern Italians
   B. Asia: Thais, Indonesians, Chinese, Koreans
   C. Africa: South Nigerian peoples, Hausa, Bantu
   D. North and South America: Eskimos, Canadian and United States Indians, Chami Indians
II. Groups among whom absorption predominates (2% to 30% malabsorbers)
   A. Europe: Danes, Finns, Germans, French, Dutch, Poles, Czechs, northern Italians
   B. Africa: Hima, Tussi, nomadic Fulani
   C. India: Punjab and New Delhi areas

*From Johnson JD et al. Gastroenterology 1977, 1299–1304. © 1977 by the American Gastroenterological Association. Reproduced with permission.

genetically controlled modulations in activities of an intestinal enzyme have stimulated intense scientific interest. The most acceptable explanation is the geographic or culture-historical hypothesis of Simoons,[18,36] which is quoted in the following paragraph.

> **. . . in the hunting and gathering stage, human groups everywhere were like most other land mammals in their patterns of lactase activity. That is, in the normal individual lactase activity would drop at weaning to low levels, which prevailed throughout life. With the beginning of dairying, however, significant changes occurred in the diets of many human groups. In some of these, moreover, there may have been a selective advantage for those aberrant individuals who experienced high levels of intestinal lactase throughout life. That advantage would have occurred only in certain situations: where milk was a specially critical part of the diet, where the group was under dietary stress, and where people did not process all their milk into low-lactose products such as aged cheese. Under those conditions, most likely to occur among pastoral groups, such aberrant individuals would drink more milk, would benefit nutritionally as a result, and would enjoy increased prospects of survival, well-being, and of bearing progeny and supporting them. In a classical mendelian way, then, the condition of high intestinal lactase activity throughout life would come to be typical of such a group.**

A unique pattern of development of sucrase-isomaltase has been observed in Greenland Eskimos: in 10% of individuals the enzyme is congenitally deficient. However, symptoms due to maldigestion of the disaccharide substrates of these enzymes are unusual.[37]

Epidemiology and Etiology

Deficiencies of Disaccharidases (General). Deficiencies of disaccharidases may be hereditary. Characteristically in hereditary deficiencies, only one enzyme is involved, and the deficiency is total or nearly so. It is present at birth (with the exception of the adult form of lactase deficiency), is not associated with intestinal disease, and is irreversible. Secondary deficiencies usually involve all the disaccharidases, although the reduction in lactase activity may be greater than that of the others. The onset may be at any age, the deficiencies are usually associated with a disorder involving the small intestinal mucosa, and they may be reversed if the intestinal disorder is healed. Lastly, one or more disaccharides may be absorbed poorly despite normal mucosal enzyme activities; malabsorption may be due to an unphysiologic rate of presentation or to reduced contact time, such as may occur after gastrectomy and in the short bowel syndrome.

Table 104–3. HEREDITARY DISACCHARIDASE DEFICIENCIES*

Deficient Enzyme	Mechanism
Lactase	Congenital type: Present at birth (rare)
	Adult type: Develops postnatally (common in certain racial groups)
Sucrase-isomaltase	Type I: No synthesis of sucrase nor of isomaltase subunits
	Type II: Inactive sucrase subunit; high activity of isomaltase subunit

*From Hadorn et al. Clin Gastroenterol 1981; 10:671–90. Reproduced with permission.

The clinical manifestations of enzyme deficiency result from the osmotic diarrhea following ingestion of the disaccharide. The severity of the diarrhea varies with the disaccharide load, the degree of deficiency of enzyme activity, the associated intestinal disease, and possibly the intestinal microflora. The clinical diagnosis can be confirmed by direct enzyme assay of peroral jejunal mucosal biopsies or by indirect methods for detecting malabsorption of a disaccharide load. Treatment of hereditary deficiencies is usually by elimination diets; in secondary deficiencies therapy centers on healing the causative intestinal lesion.

Hereditary Lactase Deficiency, Adult (Delayed Onset) Type (HLD-A). (Primary Lactase Deficiency; Adult Lactase Deficiency; Adult Hypolactasia; Isolated Low Lactase, Acquired) (Table 104–3). HLD-A results from the genetically controlled "switching off" of synthesis by intestinal absorptive cells, which occurs in a majority of the world's populations at various ages between early childhood and early adulthood (see Table 104–2).[38] The frequency with which this occurs in whites and blacks in the United States is illustrated in Figures 104–1 and 104–2, respectively. Family studies in numerous racial and interracial groups have demonstrated that persistence of lactose absorption is inherited as a completely penetrant autosomal dominant characteristic.[38] Its opposite, HLD-A, is probably inherited as a single autosomal recessive gene.[40,41] The inheritance pattern in 5 families of predominantly American Indian origin is illustrated in Figure 104–3.[31]

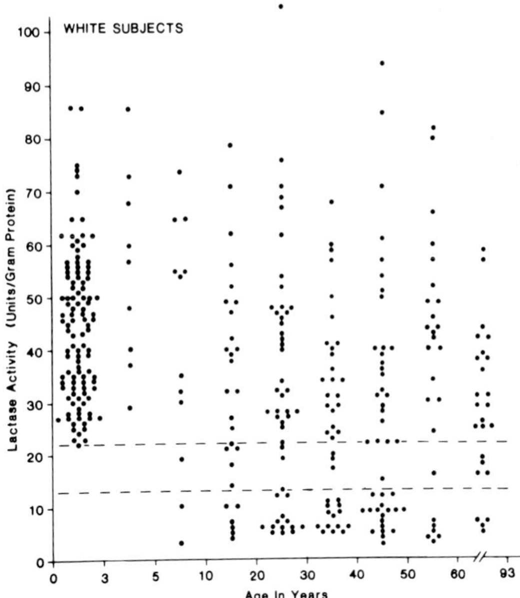

Figure 104–1. Lactase activity in normal small intestinal mucosa from 339 white subjects. (From Welsh JD et al. Gastroenterology 1978; 847–55. © 1978 by the American Gastroenterological Association. Reproduced with permission.)

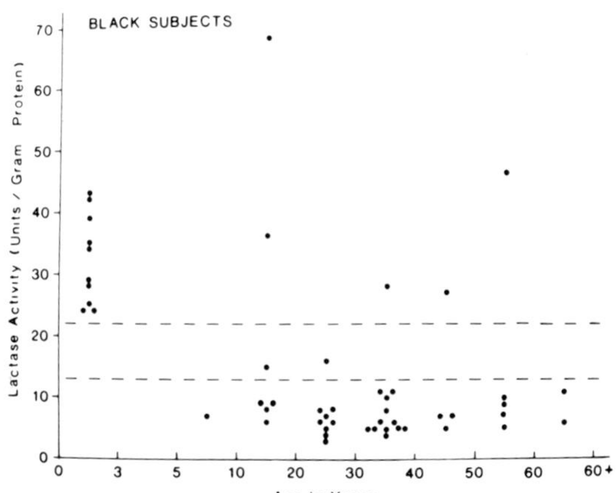

Figure 104–2. Lactase activity in normal small intestinal mucosa from 53 black subjects. (From Welsh JD et al. Gastroenterology 1978; 847–55. © 1978 by the American Gastroenterological Association. Reproduced with permission.)

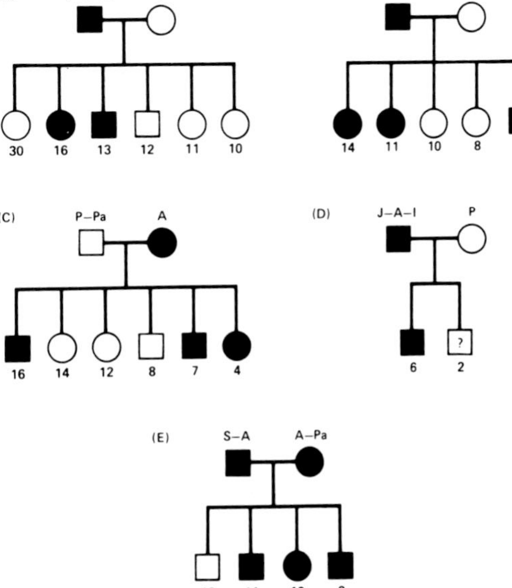

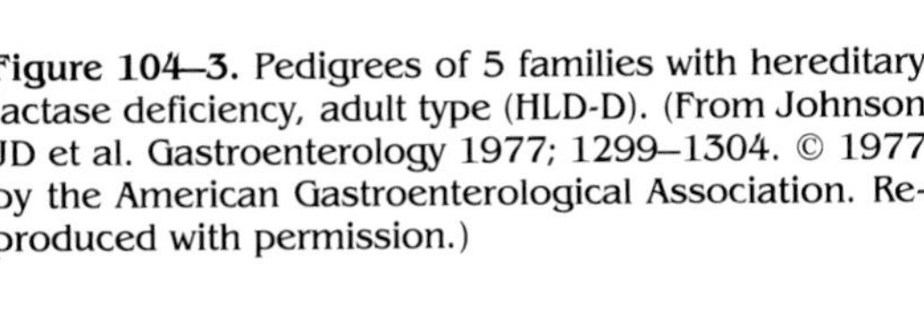
Figure 104–3. Pedigrees of 5 families with hereditary lactase deficiency, adult type (HLD-D). (From Johnson JD et al. Gastroenterology 1977; 1299–1304. © 1977 by the American Gastroenterological Association. Reproduced with permission.)

Because HLD-A is associated with a degree of residual lactase activity, which ranges widely but averages 10% of normal values, control by a regulatory gene has been inferred.[42]

Hereditary Lactase Deficiency, Congenital Type (HLD-C) (Congenital Alactasia). This rare disorder differs from HLD-A in its low occurrence rate, onset in neonatal life, and lower levels of lactase in the mucosa. Fewer than 10 cases have been reported to date, all from northern Europe. Investigation of the properties of the lactase activity of affected persons has yielded divergent results. Studies made by Dahlqvist[42] on 4 patients isolated 3 enzymes with lactase activity, each of which was characterized by the effect of specific inhibitors; the brush border lactase, the only lactase with a digestive function, was absent and the residual activity was due to acid β-galactosidase and hetero-α-galactosidase. Dahlquist inferred that total absence of lactase in the congenital form, which does not occur in the adult form, involved a structural gene. Contrary to Dahlqvist's observations, Freiburghaus et al.,[43] utilizing a chromatographic technique, found the enzyme to be quantitatively and qualitatively similar to that in HLD-A. They concluded from their findings that the pathogenesis of the congenital and adult types was the same.

Hereditary Sucrase-Isomaltase Deficiency (HSID) (Congenital Sucrase-Isomaltase Deficiency). Sucrase and isomaltase activities are the property of a single protein with 2 subunits. Therefore, the concurrence of deficits of both enzymes is explainable as an effect of a single gene on a single protein. This is the most common of the congenital types. First recognized in 1962,[44] approximately 100 cases had been reported by 1973.[45] Its prevalence in the United States has been estimated as 0.2%.[46]

While sucrase activity is virtually absent in the mucosa of all patients with HSID, isomaltase activity is absent in only 80%; significant residual activity is detected in the remaining 20%. Hadorn et al.[40] have proposed that the larger group be designated type I and the smaller, type II.

Kindred studies have demonstrated that HSID is an autosomal recessive trait and that heterozygotes have enzyme deficiencies intermediate between patients and normal persons and may have sucrose intolerance.[47,48]

Eskimos have the highest frequency rate of HSID of any racial group[49]; in Greenland, 10% of a small study population were affected. Eskimos also have a prevalence rate of HLD-A of approximately 60%. Some Eskimo infants are affected by both disorders and in this group symptoms are often severe. It has been suggested that the genetic origins of HSID in Eskimos are mutations that survived because of the virtual absence of dietary sucrose and maltose from the traditional and unique diet of these people.

Hereditary Trehalase Deficiency. This rare disorder is characterized by diarrhea after eating young mushrooms, the major food item containing significant quantities of trehalose. A father and son were diagnosed by demonstrating a deficiency of trehalase in jejunal mucosal biopsies.[50] A third subject responded abnormally to a trehalose tolerance test.[51]

Secondary Disaccharidase Deficiency (SDD). SDD, as defined previously, is associated with a disorder of the small intestine involving diffuse mucosal injury caused by several mechanisms and resulting in reduced activity of all of the disaccharidases. The degree of enzyme deficiency is approximately proportional to the severity of the intestinal lesion, but is seldom absolute. The various enzyme activities are reduced in parallel, except lactase, which is reduced relatively more than the others. Therefore, in minimal deficiency states the other enzymes may be at low normal levels and lactase the only one below normal. Diarrhea follows the ingestion of dietary disaccharides above threshold levels. If the intestinal lesion is completely healed, all enzymes eventually become normal and dietary disaccharides are then well tolerated. Specific disorders frequently associated with SDD are listed in Table 104–4.

Acute Infectious Enteritis and Prolonged Diarrhea. Children less than 2 years old are uniquely vulnerable to repeated episodes of acute infectious enteritis. These are often associated with mucosal injury and multiple defects in mucosal function, of which SDD is one.[52] SDD has been detected in patients with enteritis of both bacterial and viral etiology.[52,53] Typically, the bacteria isolated from

Table 104–4. DISORDERS OF THE SMALL INTESTINE FREQUENTLY LEADING TO SECONDARY DISACCHARIDASE DEFICIENCY

Acute enteritis—viral, bacterial, or parasitic
Nutritional disorders
Tropical sprue
Chronic alcoholism
Ulcerative colitis
Crohn's disease?
Non-tropical sprue
Stasis syndromes
Mucosal injury due to drugs and radiation

the feces are of the Enterobacteriaceae-group; the possible role of anaerobic bacteria has not been adequately investigated.

Children with SDD commonly have overgrowth of enteric microorganisms in their small intestine due to the presence of undigested disaccharides in the lumen and possibly to other factors, including stasis.[54] Bacterial overgrowth may perpetuate the mucosal injury and resultant SDD and provides a rationale for dietary restriction of carbohydrates. The mucosal injury leads to impaired activities of disaccharidases by multiple mechanisms, among which are a reduced population of enzymatically mature absorptive cells (due to subtotal villous atrophy) and a quantitative reduction in the plasma membrane covering the microvilli.[55]

Nutritional Disorders. Infants and children with kwashiorkor have an intestinal mucosal lesion characterized by atrophy of the villi of variable severity and accumulation of lipid droplets in the cytoplasm of the absorptive cells.[57] Correlated with morphologic abnormalities are multiple deficits of mucosal function leading to malabsorption of major dietary constituents, including lactose, and to steatorrhea and diarrhea. The effects of SDD may be aggravated by monosaccharide malabsorption.[57–59]

In contrast, mucosal damage is minimal in uncomplicated marasmus,[56] and SDD is infrequent in this disorder.[57] When SDD is detected, an associated infectious enteritis is likely.

Giardiasis. Infection with *Giardia lamblia* in infants and young children may be associated with intestinal villous atrophy and generalized malabsorption, including SDD.[60] The SDD may be reversed by elimination of the parasite. In adults, the intestinal lesion is usually minimal; villous atrophy and malabsorption are uncommon,[61] except in association with immunodeficiency syndromes.[62]

Chronic Alcoholism. Immediately after withdrawal from alcohol, men who are chronic alcoholics have been found to have a greater frequency of deficiency of sucrase and lactase than do non-alcoholics.[63] Lactase suppression is much more profound than suppression of sucrase and occurs with much greater frequency and severity in black as compared with white alcoholics. The histology of the jejunum in alcoholic patients with enzyme deficiencies may be within normal limits, although a rise in the mitotic index during continued abstinence is evidence for regenerative repair after injury. Disaccharidase deficiency is one of many changes in intestinal structure and function in chronic alcoholism.[64]

Inflammatory Bowel Disease. The longstanding clinical impression that milk ingestion may worsen the course of *ulcerative colitis* has been confirmed.[65] Thus, a controlled dietary trial has demonstrated that patients on a milk-free diet relapsed less frequently than when their diet included milk.[66] These results were considered to be consistent with allergy to milk proteins, but an attempt to demonstrate antibodies in the serum of milk-sensitive patients was unsuccessful.[67] Subsequently, apparent milk sensitivity was found to correlate with lactose intolerance,[68] but no increase in the frequency of lactase deficiency was found in either adults or children with ulcerative colitis when compared with control subjects of similar ethnic origin.[69,71]

Attempts to determine whether the severity of ulcerative colitis correlates with the degree of mucosal lactase deficit have yielded conflicting results. Two investigations led to a positive correlation, and in one of these, serial biopsies in the lactase-deficient group showed improvement in enzyme activity after remission of the disease in approximately one-half; in the remaining patients, lactase deficiency persisted.[72] By contrast, a third study demonstrated no correlation between lactase deficiency and disease activity; moreover, adding lactose to the diet had no effect on the course, regardless of enzyme status.[68]

Crohn's Disease (Chapter 127). Crohn's disease involving the small intestine may also be associated with lactose intolerance.[71,73] There is no evidence, however, that this is correlated with disease activity or that its frequency is greater than that in individuals who do not have Crohn's disease but who are of similar genetic constitution.

Celiac Sprue (Non-tropical Sprue, Gluten-Sensitive Enteropathy) (Chapter 105). Lactose intolerance has been observed in patients of all ages, and symptoms attributed to celiac sprue have improved when dietary lactose, as well as gluten, was restricted.[74] Mucosal disaccharidase deficits, correlating approximately with disease severity, have been demonstrated in all patients investigated; lactase and trehalase are more severely affected than sucrase and maltase.[74–78] The intestinal lesion of celiac sprue, with villous atrophy and lack of differentiated absorptive epithelial cells, is a likely mechanism for enzyme abnormalities but does not explain the non-parallel deficits. Following improvement of the mucosal injury by gluten withdrawal, disaccharidase activities return toward normal, although more slowly in adults than in children. Lactase and trehalase abnormalities may persist for years.

Tropical Sprue (Chapter 106). Lactose intolerance has not been reported in patients with tropical sprue, possibly because milk drinking is uncommon in areas where tropical sprue is prevalent. Moderate deficits in sucrase and maltase activities have been demonstrated, which approached normal after antibiotic therapy. Instances of severe lactase deficiency persisting after the intestinal lesion had apparently healed[79,80] probably represent HLD-A, which is found in the majority of most tropical populations.

Stasis Syndromes (Chapter 107). Disaccharidase deficit in the mucosa adjacent to a blind intestinal loop in man has rarely been documented[79] and its clinical consequences may be trivial. In experimental blind intestinal loops in rats, however, maltase, sucrase, and lactase activities were found to be reduced in mucosa from the blind loop and an adjacent distal segment.[81] The extent of enzyme change paralleled the degree of bacterial proliferation; antimicrobial therapy reversed abnormal activities of sucrase and maltase, but not lactase. The differential loss of the various disaccharidases may be explained by differential susceptibility to their removal from intestinal membranes by intraluminal bacterial proteases.[82,83]

Iatrogenic Causes. In man, colchicine,[84] neomycin,[85,86] kanamycin,[86] and aminosalicylic acid[87] have been shown to induce malabsorption, mucosal damage, and reversible disaccharidase deficiencies. In rodents, doses of colchicine below that causing detectable histopathologic changes led to deficits in lactase and sucrase, but not in other mucosal enzymes.[88,89] This experimental model is another example of mucosal injury resulting in a biochemical lesion without a morphologic correlate.

When patients are deprived of food without nutritional support, a striking reduction in the rate of epithelial cell renewal leads to a reduction in the mucosal mass in the proximal small intestine and to decreases in disaccharidase activity and height of villi.[90] These changes are reversed after several days of re-feeding. In the rat, these changes are related directly to absence of food in the gut lumen and are not prevented by parenteral alimentation and maintenance of nitrogen balance.[91] If the rat model is relevant, it may be assumed that when a patient resumes oral intake after total parenteral nutrition, several days will be required for return of normal intestinal function, including disaccharide digestion.

Radiotherapy to the abdomen in total doses of 2600 to 6000 rads may be followed by moderate decreases in disaccharidase activities associated with morphologic evidence of mucosal damage.[92]

Changing Concepts. While there is no evidence to support a causal relationship between reduced milk intake prompted by lactase deficiency and the development of *osteoporosis*,[93] the frequency of HLD-A in osteoporotic women is greater than in appropriate controls.[94]

An extensive study has corrected previous erroneous conclusions and established that disaccharidase deficiency is not associated with *mucoviscidosis*.[95] In fact, in those patients with associated pancreatic insufficiency, disaccharidase activities are usually increased, similar to the findings in chronic pancreatitis.[31] *Diabetes* that is not associated with chronic pancreatitis does not affect disaccharidase activities.[31]

Relative Disaccharidase Deficiency. Disaccharide malabsorption may develop despite normal mucosal enzyme content when the rate of delivery exceeds the rate of hydrolysis. This may occur when these sugars move through the lumen at faster than physiologic rates, as in the postgastrectomy dumping syndrome,[96] or when their concentration is high, as when certain liquid nutritional supplements are ingested.[97] Malabsorption may also occur when the absorptive surface is quantitatively reduced, as in the short bowel syndrome.[98]

Clinical Aspects

Hereditary Lactase Deficiency, Adult (Delayed Onset) Type (HLD-A). Malabsorption of lactose results when the dietary lactose load exceeds the hydrolytic capacity of the mucosal enzyme. The amount recovered from the distal ileum after an oral load of 12.5 g (equivalent to 1 glass of milk) ranges from 42% to 75% in these patients, compared with 0% to 8% in controls.[99] As a consequence of the retention of lactose in the jejunum, osmotic forces move water and sodium from the extracellular space into the lumen, increasing the volume of chyme,[100,101] stimulating intestinal motor activity, and speeding transit.[102,103] Upon reaching the colon, unabsorbed lactose is metabolized by the bacterial flora to CO_2 and short-chain fatty acids (chiefly acetate, butyrate, and propionate), reducing the pH of the feces. Mild steatorrhea may result from intestinal hurry in children, and diarrhea occurs if the volume of chyme exceeds the absorptive capacity of the colon.

Symptoms. There is probably a variable time lag between the onset of HLD-A and the first recognition of symptoms related to lactose-containing foods. In whites, the age at which this occurs ranges from 5 to 70 years, the peak incidence being in the third and fourth decades.[107] Symptoms begin about an hour after the ingestion of a threshold quantity of lactose in food or beverage. The affected individual develops moderate *cramping, abdominal distress,* and *distention.* This may be relieved in a short time by *expulsion of liquid stool* and *flatus.* The pattern and severity of symptoms will vary according to the amount and frequency of lactose consumed. In children, abdominal cramping may be the only complaint.[109] In otherwise healthy adults, distress and diarrhea are usually mild to moderate. Weight loss is uncommon and dehydration and electrolyte disorders are rarely due to HLD-A alone.

The threshold amount of lactose ranges from 3 to 90 g.[110] An increased amount may be tolerated when gastric emptying is slowed (as when lactose is diluted by a meal), when increased fat is consumed (whole compared with skim milk), or when osmolarity is increased (chocolate compared with plain milk).[111] Children and adolescents generally tolerate larger amounts of lactose than older adults.[112] It might be anticipated that individuals who recognize the causal role of milk would reduce their consumption, but estimates of dietary lactose in lactase-deficient compared with lactase-sufficient individuals have demonstrated no consistent difference.[113]

Differential Diagnosis. The clinical manifestations of HLD-A may resemble those of HLD-C, SDD, allergy to cow's milk, glucose-galactose malabsorption, and the irritable colon syndrome. HLD-C is symptomatic in neonatal life when the infant is first fed milk, while HLD-A becomes symptomatic after age 2 years. Mucosal assay usually reveals lower activity of lactase in HLD-C, compared with HLD-A. SDD is associated with the clinical and pathologic features of the primary disease; not only lactose but other disaccharides may be malabsorbed. The disorder reverses as the primary disease is controlled. Allergy to cow's milk occurs most commonly in infants who were not initially breast-fed. There is normal tolerance to lactose. Symptoms are relieved by replacing cow's milk with a substitute. Glucose-galactose malabsorption, a rare congenital autosomal recessive disorder believed due to absence of membrane binding sites for these actively transported sugars, is first manifested in neonatal life by diarrhea and glycosuria following milk feedings. Lactose, glucose, and galactose are malabsorbed, but fructose is absorbed normally.[114] Before the diagnosis of the irritable colon syndrome should be accepted, a dietary history should be obtained in regard to lactose-containing foods and beverages (Chapters 14, 134). In patients consuming substantial amounts of lactose, HLD-A should be suspected as the cause of symptoms.

Hereditary Lactase Deficiency, Congenital Type (HLD-C). Although the derangements are qualitatively similar to those in HLD-A, they are quantitatively so much greater that survival and growth are threatened. This difference is attributable in part to less mucosal enzyme activity but perhaps even more to the onset of clinical manifestations in neonatal life.

Symptoms. Whenever lactose-containing diets are fed, *diarrhea*, evidence of *abdominal pain, vomiting*, and the consequences of *dehydration* and *metabolic acidosis* occur and persist until dietary lactose is withdrawn.

Differential Diagnosis. The clinical manifestations of HLD-C occurring during neonatal life may resemble infant colic, allergy to cow's milk, glucose-galactose malabsorption, and lactose intolerance without lactase deficiency. Infant colic is manifested by behavior indicating abdominal distress with or without diarrhea; this occurs without regard to the lactose content of the diet and the infant develops normally. The distinguishing features of allergy to cow's milk and glucose-galactose malabsorption are described in the preceding discussion of the differential diagnosis of HLD-A. Lactose intolerance without lactase deficiency is extremely rare. Symptoms include vomiting as well as diarrhea, and the laboratory features are lactosuria, aminoaciduria, and xylose malabsorption.[115]

Hereditary Sucrase-Isomaltase Deficiency (HSID). Symptoms usually begin when sucrose-containing infant formulas or other foods are first consumed; the addition of dextrin or starch has similar effects. *Diarrhea* may be severe in young infants and associated with dehydration and malnutrition. Rarely, *steatorrhea* occurs owing to rapid intestinal transit.[47] Symptoms may become less severe in middle childhood, but persist in adulthood if the cause is not recognized.

Secondary Disaccharidase Deficiency (SDD). Almost all disorders leading to SDD cause symptoms, such as diarrhea, which may be indistinguishable from those of HLD-A. In patients with an intestinal disorder, exacerbation of symptoms by ingestion of carbohydrates, especially lactose, may be a clue that SDD has developed. More subtly, the patient's diarrhea may persist despite appropriate specific therapy while the patient is regularly consuming significant amounts of carbohydrate.

Diagnosis

Hereditary Lactase Deficiency, Adult (Delayed Onset) Type (HLD-A). Laboratory confirmation is not indicated in every patient. The disorder is benign and a symptomatic response to dietary treatment is often adequate corroboration. When indicated, the selection of the laboratory method will depend upon the patient, the purpose, the cost, and the facilities available. The most commonly used methods are the disaccharide tolerance and the breath hydrogen test.

The *disaccharide tolerance tests* estimate enzyme activity by measuring the rise in the level of a product, usually glucose, after administering a standard oral loading dose of disaccharide. For assessing lactase activity, an oral dose for adults of 50 or 100 g of lactose (for children 1 g/kg) in a flavored solution is administered. Blood samples, venous or capillary,[116] obtained prior to and 15, 30, 60, 90, and 120 minutes afterward, are tested for glucose. A maximum rise of less than 20 mg/dl above the fasting level is abnormal and usually indicates lactase deficiency (Fig. 104–4).[117] A maximal increment between 20 and 25 mg/dl is considered an equivocal value in some laboratories and an indication to repeat the test. The patient should be observed for 4 hours after lactose administration. If abdominal cramps, distention, and diarrhea develop, the diagnosis of lactase deficiency becomes more firm (Table 104–5).[118] However, approximately 15% of lactase-sufficient persons will have similar symptoms. If secondary disaccharidase deficiency is likely, the test is repeated with the same doses of sucrose and maltose. It is not necessary to test for tolerance to a mixture of glucose and galactose,[117] except in the rare circumstance in which glucose-galactose malabsorption is suspected.

A modification of the standard lactose tol-

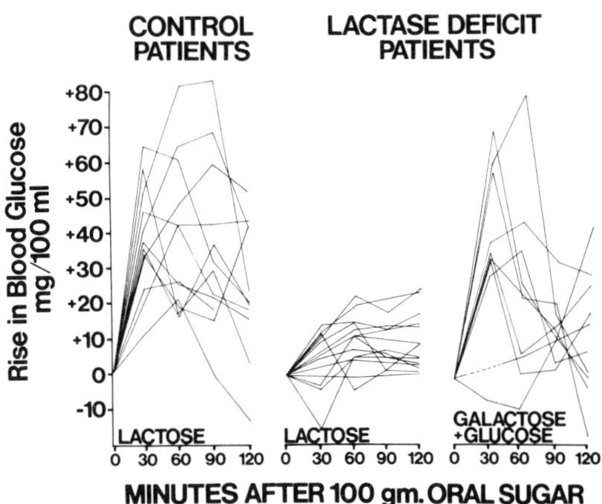

Figure 104–4. Increments of blood sugar over fasting level after oral loads of 100 g of lactose and 100 g of glucose-galactose in control and lactase-deficient patients. (From Dunphy J, et al. Gastroenterology 1965; 49:12. © 1965, Williams & Wilkins, Baltimore. Reproduced with permission.)

erance test involves testing the blood for galactose instead of glucose. To prevent conversion of galactose derived from lactose hydrolysis to glucose by a hepatic enzyme, administration of ethanol, an inhibitor of the enzyme, is required. Results are similar to those of the standard test.[119] However, testing the blood for galactose is not as readily available as the standard test and some patients, including children, should not be given ethanol.

The tolerance tests are simple and inexpensive and require only readily available laboratory methods. The results cannot be interpreted, however, in the presence of a high fasting blood glucose value, as occurs in diabetes mellitus. Obtaining blood samples is moderately invasive, and therefore objectionable in infants and children.

The *breath hydrogen test* is described in Chapter 27. When undigested lactose is metabolized by colonic bacteria, one of the products is hydrogen, part of which is transported to the lungs and excreted. Its concentration in the expired air may reach 4 ppm or higher and can readily be determined by gas chromatography (Fig. 104–5).[19] The patient ingests the test disaccharide, usually in the same amounts as for the tolerance tests, and expired air samples are obtained at intervals.[120] Gas samples can be stored in rubber stoppered tubes for several days for convenience. Test results can be affected by pulmonary disease or by treatment with antibiotics, which may reduce the lactose-fermenting colon bacteria. The technique is particularly suitable for infants and children.[121]

Table 104–5. SYMPTOMS WITH LACTOSE TOLERANCE TESTS, BASED ON 104 CASES*

	Lactose Normal (%)	Lactose Deficient (%)
Cramps	9.9	45.4
Diarrhea	7.0	36.4
Distention	4.2	18.2
One or more of above symptoms	15.5	66.7
None of the above symptoms	84.5	33.3

*From Littman A et al. Israel J Med Sci 1968; 4:110–6. Reproduced with permission.

Peroral jejunal mucosal biopsy and enzyme assay make possible direct determination of the activities of all the disaccharidases on a small (usually 3 to 10 mg) sample of jejunal mucosa obtained at the duodenojejunal angle (ligament of Treitz). Another portion of the biopsy fragment, or a second biopsy, can be processed for histopathologic examination, which may be of crucial importance in detecting intestinal disorders causing secondary disaccharidase deficiency.

The most widely used assay procedure is that of Dahlqvist.[16] The lower limit of normal for lactase activity has been variously determined, so that each laboratory must develop its own range of normal enzyme values (Table 104–6). The normal lactase values established by Welsh[107] are representative: more than 1 IU/g wet weight or 13 IU/g protein and a sucrose/lactose ratio of less than 4. The disadvantages of the mucosal assay method are that an invasive biopsy procedure is in-

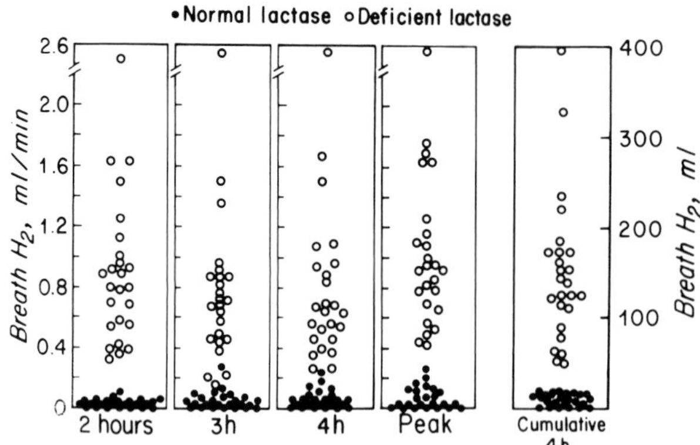

Figure 104–5. Breath hydrogen excretion after a 50-g oral lactose load. (From Newcomer et al. N Engl J Med 1975; 293:1232–6. Reprinted by permission of the New England Journal of Medicine.)

volved and a specialized biochemistry laboratory is needed. However, it is the most definitive method.

Hereditary Sucrase-Isomaltase Deficiency (HSID). Laboratory confirmation is usually obtained by demonstrating a blunted response to sucrose and isomaltase challenge as estimated by blood glucose increment or increases in breath hydrogen. Testing separately for tolerance to each disaccharide should more readily differentiate patients with type I from those with type II deficiency.[40] If the test results are equivocal or do not correlate with the patient's symptoms, mucosal enzyme assay should be considered.

Secondary Disaccharidase Deficiency (SDD). Laboratory aids are directed at establishing the deficiency of one or more disaccharidases associated with an intestinal disorder known to be etiologic. Eventually, confirmation is obtained by amelioration of the enzyme abnormality if the intestinal disorder improves. The demonstration of a deficiency in 3 enzymes is prima facie evidence for SDD; however, SDD may be associated with a deficiency of lactase alone. The histopathologic demonstration of a diffuse mucosal lesion in biopsy material is corroborative, particularly if characterized by villous atrophy. The methods for demonstrating SDD are similar to those described for the diagnosis of HLD-A. For tolerance or breath hydrogen testing, oral loads of sucrose and maltose, as well as lactose, should be utilized.

Table 104–6. JEJUNAL DISACCHARIDASE ACTIVITIES IN NORMAL ADULTS: RANGE OF AVERAGE VALUES*

Enzyme	Activity†
β-Galactosidase; lactase	44–96
α-Glucosidase; glycoamylase	180–540
Sucrase	82–157
Isomaltase	80–144

*From 5 laboratories.[28,29,30,65,87]

†Expressed as International Units (M substrate hydrolyzed/minute) per g protein. Values expressed as per g wet weight will be approximately 1/7 to 1/10 smaller.

Treatment

Hereditary Lactase Deficiency, Adult (Delayed Onset) Type (HLD-A). One of 2 approaches should be selected: (1) reduce dietary lactose below threshold levels, accepting the nutritional consequences; or (2) substitute low-lactose milk for unmodified milk, thus retaining its nutritional benefits. The first approach is usually selected for most adults, whose lactose tolerance is usually about 12 g/day or more.[122] In this group, controlling the consumption of whole milk in its various forms and maintaining adequate nutrition by substituting processed low-lactose dairy products may be convenient. The second approach may be selected for (1) children and adolescents with high nutritional requirements, particularly for calcium, riboflavin, and vitamin A; and (2) adults whose lactose tolerance is less than approximately 12 g/day or adults who enjoy milk.

If dietary control is selected and the patient is an adult, a detailed dietary history will disclose the major sources of lactose (Table 104–7).[123] Symptomatic relief will usually be

Table 104–7. LACTOSE CONTENT OF MILK, MILK PRODUCTS, AND SUBSTITUTES

Product	Unit	Lactose (Approx.) (g/unit)
Milk	1 C—244 g	11
Low fat milk, 2% fat	1 C—244 g	9–13
Skim milk	1 C—244 g	12–14
Chocolate milk	1 C—244 g	10–12
Dried whole milk	1 C—128 g	48
Non-fat dry milk, instant	1½ C—91 g	46
Buttermilk	1 C—245 g	9–11
Whipped cream topping	1 T—3 g	0.4
"Half and half" cream	1 T—15 g	0.6
Low fat yogurts	8 oz—227g—258g	11–15
Cheese:		
Blue	1 oz—28 g	0.7
Camembert	1 oz—28 g	0.1
Cheddar	1 oz—28 g	0.4–0.6
Colby	1 oz—28 g	0.7
Cream	1 oz—28 g	0.8
Cheese, pasteurized, processed:		
American	1 oz—28 g	0.5
Swiss	1 oz—28 g	0.4–0.6
Cottage cheese	1 C—210 g	5–6
Cottage cheese, low fat, 2% fat	1 C—226 g	7–8
Butter	2 pats—10 g	0.1
Oleomargarine	2 pats—10 g	0
Ice cream, vanilla, regular	1 C—133 g	9
Ice milk, vanilla	1 C—131 g	10
Sherbet, orange	1 C—193 g	4
Ice, orange	100 g	0

From Welsh JD. Am J Clin Nutr 1978; 31:1499–503. Reproduced with permission.

achieved by instructing the patient to eliminate these sources and to substitute foods containing no lactose. Less commonly, if the persistence of symptoms indicates extremely low lactose tolerance, of the order of 3–8g/day, further inquiry should be directed to sources of small amounts of lactose, such as prepared foods (french fried potatoes, puddings, pie fillings), dried foods (soups, instant potatoes), and excipients in tablets and capsules.[124] Tolerance to lactose-containing foods is increased when relatively small amounts are taken with other foods and distributed among the daily meals. Therapeutic diets for infants and children should be adapted to their needs and food preferences. Lactose-free formula diets for infants are available.[124]

Low-lactose milk is available in some localities. It can be prepared by adding yeast lactase (LactAid, SugarLo Co.) to milk and refrigerating for 24 hours; 70% to 90% hydrolysis can be obtained, depending on the amount of enzyme added.[125] Clinical experience has confirmed the expected improvement in milk tolerance resulting from lactase pre-treatment.[126,127] Objectively, the rise in blood glucose levels after ingesting 8 ounces of enzyme-digested milk was tripled.[127]

Hereditary Sucrase-Isomaltase Deficiency (HSID). An effective elimination diet should exclude foods with a sucrose content above 2%.[45] Since this restriction is permanent, the diet prescribed must be adequate and should be altered periodically according to the patient's requirements.

Secondary Disaccharidase Deficiency (SDD). Treatment consists principally of reducing the dietary intake of malabsorbed sugars to subthreshold levels, combined with specific therapy for the primary disorder. In practice, control of dietary lactose usually suffices; sucrose and maltose will be tolerated unless maltase and sucrase deficiency is severe.[53] As the primary disorder improves, restriction of dietary lactose should be eased, adjusting to the improved tolerance.

References

1. Davidson M. Disaccharide intolerance. Pediatr Clin North Am 1967; 14:93–107.
2. Kretchmer N. Lactose and lactase—a historical perspective. (Memorial lecture.) Gastroenterology 1971; 61:805–13.
3. Berk JE. Intestinal carbohydrate dyspepsia. *In:* Bockus H, ed. Gastroenterology. 3rd Ed. Philadelphia: WB Saunders, 1974: 335.
4. Rohmann F, Lappe J. Ueber die Lactase des Dünndarms. Berichte Deutsch Chem Gesellschaften 1895; 28:2506.
5. Mendel LB, Mitchell PH. Chemical studies on growth. I. The inverting enzymes of the alimentary tract, especially in the embryo. Am J Physiol 1907; 20:81–96.
6. Plimmer RHA. On the presence of lactase in the intestines of animals and on the adaptation of the intestine to lactose. J Physiol (Lond) 1907; 35:20–31.
7. Durand P. Lattosuria idiopatica in una paziente con diarrea cronica ed acidosi. Minerva Pediatr 1958; 10:706–11.
8. Holzel A, Schwarz V, Sutcliffe KW. Defective lactose absorption causing malnutrition in infancy. Lancet 1959; 1:1126–9.
9. Holzel A, Mereu T, Thomson, ML. Severe lactose intolerance in infancy. Lancet 1962; 2:1346–8.
10. Weijers HA, van de Kamer JH, Dicke WK, Ijsseling J. Diarrhoea caused by deficiency of sugar-splitting enzymes. I. Acta Paediatr 1961; 50:55–71.
11. Cevini G, Giovannini M, Carreddu P. Alterazioni della digestione e dell' assorbimento intestinale die glucidi nei disturbi acuti e cronici della nutrizione del lattante. Minerva Pediatr 1962; 14:831–5.
12. Auricchio S, Rubino A, Landholt M, Semenza G, Prader A. Isolated lactase deficiency in the adult. Lancet 1963; 2:324–6.

13. Haemmerli UP, Kistler HJ, Ammann R, Auricchio S, Prader A. Lactase mangel der Dunndarmmucosa als Ursache gewisser Formen erworbener Milchintoleranz beim Eruachsenen. Helv Med Acta 1963; 30:693–705.
14. Dahlqvist A, Hammond JB, Crane RK, Dunphy JV, Littman A. Intestinal lactase deficiency and lactose intolerance in adults: Preliminary report. Gastroenterology 1963; 45:488–91.
15. Dahlqvist A. Specificity of the human intestinal disaccharidases and implications for hereditary disaccharidase intolerance. J Clin Invest 1962; 41:463–70.
16. Dahlqvist A. Method for assay of intestinal disaccharidases. Analyt Biochem 1964; 7:18–25.
17. Bayless TM, Rosensweig NS. A racial difference in incidence of lactase deficiency. JAMA 1966; 197:968–72.
18. Simoons FJ. Primary adult lactose intolerance and the milking habit: A problem in biological and cultural interrelations. II. A culture historical hypothesis. Am J Dig Dis 1970; 15:695–710.
19. Bond JH, Levitt MD. Use of pulmonary hydrogen (H_2) measurements to quantitate carbohydrate absorption: Study of partially gastrectomized patients. J Clin Invest 1972; 51:1219–25.
20. Rand AG, Linklater PM. The use of enzymes for the reduction of lactose levels in milk products. Amst J Dairy Technol 1973; 28:63–7.
21. Gray CM, Fogel MR. Nutritional aspects of dietary carbohydrates. *In:* Goodhart RS, Shils ME, eds. Modern Nutrition in Health and Disease. Philadelphia: Lea & Febiger, 1980.
22. Marston R, Friend B. Nutritional review, national food situation. Economic Research Service, US Dept of Agriculture, November 1976; publication no (NFS) 158–25.
23. Crane RK. A concept of the digestive-absorptive surface of the small intestine. *In:* Code CF, ed. Handbook of Physiology. Sec. 6, Vol 5, Alimentary Canal. Baltimore: Waverly Press, 1968: 2535.
24. Gitzelmann R, Bachi T, Binz H, Lindenmann J, Semenza G. Localization of rabbit intestinal sucrase with ferritin antibody conjugates. Biochem Biophys Acta 1970; 196:20–8.
25. Gray CM, Santiago NA. Disaccharide absorption in normal and diseased human intestine. Gastroenterology 1966; 51:489–97.
26. Alpers DH, Cote MN. Inhibition of lactose hydrolysis by dietary sugars. Am J Physiol 1971; 221:865–8.
27. Rosensweig NS, Herman RH. Time response of jejunal sucrase and maltase activity to a high sucrose diet in normal man. Gastroenterology 1969; 56:500–5.
28. Newcomer AD, McGill DB. Distribution of disaccharidase activity in the small bowel of normal and lactase-deficient subjects. Gastroenterology 1966; 51:481–8.
29. Alpers DH, Tedesco FJ. The possible role of pancreatic proteases in the turnover of intestinal brush border proteins. Biochem Biophys Acta 1975; 401:28–40.
30. Seetharam B, Perillo R, Alpers DH. The effect of pancreatic proteases on intestinal lactase activity in man. Gastroenterology 1980; 79:728–32.
31. Arvanitakis C, Olsen WA. Intestinal mucosal disaccharidases in chronic pancreatitis. Am J Dig Dis 1974; 19:417–21.
32. Auricchio S, Rubino A, Murset G. Intestinal glycosidase activities in the human embryo, fetus, and newborn. Pediatrics 1965; 35:944–54.
33. Antonowicz I, Lebenthal E. Developmental pattern of small intestinal enterokinase and disaccharidase activities in the human fetus. Gastroenterology 1977; 72:1299–303.
34. MacLean WC Jr, Fink BB. Lactose malabsorption by premature infants: Magnitude and clinical significance. J Pediatr 1980; 97:383–8.
35. Johnson JD, Kretchmer N, Simoons FJ. Lactose malabsorption: Its biology and history. *In:* Schulman I, ed. Advances in Pediatrics. Vol 21. Chicago: Year Book Medical Publishers, 1974: 197.
36. Simoons FJ. Geographic patterns of primary adult lactose malabsorption: A further interpretation of evidence for the old world. *In:* Paige DM, Bayless TM, eds. Lactose Digestion: Clinical and Nutritional Implications. Baltimore: Johns Hopkins University Press, 1981: 23.
37. McNair A, Gudmand-Høyer E, Jarnum S, Orrild L. Sucrose malabsorption in Greenland. Br Med J 1972; 2:19–21.
38. Johnson JD. The regional and ethnic distribution of lactose malabsorption: Adaptive and genetic hypotheses. *In:* Paige DM, Bayless TM, eds. Lactose Digestion: Clinical and Nutritional Implications. Baltimore: Johns Hopkins University Press, 1981: 11.
39. Welsh JD, Poley JR, Bhatia M, Stevenson DE. Intestinal disaccharidase activities in relation to age, race, and mucosal damage. Gastroenterology 1978; 75:847–55.
40. Hadorn B, Green JR, Sterchi EE, Hauri HP. Biochemical mechanisms in congenital enzyme deficiencies of the small intestine. Clin Gastroenterol 1981; 10:671–90.
41. Isokoski M, Sahi T, Vallako K, Tamm A. Epidemiology and genetics of lactose malabsorption. Ann Clin Res 1981; 13:164–8.
42. Dahlqvist A. The basic aspects of the chemical background of lactase deficiency. Postgrad Med J 1977; 53:57.
43. Freiburghaus AU, Schmitz J, Schindler M, Rotthauwe HW, Kuitunen P, Launiala K, Hadorn B. Protein patterns of brush border fragments in congenital lactose malabsorption and in specific hypolactasia of the adult. N Eng J Med 1976; 294:1030–2.
44. Auricchio S, Dahlqvist A, Mürset G, Prader A. Intestinal isomaltase deficiency in patients with hereditary sucrose and starch intolerance. Lancet 1962; 1:1303.
45. Ament ME, Perera DR. Sucrase-isomaltase deficiency—a frequently misdiagnosed disease. J Pediatr 1973; 83:721–7.
46. Peterson ML, Herber R. Intestinal sucrase deficiency. Trans Assoc Am Phys 1967; 80:275–83.
47. Anderson CM, Messer M, Townley RRW, Freeman M. Intestinal sucrase and isomaltase deficiency in two siblings. Pediatrics 1963; 31:1003–10.
48. Kerry KR, Townley RRW. Genetic aspects of sucrase-isomaltase deficiency. Aust Paediatr J 1965; 1:223–35.
49. Bell RR, Draper HH, Bergan JG. Sucrose, lactose and glucose intolerance in Northern Alaskan Eskimos. Am J Clin Nutr 1973; 26:1185–90.
50. Madžarovová-Nohejlova J. Trehalase deficiency in a family. Gastroenterology 1973; 65:130–3.
51. Bergoz R. Trehalase malabsorption causing intolerance to mushrooms. Gastroenterology 1971; 60:909–12.
52. Gall DG, Hamilton JR. Infectious diarrhea in infants and children. Clin Gastroenterol 1977; 6:431–44.
53. Lifshitz F. Carbohydrate problems in pediatric gastroenterology. Clin Gastroenterology 1977; 6:415–29.
54. Coello-Ramirez P, Lifshitz F. Enteric microflora and carbohydrate intolerance in infants with diarrhea. Pediatrics 1972; 49:233–42.
55. Phillips AD, Arigao S, Sacks J, Rice SJ, France NE, Walker-Smith JA. Microvillous surface area in secondary disaccharidase deficiency. Gut 1980; 21:44–8.
56. Brunser O. Effects of malnutrition on intestinal structure and function in children. Clin Gastroenterol 1977; 6:341–53.
57. James WPT. Jejunal disaccharidase activity in children with marasmus and with kwashiorkor: Response to treatment. Arch Dis Child 1971; 46:218–20.
58. James WPT. Sugar absorption and intestinal motility in children when malnourished and after treatment. Clin Sci 1971; 39:305–18.
59. Prinsloo JG, Wittmann W, Pretorius PJ, Kruger H, Fellingham SA. Effect of different sugars on diarrhoea of acute kwashiorkor. Arch Dis Child 1969; 44:593–9.
60. Cortner JA. Giardiasis, a cause of celiac syndrome. J Dis Child 1959; 98:311.
61. Hoskins LC, Winawer SJ, Broitman SA, Gottlieb LS, Zamcheck N. Clinical giardiasis and intestinal malabsorption. Gastroenterology 1967; 53:265–79.
62. Ament EM, Rubin CE. Relation of giardiasis to abnormal intestinal structure and function in gastrointestinal immunodeficiency syndromes. Gastroenterology 1972; 62:216–26.

63. Perlow W, Baraona E, Lieber CS. Symptomatic intestinal disaccharidase deficiency in alcoholics. Gastroenterology 1977; 72:680–4.
64. Wilson FA, Hoyumpa AM Jr. Ethanol and small intestinal transport. Gastroenterology 1979; 76:388–403.
65. Truelove SC. Ulcerative colitis provoked by milk. Br Med J 1961; 1:154–60.
66. Wright R, Truelove SC. A controlled therapeutic trial of various diets on ulcerative colitis. Br Med J 1965; 2:138–41.
67. Wright R, Truelove SC. Circulating antibodies to dietary proteins in ulcerative colitis. Br Med J 1965; 2:142–4.
68. Cady AB, Rhodes J, Littman A, Crane RK. Significance of lactase deficit in ulcerative colitis. J Lab Clin Med 1967; 70:279–86.
69. Newcomer AD, McGill DB. Incidence of lactase deficiency in ulcerative colitis. Gastroenterology 1967; 53:890–3.
70. Tandon R, Mandell H, Spiro HM, Thayer WR. Lactose intolerance in Jewish patients with ulcerative colitis. Am J Dig Dis 1971; 16:845–8.
71. Kirschner BS, DeFavaro MV, Jensen W. Lactose malabsorption in children and adolescents with inflammatory bowel disease. Gastroenterology 1981; 81:829–32.
72. Pēna AS, Truelove SC. Hypolactasia and ulcerative colitis. Gastroenterology 1973; 64:400–4.
73. Beeken WL. Absorptive defects in young people with regional enteritis. Pediatrics 1973; 52:69–74.
74. Arthur AB, Cottom DG, Clayton BE, Seakins JWT, Platt JW. Importance of disaccharide intolerance in the treatment of celiac disease. Lancet 1966; 1:172–4.
75. Berg NO, Dahlqvist A, Lindberg T, Nordén A. Intestinal dipeptidases and disaccharidases in celiac disease in adults. Gastroenterology 1970; 59:575–82.
76. Lifshitz F, Holman G. Familial celiac disease with intestinal disaccharidase deficiencies. Am J Dig Dis 1966; 11:377–88.
77. Pēna AS, Truelove SC, Whitehead R. Disaccharidase activity and jejunal morphology in celiac disease. Q J Med 1972; 41:457–76.
78. Plotkin GR, Isselbacher KJ. Secondary disaccharidase deficiency in adult celiac disease (non-tropical sprue) and other malabsorption states. N Engl J Med 1964; 271:1033–9.
79. Desai HG, Chitre AV, Parekh DV, Jeejeebhoy KN. Intestinal disaccharidases in tropical sprue. Gastroenterology 1967; 53:375–80.
80. Gray GN, Walter WM Jr, Colver EH. Persistent deficiency of intestinal lactase in apparently cured tropical sprue. Gastroenterology 1968; 54:552–8.
81. Giannella RA, Rout WR, Toskes PP. Jejunal brush border injury and impaired sugar and amino acid uptake in the blind loop syndrome. Gastroenterology 1974; 67:965–74.
82. Jonas A, Krishnan C, Forstner G. Pathogenesis of mucosal injury in the blind loop syndrome: Release of disaccharidases from brush border membranes by extracts of bacteria from intestinal blind loops in rats. Gastroenterology 1978; 75:791–5.
83. Sherman P, Wesley A, Forstner G. Sequential loss of disaccharidase activities in the experimental blind loop syndrome. Gastroenterology 1982; 82:1178 (Abstract).
84. Race TF, Paes IC, Faloon WW. Intestinal malabsorption induced by oral colchicine. Clin Res 1966; 14:480.
85. Cain GD, Reiner EG, Patterson M. Effects of neomycin on disaccharidase activity of the small bowel. Arch Intern Med 1968; 122:311–4.
86. Paes IC, Searl P, Rubert MW, Faloon WW. Intestinal lactase deficiency and saccharide malabsorption during oral neomycin administration. Gastroenterology 1967; 53:49–58.
87. Halsted CH, McIntyre PA. Intestinal malabsorption caused by aminosalicylic acid therapy. Arch Intern Med 1972; 130:935–9.
88. Herbst JJ, Hurwitz R, Sunshine P, Kretchmer N. Effect of colchicine on intestinal disaccharidases: Correlation with biochemical aspects of cellular renewal. J Clin Invest 1970; 49:530–6.
89. Cohen MI, McNamara H. The effect of colchicine on guinea pig intestinal enzyme activity. Am J Dig Dis 1970; 15:247–50.
90. Knudsen KB, Bradley EM, Lecocq FR, Bellamy HM, Welsh JD. Effect of fasting and refeeding on the histology and disaccharidase activity of the human small intestine. Gastroenterology 1968; 55:46–51.
91. Levine GM, Deren JJ, Steiger E, Zinno R. Role of oral intake in maintenance of gut mass and disaccharidase activity. Gastroenterology 1974; 67:975–82.
92. Tarpila S. Morphological and functioning response of human small intestine to ionizing radiation. Scand J Gastroenterol 1971; 6(Suppl 12):9–52.
93. Neale G. The diagnosis, incidence and significance of disaccharidase deficiency in adults. Proc Roy Soc Med 1968; 61:1099–104.
94. Newcomer AD, Hodgson SF, McGill DB, Thomas PJ. Lactase deficiency: Prevalence in osteoporosis. Ann Intern Med 1978; 89:218–20.
95. Antonowicz I, Lebenthal E, Shwachman H. Disaccharidase activities in small intestinal mucosa in patients with cystic fibrosis. J Pediatr 1978; 92:214–9.
96. Bergoz R, de Peyer R. Lactose intestinale et consummation de lait avant et apres gastrectomie. Schweiz Med Wochenschr 1979; 109:605–6.
97. Walike BC, Walike JW. Relative lactose intolerance: A clinical study of tube-fed patients. JAMA 1977; 238: 948–51.
98. Bond JH, Bradley E, Currier B, Buchwald H, Levitt MD. Colonic conservation of malabsorbed carbohydrate. Gastroenterology 1980; 78:444–7.
99. Bond JH, Levitt MD. Quantitative measure of lactose absorption. Gastroenterology 1976; 70:1058–62.
100. Launiala K. The mechanism of diarrhea in congenital disaccharide malabsorption. Acta Paediatr Scand 1968; 57:425–32.
101. Christopher NL, Bayless TM. Role of the small bowel and colon in lactose-induced diarrhea. Gastroenterology 1971; 60:845–52.
102. Bond JH, Levitt MD. Investigation of small bowel transit time in man utilizing pulmonary hydrogen (H_2) measurements. J Lab Clin Med 1975; 85:546–55.
103. Debongnie JC, Newcomer AD, McGill DB, Phillips SF. Absorption of nutrients in lactase deficiency. Dig Dis Sci 1979; 24:225–31.
104. Bond JH, Levitt MD. Fate of soluble carbohydrate in the colon of rats and man. J Clin Invest 1976; 57:1158–64.
105. Ruppin H, Bar-Meir S, Soergel KH, Wood CM, Schmitt MG. Absorption of short chain fatty acids by the colon. Gastroenterology 1980; 78:1500–7.
106. Phillips SF. Lactose malabsorption and gastrointestinal function: Effects on gastrointestinal transit and the absorption of other nutrients. *In:* Paige DM, Bayless TM, eds. Lactose Digestion: Clinical and Nutritional Implications. Baltimore: Johns Hopkins University Press, 1981: 51.
107. Welsh JD. Isolated lactase deficiency in humans: report on 100 patients. Medicine 1970; 49:257–77.
108. Bayless TM, Huang SS. Recurrent abdominal pain due to milk and lactose intolerance in school-aged children. Pediatrics 1971; 47:1029–32.
109. Barr RG, Levine MD, Watkins JB. Recurrent abdominal pain of childhood due to lactose intolerance: A prospective study. N Engl J Med 1979; 300:1449–52.
110. Bedine MS, Bayless TM. Intolerance of small amounts of lactose by individuals with low lactase levels. Gastroenterology 1973; 65:735–43.
111. Welsh JD, Hall WH. Gastric emptying of lactose and milk in subjects with lactose malabsorption. Am J Dig Dis 1977; 22:1060–3.
112. Newcomer HD, Thomas PJ, McGill DB, Hoffman AF. Lactase deficiency: A common genetic trait of the American Indian. Gastroenterology 1977; 72:234–7.
113. Newcomer AD. Immediate symptomatic and long-term nutritional consequences of hypolactasia. *In:* Paige DM, Bayless TM, eds. Lactose Digestion: Clinical and Nutritional Implications. Baltimore: Johns Hopkins University Press, 1981: 124.
114. Ekus LJ, Hillman RE, Patterson JH, Rosenberg LE. Renal

and intestinal hexose transport in familial glucose-galactose malabsorption. J Clin Invest 1970; 49:576–85.
115. Derling S, Mortonsen O, Sonergeerd C. Lactosuria and aminoacidurea in infancy. A newborn error of metabolism? Acta Paediatr 1960; 49:281.
116. McGill DB, Newcomer AD. Comparison of venous and capillary blood samples in lactose tolerance testing. Gastroenterology 1967; 53:371–4.
117. Dunphy JV, Littman A, Hammond JB, Forstner G, Dahlqvist A, Crane RK. Intestinal lactose deficit in adults. Gastroenterology 1965; 49:12–21.
118. Littman A, Cady A, Rhodes J. Lactase and other disaccharidase deficiencies in a hospital population. Israel J Med Sci 1968; 4:110–6.
119. Isokoski M, Jussila J, Sarna S. A simple screening method for lactose malabsorption. Gastroenterology 1972; 62:28–32.
120. Newcomer AD, McGill DB, Thomas PJ, Hoffman AF. Prospective comparison of indirect methods for detecting lactase deficiency. N Engl J Med 1975; 293:1232–6.
121. Barr RG, Watkins JB, Perman JA. Mucosal function and breath hydrogen excretion: Comparative studies in the clinical evaluation of children with non-specific abdominal complaints. Pediatrics 1981; 68:526–33.
122. Lisker R, Aguilar L, Zavala C. Intestinal lactase deficiency and milk drinking capacity in the adult. Am J Clin Nutr 1978; 31:1499–503.
123. Welsh JD. Diet therapy in adult lactose malabsorption: Present practices. Am J Clin Nutr 1978; 31:1499–503.
124. The Medical Letter 1981; 23:67 (July 24).
125. Cheng AHR, Brunser O, Espinoza J, Fones HL, Monkeberg F, Chichester CO, Rand G, Hourigan AG. Long-term acceptance of low-lactose milk. Am J Clin Nutr 1979; 32:1989–93.
126. Turner SJ, Daly T, Hourigan JA, Rand AG, Thayer WR. Utilization of a low-lactose milk. Am J Clin Nutr 1976; 29:739–44.
127. Paige DM, Bayless TN, Huang SS, Wexler R. Lactase hydrolyzed milk. Am J Clin Nutr 1975; 28:818–22.

Chapter 105

Gluten-induced Enteropathy (Celiac Disease)

W. T. Cooke • G. K. T. Holmes

The first description of sprue is attributed to Aretaeus the Cappadocian, who lived in the second century AD.[1] He described the characteristic stool and recognized the chronicity of the condition, noting that the disorder was more common in women than in men and that children could also be affected. However, it was not until 1888 that Gee[2] produced his classic paper "On the Coeliac Affection," in which he delineated with great precision the features of what would now be regarded as celiac disease in childhood. Gee clearly regarded this disorder and tropical sprue, which was already well documented, as the same disease. The confusion was to continue for several years, being perpetuated by Thaysen[3] in his influential monograph published in 1932, in which he declared that tropical sprue, non-tropical sprue, and Gee-Herter disease should all be grouped under the term "idiopathic steatorrhoea." During this period the clinical, metabolic, and radiologic features of non-tropical sprue were becoming better established.[4,5] The views of Thaysen were increasingly questioned, and in 1954 Paulley[6] demonstrated definite abnormalities in the jejunal mucosa in patients. With the introduction of jejunal biopsy and the discovery of the role of gluten, it became clear that celiac disease and non-tropical sprue were identical conditions and that tropical sprue was a separate and distinct entity.

Definition

Celiac disease requires definition to allow evaluation of clinical data, diagnostic methods, treatments, and research results. Its definition over the last 30 years has revolved around the clinical reactions and responses of the jejunal mucosa to gluten withdrawal and challenge. Two definitions have gained popularity in adult practice: the first, as expressed by Rubin et al.,[7] is "the demonstration of a characteristic flat mucosal lesion by suction biopsy of the proximal small intestine" and "the demonstration of a dramatic clinical response to the removal of gluten from the diet"; the second, as stated by Booth,[8] is "a condition in which there is an abnormal jejunal mucosa which improves morphologically when treated with a gluten-free diet and which again shows abnormalities when gluten is reintroduced."

The European Society for Paediatric Gastroenterology (ESPGAN)[9] proposed a further definition for childhood celiac disease: (1) it is a permanent condition; (2) there is a flat mucosa in the upper small intestine; (3) a gluten-free diet results in the complete restoration of normal mucosal architecture; and (4) reintroduction of gluten into the diet will be followed by mucosal abnormalities. It was stated that a gluten-free diet should not contain wheat, barley, rye, or oats.

However, there are clearly problems with these definitions.[10] What constitutes an acceptable clinical and morphologic response has not been defined in quantitative terms. Also, there is no standardized procedure for a gluten challenge either in the amount of gluten administered or for how long. Nor are the morphologic criteria for relapse specified. Indeed, sensitivity to gluten among celiac patients, particularly adults, is so variable that it would be virtually impossible to standardize the test. This is reflected in the widely differing regimens that different workers have used. Although there is usually a clear-cut response to the administration of gluten within 6 months to 1 year in children, in some instances the response may be delayed much longer.[11] Therefore it cannot be stated that if a normal diet has not produced a positive result in 2 years, the patient cannot have celiac disease.[12] This has made the concept of transient gluten intolerance difficult to evaluate, for it is not certain whether patients so labeled will present in later life with celiac disease. While a positive result can be taken as proving the diagnosis, a negative one cannot immediately refute it. In any event, gluten challenge is rarely used to establish the diagnosis in adults and even in children is carried out only in a minority of patients.

It can be assumed that the transition from normal mucosa to flat mucosa to normal mucosa as gluten is added to and removed from the diet may take weeks, months, or even years to evolve. The first abnormality to occur in the mucosa on exposure to gluten is an increase in inflammatory cells, followed by progressive shortening of the villi and elongation of the crypts. An even more dense infiltrate develops and finally the flat mucosa results. A jejunal biopsy could be done at any point in this process, so that it is theoretically possible to detect an early lesion. Support for the concept of a mild or early lesion comes from several sources. Thus, children on a gluten-containing diet are described who have normal jejunal mucosa, which later becomes flat.[13,14] In patients with dermatitis herpetiformis the increased number of intra-epithelial lymphocytes in otherwise normal biopsies decreases when a gluten-free diet is instituted; this is taken to indicate celiac disease.[15] Of major importance in this respect is the observation that if patients with dermatitis herpetiformis and apparently normal villi are subjected to a heavy gluten load, a flat mucosa results.[16] Finally, family studies of celiac disease have revealed many individuals with mild mucosal abnormalities who may well be potential celiacs.[17]

With regard to the specificity of the lesion characteristic of untreated celiac disease, one stumbling block has been that all too often only the "flatness" of the mucosa has been considered. Excluded from consideration are the many other features of the mucosa, such as the state of the epithelium, the nature of the cellular infiltrate, and the mitotic activity in the crypts. When all these features are carefully considered, *a flat jejunal biopsy obtained from a white adult in the Western World is almost always indicative of celiac disease.* There are very few disorders with biopsy findings indistinguishable from those of celiac disease, although tropical sprue, soy protein intolerance, cow's milk protein intolerance, and infantile gastroenteritis may cause some diagnostic problems.

In summary, it must be conceded that there is no satisfactory definition of celiac disease, but from the practical point of view, the diagnosis in the majority of patients is relatively easy. Nearly all patients will have flat jejunal biopsies and most will show clinical and morphologic improvement on a gluten-free diet.

Epidemiology

Geographic Distribution and Prevalence. Celiac disease has been considered a disorder of Europe, North America, and Australia, but is now known to occur in many other parts of the world. Its prevalence is not known for certain, but in England it is probably higher than the figure often quoted of 1 in 2000 of the population. In an analysis based on the number of children who were recommended for special diets in England and Wales in the years 1946 to 1948, the average number of *new cases* per year was 92, an occurrence rate of 1 in 8000. The corresponding figure for Scotland was 1 in 4000. Other studies of children in the United Kingdom have suggested a prevalence rate lying between 1 in 2000, 1 in 6000, 1 in 1778, 1 in 1850, and 1 in 1100.[18]

In the West of Ireland figures are much higher than for Britain, with a prevalence rate of 1 in 303.[18] Approximately 2 children for every adult are diagnosed in Ireland. In France, in the Paris area, the frequency appears to be less than that in England (0.52 per 100,000 per year in the general population, with about 10 children for every adult). In Austria, the incidence has been quoted as 1 in 403 in girls and 1 in 636 in boys. In Switzerland, it is reported as 1 in 890; in Norway, 1 in 1143; and in Sweden, variously as 1 in 6500, 1 in 3700, 1 in 982, and 1 in

1700.[19,20] There are no figures on which to make an accurate assessment of the frequency in the United States. The apparent scarcity of celiac disease in the United States is surprising, since large numbers of Europeans have formed the immigrant population for several centuries.

Celiac disease occurs in non-white peoples. It has been reported from the wheat-eating areas of Bengal and the Punjab, as opposed to the predominantly rice-eating areas of Southern India. Indian and Pakistani children with celiac disease have been recorded in England. The disorder has also been found in blacks, Arabs, Cubans, Mexicans, Spaniards, Brazilians, Sudanese, and Cantonese. The frequency of celiac disease in tropical countries is at present uncertain.[21]

Sex and Age Distribution. Celiac disease is more common in women than in men, in a ratio of 1.3:1. The disorder may present at any age after the introduction of cereals into the diet. In a series of 157 children with celiac disease seen in Glasgow, Scotland between 1964 and 1970, 50% were diagnosed before the age of 2 years.[22] Because of the natural remission that occurs during adolescence, it is most unusual for a patient to present during this period. A bimodal distribution has been observed, with an early peak in the fourth decade, mainly in women, and a later peak in the sixth and seventh decades, mainly in men. A similar bimodal distribution was noted among more than 1000 patients joining the Coeliac Society of the United Kingdom over a period of 1 year. The frequency in childhood may be declining owing to changes in infant feeding practices and the later introduction of cereals into the diet. The diagnosis appears to be made much more frequently in children than in adults, in whom estimates are difficult to come by. Nevertheless, the diagnosis should not be overlooked in the elderly, for as many as 27% of patients may present in the seventh decade of life.[23]

Familial Occurrence. The first attempt at a systematic family study of celiac disease was that carried out by Davidson and Fountain in 1950. They obtained a history of steatorrhea or symptoms suggestive of malabsorption in 8.2% of relatives of 205 children with celiac disease. A number of series followed based only on clinical information, but confirming these findings. MacDonald and colleagues, in 1965, carried out the initial study in which jejunal biopsy was used in 96 relatives of 17 index patients. Four of 31 siblings had celiac disease, and 5 of 26 children of the index patients were affected; none of the parents were affected.

Stokes and his colleagues,[17] in an extensive study, found that 35 of 182 first-degree relatives had a flat biopsy. Of these, 12 were asymptomatic. Nevertheless, all those who accepted a gluten-free diet noticed a marked improvement in energy and well-being. In addition, 6 relatives with less severe changes in the jejunal mucosa improved clinically on a gluten-free diet and were also considered to have celiac disease. This gave an overall familial frequency of 22% for those biopsied and 12% for all the available living first-degree relatives. There were higher percentages than normal of relatives with HLA-B8 antigen and anticonnective tissue antibodies among those with nonspecific biopsy appearances. This suggests that the series contained a number of potential celiac patients who might manifest the full syndrome at a future date.

Studies of Twins. The occurrence of celiac disease in twins has centered on discordance in monozygotic twins.[24] Because of the identical genetic make-up of these individuals, it is certain that each twin has the celiac trait. Hence, other influences, such as additional dietary gluten, intestinal infection, or other stresses, are necessary to provoke overt disease. These examples highlight the interplay of genetic and environmental factors in the etiology of celiac disease. Concordance in identical twins is well documented.[21]

Blood Groups. The frequency of ABO, Rhesus, P_1, and MN antigens in celiac patients is similar to that in the general population.

Pathology

Small Intestinal Biopsy. Various devices for obtaining jejunal biopsies have been developed,[25] and specially modified instruments are available that can be safely used in children.[27] These instruments and the techniques for obtaining a biopsy with their use are discussed in detail in Chapters 47 and 103.

Celiac disease may be diagnosed reliably by duodenoscopy and biopsy. Although specimens obtained by the endoscopic forceps are much smaller than those obtained by conventional capsules, they are usually quite adequate for histologic assessment. In addition, this technique allows the upper gastrointestinal tract to be inspected for other lesions.[28] Biopsies obtained by endoscopic forceps are too small to orientate and may be submitted to the laboratory floating freely in fixative. Small intestinal biopsies only rarely cause complications, e.g., bleeding, perforation, retention of the capsule, ileus, intramural jejunal hematoma, and the postbiopsy syndrome consisting of low-grade fever, diffuse abdominal pain, and rebound tenderness. Young children and the elderly, however, are at special risk.[29]

Morphologic Appearances of Jejunal Mucosa. The structural changes found in the malabsorption syndromes are described in Chapter 103. Those characteristically noted in celiac disease are also discussed here in greater detail because of their importance in this disease.

Dissecting Microscopy. Digitate villi, leaf forms, and ridges may be found in normal subjects, (Fig. 105–1). Digitate villi have a characteristic finger-like appearance with a height usually about 3 times greater than their width. Leaf forms are more flattened from side to side, whereas ridges are shorter than either the villi or the leaf forms but have more extensive long axes. Convolutions are extremely long ridges that have fused and buckled and show a striking resemblance to the surface of the brain. In tropical areas, a fully convoluted pattern may be found in more than 5% of the normal population; malnutrition and infection undoubtedly play an important part in its development. Such an appearance would not fall within the normal range in persons living in temperate zones.

In celiac disease, the jejunal mucosa may be flat and featureless. More usually, it presents a mosaic pattern, the surface being intersected by deep depressions that leave elevated mounds. Some 8 to 40 crypt openings are found on each mound (Fig. 105–2).

Examination by stereomicroscopy and transmission microscopy should be regarded as complementary procedures. The dissecting microscope quickly and easily allows the whole specimen to be assessed for mucosal patchiness.

Transmission Microscopy. An overall impression of the mucosa may be obtained under the light microscope at low magnification. Normally, the villi constitute 65% to 80% of the total mucosal thickness, while the crypts make up the remainder. At higher magnification the epithelium is seen to be made up of tall columnar cells with a well-marked brush border and a basally situated nucleus. The crypts are lined by undifferentiated cells that, by a process of division, migration, and maturation, replace the mature absorptive cells that are continually being lost from the tips of the villi. In celiac disease, while there may be depressions on the surface corresponding to the edge of mosaics, there are no structures identifiable as villi (Fig. 105–3). The crypts are hypertrophied and sometimes branched and the num-

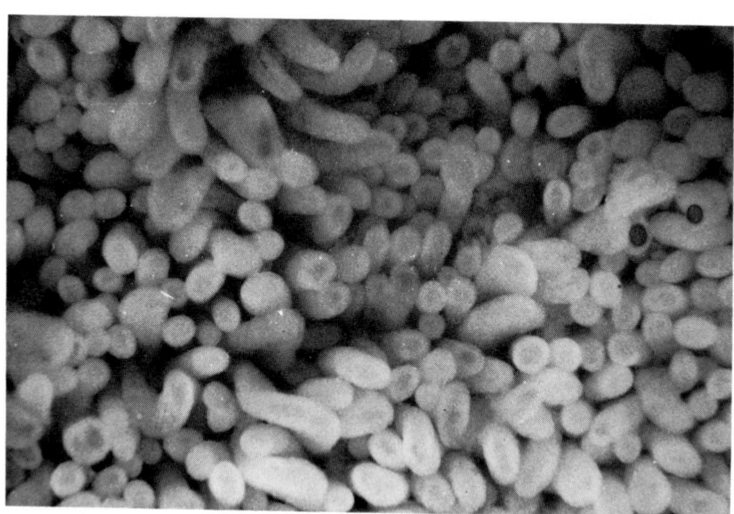

Figure 105–1. Dissecting microscope view of normal jejunal mucosa showing digitate and leaf shaped villi.

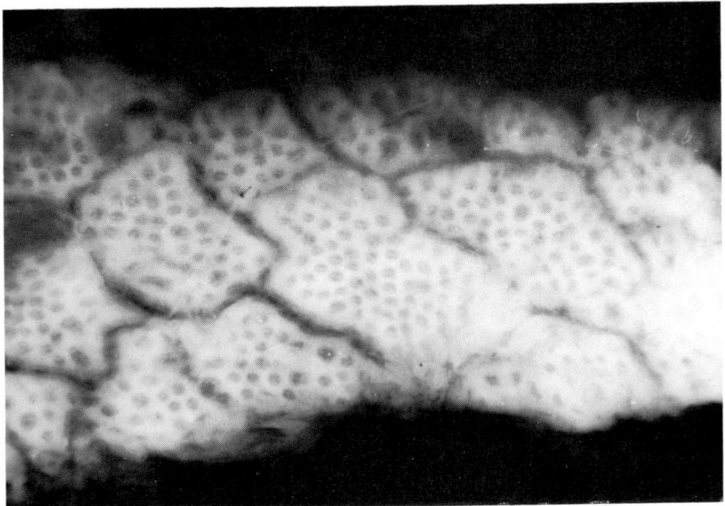

Figure 105–2. Dissecting microscope view of flat, mosaic jejunal mucosa in untreated celiac disease.

bers of mitoses are increased. The total mucosal thickness is normal. The epithelial cells are cuboidal and may appear stratified. The brush border is poorly developed or absent, and under the electron microscope the microvilli show varying degrees of abnormalities ranging from shortening to complete absence (Fig. 105–4).

Paneth Cells. Paneth cells have a characteristic morphology and are found almost exclusively at the bases of the crypts. Their function is unclear, but they secrete immunoglobulin and lysozyme. Estimates of their numbers in celiac disease have given conflicting results. Paneth cell deficiency has been reported in patients who have responded poorly to a gluten-free diet, but this is disputed. Because of the mucosal disorganization in celiac disease, Paneth cells may more readily discharge their contents into the crypt lumen. As a consequence, their recognition may be difficult, and reduction in their numbers may be more apparent than real.[30]

Endocrine Cells. It has been suggested that the increased numbers of cholecystokinin (CCK) and secretin cells present in the mucosa result from an abnormality in the release mechanisms for these hormones. Some support for this view comes from the observations that celiac patients have an abnormal pancreatic exocrine response to oral stimuli, while the response to IV stimuli is normal. Enterochromaffin cells are also increased in number, along with greater tissue concentra-

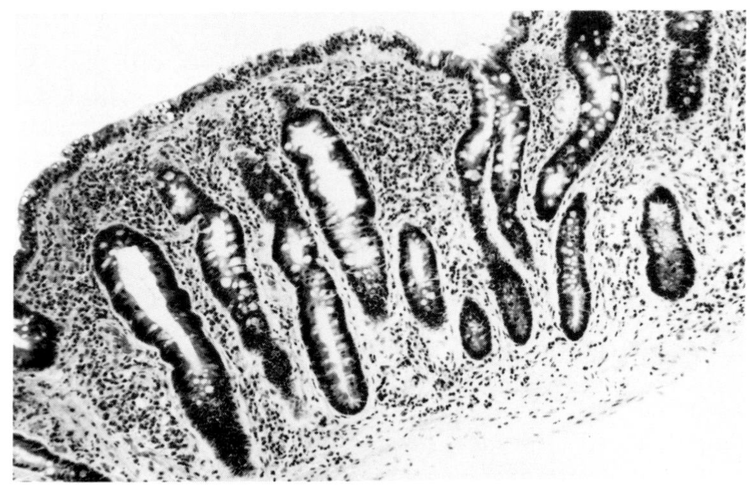

Figure 105–3. Flat jejunal mucosa in untreated celiac disease. The crypts are elongated and a dense inflammatory cell infiltrate is seen in both the lamina propria and the epithelium.

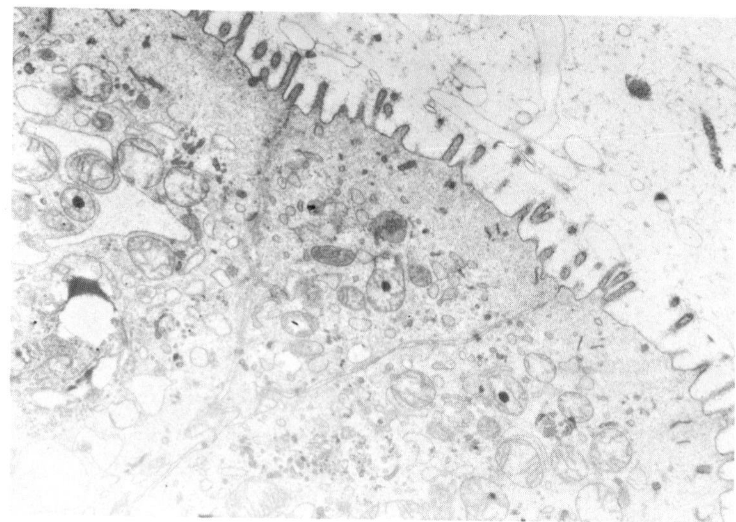

Figure 105–4. Grossly abnormal microvilli of the jejunal mucosa in untreated celiac disease. (Courtesy of Dr. M. Lucas.)

tions of 5-hydroxytryptamine in the duodenal mucosa of untreated patients.[31]

Basement Membrane. In patients with untreated celiac disease, the basement membrane varies from normal to grossly thickened and may merge with the underlying reticulin network. The significance of the thickening, which is often patchy, is unknown. Claims have been made for a specific clinical entity designated *"collagenous sprue."*[32] However, this view has not been generally accepted, as subepithelial collagenous thickening commonly occurs in celiac disease patients who respond quite normally to a gluten-free diet.[33]

Inflammatory Cell Infiltrate. A feature of the jejunal mucosa found in celiac disease is the presence of a dense inflammatory cell infiltrate. In the epithelium this is made up of lymphocytes that vary in both size and staining characteristics. Plasma cells are never seen, but eosinophils may be found occasionally. Unlike normal epithelium, in which the lymphocytes are found mainly below the level of the enterocyte nuclei, in celiac disease these cells are scattered more evenly. The infiltrate in the lamina propria is composed mainly of plasma cells. It has proved possible to quantitate these cells, and intra-epithelial lymphocyte counts have been expressed in terms of a fixed number of enterocyte nuclei or per unit length of mucosa.[34,35] These counts are high in untreated celiac disease and fall toward normal following gluten withdrawal. However, they usually remain above the normal range, even when the jejunal mucosa has returned to virtual normality.

The cells within the lamina propria can also be quantitated using a graticule in the eyepiece of a microscope and the quantity expressed as counts per square mm of tissue.[35] In patients on a normal diet, plasma cell counts are significantly increased, while lymphocytes are significantly reduced. These abnormalities tend to reverse following treatment with a gluten-free diet, but elevated plasma cell numbers usually persist. It may be that the continuing ingestion of small amounts of gluten or other allergens is responsible for the continuing changes.

Cell counts can be performed on routinely processed histologic material and have added a further dimension to the assessment of jejunal biopsies. Definitions of celiac disease need to take account of these more subtle morphologic changes.

Quantitative Assessment of Jejunal Mucosa. Subjective evaluation of jejunal biopsies is adequate for establishing the diagnosis of celiac disease and the response to treatment in the majority of patients. Nevertheless, quantitative assessment has advantages, particularly in documenting minor degrees of abnormality. Biopsies from different patients, or from the same patient on different occasions, may be compared with greater accuracy and effects of treatment can be monitored more precisely.

Early attempts at quantification relied on

linear measurements of such features as mucosal thickness, villous height, and crypt depth. Minor degrees of villous abnormality are reflected in a surface-to-volume ratio obtained by using a template. Television image analysis also derives a ratio for the areas occupied by the surface and crypt epithelium. Image tracing techniques employing a mini-computer allow computation of several indices for detecting minor changes. However, the clinical relevance of these sophisticated methods is far from clear, and in the majority of instances these procedures achieve little more than does routine histologic assessment.

Formation of the Flat Mucosa. The flat jejunal mucosa of celiac disease has been considered a consequence of chronic inflammation or the progressive fusion of villi following injury, but such hypotheses are now of only historical interest. Villous atrophy can be induced experimentally in animals by arresting cell division in the mucosa. This mechanism, however, cannot also account for the biopsy appearances in celiac disease, since most workers have found increased mitotic activity in the crypts. Furthermore, the increased loss of DNA into the bowel lumen and evidence from organ culture studies of epithelial cell proliferation and migration along the villi[36] point to increased cellular activity in the mucosa in untreated celiac disease. Both the proliferative and maturation compartments of the epithelium increase so that, overall, *celiac mucosa produces 6 times more cells per hour than does normal mucosa.*[37] The hyperactivity of the mucosa may be regarded as a compensatory mechanism for replacing damaged enterocytes.

The Distribution of Mucosal Lesions. The most severe lesions in celiac disease are to be found in the proximal small intestine, but within this area the mucosal changes are patchy. When multiple jejunal biopsies are taken, the specimens will differ by one or more histologic grades in 1 in 5 patients.[38] In celiac disease and dermatitis herpetiformis, differences of 2 or more grades were found in 25% of the patients assessed by dissecting microscopy and in 10% assessed by histologic studies.[39] Furthermore, patchiness was similar for the 2 conditions. These observations emphasize that multiple biopsies may be necessary to detect a mucosal abnormality or to assess the response of patients to treatment with a gluten-free diet.

Autopsy studies have revealed that the extent of involvement of the intestine with flat, mosaic mucosa varies considerably. In untreated patients, as little as 14% of the proximal small bowel may be flat, with more distal areas showing less severe change or normal mucosa. Only rarely does the entire small intestine show extensive, severe abnormalities. Again, patchiness of the lesions has been observed.[40]

Pathogenesis

The Role of Gluten. It has been recognized for over 30 years, since the classic observations made in Holland by Dicke, Weijers, and Van de Kamer,[41,42] that the etiology of celiac disease is inextricably bound to cereal consumption and, in particular, to gluten and its constituent fractions. Research has been aimed at identifying a specific factor in wheat that is harmful to celiac patients and determining how this factor produces its damaging effects. This has necessitated extensive investigation of the very complex chemistry of cereal proteins and has also required the development of methods whereby gluten and its subfractions could be tested in a clinical setting.

Chemistry of Wheat Protein. Wheat flour contains 7% to 15% protein, of which 90% is *gluten.* Gluten itself consists of a heterogeneous group of proteins that still have not been completely characterized. Extraction of gluten with ethyl alcohol separates the protein in a soluble fraction, *gliadin,* and an insoluble part, *glutenin.* When only a single wheat variety is used as the source, gliadin contains about 40 different components. These can be divided into 4 groups: α-, β-, γ-, and ω-gliadins, depending on electrophoretic mobility in starch gel. The molecular weights are not known for certain because of technical difficulties involved in separating the components. For α-gliadin the molecular weight probably lies between 30,000 and 50,000.

The Toxic Fraction. Frazer and his colleagues[43] showed that a soluble peptic-tryptic digest of gluten, designated gluten fraction III, was harmful to patients with celiac disease. Gluten fraction III has since been used extensively in many investigations of the disorder. Gliadin is rendered nontoxic by exhaustive digestion with crude papain. This action has been attributed to the presence of the enzyme glutamine cyclotransferase, which promotes the conversion of *N*-glutamyl peptides to pyrrolidone carboxyl peptides.[44] However, the intestinal mucosa does not contain this enzyme and the detoxicating mechanism in vivo is almost certainly unlike that of crude papain. Furthermore, there is evidence that *N*-pyrrolidone carboxyl peptides are harmful to patients with celiac disease. Thus, Bronstein and his group[45] digested gliadin sequentially with pepsin, trypsin, pancrelipase (Cotazym), and intestinal peptidase. The ultrafiltrates of these digests, containing smaller peptides, were shown to be toxic, as indicated by an increase in fecal fat excretion in feeding experiments. It was believed that the harmful fractions contained *N*-pyrrolidone carboxyl peptides. The toxic peptide, if such exists, may have a molecular weight of less than 1000 and so be composed of 6 to 8 amino acids.[46]

Gliadin has also been separated into components by ion exchange chromatography. Of these, fraction 9 is the most toxic. This fraction was shown (1) to inhibit morphologic improvement of duodenal mucosa from patients with untreated celiac disease in organ culture; (2) to yield the highest agglutination titers with sera from untreated patients; and (3) to disrupt rat liver lysosomes.[47]

Because of the great complexity of gluten and the difficulties of testing potentially harmful fractions, a specific toxic substance has still to be identified.

The Missing Enzyme Hypothesis. Frazer[48] suggested more than 20 years ago that the prime defect in celiac disease might be the absence of a peptidase from the jejunal mucosa. The absence of this peptidase would result in the maldigestion of gluten with accumulation of harmful peptides. This was deduced from observations that wheat protein was injurious to celiac patients, but was rendered innocuous following incubation with hog intestinal mucosa. While many enzyme activities are altered in the damaged mucosa obtained from newly diagnosed patients, these return to normal following gluten withdrawal and the restoration of mucosal architecture. There may be some exceptions with respect to enzymes in the brush border (e.g., β-glucosidase), in which activity remains reduced even when jejunal histology has returned to near normal.[49] Whether this reflects a basic defect in the brush border or, as is more likely, a very slow response following treatment, is still unclear.

Peptidase Deficiency. Through the years, a peptidase deficiency has been sought by means of several techniques. The measurement of plasma amino acids in celiac disease does not provide any evidence that gluten digestion is specifically impaired. The reduced ability of jejunal mucosa from untreated patients to release proline, glutamine, and other amino acids from a digest of gluten is clearly a secondary phenomenon, since after treatment with a gluten-free diet or steroids, amino acid release reverts to normal. Peptidases have also been studied by starch gel electrophoresis and analytical subcellular fractionation, but without providing any evidence of an enzyme deficiency in patients fully treated with a gluten-free diet. In any event, the peptide hydrolases have such broad specificity that even if one were missing its absence would be unlikely to result in such severe changes as are found in celiac disease.[50]

Carbohydrase Deficiency. Other approaches to the problem of etiology have led to the suggestion that the toxicity of gluten may lie not in a particular sequence of amino acids but in a side-chain substituent, such as a glycoprotein.[51] Thus, the removal of a carbohydrate component should render gluten innocuous to celiac patients while leaving the peptide chain intact. An enzyme system from *Aspergillus niger* achieves this. Gliadin so treated has been tested in feeding experiments and appears not to harm patients. It was suggested, therefore, that carbohydrase present in the microbial extract was responsible for detoxifying gliadin. Characterization of the enzymes, however, has not been completed and this work awaits confirmation.

Disaccharidase Deficiency. In untreated celiac disease, brush border enzymes are particularly reduced. Since concentrations improve following treatment with a gluten-free diet, this has been regarded as a secondary effect. However, lactase levels remain low even though the mucosa has returned to normal morphologically.[52] It has been suggested that an underlying lactase deficiency may precipitate the disorder, and perhaps this enzyme is important in the pathogenesis of the disease.

The Immunologic Hypothesis. The view that celiac disease may be an immunologic disorder has gradually gained ground over the last decade and is supported by both clinical observations and experimental data. Thus, an occasional patient may develop a severe reaction to ingested gluten suggestive of a hypersensitivity reaction and termed *"gliadin shock."*[53] Also, there appears to be an increased occurrence of disorders associated with celiac disease that themselves have an immunologic basis.[54] In addition, the cellular infiltrate of plasma cells and lymphocytes in the jejunal mucosa suggests an immunologic disturbance. The lymphoid tissues are abnormal, with enlarged fleshy mesenteric nodes, while the peripheral lymph nodes are small and fibrotic. The occurrence of hyposplenism may reflect impaired immunity and the increased frequency of autoimmunity found in celiac disease.[55] Finally, the increased prevalence of malignancy, particularly lymphoma, observed in celiac disease may be due to defective immune surveillance mechanisms.[56]

The Local Immune System. The first point of contact for ingested gluten in the small bowel is with the epithelium. It would seem logical to propose, therefore, that the basic defect in celiac disease may be an abnormality in the binding of gluten to the surface membrane of the enterocytes. Alternatively, interaction between gluten and the intraepithelial lymphocytes may be the prime event. In this regard, the local immune system in the mucosa has been implicated as an etiologic factor. IgA and IgM synthesis is increased in the jejunal mucosa of celiac patients consuming either a normal diet or a gluten-free diet, followed by gluten challenge; antigliadin antibody can also be demonstrated.[57] It is not known whether the synthesis of these locally produced antibodies represents a primary pathologic abnormality or a secondary event. Their role has still to be determined.

Type I Hypersensitivity Reactions. An increase in IgE-containing cells has been observed in the jejunal mucosa of untreated celiac patients and in many patients treated with a gluten-free diet.[58] A significant increase in IgE cells following gluten challenge, with mast cell degranulation and increased eosinophil counts in the post-challenge biopsies, has also been demonstrated. In addition, gluten challenge is associated with increased histamine and 5-hydroxytryptamine in the mucosa.[59] These observations suggest that type I hypersensitivity reactions may be of importance in the etiology of celiac disease. A few patients with food allergy are sensitive to cereals, but jejunal biopsies have not been carried out in these cases. In patients with celiac disease, radioallergosorbent (RAST) studies using a variety of cereal antigens have been negative, even when the serum IgE levels were elevated.[60] Cereals can undoubtedly produce symptoms in some patients without celiac disease by mechanisms that are not understood, although in some, type I hypersensitivity has been demonstrated. It is doubtful whether this mechanism has any relevance in the pathogenesis of celiac disease.

Immune Complexes. The small intestinal mucosa may be damaged by immune complexes. While these complexes may represent nothing more than the end result of tissue damage, they could be of importance in pathogenesis. Following gluten challenge they appear to be deposited in the subepithelial tissues of the mucosa and produce cytopathologic damage, which precedes changes in the enterocytes.[61] Immune complexes arising in the damaged mucosa may also be deposited in tissues and organs elsewhere. The disturbances they incite at these sites could account for the many different immunologic disorders found in association with celiac disease. Support for this suggestion comes from observations made in patients with dermatitis herpetiformis, in whom immune complexes have been detected in the circulation and may play a part in producing the characteristic skin lesions.

Cell-Mediated Mechanisms. It has been demonstrated by several techniques that lymphocytes from patients with celiac disease are sensitized to gluten. The question that arises is whether such cells play any part in producing the flat biopsy characteristic of this disease. Thymus-dependent mechanisms are involved in the rejection of allografts of mouse small intestine.[62] While the process of rejection bears some resemblance to the mucosal changes found in untreated celiac disease, there are some important differences. For example, the epithelium is well preserved and intraepithelial lymphocytes are absent from the mucosa in about one quarter of the grafts. By contrast, an abnormal epithelium infiltrated with lymphocytes is a characteristic finding in celiac disease. In addition, antigen within the mucosa is probably removed rapidly under normal circumstances, and it is not clear how gluten could remain at this site sufficiently long for cell-mediated reactions to occur. It is possible, however, that gluten is held in immune complexes or macrophages.

Another puzzle is why the reactions should be so localized in the gut, since skin tests have not shown convincing evidence of delayed hypersensitivity. Positive skin tests, rather, have been of the Arthus type.[63] One thought is that celiac patients may have a population of lymphocytes directed against their own jejunal mucosa. It has also been suggested that celiac disease results from a graft-versus-host–like reaction localized to the small bowel wall.[64]

If celiac disease is due to immunologic mechanisms, it is likely that several types are involved. Thus, the interaction of gluten with the intra-epithelial lymphocytes could stimulate antibody formation. This, in turn, could damage the epithelium, and render it permeable to macromolecules, such as gluten. As a consequence, complexes form in the lamina propria, particularly around the basement membrane, and cause further mucosal damage. Gluten held in macrophages or complexes may sensitize lymphocytes and result in delayed hypersensitivity reactions that perpetuate the lesion. However, immunologic experiments have not fully reproduced the mucosal changes seen in well-established celiac disease and the primary event whereby patients are immunized to gluten remains unidentified.

The Lectin Hypothesis. A suggestion regarding the etiology of celiac disease has been advanced by Weiser and Douglas[65] based on the ability of lectins to react with cell membranes. Lectins are proteins and glycoproteins that are widely distributed in the plant kingdom and have a number of potent biologic properties. For example, they preferentially agglutinate tumor cells and epithelial cells from the intestine of the human fetus and can differentiate virally transformed and nontransformed cells in tissue culture. The effect of lectins on cells is thought to be due to the specificity that they have for a carbohydrate component of the cell membrane, a reaction analogous to the binding of an antigen and its antibody.

The biosynthesis of the glycoproteins of the cell membranes is dependent upon a series of glycosyltransferases. Through their action, sugars are added in a specific sequence to the oligosaccharide chains that grow at the non-reducing ends or branch points. Some chains will be incomplete, and their numbers are increased in intestinal tumor cells, normal crypt intestinal cells, and virally transformed cells. Immature intestinal cells show increased binding and susceptibility to agglutination by a plant lectin, concanavalin A, which can lead to cell death.

These observations led Weiser and Douglas to suggest that "gluten, or a fraction thereof, would bind to altered, exposed, incomplete cell-surface-membrane glycoproteins and act as a toxic lectin." This reaction would kill villous absorption cells, which would result in increased cell turnover and lengthened crypts in the mucosa, characteristic findings in celiac disease. A cycle of increasing pathologic change would be set up, since immature cells have more incomplete glycoproteins on the surface membrane and consequently are more susceptible to damage by gluten. This hypothesis helps to explain why some patients may have a normal jejunal mucosa at certain times in life; there could be a phase when cells composing the epithelium are well differentiated and relatively resistant to damage by gluten and when cell losses are easily replaced. A period of stress, such as an enteric infection or an unusually high gluten intake, could upset this delicate balance. The mucosa would then be unable to compensate for cell loss and obvious morphologic damage would result.

This hypothesis offers new approaches to the study of celiac disease and perhaps other enteropathies, such as soy protein intolerance. It centers attention on defects of glycoprotein synthesis in the cell membrane as the primary abnormality.

The Constitutional Hypothesis. Celiac disease is considered to be a life-long inherited condition. Since many patients do not develop symptoms until late in life, however, both constitutional factors and external influences must be important and operating together cause the disorder to become manifest. The relative contributions of these 2 influences must differ considerably in different individuals, as evidenced by the variable clinical picture of celiac disease. Thus, those who develop overt celiac disease in childhood may have a particularly strong predisposing constitutional make-up, whereas those who develop the disease later in life may have a weak inherited background and require a prolonged heavy gluten load or other stresses to precipitate symptoms. There is an increased prevalence of celiac disease among first-degree relatives of celiac patients. The older the proband, the greater is the frequency. When the proband is a child, the prevalence rate among first-degree relatives is about 5%; when the proband is an adult, the rate is about 19%. These observations support the view of an interplay between a constitutional factor and external influences, with exposure to gluten in particular playing an increasingly important role as time passes.

With regard to constitutional factors, the HLA antigens, particularly HLA-B8, have aroused considerable interest. Approximately 75% of celiac patients have this antigen, as compared with about 20% of the general population.[66] The HLA antigens are inherited and are not the result of disease. However, other factors must be involved because family studies have shown conclusively that celiac disease is inherited independently of HLA-B8 while 20% of the normal population have this antigen but do not have celiac disease. Furthermore, celiac patients with and without HLA-B8 are identical, both in terms of clinical presentation and response to a gluten-free diet. There also is increased frequency of HLA-Dw3, DRw3, and gluten-sensitive enteropathy (GSE)–associated B cell antigens. In an important family study, celiac disease appeared to occur when the family member was homozygous for the GSE-associated antigen and also carried the HLA-Dw3 antigen(s) or an antigen usually associated with Dw3.[67] However, the observation that identical twins may be discordant for the disease[24] would indicate that genetic make-up alone is insufficient to induce the disorder.

Pathophysiology

The reduction in the surface area of the intestine as a consequence of the intestinal changes that characterize celiac disease very likely does not play a major role with respect to intestinal absorption in most patients with this disease. Usually a flat biopsy is found only in the upper jejunum and involvement of the entire length of the intestine is rare. Much more important are the enzyme changes in the damaged epithelial absorptive cells and the alterations in the microclimate and glycocalyx.

Intraluminal pH. The intraluminal pH in the upper jejunum in patients with untreated celiac disease is more alkaline than in normal subjects (i.e., about 7.5, with return to the normal of about 7.1 after treatment with a gluten-free diet).[68]

Bacterial Flora. The upper intestinal tract in many celiac patients is sterile. Those with abnormal bacterial counts have a variety of gram-negative and anaerobic organisms; following gluten withdrawal, these organisms tend to return to insignificant numbers. There is no relationship between intestinal infection and the degree of steatorrhea, intestinal pH, vitamin B_{12} absorption, or serum folic levels. Despite such observations, claims for clinical improvement following treatment with antibiotics have been made.

Epithelial Cells. The covering of the intestinal mucosa is formed by a sheet of epithelial cells, which also line the elongated crypts. There is a markedly increased turnover of these cells in celiac disease, with approximately a 3-fold increase in the number of proliferating cells and a doubling of the rate of cell division. The crypt cells in celiac patients are essentially the same as those in normal subjects except that they cover one third or more of the elongated crypts in patients with untreated celiac disease. The microvilli are sparse and irregular and the terminal web is virtually absent. Epithelial cells from the middle third of the elongated crypts show varying degrees of morphologic differentiation. The epithelial cells lining the upper third are well differentiated, being tall and columnar with a clearly marked terminal web.

The surface epithelial cell is strikingly abnormal with a reduction in height due to a cuboidal rather than a columnar shape. The majority of surface epithelial cells show degenerative changes, such as an incompletely developed terminal web, variability in staining or electron density, swelling of the mitochondria and endoplasmic reticulum, loss of organelles, and prominence of lysosomal structures.[69] The microvilli are nearly always abnormal, being short, irregular in shape and size, and fused or missing. The glycocalyx is often thinner than normal, irregular, or absent.

The Glycocalyx. Filamentous extensions from the trilaminar membrane of the microvilli constitute the glycocalyx, which is also known as the fuzzy coat or fuzz (Fig. 105–5). It is not merely a protective layer of mucus, as once thought, but a polysaccharide structure. Hence, the term "glycocalyx," a Greek word meaning a sweet husk. It is readily seen by light microscopy when stained by periodic acid–Schiff and may be as much as 0.7 μ thick on intestinal absorptive cells. The fibrils become longer and more dense as cells move up from the crypts to the luminal surface. Studies on the composition of the glycocalyx show that this area is subject to dynamic stresses and changes and that a viable epithelial cell is essential for its maintenance and survival. The glycocalyx is thought to be composed of glycoproteins, comprising a polypeptide chain and pendant carbohydrate side-chains. Its functions are considerably greater than just a protective covering for the "underlying plasmalemma from variation in pH and the various enzymes in the bowel lumen."[69a] The glycocalyx is the point at which the initial phase of digestion and absorption takes place. The differences between the glycocalyx of the cells of the villus and the crypt are important, both in normal subjects and in patients with conditions such as celiac disease. In the crypts, the microvilli are shorter and less numerous and regular than those on the absorptive cells, and the glycocalyx is less distinct. The Golgi apparatus in the crypt cells is poorly developed, there is no well-developed terminal web, and only a slow rate of glycoprotein synthesis with incomplete surface glycoproteins is present, as demonstrated by increased glycosyl transferase activities. Such findings become particularly significant when considering celiac disease, in which the immature crypt cells are so greatly increased in number.

The Microclimate. One of the most important functions of the glycocalyx is to provide a suitable climate for the passage of neutral species from the environment of the intestinal lumen, with its acid pH, through the phospholipid terminal web, with its negative charge, to the absorptive cell, with its more neutral pH. Such neutral species readily pass cell membranes by simple diffusion, while those in ionic form in solution require an active mechanism or pump to achieve absorption. Weak acids, such as folic acid, may be completely ionized at pH 7 and hence, by pushing the pH toward acidity and lower pKa values, would increase absorption by passive diffusion. This partition hypothesis applies to a number of drugs and water-soluble vitamins and requires the existence of an acid layer on the surface of the epithelium.[70]

The provision of a retaining layer for hydrogen ions is a function ascribed to the glycocalyx to maintain the more acid microclimate. The glycocalyx is probably kept more acid than the intestinal contents by the hydrolysis of adenosine triphosphate (ATP) brought about by mucosal adenosine triphosphatase (ATPase), both being present in the

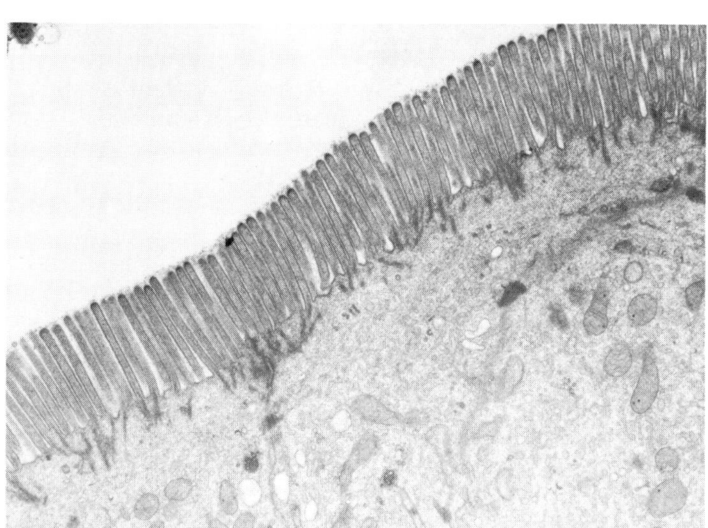

Figure 105–5. Normal jejunal microvilli showing the glycocalyx on the surface. (Courtesy of Dr. M. Lucas.)

epithelial cells down the length of the small intestine in decreasing concentrations distally. The pH of the microclimate (calculated to lie between 4.8 and 5.2) is found to be 5.9 by direct measurement. In celiac disease, the pH of untreated jejunal mucosa is about 6.5, significantly different from that of normal subjects or treated celiac patients.[71] Such a finding readily explains the impaired absorption of a number of substances in untreated celiac disease and the consequent development of many deficiencies as a secondary effect of gluten toxicity.

Enzymes. Padykula and her colleagues[72] regarded the abnormalities found in untreated celiac disease to be a reflection of the rate of change from immature cells to mature cells, resulting in impaired synthesis of the various enzymes in the absorptive cell. All such changes returned to normal on treatment with a gluten-free diet. More refined investigation of the enzyme content was made possible by the analytical subcellular fractionation technique. In the untreated celiac patient, brush border enzymes are grossly reduced to as little as 10% of normal.[49] Increase of some lysosomal enzymes occurs and reflects increased lysosomal fragility.[73] The enzymes in the basal and lateral cell membranes and in the endoplasmic reticulum appear to be relatively unchanged. In general, enzyme activities return to normal following treatment with a gluten-free diet. Exceptions are certain brush border enzymes, particularly β-glucosidase, which remains abnormal even in patients with apparently normal jejunal histology.[49]

Ever since the missing peptidase hypothesis was put forward, considerable interest has been displayed in the distribution of the peptidases in the mucosa. These occur in the brush border, cytosol and lysosomal areas of the absorptive cell, and exist in multiple molecular form. The brush border contains at least 5 peptidases. Considerably more work is necessary, however, to determine the number of peptidases in the intestinal mucosa and their function, for there is considerable overlap between all these enzymes.[50]

Disaccharidase concentrations in the mucosa of the untreated celiac patient are almost invariably reduced. They return to normal levels upon gluten exclusion, with the possible exception of lactase. Whether lactase levels ever return completely to normal is unclear, particularly in the elderly.[52,74]

Immunologic Changes. Many immunologic phenomena occur in celiac disease, some of which may have a bearing on etiology, as discussed later. However, it seems likely that the majority of these changes represent nothing more than gluten and other antigens crossing the damaged mucosal barrier and reaching the immune system.

Immunoglobulins and Immunoglobulin-containing Cells. It is generally accepted that IgM-containing cells are increased in the lamina propria of the jejunal mucosa in children and adults with both treated and untreated celiac disease.[75] There is less agreement about IgA cells. The large numbers of IgA cells reported by some is in keeping with the high concentration of IgA found in the intestinal juice. Also, increased synthesis of IgA by jejunal mucosa has been demonstrated in tissue culture. The excess of IgM cells appears to be localized to the gut, for normal numbers are found in the bone marrow and rectum. IgM cells are increased in IgA-deficient subjects. In celiac disease, the increased IgM cellular infiltrate may therefore be a compensatory mechanism for impaired IgA response. However, the synthesis rate of IgM is reduced and low serum levels occur, so that the compensation is incomplete. IgG and IgE cells are increased in number, while IgD cells are only rarely seen.[58,76]

Serum levels of IgM are reduced, while IgA is elevated in untreated patients. These abnormalities tend to reverse following gluten withdrawal. Increased levels of IgA may indicate an associated milk sensitivity; a rising value has been associated with developing lymphoma, although this is not a consistent finding.

Twenty to 50% of patients with hypogammaglobulinemia have a sprue-like syndrome with diarrhea, steatorrhea, protein-losing enteropathy, and a whole range of malabsorption problems. Many patients with acquired hypogammaglobulinemia have jejunal mucosal lesions indistinguishable from those found in patients with celiac disease, apart from the virtual absence of plasma cells. Also, some patients with hypogammaglobulinemia respond to a gluten-free diet. IgA deficiency is about 10 times more common in patients with celiac disease than in the general population and is without obvious significance.

Antibodies. Antibodies to wheat and gluten extract are present in the serum and intestinal juice of patients with celiac disease, but are also found in healthy subjects and those with other gastrointestinal disorders.[77] An antibody of the IgG class against reticulin antigens is present in the serum of about one third of patients with adult celiac disease and in approximately one fifth of those with dermatitis herpetiformis. It is also present in children with celiac disease. This antibody is not specific for celiac disease; it also occurs in Crohn's disease and some other conditions. IgA antireticulin antibodies have similarly been detected and appear to be specific for celiac disease.[78] Exactly what these antibodies are directed against is uncertain. Inasmuch as they are not absorbed by human reticulins, collagen, or elastin, the more general term "connective tissue antibody" has been applied. There is evidence of abnormal IgM and IgG responses in celiac patients following immunization, while IgA response to polio vaccine is enhanced.

Immune Complexes. Morphologic abnormalities have been observed to occur in the jejunal mucosa of celiac patients 2 to 96 hours after gluten challenge.[61] These are noted mainly in the subepithelial region and consist of mucosal swelling, widening of the connective tissue spaces, an increase in fibrous tissue, swelling of the endothelium, and infiltration by lymphoid cells, eosinophils, mast cells, and polymorphonuclear leukocytes (Fig. 105–6). These changes (together with

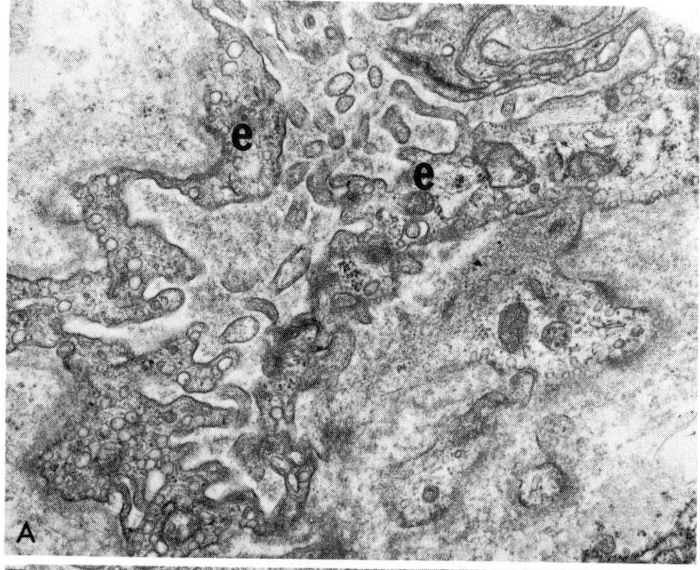

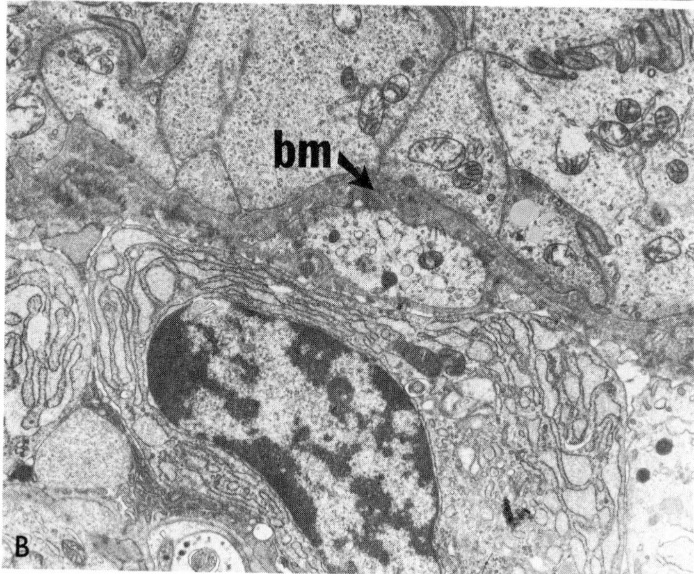

Figure 105–6. Transmission electron micrographs of jejunal mucosa from celiac patients in remission. *A,* 15 hours after gluten challenge showing endothelial swelling (e) with edema of connective tissue. *B,* 48 hours after challenge; thickening of the enterocyte basement membrane (bm) is evident. (Courtesy of Dr. Margot Shiner.)

results from immunofluorescence studies demonstrating the early deposition of complement and immunoglobulin in the region of the basement membrane, and the consumption of complement from serum after gluten challenge) suggest that a local Arthus type immunologic reaction is occurring in the intestinal mucosa. After gluten challenge, complement breakdown products and soluble antigen-antibody complexes can be found in the serum of some patients. The antigen in these complexes has not been identified, but is presumed to be gluten or a subfraction of gluten.

Cell-Mediated Reactions. While lymphocytes from some patients with celiac disease show reduced transformation to nonspecific mitogens, such as phytohemagglutinin, the responses generally are probably little different from normal.

Peripheral blood and mesenteric lymph node lymphocytes are sensitized to gluten. This has been shown by stimulating cells with gluten in vitro[79] and also by the leukocyte migration inhibition test.[80] Further evidence is added by assay of leukocyte migration inhibition factor in culture medium supporting the growth of jejunal mucosa or lymphocytes in the presence of gluten.

Clinical Aspects

Early reports of the disorder were largely concerned with the grosser manifestations of the disease and tended to neglect the relatively mild symptom expressions that feature celiac disease as it is recognized today. Many patients have virtually no symptoms or only nonspecific complaints. Diagnosis in them must be made by a greater awareness of the wide clinical spectrum of the disorder and appreciation of the significance of minor abnormalities encountered in hematologic and biochemical investigations.

Presentation. The classic presentation of celiac disease in childhood is the insidious onset of ill health with failure to thrive after the introduction of cereals into the diet. The affected infant stereotypically is anorexic and appears apathetic, pale, and wasted; examination discloses generalized hypotonia and abdominal distention; stools are soft, bulky, clay-colored, and offensive.[22] However, many children under 4 years of age present acutely. In the very young, the predominant symptom may be vomiting, often effortless and of large volume, that is usually associated with abdominal distention and little or no diarrhea. In older children, abdominal pain may be so severe that the occasional child undergoes laparotomy because of the mistaken diagnosis of intestinal obstruction, particularly when constipation is also present. These older children may present with varied symptoms, including anemia, rickets, and failure to grow normally. Indeed, unexplained short stature is a reason for jejunal biopsy even in the absence of gastrointestinal symptoms.[81]

The earlier presentation of celiac disease noted in recent years is related to the practice of introducing gluten in the form of cereals at an increasingly early age. Probably as many as half of the children with celiac disease have the onset of their disorder in the first 6 months of life; by this time as many as 90% will have been introduced to cereals. It is of interest that the frequency of diagnosis of celiac disease among young children has dropped in the British Isles since 1974, when there was a change to more breast feeding and delay in the introduction of cereals into the diet.

Adult and adolescent patients with celiac disease fall into 3 groups as regards the clinical picture with which they present: (1) those in whom diarrhea, usually severe, is the main feature; (2) those with constitutional disturbances, such as lassitude, loss of weight, glossitis, or symptoms of anemia; and (3) those with such varied symptoms as neuropathy, problems related to osteomalacia, (such as bone pain, spontaneous fractures, or myopathy), skin complaints, bleeding diatheses, psychiatric disturbances, or infertility. Many of the older patients will have had continuous or episodic ill health for many years and, never having been well, come to accept their state as normal. This acceptance of ill health or loose stools may have dire consequences. Notably, it may lead to misdiagnosis and delay when acute symptoms bring the patient to seek medical attention, for the long-standing history is often overlooked. It is particularly important to probe the early history of adult patients for disturbances in childhood, such as failure to grow, anemia, rickets, and poor attendance at school for health reasons. Also important is attention to the habits and to minor abnormalities in the hematologic and biochemical findings.

The stress of pregnancy in a patient with smoldering celiac disease may result in persistent diarrhea or a macrocytic anemia that does not resolve after delivery. Recurrent aphthous stomatitis can be the sole symptom. While stomatitis is due to celiac disease in only a minority of patients with this manifestation, it is important to identify them, for the ulceration will readily respond to a gluten-free diet. Similarly, patients with dermatitis herpetiformis, in whom intestinal symptoms are often absent, must be regarded as potential celiacs; 30% will have a flat jejunal biopsy characteristic of celiac disease and usually both the rash and the intestinal abnormalities respond to a gluten-free diet.

Among the more unusual presentations is pericarditis, which is responsive to gluten withdrawal.[82] In a few patients who are hospitalized for other disorders, celiac disease is suspected from the presence of laboratory abnormalities. This occurred in 3 of our patients who were admitted for myocardial infarction, pneumonia, and repair of an inguinal hernia, respectively. Each had a mild macrocytic anemia due to folic acid deficiency, and further investigation led to the additional diagnosis of celiac disease. Lastly, it behooves all who treat celiac disease to be aware of its high prevalence among the relatives of patients. In our own experience, a few probing questions to relatives accompanying patients has led to the diagnosis of celiac disease in individuals previously not suspected of having this disease.

Manifestations. To the foregoing discussion of the symptoms of celiac disease in infancy and childhood, it may be emphasized here that failure to thrive with weight loss, vomiting, abdominal pain and distention, irritability, and diarrhea are all common manifestations.

A wide variety of symptoms affect adults with celiac disease. These can readily be demonstrated following a gluten challenge in patients who are well controlled on a gluten-free diet. Some will react simply by feeling vaguely unwell for a few hours to a few weeks. In most, the common symptoms are malaise, anorexia, nausea, abdominal distention, loose stools, and weight loss. Others have no symptoms despite histologic damage to the jejunal mucosa. Occasionally the reaction to gluten can be violent, as in "gluten shock,"[42] an abnormally violent reaction appearing 3 to 6 hours after administration of any form of wheat and characterized by severe abdominal pain, vomiting, pallor, and sometimes even slight shock.

Symptoms may be due directly to gluten, develop secondary to the small intestinal damage caused by gluten, or result from both.

Lassitude. Of the symptoms directly due to gluten, lassitude is probably the most common. It is often attributed to mild psychiatric disturbances, but its persistence after diarrhea has abated or anemia has been corrected suggests otherwise. Furthermore, its recurrence in patients on a gluten-free diet following either the deliberate or the inadvertent consumption of gluten clearly associates it with gluten ingestion. Despite the common complaint of always feeling tired, patients nevertheless are often able to perform heavy physical duties. Bouts of excessive weariness tend to be experienced for 2 to 3 weeks at a time. Others complain of lassitude in the evening, rendering them incapable of physical activity even though they are mentally alert.

Menstruation and Fertility. Disturbances in menstruation and fertility are common in untreated celiac disease and are largely relieved by exclusion of gluten from the diet.[83] Menarche is significantly delayed and the menopause occurs earlier in untreated women than in treated patients or the normal population. Amenorrhea or oligomenorrhea is frequent. Though celiacs can have children, as a group they are relatively infertile. While there is no significant difference in the time for conception of those on a gluten-free diet and those who are untreated, conception may take place dramatically, after years of infertility, soon after the commencement of a gluten-free diet. The mechanism whereby gluten exerts these effects is not known.

Short Stature. This manifestation appears to be directly related to gluten ingestion and not simply a result of malnutrition, as gastrointestinal symptoms may be absent.[81] The resumption of normal growth is a standard method of assessing the effects of a gluten-free diet. However, tall patients are also encountered.

Mood and Mental Change. Celiac patients as a whole are a relatively intelligent group and not particularly liable to neurotic symptoms. Nevertheless, the mood and mental changes that precede the exclusion of gluten from the diet are well known and form a characteristic set of symptoms. Depression, in particular, is a prominent feature of childhood celiac disease, and approximately 1 in 10 of our own adult patients, mainly women, have needed treatment for depression. Terms that have been applied to these mental changes include irritable, schizoid, depressive, querulous, obsessional neurotic, paranoid, and delusional. While the changes in mood are clearly the result of gluten toxicity in the majority of patients, both potassium and magnesium deficiency may also be responsible.

Recurrent Aphthous Ulcers. These have been associated traditionally with intestinal disturbances and are relatively common in celiac disease. The ulcers may occur without any other abnormality in the mouth, and there are no specific features that distinguish the aphthous ulcers associated with celiac disease from those occurring for other reasons.[84] They are important in celiac disease because they may be the only manifestation. Their direct relationship to gluten is demonstrated by their disappearance after a gluten-free diet. Furthermore, gluten appears to be related to aphthous ulceration in some nonceliac patients.

Bowel Disturbance. This is present in most patients, commonly as loose stools for a few days 3 or 4 times a year. Attacks are often confined to the early morning, with the remainder of the day being undisturbed. The number of stools varies, but is commonly 3 to 4 a day and rarely more than 8. The stools during attacks may be paler than normal, sometimes offensive, and sometimes frothy. Normal-colored, formed stools containing excess fat are relatively common. Attacks can occur suddenly, with frequent, loose, watery stools, as may happen when the precipitating factor causing relapse is infective. Untreated patients commonly complain of nocturnal diarrhea and an appreciable number are incontinent at night.[85] Inasmuch as bowel function is easily disturbed by emotional factors, it should be cautioned that celiac patients may mistakenly be regarded as having functional or nonorganic bowel disturbance.[86]

While an increase in frequency is the most common abnormality of bowel action, many patients will deny any disturbance of bowel habit whatsoever and some will even be constipated. The colon in the latter tends to be large and capacious.[4] Fecal impaction is present in some children when they are first seen, and Hirschsprung's disease may be mistakenly diagnosed.[87]

Appetite. Anorexia is a complaint in from 16% to 41% of patients.[21] Bulimia has also been noted, with patients failing to gain weight even on an intake of 6000 to 7000 calories/day.

Glossitis. Inflammation of the tongue occurs in most untreated patients. It is severe in approximately one third, mild or transitory in another third, and moderate in the remainder. The glossitis is indistinguishable from that seen in other nutritional deficiency states. The whole tongue may be fiery red, often with buccal ulceration. In mild cases, the tongue is only red, smooth, and sore, with absence of papillae along the edges and on the tip. The onset can be extremely rapid so that within 48 hours the tongue and palate are fiery red. Rarely, this extends to the pharynx and esophagus, making swallowing difficult and restricting food intake. In those patients in whom the glossitis is troublesome, other body surfaces may be involved, leading to perianal soreness and excoriation and, occasionally, to dyspareunia. Angular stomatitis occurs in approximately half the untreated patients. Marked cheilosis is present in some. All of these manifestations are likely to disappear on a gluten-free diet, although occasionally glossitis persists if the serum folic acid levels are low.

Abdominal Pain. Moderate or severe abdominal pain occurs in 5% to 43% of patients.[21] The pain may be due to nonceliac complications, and intestinal radiologic examination is mandatory to help establish the cause.

Celiac patients, particularly when they have frequent stools, are at risk of incurring electrolyte depletion, which can lead not only to muscle weakness but also to varying degrees of intestinal dilatation and abdominal distention and rarely to volvulus (Chapter 122). Transient intussusceptions associated with colicky abdominal pain are not uncommon in children and may also occur in adults (Chapter 22). Constant and severe pain may attend mesenteric adenitis. Painful attacks are particularly liable to occur in patients who have only recently begun a gluten-free diet and consciously or inadvertently ingest gluten. Perseverance with diet leads to cessation of the attacks.

The prevalence of cholelithiasis is not increased in celiac disease, despite sluggish emptying of the gallbladder. Peptic ulceration is relatively uncommon, but operations for suspected ulcers have led to diarrhea and the diagnosis of celiac disease. Attacks of acute pancreatitis are rare. Two patients have been reported with pancreatic lithiasis[88] and pancreatic dysfunction may underlie persistent steatorrhea unresponsive to treatment in both adults and children.[89]

Hemorrhagic Manifestations. The frequency of hemorrhagic manifestations varies between 10% and 31% of patients.[21] Most of these are due to vitamin K deficiency and are readily corrected by vitamin K administration. Bleeding into the skin and mucous membranes, often with extensive confluent hemorrhages, is most common. Hematuria and bleeding into the gastrointestinal tract are more serious and potentially fatal. Retroperitoneal hemorrhage may present as an acute abdominal emergency. Other manifestations are hemarthroses and bleeding from the uterus. In a rare patient, disseminated intravascular coagulation may occur.[90]

Bone and Calcium Upsets. Among a group of celiac patients investigated by bone biopsy, radiology, and biochemistry, 63% were found to have some disturbance of bone metabolism (osteoporosis and osteomalacia).[91] Symptoms of rickets and osteomalacia are insidious in onset and are usually quite severe before the underlying diagnosis is made. The main symptom is bone pain, which affects between 2% and 38% of patients in reported cases.[21] "Rheumatism" is a common complaint; the term is used to refer to bone pain, often with alterations of gait and sometimes associated with pseudofractures of the neck of the femur or the pelvic bones. Fractures of the ribs and even the wings of the scapulae are not uncommon. Joint swelling in association with deficiency of vitamin D and osteomalacia may be diagnosed as rheumatoid arthritis. Rickets in most children with celiac disease does not cause significant growth deficit. Vitamin D deficiency is also accompanied by muscle weakness, and myopathy affecting the proximal muscles of the legs can sometimes be the most prominent feature, resulting in a characteristic waddling gait. At one time, cure was considered impossible unless gluten was removed from the diet, for it was thought that gluten blocked the effect of vitamin D. The main reason, however, is depressed absorption of vitamin D due to alteration in the pH of the microclimate secondary to the mucosal damage caused by gluten.[92]

The serum levels of alkaline phosphatase and vitamin D are the most important laboratory measurements. Calcium and phosphorus levels are often normal and are thus quite unreliable as diagnostic aids. By far the most common cause of increased alkaline phosphatase activity in celiac disease is osteomalacia. In the rare case, usually with magnesium deficiency in addition, serum alkaline phosphatase activity may be normal. Serum vitamin D levels, of course, are low. Bone biopsy in osteomalacia shows increased amounts of osteoid together with increased bone scores; in osteoporosis, bony matrix is scanty.

In our experience, the administration of oral calciferol, with or without gluten withdrawal, rarely fails to cure even the most severe cases of osteomalacia. Nevertheless, in a few patients osteomalacia persists despite a gluten-free diet and administration of calciferol and responds only to 25-hydroxy vitamin D.[93]

Nocturnal Diuresis. Many untreated celiac patients have nocturnal diuresis. Occasionally, it is the reason for their seeking advice. The patient may have to rise 4 or 5 times during the night to pass urine. Even when fluid intake is restricted, as much as 4 ml/minute of urine may be passed between midnight and 1 AM. The normal rhythms of water and electrolyte excretions are disrupted in a random fashion. Since poor diuresis follows the ingestion of a water load in most celiac patients, nocturnal diuresis was thought to be due to the retention of large volumes of water in the lumen of the small intestine during the abnormally long period necessary for the digestion of food. Though there is indeed impaired absorption of water from the intestine, the degree of impairment does not account for the very much greater impaired diuresis.[94] If a similar water load is administered at midnight under suitably controlled conditions with regard to food ingestion, exercise, and posture, normal diuresis follows. The abnormal diuresis is not related to the total body potassium stores, and though tubular nephropathy due to potassium depletion can be demonstrated in some celiac patients, the disturbance appears to be more fundamental than any of the suggested mechanisms.[95] The disappearance of nocturnal diuresis can be regarded as a measure of satisfactory response to gluten withdrawal.

Objective Features

Physical Characteristics. Approximately half of adult patients have lost weight when they are first seen and in one series an average loss of 12 kg was noted.[85] The majority of children newly diagnosed celiac disease are below the 50th percentile for weight and are often below the 3rd percentile. An occasional patient, either in adult or pediatric practice, may be grossly overweight at presentation.[96] Though hypoplasia of dental enamel has been described, delay in eruption of the teeth is uncommon and dental caries is rare. The hair tends to be of fine texture and fair in color, and celiac patients with black hair, unless they are Asian, are uncommon. Premature graying is often noted. The beard in the untreated patient grows poorly and shaving may be necessary only 2 or 3 times a week. Axillary hair may disappear. All these features improve with a gluten-free diet, often with some return of color to the hair.

The frequency of finger clubbing is appreciable, affecting as many as 1 in 5 children or adults, and is no greater in those with malignant complications. The reason for finger clubbing is not clear, but it disappears with a gluten-free diet. Koilonychia is not as common and responds to iron therapy. Dermal and epidermal ridge atrophy is claimed to be present, even in treated patients.[97] This finding is not specific for celiac disease; it is found in liver disorders and is also related to occupation. It does not occur in child celiacs or in patients with dermatitis herpetiformis. Edema of the legs in untreated patients is not uncommon, particularly in those in poor general condition. Abdominal distention and dilatation of the intestinal tract make the detection of ascites particularly difficult. The abdomen tends to feel "doughy." An intermittent chylous ascites has been reported, which clears on treatment with a gluten-free diet.

Disorders of the Skin. Skin lesions occur commonly in celiac disease. As many as 1 in 5 patients will have consulted a dermatologist for supposed *seborrheic dermatitis* at some time prior to the diagnosis of celiac disease. *Atopic eczema* is slightly more common than in the general population and sometimes is dramatically cured by a gluten-free diet. Among other skin lesions, one simulating *psoriasis* is fairly common, tending to deteriorate when the celiac condition relapses. An extensive *exfoliative dermatitis* also occurs occasionally. Some patients develop *generalized pigmentation* resembling that seen in Addison's disease, even to the extent of having buccal involvement. Seven of the 10 patients reported by Thaysen[98] had a patchy symmetrical pigmentation on the cheeks and forehead. The majority of untreated celiac patients sunburn easily, pigmentation being particularly marked on the forearms, neck, and face, and contrasting sharply with the pallor of the palms and unexposed surfaces. In more severe examples, the parchment-like epithelium is cracked and pigmented, changes suggestive of mild *pellagra*, especially when associated with glossitis and cheilosis.

There are, in addition, a number of rare skin disorders which occur in association with celiac disease, but for which no etiologic relationship or response to a gluten-free diet has yet been established. These include primary cutaneous amyloid, cutaneous vasculitis, nodular prurigo, acquired ichthyosis and epidermal necrolysis, pityriasis rubra pilaris, and mycosis fungoides. (A separate discussion of dermatitis herpetiformis follows later.)

Cardiovascular Disorders. It has often been assumed that cardiovascular disorders are few in celiac patients. Many have called attention to the low blood pressure that occurs and our own experience supports this. In a survey of 100 patients, apart from 3 with moderate hypertension, 45 had a systolic pressure less than 105 mm Hg and 20 had a systolic pressure of less than 95 mm Hg. Hypotension is not associated with anemia or electrolyte depletion. The frequency of coronary artery disease is thought to be low.[99] In one of our earlier surveys of 76 autopsies, 9 deaths were due to coronary thrombosis; in another later series with a younger mean patient age, only 4 of 63 deaths were due to this cause. The prevalence of ischemic heart disease among 314 patients with biopsy-proven celiac disease was 5% and cerebrovascular disease affected 3.1%.

Splenic Atrophy. As discussed later, splenic atrophy has been found in many patients at operation or autopsy and appears to be part and parcel of a generalized reduction of the lymphoreticular tissues. Unexplained splenomegaly is also encountered.

Laboratory Findings

Steatorrhea. "Steatorrhea," as now used, refers to feces in which there is excess fat, whether visible or not. Methods for detecting steatorrhea are discussed in greater detail in

Chapters 24 and 101 and only certain aspects will be noted here.

Microscopic examination has limited use.[100] The percentage of fat in a single specimen of stool is also unreliable. Various markers have been used, but such methods are inaccurate when checked against quantitative balance studies and have not gained wide acceptance. Increasing use is now being made of the absolute amounts of fat excreted in a given time. This approach does not require precise determination of the amount of fat that is ingested and uses fats normally found in the daily diet.

The normal mean daily fat intake in Great Britain varies between 60 and 90 g, but is somewhat higher in the United States (about 100 g). Alteration in dietary fat from 50 up to 150 g/day makes little difference in mean excretion of fat, increasing it by not much more than 2 g/day in the normal subject. The upper limit of normal daily fat excretion is usually set at 6 to 7 g. A minimum of 3 days, and preferably more, should be allowed for the fecal collection. The estimation of fecal fat is a relatively crude tool, readily subject to errors of collection and measurement and associated with a considerable variation in day-to-day excretion. *As many as 30% of celiac patients may have no steatorrhea at the time of presentation when fecal fat is so measured.* The test can be misleading too as an index of clinical improvement, inasmuch as a variation of 2 to 4 g daily has little significance.

Although it is a more pleasant way of assessing for steatorrhea, the use of radioisotopic methods has not proved to be as dependable as quantitative fecal fat determination.[101, 102]

To sum up, the presence of steatorrhea suggests the possibility of celiac disease, but other causes require consideration. *The absence of steatorrhea does not exclude the diagnosis.*

Carbohydrates

Glucose. A rise in blood glucose of less than 40 mg/dl after a glucose load has been regarded as abnormal, and a flat glucose tolerance test as characteristic of celiac disease. However, a sizable proportion of the normal population also has flat curves. Treatment with a gluten-free diet returns low curves to normal, and a normal or high normal curve in an untreated patient may be transformed into a frankly diabetic curve.

The reason for a low blood glucose curve in celiac disease is almost certainly impaired intestinal absorption due to many factors, including reduced glucose flux influenced by reduced ATPase in the intestinal mucosa. Insulin production is not impaired, as the responses to IV insulin in celiac patients and normal subjects are identical. However, there is some delay in insulin response in the untreated patient, which improves following gluten withdrawal. During the early period after ingestion, intestinal hormones such as gastric inhibitory polypeptide (GIP) are thought to exert their insulinotropic effect. The early response of this hormone is impaired in celiac disease and improves following treatment with a gluten-free diet.[103] These effects appear to be secondary to the damage caused by gluten to the intestinal mucosa.

Lactose. An abnormal test is characterized by a rise of glucose of less than 20 mg/dl following an oral load of lactose (50 g/m^2 of body surface or a standard dose of 100 g). However, such flat curves are also found in about 30% of normal subjects. *There is almost always some degree of lactose intolerance in celiac disease,* depending, it is thought, on the degree of mucosal damage. Following treatment, this intolerance tends to disappear in all but those with a constitutional alactasia. Lactosuria also follows an oral load in untreated celiacs, but it is not sufficiently specific to allow its use as a diagnostic test.

D-Xylose. This aldopentose, which is absorbed virtually entirely in the upper small intestine and is excreted in the urine almost completely in the first 5 hours after ingestion, has been employed as a screening test for celiac disease using either a 5 g or a 25 g oral dose. Approximately 95% of patients with celiac disease have abnormal urinary excretion values, i.e., $<$4.2 g in 5 hours after an oral dose of 25 g, or $<$17% of the oral dose. With 5 g loads, as used in children, the excretion varies between 15 and 25% of the oral dose in 5 hours. Because a number of adults have normal results, many question the value of the test. It also appears of little use in differentiating celiac from normal children.[104,105]

Somewhat similar views have been expressed on the use of peak plasma values as a diagnostic or screening test, though some have claimed that adjustment for surface area improves the sensitivity.[106] The use of D-xylose absorption as a means of assessing the toxicity of gluten fractions must also be viewed with some reservations.

Other Carbohydrates. The search for a

screening test based on intestinal permeability has given some promising results. The simultaneous administration of either L-rhaminose and lactulose or mannitol and cellobiose as probe molecules has allowed calculation of excretion ratios that appear to give good differentiation of healthy subjects and untreated celiac patients.[107]

Amylase. Celiac patients may have elevated serum amylase activities. In some cases, hyperamylasemia is due to the presence of a macroamylase in the serum, the significance of which is not clear (Chapter 220). Macroamylasemia has been noted to disappear following gluten withdrawal.[108]

Albumin. In early reports of celiac disease, as many as half or even four fifths of patients had hypoalbuminemia, reflecting the high proportion of seriously ill patients coming to diagnosis at that time. With earlier diagnosis, this is much less of a feature. Thus, in a recent analysis of 132 of our patients, the mean serum albumin level at presentation was 41 g/liter, rising on gluten withdrawal to 44 g/liter. Both reduced protein synthesis and loss into the gastrointestinal tract contribute to hypoalbuminemia. The intestinal loss, which ceases following a gluten-free diet, is probably the main factor and usually is compensated for by increased synthesis. Only when some complication supervenes is the body unable to keep pace with adequate replacement.

In clinical practice, a low serum albumin level should be regarded as an indicator of a superimposed complication, such as a gastrointestinal infection, lymphoma, carcinoma, or benign ulceration of the intestinal tract. Severe hypoalbuminemia is also a complication of dapsone treatment of dermatitis herpetiformis.[109] Serum albumin levels should be regarded as one of the essential determinations at follow-up examinations of celiac patients.

Gastrointestinal Hormones. The gross mucosal abnormalities found in celiac disease affect the production and release of the gastrointestinal hormones (Chapter 241). In untreated patients, the release of secretin in response to acid infused into the duodenum is impaired, as is cholecystokinin following a fatty meal. The grossly elevated levels of enteroglucagon, and the response to oral glucose or a test breakfast, are probably unique to celiac disease. Indeed, the characteristic hormone profile may have implications as a screening or diagnostic test.[110]

Hematologic Elements

Hemoglobin. The characteristic blood picture in adult celiac disease is a hypochromic, macrocytic anemia of mild degree. About half the male patients will have a hemoglobin concentration of less than 13 g/dl, and a similar proportion of women will have a concentration of less than 12 g/dl when first seen. Severe anemia is relatively uncommon and should always raise the suspicion of a superimposed complication, such as malignancy.

Red Blood Cells. There are a number of features in the peripheral blood films that suggest the diagnosis: target cells, Howell-Jolly bodies, siderocytes, irregularly contracted and crenated cells, Heinz bodies, microspherocytes, and occasional erythroblasts. Circulating nucleated red cells, pale ring-like cells, and cells containing nuclear fragments are suggestive of splenic atrophy, a common cause of which is celiac disease.[111] The great differences in size and shape of the cells, together with variation in the degree of hemoglobinization, gives rise to one characteristic red cell picture, i.e., dimorphic anemia.

In children, the predominant picture is that of a hypochromic, microcytic anemia responding only slowly to iron therapy. A similar type of hypochromic anemia is also occasionally found in adults.

Thrombocytes (Platelets). Thrombocytes are increased in about half the patients with untreated celiac disease and return to normal levels on treatment with a gluten-free diet.[112] However, the platelet count occasionally is considerably diminished in the presence of severe granulocytopenia.

White Blood Cells. Total white blood cell counts usually vary between 5000 and 8000 cells/mm^3. Approximately 10% of patients have total white cell counts of less than 3500 cells/mm^3 when first seen, and about the same percentage have either neutropenia, with less than 3000 cells/mm^3, or lymphopenia with less than 1500 lymphocytes/mm^3. Counts less than 500/mm^3 are sometimes encountered and, if associated with the appearance of primitive cells in the circulation, may raise the possibility of leukemia.[113]

The mean lymphocyte count of those on a gluten-free diet is significantly lower than for those on a normal diet, but neither is different from the values in a normal population. T cell numbers in untreated patients are significantly lower than in treated individuals or controls, but B cells show no differences.[114]

Sternal Marrow. Most untreated adult patients with celiac disease have megaloblastic erythropoiesis of some degree. Approximately 45% have pure megaloblastic marrows and 52% have megaloblastosis combined with lack of iron; in the remaining few the changes are those of pure iron deficiency.[115]

Folate Derivatives. The level of the major folate compound in the serum, i.e., 5-methyltetrahydrofolate, is usually reduced in celiac disease. All of one group of 163 celiac patients had serum levels below the lower limit of normal, and in 140 of these, the values indicated serious folate deficiency. Red cell folate, not considered to be as sensitive a test as the serum level, was nevertheless low in 85% of the patients.[115] Our own survey showed that 60% of patients when first seen had levels lower than 3 ng/ml (the lower limit of normal for our laboratory).

Vitamin B_{12}. The mean serum vitamin B_{12} level falls within the normal range in celiac disease. In our series, only 14% of the patients had values below the normal limit at presentation. The frequency of malabsorption of vitamin B_{12} varies from our own rate of 20% to as much as 53%. The absence of intrinsic factor in proven celiac disease is very rare; only 2 patients appear to have been described in the literature.[21] Some improvement in absorption results from treatment with a gluten-free diet. It should also be noted that many patients with low vitamin serum B_{12} and low serum folic acid levels will have their serum levels of vitamin B_{12} restored by folic acid treatment alone.

Iron. Iron deficiency is common in celiac disease, but with the high occurrence rate of megaloblastosis in untreated patients, the initial serum iron level in a given patient may not immediately reflect this. Iron deficiency anemia responds slowly to iron therapy. The deficiency is thought to be caused by both impaired absorption and increased iron loss into the intestinal tract.[116]

Pyridoxine. Low serum levels of pyridoxine occur in approximately half of untreated celiac patients, and pyridoxal phosphate concentrations are low in the duodenal mucosa of child celiacs.[117] Pyridoxine is involved in a number of important metabolic processes, particularly in the metabolism of serotonin and its precursor, 5-hydroxytryptophan. The most sensitive index of serotonin production is the excretion of 5-hydroxyindoleacetic acid (5-HIAA). This is greatly increased from the normal range of 1.7 to 8.5 mg/day in normal subjects to between 9 and 21 mg/day in untreated celiac patients. This difference is removed on treatment with a gluten-free diet.[118] Nevertheless, a tryptophan load administered to treated celiac patients still results in increased excretion of 5-HIAA; restoration to normal follows the administration of IM pyridoxine.

Indican. Measurement of urinary indican excretion has been used to detect bacterial overgrowth in the intestinal tract. Indican results from the intraluminal degradation of tryptophan to indole by bacterial tryptophanase. Indole is readily absorbed, hydroxylated, and conjugated in the liver and is excreted in the urine as indoxy-sulfate or indican. Indicanuria is not uncommon in celiac disease, but it does not necessarily indicate bacterial overgrowth. False positive and false negative results occur sufficiently often to render its measurement of little clinical value.

Sodium and Potassium. All patients with persistent or recurring loose stools are at risk of developing potassium depletion. This is particularly so in those with untreated celiac disease, in whom there is an increased excretion of potassium of endogenous origin, even in patients who are passing formed stools. Thus, in one group of patients, the total body potassium was 60% of normal. The deficit appears to arise from a combination of loss of muscle mass and intracellular depletion of potassium.[119] It must be emphasized that serum levels of potassium are an unreliable indicator of potassium stores.

Sodium is not affected in the same way, and the total body sodium remains relatively constant. The distribution of sodium is altered, however, with more in the cells and less in the extracellular space.

Magnesium. In disorders associated with steatorrhea, excessive fecal loss of magnesium may occur. Untreated celiac patients are particularly liable to develop this deficiency. Low serum magnesium values are associated with other losses, particularly of potassium and calcium. Low serum calcium levels in some instances will be restored to normal by magnesium therapy alone.

Zinc and Copper. Zinc is primarily absorbed in the upper small intestine and is demonstrable in all tissues, either as a zinc metalloenzyme or a zinc protein complex.

Zinc deficiency has a direct effect upon the metabolism of nucleic acids, with resultant inhibition of collagen and protein synthesis. In man, loss of appetite and smell have been described; inhibition of growth and development and infertility have also been attributed to zinc deficiency. The mean serum level of zinc in celiac patients tends to be lower than in control subjects; irrespective of the plasma albumin level.[120] Zinc therapy has been claimed to benefit "non-responsive" celiac disease, but this has not been confirmed by improvement in jejunal morphology or in the epithelial lymphocyte count.[121]

The role played by copper is not known. Low values have been described in celiac disease in conjunction with low ceruloplasmin levels. Anemia may also be caused by copper deficiency induced by zinc therapy.

Roentgen Aspects

The radiologic manifestations of celiac disease are discussed in Chapter 102. Suffice it here, therefore, to stress the principal features. The most constant of the roentgen features is dilatation of the small intestine (Fig. 105–7). Straightening of the valvulae conniventes, thickening of the mucosal folds, and increasing separation between these folds are also common. Superimposed upon dilatation and thickening of the mucosal folds are varying degrees of flocculation, segmentation, and clumping of barium, which are particularly relevant when they occur early in the examination (Fig. 105–8). These features, however, are not specific for celiac disease. Moreover, electrolyte disturbances, particularly potassium depletion; renal or cardiac failure; and other conditions encountered in seriously ill patients may give rise to some dilatation of the intestine and to secretion of mucus, which is one of the factors causing flocculation.

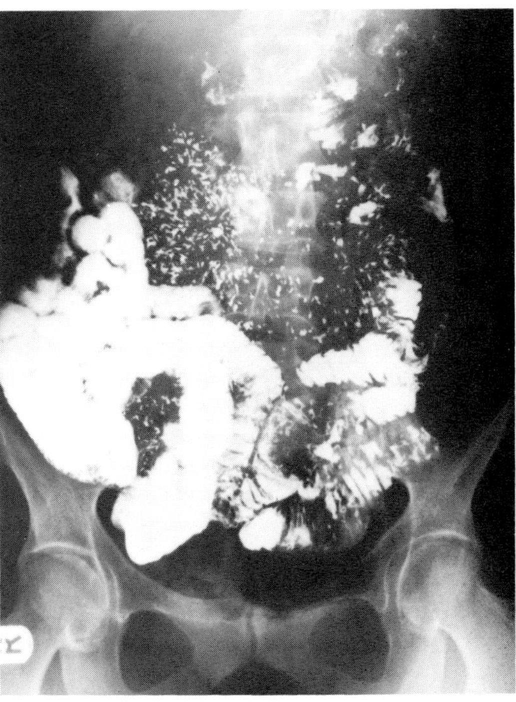

Figure 105–8. Flocculation, segmentation, and clumping of barium in the upper small bowel of a patient with untreated celiac disease. The lumen is widened.

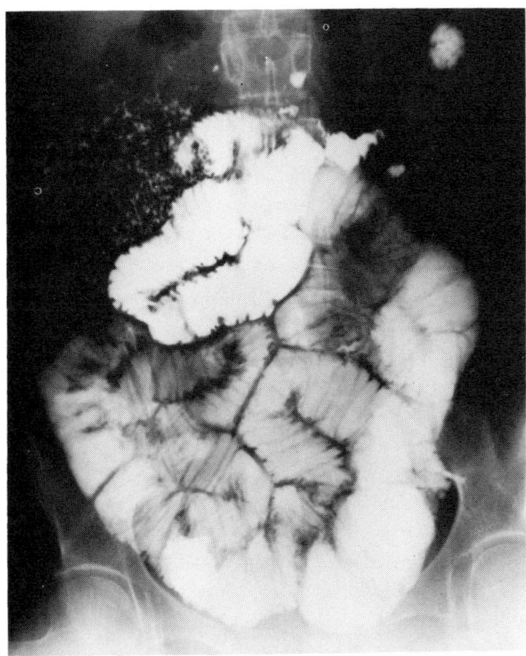

Figure 105–7. Barium in the small bowel of a patient with untreated celiac disease showing coarsening of the valvulae and widening of the lumen. In some of the loops, barium has become diluted and appears less dense.

It must be emphasized that as many as 23% of children with celiac disease[122] and 12% of adult patients have no significant intestinal radiologic abnormality.[123] Nevertheless, radiologic examination in suspected celiac disease is important to exclude other disorders or complicating lesions such as malignancy or stricture.

Dilatation of the colon, one of the earliest radiologic features to which attention was directed, is relatively common. A dilated and often redundant colon is one of the factors making the untreated celiac patient prone to the development of volvulus.

Complications

The 3 main complications of celiac disease are malignancy, neuropathy, and ulcerative jejunoileitis. Why these should arise is still unexplained.

Malignancy. The precise frequency of malignancy among patients with celiac disease is unknown for 2 main reasons: (1) the prevalence of celiac disease itself is uncertain, inasmuch as many patients with only minor symptoms are undiagnosed; and (2) unless autopsies are regularly carried out, the presence of malignancy is likely to be underestimated because diagnosis is only established by postmortem examination in about one third of the cases.[124] Still another limiting factor is failure to investigate for associated celiac disease in patients with a diagnosis of abdominal lymphoma. This need is underscored by the findings in one report in which 7 patients who presented with primary abdominal lymphoma were shown to have either celiac disease or dermatitis herpetiformis.[125]

With these reservations, the prevalence of malignancy may be estimated from the data obtained in 2 series of patients who were followed for many years.[56] A significantly increased frequency of lymphoma was demonstrated in both men and women. Also found was an increased frequency of carcinoma of the gastrointestinal tract, particularly of the esophagus in men. In absolute figures, malignancy was the cause of nearly half the deaths.

The risk of malignancy appears to be somewhat greater in men than in women. There also appears to be an increased frequency of malignancy in first-degree relatives. For example, an analysis of 1329 relatives of 139 patients with celiac disease showed an overall increase in cancer deaths; in men this was attributed to carcinoma of the esophagus, bladder, and brain and in women to carcinoma of the breast.[126]

There are no long-term studies on the prevalence of malignancy in dermatitis herpetiformis, but a number of reports suggest that malignancy is increased.

Lymphoma. Lymphoma affecting the small intestine is fully reviewed in Chapter 112. Because of the importance of lymphoma as a complication of celiac disease, the features are noted here as well.

Age and sex. The numbers of men and women with celiac disease complicated by lymphoma are approximately equal. It has been observed in a patient who was only 29 years old, but few develop the complications under the age of 40. The peak incidence is in the seventh decade, with mean ages in 3 published series of 47, 55, and 61 years, respectively.[21] Celiac patients who are newly diagnosed when more than 50 years of age should be followed closely, for they have a 1 in 10 chance of harboring a lymphoma.[127]

Clinical features. Early clinical features such as weight loss, malaise, and diarrhea are nonspecific and indistinguishable from those of uncomplicated celiac disease in relapse. Such symptoms occurring in a celiac patient who has been under good control on a gluten-free diet are all too often mistakenly attributed to dietary indiscretion. The most common symptom is weight loss. This occurs in most, but not all, patients and is usually the first symptom. Loss of energy occurs in about two thirds, and abdominal pain in about half the patients. One of the most striking symptoms is the profound muscle weakness that affects about half the patients. It involves the voluntary muscles and becomes more marked as the illness progresses, leading ultimately to almost total inability to walk or perform other motor functions. Apart from lymphoma, such marked muscle weakness is seen only in celiac patients who have developed osteomalacia or neuropathy. Rarely, lymph gland enlargement alerts the patient to seek medical attention. The onset is insidious in the majority. In a few it is acute, owing to such phenomena as intestinal perforation, obstruction, hemorrhage, or an opportunistic infection.

Physical signs are also vague and nonspecific. Lymphadenopathy and hepatomegaly tend to appear late when malignancy is widely disseminated. Skin rashes sometimes represent infiltration with lymphoma. Finger clubbing has been linked with malignancy, but it is doubtful whether this finding is any more frequent in lymphoma than in uncomplicated celiac disease. It must be stressed that the presence of lymphoma is often strongly suspected for some time before it is possible to make a definitive diagnosis.

Laboratory data. Patients with lymphoma are unable to maintain normal hematologic and biochemical indices. The most common findings are a low hemoglobin value, raised sedimentation rate, and low serum albumin and serum iron levels. In about half the patients the serum alkaline phosphatase activity is raised. The origin of the phosphatase is nearly always bone and is indicative of osteomalacia. The development of rising alkaline phosphatase values in a patient with celiac disease who is receiving a gluten-free diet, and even calciferol, indicates some additional complication, usually malignancy with spread to the liver.

Serum globulin is increased in about half the patients. A progressive rise in serum IgA is sometimes noted and should arouse suspicion of lymphoma, but increased levels of serum IgA are also found in many untreated celiac patients for other reasons. Steatorrhea is not found universally, but is usually present in those who have diarrhea. Serum lysozyme levels may be raised in gastrointestinal lymphoma,[128] but elevated levels can also be found in celiac patients who have not developed malignancy even after long periods of observation.

Macrocytic anemia, together with a megaloblastic bone marrow, is frequent. In about one third of the patients the total white blood cell count is reduced because of lymphopenia, neutropenia, or a combination of both. Of those with neutropenia, the bone marrow is likely to be infiltrated by lymphoma. A raised white blood cell count due to an absolute rise in neutrophils is invariably associated with gut involvement and intestinal perforation.

RADIOLOGIC FINDINGS. Multiple, irregular, narrow segments are characteristic of small gut lymphoma, but such appearances are rare (Fig. 105–9). Most barium studies reveal only a "malabsorption" pattern; some are completely normal, although subsequent pathologic examinations of the gut reveal involvement with tumor.

DIAGNOSIS. Confirmation of the diagnosis must be by biopsy of lymph nodes, liver, or other tissues. When suspicion is strong, laparotomy must be seriously considered, in part as well because laparotomy sometimes reveals other conditions amenable to treatment, such as intestinal ulceration, diaphragms, or strictures.

It has to be decided whether those patients in whom both celiac disease and lymphoma present together, or within a short time of each other, have 2 disorders or merely a primary abdominal lymphoma bringing about change in the intestinal mucosa similar to that seen in celiac disease. In our view, such patients should always be regarded as having celiac disease complicated by lymphoma because there is usually a long history compatible with celiac disease. Occasionally, lymphoma may be diagnosed before the appearance of celiac symptoms. Jejunal biopsy is advisable in such patients, for if they also have celiac disease, a gluten-free diet may temporarily ameliorate symptoms.[125]

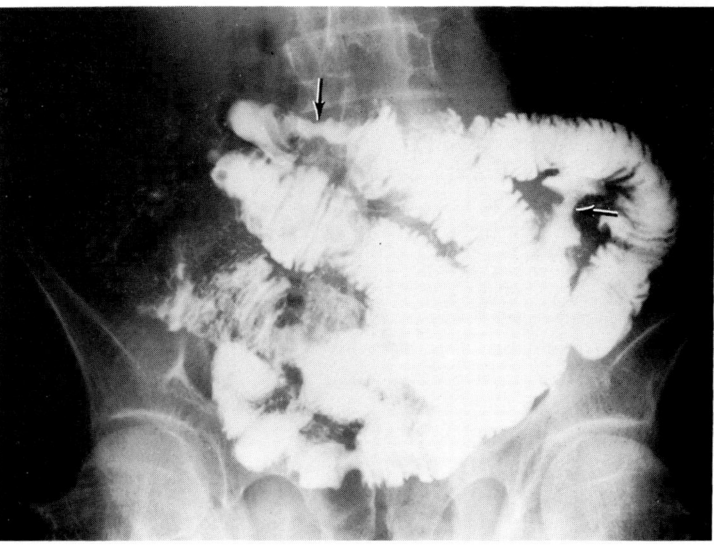

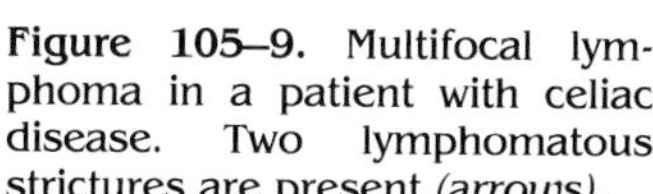

Figure 105–9. Multifocal lymphoma in a patient with celiac disease. Two lymphomatous strictures are present *(arrows)*.

TREATMENT AND PROGNOSIS. Patients with lymphoma who are not terminal show both clinical and jejunal morphologic response to gluten withdrawal. This is short lived, unfortunately, because the usual period of survival from diagnosis to death is less than 1 year. Results of treatment by surgery, radiotherapy, or chemotherapy are depressing, but an occasional patient may survive for many years.

PATHOLOGY. The lymphoma complicating celiac disease has been referred to by many different names. This has hampered classification, but the term *malignant histiocytosis* is coming into more general use.[129] It has been claimed that the complicating lymphoma is a reticulosarcoma, which is preceded by a stage of progressive hyperplasia.[130] In this phase, there is a superficial resemblance of Hodgkin's disease. In Hodgkin's disease, however, the cellular proliferation includes Sternberg-Reed cells, lymphoid cells, fibroblasts, and eosinophils, but cells of the histiocytic series are not found.

The transition to sarcoma may take place either in the mesenteric nodes or in the intestinal mucosa. In a small percentage of patients, the lymphoma does not involve the intestinal mucosa. Only painstaking histologic examination of the gut at autopsy will reveal tumor in some patients, since it may be confined to microscopic foci. Plasma cells in the lamina propria of the jejunal mucosa are fewer in biopsies from patients who develop lymphoma than in biopsies from patients who do not develop this complication, and this phenomenon may be present for as long as 10 years prior to the diagnosis of malignancy.[131] Malignant cells can sometimes be found in peroral jejunal biopsies of patients with celiac disease who develop lymphoma, though careful review of our own cases failed to reveal any such example. This contrasts with *Mediterranean lymphoma,* in which abnormal cells are found in the jejunal mucosa in a significant proportion of patients.

Carcinoma

CLINICAL FEATURES. Carcinoma has been shown to occur at many sites in celiac disease but is particularly common within the esophagus, pharynx, stomach, and rectum. The development of carcinoma may exacerbate or provoke the symptoms of celiac disease. Thus, celiac patients who relapse unexpectedly after a period of good health on a gluten-free diet, or who do not respond to gluten withdrawal, need careful assessment from this point of view.

Carcinoma of the small bowel, in particular the duodenum and upper jejunum, has been reported in a number of patients.[132] Whether it is statistically increased in frequency is not known, but it would appear likely that this is the case. Its presenting features are abdominal pain, anemia, occult gastrointestinal bleeding, an abdominal mass, and associated symptoms of obstruction. Bleeding from the tumor itself is the main factor contributing to the anemia.

AGE AND SEX. Carcinoma of the intestinal tract affects men more than women, particularly carcinoma of the esophagus and small intestine. The average age of patients is between 55 and 60 years.

TREATMENT AND PROGNOSIS. The results of treating carcinoma are similar in celiac and nonceliac patients. Occasionally, resection of small intestinal carcinoma, if the diagnosis is made early, will lead to long-term survival.

There is no evidence that a gluten-free diet is in any way protective in either preventing or reducing the incidence of malignant complications.[56] The suggestion that those celiacs who show less than optimum response to diet are also more liable to develop malignancy could not be supported in one large study.[56] It is possible that gluten withdrawal may prevent malignant complications, but the final answer can only come from an analysis of large numbers of celiac patients who have been on a gluten-free diet since infancy. Nevertheless, it is prudent to insist upon a gluten-free diet for all celiacs at any age.

Malignancy and Flat Jejunal Biopsy. The association of malignancy and a biopsy characteristic of celiac disease could be explained if the metabolic changes of the malignancy itself were responsible for the mucosal changes. No real support for this hypothesis has been adduced, but the possibility is particularly relevant in those patients in whom a diagnosis of lymphoma and celiac disease is made at approximately the same time. Most of these patients will be found to have long histories suggestive of celiac disease. Furthermore, the development of lymphoma in a treated celiac patient does not lead to the production of a flat biopsy. Nevertheless, the possibility that the metabolic derangements associated with malignancy produce a flat biopsy in patients who already have the celiac trait cannot be dismissed entirely. It is reasonable, therefore, to regard such patients as having celiac disease complicated by malignancy.

Etiology. Several mechanisms could be responsible for the increased prevalence of malignancy in celiac disease. The jejunal mucosa itself may represent a premalignant state for the development of either carcinoma or lymphoma. There are changes in the mucosa that are similar to those found in other precancerous conditions: increased mitotic activity in the crypts and irregularity and increased basophilia of the surface epithelium. Also, the increased number of mitoses among the lymphoid cells may increase the chance of malignant cells arising. Mechanisms that are more general than the local features are necessary to explain the occurrence of malignancy not involving the bowel. For example, carcinogens may penetrate the damaged jejunal mucosa more easily, and the mucosa itself may be deficient in carcinogen detoxifying mechanisms. Tobacco and alcohol consumption do not appear to play any part in the increase of carcinoma of the esophagus in celiac disease.

It is recognized that an immature or abnormally developed immune system, or one altered in various ways, may predispose to the development of malignant change. This may be relevant in celiac disease, in which both humoral and cellular immunologic disturbances have been described. Lymphocytes from patients with celiac disease have an appreciable diminution of proliferative and cytotoxic capacity as compared with normal lymphocytes. This deficiency is related to an intrinsic cellular defect as well as an inhibiting factor in the serum of celiac patients. Lymphomas may arise when oncogenic viruses are activated immunologically. In this context, the association of the Epstein-Barr virus with 2 human malignancies may be particularly relevant,[133] because the immunologic disturbances found in celiac disease could provide the environment under which oncogenic viruses may flourish.

Intestinal Ulceration. This condition is characterized by chronic multiple, apparently benign ulcers, most frequently found in the jejunum, occasionally in the ileum, and rarely in the colon.[134] It appears in the literature under a number of names, e.g., *intestinal ulceration, chronic non-granulomatous ulcerative enterocolitis, ulcerative jejunitis,* and *chronic ulcerative non-granulomatous jejunitis.* The disorder affects mainly those in the fifth and sixth decades of life.

Presenting Symptoms. Fever, lassitude, anorexia, weight loss, abdominal pain, and diarrhea are the usual clinical expressions, similar to untreated celiac disease or malignancy complicating celiac disease. The ulcers may be complicated by hemorrhage, perforation, or stricture formation, often one of these is the initial manifestation of the disease.

Laboratory Findings. Anemia, both microcytic and macrocytic, is common, as is steatorrhea and protein-losing enteropathy with associated low serum albumin levels. The majority of patients have a flat jejunal biopsy similar to that found in celiac disease.

Gluten-free Diet. Many of these patients benefit initially from a gluten-free diet. With the onset of ulceration, the response to this diet may end and at this stage the diagnosis of unclassified sprue or refractory sprue is likely to be applied.

Etiology. Whether this condition is related to celiac disease is disputed. Some workers take the view that most, if not all, of those with an initial flat jejunal biopsy are suffering basically from celiac disease.[134] Others regard the condition as a disorder of unknown cause with an uncertain relationship, if any, to celiac disease.[135] It is clear, however, that about half the patients reported in some series fulfill the diagnostic requirements for celiac disease (flat jejunal biopsy and clinical and jejunal morphologic response to gluten withdrawal). Another group with progressive malabsorption unresponsive to a gluten-free diet have been regarded as not having celiac disease. Both groups, however may present with the complications of ulceration, hemorrhage, and perforation or stricture formation. We agree with the view that both these groups, irrespective of the response to gluten withdrawal, have celiac disease complicated by intestinal ulceration.[134]

It seems probable that ulcerative jejunitis, intestinal pseudolymphoma, and malignant lymphoma when associated with villous atrophy are all one condition, i.e., *malignant lymphoma,* and should be designated malignant histiocytosis.[129] There is the occasional patient with normal villi in whom no evidence of a relationship to celiac disease exists and in whom no cause has been demonstrated, but who could have a diffuse form of Crohn's disease. It is of interest that gluten sensitivity in this condition (as assessed by alkaline phosphatase activity of the jejunal mucosa in organ culture) persists in spite of apparent clinical nonresponsiveness to gluten withdrawal. However, jejunal IgA synthesis does not decrease after gluten restriction, as occurs in uncomplicated celiac disease. This would suggest that the local immune system plays some part in the etiology.[136]

Prognosis and Treatment. In general, the outlook is poor. Of a series of 33 patients with small intestinal ulceration and malabsorption, 24 died of complications, 16 within 7 months of the onset of the symptoms referable to the ulcers.[137] A number of patients have been treated by resection of the ulcerated area with good results, but because of the chance that there is underlying lymphoma, prognosis must remain guarded.

One of our patients who had a good clinical and morphologic response to a gluten-free diet for some years developed abdominal pain and vomiting. A short length of strictured and ulcerated small bowel was resected without any evidence of lymphoma or Crohn's disease (Fig. 105–10). She required steroids for 2 years in addition to a gluten-free diet, but since then has remained in excellent health for 11 years on diet alone.

Steroid therapy has been used successfully in some patients.

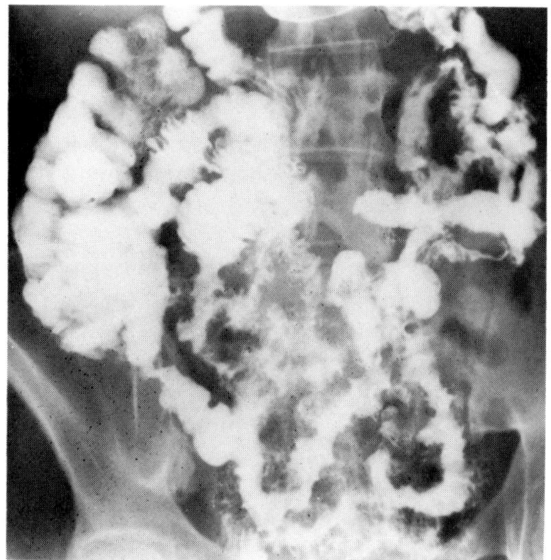

Figure 105–10. Barium appearances of benign ulcerations with diffuse edema and stricture formation in a patient with a celiac disease.

Neuropathy. The prevalence of neuropathic complications is uncertain, but may well lie between 5% and 8% in celiac patients followed for more than 10 years. They occur more often in men than in women, and in our group the age of onset was from 23 to 68 years.

Etiology. The cause of these neurologic complications is not known, but it is likely that there are a number of factors acting singly or in combination.

The clinical course, together with the destruction of Purkinje cells and sparing of other types, are features resembling those in certain viral infections, such as poliomyelitis or the spongiform slow virus type encephalopathies. Indeed, analogies to the neuropathy of celiac disease were made in one of the early descriptions of kuru at a time when infection had been dismissed as a cause for that disorder. There is undoubtedly some defect in the immunologic status of celiac patients, and while there is no evidence to suggest that they are more prone to commonly encountered infections, they may react abnormally to some other more unusual types. Thus, it is suggested that a basic protein formed as a by-product of viral synthesis may become a myelinotoxic antigen by triggering an immune response of lymphocytes.[138]

There is little or no evidence to link vitamin B_{12} deficiency with the neurologic complications of celiac disease. Absence of intrinsic factor is excessively rare, while the neuropathy may appear in patients already receiving vitamin B_{12} therapy.[139] Nor is there adequate evidence that folic acid deficiency plays any part in the neuropathy of celiac disease. Similarly, while there may be a fundamental disturbance of pyridoxine metabolism in celiac disease, no convincing evidence of a beneficial role for pyridoxine in this complication has been adduced.[139]

Pathology. There is great variation in the character and distribution of lesions within the nervous system. Atrophy and focal loss of neurons are common findings. Cortical or cerebellar atrophy may be sufficiently marked to be recognized macroscopically, while histologically the nerve cells are replaced by a retiform network of glial fibers. In the spinal cord, the lesions tend to be patchy and nonsystematized, with spongy demyelination of the posterior and posterolateral columns associated with varying degrees of axonal degeneration.

In the peripheral nerves, light microscopy shows collateral branching and reinnervation together with diffuse swelling of the terminal axons, most marked distally. Electron microscopy shows gross disorganization of the internal structure of the terminal axonic expansions with changes in the relationship of neurofibrils and synaptic vesicles. There is replacement and possibly lysis and phagocytosis of degenerating axoplasm by Schwann cells, a remarkable "frog spawn–like" cytoplasm in relation to the degenerating axonic expansions, and fibrous long-spacing collagen in the intramuscular nerve bundles.[140] Patchy focal demyelination of peripheral nerves without cellular response or leukocytic infiltration is sometimes seen.

Clinical Presentation. A rapidly developing sensory ataxia, referred to as a "progressive, crippling, myeloradiculoneuropathy (pseudotabes),"[141] is the most prominent feature in the majority of patients. Commonly associated with it are numbness, tingling, pain, and weakness of the legs. Though symptoms referable to the arms are less common and milder, some patients may find difficulty in writing or dressing. Dysarthria, dysphonia, diplopia, or palatal myoclonus occasionally occurs. Other patients may experience episodes of unconsciousness that, when associated with lateralizing signs, may simulate many intracranial lesions. Both focal and generalized epilepsy may be encountered, with an overall frequency varying between 3% and 5% of all celiac patients. While such symptoms usually occur in patients already under medical observation for celiac disease, occasionally they are the presenting feature.

Objectively, ankle jerks are diminished earlier and more markedly than are knee jerks, though brisk reflexes can occur. Plantar reflexes are invariably flexor; extensor responses are rarely found. Sensory impairment of the "glove and stocking" variety is common, with muscle power usually diminished. Incoordination is invariably present, and in some patients definite signs of cerebellar dysfunction are found. Optic atrophy can occur.[139]

It is of interest with regard to neurologic alterations in celiac disease to note that acute infective polyneuritis, syringomyelia, amyotrophic lateral sclerosis, and progressive multifocal leukoencephalopathy have all been described in association with this disorder.

Prognosis and Treatment. Most patients follow a progressive downhill course with a fatal outcome ascribable to the neurologic disturbance itself. Nevertheless, long-term survival is encountered, as evidenced by one of our patients who was originally seriously ill with seizures and severe incoordination of the legs but is alive 16 years later. Although still suffering from incoordination of the legs, he has been free of seizures on a strict gluten-free, milk-free diet and has been engaged in regular work for the past 14 years. Most of the survivors have residual neurologic changes.

While gluten withdrawal is strongly advocated, neuropathy has appeared in patients on a gluten-free diet.[139] Evidence of a beneficial role for corticosteroids is inconclusive. In an occasional patient, such as those with chronic inflammatory neuromuscular disorders, some useful effect may be seen.[142] On the other hand, the onset of serious neuropathy has followed or appeared during corticosteroid treatment.[139] Nevertheless, if faced with rapidly progressing neuropathy in a celiac patient, serious consideration should be given to the use of corticosteroids or adrenocorticotropin. We have used ACTH (Acthar Gel), 40 units IM daily for 3 to 7 days, followed by 20 units daily until the condition stabilizes or remits. Ten units daily should be given for a further 2 to 3 months, reducing the administration to alternate days for a similar period prior to stopping therapy.

Mental Disorders. Apart from mood changes produced by gluten, more serious mental disturbances are encountered in a proportion of celiac patients.

Organic Dementia. A progressive mental deterioration is seen in some patients. There is impairment of recent memory and intellectual capacity, together with depression, emotional instability, and periods of confusion.

In a few patients, arrest of the steady downhill course may be brought about by a strict gluten-free diet.

Schizophrenia. A relationship between schizophrenia and celiac disease has been postulated.[143] The frequency of this disorder in celiac disease is not known, but it is at least 10/1000 celiacs as compared with 4.7/1000 persons in the general population. In Ireland, where the frequency of both schizophrenia and celiac disease is high, possible linkage of the 2 disorders has not been confirmed. Much of the evidence for an association between these disorders is circumstantial. The prevalence of schizophrenia diminished during the World War II years in those countries in which cereal supplies were limited and is highest where wheat and rye consumption is greatest.[143] A beneficial effect of a cereal-free, milk-free diet has been demonstrated in schizophrenia, together with an exacerbation of the major symptoms when gluten is restored to the diet. The changes in the morphology of the motor end plates of schizophrenic patients are similar to those seen in the neuropathy of celiac disease. In celiac patients with schizophrenia, there is a clear relationship between dietary gluten exclusion and mental well being, although it is not always easy to persuade these patients to resume their diet on relapse.

Associated Diseases

Many disorders have been found in association with celiac disease. While these disorders themselves could be responsible for producing a flat jejunal biopsy, the weight of evidence is against this view. For example, long histories compatible with celiac disease are often elicited, and in many instances clinical remission and morphologic improvement in the jejunal mucosa follow gluten withdrawal.[21]

Immunologic Disorders. The disturbed immunity in celiac disease has been considered to predispose to an association with disorders that are also suspected of having an immunologic etiology.[54] In this category the most common associations are diabetes mellitus, pulmonary disorders, liver disorders, and thyroid disease.

Diabetes Mellitus. The prevalence of diabetes mellitus in celiac disease may be greater than can be accounted for by chance.[144] Diarrhea is seen in both disorders, and in both it may be intermittent and troublesome at night (Chapter 252). When diarrhea in a diabetic is due to celiac disease, however, there is often a long history of bowel disturbance dating back to childhood. Other features of untreated celiac disease such as poor nutrition, abdominal distention, and mouth ulceration may also be present. With exacerbation of the diarrhea there may be troublesome hypoglycemic episodes. A gluten-free diet enables the diabetes to be more easily controlled, but insulin requirements may increase.

Pulmonary Disorders. Diffuse lung disease occurs in association with celiac disease. Some patients with fibrosing alveolitis have serum antibodies to avian-derived antigens, suggesting the possibility that the pulmonary disorder in them is bird fancier's lung.[145] Farmer's lung has also been reported in celiac disease.

Liver Disorders. Hepatic injury may be common in celiac disease, as judged by the levels of aspartate aminotransferase and alanine aminotransferase.[146] Primary biliary cirrhosis would appear to occur more commonly than by chance.

Non-immunologic Disorders. Many other disorders occur only coincidentally with celiac disease, since celiac patients may develop much the same conditions as the general population.

Cystic Fibrosis. The overlapping clinical picture of celiac disease and cystic fibrosis (Chapter 226) makes it difficult to untangle the 2 disorders. The persistence of symptoms in a young patient with suspected celiac disease following gluten withdrawal should raise the possibility of cystic fibrosis. Also, children with cystic fibrosis should be considered for jejunal biopsy when failure to thrive and grow is disproportionate to the pulmonary problems. Both disorders have occurred within the same sibship.

Dermatitis Herpetiformis

Dermatitis herpetiformis is an important associated disorder or complication of celiac disease (Chapter 18). There is strong evidence that the changes in the intestinal mucosa and the immunologic findings in the majority of patients are identical with those found in celiac disease. Furthermore, gluten has a close relationship with the skin rash.

Clinical Features. Dermatitis herpetiformis is characterized by papulovesicular lesions usually located symmetrically on the elbows, knees, buttocks, sacrum, face, scalp, neck, trunk, and sometimes within the mouth.[147] The predominant symptoms are itching and burning, which may be so severe as to cause pain; rupture of the blisters leads to rapid relief. The average case is relatively mild, and the lesions are sparse in the affected areas. The earliest abnormality is a small erythematous macule, 2 to 3 mm in diameter, which quickly develops into an urticarial papule. At this stage, small vesicles appear that may coalesce and, with scratching, rupture and rapidly dry up. Scarring and pigmentation may result (Fig. 105–11). The vesicles are rarely pustular. Sometimes solitary vesi-

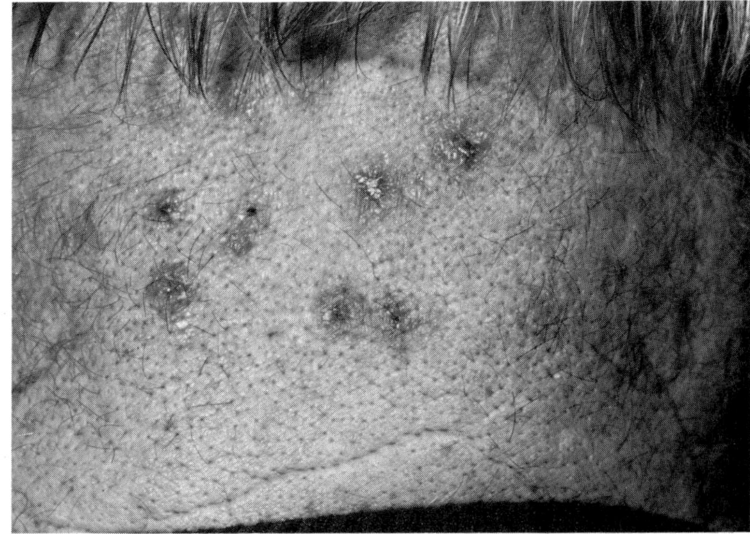

Figure 105–11. The rash of dermatitis herpetiformis seen on the back of the neck.

cles arise in apparently normal skin, and this is particularly so in celiac disease. Though the lesions tend to come out in crops, all stages can usually be seen at any one time. The blisters take 7 to 10 days to involute. The liability to attacks is thought to remain for life. Spontaneous remission, if it occurs at all, is thought to be rare. The rash occurs at any age, though it is uncommon in childhood. It may appear for the first time in a celiac patient who has made both a clinical and a morphologic response to gluten withdrawal.

Symptoms of diarrhea, lassitude, abdominal pain, and distention, all common in celiac disease, are unusual in patients with dermatitis herpetiformis even though steatorrhea may be present in some and the majority have low serum values for iron and folic acid.[148] Severe hypoproteinemia may occur in patients under therapy with dapsone. Lowering of serum protein levels is due partly to protein loss into the intestinal tract and partly to interference with the production of albumin by dapsone. As with celiac disease, the frequency of occurrence of lymphoma is probably increased, but this has not been proved statistically.

Jejunal Mucosa. The jejunal mucosa in dermatitis herpetiformis is flat in about one third of patients, is apparently normal in one third, and shows intermediate changes in the remainder. Many of the macroscopically normal biopsies have increased numbers of intra-epithelial lymphocytes. These cells return to normal values following gluten withdrawal.[15] Of importance for the diagnosis of celiac disease is the observation that giving extra gluten to patients with dermatitis herpetiformis whose jejunal mucosa is apparently normal causes the mucosa to become flat.[16] The mucosal lesions, as in celiac disease, may be patchy.[39]

Immunology. The demonstration of IgA deposits in the skin of patients with dermatitis herpetiformis has become the most important diagnostic finding. Such deposits can be detected in 95% to 100% of patients[148] (Fig. 105–12). The granular or speckled IgA deposits are located with the microfibrillar bundles in the dermal papillary tips. Linear IgA is associated with the anchoring fibrils along the basement membrane. Deposits of this type are not found in either celiac patients or normal subjects. Other immunologic phenomena, including the increased frequency of HLA-B8, are similar to those found in celiac disease.

Gluten Withdrawal and Dapsone

Jejunal Mucosa. The response of the jejunal mucosa to gluten withdrawal in dermatitis herpetiformis is essentially similar to that noted in celiac disease. In general, all those whose skin rash responds well will show improvement in jejunal morphology. The converse, improvement in the mucosal lesions associated with improvement of the skin, does not hold.

Skin Lesions. A gluten-free diet has been

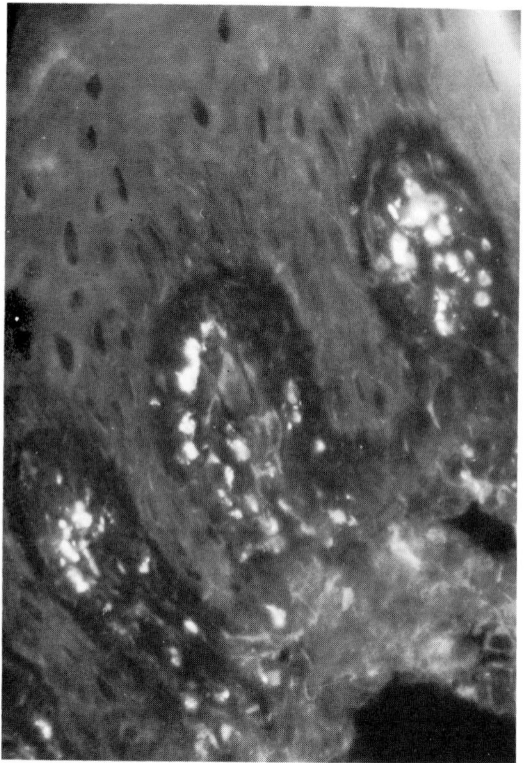

Figure 105–12. Dermatitis herpetiformis showing granular deposits of IgA in the dermal papillae. These are seen as the fluorescent (white) areas.

shown to permit a reduction of the dosage of dapsone in 93% of patients, as compared with 16% of controls.[149] Furthermore, approximately one third of the patients were ultimately able to dispense with dapsone completely. Though the rash in most patients is benefited by a gluten-free diet, a small minority obtain no relief despite morphologic improvement of the jejunal mucosa.

Etiology. There is at present no satisfactory explanation for the mode of action of gluten in dermatitis herpetiformis. It has been suggested that antibodies formed in the gut as a result of stimulation by gluten fix to the skin of patients. While there are circulating immune complexes in both celiac disease and dermatitis herpetiformis, the complexes have not been shown to contain IgA. Neither has gluten been demonstrated in the skin. Antireticulin antibodies have also been suggested as the means whereby IgA is deposited on the reticulin fibers in the skin, but reticulin antibodies are mainly IgG. In any event, whatever the mechanism, IgA is found in both involved and uninvolved skin in dermatitis herpetiformis, so that additional influences must be present to produce the rash.

Confirmation of Diagnosis of Celiac Disease

Unfortunately there is no specific immunologic or biochemical test for celiac disease. As a general rule, *a flat jejunal biopsy from a white adult in the Western World is almost certain to indicate celiac disease,* although other disorders can be associated with the same change (tropical sprue, soy protein intolerance, cow's milk protein intolerance, and gastroenteritis in infancy).

It has been claimed that organ culture techniques will help differentiate the flat mucosa of celiac disease from that of other causes.[150] This test is based on the findings that improvement in biopsies cultured in a gluten-free medium is inhibited by the addition of gluten fractions. An accuracy of over 85% has been reported in classifying gluten-sensitive lesions, but doubt has been cast on the value of this investigation.[151] The measurement of enterocyte height of mucosa in culture appears to be a promising approach. Skin tests have proved to be of no clinical value.

Differential Diagnosis

In the differential diagnosis of celiac disease consideration must be given to other disorders associated with malabsorption (pancreatogenous steatorrhea, Crohn's disease, contaminated bowel syndrome, and postgastrectomy states), disorders with jejunal changes and gastrointestinal symptoms (eosinophilic gastroenteritis, intestinal lymphangiectasia, and Mediterranean lymphoma), and jejunal mucosal damage induced by some drugs or therapeutic x-rays. These conditions usually are easily distinguished. A number of other conditions, however, require particular consideration.

Refractory Sprue (Non-responsive Celiac Disease). These patients have all the characteristics of celiac disease, including a flat jejunal biopsy, but fail to respond to a gluten-free diet.[7] The terms "refractory" and "non-responsive" are unfortunate, for they are often applied indiscriminately to patients who have not adhered strictly to the diet, to patients who have not been followed for long enough, to those who have not had full morphologic assessment of the jejunal mucosa with cell counts and enzyme assays before and after gluten withdrawal, and to those in whom the effects of other protein or nonprotein factors have not been fully considered.[152] Some prove to be celiac patients in whom the complication of lymphoma subsequently appears.

IgA Deficiency. The majority of patients with selective IgA deficiency have no intestinal abnormalities. In some, however, flat jejunal biopsies have been reported and in these, responses to a gluten-free diet confirm celiac disease.

Lymphoma. Lymphoma itself has been claimed to be a cause for a flat jejunal biopsy and associated malabsorption. Accumulated evidence, however, indicates that patients with these features have celiac disease complicated by malignant histiocytosis.

Collagenous Sprue. It has been alleged that "collagenous" sprue is a distinct disorder associated with progressive malabsorption and deposits of hyalin material (thought to be collagen) in the subepithelial layer of the intestinal mucosa.[32] The presence of this material has been considered to indicate a poor prognosis. However, collagen deposition occurs in a substantial number of patients with untreated celiac disease and disappears on gluten withdrawal in nearly every case within 6 months. Moreover, follow-up observations for more than 20 years in 22 such patients showed that the outlook in patients with collagen deposition was no different from that in a matched group without collagen deposits.

Cow's Milk Protein Intolerance. Intolerance to cow's milk protein is a temporary condition encountered in early infancy.[153] The jejunal mucosal abnormality is similar to that found in celiac disease but in general is less severe, and the lymphocytic epithelial infiltration is not as marked. Diagnosis is made difficult by the fact that children with untreated celiac disease may be intolerant to milk and will not achieve full remission until milk is withdrawn. Infants have been reported in whom cow's milk protein intolerance is present and in whom the administration of gluten produces clinical symptoms, but not morphologic changes in the jejunal mucosa.[154] It has also been demonstrated that the flat jejunal mucosa of such patients will revert to normal on withdrawal of milk and while they are still ingesting gluten.

Soy Protein Intolerance. Soy protein has been used in the treatment of celiac disease as a replacement for gluten and also as a substitute for milk protein in cow's milk intolerance. There are, however, a few reports in which it has been demonstrated that soy protein itself may cause serious clinical illness and changes in the mucosa, "identical with that seen in celiac disease."[155] Patients with soy protein intolerance appear to tolerate gluten, though some also have an associated cow's milk protein intolerance.

Tropical Sprue. Tropical sprue and celiac disease were first believed to be essentially the same disorder (Chapter 106). Jejunal biopsy changes in patients with tropical sprue do not differ appreciably from the appearance of the jejunum in apparently normal individuals living in the same area. A flat biopsy may be found in an occasional patient, but the mucosa is thinner than that encountered in celiac disease and the lipid is confined more to the region of the basement membrane.[156] Treatment with folic acid or antibiotics leads to clinical and morphologic improvement, whereas a gluten-free diet is without benefit. It must be remembered that natives of tropical countries may have celiac disease.[157]

Non-celiac Gluten-sensitive Diarrhea. This condition has been described in infants and young children, but also occurs in adults. Ingestion of gluten by these patients is associated with diarrhea and vomiting; dermatitis, rhinitis, and bronchitis may also appear. Blood and mucus may be found in the stools. The jejunal mucosa remains normal or only mildly edematous.[154] The abdominal pain, diarrhea, vomiting, headaches, and malaise described by adult patients are dramatically relieved on withdrawal of gluten. The jejunal morphology shows a slight increase of intra-epithelial lymphocytes, which return to normal on a gluten-free diet. The biochemical and immunologic defects common in celiac disease are not present.[158]

Transient Gluten Intolerance. It is implicit in many of the definitions of celiac disease that following gluten challenge, the jejunal mucosa deteriorates within a relatively short time. Indeed, the criteria laid down by the ESPGAN imply that if the mucosa is normal after 2 years, the disorder was not celiac disease.[9,12] Under these circumstances, the diagnosis of transient gluten intolerance has been applied in childhood. It is now clear, however, that relapse may occur much later than 2 years and that patients diagnosed as suffering from transient gluten intolerance will require long term follow-up. They may well present with celiac disease in later life.[159]

Parasitic Disease. A number of parasitic

disorders (giardiasis, strongyloidiasis, coccidiosis, and hookworm disease) have been associated with clinical symptoms of malabsorption and with changes in jejunal morphology including, in rare cases, flat biopsies (Chapter 232). When this occurs in giardiasis, it appears to reflect celiac disease[160] or immunoglobulin deficiency.

Treatment

Gluten-free Diet. The mainstay of therapy for celiac disease is the gluten-free diet, which restores the majority of patients to normal in all respects. *Improvement in well-being is often noted within 48 hours of starting the diet, but full remission may take weeks or months to achieve.* Patients with continued ill health and recurring symptoms are nearly always taking gluten, either deliberately or accidentally. This is often a problem in the early stages of treatment or when eating away from home. Difficulties are also encountered when foods regarded as gluten-free contain gluten, as may happen with processed foods. Apart from failure to maintain a proper diet more or less permanently, patients may fail to respond to gluten withdrawal because of the development of complications, such as malignancy or intestinal ulceration. However, 15% to 20% of celiac patients still remain who do not completely respond, be it clinically with a good morphologic response, morphologically with a good clinical response, or only partially in either respect. Other cereals and foods and trace elements require consideration in these patients. The recognition of these possibilities has made the patient who deteriorates and dies unaccountably very rare indeed.

The acceptance of a gluten-free diet by the patient is largely conditioned by initial explanation of the need for the diet and its implications in practical terms. Unfortunately, there are still some physicians who are not convinced of the necessity for the diet or that it should be continued indefinitely. They believe that celiac disease is a disorder confined to childhood and, occasionally, even refuse to prescribe gluten-free products. Special efforts must be made to ensure that young patients, particularly teenagers, do not regard themselves as handicapped and different from others. A powerful argument to them is the importance of a gluten-free diet in ensuring full physical and intellectual development in these important years. With parental support and cooperation, there should be little difficulty with teenagers.

It is not a kindness to withhold dietary treatment from the elderly. To do so denies them many years of health and enjoyment. A gluten-free diet is advised for *all* patients, including those who may be asymptomatic and discovered as a result of family studies, for example. Since a single dietary transgression may not be followed by any obvious ill effects, patients are easily tempted to ingest more gluten. The results of such action may not be evident for months or even years later. It must be stressed from the outset that a gluten-free diet will need to be maintained strictly throughout life. If the physician does not believe and emphasize this, the patient will be unlikely to continue with the diet.

Wheat flour is incorporated in a number of manufactured foods and is also used in many cooking procedures. This is not always suspected by patients, particularly those who are newly diagnosed (Table 105–1). In most instances, these foods can be identified from descriptions on their containers. In any event, celiac societies established in many countries* produce lists of gluten-free products in addition to giving advice about many other aspects of diet and cooking. Inasmuch as gluten-free flour does not contain glutenin, which is responsible for the viscoelastic properties of wheat flour, instruction in cooking with gluten-free materials is an important contribution to diet acceptability.

Rye, Barley, and Oats. The evidence for excluding rye from the diet of celiac patients is strong. In some patients, barley is also toxic. Oats are less likely to cause problems, while maize and rice appear to be harmless.

Milk, Eggs, and Other Foods. A sizable number of patients are milk intolerant and will attain full clinical and morphologic remission only when milk, in addition to gluten, is withdrawn from the diet. Eggs may also have to be excluded in some patients. The importance of other foods is emphasized by the patient who responded only partially to a gluten-free diet and needed the exclusion as well of egg yolk, egg white, chicken, and tuna fish to obtain full clinical remission.[152]

---

*Australia, Austria, Canada, Eire, Finland, France, Holland, Italy, New Zealand, Poland, South Africa, Spain, Sweden, Switzerland, United Kingdom, United States, and West Germany.

Table 105–1. FOODS ALLOWED AND PROHIBITED IN CELIAC DISEASE

	Foods Allowed		Foods Not Allowed
Cereals	Cornflour, custard powder, arrowroot, maize, millet, tapioca, sago, rice, Cornflakes, Rice Krispies, gluten-free bread, gluten-free biscuits, gluten-free starch, soya bran	Cereals	Wheat and wheat flour, bread, pastry, biscuits, noodles, macaroni, semolina, Shredded Wheat, All Bran and commercial bran, Puffed Wheat, Weetabix, porridge, groats, barley, rye, Ryvita and rye bread, Lemon and Barley, pearl barley
Meat	Fresh, smoked, and frozen	Meat*	Sausages, pre-cooked meals, meat pies
Fish	Fresh, smoked, frozen, and tinned	Fish	Battered, breadcrumbed, and fish in sauce
Cheese	All plain cheeses, cream and curd cheeses	Cheese	Spreads*
Milk	Fresh, tinned, dried; cream, plain yogurt	Milk products	Flavored yogurt,* ice cream,* batters, pancakes, Yorkshire pudding
Fats	Margarine, butter, lard, and cooking oils		
Eggs			
Fruits	Fresh, frozen, tinned, and dried; juices	Fruits	Pies and flans and crumbles
Nuts			
Vegetables	Fresh, frozen, tinned, dried	Vegetables	Tinned, vegetables in sauce, tomato juice from vending machine, instant potatoes*
Sauces and gravies, condiments	Bovril, Marmite, salt, pepper, herbs, vinegar, spices, monosodium glutamate	Sauces and gravies	Oxo, Bisto, Bovril from vending machine
Beverages	Tea, coffee, alcohol	Beverages	Home-made beers
Preserves	Jam, marmalade, jelly, honey, golden syrup, molasses, black treacle	Preserves	Peanut butter*
Sweets/ candies	Boiled sweets	Sweets/ candies	Unwrapped sweets, chocolate*

*Check with manufacturers

Trace Elements

Zinc. The administration of zinc to patients with celiac disease who have failed to respond to withdrawal of gluten has been claimed to result in sustained improvement in well being, intestinal function, and nutritional status.[161] However, not all have found such striking effects. Zinc deficiency, which is relatively common in celiac disease, may be responsible for the lack of appetite and taste noted in untreated celiac disease; both are readily corrected by administration of zinc sulfate, 220 mg 3 times per day by mouth.

Magnesium. Magnesium deficiency in the untreated celiac patient may need specific replacement in addition to gluten withdrawal, particularly in those with severe diarrhea. In the acute state, magnesium chloride, 0.5 mEq/kg body weight in 0.6% dextrose or

0.9% saline may be given IV over 60 to 90 minutes. Alternatively, magnesium hydroxide, 10 ml of an 8% solution given 3 times per day daily by mouth (equivalent to 83 mEq or 1 g of magnesium per day) is well absorbed.

Hematinics. Treatment with a gluten-free diet will lead to the restoration of normal hematologic values in most patients. Folic acid (5 to 10 mg daily) and iron are usually given to hasten the process. Even though there is no good evidence that pyridoxine is a factor in the anemia of celiac disease, it may be tried in daily doses of 200 to 400 mg by mouth in those patients with anemia unresponsive to other treatment. Vitamin B_{12} deficiency is relatively uncommon and is best treated with hydroxycobalamin, 1 mg IM every 2 to 3 months.

Vitamin D. The institution of a gluten-free diet leads to improvement in the absorption of vitamin D. Still, osteomalacia may appear in patients who are on a gluten-free diet. Consequently, the administration of calciferol is often necessary to effect a cure (1.25 mg or 50,000 units daily). Calciferol may be given for many months without side effects, but the serum calcium level should be monitored regularly. Occasionally, osteomalacia may persist despite calciferol and a gluten-free diet. In such instances, 25-hydroxy vitamin D is required (20 μg daily).[93]

Steroid Therapy. The necessity for steroid therapy is rare. Its use has been suggested when the serum levels of albumin are low in order to bring associated protein-losing enteropathy under control. Azathioprine has also been used to induce remission in a nonresponsive celiac and to act as a steroid-sparing agent.[162]

In general, there are 3 indications for steroids: (1) the patient's refusal or inability to tolerate a gluten-free diet despite deteriorating health; (2) the presence of complicating disorders, such as chronic active hepatitis or ulcerative jejunitis; and (3) the inability to maintain health despite a strict milk-free and gluten-free diet. Apart from an earlier short-term study,[163] we have used steroids in only 6 patients among 500 treated patients equally divided into the 3 foregoing categories.

Prognosis

Before the gluten-free diet was introduced, the outlook for celiac patients was poor, with mortality rates in published series ranging between 5% and 30%. After use of the gluten-free diet was adopted, mortality fell considerably. For a group of 485 children attending Great Ormond Street Children's Hospital, London, and reviewed in 1969,[164] the mortality rate was only 0.4%. Our own statistics show that for a group of adult patients, the mortality rate against a matched control population is approximately twice normal.[56]

References

1. Aretaeus. On the coeliac affection. Quoted by Major RH. *In:* Classic Descriptions of Disease. 3rd Ed. Springfield, Ill: Charles C Thomas, 1945:600–1.
2. Gee S. On the coeliac affection. St. Bartholomews Hosp Rep 1888; 24:17–20.
3. Thaysen TEH. Non-tropical Sprue. A Study in Idiopathic Steatorrhoea. London: Oxford University Press, 1932.
4. Bennett TI, Hunter D, Vaughan JM. Idiopathic steatorrhoea (Gee's disease). A nutritional disturbance associated with tetany, osteomalacia and anaemia. Q J Med 1932; 1:603–77.
5. Snell AM. Tropical and non-tropical sprue (chronic idiopathic steatorrhea). Their probable interrelationship. Ann Intern Med 1939; 12:1632–69.
6. Paulley JW. Observations on the aetiology of idiopathic steatorrhoea and lymph node biopsies. Br Med J 1954; 2:1318–21.
7. Rubin CE, Eidelman S, Weinstein WM. Sprue by any other name. Gastroenterology 1970; 58:409–13.
8. Booth CC. Definition of adult coeliac disease. *In:* Hekkens WTJM, Pena AS, eds. Coeliac Disease. Leiden: Stenfert Kroese, 1974: 17–22.
9. Meeuwisse GW. Diagnostic criteria in coeliac disease (Round table discussion. European Society for Paediatric Gastroenterology and Nutrition) (ESPGAN). Acta Paediatr Scand 1970; 59:461–3.
10. Cooke WT, Asquith P. Introduction and definition. Celiac disease. Clin Gastroenterol 1974; 3:3–10.
11. McNicholl B, Egan-Mitchell B, Fottrell PF. Variability of gluten tolerance in treated childhood coeliac disease. Gut 1979; 20:126–32.
12. McNeish AS, Harms HK, Rey J, Shmerling DH, Visakorpi JK, Walker-Smith JA. The diagnosis of coeliac disease. A commentary on the current practices of members of the European Society for Paediatric Gastroenterology and Nutrition (ESPGAN). Arch Dis Child 1979; 54:783–6.
13. Egan-Mitchell B, Fottrell PF, McNicholl B. Early or precoeliac mucosa: Development of gluten enteropathy. Gut 1981; 22:65–9.
14. Rolles CJ, Kyaw-Myint TB, Wai-Kee S, Anderson CM. The familial incidence of asymptomatic coeliac disease. *In:* McConnell RB, ed. The Genetics of Coeliac Disease. Lancaster: MTP Press, 1981:235–43.
15. Fry L, Seah PP, McMinn RMH, Hoffbrand AV. Lymphocytic infiltration of epithelium in diagnosis of gluten sensitive enteropathy. Br Med J 1972; 3:371–4.
16. Weinstein WM. Latent celiac sprue. Gastroenterology 1974; 66:489–93.
17. Stokes PL, Ferguson R, Holmes GKT, Cooke WT. Familial aspects of coeliac disease. Q J Med 1976; 45:567–82.
18. Mylotte M, Egan-Mitchell B, McCarthy CF, McNicholl B. Incidence of coeliac disease in the West of Ireland. Br Med J 1973; 1:703–5.
19. Houdenak N. Prevalence and clinical picture of adult gluten-induced enteropathy in a Norwegian population. Scand J Gastroenterol 1980; 15:401–4.
20. Stenhammar L, Johansson CG. The incidence of coeliac disease in children in South-East Sweden. Acta Paediatr Scand 1981; 70:379–81.
21. Cooke WT, Holmes GKT. Coeliac Disease. Edinburgh: Churchill Livingstone, 1983.
22. McNeish AS, Anderson CM. Coeliac disease. The disorder in childhood. Clin Gastroenterol 1974; 3:127–44.

23. Swinson CM, Levi AJ. Is coeliac disease underdiagnosed? Br Med J 1980; 4:1258–60.
24. Lord C, MacGregor GA. Coeliac disease in identical twin infants. Postgrad Med J 1981; 57:658–9.
25. Bolt RJ. Methods of small bowel biopsy. JAMA 1964; 188:40–1.
26. Kilby A. Paediatric small intestine biopsy capsule with two ports. Gut 1976; 17:158–9.
27. Gaze H, Rolles C, Signer E, Sagaro E. Premedication for jejunal biopsy in childhood using intravenous diazepam and metoclopramide. Arch Dis Child 1974; 49:322–4.
28. Holdstock G, Eade OE, Isaacson P, Smith CL. Endoscopic duodenal biopsies in coeliac disease and duodenitis. Scand J Gastroenterol 1979; 14:717–20.
29. Linaker BD, Calam J. Jejunal biopsy with the Watson capsule and perforation in the elderly. Gastroenterology 1978; 75:723–5.
30. Scott H, Brandtzaeg P. Enumeration of Paneth cells in coeliac disease: Comparison of conventional light microscopy and immunofluorescence staining for lysozyme. Gut 1981; 22:812–6.
31. Sjolund K, Alumets J, Berg NO, Hakanson R, Sundler F. Enteropathy of coeliac disease in adults: Increased number of enterochromaffin cells in the duodenal mucosa. Gut 1982; 23:42–8.
32. Weinstein WM, Saunders DR, Tytgat GN, Rubin CE. Collagenous sprue—an unrecognized type of malabsorption. N Engl J Med 1970; 283:1297–1301.
33. Bossart R, Henry K, Booth CC, Doe WF. Subepithelial collagen in intestinal malabsorption. Gut 1975; 16:18–22.
34. Ferguson A, Murray D. Quantitation of intraepithelial lymphocytes in human jejunum. Gut 1971; 12:988–94.
35. Holmes GKT, Asquith P, Stokes PL, Cooke WT. Cellular infiltrate of jejunal biopsies in adult coeliac disease in relation to gluten withdrawal. Gut 1974; 15:278–83.
36. Trier JS, Browning TH. Epithelial cell renewed in cultured duodenal biopsies in celiac sprue. N Engl J Med 1970; 283:1245–50.
37. Watson AJ, Wright NA. Morphology and cell kinetics of the jejunal mucosa in untreated patients. Clin Gastroenterol 1974; 3:11–31.
38. Roy-Choudhury DC, Cooke WT, Banwell JG, Smits BJ. Multiple jejunal biopsies in adult celiac disease. Am J Dig Dis 1967; 12:657–63.
39. Scott BB, Losowsky MS. Patchiness and duodenal-jejunal variation of the mucosal abnormality in coeliac disease and dermatitis herpetiformis. Gut 1976; 17:984–92.
40. Thompson H. The small intestine at autopsy. Clin Gastroenterol 1974; 3:171–81.
41. Dicke WK, Weijers HA, Van de Kamer JH. Coeliac disease. II. The presence in wheat of a factor having a deleterious effect in cases of coeliac disease. Acta Paediatr 1953; 42:34–42.
42. Van de Kamer JH, Weijers HA, Dicke WK. Coeliac disease. IV. An investigation into the injurious constituents of wheat in connection with their action on patients with coeliac disease. Acta Paediatr 1953; 42:223–31.
43. Frazer AC, Fletcher RF, Ross CAC, Shaw B, Sammons HG, Schneider R. Gluten-induced enteropathy. The effect of partially digested gluten. Lancet 1959; 252–5.
44. Messer M, Anderson CM, Hubbard L. Studies on the mechanisms of destruction of the toxic action of wheat gluten in coeliac disease by crude papain. Gut 1964; 5:295–303.
45. Bronstein HD, Haeffner LJ, Kowlessar OD. Enzymatic digestion of gliadin: The effect of the resultant peptides in adult coeliac disease. Clin Chim Acta 1966; 14:141–55.
46. Krainick HG, Mohn G, Fischer HH. Further studies on the harmful effects of wheat flour in coeliacs. II. The action of the enzymatic breakdown products of gliadin. Helv Paediatr Acta 1959; 14:124–40.
47. Townley RRW, Bhathal PS, Cornell HJ, Mitchell JD. Toxicity of wheat gliadin fractions in coeliac disease. Lancet 1973; 1:1363–4.
48. Frazer AC. Discussion on some problems of steatorrhoea and reduced stature on the growth defect in coeliac disease. Proc R Soc Med 1956; 49:1009–13.
49. Peters TJ, Jones PE, Wells G. Analytical subcellular fractionation of jejunal biopsy specimens: Enzyme activities, organelle pathology and response to gluten withdrawal in patients with coeliac disease. Clin Sci Mol Med 1978; 55:285–92.
50. Sterchi EE, Woodley JF. Peptidases of the human intestinal brush border membrane. *In:* McNicholl B, McCarthy CF, Fottrell PF, eds. Perspectives in Coeliac Disease. Lancaster: MTP Press, 1978:437–49.
51. Phelan JJ, Stevens FM, McNicholl B, Fottrell PF, McCarthy CF. Coeliac disease: The abolition of gliadin toxicity by enzymes from *Aspergillus niger*. Clin Sci Mol Med 1977; 53:35–43.
52. McNicholl B, Egan-Mitchell B, Stevens F, Keane R, Baker S, McCarthy CF, Fottrell PF. Mucosal recovery in treated childhood celiac disease (gluten sensitive enteropathy). J Pediatr 1976; 89:418–24.
53. Krainick HG, Debatin F, Gauter E, Tobler R, Velasco JA. Additional research on the injurious effect of wheat flour in coeliac disease. I. Acute gliadin reaction—gliadin shock. Helv Paediatr Acta 1958; 13:432–54.
54. Cooper BT, Holmes GKT, Cooke WT. Coeliac disease and immunological disorders. Br Med J 1978; 1:537–9.
55. Bullen AW, Hall R, Gowland G, Rajah S, Losowsky MS. Hyposplenism, adult coeliac disease and autoimmunity. Gut 1981; 22:28–33.
56. Holmes GKT, Stokes PL, Sorahan TM, Prior P. Waterhouse JAH, Cooke WT. Coeliac disease, gluten free diet and malignancy. Gut 1976; 17:612–19.
57. Falchuk ZM, Strober W. Gluten sensitive enteropathy: Synthesis of antigliadin antibody in vitro. Gut 1974; 15:947–52.
58. O'Donoghue DR, Swarbrick ET, Kumar PJ. Type I hypersensitivity reactions in celiac disease. Gastroenterology 1979; 76:1211.
59. Challacombe DN, Dawkins PD, Baker P. Increased tissue concentrations of 5-hydroxytryptamine in duodenal mucosa of patients with coeliac disease. Gut 1977; 18:882–6.
60. Baldo BA, Wrigley CW. IgE antibodies to wheat flour components. Studies with sera from subjects with baker's asthma or celiac condition. Clin Allergy 1978; 8:109–24.
61. Shiner M. Ultrastructural changes suggestive of immune reactions in the jejunal mucosa of coeliac children following gluten challenge. Gut 1973; 14:1–12.
62. Ferguson A, Parrott DMV. Histopathology and time course of rejection of allografts of mouse small intestine. Transplantation 1973; 15:546–54.
63. Anand BS, Truelove SC, Offord RE. Skin test for coeliac disease using a subfraction of gluten. Lancet 1977; 1:118–20.
64. Neild GH. Coeliac disease: A graft versus-host-like reaction localized to the small bowel wall. Lancet 1981; 1:811–12.
65. Weiser MM, Douglas AP. An alternative mechanism for gluten toxicity in coeliac disease. Lancet 1976; 1:567–9.
66. MacKintosh P, Asquith P. HLA and coeliac disease. Br Med Bull 1978; 34:291–4.
67. Pena AS, Mann DL, Hague NE, Heck JA, Van Leeuwen A, Van Rood JJ, Strober W. Genetic basis of gluten sensitive enteropathy. Gastroenterology 1978; 75:230–5.
68. Benn A, Cooke WT. Intraluminal pH of duodenum and jejunum in fasting subjects with normal and abnormal gastric or pancreatic function. Scand J Gastroenterol 1971; 6:313–7.
69. Rubin WL, Ross L, Sleisenger MH, Weser E. An electron microscope study of adult celiac disease. Lab Invest 1966; 15:1720–47.
69a. Rifaat MK, Iseri OA, Gottlieb LS. An ultrastructural study of the extraneous coat of human colonic mucosa. Gastroenterology 1965; 48:593–601.
70. Schanker LS, Tocco DJ, Brodie BB, Hogben CAM. Absorption of drugs from the rat small intestine. J Pharmacol Exp Ther 1958; 123:81–8.
71. Lucas ML, Cooper BT, Lei FH, Holmes GKT, Blair JA, Cooke WT. Acid microclimate in coeliac disease and Crohn's disease: A model for folate malabsorption. Gut 1978; 19:735–42.
72. Padykula HA, Strauss EW, Ladman AJ, Gardner FH. A

morphologic and histochemical analysis of the human jejunal epithelium in non-tropical sprue. Gastroenterology 1961; 40:735–65.
73. Peters TJ, Heath JR, Wansbrough-Jones MH, Doe WF. Enzyme activities and properties of lysosomes and brush borders in jejunal biopsies from control subjects and patients with coeliac disease. Clin Sci Mol Med 1975; 48:259–67.
74. Pena AS, Truelove SC, Whitehead R. Disaccharidase activity and jejunal morphology in coeliac disease. Q J Med 1972; 41:457–76.
75. Asquith P. Immunology. Clin Gastroenterol 1974; 3:213–34.
76. Baklien K, Brandtzaeg P, Fausa O. Immunoglobulins in jejunal mucosa and serum from patients with adult coeliac disease. Scand J Gastroenterol 1977; 12:149–59.
77. Ferguson A, Carswell F. Precipitins to dietary proteins in serum and upper intestinal secretions of coeliac children. Br Med J 1972; 1:75–7.
78. Magalhaes AFN, Peters TJ, Doe WF. Studies on the nature and significance of connective tissue antibodies in adult coeliac disease and Crohn's disease. Gut 1974; 15:284–8.
79. Holmes GKT, Asquith P, Cooke WT. Cell mediated immunity to gluten fraction III in adult coeliac disease. Clin Exp Immunol 1976; 24:259–65.
80. Haeney MR, Asquith P. Inhibition of leucocyte migration by α-gliadin in patients with gastrointestinal disease: Its specificity with respect to α-gliadin and coeliac disease. *In:* McNicholl B, McCarthy CF, Fottrell PF, eds. Perspectives in Coeliac Disease. Lancaster: MTP Press, 1978: 229–41.
81. Groll A, Candy DCA, Preece MA, Tanner JM, Harries JT. Short stature as the primary manifestation of coeliac disease. Lancet 1980; 2: 1097–9.
82. Dawes PT, Atherton ST. Coeliac disease presenting as recurrent pericarditis. Lancet 1981; 2:1021–2.
83. Ferguson R, Holmes GKT, Cooke WT. Coeliac disease, fertility and pregnancy. Scand J Gastroenterol 1982; 17:65–8.
84. Ferguson R, Basu MK, Asquith P, Cooke WT. Jejunal mucosal abnormalities in patients with recurrent aphthous ulceration. Br Med J 1976; 1:11–3.
85. Green PA, Wollaeger EE. The clinical behavior of sprue in the United States. Gastroenterology 1960; 38:399–418.
86. Ross JR, Garabedian M. Systemic manifestations of gluten enteropathies and gluten sensitivity in some other diseases. *In:* Glass GBJ, ed. Process in Gastroenterology. Vol. 2. New York: Grune and Stratton, 1970; 430–49.
87. Egan-Mitchell B, McNicholl B. Constipation in childhood coeliac disease. Arch Dis Child 1972; 47:238–40.
88. Pitchumoni CS, Thomas E, Balthazar E, Sherling B. Chronic calcific pancreatitis in association with celiac disease. Am J Gastroenterol 1977; 68:358–361.
89. Regan PT, Dimagno EP. Exocrine pancreatic insufficiency in coeliac sprue: A cause for treatment failure. Gastroenterology 1980; 78:484–7.
90. Ryan FP, Timperley WR, Preston FE, Holdsworth CD. Cerebral involvement with disseminated intra-vascular coagulation in intestinal disease. J Clin Pathol 1977; 30:551–5.
91. Harris OD, Philip HM, Cooke WT, Pover WFR. 47 Ca studies in adult coeliac disease and other gastrointestinal conditions with particular reference to osteomalacia. Scand J Gastroenterol 1970; 5:169–75.
92. Hollander D, Muralidhara KS, Zimmerman A. Vitamin D3 intestinal absorption in vivo: Influence of fatty acids, bile salts and perfusate pH on absorption. Gut 1979; 19:267–72.
93. Hepner GW, Jowsey J, Arnaud C, Black B, Roginsky M, Fai Moo H, Young J. Osteomalacia and celiac disease. Response to 25-hydroxy vitamin D. Am J Med 1978; 65:1015–20.
94. Higgins JA, Lee PR, Scholer JF, Reitemeier RJ, Code CF, Wollaeger EE. Absorption of water and sodium from the small intestine of patients with non-tropical sprue. J Clin Invest 1957; 36:265–9.
95. Cooke WT. Water and electrolyte upsets in the steatorrhea syndrome. J Mt Sin Hosp 1957; 24:221–31.
96. Owen DA, Thorlakson TK, Walli JE. Celiac disease in a patient with morbid obesity. Ann Intern Med 1980; 140:1380–3.
97. David TJ, Ajdukiewicz AB, Read AE. Dermal and epidermal ridge atrophy in celiac sprue. Gastroenterology 1973; 64:539–44.
98. Thaysen TEH. Ten cases of idiopathic steatorrhoea. Q J Med 1935; 4:359–95.
99. Whorwell PJ, Foster KJ, Alderson MR, Wright R. Death from ischaemic heart disease and malignancy in adult patients with coeliac disease. Lancet 1976; 2:113–4.
100. Drummery GD, Benson JA, Jones CM. Microscopical examination of the stool for steatorrhea. N Engl J Med 1961; 264:85–7.
101. Tuna N, Mangold HK, Mosser DG. Re-evaluation of the I^{131} triolein absorption test. J Lab Clin Med 1963; 61:620–8.
102. Newcomer AD, Hofmann AF, Dimagno EP, Thomas PJ, Carlson GL. Triolein breath test. A sensitive and specific test for fat malabsorption. Gastroenterology 1979; 76:6–13.
103. Cooper BT, Walsh CH, Holmes GKT, Wright AD, Cooke WT, Bloom SR. GIP and insulin responses to oral glucose in coeliac patients before and after treatment. Scand J Gastroenterol 1981; 16:411–5.
104. Lamabadusuriya SP, Packer S, Harries JT. Limitations of xylose tolerance test as a screening procedure in childhood coeliac disease. Arch Dis Child 1975; 50:34–9.
105. Sladen GE, Kumar PJ. Is the xylose test still a worthwhile investigation? Br Med J 1973; 3:223–6.
106. Haeney MR, Culank LS, Montgomery RD, Sammons HG. Evaluation of xylose absorption as measured in blood and urine: A one-hour screening test in malabsorption. Gastroenterology 1978; 75:393–400.
107. Cobden I, Rothwell J, Axon ATR. Intestinal permeability and screening tests for coeliac disease. Gut 1980; 21:512–8.
108. Hodgson HJF, Whitaker K, Cooper BT, Baron JH, Freeman HGM, Moss DM, Chadwick VS. Malabsorption and macroamylasemia. Response to gluten withdrawal. Am J Med 1980; 69:451–7.
109. Kingham JGC, Swarbrick ET, Swain P, Walker JG, Dawson AM. Dapsone and severe hypoalbuminaemia. A report of two cases. Lancet 1979; 2:662–4.
110. Besterman HS, Bloom SR, Sarson DL, Blackburn AM, Johnson DI, Patel HR, Stewart JS, Modigliani R, Guerin S, Mallinson CN. Gut-hormone profile in coeliac disease. Lancet 1978; 1:785–8.
111. Marsh GW, Stewart JS. Splenic function in adult coeliac disease. Br J Haematol 1970; 19:445–57.
112. Nelson EW, Ertan A, Brooks FP, Cerda JJ. Thrombocytosis in patients with celiac sprue. Gastroenterology 1976; 70:1042–4.
113. Mann JG, Brown WR, Kern F. The subtle and varied clinical expressions of gluten induced enteropathy (adult celiac disease, non-tropical sprue). An analysis of 21 consecutive cases. Am J Med 1970; 48:357–66.
114. Bullen AW, Losowsky MS. Lymphocyte subpopulations in adult coeliac disease. Gut 1978; 19:892–7.
115. Hoffbrand AV. Anaemia in adult coeliac disease. Clin Gastroenterol 1974; 3:71–89.
116. Kosnai I, Kuitunen P, Siimes MA. Iron deficiency in children with coeliac disease on treatment with a gluten free diet. Arch Dis Child 1979; 54:375–8.
117. Reinken L, Zieglauer H, Berger H. Vitamin B_6 nutrition of children with acute celiac disease, celiac disease in remission and of children with normal duodenal mucosa. Am J Nutr 1976; 29:750–3.
118. Kowlessar OD, Haeffner LJ, Benson GD. Abnormal tryptophan metabolism in patients with adult coeliac disease with evidence for deficiency of vitamin B_6. J Clin Invest 1964; 43:894–903.
119. Flear CTG, Cawley R, Quinton A, Cooke WT. The simultaneous determination of total exchangeable sodium and potassium and its significance with particular reference to congestive cardiac failure and the steatorrhoea syndrome. Clin Sci 1958; 17:81–104.
120. Solomons NW, Rosenberg IH, Sandstead HH. Zinc nutrition in celiac sprue. Am J Clin Nutr 1976; 29:371–5.
121. Jones PE, Peters TJ. Oral zinc supplementation in nonresponsive coeliac disease: Effect on jejunal morphology, enterocyte production and brush border disaccharidase activities. Gut 1981; 22:194–8.

122. Carswell F, Ferguson A. Food antibodies in serum—a screening test for coeliac disease. Arch Dis Child 1972; 47:594–6.
123. Burrows FGO, Toye DKM. Barium studies. Clin Gastroenterol 1974; 3:91–107.
124. Cooper BT, Holmes GKT, Ferguson R, Cooke WT. Coeliac disease and malignancy. Medicine 1980; 59:249–61.
125. Freeman HJ, Weinstein WM, Shnitka TK, Piercy JRA, Wensel RH. Primary abdominal lymphoma. Presenting manifestation of celiac sprue, or complicating dermatitis herpetiformis. Am J Med 1977; 63:585–94.
126. Stokes PL, Prior P, Sorahan T, McWalter RJ, Waterhouse JAH, Cooke WT. Malignancy in relatives of patients with coeliac disease. Br J Prev Soc Med 1976; 30:17–21.
127. Cooper BT, Holmes GKT, Cooke WT. Lymphoma risk in coeliac disease of later life. Digestion 1982; 23:89–92.
128. Hodges JR, Isaacson P, Eade OE, Wright R. Serum lysozyme levels in malignant histiocytosis of the intestine. Gut 1979; 20:854–7.
129. Isaacson P, Wright DH. Malignant histiocytosis of the intestine. Its relationship to malabsorption and ulcerative jejunitis. Hum Pathol 1978; 9:661–77.
130. Whitehead R. Primary lymphadenopathy complicating idiopathic steatorrhoea. Gut 1968; 9:569–75.
131. Ferguson R, Asquith P, Cooke WT. The jejunal cellular infiltrate in coeliac disease complicated by lymphoma. Gut 1974; 15:458–61.
132. Holmes GKT, Dunn GI, Cockel R, Brookes VS. Adenocarcinoma of the upper small bowel complicating coeliac disease. Gut 1980; 21:1010–16.
133. Ziegler JL, Magrath IT, Gerber P, Levine PH. Epstein-Barr virus and human malignancy. Ann Intern Med 1977; 86:323–36.
134. Baer AN, Bayless TM, Yardley JH. Intestinal ulceration and malabsorption syndromes. Gastroenterology 1980; 79:754–65.
135. Mills PR, Brown IL, Watkinson G. Idiopathic chronic ulcerative enteritis. Report of five cases and review of the literature. Q J Med 1980; 49:133–9.
136. Klaeveman HL, Gebhard RL, Sessoms C, Strober W. In vitro studies of ulcerative ileojejunitis. Gastroenterology 1975; 68:572–82.
137. Bayless TM, Baer A, Yardley JH, Hendrix TR. Intestinal ulceration, flat mucosa and malabsorption: Report of registry of 33 patients. *In:* McNicholl B, McCarthy CF, Fottrell PF, eds. Perspectives in Coeliac Disease. Lancaster: MTP Press, 1978:311–12.
138. Kepes JJ, Chou SM, Price LW. Progressive multifocal leukoencephalopathy with a 10 year survival in a patient with non-tropical sprue. Neurology 1975; 25:1006–12.
139. Cooke WT, Smith WT. Neurological disorders associated with adult coeliac disease. Brain 1966; 89:683–722.
140. Cooke WT, Johnson AG, Wolff AL. Vital staining and electron microscopy of the intramuscular nerve endings in the neuropathy of adult coeliac disease. Brain 1966; 89:663–82.
141. Sencer W. Neurologic manifestations in the malabsorption syndrome. J Mt Sin Hosp 1957; 24:331–45.
142. Bernier JJ, Buge A, Rambaud JC, Rancurel G, Hauw JJ, L'Hirondel C, Denvil D. Chronic inflammatory neuromuscular disorders associated with treated coeliac disease. *In:* McNicholl B, McCarthy CF, Fottrell PF, eds. Perspectives in Coeliac Disease. Lancaster: MTP Press, 1978: 495–7.
143. Dohan FC. Cereals and schizophrenia: Data and hypothesis. Acta Psychiatr Scand 1966; 42:125–52.
144. Walsh CH, Cooper BT, Wright AD, Malins JM, Cooke WT. Diabetes mellitus and coeliac disease: A clinical study. Q J Med 1978; 47:89–100.
145. Editorial. Coeliac lung disease. Lancet 1978; 1:917–18.
146. Hagader B, Berg NO, Brandt L, Norden A, Sjolund K, Stenstam M. Hepatic injury in adult coeliac disease. Lancet 1977; 1:270–2.
147. Alexander JOD. Dermatitis Herpetiformis. Philadelphia: WB Saunders, 1975:11–73.
148. Katz SI, Strober W. The pathogenesis of dermatitis herpetiformis. J Invest Dermatol 1978; 70:63–75.
149. Reunala T, Blomqvist K, Tarpila S, Halme H, Kangas K. Gluten-free diet in dermatitis herpetiformis. I. Clinical response of skin lesions in 81 patients. Br J Dermatol 1977; 97:473–80.
150. Falchuk ZM, Gebhard RL, Sessoms C, Strober W. An in vitro model of gluten-sensitive enteropathy. Effect of gliadin on intestinal epithelial cells of patients with gluten-sensitive enteropathy in organ culture. J Clin Invest 1974; 53:487–500.
151. Hauri HP, Kedinger M, Haffen K, Gaze H, Hadorn B, Hekkens W. Re-evaluation of the technique of organ culture for studying gluten toxicity in coeliac disease. Gut 1978; 19:1090–8.
152. Baker AL, Rosenberg IH. Refractory sprue: Recovery after removal of non-gluten dietary protein. Ann Intern Med 1978; 89:505–8.
153. Walker-Smith J, Harrison M, Kilby A, Philips A, France N. Cow's milk-sensitive enteropathy. Arch Dis Child 1978; 53:375–80.
154. Nussle D, Bozic C, Cox J, Deleze M, Roulet M, Fete R, Megevand A. Non-coeliac gluten intolerance in infancy. *In:* McNicholl B, McCarthy CF, Fottrell PF, eds. Perspectives in Coeliac Disease. Lancaster: MTP Press, 1978: 277–86.
155. Ament ME, Rubin CE. Soy protein. Another cause of the flat intestinal lesion. Gastroenterology 1972; 62:227–34.
156. Schenk EA, Samloff M, Klipstein FA. Morphologic characteristics of jejunal biopsy in celiac disease and tropical sprue. Am J Pathol 1965; 47:765–81.
157. Misra RC, Kasthuri D, Chuttani HK. Adult coeliac disease in the tropics. Br Med J 1966; 2:1230–2.
158. Cooper BT, Holmes GKT, Ferguson R, Thompson RA, Allen RN, Cooke WT. Gluten sensitive diarrhea without evidence of celiac disease. Gastroenterology 1980; 79:801–6.
159. Walker-Smith J. Diseases of the Small Intestine in Childhood. 2nd Ed. Tunbridge Wells: Pitman Medical, 1979: 160–9.
160. Cameron AH, Astley R, Hallowell M, Rawson AB, Miller CG, French JM, Hubble DV. Duodeno-jejunal biopsy in the investigation of children with coeliac disease. Q J Med 1962; 31:125–140.
161. Love AHG, Elmes M, Golden MK, McMaster D. Zinc deficiency and coeliac disease. *In:* McNicholl B, McCarthy CF, Fottrell FP, eds. Perspectives in Coeliac Disease. Lancaster: MTP Press, 1978: 335–42.
162. Hamilton JD, Chambers RA, Wynn-William A. Role of gluten, prednisone and azathioprine in non-responsive coeliac disease. Lancet 1976; 1:1213–6.
163. Cooke WT. The effect of corticotrophin in idiopathic steatorrhoea. Lancet 1953; 2:425–8.
164. Sheldon W. Prognosis in early adult life of coeliac children treated with a gluten free diet. Br Med J 1969; 2:401–4.

Chapter 106

Tropical Sprue

Thomas W. Sheehy

History

Although Hillary is usually credited with the first clinical description of tropical sprue (1766), the condition was actually described by Ketelaer in the Dutch East Indies a century earlier (1672).[1, 2] Neither work was appreciated and another century was to pass before the disease was described again with authority. Throughout the 19th century, reports of "an affliction of the bowel peculiar to Europeans long resident in the tropics" were made by physicians stationed in various parts of Asia. Recently, these writings were ably summarized by Cook.[3] During this era, the disease was variously labeled as aphthae tropica, diarrhea alba, Hill diarrhea, white flux, Ceylon sore mouth, psilosis lingua, and sprouw. In 1880, Manson published an authoritative clinical account of tropical sprue, in which he anglicized the Dutch term "indische sprouw" to "sprue."[4] In the same year, Van Der Burg reported the presence of sprue among the natives of Batavia.[5] His clinical description of the disease corresponded closely with Manson's, but his concept regarding its etiology differed. Van Der Burg believed that the essential lesion was a gastric catarrh that led to secondary atrophy of the intestine, whereas Manson thought that the disease primarily affected the small intestine and led to atrophy of its mucosa. In his first edition of "Tropical Diseases" (1898), Manson wrote that tropical sprue was the result of congestion and erosion of the gut with destruction of the villi.[6] In 1912, his son-in-law, Manson-Bahr, illustrated the mucosal lesion of tropical sprue as it existed in the ileum and stated "there is general atrophy of the villi due to fibrosis and a diffuse round cell infiltration of the whole of the mucosa."[7] In the same period, other observers (LeDantec, Thin, and Wethered) independently recognized that attenuation of the small intestinal mucosa was a consistent feature and interpreted this to mean that the disease process primarily affected the mucous membrane of the ileum, where it destroyed the villi and crypts and led to cystic dilation of the lamina.

By the turn of this century, tropical sprue was recognized as a clinical entity prone to afflict European expatriates residing in India, China, Ceylon and the Philippines, the Dutch East Indies, and parts of the Caribbean, i.e., Puerto Rico and Cuba. The clinical picture was reasonably well known. More importantly, the intestinal lesion had been identified and reconfirmed beyond doubt.[8, 9] Unfortunately, the concept of a mucosal lesion as an inherent part of the disease was soon to be disputed and then discarded. This began with Faber's observations on postmortem autolysis of the bowel in 1904 and culminated with Thaysen's classic review in 1932.[10] In this otherwise authoritative treatise, Thaysen separated tropical sprue from idiopathic steatorrhea but, on the basis of a single autopsy, he pronounced the small bowel mucosa as normal in tropical sprue. Assailing Manson-Bahr's description of the intestinal lesion, Thaysen stated emphatically that "in well preserved material, the intestinal epithelium of the villi as well as that of the Lieberkuhn crypts show nowhere . . . degeneration or atrophy." A brief glance at the photomicrographs in Thaysen's report is sufficient to convince anyone familiar with small bowel disease that the intestinal mucosa of his patient had the classic lesion now known to accompany tropical sprue. Even so, Thaysen's reputation as a pathologist was so great that his viewpoint was immediately and almost universally accepted. For decades thereafter, earlier evidence that tropical sprue was associated with a significant intestinal lesion was either forgotten or attributed to postmortem autolysis.

Despite this setback, tropical sprue remained the subject of intensive interest both in the Far East and the Caribbean. World War II stimulated investigations dealing with its etiology, pathogenesis, and treatment. Throughout the campaigns in India and Burma, tropical sprue ranked as a major medical and logistical problem. For the first time, its importance as a disabling disease and one capable of reaching epidemic proportions was recognized.[11–15] Between 1943 and 1946, it accounted for one eighth of all the medical evacuees from the British Army in India.[16] This enormous logistical strain was compounded by the fact that the average patient required almost 1 year of hospitalization before evacuation to England.[16] Field experience soon shattered older beliefs that tropical sprue was acquired by Europeans only after long residence in the tropics and that natives were immune to the disease. Newly arrived British troops fell prey to the disease within months, and sometimes weeks, of their arrival.[11,12,16] A seasonal pattern was recorded in Assam and Burma (as it was recently in Puerto Rico), with the largest number of cases occurring between April and June, shortly before the rainy season and during the fly season.[11,16] The disease also reached epidemic proportions among certain native regiments.[16,17] Since many of these troops subsisted on marginal rations, poor nutrition was held to be partially responsible for their disease.[16]

Definition and Classification

Tropical sprue is a complex disease that is not easily defined. In 1898, Manson defined tropical sprue as "an extremely chronic and insidious disease peculiar to warm climates; the principal symptoms of which are referable, first, to a remitting inflammation of the mucous membrane of the mouth and alimentary canal generally; second, to diarrhea and irregular action of the bowels; and third, to anemia and general atrophy."[6] Diarrhea, glossitis, weight loss, and aphthous ulcers were the clinical sine qua nons of the disease. In the Caribbean area, the definition was expanded to include the presence of nutritional deficiency and megaloblastic anemia. Later, Perez-Santiago and Butterworth[18] suggested that in addition to the usual clinical findings, a megaloblastic bone marrow and malabsorption for at least 2 test substances be required for diagnosis. With the advent of peroral intestinal biopsy and rediscovery of the mucosal lesion, it was recommended that morphologic abnormalities of the small intestinal mucosa be included as well among the integral components of the disease.

In recent years it has become customary to refer to tropical sprue as a member of the tropical malabsorption (TM) syndromes.[19] Tomkins and his associates have classified tropical sprue as a type of "infective malabsorption" (IM) that occurs in the tropics.[19] They subdivided the infective malabsorption syndrome into two major types: "parasitic" (e.g., giardiasis) and "non-parasitic" (e.g., tropical sprue). Both types are subdivided into "mild" and "severe" forms on the basis of absorption tests. Non-parasitic malabsorption is mild if one test of absorption function (e.g., xylose) is abnormal and whether or not the patient is symptomatic. It is severe if there is malabsorption of 2 or more substances (i.e., vitamin B_{12}, xylose, or xylose and fat). The *severe form* of TM is synonymous with *tropical sprue*, the *mild form* with *tropical enteropathy*.

This rather cumbersome classification resulted from the finding that many asymptomatic tropical residents, children as well as adults, and expatriates living in the tropics several months or more, have tropical enteropathy. This is not associated with parasitism or malnutrition and is without the classic features of tropical sprue.[20–22] These individuals absorb vitamin B_{12} and/or xylose poorly and have structural mucosal lesions in their small bowel similar to those found in classic sprue. Some believe that this entity is a subclinical form of tropical sprue; others consider it the result of repeated bacterial insults to the jejunum. At present, its exact relation to tropical sprue is not certain.

Tropical enteropathy is distinguished from tropical sprue by several parameters. Most of those affected are asymptomatic, their subclinical malabsorption varies in severity from time to time, and response to treatment is variable. In expatriates who return to temperate climates, intestinal function and appearance return to normal within 6 to 12 months. By contrast, patients with tropical sprue have gastrointestinal symptoms; their intestinal lesion grows steadily worse, usually leading to secondary nutritional anemia and malnutrition; and they respond well to specific therapy.[20–23]

Frequency

Tropical Sprue. The frequency of tropical sprue is not certain. Stefanini estimated an annual incidence of 3.5% for his fellow Italian prisoners of war in India.[24] British experiences in the same area and at the same time suggest a much higher incidence. An annual incidence of 6% was estimated amoung North Americans living temporarily in Puerto Rico.

In some endemic areas, the disease is no longer seen with its former frequency. Between 1927 and 1953, the frequency of tropical sprue among the hospitalized population of Cuba decreased from 2.0% to 0.4% while in Puerto Rico, the annual death rate due to tropical sprue dropped from 7.4 to 0.3/100,000 population.[25] Between 1953 and 1961, there were 77 "casos de merte" due to sprue reported in Puerto Rico. The decline in morbidity and mortality in Puerto Rico stems from improved medical care, better nutrition, educational advances, a better standard of living, and specific therapy. The prophylactic use of vitamins and antibiotics, a common practice in these islands, may mask or even cure the disease. The absence of these factors in poorer countries, e.g., Haiti, allows the disease to flourish.

Tropical Enteropathy. The frequency of tropical enteropathy is much higher. In 1956, impaired xylose absorption was found in 59 of 190 (31%) healthy asymptomatic Puerto Rican inductees into the US Army.[26] A decade later, Lindenbaum[21] observed that 40% of a group of healthy Pakistanis had subnormal absorption of D-xylose, while 20% had malabsorption of vitamin B_{12}. Peace Corps volunteers living in Pakistan for 6 to 20 months had similar findings. A survey of Amercian soldiers living for 6 months in Viet Nam, and subsisting for a large part on the native economy, revealed tropical enteropathy in 12%.[20]

Tropical malabsorption is now considered a major health problem in developing countries such as India, Viet Nam, Cambodia, Haiti, Santa Domingo, Iran, Central and South Africa, Indonesia, Colombia, and Venezuela. In some countries, it accounts for loss of 10% of the available food supply.

Etiology and Pathogenesis

One of the more unusual and fascinating features of tropical sprue is its distribution (Fig. 106–1). Why the disease is endemic in certain tropical countries and not in others has never been explained satisfactorily. The argument that some countries lack diagnostic facilities is no longer tenable. While it may explain the late discovery of tropical sprue in Africa, it does not apply to the situation in Southeast Asia and the Caribbean. Sprue has been known to exist in Puerto Rico and Cuba for over 70 years. More recently it has been found in Haiti and Santa Domingo but, strangely enough, it is absent from Jamaica, where it has been sought for several decades.

Abnormal Metabolites. In 1952, it was suggested by Fraser that tropical sprue in Hong Kong resulted from intestinal sensitivity to substances produced by oxidative rancidity of unsaturated long-chain fatty acids. Presumably, oxidation of the unsaturated fats resulted from inadequate refrigeration in the warm climate and the rancidity was accelerated by repeatedly reheating the fat for frying.[27] While studying the etiology of sprue in Hong Kong, Webb[28] observed that British servicemen who acquired the disease invariably had their food prepared with unsaturated fats. By contrast, not a single case of tropical sprue developed among 3000 Gurkas who prepared their food with "ghee," a milk derivative. Also, the occurrence rate of tropical sprue in Hong Kong fell strikingly after the introduction of refrigeration.

The prevalence of tropical sprue in Puerto Rico, Haiti, Cuba, and Santa Domingo has been attributed to the use of pork (lard) drippings for deep fat frying. These are high in unsaturated fatty acids. The absence of sprue in Jamaica is thought to be due to the use of vegetable oils, i.e., coconut and palm oil, and to a preference for broiling. These oils are more saturated and resistant to the oxidative changes induced by reheating.[28]

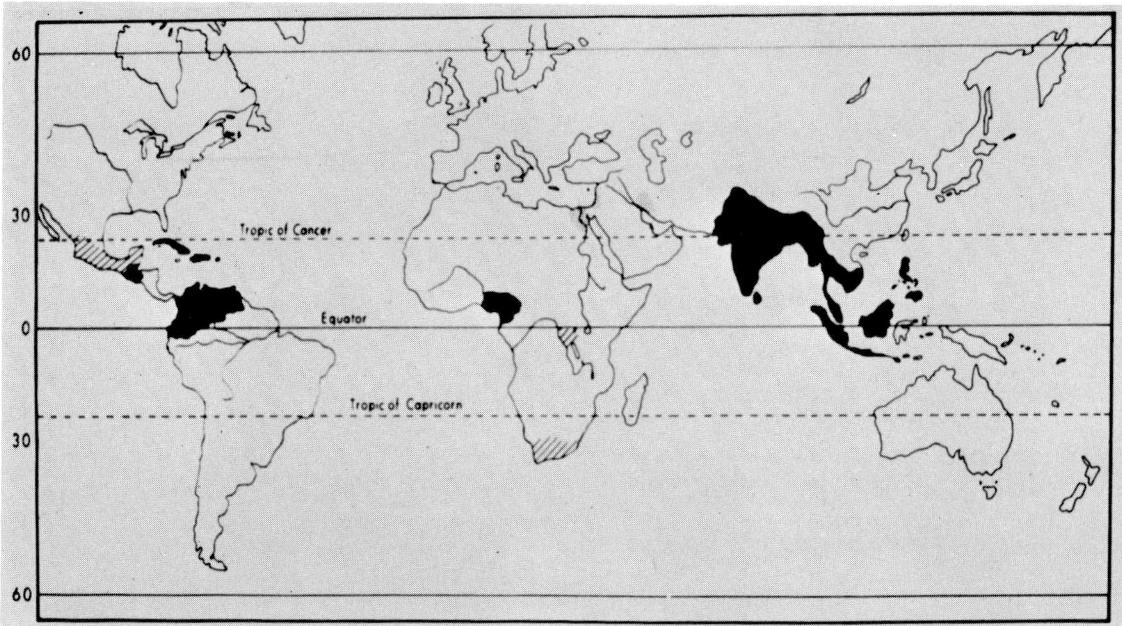

Figure 106–1. Geographic distribution of tropical malabsorption. Black indicates those areas where overt tropical sprue occurs; cross hatching, areas where a disorder resembling sprue occurs; and stippling, areas where only subclinical abnormalities of small intestinal structure or function have been observed.

The seasonal occurrence of sprue in Puerto Rico has also been attributed to dietary changes that take place during the month-long Christmas season; the intake of pork and foodstuffs prepared by deep frying in pork drippings is increased markedly at this season.[29]

Although the etiologic importance of rancid fat is not clear, the capacity for dietary factors to influence the gut flora and the fatty acid composition of the succus entericus is well known. Fatty acids are thought to play a role in balancing the intestinal flora;[31] the normal small intestinal flora retards colonization by enteric pathogens by producing short-chain fatty acids.[32, 33] In turn, normal flora growth is inhibited by long-chain unsaturated fatty acids.[34] Interestingly, the long-chain unsaturated fat, linoleic acid, a principal component of "pork drippings," increases the production of *Klebsiella pneumoniae*, the most common microorganism isolated from the jejunal aspirates of sprue patients.[35] An increased dietary intake of unsaturated fatty acids may also alter the jejunal milieu sufficiently to allow colonization by coliform bacteria.[29]

Gluten. Discovery of the deleterious effect of wheat and other cereal products in celiac disease led to investigation of the role of gluten in tropical sprue. Appreciable improvement in sprue patients fed a gluten-free diet has been noted.[36] However, improvement in the patients studied may have resulted from additional folate in their diet. It has also been claimed that gluten (30 g/day) increases the intestinal abnormality of sprue patients. On the other hand, antibodies to gliadin have never been found in patients with sprue,[37] and the weight of evidence leads to the conclusion that *gluten plays no essential role in the etiology of tropical sprue.*

Infectious Theory. The belief that tropical sprue has an infectious origin dates to the last century.[3] Thin, in 1897, suggested that the high fecal bacterial content of sprue patients had etiologic significance. Kiener and Kelsch (1884) believed that sprue resulted from an intestinal lesion from which infection spread. Galloway (1905) and Rogers (1913) were certain that specific microorganisms induced the disease. Begg[8] (1912) treated his patients with santonin, a non-absorbable germicide. Kolbrugge's earlier description (1901) of a yeast that invaded the mucosa led several investigators to follow this lead. Ashford became an enthusiastic exponent of this theory and, in 1915, described *"Monilia psilosis"* as the etiologic factor.[38] With remarkable foresight, Low (1928) predicted that the most likely etiologic factor was a gastrointestinal toxin.[39]

Evidence in support of an infectious etiology includes the epidemic nature of the disease, its ability to affect visitors to endemic areas (Fig. 106–2), the existence of "sprue" houses, wherein many of the residents have sprue, and the success of certain antibiotics and sulfonamide preparations in treating the disease.

The disease was epidemic among British forces in India, often incapacitating troops shortly after their arrival.[11–15] In one Royal Air Force unit, 10% of the personnel became ill within 3 weeks of landing in Burma.[12] Dysentery or gastroenteritis often preceded the onset of tropical sprue. This observation was more recently confirmed in India and the Philippines.[40, 41] Following an epidemic of acute diarrhea in Southern India, 5% to 10% of the 100,000 patients failed to recover and over the course of the next year, acquired the clinical and hematologic features of tropical sprue. Seasonal epidemics of acute gastroenteritis among Americans stationed in the Philippines also appear to have precipitated sprue in many, and the malabsorption and diarrhea of those affected responded to combined therapy with folic acid and tetracycline. Attempts to isolate a causative agent were unsuccessful in both of these outbreaks. Efforts to transmit the disease encountered in the Philippines to human volunteers also failed.[40, 41]

Therapeutic responses similarly suggest an infectious etiology. In India, Keele and Bound[11] found that sulfaguanidine helped to control the diarrhea and often led to clinical improvement. French et al.[42] observed that tetracycline and chloramphenicol resulted in the clinical remission of 6 of 7 patients with the disease. In Puerto Rico, the same antibiotics given for only 2 weeks led to clinical, hematologic, and some histologic bowel improvement in 6 of 12 patients.[43] Two patients maintained on tetracycline for 2 months had complete hematologic and gastroenterologic recovery. Follow-up studies in the same laboratory confirmed the observation that prolonged tetracycline therapy (500 mg daily for 6 months) led to clinical cure along with correction of the anemia, elimination of malabsorption, and remarkable improvement in the intestinal morphology of 16 of 17 pa-

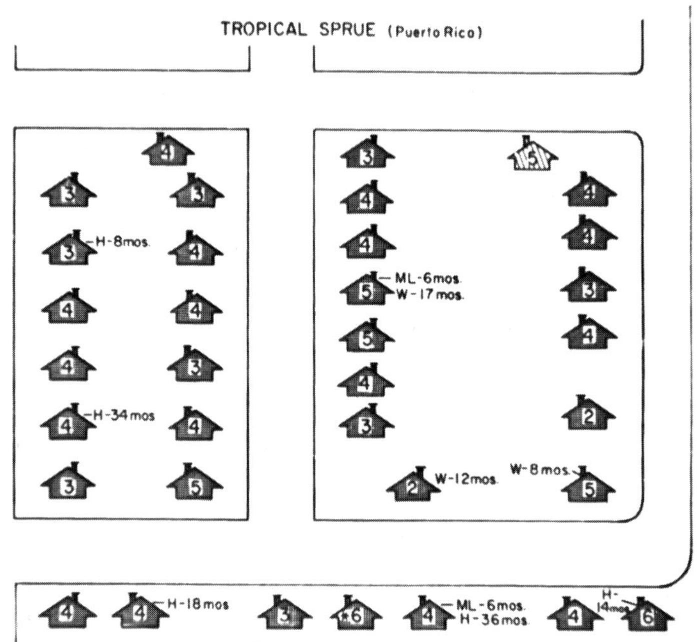

Figure 106–2. Tropical sprue developed over a 2-year period in 10 of the 78 adult Americans living in this military compound in Puerto Rico.

tients.[44] Improvement in the jejunal mucosa occurred within 2 weeks of treatment; improved intestinal absorption and weight gain were evident within 4 weeks and hematologic recovery occurred after 4 to 8 weeks of tetracycline. The combination of folic acid therapy and antibiotics hastened recovery. Tetracycline therapy rapidly returned vitamin B_{12} absorption to normal, sometimes within 48 hours of treatment. [45] These results differ considerably from those observed with folate therapy alone. The latter usually led to excellent hematologic improvement, but it often failed to eliminate the bowel lesion or to improve vitamin B_{12} absorption; less than one third of those treated with folate alone recovered their ability to absorb vitamin B_{12} normally.[46]

Perhaps the most significant finding in support of the infectious etiology was the isolation of enterotoxigenic microorganisms from jejunal isolates. Working in Calcutta, Gorbach et al.[47] found that colonization of the small intestine with coliform bacteria was common in both mild and severe untreated tropical sprue. In the same study, healthy adult Westerners and Pakistanis were found to harbor an autochthonous small intestinal flora dominated by streptococci and lactobacilli; they had no enterobacteria in their proximal small bowel. Subsequently, others[48–50] in different parts of the world also recovered enterobacteria from the jejunal isolates of patients with tropical sprue. These microorganisms were qualitatively and quantitatively different from those found in healthy individuals. The coliform organisms isolated from 10 of 11 patients examined by Klipstein and his group[49] included *Klebsiella pneumoniae* (7 patients), *Enterobacter cloacae* (2 patients), and *Escherichia coli* (1 patient). Similar organisms were recovered from small bowel isolates and jejunal biopsies of expatriates returning to London with tropical sprue.[51] Concentrations of enterobacteria ranging from 10^3 to 10^8 per ml of fluid or per gram of mucosa were found in both jejunal fluid and mucosa of these patients [51] (Table 106–1).

The enterobacteria recovered are non-invasive. Unlike microorganisms that cause "acute adult gastroenteritis" and are flushed from the upper jejunum within 1 or 2 weeks, these enterobacteria somehow manage to retain a foothold for prolonged periods. Preliminary studies suggest that they are capable of adhering to tissue culture cells and that long-chain fatty acids increase their production by suppressing the normal flora.[35,52] They are toxigenic but without the virulence of enterotoxigenic *E. coli* or *Vibrio cholerae*.[49] In animal experiments, these enterobacteria are capable of inducing mucosal lesions, of increasing mucosal water and electrolyte secretion, and of impairing xylose and glucose absorption.[23, 53, 54] In some, but not all, patients, they cause a net jejunal secretory state for water and electrolytes.[54, 55] They also elaborate ethanol as one of their metabolic products. Whether the concentration of alcohol present in the jejunum of sprue patients is sufficient to be deleterious to enzymes or to impair jejunal absorption is not yet clear.[54,56]

Klipstein et al.[54] claim that the basic defect in tropical sprue is an inability to expel contaminating coliform bacteria. This idea is reminiscent of Ashford's earlier proposal regarding *Monilia psilosis* and one that may have merit. Small bowel transit is delayed in tropical sprue, but stasis is not a major etiologic factor in the disease.[54] Nor is the immunologic system at fault.[57] Perhaps the acute gastroenteritis that so often preceeds the onset of sprue alters the mucosa sufficiently to allow enterobacteria to gain a foot-

Table 106–1. ENTEROBACTERIA ISOLATED FROM JEJUNAL LUMINAL FLUID OR MUCOSA

	Gorbach et al.[45] **1970**	**Bhat et al.**[48] **1972**	**Klipstein et al.**[49] **1973**	**Tomkins et al.**[50] **1975**
Controls	0/13	6/12	2/9	1/8
Patients with malnutrition	4/7	—	—	—
Patients with tropical sprue	14/15*	23/33*	10/11†	15/16‡

*Indians (+)/total
†Puerto Ricans
‡European travelers

hold and subsequently injure the jejunal mucosa by an enterotoxin that they elaborate.

Loss of the gastric acid barrier is not considered to be etiologically important. About one fourth to one third of patients have achlorhydria and many have atrophic gastritis.[58, 59] However, neither of these changes is universal.

Although present evidence overwhelmingly favors a bacterial etiology, there are some concerns: (1) no single bacteriologic species has been found to be responsible for all cases, although the number of species isolated is limited; (2) the enterotoxins have not yet been clearly shown to cause mucosal lesions in man; (3) the relationship between colinization and morphologic changes is unsettled; and (4) not all observers have been able to isolate enterotoxigenic bacteria from their patients.[50]

The epidemic nature of sprue in Southeast Asia is highly suggestive of a viral etiology. Viruses can cause acute gastroenteritis and 2 of them, the Norwalk agent and rotavirus, induce significant mucosal lesions.[51] Particles suggestive of a rotavirus have been observed in jejunal biopsies studied by electron microscopy. Corona-like viruses have also been identified in the feces of patients with sprue, but similar viruses were also isolated in the feces of control subjects. To date, therefore, viruses have not been shown to play a definitive role in the disease.[60, 61]

Nutritional Deficiency. Nutritional deficiency is commonplace in advanced tropical sprue. The disease is prevalent where malnutrition is rife, and multiple deficiencies are prone to occur in the course of the disease. These observations, and the almost miraculous clinical improvement observed in sprue patients when liver therapy and later folic acid became available, led to the belief that a nutritional or folate deficiency caused the disease. This is easy to understand, for previous to the introduction of liver therapy, the average life span for a patient with tropical sprue was estimated to be 2 years.[62, 63] Folate therapy eliminated this grim prognosis and led to a remarkable clinical improvement.[63, 64]

Today, the idea that nutritional deficiency is etiologically responsible for tropical sprue is not given great weight. Even in the earliest phase of the disease, when there is evidence of neither nutritional deficiency nor anemia, an intestinal lesion is present.[65] It seems instead that the nutritional deficiencies associated with sprue are usually secondary to the intestinal lesion. Once gastrointestinal symptoms begin, nutritional deficiencies (notably of folate) occur, and anemia develops in its wake.

Sprue patients quickly realize that food and certain beverages, particularly alcohol, aggravate their intestinal symptoms and diarrhea.[66] Consequently, they try to avoid food, eat less, and a vicious circle subsequently results. Alcoholics do poorly and without treatment develop an intractable form of the disease.[67] The effect of alcohol is understandable. Alone, it can cause steatorrhea and impair the absorption of thiamine, folate, and vitamin B_{12}.[68, 69] Poverty, famine, and chronic parasitism among the native populace hasten this clinical cycle.

The presence of folate deficiency in tropical sprue provided impetus for the study of folate metabolism. As a result, we now know that:

(1) man's minimal essential daily requirement for folate is 1 to 2 μg/kg of body weight or 50 to 100 μg/day;[70, 71] (2) total body stores are between 2 and 6 mg and can be depleted within 60 to 90 days on a folate-deficient diet;[72] (3) the liver is the primary storage site; (4) alcohol impairs folate absorption, transport, and metabolism[68, 69] (Chapter 156); (5) the average American diet contains about 50 μg of free folic acid and almost 200 μg of total folate activity as estimated by *Streptococcus faecalis* assay;[73] even the low income Puerto Rican diet contains enough folic acid to prevent folate deficiency in the absence of tropical sprue; (6) dietary folate consists primarily of reduced formyl and methyl folate;[74, 75] (7) these polyglutamates must be deconjugated by the intestinal enzyme "folate conjugase" (gamma glutamyl carboxypeptidase) to monoglutamates;[75, 76] (8) the absorption of monoglutamate is greatest in the proximal small intestine;[73, 75] (9) within the intestinal cell, monoglutamic acid is reduced to methylfolate (mainly 5-methyltetrahydrofolate) prior to its release into the portal circulation;[77,78] (10) mean normal absorption of tritium-labeled pteroylglutamic acid is almost 80% of an oral dose of 200 μg;[79] (11) experimental folate deficiency in rats leads to a 40% decrease in the number of intestinal epithelial cells and to villus atrophy;[51] and (12) the normal enzymatic pathway used by jejunal crypt cells for DNA synthesis depends upon the folate-dependent enzyme "thymidylate synthetase"; in folate-deficient animals, an alternate (salvage) pathway requiring "thymidine kinase" is used for DNA synthesis. The amount of "thymidine kinase" found in isolated crypt cells is 5 times normal.[51, 80]

The protein requirement of the intestinal epithelium for DNA synthesis is enormous. In untreated sprue, there is circumstantial evidence that folate deficiency compromises the capacity of the jejunal epithelium to synthesize DNA for the following reasons: (1) increased ribonucleic acid–phosphorus (RNA-P) concentrations and decreased deoxyribonu-cleic acid–phosphorus (DNA-P) levels are found in mucosal intestinal homogenates taken from untreated patients;[81] (2) the Feulgen reaction indicates that DNA fails to increase in parallel with the increasing nuclear size of the crypt cells;[82] and (3) eosin-methylene staining suggests that mature cells at the tips of the villi contain increased RNA. These changes are reminiscent of those found in the hematopoietic tissues of patients with pernicious anemia and are similar to those produced in *Lactobacillus leishmanii* by vitamin B_{12} deficiency.[83]

The hydrolysis of radioactively labeled polyglutamates as well as the absorption of pteroylglutamic acid is impaired in sprue.[84] Yet, patients respond clinically and hematologically to oral physiologic doses of folic acid and both their luminal and mucosal levels of folate conjugase, the enzyme necessary for hydrolysis, are normal or increased.[70, 85, 86] This paradox may be due to a functional folate deficiency within the crypt cells of the small intestine.[80] In untreated sprue, crypt epithelium is more megaloblastic than the bone marrow.[87, 88] Both folate and vitamin B_{12} therapy often fail to eliminate "crypt cell megaloblastosis," whereas a prompt response occurs with antibiotic therapy, sometimes within 2 or 3 days.[87] In vitro, the deoxyuridine (dU-test) fails to suppress the uptake of radioactively labeled thymidine (^{3}H-IdR) by jejunal homogenates of sprue patients who have adequate red blood cell and serum folic acid.[80] The dU-test is a sensitive indicator of cellular levels of 5,10-methylene tetrahydrofolate. Its reversal to normal in sprue homogenates following the addition of folic acid is highly suggestive of a local folate deficiency.

If "functional folate deficiency" is present in jejunal crypts of patients with tropical sprue, its disappearance following antibiotic therapy suggests that an enzyme inhibitor or a toxin is responsible for the deficiency.

Clinical Manifestations

Chronic (Classic) Tropical Sprue. Manson,[6] and later Stefanini[24] and Gardner,[89] each recognized that tropical sprue evolved clinically through 3 stages. The *first*, or *early stage*, was characterized by fatigue, asthenia, weight loss, diarrhea, and eventually steatorrhea. The *second*, or *deficiency stage*, was distinguished by the appearance of signs of nutritional and vitamin deficiencies, such as glossitis, stomatitis, cheilosis, and hyperkeratosis. The *third*, or *anemic stage*, was denoted by the evolution of macrocytic anemia and progression of the other phases of the disease. This type of progressive disease usually develops after 2 to 4 years of tropical residency and represents the classic clinical picture.

Stage 1 (Early Phase). The early phase (Stage 1) of the disease usually develops after years in the tropics. Fatigue, lassitude, and abdominal cramps precede or accompany the onset of the diarrhea. Frequently, an intolerance to food develops before the onset of diarrhea. Initially, the number of stools passed daily varies. Some patients have only 1 or 2 daily; others may have 10 or more. Generally, the stools are large or bulky, semisolid in consistency, pale in color, of fetid odor, and greasy or frothy in appearance (Fig. 106–3).

The jejunal mucosa is already involved. Grossly, it has broad leaves and/or tongue-like villi. Microscopically, the villus/crypt ratio is decreased and the lamina propria is infiltrated with lymphocytes and plasma cells.[91,92] These changes are reflected by changes in biochemical parameters, which reveal subnormal absorption of D-xylose, vitamin A, vitamin B_{12}, folate, fat, and certain sugars.

Stage 2 (Deficiency Phase). Gastrointestinal

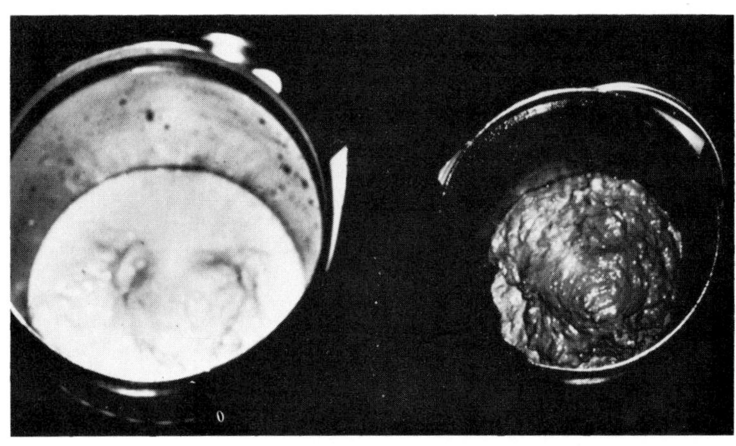

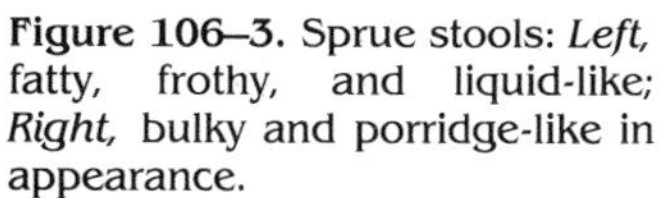

Figure 106–3. Sprue stools: *Left,* fatty, frothy, and liquid-like; *Right,* bulky and porridge-like in appearance.

symptoms dominate this phase. Over 80% of patients complain of dyspepsia, abdominal distention, epigastric fullness or burning, flatulence, and abdominal cramps or pain following the ingestion of food. Stomatitis and glossitis become pronounced as the diarrhea increases in severity. Bowel sounds are hyperactive. Feces are typically watery, frothy, yellowish, fermentative, and acid. An imperative desire to defecate or tenesmus precedes each bowel movement and stools are often passed involuntarily.

Developing vitamin deficiencies lead to cheilosis, stomatitis, glossitis, cutaneous pigmentation, eczematous or pellagroid-like rashes, and continuing weight loss. The continuing aversion to food and the persistent diarrhea and malabsorption impair the enterohepatic folate and vitamin B_{12} cycles. This leads, in turn, to rapid depletion of the body's folic acid stores and to abnormal vitamin A and B_{12} absorption. Infection with parasites, particularly those causing blood loss, may accelerate folate depletion. The result is iron deficiency and aggravation of the diarrhea.

Biochemical studies show progressive malabsorption. Sucrosuria is present. Sucrose, lactose, and maltose intolerance results from the loss of brush border disaccharidases as the mucosa deteriorates.[93–95] The jejunal mucosal lesion becomes more severe.[92] Protein-losing enteropathy may occur[96] and the mucosa is in a net secretory state for water, sodium, and chloride.[53,54] Intracellular fat transport is disturbed.[97] Small bowel barium studies indicate generalized disease in over 90% of patients. A good correlation exists between this study, intestinal biopsy changes, fecal fat, and D-xylose absorption.[90] Bone marrow examination reveals megaloblastoid hematopoiesis and occasionally frank megaloblastosis. The Schilling test is abnormal and the urinary excretion of folic acid decreases as folate deficiency ensues.

Stage 3 (Anemic Phase). The signs and symptoms of anemia dominate this stage in adults and children.[98] Usually, the anemia is megaloblastic, but it may be dimorphic owing to coexistent iron deficiency. Pancytopenia is common. Leukopenia and thrombocytopenia are often striking. Ineffective erythropoiesis leads to increased destruction of red blood cells within the bone marrow. Erythrocyte survival is shortened and an extrinsic plasma factor develops that increases the destruction of both autologous and transfused red blood cells.[99] superimposed viral infections, such as dengue fever, may lead to a sudden hemolytic crisis with hemoglobinuria, hemoglobinemia, and a precipitous fall in the hemoglobin level.

Despite their severity, hematologic changes often fail to overshadow continuing gastrointestinal manifestations and the evolving emaciation. By now, changes in the gastrointestinal mucosa may extend from the mouth to the anus and include various combinations of stomatoglossitis, atrophic gastritis with jejunitis, and occasionally even rectosigmoiditis. Flatulence, dyspepsia, meteorism, intolerance to food, abdominal distention, abdominal cramps, and diarrhea continue as nocturnal diuresis evolves.

The clinical signs and symptoms observed in 100 patients are shown in Table 106–2.

Table 106–2. COMPARISON OF MAIN SYMPTOMS AND SIGNS IN 100 PATIENTS WITH IDIOPATHIC STEATORRHEA (CELIAC DISEASE) AND 100 PATIENTS WITH TROPICAL SPRUE

Symptoms and Signs	Idiopathic Steatorrhea (%)	Tropical Sprue (%)
Lassitude	96	97
Weight loss	97	96
Diarrhea	80	95
Flatulence	59	98
Glossitis	90	90
Nausea and vomiting	37	15
Abdominal discomfort	31	90
Skin lesions	20	60
Tetany	50	0
Purpura	10	
Clubbing of fingers	17	2
Splenomegaly	11	3
Pigmentation	42	—
Anemia	95	100
Macrocytosis	63	95

The tongue may be smooth and fiery red, owing to nicotinic acid or riboflavin deficiency, or pale gray and shiny owing to papillary atrophy and anemia. The skin becomes coarse, and often a pellagroid or eczematous-like rash covers the ankles and wrists. Brownish pigmentation is common over sun-exposed areas, but the buccal mucosa is spared. As muscle wasting and weight loss progress, the resulting emaciation gives rise to hippocratic facies with prominent zygomatic arches, sunken cheeks, and triangular facies (Fig. 106–4). Pyrexia occurs in 30% to 60% of the cases. The temperature rises to 100 or 101°F in the afternoon and returns to normal by early morning.

The heart is seldom enlarged, but circulation time is shortened and venous pressure is elevated because of high cardiac output. Flow murmurs and sinus tachycardia are common. The systolic blood pressure ranges from 75 to 100 mm Hg and the diastolic pressure from 40 to 65 mm Hg. If anti-anemia treatment is not available, congestive heart failure eventually develops.

Abdominal distention increases and often becomes subumbilical, the area between the umbilicus and the symphysis pubis assuming a dome shape (Fig. 106–5). Body organs, including the liver and spleen, grow smaller as starvation progresses. Paresthesias with numbness and tingling of the tips of the fingers and toes, diminution of the deep tendon reflexes, and reduction of vibratory sensation occur in 5% to 10% of patients.

Without supportive care, electrolyte disturbances appear, particularly hypokalemia, and sometimes cause cardiac arrhythmias. Tetany is rare, occurring in less than 2% of patients. Confusion and irrational behavior may arise as a result of "megaloblastic madness" (the dementia that often accompanies severe vitamin B_{12} or folate deficiency) and/or electrolyte disturbances.

Laboratory Findings. Megaloblastic anemia is present and is often severe. The packed bone marrow oozes through the aspiration needle. The prothrombin time may be prolonged, but bleeding and clotting times are normal. Hypochlorhydria is present in 10% to 40% of patients and achlorhydria is found in another 15% to 30%. Hypokalemia is common and the urinary potassium level is decreased. Hypocalcemia is seldom encountered. Hypoglycemia is uncommon but hypocholesteremia is an almost invariable

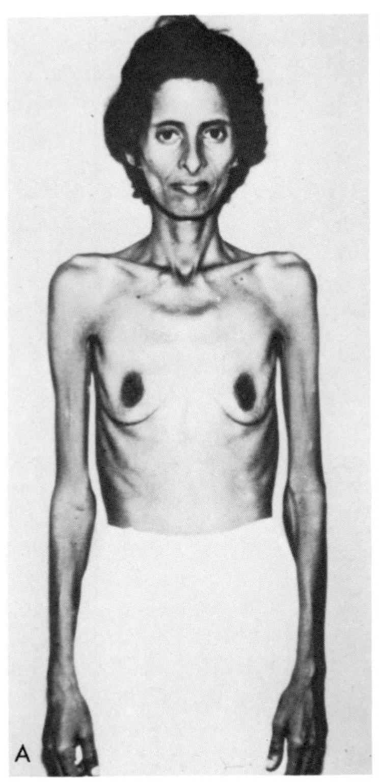

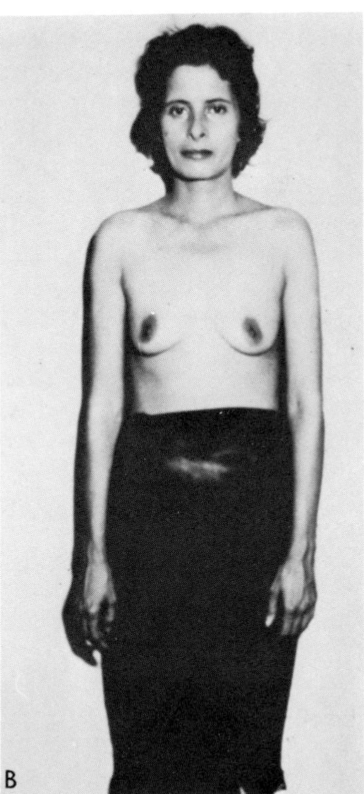

Figure 106–4. *A,* Emaciation and triangular (hippocratic) facies induced by classic sprue in a native Puerto Rican. *B,* Marked improvement following folic acid therapy plus tetracycline.

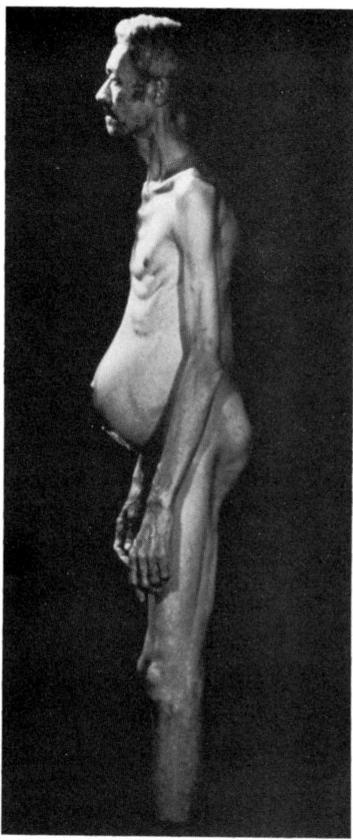

Figure 106–5. This patient exhibits a form of abdominal distention seen with tropical sprue.

finding. Blood urea nitrogen, uric acid, and creatinine levels are usually within normal limits.[66] Hypoproteinemia is found in 5% to 20% of patients. Serum bilirubin levels, although elevated, are rarely above 2 mg/dl. Liver function studies are usually normal, as are liver biopsies; hepatic lipofuscin is present in amounts similar to that observed in pellagra and chronic malnutrition.[84, 100]

Acute Tropical Sprue. Tropical sprue can develop "acutely," within a matter of weeks or months.[90] The "overlander syndrome," for example, refers to Europeans traveling to India via the Middle East who fall ill with sprue on tour or shortly after their return to Europe. "Military sprue" refers to servicemen who acquire the disease within weeks or months after their arrival in the tropics.[20,21] The shortest acquisition time I have observed was 2 weeks.

In the "acute" variety, the classic phases of sprue are telescoped or accelerated and clinical findings are related to the stage of evolution. Length of stay in the tropics is irrelevant. The onset is rapid, sometimes within weeks of arrival, and often follows an episode of acute gastroenteritis with the initial diarrhea quickly evolving into steatorrhea. Response to therapy is usually prompt. In contrast, the chronic type, or classic sprue, is more insidious in onset, is more likely to evolve after years in the tropics, afflicts the native populace more commonly, and is more resistant to treatment.

Clinical Features. Table 106–3 compares the symptoms and physical findings of American and British military personnel with acute tropical sprue. The average duration of symptoms before diagnosis was 2 to 8 weeks. Over 50% of patients could date the exact time of onset. Three forms of presentation were recorded: (1) 25% experienced gastrointestinal symptoms within a few days of "flu-like" illness manifested by systemic weakness, myalgia, fever, and nausea; (2) 25% claimed their illness began with an acute attack of diarrhea that was soon accompanied by asthenia, weakness, and anorexia; and (3) the remainder had similar symptoms but their diarrhea developed gradually over a period of several weeks or months.

Symptoms of progressive weakness and lassitude occurred in 90% of patients, nausea in 87%, abdominal cramping in 50%, and flatulence and alcohol intolerance[1] in 33%. Alcohol intolerance often occurs early and may also be the last symptom to disappear following appropriate treatment.

Physical Findings. European and American military personnel and tourists with acute tropical sprue have few physical findings, perhaps because most are young and in the prime of life.[28, 85] However, the longer the duration of disease, the more numerous the physical findings. After 2 to 3 months, glossitis, signs of weight loss, skin lesions, low-grade fever, and signs of anemia are encountered. The young helicopter gunner shown in Figure 106–6 is an example of a patient with the acute military variety. His disease began 1 month after arriving in Southeast Asia, starting with intermittent diarrhea and leading to malabsorption, severe wasting, and megaloblastic anemia. Painful aphthous ulcers impaired his appetite.

Laboratory Findings. Absorption of D-xylose, vitamin A, and fat is impaired. Fecal fat loss ranges from 9 to 35 g/24 hours. Barium studies of the small intestine show a "deficiency pattern"; its severity correlates with the degree of mucosal injury. Grossly, the

Table 106–3. TROPICAL SPRUE IN MILITARY PERSONNEL

	Gardner[89]	Sheehy et al.[20]	O'Brien[65]
Number of cases	21	37	35
Nationality	American	American	British
Acute onset	2	28	11
Duration of symptoms less than 3 months	10	29	17
Symptoms and physical findings			
Diarrhea (+)	21	37	31
Constant	16	17	—
Intermittent	5	20	—
Lassitude	21	29	35
Weakness	21	29	35
Anorexia	21	27	—
Abdominal cramps	15	22	—
Loss of appetite	—	34	35
Dyspepsia	15	19	6
Alcohol intolerance	—	19	—
Weight Loss	21	37	42
Mean	17.9 lbs (5–30)	20.8	21.5
Fever	—	8	—
Glossitis	3	8	10
Anemia	0	2	4
Bone marrow			
Megaloblastoid	—	9	14
Megaloblastic	—	2	1
Serum folate decrease	—	12/12	17
Serum vitamin B_{12}	—	↓	↓

appearance of the jejunal mucosa ranges from broad leaves and tongues to ridges and occasionally convolutions, depending on the duration and severity of the disease. The light microscopic findings consist of villous alterations and an inflamed lamina propria.

Morphologic Alterations

Stomach. Superficial and atrophic gastritis occurs in from 30% to 70% of sprue patients.[58] Rodriguez-Olleros,[101] in a pioneering endoscopy report in 1938, observed gastric atrophy in 10 of 28 patients. Another Puerto Rican study[58] disclosed that 47% of the patients had atrophic gastritis with partial or complete replacement of their fundic glands by pyloric glands and an additional 20% had acute or chronic gastritis. Gastric biopsy specimens taken from untreated patients reveal uncommonly wide and deep foveolae, giving the surface a villiform appearance. The epithelial cells are tall and thin with a nuclear diameter of 10.2 μ (normal, 6 to 8 μ) and their chromatin networks are open instead of pyknotic.[102] Altogether, the cytologic changes are comparable to those seen in pernicious anemia. Unlike pernicious anemia, however, specific anti-anemia therapy does not lead to their rapid disappearance.[102] Serial gastric biopsies done over a period of a year following treatment in one group of patients showed no significant histologic improvements.[58] All the patients with atrophic gastritis had normal urinary uropepsin activity, but none had normal absorption of ^{57}Co-labeled vitamin B_{12} with and without intrinsic factor.[58]

Small Intestine

Gross Appearance. Normal villi are tall and cylindrical or tongue-shaped when viewed with the dissecting microscope[103, 104] (Fig. 106–7). In tropical sprue, the villi become wider and thicker as they shrink in height with progression of the disease. Coalescence of adjacent villi leads to the formation of leaf-like villi and ridges; in advanced disease,

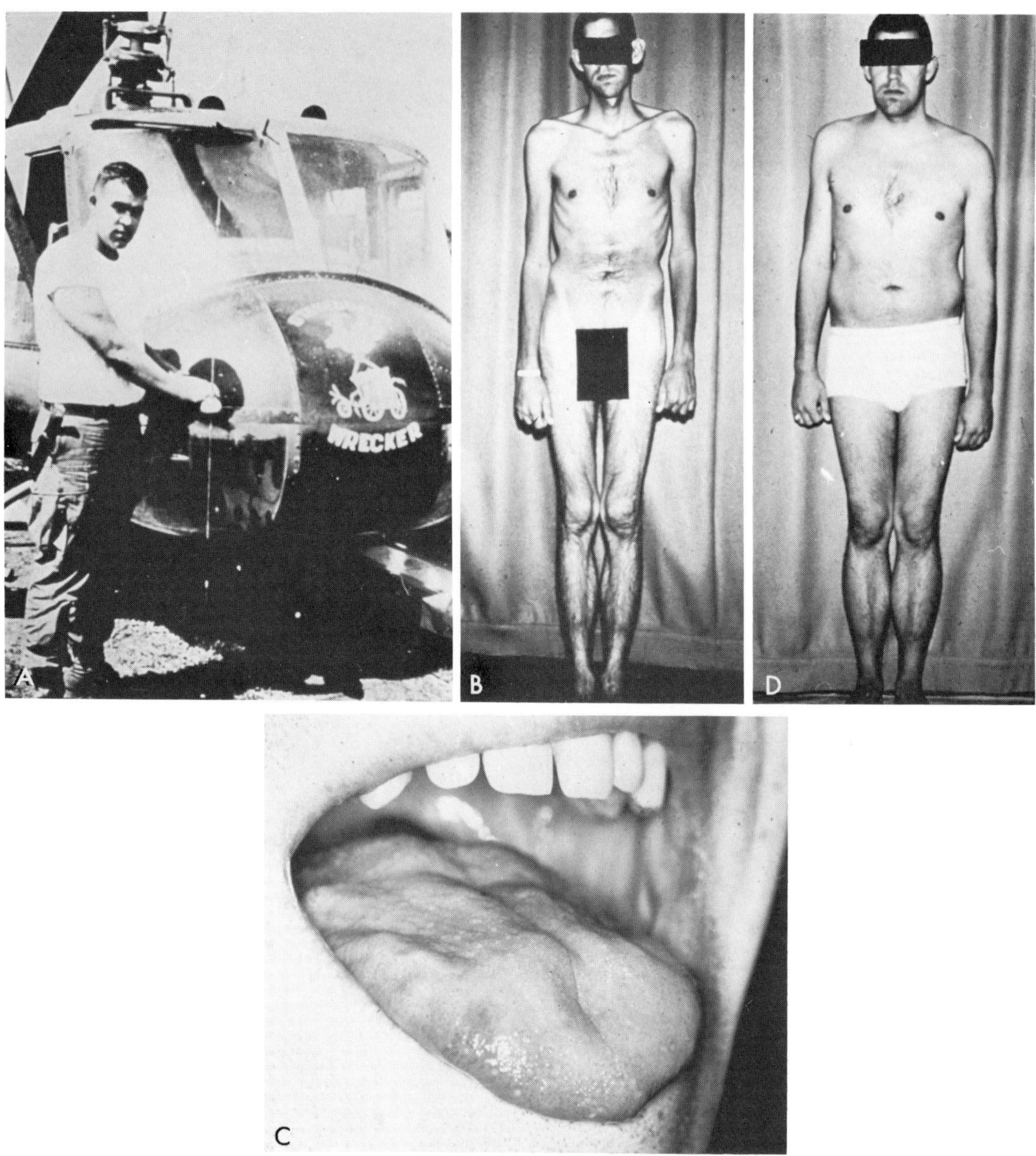

Figure 106–6. *A,* This 26-year-old helicopter crew member developed symptoms of sprue after 1 month in Southeast Asia. *B,* Five months later, malabsorption and megaloblastic anemia were present. Weight loss is evident. *C,* Aphthous ulcers and stomatitis developed after 3 months of diarrhea. *D,* Appearance after 4 months of folate and antibiotic therapy.

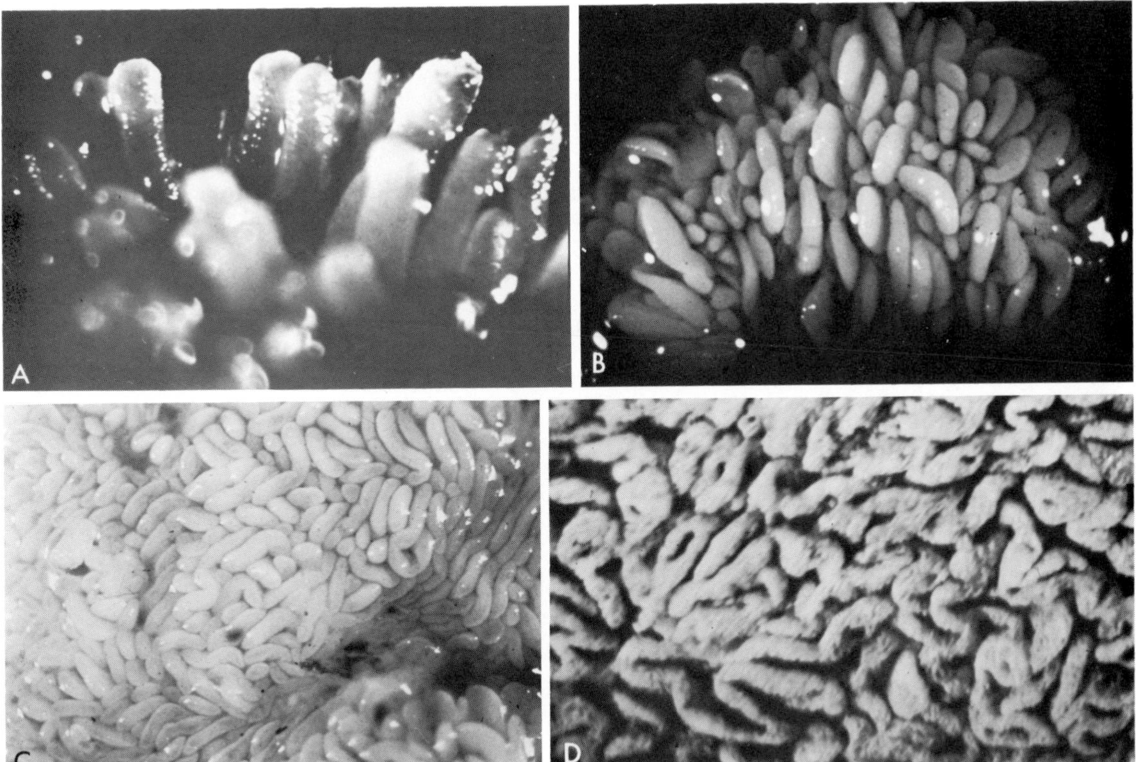

Figure 106–7. Dissecting microscope appearance of *A,* normal jejunal villi; *B,* tongue-shaped villi of early sprue; *C,* tongue and early ridge formation; and *D,* convolutions of severe sprue.

convolutions supported by submucosal blood vessels appear.

Microscopic Changes. Microscopically, the normal jejunal villi are tall, feathery-like structures surrounded by hexagonal crypts of Lieberkühn, which provide their surface epithelium.[66] Jejunal villi are ordinarily 4 to 5 times longer than their crypts, yielding a villus-crypt height ratio of 4 to 1 in 5 μ paraffin sections.[82] This ratio decreases as the disease becomes more severe. Eventually, with impaired epithelial cell production and loss of vascular support within the edematous, inflamed lamina propria, the villi shrivel (Table 106–4). Simultaneously, the epithelial cells become cuboidal in appearance. The crypts of Lieberkühn hypertrophy in a frustrated effort to replace the covering epithe-

Table 106–4. JEJUNAL MUCOSA: MEASUREMENTS OF VILLUS HEIGHT AND WIDTH IN BIOPSY SPECIMENS TAKEN FROM 100 PATIENTS WITH TROPICAL SPRUE

No. Patients	Villus Height (μ)	No. Patients	Villus Width (μ)
18	250–300	8	201–250
36	301–400	34	176–200
33	401–500	54	126–275
13	551–700	4	80–125
100		100	

Normal: height 420–875 μ; width 70–145 μ (20 controls)
Height: distance from muscularis mucosae to tip of villus

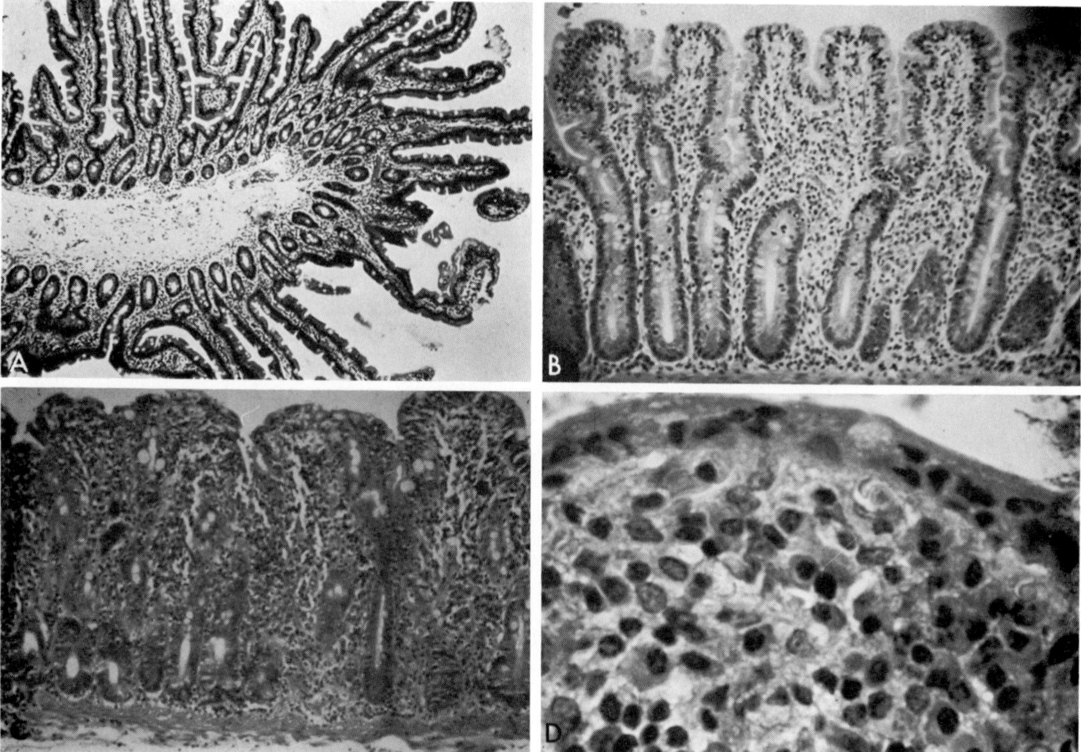

Figure 106–8. Light microscopic appearance of *A*, normal jejunal villi and crypts; *B*, abnormal villi and crypts in tropical sprue; *C*, altered villus/crypt ratio in tropical sprue; and *D*, cuboid epithelium of advanced sprue with marked lymphocytic and plasma cell infiltration of lamina propria.

lium (Fig. 106–8). The crypt cell nuclei gradually enlarge 2- to 3-fold, similar to the nuclei of the gastric cells[88, 102] (Fig. 106–9). The nuclei are pale, immature in appearance, frequently vacuolated, and have prominent nucleoli.[88, 104] This immaturity persists as the crypt cells move onto the remnants of the villi. Electron microscopy shows that the brush borders of the epithelial cells are decimated[105] (Fig. 106–10). The remaining microvilli are short, thickened, and greatly decreased in number. As a result, there is a decrease in the brush border activity of numerous enzymes, including the disaccharidases, lactic dehydrogenase, triosephosphatase, acid phosphatase, diphosphopyridine nucleotide, cytochromic oxidase, and succinic dehydrogenase.[106] The combined result of these cellular changes is a marked loss in mucosal surface area, altered digestion, a decreased absorptive capacity, and a thinning bowel wall.

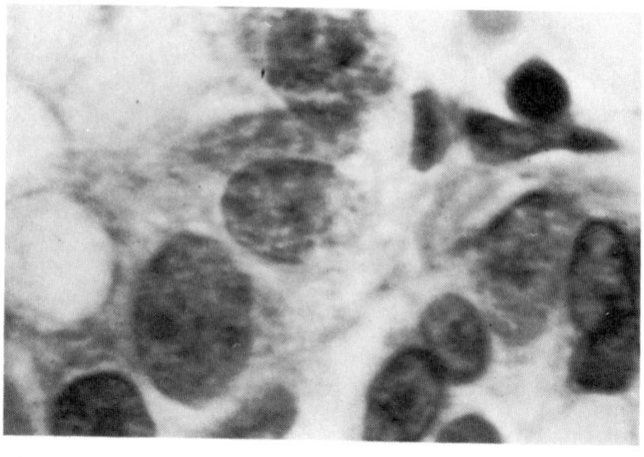

Figure 106–9. Normal and megalocytic nuclei in jejunal crypts in tropical sprue.

Intestinal Absorption

The extensive injury sustained by the intestinal mucosa, along with the enormous loss of surface area, leads to malabsorption of numerous substances. This impaired absorptive ability serves as the basis for diagnostic tests and for such clinical diagnostic features as nocturnal diuresis (Fig. 106–11) resulting from altered membrane permeability to water.

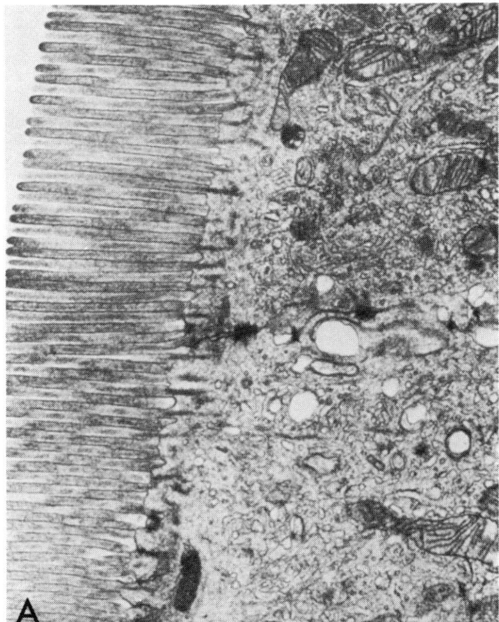

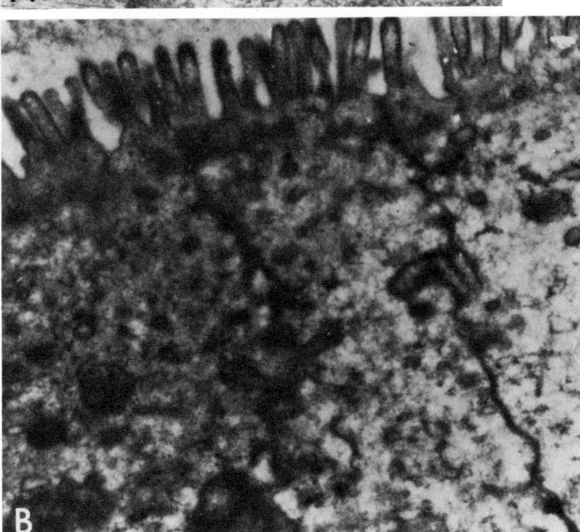

Figure 106–10. *A,* Normal microvilli and brush border, and *B,* microvilli are smaller and fewer in number in severe sprue.

Xylose. The pentose D-xylose is an excellent substance to test the functional integrity of the jejunum (Chapter 27). Using the standard 25-g oral dose, the test was found to be abnormal in 94% of 300 patients in Vellore, India, 100% of 35 patients in Haiti, and 100% of 77 patients in Puerto Rico.[107, 108]

Although less accurate, the 5-g oral dose is a useful screening test and has fewer side effects.[66] It was positive in 199 of 213 of our patients, but some claim that the dosage is inadequate to detect mild malabsorption.[109]

Vitamin A. Normally, there is a progressive rise in serum vitamin A concentration up to 7 hours postprandially.[107, 110] Fasting serum vitamin A levels in untreated sprue patients range from 10 to 40 μg/dl and in those treated with folic acid from 15 to 45 μg/dl.[107] After administration of vitamin A by mouth, the serum vitamin A level in tropical sprue patients with defective intestinal absorption fails to attain a level of 125 μg/dl at 5 to 7 hours. This test is a screening test and is helpful in assessing therapy. However, it tends to return to normal more rapidly than other tests of absorption.

Folate. Perfusion studies with radiolabeled folate in untreated sprue patients have

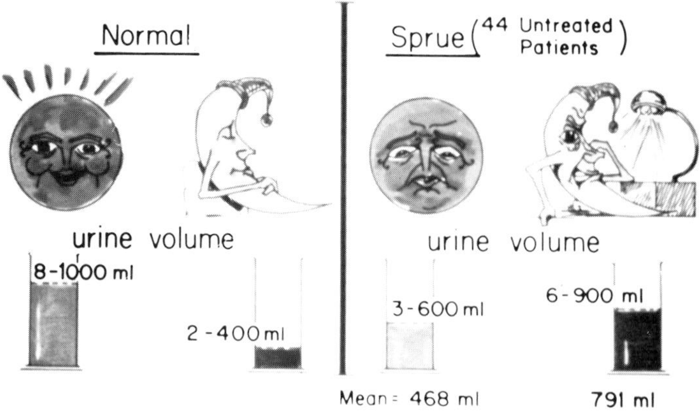

Figure 106–11. Nocturnal diuresis in tropical sprue. The ratio of night-to-day urine volumes ranged from 0.85 to 2.70 (mean 1.70).

shown that the hydrolysis of polyglutamate folate is decreased and the absorption of its digestive product, folic acid, is impaired.[84] Both improve following a 6 month course of tetracycline. Although urinary folate excretion tests and radioisotope serum folate tolerance tests are useful for detecting folate absorption and deficiency, they are seldom used clinically.[111] Plasma clearance of tritium-labeled folate is extremely rapid in the folate-depleted patient; 50% of an IV dose disappears from the plasma within 3 minutes. Patients with classic tropical sprue associated with megaloblastic anemia almost always have folate deficiency. In contrast, patients with tropical enteropathy seldom have low folate levels.

Vitamin B_{12}. Serum vitamin B_{12} levels are low in patients with untreated sprue and malabsorption of the vitamin, with and without intrinsic factor, is common.[112] In expatriates, vitamin B_{12} levels are normal early in the disease but fall within months as the disease progresses.[92] Such a rapid fall suggests impairment of the enterohepatic cycle for vitamin B_{12}. Young servicemen newly arrived in the tropics should have sufficient stores of vitamin B_{12} to last for at least 5 years. Yet, their vitamin B_{12} levels may fall within months of the disease onset. Moreover, their ability to absorb the vitamin often fails to improve with folate therapy, even in the face of hematologic recovery.

Intrinsic factor deficiency occasionally occurs in tropical sprue but is not the usual cause for impaired vitamin B_{12} absorption;[51] addition of intrinsic factor to vitamin B_{12} in the Schilling test does not improve vitamin B_{12} absorption.[84] In jejunal aspirates from untreated patients, the amount of vitamin B_{12} bound to immunoreactive intrinsic factor and to high molecular weight binders is essentially the same as in healthy individuals.[113] Although bacterial binding of the vitamin does not appear to be a factor in compromising vitamin B_{12} absorption, a correlation has been observed between impaired vitamin B_{12} absorption and the concentration of bacterial flora in the jejunum of untreated patients.[84] In some patients, improved vitamin B_{12} absorption occurs within 48 hours of the start of antibiotic therapy, before new epithelial cells can be restored to the villi.[114] This is not a universal finding, however, for most patients require months of antibiotic therapy before they completely recover their ability to absorb the vitamin normally.[114, 115] Together, these findings suggest that an ileal lesion is responsible for malabsorption of vitamin B_{12}. This lesion may be aggravated or even induced by an abnormal bacterial flora or toxin.

Fat. On a diet containing 50 to 100 g of fat, daily fecal fat loss is usually below 6 g[116, 117] (Chapter 27). *Steatorrhea* is defined as a daily fecal fat loss of greater than 6 g. Steatorrhea occurs in 95% or more of patients with tropical sprue due to impaired fat absorption.[66,84] It is present even in the early stage of the disease. Servicemen with symptoms of less than 2 months' duration had an average daily fecal fat loss of 14.4 g daily; those with symptoms of 4 months or more had an average daily fecal fat loss of 21.2 g.[92] In severe sprue, fecal fat may exceed 50 g daily, but ordinarily it seldom exceeds 20 g.[66] Figure 106–12 relates the D-xylose (5 g) test, the vitamin A tolerance test, the serum carotene level, and the findings on jejunal biopsy to steatorrhea in 100 patients with tropical sprue.

Exogenous fat is probably digested reasonably well by pancreatic lipase in patients with tropical sprue, but the absorption of long-chain unsaturated fatty acids is seriously impaired. In contrast, medium-chain fatty acids are absorbed normally. Indeed, a diet with less than 20 g of fat or one consisting of short-chain fatty acids can often abolish the steatorrhea.[118, 119] The intracellular transport of fat also appears to be faulty. In the fasting patient, lipid droplets are found in and immediately below the epithelium but not in the intercellular spaces.[120] This pattern differs from that observed in normal individuals and in untreated celiac patients. Normally, lipid droplets accumulate in the lower half of the lamina propria; in celiac disease, lipid accumulates within the epithelial cells.[120] The lipid lesion of tropical sprue is comparable to the microscopic lesion seen in rats with experimental essential fatty acid deficiency.[121] However, unequivocal evidence for essential fatty acid deficiency in tropical sprue is lacking, even in patients subsisting on less than 20 g of fat daily.[122] The finding that stearic acid is poorly converted to triglyceride within the epithelium, along with the epithelial fat pattern, suggests that either triglyceride resynthesis is impaired or chylomicron synthesis is abnormal. Either of these, in conjunction with surface loss and mucosal injury, would account for the steatorrhea.[122] Bile salt deconjugation is not causally involved in sprue, even though jejunal bile salt concentrations are reduced.[122, 123] (Chapter 92).

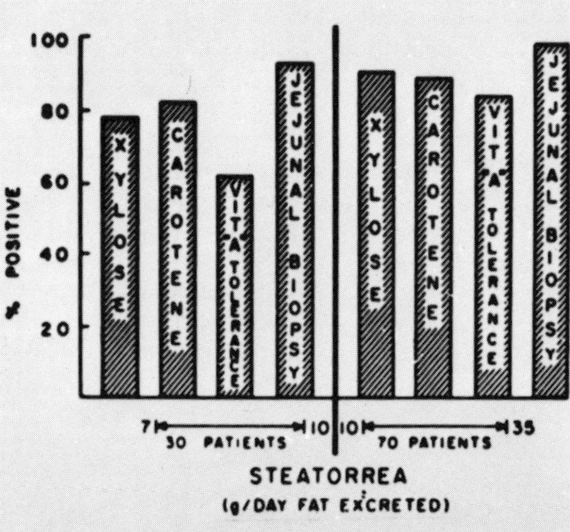

Figure 106–12. Correlation of various absorption studies with steatorrhea (as determined by 72-hour fecal fat analysis in 100 patients with tropical sprue).

The theoretical and technical aspects of *tests for fat absorption* are discussed in Chapters 27 and 92. The only comment with respect to these that will be made here concerns the simple method of microscopically examining a Sudan III–stained fecal smear. This examination was positive in 81% of 150 of our tropical sprue patients with fecal fat loss greater than 12 g/24 hours. [66] Its accuracy, however, is the least in those with mild steatorrhea.[124]

Protein. Protein deficiency is a prominent feature in many tropical sprue patients and hypoalbuminemia is common. The hypoalbuminemia is often due to a combination of factors, including an inadequate diet, impaired protein absorption, excessive protein loss into the bowel, reduced hepatic synthesis, and duration and severity of the disease. In endemic areas, the diet is often suboptimal for protein as well as for fat.[121]

In normal individuals, glycine reaches a peak serum concentration 17 times the fasting value after an oral loading dose.[125] In those with untreated tropical sprue, the glycine absorption is poor and is comparable to the pattern seen with anatomic loss of a large section of the small intestine. Branched-chain amino acids, methionine, leucine, and valine are all absorbed poorly [126]; absorption of the dipeptide glycylglycine is impaired even more.[127] This is not surprising in view of the brush border and enzymatic changes observed in tropical sprue. Normally, glycylglycine is absorbed intact and undergoes hydrolysis intracellularly, where 85% to 90% of glycylglycine hydrolase exists.[128] The remainder is present in the brush border.

Azotorrhea is also common. More than 3 g of fecal nitrogen/24 hours is observed in 25% to 50% of patients.[129] Rubini[130] observed azotorrhea of greater than 6 g/day in 30% of 41 untreated tropical sprue patients on regular diets. A significant correlation was found between the degree of azotorrhea and steatorrhea ($p < 0.001$), but correlation between the degree of diarrhea and azotorrhea was even better.

Excess protein loss from the jejunal mucosa has been shown in 2 studies using ^{51}Cr-labeled albumin and [131]PVP.[96, 131] However, no correlation was detected between the intestinal protein loss and the degree of hypoalbuminemia.

The emaciation accompanying severe sprue leads to a decrease in hepatic size and albumin synthesis. Jeejeebhoy et al.[132] reported reduced hepatic synthesis of albumin in 20 of 37 sprue patients. The hypoalbuminemia in these patients appeared to be related to the severity of malabsorption.

Disaccharides. Carbohydrate absorption is substantially impaired in patients with tropical sprue, as demonstrated by oral tolerance tests. *Lactose* intolerance is almost universal.[94] *Sucrose* intolerance occurs in 50% to 75% of patients. *Galactose* intolerance is even more common. *Glucose* tolerance is subnormal in 50% to 80% of untreated patients.[94, 133] These abnormalities in sugar tolerance in part reflect decreased disaccharidase activity in the jejunal mucosa of treated and many untreated patients.[95] Lactase is invariably absent in jejunal mucosa aspirates. Sucrase activity is substantially reduced in most, and maltase activity is subnormal in 70%. Treatment with folate leads to a prompt recovery of maltase and sucrase activity, but lactase recovery requires prolonged therapy and in 15% to 20% of patients recovery never occurs.[95, 134]

Vitamin B_6. Increased urinary excretion of 5-hydroxyindoleacetic acid, 3-indoleacetic acid, and xanthurenic acid occurs in tropical sprue.[135] All 3 are metabolites of tryptophan. Xanthurenic aciduria occurs with both pyridoxine and riboflavin deficiency. In tropical sprue, it occurs without either deficiency and pyridoxine administration does not consistently lower urinary xanthurenic acid excretion.[136] Pyridoxine absorption is normal, as assessed by both microbiologic and radioisotope studies.

Iron. The absorption of radioactive iron as assessed by fecal excretion is usually normal. However, the uptake of radioactive iron and its incorporation into red blood cells varies with the state of folate and iron stores.[46] In the severely anemic patient, such uptake may be less than 20%, but with the administration of folic acid, radioactive iron is incorporated into 90% or more of the red blood cells within 5 to 7 days.

Calcium and Magnesium. Haddoch and Vazquez[137] believe that the reduced absorption of radionuclide-labeled calcium is due to impaired absorption and to a deficiency of vitamin D. They observed hypocalcemia in 10 of 26 patients. Folate therapy restored both calcium and vitamin D serum levels to normal despite the persistence of steatorrhea. Hypomagnesemia is more apt to occur in association with hypocalcemia and is corrected by restoration of calcium levels to normal with either supplemental calcium and vitamin D or folic acid therapy.

Differential Diagnosis

Tropical sprue must be differentiated from parasitic causes of tropical malabsorption such as *Giardia lamblia, Strongyloides stercoralis, Isospora belli, Capillaria philippinesis,* and the fluke *Metagonimus yokogawai* (Chapter 232). Giardia, a parasite that commonly afflicts travellers,[138] may impair vitamin B_{12} absorption and cause mucosal changes in expatriates. It may even exacerbate the steatorrhea observed in chronic pancreatitis.[139] Bacterial overgrowth of the small intestine with *Klebsiella* also occurs in giardiasis, and this is the same organism isolated in many sprue patients.[140] Giardia may additionally interfere with tetracycline therapy.

Shigellosis, salmonellosis, and amebiasis are common causes of tropical diarrhea. Hence, stool cultures as well as stool examinations for ova and parasites are mandatory. Tuberculous enteritis and schistosomiasis are extremely common in certain parts of Asia and Africa. Inflammatory bowel disorders, such as Crohn's disease (regional enteritis) and ulcerative colitis, must also be considered. Gluten enteropathy occurs in the tropics and, occasionally, tropical sprue develops in such patients.

Vitamin B_{12} deficiency per se can cause malabsorption of xylose and induce jejunal mucosal abnormalities, the so-called "megaloblastic gut."[115] Ordinarily, pernicious anemia can be ruled out by the correction of vitamin B_{12} malabsorption with intrinsic factor. Therapy usually restores absorption to normal and eliminates the anemia. However, in some patients, treatment with vitamin B_{12} for 2 to 8 weeks is necessary to restore the Schilling test to normal.[115]

Treatment and Prognosis

Supportive therapy is required for individuals with electrolyte depletion, protein deficiency, or dehydration. Despite severely depressed hemoglobin levels, most patients do not need blood transfusions for their anemia. Many are surprisingly sensitive to dietary folate, some developing a reticulocyte response after 1 or 2 weeks on a nutritious diet without supplemental folic acid.[66, 129, 141] Most, however, require specific anti-anemia therapy. Treatment with pharmacologic doses of folic acid leads to clinical and hematologic improvement. Within 48 to 72 hours, the patient develops a tremendous sense of well-being and soon thereafter a ravenous appetite.[66, 141] Amazingly, patients with "megaloblastic madness" who are given parenteral folate become rational within 48 to 72 hours.[66] Simultaneously, cheilosis and glossitis are eliminated. After 7 to 10 days, a prompt reticulocytosis is observed and erythrokinetic studies reveal a return of effective erythropoiesis.[99]

Patients with protein deficiency often develop refeeding edema after 1 or 2 weeks of folic acid therapy. Such edema may be preceded by a rise in the serum ferritin level.[143] Diarrhea generally begins to abate within the first week of treatment, but steatorrhea fails to clear in a large number of patients. In some, serial observations reveal rapid morphologic improvement in the bowel mucosa and in brush border enzymatic activity.[20, 23, 51, 81] In most, however, particularly in those with disease of long duration, folate therapy does not relieve the malabsorption, and their intestinal structural abnormalities persist despite years of folate therapy.[20, 23, 51, 64, 144]

The success of folic acid therapy depends to a degree on the duration of the disease and the length of treatment. Military personnel in the Caribbean and Southeast Asia respond effectively to folate therapy if their symptoms are of short duration. However, those with symptoms for 4 to 6 months require longer therapy and usually antibiotics for complete jejunal healing.[20]

For treatment, 5 mg of folic acid, orally, is prescribed for 1 year. For patients with symptoms for 4 or more months and for those with subnormal vitamin B_{12} levels, parenteral therapy with 100 mg of vitamin B_{12} daily for 7 days is added to the treatment regimen. Larger loading doses are not given, since most of the vitamin would be lost in the urine. Thereafter, vitamin B_{12}, 100 mg IM, is given monthly along with oral folic acid.

Antibiotics. Earlier reference was made to the inital studies of antibiotics in the treatment of sprue.[42–45] Both expatriates and local citizens respond to tetracycline therapy with improvement in their jejunal morphology, intestinal absorption, and hematologic parameters. Short-term therapy (2 to 4 weeks) is less successful than more prolonged administration of tetracycline (6 months).[44, 145] The latter is consistently effective in untreated patients and those who do not respond to vitamin B_{12} or folate. Poorly absorbed sulfonamides are apparently as effective as tetracycline in bringing about clinical and morphologic improvement.[146]

Following administration of antibiotics, gastrointestinal symptoms improve within a matter of weeks. Simultaneously, improvement occurs in the intestinal mucosa, particularly in the architecture of the villi. The surface epithelium returns to a columnar status and brush border enzymatic activity and morphology improve. The secretory pattern of water and electrolyte loss returns to normal, and tests for malabsorption improve as the steatorrhea declines. Clinical recovery differs somewhat from that observed with folate therapy. The marvelous sense of well-being so delightfully exhibited following folate therapy and the remarkable recovery of appetite are often delayed with antibiotic therapy.

Antibiotic therapy consists of either tetracycline, 500 mg 4 times daily for 1 month and then twice daily for an additional 5 to 11 months, or succinylsulfathiazole (Sulfasuxidine), 4 g daily for 1 month followed by 2 g daily for 5 months.

Since tropical sprue has a tendency to recur in patients with long-standing disease and response to therapy in such cases is much slower, combination therapy is preferable for these patients. Both folate and antibiotic therapy should be given therefore, to patients who have experienced symptoms for more than 4 months. In endemic areas, some patients may have a relapse or recurrence of their disease following discontinuation of combined therapy. Rickles et al.[144] evaluated 17 Puerto Ricans 5 years after long-term antibiotic treatment and found over 50% had recurrence of malabsorption.

REFERENCES

1. Hillary W. Observations on the Changes of the Air and the Concomitant Diseases in the Islands of Barbadoes. 2nd Ed. London: Hawkes, Clorhe, Collins, 1766.

2. Ketelaer V. Commentarius Medicus. de Apthis Nostratibus seu Belgarum Sprouw. Lugde Bat 1672.
3. Cook GC. Tropical sprue: Implications of Manson's concept. J Coll Phys Lond 1978; 12:329–49.
4. Manson P. Notes on sprue. China: Imperial Customs. Medical Report: 1879–1880; 19:33–7.
5. Van Der Berg CL. Indische Sprouw: Eene monographie, Batavia, Ernst, 1880. China: Imperial Customs. Medical Report: 1883–1884; 27:55.
6. Manson P. Tropical Diseases: A Manual of the Diseases of Warm climates. London: Cassell & Co, Ltd, 1898: 322–37.
7. Bahr PH. Report Researches on Sprue in Ceylon. 1912–1914. London: Cambridge, 1915: 62–74.
8. Begg C. Sprue: Its Diagnosis and Treatment. Bristol: Wright & Sons, 1912.
9. Brown WB. Sprue and Its Treatment. London: John Bale, Sons & Danielson, 1908.
10. Thaysen TEH: Non-Tropical Sprue: A Study of Idiopathic Steatorrhoea. London: Humphrey Milford, 1932.
11. Keele KD, Bound JP. Sprue in India: A clinical survey of 600 cases. Br Med J 1946; 1:77–81.
12. Leishman AWD. Thoughts on sprue after experience in India. Lancet 1945; 2:813–5.
13. Elder HAA. Clinical features, diagnosis and treatment of sprue. J Trop Med Hyg 1947; 50:212–8.
14. Ayrey F. Outbreaks of sprue during the Burma campaign. Trans Soc Trop Med Hyg 1947; 41:377–406.
15. Keele KD: Study of the onset and cyclic development of the sprue syndrome. Br Med J 1946; 2:111–4.
16. Walters JH. Dietetic deficiency syndromes in Indian soldiers. Lancet 1947; 1:861–5.
17. Woodruff AW. Aetiological and prognostic features of tropical sprue. Trans Soc Trop Med Hyg 1949; 42:605–12.
18. Perez-Santiago E, Butterworth CE. Definition and diagnosis of sprue. Am J Dig Dis 1957; 2:225–35.
19. Tomkins AM, Wright SG, Drasar BS. Bacterial colonization of the upper intestine in mild tropical malabsorption. Trans Soc Trop Med Hyg 1980; 74:752–5.
20. Sheehy TW, Cohen WC, Wallace DK, Legters L: Tropical sprue in North Americans. JAMA 1965; 194:1069–76.
21. Lindenbaum J: Small intestine dysfunction in Pakistanis and Americans resident in Pakistan. Am J Clin Nutr 1968; 21:1023–9.
22. Klipstein FA, Beauchamp I, Corcino JJ. Nutritional status and intestinal function among rural populations of the West Indies. II. Barrio Nuevo, PR. Gastroenterology 1972; 63:758–67.
23. Klipstein FA: Tropical sprue in travelers and expatriates living abroad. Gastroenterology 1981; 80:590–600.
24. Stefanini M. Clinical features and pathogenesis of tropical sprue. Medicine 1948; 27:379–427.
25. Milanes F. Changes in the epidemiology and clinical behavior of sprue occurring in Cuba during the 3 decades 1927–1957. Arch Hosp Univ 1960; 12:125–44.
26. Tropical Sprue: Studies of the U.S. Army's sprue team in Puerto Rico. US Army Medical Science Publication 1958; 5:55–6.
27. French JM. The aetiology and mechanism of steatorrhoea. Postgrad Med J 1955; 31:299–309.
28. Webb JF. The aetiology of tropical sprue as seen in Hong Kong and its relation to celiac disease. J Army Med Corps 1972; 118:1–12.
29. Klipstein FA, Corcino J J. Seasonal occurrence of overt and subclinical tropical malabsorption in Puerto Rico. Am J Trop Med Hyg 1974; 23:1189–96.
30. Smith HW. Observations on the flora of the alimentary tract of animals and factors affecting its composition. J Pathol Bacteriol 1965; 89:95–122.
31. Hentges DJ. Enteric pathogen and normal flora interactions. Am J Clin Nutr 1970; 23:1451–6.
32. Levison ME. Effect of colon flora and short-chain fatty acids on growth in vitro of *Pseudomonas aeruginosa* and *Enterobacteriaceae*. Infect Immun 1973; 8:30–5.
33. Mickelson MJ, Klipstein FA. Enterotoxigenic intestinal bacteria in tropical sprue. IV. Effect of linoleic acid on growth interrelationships of *Lactobacillus acidophilus* and *Klebsiella pneumonia*. Infect Immun 1975; 1121–6.
34. Galbraith H, Miller TB, Paton AM, Thompson JK. Antibacterial activity of long chain fatty acids and the reversal with calcium, magnesium, ergocalciferol and cholesterol. J Appl Bacteriol 1971; 34:803–13.
35. Klipstein FA, Corcino JJ. Sprue again. Lancet 1975; 2:180 (Letter). 36. Cancio M, Rodriquez-Molina R, Asenjo CF. Gluten and tropical sprue. Am J Trop Med Hyg 1961; 10:782–9.
37. Bayless TM, Partin JS, Partin JC. Serum precipitins to milk, gluten and rice in tropical sprue. Johns Hopkins Med J 1967; 120:310–16.
38. Ashford BK. Amonilia found in certain cases of sprue: Preliminary note. JAMA 1915; 64:810–11.
39. Low GC. Sprue: analytical study of 150 cases. J Med 1928; 21:523–34.
40. Baker SJ, Mathan VI. An epidemic of tropical sprue in southern India. II. Epidemiology. Ann Trop Med Parasitol 1970; 64:453–67.
41. Dean AG, Jones TC. Seasonal gastroenteritis and malabsorption at an American military base in the Philippines. I. Clinical and epidemiologic investigations of the acute illness. Am J Epidemiol 1972; 95:111–27.
42. French JM, Gaddie R, Smith NM. Tropical sprue: A study of seven cases and their response to combined chemotherapy. J Med 1956; 25:333–51.
43. Sheehy TW, Perez-Santiago E. Antibiotic therapy in tropical sprue. Gastroenterology 1961; 41:208–14.
44. Guerra R, Wheby MS, Bayless TM. Long-term antibiotic therapy in tropical sprue. Ann Intern Med 1965; 63:619–34.
45. Gorbach SL, Banwell JC, Jacobs B, Chatterjee BD, Mitra R, Ghua-Maxumder DN. Tropical sprue and malnutrition in West Bengal. I. Intestinal microflora and absorption. Am J Clin Nutr 1970; 23:1545–58.
46 Sheehy TW, Perez-Santiago E, Rubini ME. Tropical sprue and vitamin B_{12}. N Engl J Med 1961; 265:1232–6.
47. Gorbach SL, Mitra R, Jacobs B, Banwell JG, Chatterjee BD, Mazumder DNG. Bacterial contamination of the small bowel in tropical sprue. Lancet 1969; 1:74–7.
48. Bhat P, Shantakumari S, Rajan D, Mathan VI, Kapadia CR, Swarnabi C, Baker, SJ. Bacterial flora of the gastrointestinal tract in southern Indian control subjects and patients with tropical sprue. Gastroenterology 1972; 62:11–21.
49. Klipstein FA, Holdeman LV, Corcino JJ, Moore WEC: Enterotoxigenic intestinal bacteria in tropical sprue. Ann Intern Med 1973; 79:632–41.
50. Tomkins AM, Drasar BS, James WPT. Bacterial colonisation of jejunal mucosa in acute tropical sprue. Lancet 1975; 1:59–62.
51. Tomkins A. Tropical malabsorption: Recent concepts in pathogenesis and nutritional significance. Clin Sci 1981; 60:131–7.
52. Drasar BS, Agostini C, Clarke D, Mann G, Mhuala F, Montgomery F, Tomkins AM. Adhesion of enteropathogenic bacteria to cells in tissue culture. Dev Biol Stand 1980; 46:83–9.
53. Klipstein FA, Horowit IR, Engert RF, Schenk EA. Effect of *Klebsiella pneumoniae* enterotoxin on intestinal transport in the rat. J Clin Invest 1975; 56:799–807.
54. Klipstein FA, Engert RF, Short HB. Enterotoxigenicity of colonising coliform bacteria in tropical sprue and blind-loop syndrome. Lancet 1978; 2:342–4.
55. Banwell JG, Gorbach SL, Mitra R, Cassells JS, Guha-Mazumder DN, Yardley TJ. Tropical sprue and malnutrition in West Bengal. II. Fluid and electrolyte transport in the small intestine. Am J Clin Nutr 1970; 23:1559–68.
56. Greene HL, Stifel FB, Herman RH, Herman YF, Rosensweig NS. Ethanol-induced inhibition of human intestinal enzyme activites: Reversal by folic acid. Gastroenterology 1974; 67:434–40.
57. Haeney MR. Myelomatosis, amyloidosis, Whipple's disease, tropical sprue and intestinal lymphangiectasia. *In*: Asquith P, ed. Immunology of the Gastrointestinal Tract. New York: Churchill Livingstone, 1979:316–40.
58. Baker SJ, Mathan VI. Tropical sprue in southern India. *In*: Tropical Sprue and Megaloblastic Anemia. London: Churchill Livingstone, 1971: 189–260.
59. Floch MH, Thomassen RW, Cox RS Jr, Sheehy TW. The

gastric mucosa in tropical sprue. Gastroenterology 1963; 44:567–77.
60. Davidson GP, Barnes GL. Structural and functional abnormalities of the small intestine in infants and young children with rotavirus enteritis. Acta Paediatr Scand 1979; 68:181–6.
61. Mathan M, Mathan VI, Swaminathan SP, Yesudos S, Baker SJ. Pleomorphic virus-like particles in human feces. Lancet 1975; 1:1068–9.
62. Rodriguez-Molina R. Sprue in Puerto Rico. Puerto Rico J Pub Health 1941; 17:134–51.
63. Rodriguez-Molina R. Sprue in Puerto Rico: Ten years later. Puerto Rico J Pub Health 1943; 18:314–40.
64. Sheehy TW, Baggs BH, Perez-Santiago E, Floch MH. Prognosis in tropical sprue. Ann Intern Med 1962; 57:892–908.
65. O'Brien W. Acute military tropical sprue in Southeast Asia. Am J Clin Nutr 1968; 21:1007–12.
66. Sheehy TW, Floch MH. The Small Intestine—Its Function and Diseases. Harper & Row, New York: 1964: 74–6.
67. Manson-Bahr P, Willoughby H. Studies on sprue with special reference to treatment: Based on an analysis of two hundred cases. Q J Med 1930; 232:411–42.
68. Hillman RS, McGuffin R, Campbell C. Alcoholic interference with the folate enterohepatic cycle. Trans Assoc Am Phys 1977; 90:145–56.
69. Halsted CH, Robles EA, Mezey E. Decreased jejunal uptake of labeled folic acid (3 H-PGA) in alcoholic patients: Roles of alcohol and nutrition. N Engl J Med 1971; 285:701–6.
70. Sheehy TW, Rubini ME, Perez-Santiago E, Santini R Jr, Haddock J. Effect of "minute" and "titrated" amounts of folic acid on the megaloblastic anemia of tropical sprue. Blood 1961; 18:623–36.
71. Herbert V. Experimental nutritional folate deficiency in man. Trans Assoc Am Phys 1962; 75:307–20.
72. Herbert V. A palatable diet for producing experimental folate deficiency in man. Am J Clin Nutr 1963; 12:17–20.
73. Butterworth CE Jr. The availability of food folate. Br J Haematol 1968; 14:339–43.
74. Santini R Jr, Brewster C, Butterworth CE Jr. The distribution of folic acid active compounds in individual foods. Am J Clin Nutr 1964; 14:205–10.
75. Rosenberg IH, Godwin HA. The digestion and absorption of dietary folate. Gastroenterology 1971; 60:445–63.
76. Butterworth CE Jr, Baugh CM, Krumdieck C. A study of folate absorption and metabolism in man utilizing carbon-14-labeled polyglutamates synthesized by the solid phase method. J Clin Invest 1969; 48:1131–42.
77. Corcino JJ, Klipstein FA. Pteroylglutomic acid malabsorption in tropical sprue. Blood 1975; 45:577–80.
78. Brown JP, Scott JM, Foster FG, Weir DG. Ingestion and absorption of naturally occurring pteroylmonoglutamates (folates) in man. Gastroenterology 1973; 64:223–32.
79. Tomkins AM, Badcock J, James WP. Altered morphology and pathways of DNA synthesis in small intestinal epithelium in dietary folate deficiency. Proc Nutr Soc 1976; 35:144A.
80. Tomkins AM. Folate malnutrition in tropical diarrhoeas. Trans Soc Trop Med Hyg 1979; 73:498–502.
81. Sheehy TW, Guardiola-Rotger A. Nucleoprotein changes in the intestinal mucosa of patients with tropical sprue. J Indian Med Assoc 1965; 12:5359–62.
82. Swanson VL, Thomassen RW. Pathology of the jejunal mucosa in tropical sprue. Am J Pathol 1965; 46:511–51.
83. Beck WS, Hood, S, Barnett BH. The metabolic functions of vitamin B_{12}. I. Distinctive modes of unbalanced growth behavior in *Lactobacillus leichmannii.* Biochim Biophys Acta 1962; 55:455–69.
84. Corcino JJ, Reisenauer AM, Halsted CH. Jejunal perfusion of simple and conjugated folates in tropical sprue. J Clin Invest 1976; 58:298–305.
85. Santini R Jr, Berger FM, Berdasco G, Sheehy, TW, Aviles J, Dvaila I. Folic acid activity in Puerto Rican diets. J Am Diet Assoc 1962; 41:562–7.
86. Klipstein FA. Intestinal folate conjugase activity in tropical sprue. Am J Clin Nutr 1967; 20:1004–9.
87. Butterworth CE Jr, Perez-Santiago E. Jejunal biopsies in sprue. Ann Intern Med 1958; 48:8–29.
88. Wheby MS, Swanson V, Bayless T. Jejunal crypt cell and marrow morphology in tropical sprue. Ann Intern Med 1968; 69:427–34.
89. Gardner FH. Tropical sprue. N Engl J Med 1958; 258:791–6.
90. Tomkins AM, James WPT, Cole ACE, Walters JJ. Malabsorption in overland travelers to India. Br Med J 1974; 1:380–4.
91. Sheehy TW, Cohen WH, Brodsky JP. The intestinal lesion in the initial phase of tropical (military) sprue. Am J Dig Dis 1963; 8:826–36.
92. O'Brien W, England, MWJ. Military tropical sprue from southeast Asia. Br Med J 1966; 2:1157–62.
93. Santini R Jr, Aviles J, Sheehy TW. Sucrase activity in the intestinal mucosa of patients with sprue and normal subjects. Am J Dig Dis 1960; 5:1059–62.
94. Sheehy TW, Anderson PR, Baggs BE. Carbohydrate studies in tropical sprue. Am J Dig Dis 1966; 11:461–73.
95. Sheehy TW, Anderson RP. Disaccharidase activity in normal and diseased bowel. Lancet 1965; 2:1–4.
96. Rubini ME, Sheehy TW, Meroney, WH, Louno J. Exudative enteropathy. II. Observations in tropical sprue. J Lab Clin Med 1961; 58:902–7.
97. Schenk, EA, Samloff IM, Klipstein FA. Morphology of small bowel biopsies. Am J Clin Nutr 1968; 21:944–61.
98. Santiago-Borrero PJ, Maldonada N, Horta E. Tropical sprue in children J Pediatr 1970; 76:470–9.
99. Sheehy TW, Rubini ME, Baco Dapena R, Perez-Santiago E. Erythrokinetics in the megaloblastic anemia of tropical sprue. Blood 1960; 15:761–71.
100. Floch MH, Thomassen RW, Guerra R, Cox RS Jr, Sheehy TW, Plough IC. The structural and functional status of the liver in tropical sprue. Am J Dig Dis 1963; 8:344–52.
101. Rodriguez-Olleros A. The stomach in tropical sprue. Puerto Rico Public Health 1938; 13:503–21.
102. Gardner FH. Observations on the cytology of gastric epithelium in tropical sprue. J Lab Clin Med 1956; 47:529–39.
103. Suarez RM, Spies TD, Suarex RM Jr. The use of folic acid in sprue. Ann Intern Med 1947; 26:642–77.
104. Butterworth CE Jr, Perez-Santiago E. Jejunal biopsies in sprue. Ann Intern Med 1958; 48:8–29.
105. Mathan M, Mathan VI, Baker SJ. An electron-microscopic study of jejunal mucosal morphology in control subjects and in patients with tropical sprue in Southern India. Gastroenterology 1975; 68:17–32.
106. Schenk EA, Samloff IM, Klipstein FA. Morphologic characteristics of jejunal biopsies in celiac disease and in tropical sprue. Am J Pathol 1965; 47:765–81.
107. Gardner FH, Perez-Santiago E. Oral absorption tolerance tests in tropical sprue. Arch Intern Med 1956; 98:467–74.
108. Lindenbaum J. Small intestinel dysfunction in Pakistanis and Americans resident in Pakistan. Am J Clin Nutr 1968; 21:1023–9.
109. Mehta SK, Khurana KK, Mysorekar NR, Chhuttani PN. Evaluation of d-xylose absorption in tropical sprue in North India. India J Med Res 1971; 59:552–9.
110. Kagan BM. The vitamins. *In*: Wohl MC, Goodhart RS, eds. Modern Nutrition in Health and Disease. 2nd Ed. Philadelphia: Lea and Febiger, 1960: 288–321.
111. Sheeny TW, Santini R Jr, Guerra R, Angel R, Plough IC. Tritiated folic acid as a diagnostic aid in folic deficiency. J Lab Clin Med 1963; 61:650–9.
112. Rodriguez-Rosado AL, Sheehy TW. The role of calcium in the intestinal absorption of vitamin B_{12} in tropical sprue. Am J Med Sci 1961; 242:548–50.
113. Kapadia CR, Bhat P, Jacob E, Baker SJ. Vitamin-B_{12} absorption; A study of intraluminal events in control subjects and patients with tropical sprue. Gut 1975; 16:988–93.
114. Tomkins AM, Smith T, Wright SG. Assessment of early and delayed responses in vitamin-B_{12} absorption during antibiotic therapy in tropical malabsorption. Clin Sci 1978; 55:533–9.
115. Lindenbaum J. Aspects of vitamin B_{12} and folate metabolism in malabsorption syndromes. Am J Med 1979; 67:1037–48.
116. Stier LB, Taylor DD, Pace JK, Eisen JN. Metabolic patterns in preadolescent children. IV. Fat intake and excretion. J Nutr 1961; 73:347–51.

117. Jones FA, Gummer JWP. Clinical Gastroenterology. Springfield, Ill: Charles C. Thomas, 1960.
118. Asenjo CF, Rodriquez-Molina R, Cancio M, Bernabe RA. Influence very low-fat diets, with and without gluten, on the endogenous-fecal-fat excretion of patients with tropical sprue. Am J Trop Med 1958; 7:347–52.
119. Cancio M, Menendez-Corrado R, Asenjo CF. Effect of fatty acid structure on absorption of fats by sprue patients. Bol Asoc Med PR 1967; 59:155–60.
120. Brunsen O, Eidelman S, Klipstein FA. Intestinal morphology of rural Haitians: A comparison between overt tropical sprue and asymptomatic subjects. Gastroenterology 1970; 58:655–68.
121. Tiruppathi C, Hill PG, Mathan VI. Plasma lipids in tropical sprue. Am J Clin Nutr 1981; 34:1117-20.
122. Bevan G, Engert R, Klipstein F A. Bile salt metabolism in tropical sprue. Gut 1974; 15:254–9.
123. Kapadia C R, Radhakrishnan A N, Mthan VI, Baker S J. Studies on bile salt deconjugation in patients with tropical sprue. Scand J Gastroenterol 1971; 6:29–31.
124. Simko V. Fecal fat microscopy: Acceptable predictive value in screening for steatorrhea. Am J Gastroenterol 1981; 75:204–8.
125. Butterworth CE Jr, Santini R Jr, Perez-Santiago E. The absorption of glycine and its conversion to serine in patients with sprue. J Clin Invest 1958; 37:20–7.
126. Klipstein FA, Corcino JJ. Malabsorption of essential amino acids in tropical sprue. Gastroenterology 1975; 68:239–44.
127. Hellier MD, Ganapathy V, Gammon A, Mathan VI, Radhakrishnan AN. Impaired intestinal absorption of depeptide in tropical sprue patients in India. Clin Sci 1980; 58:431–3.
128. Adibi SA. Intestinal absorption of amino acids and dipeptides. Viewpoints Dig Dis 1978; 10:1–4.
129. Klipstein FA, Corcino JJ. Factors responsible for weight loss in tropical sprue. Am J Clin Nutr 1977; 30:1703–8.
130. Rubini ME. Personal communication.
131. Vaish SK, Ignatius M, Baker SJ. Albumin metabolism in tropical sprue. Q J Med 1965; 34:15–32.
132. Jeejeebhoy KN, Samuel AM, Singh B, Nadkanni GC, Desai HB, Bonkan AV, Mani LS. Metabolism of albumin and fibrinogen in patients with tropical sprue. Gastroenterology 1969; 56:252–67.
133. Jeejeebhoy KN, Desai HB, Verghese RV. Milk intolerance in tropical malabsorption syndrome. Lancet 1964; 2:666–8.
134. Desai HB, Chitre AV, Parekh DV, Jeejeebhoy KN. Intestinal disaccharidases in tropical sprue. Gastroenterology 1967; 53:375–80.
135. Weissbach H, King W, Sjoerdsma A, Udenfriend S. Formation of indole-3-acetic acid and tryptamine in animals: A method for estimation of indole-3-acetic acid in tissues. J Biol Chem 1959; 234:81–6.
136. Sigler MH, Sheehy TW, Santini R Jr, Rubini ME. Xanthurenic aciduria in tropical sprue. Am J Med Sci 1962; 244:197–201.
137. Haddoch L, Vazquez MC. Antirachitic activity of the sera of patients with tropical sprue. J Clin Endocrinol 1966; 26:859–66.
138. Goldsmith RS. Chronic diarrhea in returning travelers: Intestinal parasitic infection with the fluke—*Metagonimus yokogawai*. South Med J 1978; 71:1513–15.
139. Sheehy TW, Holley, HP Jr. Giardia-induced malabsorption in pancreatitis. JAMA 1975; 233:1373–5.
140. Wright SG, Tomkins AM, Ridley DC. Giardiasis: Clinical and therapeutic aspects. Gut 1977; 18:343–50.
141. Chuttani HK, Kasthuri D, Misra RC: 1968 Courses and prognosis of tropical sprue. J Trop Med Hyg 1968; 71:96–9.
142. Klipstein FA, Corcino JJ. Factors responsible for weight loss in tropical sprue. Am J Clin Nutr 1977; 20:1703–8.
143. Srikantia SG, Gapalan C. Role of ferritin in nutritional edema. J Appl Physiol 1959; 14:829–33.
144. Rickles FR, Klipstein FA, Tomasinin J, Corcino JJ, Maldonado N. Long-term follow-up of antibiotic-treated tropical sprue. Ann Intern Med 1972; 76:203–10.
145. Klipstein FA. Antibiotic therapy in tropical sprue: the role of dietary folic acid in the hematologic remission associated with oral antibiotic therapy. Ann Intern Med 1964; 61:721–8.
146. Maldonado N, Horta E, Guerra R, Perez-Santiago E. Poorly absorbed sulfonamides in the treatment of tropical sprue. Gastroenterology 1969; 57:559–68.

Chapter 107

Bacterial Overgrowth Syndromes

Charles E. King • Phillip P. Toskes

Alterations in one or more of the mechanisms controlling the content of bacteria in the small intestine can lead to a qualitative and quantitative change in the flora. By various means, this overgrowth of bacteria can lead secondarily to disturbed absorption or metabolism of intestinal contents (both ingested nutrients and endogenous secretions). In the early part of the 20th century, it was recognized that an anemia resembling pernicious anemia occurred in the setting of small intestinal strictures and that surgical removal of these strictures corrected the anemia. It was later appreciated that other conditions, such as small bowel diverticula and surgical blind pouches, could lead not only to anemia but also to fat malabsorption. These clinical abnormalities were thought to be due to stasis and consequent bacterial overgrowth. Because the most apparent settings of bacterial overgrowth were those of intestinal blind loops, the entity of surgically or antibiotic-correctable malabsorption became most widely known as the *"blind loop syndrome."*[1] As further awareness and identification of bacterial overgrowth evolved, it was recognized that disturbances of motor function of the small intestine and consequent bacterial overgrowth may occur as frequently in the absence of anatomic blind loops as with them. Thus, the syndrome is now frequently called the *"stasis"* or *"stagnant loop syndrome."*[2] Focus on the primary pathophysiologic event has encouraged a trend toward use of the term *"bacterial overgrowth syndrome."* In addition, studies over the past decade have clearly demonstrated that altered assimilation of nutrients in the setting of small intestine bacterial overgrowth may occur as a result of both bacterial metabolism of luminal contents and damage to the small intestinal absorptive cells. With this expanded knowledge of the pathophysiologic mechanisms plus more frequent identification of the syndrome, a better appreciation of the clinical significance of this entity has developed.

Pathogenesis

Maintenance of the normally sparse small bowel flora relies predominantly on a combination of: (1) the gastric acid killing of ingested bacteria; (2) the presence of normal motor activity of the small intestine unimpeded by localized blind loops, inflammatory or postoperative strictures, or abnormal connections between loops of bowel (allowing recirculation of bowel contents); and (3) the presence of a normally functioning ileocecal valve, preventing undue reflux of colonic contents into the small intestine. Some of the causes of bacterial overgrowth are associated with diffuse stagnation of contents (e.g., small bowel strictures, Kock continent ileostomy pouches, scleroderma, intestinal pseudo-obstruction, diabetic autonomic neuropathy) (Figs. 107–1 and 107–2).[2–7] Other conditions have localized areas of stagnation (e.g., small bowel diverticula, afferent loop of a gastrojejunostomy) in which bacterial proliferation occurs in the localized area with secondary contamination of otherwise normal small bowel distal to the stagnant area (Figs. 107–3 and 107–4).[1,8] Frequently, more than one predisposing factor is seen, such as the patient who underwent partial gastrectomy and who now has both achlorhydria and a stagnant afferent loop, or the patient with small intestinal Crohn's disease who

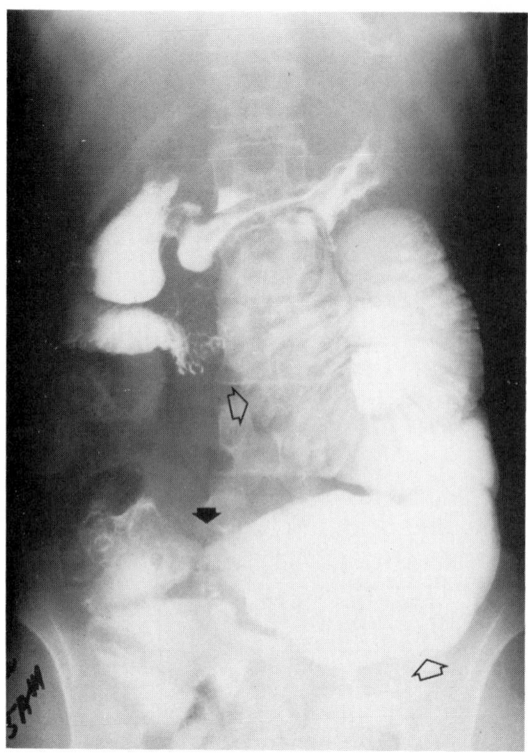

Figure 107–1. Stricture in proximal ileum *(solid arrow)* with proximal dilated small bowel loops *(open arrows)* in a patient with Crohn's disease and clinically important malabsorption due to bacterial overgrowth. (Courtesy of Dr. Juri Kaude.)

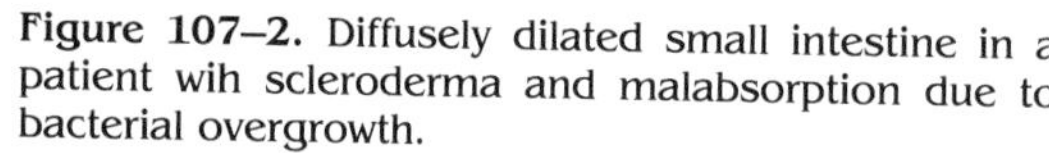

Figure 107–2. Diffusely dilated small intestine in a patient wih scleroderma and malabsorption due to bacterial overgrowth.

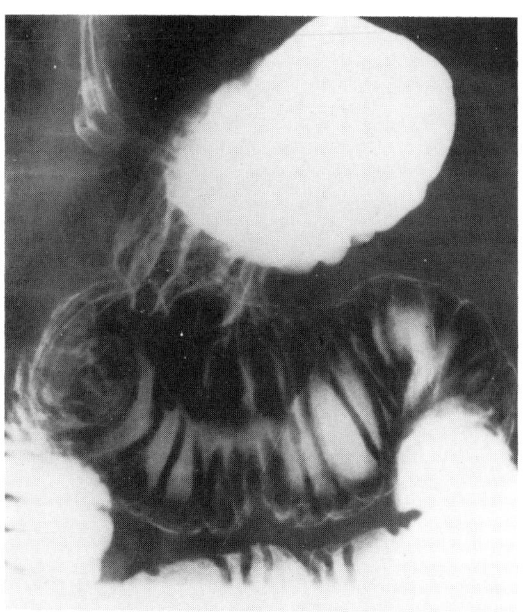

Figure 107–3. Gastrojejunal (Billroth II) anastomosis following partial gastrectomy, a frequent setting for bacterial overgrowth due to hypochlorhydria and afferent loop stasis with secondary "seeding" of the small bowel distal to the anastomosis.

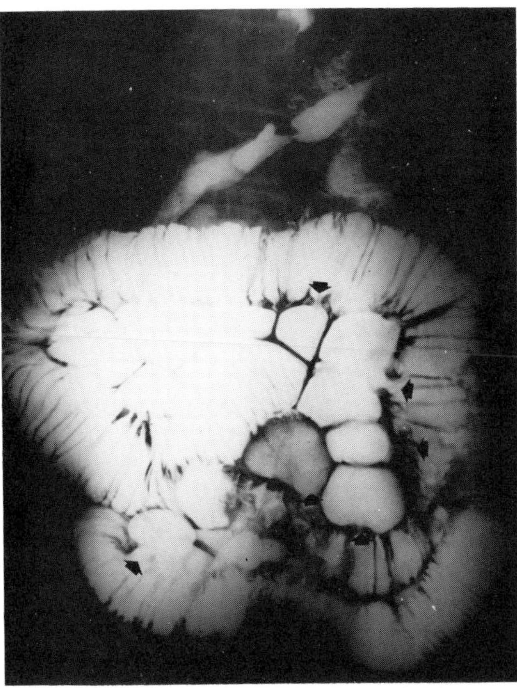

Figure 107–4. Multiple small intestine diverticula *(arrows)*, each of which serves as a stagnant reservoir of proliferating bacteria that constantly contaminate the otherwise normal small intestine.

has both small intestinal strictures and ileocecal valve dysfunction (or surgical absence) or enteroenteric recirculating fistuals (Fig. 107–5).[1,9] *Old age* and/or *malnutrition* are additional factors that have been noted to predispose to bacterial overgrowth.[10] Table 107–1 lists the disorders known to be associated with small intestine bacterial overgrowth.

Pathophysiology

The most evident and longest appreciated pathophysiologic event leading to malabsorption as a result of bacterial overgrowth is that of intraluminal bacterial assimilation or metabolism of intestinal contents. In this regard, cobalamin (vitamin B_{12}) malabsorption has received intense evaluation (Chapter 96). Studies by Donaldson[11] documented that uptake of cobalamin by bacteria made the vitamin unavailable to the host. No deleterious effect of bacteria on either gastric intrinsic factor (IF) or the ileal receptor for the IF-cobalamin complex has been noted. Giannella et al.[12] demonstrated that aerobic bacteria had an affinity for cobalamin that ap-

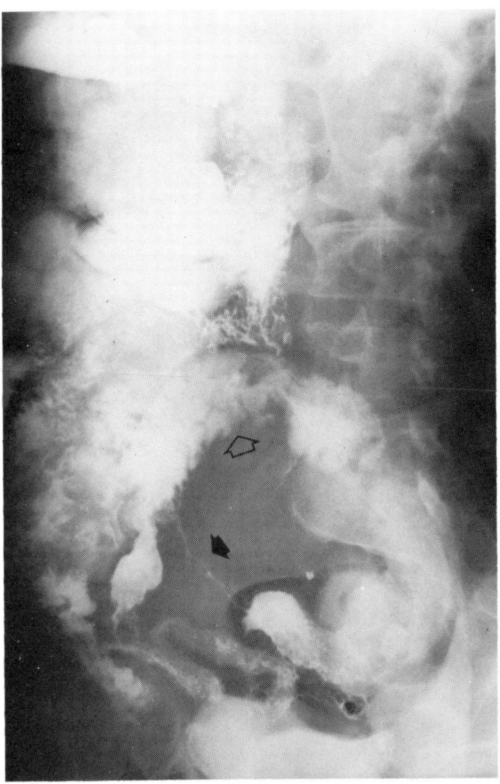

Figure 107–5. Classic ileal "string sign" *(solid arrow)* with secondarily obstructed proximal small intestine *(open arrow)* in Crohn's diease. Bacterial overgrowth occurred as a result of both small bowel stagnation and recirculation of small bowel contents due to enteroenteric fistula. (Courtesy of Dr. James Weaver.)

Table 107–1. DISORDERS ASSOCIATED WITH SMALL INTESTINE BACTERIAL OVERGROWTH*

- A. Gastric proliferation
  - 1. Achlorhydria
  - 2. Gastric atony or outlet obstruction
- B. Small intestinal stagnation
  - 1. Anatomic
    - a. Afferent loop of gastrojejunostomy
    - b. Duodenal/jejunal diverticulosis
    - c. Surgical blind loop (end-to-side enteroenterostomy)
    - d. Surgical recirculating loop (side-to-side anastomosis)
    - e. Obstruction (stricture, adhesion, cancer)
  - 2. Motor
    - a. Scleroderma
    - b. Idiopathic intestinal pseudo-obstruction
    - c. Diabetic autonomic neuropathy
    - d. Derangements of interdigestive motor complex
  - 3. Abnormal communication between upper and lower gastrointestinal tract
    - a. Gastrocolic or jejunocolic fistula
    - b. Resection of ileocecal valve

*Modified from King and Toskes.[2]

proached that of gastric IF, although prior complexing of cobalamin with IF greatly decreased the amount of cobalamin bound by aerobic bacteria. We have demonstrated the predominant importance of anaerobic bacteria for the cobalamin malabsorption occurring in the presence of bacterial overgrowth.[13] In contrast to the "protection" of cobalamin by IF against uptake by aerobic bacteria, anaerobic bacteria were shown to take up cobalamin equally well in the presence or absence of IF complexed to the cobalamin. Likewise, antimicrobial therapy (metronidazole) directed against anaerobic bacteria corrected the cobalamin malabsorption in the experimental rat blind loop syndrome, whereas therapy directed against aerobic members of the overgrowth flora did not.

Study of fat malabsorption has revealed that altered bile acid metabolism (due to intraluminal bacterial deconjugation of solubilizing conjugated bile salts) is a major pathophysiologic event. Both Kim and associates[14] (in experimental studies with dogs) and Tabaqchali and co-workers[15] (in humans) noted improvement in overgrowth-related steatorrhea with the feeding of conjugated bile salts, suggesting that deficiency of conjugated bile salts may be important. However, fat malabsorption occurring with bacterial overgrowth frequently exceeds that seen with complete biliary diversion or therapy with bile acid–binding resins, an argument against simple bile acid deficiency as the sole cause for fat malabsorption. Moreover, support for the importance of inhibition of absorption by deconjugated bile salts has been presented. Thus, Donaldson[16] noted inhibition of uptake and esterification of fatty acid by deconjugated bile salts, and this was confirmed in vivo by the studies of Ament et al.[17] Evidence from our laboratory regarding the importance of mucosal injury in fat malabsorption supports the role of toxic factors, including deconjugated bile salts.[18] Our observations of continuing severe steatorrhea despite antibiotic control of the bacterial overgrowth and of steatorrhea exceeding oral intake of fat (suggesting a "fat-losing enteropathy") both point to gut damage as an important factor.[19] The electron microscopic study of Ament et al.[17] demonstrated diminished uptake and re-esterification of fatty acids and decreased exit of chylomicrons from jejunal enterocytes of human subjects with the blind loop syndrome, all manifestations of significant mucosal dysfunction.

Malassimilation of carbohydrate occurs as a result of both intraluminal bacterial fermentation and maldigestion and malabsorption due to gut damage. The importance of intraluminal metabolism of carbohydrate has been demonstrated by our study of xylose catabolism in the experimental rat model. In this study, diminished levels of xylose absorption (as judged by urinary xylose excretion) were accounted for by intraluminal bacterial fermentation (as manifested by excess breath excretion of labeled CO_2 following oral administration of labeled xylose).[20] These studies support the findings of Goldstein and associates,[21] who reported that antibiotic therapy for patients with bacterial overgrowth led to increased recovery of luminally perfused xylose (combined gut lumen and urine levels), implying less bacterial catabolism following antibiotic therapy. In both our studies and that of Goldstein et al., complete restoration to normal of urine xylose excretion was at times delayed, implying that an element of slowly reversible gut damage (and diminished xylose absorption) participated in the xylose malabsorption.[19–22]

Absorption of other sugars has been less well studied in the setting of bacterial overgrowth. However, we have noted the frequent occurrence of diminished enterocyte brush border levels of 2 disaccharidases (lactase and sucrase) along with clinical lactose intolerance in human subjects with small intestine bacterial overgrowth.[19] Thus, although intraluminal bacterial catabolism of sugars is a major determinant of carbohydrate malabsorption in this setting, functional abnormalities of the mucosa play an important additive part.

Patients with bacterial overgrowth at times have depressed serum protein levels and/or severe protein malnutrition despite adequate dietary intake. Investigation has shown that both intraluminal bacterial catabolism and mucosal injury are etiologic factors. We have demonstrated intraluminal bacterial catabolism in studies of the metabolism of ^{14}C-taurine, an aminosulfonic acid that undergoes limited metabolism by mammalian tissue.[23] Importance of gut damage as an etiologic factor for disturbed assimilation of protein has been demonstrated in humans with diminished brush border and luminal enterokinase levels and in the rat model with diminished brush border peptidase levels and diminished in vitro uptake of amino acid.[24–26] We have also demonstrated a significant protein-losing enteropathy in both the experimental rat and the human bacterial overgrowth syndrome, an abnormality that was only slowly (and at times incompletely) reversible with adequate therapy for the overgrowth.[27] Any excessive protein loss to the gut lumen would have an additive effect in leading to protein deficiency if concomitant derangements in protein digestion or absorption were present, since compensatory reabsorption of the secreted protein would be less available.

Just as with all forms of nutrient malabsorption, excess fecal water and electrolyte excretion, manifested as diarrhea, may be seen with the bacterial overgrowth syndromes. Increased colonic secretion of water and electrolytes secondary to colonic bacterial production of secretagogues, such as hydroxy fatty acids (from malabsorbed fat), osmotically active organic acids and ethanol (from malabsorbed carbohydrate), and deconjugated bile salts (from malabsorbed conjugated bile salts) are well-known causes of diarrhea in the setting of malabsorption. In small intestine bacterial overgrowth, water and electrolyte secretion may also occur in the small intestine as well as in the colon, inasmuch as similar secretagogues may be produced by action of the small bowel overgrowth flora on the luminal contents.[28–30] In fact, diarrhea without major nutrient malabsorption is seen at times in the setting of bacterial overgrowth, probably as a reflection of small bowel secretion of water and electrolytes. We have also noted that the abnormal flora leads to antibiotic-reversible alterations in the myoelectric activity of the smooth muscle of the small bowel, suggesting that alterations in motility may contribute to the diarrhea.[31]

In addition to the deleterious effects that malabsorption may play in drug absorption, the development of bacterial overgrowth has interesting and important implications with respect to drug metabolism. The normal gastrointestinal flora participates in the metabolism of several drugs because bacteria possess certain metabolizing enzymes that are not present in gut secretions or in host enterocytes.[32] If the drug metabolism is altered because of "premature" metabolism (by bacteria in the small intestine), increased or decreased effect of the drug may be seen. For example, bacterial overgrowth may diminish the effectiveness of L-dopa or sulfasalazine therapy.[33] Although drug absorption has been only sparsely studied in the bacterial overgrowth syndromes, the potential impact that the disease and/or its treatment could play in drug metabolism is significant.

Mucosal Injury

It was felt for many years that malabsorption in the bacterial overgrowth syndrome was due solely to alterations in the luminal environment. Over the past decade, however, morphologic and functional studies have demonstrated mucosal injury to be an important additional pathophysiologic mechanism.[17,23–27] Injury is seen at the light microscopic level as a patchy broadening and flattening of the villi (Fig. 107–6). Electron

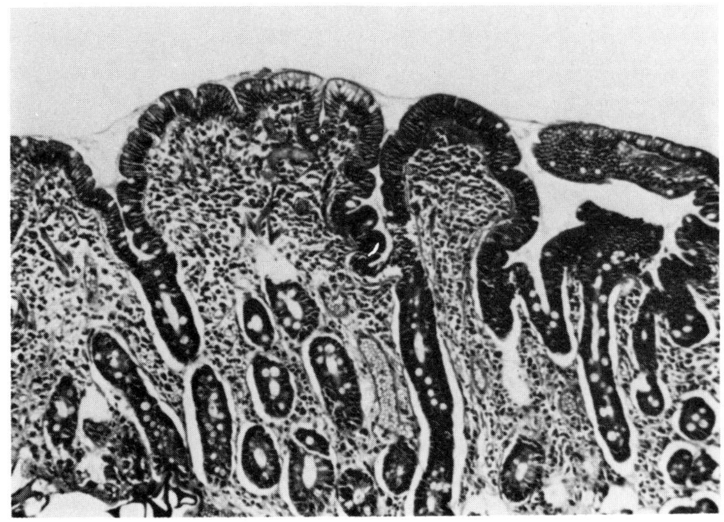

Figure 107–6. Shortened, broadened villi in a subject with bacterial overgrowth and severe malabsorption. (From King CE, Toskes PP. *In*: Bushkin FL, Woodward ER. Postgastrectomy Syndromes. Philadelphia: WB Saunders, 1976. Reproduced with permission.)

microscopy has revealed degenerative changes of the microvilli, disruption of the terminal web, and swelling of endoplasmic reticulum and mitochondria. Histochemical and biochemical studies in the experimental rat model have revealed a loss of enzyme activity in the brush border, endoplasmic reticulum, and mitochondria.[26] We have also noted diminished brush border enzyme activities in humans with bacterial overgrowth that have slowly or incompletely reversed with therapy.[19] Functional abnormalities of the damaged mucosa have been noted with respect to loss to the lumen of serum protein, fat, and hemoglobin iron.[17, 19, 27]

Development of the mucosal injury may occur as a result of: (1) toxic effects of metabolic by-products of bacterial interactions with luminal contents; and/or (2) direct action on the mucosa of bacteria or toxins released by bacteria.[2] Deconjugated bile salts are the metabolic by-products that have been studied the most as potential toxins in the bacterial overgrowth syndromes. They have been shown to cause a reversible depression of small bowel absorptive function.[34] We have more recently shown that the protein-losing enteropathy in the experimental rat model is due in large part to deconjugated bile salts, since diversion of biliary secretions from the small bowel in animals with bacterial overgrowth significantly diminishes the frequency of excessive serum protein loss to the gut lumen.[18] Fewer studies have been made of other potential toxins; such as endogenously produced alcohols, volatile fatty acids, and hydroxy fatty acids. These could be chronically present in the lumen in concentrations damaging to the mucosa. In addition, release of toxins or enzymes from bacteria may be potential etiologic factors.[35, 36]

Clinical Aspects

Depending on the predisposing cause for the bacterial overgrowth, clinical manifestations may vary from virtual absence of symptoms to severe diarrhea, malnutrition, and anemia. Anatomic entities, such as small bowel diverticulosis and surgical blind loops, may be present for years before the onset of clinically apparent metabolic abnormalities. It is possible that gradual development of diminished gastric acid production with age may tip the scale to more flagrant overgrowth with consequent clinically significant disease. Patients with small bowel strictures frequently have symptoms related to partial obstruction (crampy pain, abdominal bloating) that overshadow manifestations of malabsorption and/or diarrhea. Similar findings are frequently noted in patients with primary motor abnormalities (scleroderma, intestinal pseudo-obstruction, diabetic autonomic neuropathy) in whom obstipation and/or pain may overshadow the deleterious bacterial overgrowth and nutrient malabsorption. At times, clinical deterioration of a patient with Crohn's disease or lymphoma may be due to malabsorption and malnutrition associated with bacterial overgrowth, and marked improvement may be seen following antibacterial therapy for the overgrowth flora.

Manifestations of malabsorption due to bacterial overgrowth are similar to those of other malabsorptive disorders and include significant *weight loss, diarrhea, anemia,* and development of *fat-soluble vitamin deficiency.* As noted, diarrhea may occur in the absence of major nutrient malabsorption and be related to small bowel secretion of water and electrolytes secondary to luminally produced secretagogues. The anemia is usually related to cobalamin deficiency, although iron deficiency developing as a result of mucosal injury and bleeding may lead to a dimorphic anemia. Folate deficiency is usually not seen in the bacterial overgrowth syndromes because of the production of folate by part of the overgrowth flora (surpassing the degree of bacterial folate utilization and mucosal malabsorption). In fact, an elevated serum folate level is at times a clue that small intestine bacterial overgrowth is the cause of malabsorption in an undiagnosed patient.[37]

Fat-soluble vitamin deficiency is most frequently manifested by visual disturbance (vitamin A) and osteomalacia (combined vitamin D and calcium malabsorption).[38, 39] Figure 107–7 shows the funduscopic appearance in a patient with severe fat malabsorption due to bacterial overgrowth; the yellow-white punctate lesions in the fundus are similar to the lesions seen in children with markedly restricted dietary intake of vitamin A.[39] Vitamin D and calcium malabsorption may be severe, especially when mucosal injury has led to marked fat malabsorption. Because of the precipitation of calcium with fatty acids in the lumen by soap formation, large doses of exogenous calcium may be required. Provision of added calcium may

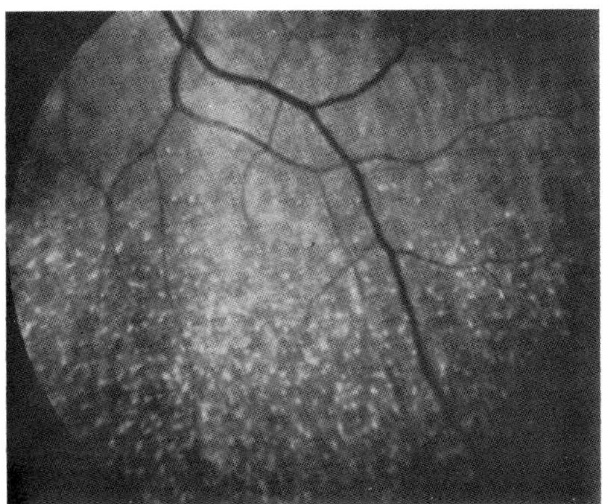

Figure 107–7. Multiple discrete yellow-white spots (most prominent in lower half of photograph) in the peripheral fundus of a subject with longstanding bacterial overgrowth and malabsorption. Funduscopic and dark adaption abnormalities improved with vitamin A therapy. (From Levy NS, Toskes PP. Published with permission from The American Journal of Ophthalmology 78:926–929, 1974. Copyright by The Ophthalmic Publishing Company.)

additionally diminish stool frequency and diarrhea. Interestingly, vitamin K deficiency occurs less frequently than would be expected for the degree of fat (and fat-soluble vitamin) malabsorption. Because the normal intestinal microflora is important for the maintenance of normal vitamin K homeostasis, it is probable that the small bowel overgrowth flora produces excess vitamin K to counterbalance in large part the vitamin K malabsorption.[32] This is similar to the findings just referred to regarding elevated serum folate levels in the bacterial overgrowth syndromes.[37]

Diagnosis

Suspicion that bacterial overgrowth may be responsible for malnutrition, malabsorption, and/or diarrhea may be aroused by a history of prior abdominal surgery leading to decreased acid secretion, blind loops, adhesions, or absence of the ileocecal valve or by a history suggestive of possible stenosis associated with Crohn's disease or lymphoma. A history of a hypomotility disorder may be obvious or subtle and may include dysphagia (to solids and liquids), markedly delayed gastric emptying (e.g., vomiting of food ingested many hours previously), abdominal bloating, and/or obstipation. When predisposition for overgrowth is simply related to malnutrition and/or old age, historical keys to detecting the condition may be very subtle.

The classic "gold standard" for diagnosing bacterial overgrowth is an appropriately obtained, well-handled small intestinal aspirate for aerobic and anaerobic microbiologic culturing. The aspiration tube should be of small caliber to allow discarding of juice equal to 2 to 3 times the tube volume (rinsing away contaminating organisms from the throat and stomach) prior to anaerobic collection of the aspirate for culture. Unless the specimen is to be cultured immediately, it should be placed in pre-reduced carrier media to afford optimum detection of anaerobic bacteria. Processing by the microbiologic laboratory should include both aerobic and anaerobic culturing on various media to allow identification of at least the genus of all organisms present from anaerobic culture and all aerobic organisms in concentrations $>10^4$/ml. Cultures should be considered suspicious if $>10^3$ organisms/ml are present (especially when anaerobes are identified) and clearly abnormal when $>10^5$ organisms/ml are seen.[32]

Because adequate microbiologic culturing demands meticulous specimen collection and evaluation and because there is a long delay before test results are available, alternative methods to screen for or identify the syndrome have been sought over the years. Some of the methods suggested still require small bowel intubation and analysis of fresh or incubated aspirates for the presence of deconjugated bile salts or volatile fatty acids.[15, 30, 40, 41] To bypass small bowel intubation, analysis of the urine for excess excretion of indican or other bacterial metabolites has been suggested. The major problem with using urinary excretion tests to identify small intestine bacterial overgrowth is that they do not reliably identify the site of bacterial production of the measured metabolite (i.e., small bowel versus colonic bacterial production) and thus do not differentiate bacterial overgrowth from other malabsorption disorders.[52]

The most successful alternatives to small bowel intubation in identifying bacterial overgrowth have been the *carbon isotope* and *hydrogen breath tests*[43] (Chapter 27). These tests involve measurement of labeled CO_2 in the breath after administration of ^{14}C- or ^{13}C-labeled substrates or of hydrogen after the oral intake of non-labeled fermentable substances. They afford specific detection of small intestinal processes by analysis of the breath soon after the oral dose has been administered (at times when the test substrate is in contact with small intestinal but not colonic bacteria). Although the ^{14}C-bile acid breath test was one of the earliest breath tests developed to aid in detecting bacterial overgrowth, it is difficult to use the test to differentiate ileal malabsorption of bile salts from small intestine bacterial overgrowth unless concurrent fecal analysis for labeled bile acid content is employed.[44] Because the sensitivity of the bile acid breath test is only 65% to 70%, it is infrequently used alone to detect bacterial overgrowth.[45–47]

The one-gram ^{14}C-D-xylose breath test has afforded much better specificity and sensitivity in detecting bacterial overgrowth.[22, 47, 48] This test utilizes a test probe absorbed in the proximal small intestine (as contrasted to the ileal absorption of conjugated bile salt, which is the test probe in the bile acid breath test). This affords better specificity in distinguishing abnormal labeled CO_2 generation by bacteria of the small intestine overgrowth flora from that by the normal and luxuriant colonic flora. In addition, sensitivity in detecting overgrowth is better, owing to reduced contact of the test probe with the colonic flora. This minimizes the "dirty background" of labeled CO_2 against which small bowel bacterial CO_2 generation must be measured. The sensitivity of the one-gram xylose breath test (>95%) in detecting bacterial overgrowth is much greater than that of the bile acid breath test (60% to 70%) and better than a single jejunal culture.[47, 48] The last obtains because the xylose breath test detects excessive bacteria throughout the small intestine, while a single jejunal culture is from only one location that may not be representative.[48] The short duration of the xylose breath test (analysis at 30 and 60 minutes after administration of 1 g of xylose and 5 to 10 μCi of ^{14}C-D-xylose in 500 ml of water) and the immediate availability of breath test results are in contrast with the delay (3 to 6 days depending on the complexity of the flora) necessary for aerobic and anaerobic microbiologic analysis.

Analysis of the long-term maximum radiation exposure derived from administration of ^{14}C-xylose and ^{14}C-cholylglycine has shown that dosimetry is in the same range as plain chest or abdominal x-rays and much below that used for fluoroscopic jejunal tube placement or contrast x-rays.[49] However, extending breath analysis to the diagnostic workup of children and reproductive-age females has required a search for non-radioactive alternatives. The test is currently available only as a radioisotopic $^{14}CO_2$ procedure. However, evaluation of a stable-isotopic ^{13}C-xylose breath test for bacterial overgrowth is in process. A ^{13}C-bile acid breath test has been developed, but its sensitivity and specificity have the same deficiencies in detecting bacterial overgrowth as the ^{14}C-bile acid breath test.[50] Although not yet tested in humans, ^{13}C-taurine has potential utility, since studies with ^{14}C-taurine in the experimental rat model have shown excellent distinguishing of normal rats from rats with bacterial overgrowth; the sensitivity of this test is due to absent tissue metabolism and modest bacterial catabolism of the substrate.[23]

Alternative non-radioactive testing with *glucose-*H_2 and *lactulose-*H_2 *breath tests* has been reported. With H_2 breath analysis after the administration of 50 g of glucose, a false-negative rate similar to that of the bile acid breath test (30% to 40%) was seen.[45] We have noted better sensitivity in detecting overgrowth with an 80-gram glucose-H_2 breath test in preliminary studies (approximately 80% to 85%), probably because of better contact of the overgrowth flora with the avidly absorbed glucose.[51] Higher doses of glucose would have the risk of diminished specificity based on the observation of Bond and Levitt[52] that the frequency of glucose malabsorption (colonic bacterial fermentation of malabsorbed substrate) is high when 100 g of glucose is administered to subjects with partial gastrectomy (a frequent clinical setting in which evaluation for bacterial overgrowth is desirable).[1, 2, 52] Although a 10-gram lactulose-H_2 breath test was reported to detect abnormal H_2 production in 8 of 9 patients with bacterial overgrowth, further evaluation with specific attention paid to separating small bowel from colonic bacterial catabolism of non-absorbed lactulose is necessary.[53] Table 107–2 summarizes the positive and negative aspects of the various procedures available for diagnosing bacterial overgrowth.

Treatment

Management of patients with bacterial overgrowth involves consideration of the contributory surgical, medical, and nutritional factors. If there is a surgically correctable

Table 107–2. DIAGNOSTIC PROCEDURES FOR BACTERIAL OVERGROWTH*

Procedure	Simplicity	Sensitivity	Specificity (Small Bowel vs Colon)	Tissue Production of Metabolite	Safety
Culture	Poor	Good	Excellent	—	Good
Urine tests	Excellent	Fair	Poor	—	Excellent
Breath tests					
^{14}C-xylose	Excellent	Excellent	Excellent	Small	Good
^{14}C bile acid (also ^{13}C)	Excellent	Fair	Poor	Moderate	Good
Lactulose-H_2	Excellent	Fair–good	Unknown	None	Excellent
Glucose-H_2	Excellent	Fair–good	Unknown	None	Excellent

*Modified from King and Toskes.[43]

cause for the overgrowth (e.g., gastrojejunocolic fistula, isolated small bowel diverticulum) and if nutrient malabsorption is present, surgical intervention is appropriate. Since most causes of overgrowth cannot be corrected surgically (e.g., primary motor disorders, multiple diverticula), therapy is lifelong and directed toward antibacterial and nutritional needs. Because of the risk of an allergic or adverse drug reaction or the development of an antibiotic-resistant flora, antibiotic therapy should be reserved for times when weight loss and/or diarrhea due to malabsorption becomes clinically significant. While intermittent therapy may be beneficial in preventing development of mucosal injury, antibiotic therapy should be therapeutic rather than prophylactic. Response to antibiotic therapy in the patient with only diarrhea is at times difficult to judge because of the 10% to 20% frequency rate of diarrhea secondary to antibiotic therapy. Thus, whereas it is important for clinicians to think of breath tests and jejunal cultures to detect the presence of bacterial overgrowth, treatment with antibiotics may be undertaken after appropriate consideration of both the patient's status and the means by which response to therapy will be gauged.

Choice of the antibiotic to employ should, of course, be based on the sensitivity of the organisms recovered from the jejunal culture. However, the multitude of organisms with varying sensitivities present in the flora frequently makes this approach impractical. Usually, an oral broad-spectrum antibiotic, such as tetracycline 250 to 500 mg 4 times a day, is given for a 7 to 10 day period. Clinical improvement in fat and cobalamin malabsorption and diarrhea is often seen within 3 to 4 days. Lack of improvement could be due to either inadequate antibacterial therapy (resistant flora) or continuing malabsorption resulting from more slowly reversible mucosal dysfunction. If the former is present, selection of a course of an alternative broad-spectrum agent, such as chloramphenicol, 50 mg/kg/day in 4 divided doses, is reasonable. Inasmuch as anaerobes are frequently major factors in cobalamin and fat malabsorption, alternative therapy with metronidazole (Flagyl), 250 mg every 8 hours, or, rarely, clindamycin, 75 to 150 mg 4 times a day, may be indicated. At times a combination of metronidazole or clindamycin and one of the newer cephalosporins may be indicated when both severe malabsorption and antibiotic-resistant overgrowth flora are present. Response to an antibiotic may take 1 of 3 patterns: (1) most commonly, one successful course of antibiotic therapy will be followed by several months of successful remission of malabsorption; (2) less commonly, patients will have remission of malabsorption with a successful course of antibiotics, but will require intermittent therapy 1 week out of every 6 or (3) a rare patient will require an initial course of continuous antibiotic therapy for 2 to 3 months before beneficial effects are seen.

Malabsorption may at times continue despite optimum antibiotic therapy, or there may be difficulty in giving frequent courses of antibiotics because of adverse reactions or bacterial resistance. In this setting, nutritional management plays a key part in maintaining quality and quantity of life. Any unresolved fat malabsorption makes restriction of long-chain triglycerides and supplementation with better absorbed medium-chain triglycerides important in the management of calorie deficiency, diarrhea, and the tendency to formation of calcium oxalate kidney stones. Since lactase deficiency is so prevalent in the setting of bacterial overgrowth, use of a lactose-restricted diet (or one in which milk is pre-treated with lactase) is important in the management of diarrhea.[19] Supplementation with calcium carbonate, fat-soluble vitamins, and parenteral cobalamin is also frequently necessary in overall management.

Prognosis

As detection methods for bacterial overgrowth have become simpler, more patients with this disorder are being identified and more of these before the development of overgrowth-related mucosal dysfunction and/or serious malnutrition. Most patients undergo remarkable improvement in quality of life once appropriate therapy has been undertaken. A small percentage, particularly those with very slowly reversible mucosal dysfunction, have a prolonged need for intense nutritional support. These individuals have a prolonged risk of life-threatening infections and failure-to-thrive similar to that incurred by all malnourished patients.

References

1. Goldstein F, Wirts CW, Kramer S. The relationship of afferent limb stasis and bacterial flora to the production of postgastrectomy steatorrhea. Gastroenterology 1961; 40:47–55.
2. King CE, Toskes PP. Small intestine bacterial overgrowth. Gastroenterology 1979; 76:1035–55.
3. Naish JM, Capper WM, Brown NJ. Intestinal pseudoobstruction with steatorrhea. Gut 1960; 1:62–6.
4. Kahn IJ, Jeffries GH, Sleisenger MH. Malabsorption in intestinal scleroderma: Correction by antibiotics. N Engl J Med 1966; 274:1339–42.
5. Goldstein F, Wirts CW, Kowlessar OD. Diabetic diarrhea and steatorrhea. Microbiologic and clinical observations. Ann Intern Med 1970; 72:215–8.
6. Swan RW. Stagnant loop syndrome resulting from small-bowel irradiation injury and intestinal bypass. Gynecol Oncol 1974; 2:441–5.
7. Schjonsby H, Halvorsen JF, Hofstad T, Houdenak N. Stagnant loop syndrome in patients with continent ileostomy (intra-abdominal ileal reservoir). Gut 1977; 18:795–9.
8. Badenoch J, Bedford PS, Evans JR. Massive diverticulosis of the small intestine with steatorrhea and megaloblastic anemia. Q J Med 1955; 24:321–30.
9. Beeken WL, Kanish RE. Microbial flora of the upper small bowel in Crohn's disease. Gastroenterology 1973; 65:390–7.
10. Gracey M, Suharjono MD, Sunoto MD, Stone DE. Microbial contamination of the gut: Another feature of malnutrition. Am J Clin Nutr 1973; 26:1170–4.
11. Donaldson RM Jr. Malabsorption of Co^{60}-labeled cyanocobalamin in rats with intestinal diverticula. II. Studies on contents of the diverticula. Gastroenterology 1962; 43:282–90.
12. Giannella RA, Broitman SA, Zamcheck N. Vitamin B_{12} uptake by intestinal microorganisms: Mechanisms and relevance to syndromes of bacterial overgrowth. J Clin Invest 1971; 50:1100–7.
13. Welkos SL, Toskes PP, Baer H. Importance of anaerobic bacteria in the cobalamin malabsorption of the experimental rat blind loop syndrome. Gastroenterology 1981; 80:313–20.
14. Kim YS, Spritz M, Blum M, Terz J, Sherlock P. The role of altered bile acid metabolism in the steatorrhea of experimental blind loop. J Clin Invest 1966; 45:956–62.
15. Tabaqchali S, Hatzioannou J, Booth CC. Bile salt deconjugation and steatorrhea in patients with the stagnant loop syndrome. Lancet 1968; 2:12–6.
16. Donaldson RM Jr. Studies on the pathogenesis of steatorrhea in the blind loop syndrome. J Clin Invest 1965; 44:1815–25.
17. Ament ME, Shimoda SS, Saunders DR, Rubin CE. Pathogenesis of steatorrhea in three cases of small intestinal stasis syndrome. Gastroenterology 1972; 63:728–47.
18. King CE, Snook LB, Toskes PP. Development of mucosal injury in the blind loop syndrome: Effect of deconjugated bile salts on the genesis of protein-losing enteropathy. Gastroenterology 1981; 80:1192.
19. King CE, Toskes PP, Cerda JJ. Persistent mucosal injury in the human blind loop syndrome. Gastroenterology 1979; 76:1170.
20. Toskes PP, King CE, Spivey JC, Lorenz E. Xylose catabolism in the experimental rat blind loop syndrome. Studies including the use of a newly developed d-[^{14}C]-xylose breath test. Gastroenterology 1978; 74:691–7.
21. Goldstein F, Karacadag S, Wirts CW, Kowlessar OD. Intraluminal small-intestinal utilization of d-xylose by bacteria. A limitation of the d-xylose absorption test. Gastroenterology 1970; 59:380–6.
22. King CE, Toskes PP, Spivey JC, Lorenz E, Welkos S. Detection of small intestine bacterial overgrowth by means of a ^{14}C-d-xylose breath test. Gastroenterology 1979; 77:75–82.
23. King CE, Lorenz E, Toskes PP. The pathogenesis of decreased serum protein levels in the blind loop syndrome: Evaluation including a newly developed ^{14}C-amino acid breath test. Gastroenterology 1976; 70:901.
24. Rutgeerts L, Mainguet P, Tytgat G, Eggermont E. Enterokinase in contaminated small-bowel syndrome. Digestion 1974; 10:249–54.
25. Giannella RA, Rout WR, Toskes PP. Jejunal brush border injury and impaired sugar and amino acid uptake in the blind loop syndrome. Gastroenterology 1974; 67:965–74.
26. Toskes PP, Giannella RA, Jervis HR, Rout WR, Takeuchi A. Small intestinal mucosal injury in the experimental blind loop syndrome: light- and electron-microscopic and histochemical studies. Gastroenterology 1975; 68:1193–1203.
27. King CE, Toskes PP. Protein-losing enteropathy in the human and experimental rat blind-loop syndrome. Gastroenterology 1981; 80:504–9.
28. Baraona E, Pirola RC, Lieber CS. Small intestinal damage and changes in cell population produced by ethanol ingestion in the rat. Gastroenterology 1974; 66:226–34.
29. Teem MV, Phillips SF. Perfusion of the hamster jejunum with conjugated and unconjugated bile acids: Inhibition of water absorption and effects on morphology. Gastroenterology 1972; 62:261–7.
30. Prizont R, Whitehead JS, Kim YS. Short chain fatty acids in rats with jejunal blind loops. I. Analysis of SCFA in small intestine, cecum, feces, and plasma. Gastroenterology 1975; 69:1254–64.
31. Justus PG, Fernandez A, Martin JL, King CE, Toskes PP, Mathias JR. Altered myoelectric activity in the experimental blind loop syndrome. J Clin Invest 1983; 72:1064–71.
32. Donaldson RM Jr. Normal bacterial populations of the intestine and their relation to intestinal function. N Engl J Med 1964; 270:938–45, 994–1001, 1050–6.
33. Goldman P, Peppercorn MA, Goldin BR. Metabolism of drugs by microorganisms in the intestine. Am J Clin Nutr 1974; 27:1348–55.
34. Gracey M, Papadimitriou J, Burke V, Thomas J, Bower G. Effects on small-intestinal function and structure induced by feeding a deconjugated bile salt. Gut 1973; 14:519–28.

35. Jonas A, Krishnan C, Forstner G. Pathogenesis of mucosal injury in the blind loop syndrome: Release of disaccharidases from brush border membranes by extracts of bacteria obtained from intestinal blind loops in rats. Gastroenterology 1978; 75:791–5.
36. Riepe S, Goldstein J, Alpers DH. Effect of secreted Bacteroides proteases on human intestinal brush border hydrolases. J Clin Invest 1980; 66:314–22.
37. Hoffbrand AV, Tabaqchali S, Booth CC, Mollin DL. Small intestinal bacterial flora and folate status in gastrointestinal disease. Gut 1971; 12:27–33.
38. Schjonsby H. Osteomalacia in the stagnant loop syndrome. Acta Med Scand 1977; 603(Suppl):39–41.
39. Levy NS, Toskes PP. Fundus albipunctatus and vitamin A deficiency. Am J Ophthalmol 1974; 78:926–9.
40. Rosenberg IH, Hardison WG, Bull DM. Abnormal bile-salt patterns and intestinal bacterial overgrowth associated with malabsorption. N Engl J Med 1967; 276:1391–7.
41. Egger G, Kessler JI. Clinical experience with a simple test for the detection of bacterial deconjugation of bile salts and the site and extent of bacterial overgrowth in the small intestine. Gastroenterology 1973; 64:545–51.
42. Greenberger NJ, Saegh S, Ruppert KD. Urine indican excretion in malabsorptive disorders. Gastroenterology 1968; 55:204–11.
43. King CE, Toskes PP. The use of breath tests in the study of malabsorption. Clin Gastroenterol 1983; 12:591–610.
44. Pedersen L, Arnfred T, Hess Thaysen E. Rapid screening of increased bile acid deconjugation and bile acid malabsorption by means of the glycine-1-[^{14}C] cholylglycine assay. Scand J Gastroenterol 1973; 8:665–72.
45. Metz G, Gassull MA, Drasar BS, Jenkins DJA, Blendis LM. Breath-hydrogen test for small-intestinal bacterial colonisation. Lancet 1976; 1:668–9.
46. Lauterburg BH, Newcomer AD, Hofmann AF. Clinical value of the bile acid breath test: Evaluation of the Mayo Clinic experience. Mayo Clinic Proc 1978; 53:227–33.
47. King CE, Toskes PP, Guilarte TR, Lorenz E, Welkos S. Comparison of the one-gram d-[^{14}C] xylose breath test to the [^{14}C] bile acid breath test in patients with small intestine bacterial overgrowth. Dig Dis Sci 1980; 25:53–8.
48. Tillman CR, King CE, Toskes PP. Continued experience with the xylose breath test: Evidence that the small bowel culture as the gold standard for bacterial overgrowth may be tarnished. Gastroenterology 1981; 80:1304.
49. King CE, Toskes PP, Guilarte TR, Brookeman VA, Fitzgerald LT, Staley G. Safety of the ^{14}C-d-xylose and ^{14}C-cholylglycine (bile acid) breath tests: Elimination and tissue retention studies. Clin Res 1980; 28:483.
50. Solomons NW, Schoeller DA, Wagonfeld JB, Ott D, Rosenberg IH, Klein PD Application of a stable isotope (^{13}C)-labeled glycocholate breath test to diagnosis of bacterial overgrowth and ileal dysfunction. J Lab Clin Med 1977; 90:431–9.
51. King CE, Toskes PP, Ahmed EP, Harty ER. The 80 gram glucose-H_2 breath test: A quick alternative to the urine xylose screening test. Gastroenterology 1983; 84:1208.
52. Bond JH, Levitt MD. Use of pulmonary hydrogen (H_2) measurements to quantitate carbohydrate absorption. Study of partially gastrectomized patients. J Clin Invest 1972; 51:1219–25.
53. Rhodes JM, Middleton P, Jewell DP. The lactulose hydrogen breath test as a diagnostic test for small-bowel bacterial overgrowth. Scand J Gastroenterol 1979; 14:333–6.

Chapter 108

The Short Bowel Syndrome

Elliot Weser • Ernest Urban

Recent advances in anesthetic and surgical techniques have increased the survival of patients after extensive loss of intestine. This, in addition to extensive use of jejuno-ileal bypass for the treatment of obesity, has substantially increased the number of persons living with a short bowel. Proper management of these individuals is based on a thorough understanding of the pathophysiology of the shortened gastrointestinal tract.

Pathophysiology

Malabsorption. The immediate consequence of small bowel resection is a reduction of the mucosal surface that can participate in the absorption of luminal contents. Transit time through the shortened intestine is also likely to be reduced. This decreases contact time between the mucosal surface and the luminal content and thereby further contributes to maldigestion and malabsorption of nutrients. Fortunately, the small intestine has a large functional reserve. From 40% to 50% of the small bowel may be removed without major impairment of normal nutrition. However, as will be discussed later, the anatomic site of excised intestine is an important factor. The minimum length of small intestine necessary to sustain life with oral nutrition is not known. Occasional reports have appeared of extended survival after almost total loss of small bowel.[1,2] Resection of the middle-small intestine or loss of the jejunum is much better tolerated than loss of either the duodenum or the terminal ileum. In the latter instance, an accompanying loss of the ileocecal valve is an additional detrimental factor. Major factors that determine metabolic sequelae after small bowel resection are listed in Table 108–1.

Normally, the digestion and absorption of fat, protein, carbohydrate, minerals, and water-soluble vitamins, except vitamin B_{12}, occur in the duodenum and jejunum. The ileum largely represents functional reserve capacity.[3] Extensive loss of the upper small bowel, however, will concomitantly reduce cholecystokinin and secretin synthesis and release, thus decreasing hormonal stimulation of biliary and exocrine pancreatic secretions.

Loss of ileum is associated with greater metabolic deficits than loss of an equivalent length of jejunum. The ileum is the prime site for active reabsorption of conjugated bile salts, for absorption of the intrinsic factor–vitamin B_{12} complex, and possibly also for the reabsorption of hydroxy vitamin D metabolites that are excreted in bile. Studies in man and animals have shown some compensatory increases in absorption of bile salts and vitamin B_{12} by increased diffusion across the remnant jejunum.[4–6] There may also be induction of active bile salt transport in the remnant jejunum as well as the ileum.[4,5] Compensatory increase in the hepatic synthesis of bile salts occurs, but this is limited.[7] Loss of bile salts by lack of ileal reabsorption may therefore lead to a *reduction in the size of the circulating pool of bile salts* with consequent decreased small bowel luminal bile salt con-

Table 108–1. MAJOR FACTORS DETERMINING METABOLIC SEQUELAE AFTER SMALL BOWEL RESECTION

Extent of intestine resected
Anatomic site of resected intestine
Presence or absence of ileocecal valve
Functional capacities of remaining small and large bowel
Functional adaptations occurring in remaining small and large bowel
Functional capacities of the liver, gallbladder, and pancreas

centrations, reduced bile salt micelle formation, and reduced absorption of water-insoluble 2-monoglycerides, 1-lysophospholipids, fatty acids, and the fat-soluble vitamins (A, D, E, and K). Unabsorbed fats and conjugated bile salts consequently enter the large bowel in increased quantities. Bacterial action on these substrates results in the formation of hydroxy fatty acids and deconjugation of bile salts. Both interfere with water and electrolyte absorption from the large bowel,[8,9] leading to diarrhea in addition to steatorrhea.

Loss of less than 100 cm of distal ileum usually results in appreciable *diarrhea* together with modest *steatorrhea* (less than 20 g of fat/day). Both result primarily from the increased amounts of bile salts in the large bowel. Inasmuch as increased hepatic synthesis of bile salts largely compensates for the loss of bile salts from impaired absorption, steatorrhea is not prominent. More extensive ileal resections result in greater degrees of steatorrhea, as well as diarrhea, because of larger reductions in small bowel bile salt concentrations. Interruption of the enterohepatic recirculation of bile salts by intestinal resection also tends to increase the lithogenicity of bile. Inadequate absorption of *vitamin* B_{12} over a period of several years results in depletion of the body stores of the vitamin, and deficiency of vitamin B_{12} may alter intestinal mucosal cell morphology and transport functions.[10]

Malabsorption of the *fat-soluble vitamins* increases with increasing steatorrhea, and clinically evident signs of deficiencies of these vitamins may occur. Decreased serum 25-hydroxy vitamin D levels have been described in patients after intestinal resection and are attributed both to vitamin D malabsorption and to inadequate intake.[11] Quantitative enterohepatic circulation of the hydroxy products of vitamin D metabolism may also play an important role. Following the IV injection of tritiated 25-hydroxy vitamin D, significant amounts of the material appeared in intestinal aspirates of experimental animals and normal human volunteers.[12,13]

Surgical extirpation of the ileocecal valve in conjunction with the distal ileum (often together with partial colectomy) may further increase diarrhea. There are several mechanisms by which this may occur. Increased *bacterial contamination* of the already shortened small bowel may ensue,[14,15] and deconjugation of luminal bile salts in the contiguous small bowel remnant by the bacteria follows. Consequently, there is further decrease in the active reabsorption of conjugated bile salts, and increased quantities of both conjugated and already deconjugated bile salts enter the large bowel. Fat malabsorption also increases as a result of these actions.

Bacterial contamination of the remnant small bowel may result in significant bacterial metabolism of luminal vitamin B_{12}, reducing its absorption and increasing the likelihood of vitamin B_{12} deficiency. In addition, there are experimental data showing that an intact ileocecal valve prolongs transit time of small bowel luminal contents,[16] thereby potentially increasing mucosal contact time for nutrient absorption. Loss of this valve negates these effects.

The large bowel is not only important for the storage of small bowel effluent but is also an important organ for the conservation of *water* and *sodium*. Partial (or total) colectomy, which may accompany excision of the ileocecal valve, contributes to diarrhea, dehydration, hypovolemia, and electrolyte depletion. Following combined resection of the ileum and large bowel, fecal electrolytes bear a closer relationship to the length of residual large bowel than to the length of residual small bowel.[17] Additionally, preservation of increasing lengths of large bowel correlates with prolongation of total intestinal transit time.[17] Clearly, therefore, the clinical importance of the large bowel in the maintenance of fluid and electrolyte balances *cannot be overemphasized*.[18]

The large bowel is also a major site for the absorption of soluble luminal *oxalate*.[19] Normally, almost all dietary oxalate reacts with calcium within the lumen of the small bowel to form highly insoluble calcium oxalate that is not absorbed. In patients with steatorrhea, luminal calcium is sequestered by preferentially binding with unabsorbed fats and fatty acids. All patients with significant steatorrhea or with ileal disease and an intact large bowel are at risk for the absorption of an increased amount of dietary oxalate, which is then excreted in the urine.

Even though the maximum rate of absorption of *iron, calcium* and *magnesium* occurs in the duodenum, significant quantities of these ions are absorbed in the jejunum and ileum because of their greater surface area and the longer contact time between mucosa and luminal contents. Thus, extensive removal of the upper and/or lower small bowel may result in deficient absorption of these ions and consequent clinical symptoms and signs. Intestinal calcium transport is enhanced by metabolites of vitamin D. As already indicated, reduced serum levels of 25-hydroxy vitamin D have been described in patients with a short bowel.[11] In the presence of steatorrhea, luminal magnesium, as well as calcium, will bind with unabsorbed fatty acids to form insoluble soaps, thereby further decreasing their absorption. Negative metabolic balances of these ions and bone disease have been described in patients with a short bowel.[20]

Zinc and other *trace metal* concentrations in serum are not yet routinely measured in clinical situations. However, deficiencies of these substrates are likely to be present as a consequence of sequestering by combining in the intestine with unabsorbed fatty acids.[20] Limited data on serum zinc and copper concentrations after intestinal bypass surgery (for obesity) have been published.[21] It should be noted that zinc is an essential constituent of many enzyme systems and is necessary for protein synthesis.[22] Both appetite and taste are also impaired by zinc deficiency.[23]

Deficiencies of *water-soluble vitamins* (except vitamin B_{12}) and folate have been described infrequently in patients with a short bowel, probably because adequate absorption continues in all except those with minimal residual small bowel. *Folate* is of particular interest. It is normally absorbed in the proximal small intestine after deconjugation of dietary folates (primarily pteroylpolyglutamates) by the mucosa to pteroylmonoglutamates. Presumably, adequate compensatory deconjugation and transport occur. Conservation of body folate stores is undoubtedly enhanced by a quantitatively significant enterohepatic recirculation.[24] Folate deficiency in rats depresses the mucosal transport of water and electrolytes sufficiently to produce diarrhea[25] but this does not appear to have been described in man.

Massive gastric hypersecretion has been documented in some, but not all, patients shortly after extensive small bowel resection.[2, 26] The hypersecretion tends to lessen with time, and the length of small bowel lost roughly correlates with the degree of hypersecretion.[26] In man and in experimental animals, *serum gastrin levels are elevated* after intestinal resection.[27] This may result from decreased gastrin catabolism because of a reduced small bowel mass. Hormonal inhibitors of gastrin action such as secretin, cholecystokinin, and possibly other hormones (vasoactive intestinal polypeptide, gastric inhibitory peptide, enteroglucagon) may also play a role. In addition, intestinal resection results in concomitant trophic changes in the stomach, including an increased parietal cell mass.[28] The large volume of gastric juice so produced increases the volume of luminal content in the remaining bowel, diluting luminal pancreatic enzymes and bile salts and increasing peristalsis. A reduction of pH in the lumen of remnant small bowel will additionally impair the function of pancreatic enzymes in the hydrolysis of starches, protein, and fats. Bile salt micelle formation will also be inhibited. Consequently, diarrhea, steatorrhea, and peptic ulceration in the stomach, duodenum, and/or remaining small bowel, as well as breakdown of surgical anastomoses, may occur. The overall effects of post-resection gastric hypersecretion are similar to those of a patient with the Zollinger-Ellison syndrome compounded by a shortened gastrointestinal tract.

Transient increases of exocrine pancreatic secretion have been reported in laboratory animals after extensive small bowel resection,[29] but this phenomenon seems not to have been described in man. In the long term, loss of pancreatic secretory stimuli stemming from reduction in sites of cholecystokinin and secretin production could be expected to lead to *reduced pancreatic exocrine secretion*. In addition, exocrine pancreatic secretion may also be greatly reduced in the severely malnourished patient.[30] An enteropancreatic recirculation of pancreatic digestive enzymes has been postulated as the cause, but its quantitative functional significance remains in considerable doubt.[31] In experimental animals, luminal trypsin and chymotrypsin do alter pancreatic exocrine secretion, possibly by feedback inhibition.[32]

It is evident from the foregoing that malabsorption of dietary carbohydrates and proteins, in addition to fats, occurs frequently after intestinal resection and may be severe. Exogenous dietary proteins supply the amino acids necessary for albumin synthesis by the liver. Maldigestion of dietary proteins with consequent malabsorption of peptides and amino acids impairs hepatic albumin synthesis within hours.[33] The *hypoalbuminemia* may result in edema, and a kwashiorkor-like state may occur if protein-calorie malnutrition is severe enough.

Loss of small bowel is also associated with loss of brush border *disaccharidases*. This may impair luminal hydrolysis of disaccharides. Lactase is the disaccharidase most affected. Hence, ingestion of lactose in the diet may increase small bowel effluent into the colon, where bacteria ferment the undigested lactose to lactic acid. The resultant bloating, gas, and osmotic diarrhea may add appreciably to the patient's discomfort.

Intestinal adaptation is discussed subsequently, but special comment must be made here about the functional state of the remaining small and large bowel. This is of great importance in determining long-term survival, complications, and the quality of life of the patient with a short bowel. Functionally impaired or diseased intestine, such as that associated with Crohn's disease, radiation enteritis, celiac sprue, and Whipple's disease, may magnify nutrient malabsorption and increase the difficulty in maintaining adequate nutrition orally.

Intestinal Adaptation. An important element in the maintenance of nutrient absorption is adaptation of the remaining gastrointestinal tract after small bowel resection. Both morphologic and functional adaptations have been extensively studied in the large and small bowel of animals, particularly the rat.[3, 34] Controlled studies of adaptive changes in man, however, have been few and mostly indirect. The changes in man seem to bear a relationship to events in experimental animals, but total translation of animal data to man cannot be presumed. Sporadic reports in man have described dilatation of the remnant bowel[1] and, in the few studies in which proximal intestinal biopsies have been obtained, villus hyperplasia (increase in cell numbers) has been described.[35] Unlike animal studies, there was no apparent associated villus enlargement, although precise 3-dimensional morphologic studies are lacking. However, increases in villus height, particularly in the ileum, have been described, in addition to elongation of the functioning jejuno-ileum left in continuity after jejuno-ileal bypass operation for obesity.[36] The mucosal response also appears to be cellular hyperplasia and not hypertrophy. Infants and children seem to have a more favorable prognosis after bowel resection as compared with adults.[1,5] Presumably this is related to the greater potential for growth and development at that period of life.

Functional changes occur in association with the morphologic mucosal changes. In man, an obvious clinical change is gradual reduction in post-operative diarrhea or a lessening of ileostomy output. This implies functional adaptive increased water and electrolyte absorption in the remnant large and small bowel, as well as improved nutrient absorption by the small bowel. Segmental glucose absorption is increased,[37] and vitamin B_{12} absorption has been shown to adapt.[6] Gradual improvement in nitrogen balance and in fat and carbohydrate absorption has also been documented.[2]

Functional adaptation has been extensively studied in animals. Increased segmental absorption (nutrient absorption/cm intestine) in remnant bowel has been described for fat, protein, glucose, galactose, sucrose, maltose, sodium, water, bile acids, vitamin B_{12}, calcium, and zinc.[3, 34, 38, 39] The enhanced absorption may be proportional to mucosal growth, or may increase relatively more, or absorption may even decrease in spite of increased mucosal mass. Metabolic and enzyme changes have been described in the mucosa of experimental animals after intestinal resection. Specific activities (enzyme/unit weight of mucosa) may increase (Na-K-ATPase, peptide hydrolase, enterokinase, pentose phosphatase shunt enzymes, pyrimidine biosynthetic enzymes) or may be unchanged or decrease (disaccharidases, glycolytic enzymes, lipid esterifying enzymes, adenyl cyclase). It is thus apparent that morphologic and functional (transport) components of intestinal adaptation after bowel resection may occur as separate events, at least in experimental animals. This implies that different factors may regulate morphologic and functional adaptations, albeit that these factors may be sequentially interrelated for optimum responses to nutritional demands.

Mechanisms underlying adaptive changes are unclear, but are under intense study. An understanding of these mechanisms can be expected to lead to therapeutically useful maneuvers for stimulating mucosal growth and function. Table 108–2 lists possible mechanisms that affect adaptive changes.

Elevation of serum gastrin levels has al-

Table 108–2. MECHANISMS OF INTESTINAL ADAPTATION AFTER SMALL BOWEL RESECTION

Trophic effects of mucosal nutrient absorption
Trophic effects of growth factor in villi (chalone) released by luminal nutrients
Direct trophic effects by intestinal hormones released in response to intraluminal nutrients
Trophic effects of pancreatic secretions and bile salts
Trophic effects of neurovascular changes

ready been mentioned. In experimental animals, gastrin has trophic effects on gastric epithelium. DNA synthesis is stimulated, and the depth of gastric fundic glands and number of parietal cells are increased. Except for the duodenum, there is no effect on small bowel. Large bowel mucosa, however, responds to gastrin stimulation.[28, 40] Other enteric hormones have also been examined for trophism. Continuous IV infusion of cholecystokinin, together with secretin, has been observed to prevent the intestinal hypoplasia associated with total parenteral nutrition in animals with an intact intestine.[41] Chronic glucagon administration has been associated with increased transport of glucose and amino acids, and adaptive responses to starvation in rats may be inhibited by administering antiserum to glucagon.[42] In one human patient, the villus hyperplasia found in association with an enteroglucagon-secreting tumor reverted to normal following resection of the tumor.[43] Unfortunately, this morphologic growth effect has not been reproducible by the administration of exogenous glucagon.[41]

Nutrients in the lumen of the small intestine are essential for the maintenance of mucosal mass. Not only starvation, but also total parenteral nutrition with positive caloric balance, results in mucosal hypoplasia in man and experimental animals. An increase of luminal non-nutrient bulk (kaolin) in the diet does not cause mucosal growth in the small bowel, but the weight of the large bowel increases.[44] There is impressive evidence, at least in experimental animals, that active nutrient absorption of glucose and selected amino acids plays an important role in small bowel mucosal growth.[45, 46] The diarrhea that sometimes follows reintroduction of oral feedings after either starvation or total parenteral nutrition, and that improves with time, is in part attributable to mucosal hypoplasia and subsequent regrowth.

Bile and pancreatic secretions have been examined for trophic effects.[47] These secretions, which themselves contain small amounts of nutrients, may be stimulated by food in the intestinal lumen or by the IV administration of cholecystokinin and secretin. It has therefore been difficult to exclude a specific growth factor in these secretions.

Evidence suggests that there may also be an intrinsic feedback mechanism controlling the mass of intestinal mucosa. Through the operation of this mechanism, the number of functional villus cells regulates cell proliferation and maturation.[48] This suggests that an inhibitory substance (chalone) may exist in the villi that affects crypt cells.[49]

Neurovascular factors may play an as yet unclear role in intestinal adaptation. An early increase of ileal blood flow after proximal resection has been described in rats;[50] adrenergic denervation present in the remnant bowel has been associated with transiently decreased blood flow.[51] In another study, infusion of norepinephrine was associated with increased crypt cell proliferation.[52] In the rat, vagotomy and pyloroplasty result in intestinal hypoplasia followed by increased cell turnover.[53]

Unraveling these events, which must somehow all be interrelated, continues to stimulate investigative studies. As indicated earlier, clarification will most likely have important and substantial therapeutic impact.

Clinical Features

The severity of clinical findings depends on the extent and site of the small bowel resected. This may be evaluated by measuring vitamin B_{12} absorption or by the use of a bile acid breath test. Small bowel radiographs may also be useful in determining the length of remaining intestine. In addition to revealing the amount of residual gut, they often show some adaptive dilatation (Fig. 108–1). Patients with limited resections of the ileum and ileocecal junction (representing less than 30% of the total bowel length) may nevertheless have significant diarrhea and steatorrhea primarily related to the interruption of the enterohepatic circulation of bile acids and the effects of bile acids in the colon.

In patients with more extensive bowel resection, a significant decrease in absorption of all nutrients may occur. Calorie deprivation due to malabsorption usually produces

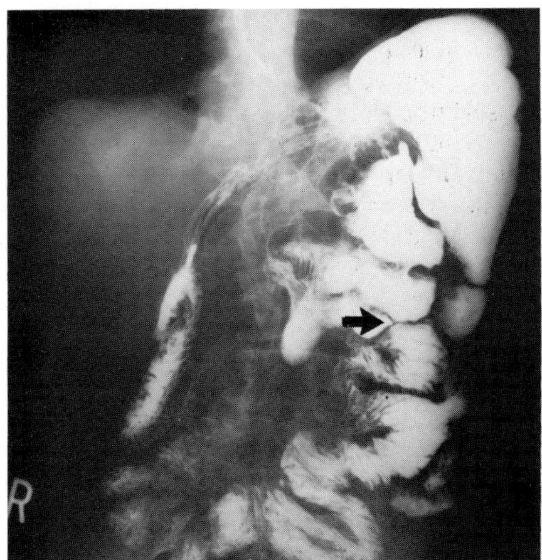

Figure 108–1. Barium study showing a surgically displaced duodeum, residual proximal jejunum, and a jejuno-transverse colostomy *(arrow)*. The patient was a 67-year-old man who underwent subtotal small bowel resection (preserving 2 feet of jejunum) and a right hemicolectomy for extensive radiation enteritis. One year previously he had an incomplete resection of a squamous cell carcinoma of the anus and irradiation of the pelvis and sacrum (6000 rads). (Courtesy of Dr. Theodore Hopens.)

severe *weight loss, lassitude, weakness,* and *fatigue* in addition to *frequent stools* daily. These and other findings are similar to the pan-malabsorption caused by other diseases of the small intestine, such as celiac disease (Chapter 105) and Whipple's disease (Chapter 109). As previously stated, malabsorption of vitamin D, calcium, and protein may in time produce metabolic bone disease (*osteomalacia* and *osteoporosis*) causing *bone pain* and *spontaneous fractures. Hypocalcemia* and *hypomagnesemia* are not uncommon and may be accompanied by tetany or carpopedal spasm. The loss of vitamin K in the stools eventually may cause significant defects in blood coagulation and result in *purpura, ecchymosis,* or *generalized bleeding. Peripheral neuropathy* and *edema* may occur secondary to B complex vitamin deficiency and hypoalbuminemia, respectively. *Anemia* is common and may be related to combined deficiencies of folic acid, vitamin B_{12}, and particularly iron, if part of the duodenum was included in the resected bowel.

In the weeks to several months following extensive small bowel resection, *gastric hypersecretion* may complicate the clinical picture. This not only may cause peptic ulcer disease but, as indicated previously, may contribute to the steatorrhea. Fortunately, gastric hypersecretion tends to be a transient phenomenon, and gastric secretion generally returns to normal after the early period following massive resection.[26]

The loss of ileum with subsequent depletion of the bile salt pool produces lithogenic bile, so that the incidence of *gallstones* in these patients may be about 3-fold greater than in the normal population.[54, 55]

Some patients with ileal or more extensive small bowel resection absorb increased amounts of oxalate from their diet. As noted earlier, this may depend upon the degree of steatorrhea, calcium sequestration, and the presence of the colon, the site where much of the oxalate is absorbed. The increase in oxalate absorption results in hyperoxaluria, which in time may produce *calcium oxalate stones* in the kidneys.[19, 56] Patients with significant steatorrhea and an ileostomy have a decreased risk of oxalate nephrolithiasis.[57]

Other complications may arise secondary to intestinal bacteria. Overgrowth of bacteria in the remaining small bowel lumen may increase the malabsorption of fat and vitamin B_{12}. The absence of the ileocecal valve more readily permits this intraluminal bacterial proliferation. Finally, bacterial fermentation of unabsorbed nutrients in the large bowel has also been postulated as the mechanism responsible for D-*lactic acidosis* in association with *neurologic manifestations.*[58]

Laboratory Findings

Abnormal laboratory findings in the short bowel syndrome might be anticipated from the losses of large volumes of intestinal fluids and electrolytes, as well as from the changes associated with pan-malabsorption. *Hypokalemia* and *depleted sodium and water states* are common. Excessive losses of fecal *calcium* and *magnesium* may be reflected by corresponding low serum concentrations of these cations. Increasing *steatorrhea* is found with increasing oral food intake, indicating unabsorbed fat of dietary origin. Low serum *prothrombin time* and *carotene* concentrations are common, as are *vitamin* B_{12} and *iron deficiency anemias,* unless these nutrients are adequately replaced. Impairment of protein absorption may eventually produce *hypoalbuminemia.* Sugar absorption tests are normally abnormal (low), whether D-*xylose absorption* or a disaccharide such as *lactose* is used as the substrate.

Treatment

Principles of treatment are outlined in Table 108–3 and logically follow an understanding of the pathophysiology of the short bowel. In patients with Crohn's disease and multiple small bowel resections, residual inflammation of the remaining bowel may further contribute to impaired absorption. If such inflammation is present, treatment with sulfasalazine and steroids should be instituted (Chapter 127 [Medical Management]).

Dietotherapy. The approach to treatment may be considered under the categories of nutritional or dietary manipulations and drug usage. In the acute period immediately following resection, patients will benefit from

Table 108–3. TREATMENT OF SHORT BOWEL SYNDROME

Diet	Drugs	Ancillary
1. Total parenteral nutrition (perioperative period)	1. Antidiarrheal agents:	1. Treat primary bowel disease (Crohn's, enteric pathogens, etc.)
	Codeine sulfate, 30–60 mg, up to 4 times daily	
2. Enteral nutrition:	Diphenoxylate hydrochloride, up to 20 mg daily in divided doses	2. Colonic infusion of electrolytes
Formula defined diets, medium chain triglycerides	Loperamide hydrochloride, 4–16 mg daily in divided doses	3. Surgical
Low saturated fat diets; try a liberal fat allowance	Deodorized tincture of opium, 10 drops, 2 or 3 times daily	
Low lactose diet; try low sucrose diet; try increased starch	2. Anticholinergic drugs:	
Low oxalate diet	Propantheline bromide, 30 mg, 2 or 3 times daily	
3. Vitamin supplementation:	Dicyclomine hydrochloride, 10–20 mg, 3 or 4 times daily	
Fat soluble:	3. H_2-blocking agents:	
Vitamin A, 25,000–50,000 IU daily; in severe deficiency, larger doses (e.g., 50,000–200,000 IU) may be necessary for short periods of time	Cimetidine, 300–600 mg, 4 times daily (adjust dosage to individual requirements)	
Vitamin D, 30,000–50,000 USP daily, depending upon initial deficiency; maintenance dose must be carefully determined for each patient and hypercalcemia avoided	Ranitidine, 150 mg, 2 or more times daily up to 6 g/day (adjust to individual requirements)	
Vitamin K (Menadione, USP), 4–12 mg daily; vitamin K_1 (Mephyton), 5–10 mg daily	4. Cholestyramine, 4–16 g daily	
Water soluble:	5. Broad-spectrum antibiotics (in divided doses, 7–14 days):	
B complex (any preparation containing the daily requirements); use 2–3 tablets daily (or equivalent in a liquid preparation)	Tetracycline, 1 g daily	
Vitamin C, 500 mg daily	Ampicillin, 2–4 g daily	
Folic acid, 5–10 mg daily	Kanamycin, 2–4 g daily	
Vitamin B_{12} (by injection), 100–1000 μg monthly	Neomycin, 1–3 g daily	
4. Mineral supplementation:	6. Pancreatic enzyme replacement:	
Calcium gluconate, 3–15 g daily	Pancrelipase (USP), 3–4 capsules during each meal (12–16 capsules daily as tolerated)	
Magnesium sulfate, 1–6 g daily (may worsen diarrhea)	Pancrease (enteric-coated microspheres of pancrelipase), 1–3 capsules during each meal	
Ferrous gluconate or sulfate, 1.8 g daily	Pancreatin, 3–4 tablets during each meal (12–16 tablets daily as tolerated)	
Zinc sulfate, 110–220 mg daily		

total parenteral nutrition and, if the resection is extensive, may not be able to undergo a rapid transition to full oral nutrition. Intestinal adaptation may require weeks or months before absorption of orally ingested nutrients can take place sufficient to supply the energy needs of the patient. In those patients with less extensive resections, usually those with a remaining long jejunal segment, enteral feedings may be well tolerated in rapid fashion.

Enteral nutrients may be started within the first week following surgery. However, parenteral nutrition should be continued until it is apparent that the patient can be sustained by the intraluminal route. Defined formula diets have been useful in implementing enteral feeding programs. These preparations have either low concentrations of or no long chain triglycerides; calories also otherwise provided through a mixture of essential amino acids, carbohydrates (usually glucose), balanced electrolytes, and other nutrients, including medium chain triglycerides.[59] Inasmuch as minimal digestion is necessary, they are theoretically better absorbed in a smaller length of intestine than regular food would be. These formulas are relatively unpalatable, however, because of their low fat content and are therefore usually administered through a small nasogastric tube. Since these solutions are hyperosmolar in full strength, they may be poorly tolerated and cause vomiting or diarrhea. Hence, they are usually initially diluted to one-fourth or one-third strength and given by slow, continuous drip over a 24-hour period; solution strength is increased in stepwise fashion.

In some patients with all or part of the colon bypassed (in addition to small bowel resection), colonic infusion of fluids and electrolytes may be useful in maintaining positive fluid and electrolyte balance, plasma volume, and normal renal function.[60]

As the patient progresses to eating more conventional foods, it has been considered useful to limit the dietary fat intake to less than 40 g/day. Absorption of fat is thought to remain severely impaired in patients with a short bowel, and ingestion of excessive quantities may result in substantial fecal losses of fluids and electrolytes (including calcium and magnesium). Recently, however, more liberal ingestion of dietary fat was shown not to be directly accompanied by such losses, and the patients overall were able to consume more calories.[61] Replacement of calcium and fat-soluble vitamin D is an important aspect of management, not only to treat or prevent hypocalcemia, but also to prevent the occurrence of metabolic bone disease. Magnesium deficiency usually responds to parenteral injections of magnesium sulfate or citrate, whereas oral magnesium therapy is often unsuccessful and may result in increased diarrhea. Measures that reduce the steatorrhea are likely to reduce the losses of magnesium in the stool. Losses of other fat-soluble vitamins may also lead to deficiencies and should be carefully monitored.

Moderate to severe steatorrhea may eventually produce vitamin K deficiency and hypoprothrombinemia, requiring periodic injections of vitamin K for correction. Although symptoms of vitamin A deficiency seem to be less common, impairment of retinal dark adaptation may cause overt symptoms or may be noted on careful eye examination. As intestinal adaptation occurs over a period of time, some improvement in fat absorption may take place and allow the patient to tolerate modest increases in dietary fat.

Water-soluble vitamins are usually sufficiently well absorbed to avoid significant deficiencies in patients with small bowel resection. These vitamins may be adequately absorbed in the ileum if the jejunum is absent. The need for substitute water-soluble vitamins is paramount, therefore, primarily in patients with extensive resections involving both the ileum and large amounts of jejunum. Large doses of *liquid oral vitamin preparations* are usually adequate to prevent or treat deficiencies of water-soluble vitamins. As noted earlier, vitamin B_{12} is actively absorbed in the ileum. Patients with ileal resection, usually greater than 6 to 8 feet, require periodic injections of *vitamin* B_{12}. Although massive oral doses of vitamin B_{12} may be absorbed by diffusion from bowel segments other than ileum, this absorption is variable and is not as reliable as that of the parenteral route. It may also be necessary to provide patients with *iron* and *calcium* supplements when the duodenum was bypassed or included in the small bowel resection, even though the extent of the resection was limited. Although these minerals are absorbed along the entire length of small bowel, their rates of absorption are maximal in the duodenum, and the absence of this segment may be just enough to cause inadequate absorption.

Patients with extensive small bowel resection may have insufficient intestinal lactase (and other disaccharidases) to hydrolyze dietary disaccharides adequately. In addition, rapid transit through the shortened bowel may increase the delivery of unabsorbed sugars to the colon, where bacterial metabolism can produce a fermentative diarrhea and contribute to the patient's symptoms. If the patient experiences symptoms of lactose intolerance (Chapter 104), *milk products should be limited.* This would additionally emphasize the need for *calcium* supplementation. In some instances, restriction of dietary sucrose and liberal allowances of starch in the form of carbohydrates have reduced jejunostomy and ileostomy fluid outputs.[62]

It was pointed out previously that some patients with a short bowel but with an intact colon may have hyperoxaluria and develop calcium oxalate kidney stones. Once on a stable diet, patients should have several determinations of 24-hour urinary *oxalate* excretion and, if elevated, should avoid foods high in oxalate (Table 108–4). *Calcium* supplementation will also help reduce oxalate absorption from the diet and reduce urinary oxalate excretion. However, excessive calcium excretion in the urine should be avoided. Although increased fluid ingestion to assure larger urinary volumes may additionally reduce the chances for developing oxalate kidney stones, it may also increase diarrhea. Whatever diet eventually proves satisfactory, the patient should be encouraged to divide his food intake into *multiple small feedings.* Large meals may exceed the absorptive capacity of remnant bowel and produce increased osmotic diarrhea.

Drug Therapy. A major goal of drug therapy is to reduce incapacitating diarrhea and permit the patient to pursue normal or near-normal activities. Effective doses of *codeine, diphenoxylate, loperamide,* and/or *anticholinergic agents* should be used to increase transit time. Liquid preparations are preferable to tablets because absorption seems more rapid or complete. Parenteral administration of anticholinergics may prove more effective than the oral route, and some patients have had successful control of their diarrhea by IM injections of propantheline.[62] Since bacterial colonization of the residual small bowel may contribute to the diarrhea (especially when the ileocecal junction is absent), courses of antibiotic therapy, such as tetracycline, ampicillin, or low doses of neomycin, may sufficiently alter the bacterial contamination to improve absorption. Bacterial culture of small bowel contents may help in selecting the appropriate initial antibiotic. A properly selected antibiotic, given for 7 to 14 days, may improve diarrhea for many weeks. Should gastric hypersecretion be present, It_2 blockers such as *cimetidine* or *ranitidine* would seem preferable to antacids and/or anticholinergic agents to control both gastric volume and acid secretion.[63, 64] Adequate doses of *pancrelipase or other pancreatic supplements* with high lipase activity, given with meals, may be useful in reducing steatorrhea. The rationale for their use is the possibility of a relative pancreatic enzyme deficiency due to inactivation or dilution of pancreatic enzymes by excessive gastric secretions, faulty stimulation of pancreatic secretion, or inadequate mixing of enzymes with ingested food.

Patients with ileal resections limited to less than 100 cm may show improvement in bile acid–induced diarrhea after treatment with *cholestyramine,* 8 to 12 g daily.[65] Cholestyramine binds unabsorbed bile acids and prevents their secretory effects in the colon. In more extensive resections, where diarrhea is additionally caused by the secretory action of hydroxy fatty acids and the osmotic effects of unabsorbed nutrients, cholestyramine is not usually helpful. By sequestering bile acids in these patients, cholestyramine may further reduce the bile acid pool and actually worsen the diarrhea and steatorrhea. Cholestyramine may also be useful in binding dietary oxalate; this decreases its absorption and leads to a reduction in urinary oxalate excretion.

Other measures have been tried in patients who respond poorly to dietary and drug management. *Surgical reversal of a bowel seg-*

Table 108–4. FOODS RELATIVELY HIGH IN OXALATE

Vegetables:
Beets, beetgreens, artichokes, green onions, parsley, okra, spinach, endive, chard, sweet potatoes, yams, sweet and green peppers, carrots, celery, rhubarb, wax beans
Fruits:
Plums, strawberries, concord grapes, raspberries, oranges, gooseberries, red currants, cranberries, blackberries, figs
Miscellaneous:
Tea, cocoa, chocolate, many cola beverages

ment or *creation of a recirculating bowel loop* has been used to improve absorption, either by increasing transit time or continuously recycling nutrients in a loop of bowel. These efforts are rarely beneficial and often produce bowel obstruction. However, re-anastomosis in continuity with any excluded intestine (small bowel or colon) may prove helpful by increasing absorption.

An increasing number of patients have been successfully managed with *long-term parenteral nutrition at home*[66] (Chapter 235). Nutrient solutions that provide all the caloric requirements of the patient are infused into an indwelling Silastic catheter inserted into the superior vena cava. Adequate provision of vitamins, trace minerals, and essential fatty acids is necessary. With increasing sophistication of this technique, special vests containing an infusion pump and solutions can be worn during the day, allowing the patient to pursue routine activities while the parenteral nutrient solution is infused. Even though there is risk of septic or thrombotic complications, this is an important development in the management of patients who cannot be adequately sustained by intraluminal nutrition.

References

1. Anderson C. Long term survival with six inches of small intestine. Br Med J 1965; 1:419–22.
2. Winawar SJ, Broitman SA, Wolochow DA, Osborne MP, Zamcheck N. Successful management of massive small bowel resection based on assessment of absorption defects and nutritional needs. N Engl J Med 1966; 274:72–8.
3. Williamson RCN. Medical progress: Intestinal adaptation. Part 1. Structural, functional and cytokinetic changes. Part 2. Mechanisms of control. N Engl J Med 1978; 298:1383–1402 and 1444–50.
4. Tilson DM, Boyer JL, Wright HK. Jejunal absorption of bile salts after resection of the ileum. Surgery 1975; 77:231–4.
5. Heubi JE, Balistreri WF, Partin JC, Schubert WK, Sucky FJ. Enterohepatic circulation of bile acids in infants and children with ileal resection. J Lab Clin Med 1980; 95:231–40.
6. Mackinnon AM, Short MD, Elias E, Dowling RH. Adaptive changes in vitamin B_{12} absorption in celiac disease and after proximal small bowel resection in man. Am J Dig Dis 1975; 20:835–40.
7. Ho KJ, Bondi JL. Cholesterol metabolism in patients with resection of ileum and proximal colon. Am J Clin Nutr 1977; 30:151–9.
8. Ammon HV, Phillips SF. Inhibition of colonic water and electrolyte absorption by fatty acids in man. Gastroenterology 1973; 65:774–9.
9. Mekhjian HS, Phillips SF, Hofman AF. Colonic secretion of water and electrolytes induced by bile acids: Perfusion studies in man. J Clin Invest 1971; 50:1569–77.
10. Arvanitakis C. Functional and morphologic abnormalities of the small intestinal mucosa in pernicious anemia. Acta Hepato-Gastroenterol 1978; 25:313–8.
11. Compston JE, Creamer B. Plasma levels and intestinal absorption of 25-hydroxy vitamin D in patients with small bowel resection. Gut 1977; 18:171–5.
12. Kumar R, Nagubandi S, Mattox VR, Londowsky JM. Enterohepatic physiology of 1,25-dihydroxy vitamin D_3. J Clin Invest 1980; 65:277–84.
13. Arnaud SB, Goldsmith RS, Lambert PW, Go VLW. 25-Hydroxy vitamin D_3. Evidence of an enterohepatic circulation in man. Proc Soc Exp Biol Med 1975; 149:570–2.
14. Isaacs PET, Kim YS. The contaminated small bowel syndrome. Am J Med 1979; 67:1049–57.
15. Simon GL, Gorbach SL. Intestinal microflora. Med Clin North Am 1982; 66:563–7.
16. Gazet JC, Kopp J. Surgical significance of ileo-cecal junction. Surgery 1964; 56:565–73.
17. Cummins JH, James WPT, Wiggins HS. Role of the colon in ileal-resection diarrhea. Lancet 1973; 1:344–7.
18. Mitchel JE, Breuer RI, Zuckerman L, Berlin J, Schilli R, Dunn JK. The colon influences ileal resection diarrhea. Dig Dis Sci 1980; 25:33–41.
19. Earnest DL. Enteric hyperoxaluria. *In*: Stollerman GH, ed. Advances in Internal Medicine. Chicago: Year Book Medical Publishers, 1978; 24:407–27.
20. Ladefoged K, Nicolaidou P, Jarnum S. Calcium, phosphorus, magnesium, zinc and nitrogen balance in patients with severe short bowel syndrome. Am J Clin Nutr 1980; 33:2137–44.
21. Atkinson RL, Dahms WT, Bray GA, Jacob R, Sandstead HH. Plasma zinc and copper in obesity and after intestinal bypass. Ann Intern Med 1978; 89:491–3.
22. Ulmer DD. Current concepts. Trace elements. N Engl J Med 1977; 297:318–21.
23. Catalanotto FA. The trace metal zinc and taste. Am J Clin Nutr 1978; 31:1098–1103.
24. Steinberg SE, Campbell CL, Hellman RS. Kinetics of the normal folate enterohepatic cycle. J Clin Invest 1979; 64:83–8.
25. Goetsch CA, Klipstein FA. Effect of folate deficiency of the intestinal mucosa on jejunal transport in the rat. J Lab Clin Med 1977; 89:1002–8.
26. Buxton B. Small bowel resection and gastric hypersecretion. Gut 1974; 15:229–38.
27. Straus E, Gerson CD, Yalow RS. Hypersecretion of gastrin associated with the short bowel syndrome. Gastroenterology 1974; 66:175–80.
28. Seelig LL, Winborn WB, Weser E. Effects of small bowel resection on the gastric mucosa in the rat. Gastroenterology 1977; 72:421–8.
29. Gelinas MD, Morin CL, Morisset J. Exocrine pancreatic function following proximal small bowel resection in rats. J Physiol 1982; 322:71–82.
30. Brand SJ, Morgan RGH. The influence of starvation on intestinal cholecystokinin-like activity and pancreatic growth. J Physiol (London) 1981; 321:469–82.
31. Toskes PP. Does a negative feedback system for the control of pancreatic exocrine secretion exist and is it of any clinical significance? J Lab Clin Med 1980; 95:11–2.
32. Green GM, Olds BA, Matthews G, Lyman RL. Protein as a regulator of pancreatic enzyme secretion in the rat. Proc Soc Ex Biol Med 1973; 142:1162–7.
33. Rothschild MA, Oratz M, Schneiber SS. Medical progress. Albumin synthesis. N Engl Med 1972; 286:748–57 and 816–21.
34. Urban E, Weser E. Intestinal adaptation to bowel resection. *In*: Stollerman GH, ed. Advances in Internal Medicine. Chicago: Year Book Medical Publishers, 1980; 26:265–91.
35. Dowling RH, Gleeson MH. Cell turnover following small bowel resection and bypass. Digestion 1973; 8:176–90.
36. Ferry OG, Backman L, Hallberg D. Morphologic changes of the small intestine following jejuno-ileal shunt in obese subjects. Acta Chir Scand 1976; 142:154–9.
37. Dowling RH, Booth CC. Functional compensation after small bowel resection in man. Lancet 1966; 2:146–7.
38. Robinson JWL, Dowling RH, Riecken EO, eds. Falk Symposium 30. Mechanisms of Intestinal Adaptation. Lancaster, Pa: MTP Press, 1982.
39. Urban E, Campbell ME. Urban E, Campbell ME. In vivo zinc transport by rat small intestine after extensive small bowel resection. Am J Physiol 1984; 247 (in press).
40. Weser E. Role of gastrin in intestinal adaptation after small bowel resection. Gastroenterology 1978; 75:323–4.

41. Weser E, Bell D, Tawil T. Effects of octapeptide-cholecystokinin, secretin and glucagon on intestinal mucosal growth in parenterally nourished rats. Dig Dis Sci 1981; 26:409–16.
42. Rudo ND, Lawrence MD, Rosenberg IH. Treatment with glucagon-binding antibodies alters the intestinal response to starvation in the rat. Gastroenterology 1975; 69:1265–8.
43. Gleeson MH, Bloom SR, Polak JM, Henry K, Dowling RH. Endocrine tumor in kidney affecting small bowel structure, motility and absorptive function. Gut 1971; 12:773–82.
44. Dowling RH, Riecken EO, Laws JW, Booth CC. The intestinal response to high bulk feeding in the rat. Clin Sci 1967; 32:1–9.
45. Spector MH, Levine GM, Deren JJ. Direct and indirect effects of dextrose and amino acids on gut mass. Gastroenterology 1977; 72:706–10.
46. Spector MH, Traylor J, Young EA, Weser E. Stimulation of mucosal growth by gastric and ileal infusion of single amino acids in parenterally nourished rats. Digestion 1981; 21:33–40.
47. Weser E, Heller R, Tawil T. Stimulation of mucosal growth in the rat ileum by bile and pancreatic secretions after jejunal resection. Gastroenterology 1977; 73: 524–9.
48. Galjaard H, VanderMeer-Fieggen W, Giesen J. Feedback control by functional villus cells on cell proliferation and maturation in intestinal epithelium. Exp Cell Res 1972; 73:197–207.
49. May RJ, Quaroni A, Kirsch V, Isselbacher KJ. A villous cell-derived inhibitor of intestinal cell proliferation. Am J Physiol 1981; 241:G520–7.
50. Touloukian RJ, Spencer RP. Ileal blood flow preceding compensatory intestinal hypertrophy. Ann Surg 1972; 175:320–5.
51. Touloukian RJ, Aghajanian GK, Roth RH. Adrenergic denervation of the hypertrophied gut remnant. Ann Surg 1972; 176:633–7.
52. Tutton PJM, Helme RD. The influence of adrenoreceptor activity on crypt cell proliferation in the rat jejunum. Cell Tissue Kinet 1974; 7:125–36.
53. Liavag I, Vaage S. The effect of vagotomy and pyloroplasty on the gastrointestinal mucosa of the rat. Scand J Gastroenterol 1972; 7:23–7.
54. Heaton KW, Read AF. Gallstones in patients with disorders of the terminal ileum and disturbed bile salt metabolism. Br Med J 1969; 3:494–6.
55. Hill GL, Mair WSJ, Goligher JC. Gallstones after ileostomy and ileal resection. Gut 1975; 16:932–6.
56. Dharmsathaphorn K, Freeman DH, Binder HJ, Dobbins JW. Increased risk of nephrolithiasis in patients with steatorrhea. Dig Dis Sci 1982; 27:401–5.
57. Dobbins JW, Binder HJ. Importance of the colon in enteric hyperoxaluria. N Engl J Med 1977; 296:298–301.
58. Stolberg L, Rolfe R, Gitlin N, Merrit J, Mann L, Linder J, Finegold S. D-lactic acidosis due to abnormal gut flora. N Engl J Med 1982; 306:1344–8.
59. Young EA, Heuler N, Russell P, Weser E. Comparative nutritional analysis of chemically defined diets. Gastroenterology 1975; 69:1338–45.
60. Rodgers JB, Bernard HR, Balint JA. Colonic infusion in the management of the short bowel syndrome. Gastroenterology 1976; 70:186–9.
61. Woolf GM, Jeejeebhoy KN. Diet for the patient with short bowel: High fat or high carbohydrate? Gastroenterology 1982; 82:1260 (abstract).
62. Greenberger NJ. State of the art: The management of the patient with short bowel syndrome. Am J Gastroenterol 1978; 70:528–40.
63. Cortot A, Fleming R, Malagelada JR. Improved nutrient absorption after cimetidine in short bowel syndrome with gastric hypersecretion. N Engl J Med 1979; 300:79–80.
64. Murphy JP, King DR, Dubois A. Treatment of gastric hypersecretion with cimetidine in the short bowel syndrome. N Engl J Med 1979; 300:80–1.
65. Hofmann AF, Poley JR. Role of bile acid malabsorption in pathogenesis of diarrhea and steatorrhea in patients with ileal resection. I. Response to cholestyramine or replacement of dietary long chain triglyceride by medium chain triglyceride. Gastroenterology 1972; 69:918–34.
66. Sheldon GF. Role of parenteral nutrition in patients with short bowel syndrome. Am J Med 1979; 67:1021–9.

Chapter 109

Whipple's Disease

William O. Dobbins, III

Historical Background

Whipple's description in 1907 of his patient is classic and can hardly be improved upon.[1] As an introduction to a discussion of this disease, it would appear to be appropriate to summarize this report and to quote from it in part.

The patient was a 36-year-old physician who was admitted to Johns Hopkins Hospital on April 12, 1907.

The illness "began insidiously, 5½ years ago with attacks of arthritis lasting 6 to 8 hours, involving nearly every joint of the body. Sometimes the joints were hot, swollen, and tender; at other times, only painful. . . . Although gradually losing weight and strength he kept at work."

There was a temporary improvement with a 5 to 6 pound gain in weight, but later "a slight evening fever developed, the temperature rising to about 100." There were occasional 'night sweats' and notable loss of strength and weight. . . . The loss of weight however, continued, and a diarrhea set in which has persisted ever since, the stools, from 3 to 4 a day on an average, of fluid or semisolid character."

In the clinical discussion, Dr. Whipple quotes Dr. W. L. Thayer, who made the prescient observation: "As one looks back upon the history of this case in connection with the remarkable observations at autopsy, it is difficult to resist the conclusion that we are here dealing with a definite and hitherto unrecognized clinical picture with which we shall meet again."

It was not until 1936 that the next acceptable case of Whipple's disease was published. However, Morgan[2] discovered a specimen of Whipple's disease in the pathologic museum at Westminister Medical School and found that the case had been recorded in the medical literature in 1895 by Allchin and Hebb in the Transactions of the Pathological Society of London. From 1908 to 1949, only 15 acceptable cases of Whipple's disease were reported. In 1949, Black-Schaffer[3] demonstrated that macrophages found within the intestinal mucosa of these patients were vividly stained by the periodic acid–Schiff (PAS) method (Fig. 109–1*A* to *D*). Yardley and Fleming[4] in 1961 obtained intestinal tissue from Whipple's original case and verified that the macrophages were indeed PAS-positive! The presence of profuse numbers of PAS-positive macrophages within the intestinal mucosa is still considered to be pathognomonic for this disease. In 1960, Cohen et al.,[5] using electron microscopy, described the presence of "virus-like" particles in the intestinal mucosa. However, it was Yardley and Hendrix[6] and Chears and Ashworth[7] who, in 1961, verified Whipple's original observation that rod-shaped organisms are found in the affected tissues—organisms that have all the structural characteristics of bacteria. In 1952, Paulley[8] described the effectiveness of antibiotics in treating Whipple's disease. He gave credit to Dr. G. Ander, the "home doctor" who elected to treat the reported patient with chloramphenicol with dramatic success. An additional 10 years of observations were required before it was uniformly accepted that antibiotics were the appropriate treatment of this disease.

The first report of the diagnosis of Whipple's disease by peroral intestinal biopsy was published in 1958 by Bolt et al.[9] Intestinal biopsy is now considered the diagnostic procedure of choice (Fig. 109–1*A* to *D*). Becker et al,[10] demonstrated, in retrospect, characterrstic changes of Whipple's disease in an

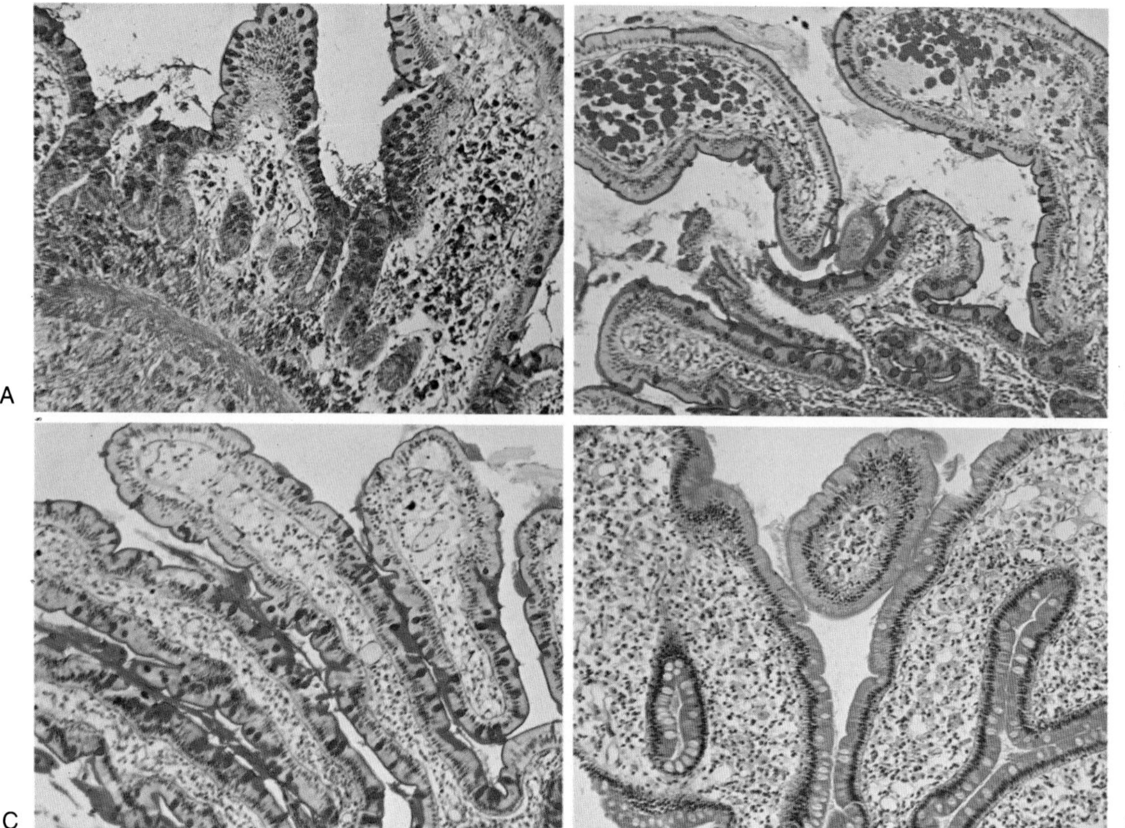

Figure 109–1. *A,* Peroral small bowel biopsy from an untreated patient (PAS preparation). Note the dilated jejunal villi containing numerous PAS-positive macrophages. Most of the characteristic PAS-positive macrophages are present above the muscularis mucosae (× 100). *B,* Same patient 6 months later, during clinical remission. PAS-positive macrophages are present in the stroma of some dilated villi, but are absent in others (× 100). *C,* Same patient 1 year later, during remission (PAS preparation). Note entirely normal villi (× 100). *D,* Peroral small bowel biopsy from an untreated patient (hematoxylin and eosin stain), showing typical club-shaped, dilated villi containing macrophages, which are not as readily apparent as when stained with PAS (× 100).

intestinal biopsy specimen obtained from a patient prior to onset of symptoms. In 1977, Moorthy et al.[11] noted that Whipple's disease may occur with minimal intestinal involvement, and in 1977, Finelli et al.[12] first demonstrated that Whipple's disease may occur in the complete absence of intestinal involvement. Since then, several reports of Whipple's disease presenting as a central nervous system illness in the absence of intestinal symptoms and/or intestinal involvement have appeared in the medical literature.

Etiology and Pathogenesis

Whipple's disease is clearly a systemic disease in which the greatest involvement occurs in the lamina propria of the small intestine and its lymphatic drainage; in the heart, with valvular lesions being particularly prominent; and in the central nervous system. Sieracki and Fine[13] emphasized the presence of systemic involvement with the finding of characteristic PAS-positive macrophages in virtually all body tissues. The PAS-positive material usually occurs in the form of small, rod-shaped masses, described as sickle-shaped (SPC cells) by Sieracki and his associates. The PAS reaction has strong affinity for glycoproteins. In this regard it should be noted that electron microscopic studies have shown that the rod-shaped masses within macrophages are actually masses of degenerating bacteria, the walls of which are apparently in part composed of glycoproteins (Fig. 109–2).

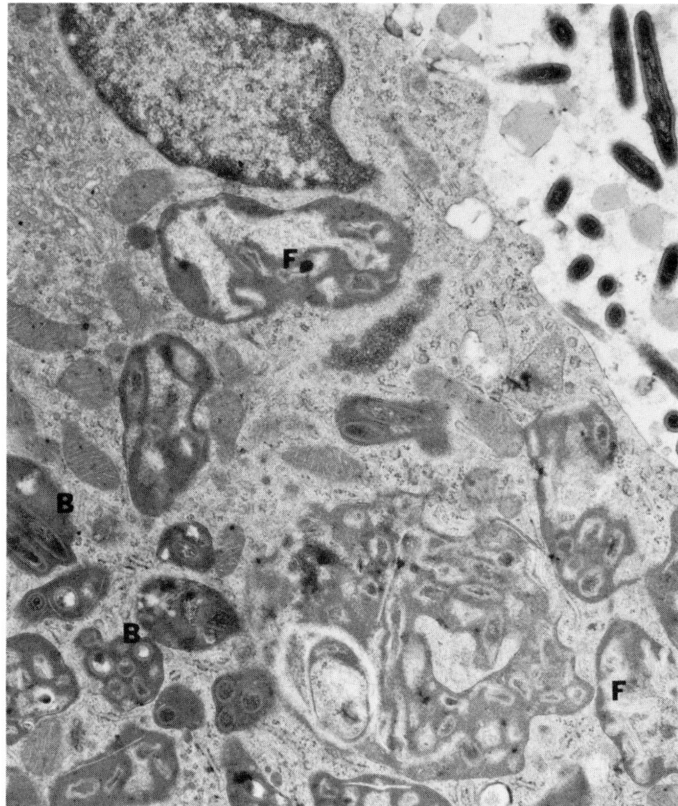

Figure 109–2. Electron micrograph of a portion of a macrophage containing numerous bacilli (B) in various stages of digestion. Note that some of the inclusions contain "fingerprint-like" structures that presumably represent terminal digestion of the bacilli within lysosomes of the macrophage. These large packages of bacilli are the "sickle-form particles" (F) described by Sieracki et al. at light microscopy (× 21,280).

Electron microscopic studies from many laboratories have documented the presence of bacilli situated both intra- and extracellularly in involved tissues. These bacilli have been remarkably uniform in appearance at electron microscopy. They are rod-shaped, approximately 0.2 μm wide by 1.5 to 2.5 μm long, and just large enough to be resolved by light microscopy. The organisms are contained within a trilaminar plasma membrane that is surrounded by a homogeneous cell wall approximately 20 nm thick (Fig. 109–3). The cell wall itself is enclosed within an outer trilaminar "membrane." This latter feature is more characteristic of gram-negative than of gram-positive bacilli. Areas of tubules or vesicles are located centrally within the bacilli, resembling mesosomes that are characteristic of gram-positive bacteria. Nucleoids can often be identified within the core of the bacilli. Binary fission is often present.

The Whipple bacillus has been found within a wide variety of cells, including macrophages, intestinal epithelial cells, lymphatic and capillary endothelial cells, smooth muscle cells, polymorphonuclear leukocytes, plasma cells, mast cells, and even intraepithelial lymphocytes.[14] The bacilli found within cells, including macrophages, often appear to be intact in structure, suggesting that these organisms behave as intracellular pathogens. Intracellular pathogens, unlike pyogenic bacteria that are rapidly digested by the macrophage after phagocytosis, may survive within the macrophage unless the cell is activated by immune mechanisms (see later).

A variety of microorganisms have been implicated in Whipple's disease. Only 3 of these microorganisms, however, deserve serious consideration because they were isolated under conditions "excluding" growth of contaminants. *Corynebacterium anaerobium*, a *Hemophilus* species, and atypical hemolytic streptococci have been cultured from intestinal tissues, surgically obtained lymph nodes, and peripheral blood. The *Hemophilus* species can be exonerated because it is gram-negative and the vast majority of the reports have indicated that the Whipple bacillus is weakly gram-positive. The *C. anaerobium* organism also probably represents a contam-

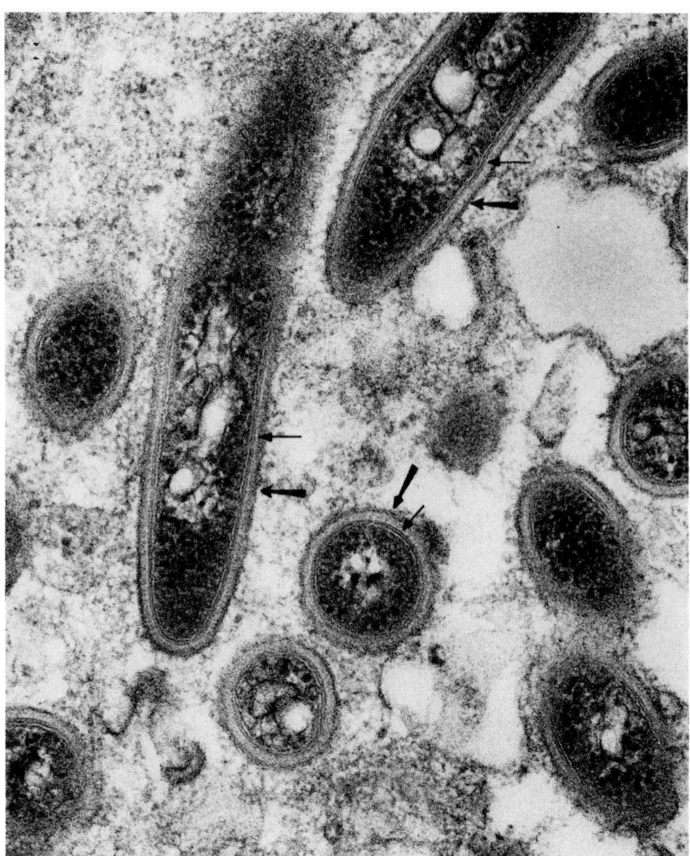

Figure 109–3. Electron micrograph showing the characteristic rod-shaped Whipple bacilli, which are approximately 0.2 μm wide by 1.5 to 2.5 μm long. Note the homogeneous cell wall outside a typical trilaminar plasma membrane *(small arrows).* Note that the cell wall itself is surrounded by a less well characterized "membrane," which has a trilaminar appearance *(large arrows).* See text for additional details (× 100,000).

inant because it has little resemblance to the Whipple bacillus when examined by electron microscopy. Only the atypical hemolytic streptococcus reported by Clancy et al.[15] has been shown by electron microscopy to be morphologically similar to the Whipple bacillus. Immunofluorescent studies have shown that the material found within macrophages in Whipple's disease has a strong antigenic similarity to material found within groups B and G streptococci. Clancy and his group[15] succeeded in culturing a cell wall–deficient alpha-hemolytic streptococcus from an axillary node. Knox et al.[16] also isolated an atypical streptococcus on culture, but the organism was not examined by electron microscopy.

The disease has not been reproduced in laboratory animals, nor has the organism been convincingly cultured in vitro. Nevertheless, the structural characteristics of the organisms found in tissues of untreated patients, the absence of these organisms after antibiotic therapy, and the uniformly good clinical result of antibiotic treatment encourage the concept of Whipple's disease as a bacterial disorder. Indeed, the likelihood is that a single bacterium, not yet defined, causes the disease. In addition, an immune deficiency (discussed later) may be operative in the pathogenesis of the disease.[17]

Pathogenesis of Steatorrhea. In patients with fat malabsorption (approximately 93% of untreated patients), response to antibiotics is prompt and dramatic, with cessation of diarrhea and steatorrhea generally within 1 to 2 weeks of therapy. The major difference in the appearance of intestinal biopsy specimens obtained prior to treatment and 1 to 2 weeks after treatment is seen within the intestinal absorptive cells. Prior to treatment, the absorptive cells generally show considerable evidence of injury and are often invaded by bacteria (Fig. 109–4). Within 1 week of treatment, the absorptive cells revert to normal appearance and there is no longer

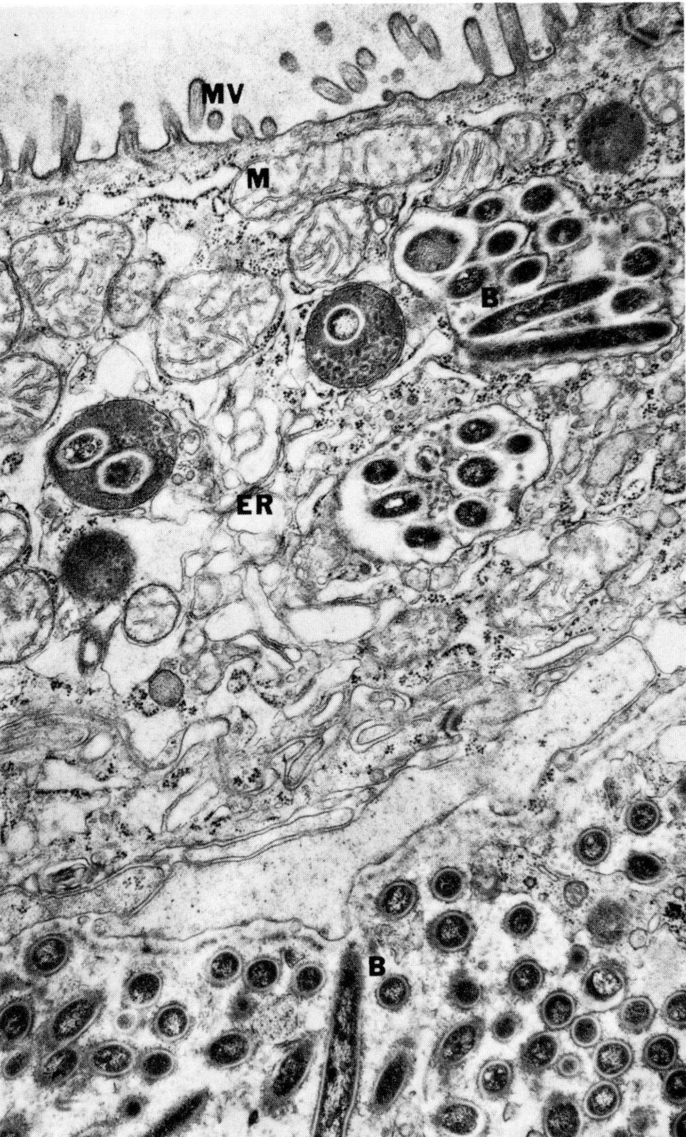

Figure 109–4. Electron micrograph showing numerous Whipple bacilli below the basal lamina of intestinal absorptive cells in the intestinal biopsy of an untreated patient. Note that the bacilli (B) have invaded the intestinal absorptive cells, resulting in marked cellular injury manifested by dilatation of the endoplasmic reticulum (ER), swollen mitochondria (M), and sparse numbers of microvilli (MV). Within 1 week of antibiotic treatment, all the abnormaliies in the intestinal absorptive cells may be reversed (× 20,000).

evidence of bacterial invasion. However, the lamina propria is still packed with macrophages, the lacteals are dilated, and there are large accumulations of fat within the lamina propria. These data suggest that the most important mechanism for fat malabsorption is injury to intestinal absorptive cells due to bacterial invasion. Further evidence that the intestinal absorptive cells are functionally abnormal is the observation that there is decreased in vitro amino acid uptake and fatty acid esterification by intestinal mucosa obtained from the untreated patient.[18]

Additional factors that may contribute to steatorrhea include a reduction in epithelial cell mass and a relative blockade to lymphatic flow due to the mesenteric lymphadenopathy and to marked infiltration of the lamina propria of the intestine by macrophages. However, obstruction to flow of chylomicrons through the lamina propria and through lacteals is not likely to be a major factor because biopsy specimens taken a few weeks after antibiotic treatment still show prominent dilatation of lacteals at a time when malabsorption is no longer present.[18]

Whipple originally called this disease "intestinal lipodystrophy" because of the striking accumulations of lipid within the lamina propria. Presumably this large accumulation of lipid results from partial obstruction to outflow of chylomicrons from the gut. It should be noted that most of these large masses of lipid are found free in the lamina propria and not within the lacteals. The prolonged retention of fat droplets following treatment is probably accounted for by the slow rate at which their triglyceride content can be solubilized and transported from the lamina propria.

Pathology

Gross. At necropsy the peritoneal surfaces are often dull gray and roughened, with fibrinous adhesions.[19] Ascites, occasionally chylous, may be found. Dilatation of the small intestine with increased thickness and rigidity of the bowel wall is usually observed. The extent of the process may be quite variable, with maximal involvement in the proximal small bowel. The mesentery is thickened and the mesenteric, periaortic, and celiac lymph nodes are markedly enlarged. The latter appear pale yellow in color, are elastic to touch, and have a sieve-like appearance on cross-section. The valvulae conniventes of the intestinal mucosa are often thickened and pale yellow in appearance. Splenomegaly is occasionally observed. Polyserositis is often evident. Gross evidence of endocarditis is found in about 25% of cases, with involvement usually of the aortic or mitral valves.

Microscopic. Typical club-shaped villi containing characteristic macrophages are almost always present in the proximal small bowel (see Fig. 109–1*A* to *D*). The appearance of these villi when stained with PAS is shown in Figures 109–1*A* and *B*. Virtually all organ systems may exhibit PAS-positive macrophages containing "sickle-form particles."[13] These characteristic macrophages are found chiefly in the gastrointestinal tract (esophagus, stomach, intestine, and colon), mesenteric and retroperitoneal nodes, heart, central nervous system, lungs, spleen, pancreas, and peripheral lymph nodes. There are minimal changes in the genitourinary tract, adrenals, joints, skin, bone marrow, and skeletal muscle. Occasional sarcoid-like granulomas have been found. Bacilli, most appropriately called Whipple bacilli, with all the structural characteristics of bacteria (see Figs. 109–2 to 109–4), have been identified by electron microscopy within the intestinal mucosa, Kupffer cells of the liver, mesenteric and peripheral lymph nodes, heart, central nervous system, eyes, and lungs.[14]

Immunopathology

There is controversy as to the role, if any, of immune deficiency in Whipple's disease.[17] Considerable evidence has been advanced for immunodeficiency in patients prior to treatment, but this must be discounted. Severe malnutrition and partial obstruction of intestinal mucosal lymphatics could account for all of the observed changes in immune function in the untreated patient. After treatment, there is no evidence for humoral immune deficiency. Secretory immunoglobulins are within normal limits. Intestinal mucosal plasma cells, although decreased before treatment, are normal in number after treatment. There are no abnormal deposits of complement or immunoglobulins within the intestinal mucosa. Circulating immune complexes, of doubtful significance, have been described in only a single patient.[17]

Lymphocytopenia is almost invariably displayed prior to treatment and the percentage of T cells is decreased both before and after treatment.[17] There is decreased responsiveness of lymphocytes to the mitogens phytohemagglutinin (PHA) and concanavalin A (Con A) before and after treatment. The cutaneous response to antigens, such as purified protein derivative (PPD), is clearly diminished before treatment, improves somewhat after treatment, but is still significantly less than that seen in normal controls. HLA typing has been reported in 15 patients. Of these, 6 (40%) were B27 positive, as compared with 10% of the normal population. The tendency for Whipple's disease to be associated with HLA B27 may be further evidence that an abnormality in the cellular immune system promotes susceptibility to the Whipple organism. There may be a subtle defect in cell-mediated immune function in the treated patient. As noted earlier, the Whipple bacillus has many characteristics of an intracellular pathogen. Such pathogens may survive within macrophages, unless the macrophage is activated. The immune response to intracellular pathogens requires interaction between T cells and macrophages, resulting in production of the lymphocyte mediators required to activate macrophages in order to destroy intracellular pathogens. This latter aspect of immune function has not been explored in this disease. Finally, the occasional clinical and bacteriologic relapse that occurs several years after adequate treatment suggests the presence of a deficient immune response to the Whipple bacillus.[17]

Epidemiology

The disease is uncommon and its exact frequency is unknown. Approximately 20 patients were described before 1950. In a review of the literature from 1950 to 1969, Maizel et al.[18] found 114 new patients, 101 males and 13 females. One of the patients was an Indian, 3 were black, and the remainder were white. To these they added 19 additional patients from Duke University Medical Center (18 males, 1 female, all white). Since 1969 there have been at least 150 additional reports of this disease. A reasonable estimate would be that about 500 cases of Whipple's disease have been observed to date, mostly in the United States, England, and continental Europe. The fact that 20 patients have been seen at Duke University Medical Center since 1936, all coming from a relatively narrow geographic area, suggests the possibility of a yet undetermined epidemiologic factor.

Approximately 88% of the patients have been white men ranging in age from 7 to 80 years. Most cases occur in the third and fourth decades. Occupation, social stratum, geographic location (whether urban or rural), and contact with livestock do not seem to be relevant. The disease has been described on 2 occasions in brothers, but there is no other evidence that it is familial.[18]

Clinical Aspects

History. The patient is usually a middle-aged white man with a history of intermittent arthritis or arthralgia involving multiple joints over a period of years. However, the actual illness most often starts gradually with diarrhea; later, gross steatorrhea develops accompanied by marked weight loss and a rapid downhill course. The exceptional patient has no diarrhea, and the illness may be characterized solely by nondescript abdominal pain and fever of varying degree. Many of the patients have occult gastrointestinal bleeding, but gross bleeding is most unusual. The arthralgias may appear 10 to 30 years prior to development of gastrointestinal symptoms and are usually migratory. Involvement of most joints has been described, those usually affected being the ankles, knees, shoulders, and wrists. The joints are sometimes swollen, contain fluid, and may be limited in motion.[20] Chronic joint deformity is unusual.

Physical Examination. Evidence of weight loss is usual. A "prominent" abdomen with tenderness to palpation is the most common abdominal finding. Enlarged abdominal lymph nodes may be palpable. Hypotension is often present and hyperpigmentation of the skin is found in approximately 50% of patients. Fever is usually low grade but, on occasion, spiking temperatures to 103° F are present. Peripheral lymphadenopathy may be present. Cardiac murmurs associated with endocarditis have been noted in 25% of patients. Ascites is uncommon, and splenomegaly and hepatomegaly occur in less than 5% of the patients. All of the manifestations of advanced malabsorption may be present in those patients diagnosed late in their clinical course.

Neurologic Abnormalities. Neurologic disorder was first described in patients who died of advanced disease and who had not received antibiotic treatment. Neurologic manifestations vary and may include personality changes, dementia, ataxia, myoclonus, hyperreflexia, paresis, and sensory loss (such as hearing loss and visual disturbances). A number of patients have also presented with neurologic and personality changes without appreciable gastrointestinal signs or symptoms.[21, 22] In these patients the recognition of Whipple's disease involving principally the central nervous system may require brain biopsy.[21] In a few such patients, systemic and neurologic symptoms recur 1 to 4 years after successful treatment with antibiotics.[22] The neurologic relapse may respond again to antibiotics, but is often irreversible.

The following neurologic changes, listed in order of decreasing frequency, are characteristically observed, either before or after antibiotic treatment:

- Personality changes, including organic psychosyndromes, memory loss, confusion, apathy, and dementia.
- Ophthalmic changes,[16] including paralysis of gaze (ophthalmoplegia), papille-

dema, and nystagmus. The retina may show histologic changes and vitreous opacities may be present.

- Hypothalamic symptoms, including insomnia, hypersomnia, hyperphagia, and polydipsia.
- Meningoencephalitis[23] manifested by fever, confusion, lapsing consciousness, and ataxia with pleocytosis and increase in protein content in the cerebrospinal fluid.
- Spastic paresis (Babinski sign present), gait disturbance, clonic movements, myoclonus, and seizures.
- Wernicke's encephalopathy and presenile dementia (with cortical atrophy).
- Posterior column disease.

Laboratory findings include nonspecific electroencephalographic (EEG) changes and changes in the cerebrospinal fluid (CSF) obtained by lumbar puncture. The latter consist of mild pleocytosis (up to 390 cells/mm^3) and slight increase in protein content. The CSF pellet may contain PAS-positive macrophages.[22]

Gross neuropathologic changes include atrophy of the cerebral cortex, dilated ventricles, varying-sized infarcts, spongy degeneration, and ependymal granulations. Histopathologically, there is widespread distribution of PAS-positive macrophages in the central nervous system, brain stem, and spinal cord in both symptomatic and asymptomatic patients. The distribution of the changes may be patchy with involvement only of the brain stem. Nodular aggregates of macrophages measuring up to 2 mm in diameter may be randomly scattered throughout the cortical and subcortical gray matter of the cerebrum, the nuclear gray matter of the brain stem, and the cortical and nuclear gray matter of the cerebellum. Nodular aggregates are found within the white matter, but they are far less numerous than those seen in the gray matter. There may be extensive involvement of the basal temporal lobe, thalamus, and hypothalamus. Other areas of involvement that have been described include the pituitary stalk, gray and white matter of the spinal cord, and the retina.

Laboratory Findings. Anemia (usually normocytic, normochromic) is present in 90% of the patients.[18] Occasional patients have iron deficiency. Megaloblastic anemia is rare. The white blood cell count is usually not elevated and the peripheral blood smear shows a normal differential count. Hypoalbuminemia, hypocholesterolemia, hypokalemia, and prolonged prothrombin times are commonly present. Steatorrhea is present in 93% of patients, decreased D-xylose absorption occurs in 78%, decreased vitamin B_{12} absorption is found in approximately 15%, and bile salt absorption is unchanged.[18]

Roentgenographic Findings. Barium studies of the upper gastrointestinal tract show coarsening of the duodenal and jejunal folds (Fig. 109–5). This is the most common roentgenographic feature, although the finding is nonspecific.[18] The duodenum and jejunum may be dilated. Similar changes may be present in the ileum, although they are less frequently seen than in the jejunum. Ileus is an uncommon observation. Enlargement of retroperitoneal lymph nodes may result in widening of the duodenal loop and displacement of the stomach, duodenum, and ureters. Mediastinal lymphadenopathy has been reported in 2 patients.

The peripheral joints may show slight demineralization and narrowing, and fusion of the sacroiliac joints has been noted. Sponta-

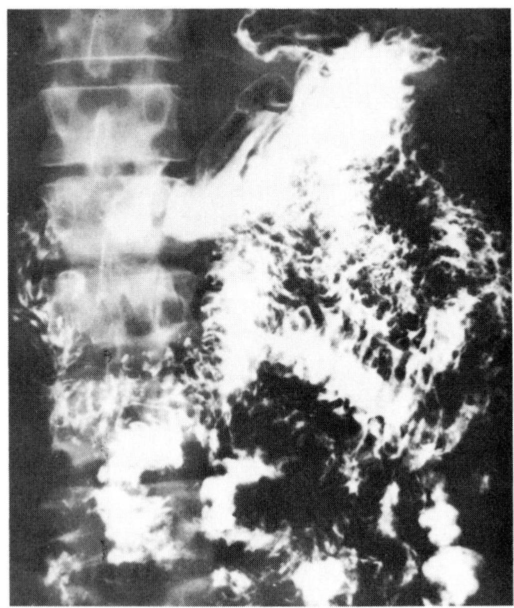

Figure 109–5. Roentgenogram obtained in an untreated patient with Whipple's disease illustrating marked coarsening of the folds of the duodenum and jejunum, a characteristic although not diagnostic finding in this disease. Following successful treatment, these folds revert to a normal appearance when studied using barium contrast media.

neous fractures and osteomalacia have not been reported in Whipple's disease.[18]

Diagnosis

This disease should be suspected in individuals with the 4 most prominent symptoms: weight loss, diarrhea, arthralgias, and abdominal pain. If the arthralgias precede the other symptoms by a period of months to years, the diagnosis deserves very serious consideration. Histologically, the most severe and consistent changes are seen in the proximal small intestine, and small bowel biopsy is the appropriate approach to diagnosis. The intestinal mucosa is characteristically filled with PAS-positive macrophages, a condition not found in any other intestinal disease. However, *PAS-positive macrophages are also found in most normal tissues and organ systems.* This is particularly the case in the rectal and colonic mucosa. Thus, only the light microscopic findings in the small intestinal mucosa are unique and may be considered diagnostic. It is very helpful to have electron microscopic confirmation of the presence of the characteristic bacilli, although these bacilli can be seen with light microscopy in appropriately prepared tissues.

The ease with which the diagnosis was made in the past has been complicated by recent observations that individuals may have Whipple's disease with minimal or *no* intestinal involvement. One individual has been reported who died of Whipple's disease and in whom multiple intestinal mucosal biopsies were normal.[24] In this unique individual, the characteristic PAS-positive macrophages were found at necropsy in the intestinal submucosa, an area not ordinarily adequately sampled by peroral biopsy. Furthermore, a number of patients with Whipple's disease have presented with neurologic and personality changes as their initial manifestation in the *absence* of significant gastrointestinal signs or symptoms.[21,22] Intestinal biopsy may demonstrate the characteristic changes of Whipple's disease in many of these individuals, but others have presented with central nervous system Whipple's disease in the complete absence of involvement of the gastrointestinal tract.[22] Indeed, brain biopsy has been utilized to establish the diagnosis in 2 such individuals.[21] Brain biopsy may be necessary to establish recurrence of disease in previously successfully treated patients who develop relapse manifested by neurologic symptoms and signs in the presence of a normal intestinal biopsy. Biopsy of a mesenteric or peripheral lymph node has occasionally been helpful in establishing the diagnosis. However, many normal lymph nodes contain PAS-positive macrophages. Hence, the presence of the characteristic bacilli demonstrated by light or electron microscopy is essential to the diagnosis in such tissues.

The characteristic changes on barium studies of the duodenum and jejunum may suggest the diagnosis of Whipple's disease, but these changes are quite nonspecific and may even be seen in normal individuals. Abdominal computed tomography (CT) scan has been utilized to demonstrate the presence of enlarged mesenteric and periaortic lymph nodes. Cerebral CT scan has been used in one individual to demonstrate the presence of a localized abnormality in the brain, leading to brain biopsy and successful diagnosis.[25]

In summary, the diagnosis is established in the vast majority of patients by small intestinal biopsy. Occasionally, biopsy of a lymph node or other tissues may permit the diagnosis in properly prepared tissues. Finally, brain biopsy may be necessary to establish the diagnosis in selected untreated patients and in treated patients who develop a neurologic relapse but in whom intestinal biopsies fail to show bacilli.

Complications

Neurologic relapse, sometimes years after apparently successful treatment, is becoming more common. In some patients there is a true relapse with involvement of the central nervous system by Whipple bacilli and with response to a second course of antibiotics. Other patients, however, appear to have progressive neurologic disease not related to invasion by Whipple bacilli. The changes in these patients are thought to be a complication (diffuse fibrosis?) of the original successfully treated infection. Aortic valvular insufficiency has been reported, both as an initial complication of Whipple's disease and as a late manifestation of bacterial endocarditis.[26] Mitral valvular disease occurs more frequently than does aortic valvular disease and may occasionally result in the development of mitral stenosis or insufficiency.

Treatment

Antibiotics are the treatment of choice.[27] Patients have been reported to respond favorably to chloramphenicol, tetracycline, chlortetracycline, ampicillin, penicillin, trimethoprim-sulfamethoxazole, and doxycycline. The appropriate duration of therapy has never been determined, but because occasional patients have had early relapses after only several weeks to a few months of treatment, it is generally held that treatment should be maintained for 1 year. The approach recommended by the Duke University groups seems to be the most reasonable initial approach to treatment. They recommend 1.2 million units of procaine penicillin G and 1 g of streptomycin daily for 10 days to 2 weeks, followed by tetracycline, 1 g daily, for 10 to 12 months.[18] Occasional patients have had relapses while being treated with tetracycline and have then responded to a different antibiotic, such as ampicillin.

Intestinal biopsies obtained during antibiotic treatment show improvement in the appearance of the surface epithelium within 1 week. Free bacilli have been reported to persist within the lamina propria for up to 9 weeks. The PAS-positive macrophages clear at a much slower rate, so that even at 6 months and 1 year the lamina propria often contains prominent macrophages even though free bacilli are no longer identifiable. The PAS-positive macrophages may persist within the lamina propria for as long as 11 years after successful treatment.[28] Thus, duration of therapy cannot be determined by the presence or absence of PAS-positive macrophages, but should be based upon the presence or absence of free bacilli as determined by appropriately performed light microscopy or by electron microscopy. A routine of 1 year of therapy using a safe antibiotic, such as tetracycline, should suffice in the majority of patients and routine follow-up intestinal biopsies are probably not necessary.

Within days of institution of appropriate therapy, the patient experiences a sense of well-being: the appetite returns, the diarrhea ceases, the fever subsides, and a gradual gain in weight is observed. Within weeks to months, all the abnormal laboratory data should revert to normal, and the patient should return to normal weight.

As more and more successfully treated patients are being followed for long periods of time, it is becoming apparent that many of these patients will have clinical relapses, both in the presence and in the absence of intestinal symptoms. As stated earlier, central nervous system relapses have become the major concern in recent years.[21, 22] Thus, all treated patients should be followed by careful clinical evaluation on at least a yearly basis. There is no real value in repeating intestinal biopsies at periodic intervals. If a relapse is suspected, intestinal biopsy should be obtained and the presence or absence of free bacilli determined. Rarely, a brain biopsy or lymph node biopsy will be necessary in order to establish the presence of free bacilli, indicating relapse of disease. An empiric trial of antibiotics may be more appropriate than a brain biopsy, however, especially since the histopathologic changes in the brain are generally patchy. A good response of a relapse to antibiotics requires at least an additional year of antibiotic treatment.

Prognosis

Prior to the antibiotic era, Whipple's disease was uniformly fatal. During the first decade of antibiotic therapy, it appeared that such therapy was invariably successful and that virtually all patients were cured with the initial course of treatment. Occasional patients who relapsed during or following treatment were reported as curiosities. During the past 5 to 10 years, there have been an increasing number of reports of individuals who have required more than one antibiotic for successful treatment, and even of some who have failed to respond to antibiotics.[27]

Unsolved Problems

The consistent presence of bacilli in the small intestine and lymph nodes of patients with Whipple's disease prior to treatment and the absence of these bacilli after antibiotic administration have been repeatedly confirmed. Yet, the suspect bacillus has never been convincingly cultured and the disease has not been reproduced in animals. Nevertheless, the structural characteristics of the organism in the untreated patient, the absence of bacilli after antibiotic therapy, and the generally good clinical result of antibiotic treatment are powerful evidence that the disorder is fundamentally a bacterial disease.

The riddle is not confined to inability to culture the organism. Why are the great majority of these patients middle-aged white males? Why is the disease found predominantly in the United States and Northern Europe? Why was there such a clustering of patients reported in one large series from a small geographic area?[18] Why are there conflicting data in regard to immune function (particularly T cell function)? Is the macrophage functionally normal in these patients? Finally, why are the intestinal lamina propria, the endocardium, and the central nervous system most susceptible to bacillary involvement?

References

1. Whipple GH. A hitherto undescribed disease characterized anatomically by deposits of fat and fatty acids in the intestinal and mesenteric lymphatic tissues. Bull Johns Hopkins Hosp 1907; 18:382–91.
2. Morgan AD. The first recorded case of Whipple's disease? Gut 1961; 2:370–2.
3. Black-Schaffer B. Tinctoral demonstration of glycoprotein in Whipple's disease. Proc Soc Exp Biol Med 1949; 72:225–7.
4. Yardley JH, Fleming WH. Whipple's disease: A note regarding PAS-positive granules in the original case. Bull Johns Hopkins Hosp 1961; 109:76–9.
5. Cohen AS, Schimmel EM, Holt PR, Isselbacher KJ. Ultrastructural Abnormalities in Whipple's disease. Proc Soc Exp Biol Med 1960; 105:411–4.
6. Yardley JH, Hendrix TR. Combined electron and light microscopy in Whipple's disease. Bull Johns Hopkins Hosp 1961; 109:80–98.
7. Chears WC, Ashworth CT. Electron microscopic study of the intestinal mucosa in Whipple's disease. Gastroenterology 1961; 41:129–38.
8. Paulley JW. A case of Whipple's disease (intestinal lypodystrophy). Gastroenterology 1952; 22:128–33.
9. Bolt RJ, Pollard HM, Standaert L. Transoral-bowel biopsy as an aid in the diagnosis of malabsorption states. N Engl J Med 1958; 259:32–4.
10. Becker FF, Hearst WM, Tesler, MA, Dumont AE. Intestinal lipodystrophy (Whipple's disease): Demonstration of anatomic alteration before onset of symptoms. JAMA 1965; 194:559–61.
11. Moorthy S, Nolley G, Hermos JA. Whipple's disease with minimal intestinal involvement. Gut 1977; 18:152–5.
12. Finelli PF, McEntee WJ, Lessel S, Morgan TF, Copetto J. Whipple's disease with predominantly neuroophthalmic manifestations. Ann Neurol 1977; 1:247–52.
13. Sieracki JC, Fine G. Whipple's disease: Observation on systemic involvement. I. Gross and histologic observation. Arch Pathol 1959; 67:81–93.
14. Dobbins WO III, Kawanishi H. Bacillary characteristics in Whipple's disease: An electron microscopic study. Gastroenterology 1981; 80:1468–75.
15. Clancy RL, Tomkins WAF, Muckle TJ, Richardson H, Rawls WE. Isolation and characterization of an aetiological agent in Whipple's disease. Br Med J 1975; 3:568–70.
16. Knox DL, Bayless TM, Yardley JH, Charache P. Whipple's disease presenting with ocular inflammation and minimal intestinal symptoms. Johns Hopkins Med J 1968; 123:175–82.
17. Dobbins WO III. Is there an immune deficit in Whipple's disease? Dig Dis Sci 1981; 26:247–52.
18. Maizel H, Ruffin JM, Dobbins WO III. Whipple's disease: A review of 19 patients from one hospital and a review of the literature since 1950. Medicine 1970; 49:175–205.
19. Enzinger FM, Helwig EB: Whipple's disease—a review of the literature and report of fifteen patients. Virchows Arch Pathol Anat 1963; 336:238–68.
20. LeVine ME, Dobbins WO III. Joint changes in Whipple's disease. Sem Arth Rheum 1973; 3:79–93.
21. Johnson L, Diamond I. Cerebral Whipple's disease: Diagnosis by brain biopsy. Am J Clin Pathol 1979; 74:486–90.
22. Feurle GE, Volk B, Waldherr R. Cerebral Whipple's disease with negative jejunal histology. N Engl J Med 1979; 300:907–8.
23. Schmitt BP, Richardson H, Smith E, Kaplan R. Encephalopathy complicating Whipple's disease. Ann Intern Med 1981; 94:51–2.
24. Kuhajda FP, Belitsos NJ, Keren DR, Hutchins GM. A submucosal variant of Whipple's disease. Gastroenterology 1982; 82:46–50.
25. Grossman RI, Davis KR, Halperin J. Cranial computed tomography in Whipple's disease. J Comp Assist Tomog 1981; 5:246–8.
26. Bostwick DG, Bensch KG, Burke JS, Billingham ME, Miller DC, Smith JC, Keren DF. Whipple's disease presenting as aortic insufficiency. N Engl J Med 1981; 305:995–8.
27. Bayless TM. Whipple's disease: Newer concepts of therapy. Adv Intern Med 1970; 16:171–89.
28. Martin FF, Vilseck J, Dobbins WO III, Buckley CE III, Tyor, MP: Immunological alterations in patients with treated Whipple's disease. Gastroenterology 1972; 63:6–18.

Chapter 110

Protein-losing Gastroenteropathies

Thomas A. Waldmann

Definition and History

The gastrointestinal tract plays a major role in the homeostasis of the plasma proteins in both normal and pathologic states. The small intestine has been shown to be a significant site of synthesis of serum proteins, including certain lipoproteins, complement components, and immunoglobulins. In addition, the intestinal mucosa is responsible for the absorption of products of protein digestion and, under certain circumstances, can absorb intact plasma proteins. For example, IgG antibodies are transported across the gastrointestinal tract of neonatal rats by a saturable transport process that involves binding by cell surface receptors specific for IgG on the enterocytes of the small intestine.[14,54] Finally, the gastrointestinal tract plays a part in the catabolism of plasma proteins, especially in disease states. A major development has been the demonstration that excessive loss of serum proteins into the gastrointestinal tract is a common disorder that plays a role in the pathogenesis of the hypoproteinemia associated with gastrointestinal diseases.[47,53,56,98] The term *protein-losing gastroenteropathy* was introduced to denote this abnormal condition.

For many years it was assumed that the hypoproteinemia occurring in patients with gastrointestinal diseases was secondary to impairment of synthesis of these proteins. Subsequently, Albright and co-workers,[1] studying the fate of infused albumin with a complex balance technique, showed that excessive catabolism rather than defective synthesis could explain the hypoalbuminemia of patients with idiopathic hypoproteinemia. Studies of metabolic turnover using radioiodinated albumin in patients with this syndrome confirmed that an increased fractional rate of albumin catabolism rather than decreased synthesis was the cause of the hypoproteinemia.[80] However, these experimental approaches could not demonstrate the mechanism or site of the excessive protein catabolism. This demonstration was first provided by Citrin and co-workers,[17] who showed that a patient with giant hypertrophy of the gastric mucosa and associated hypoalbuminemia lost excessive amounts of albumin into the gastrointestinal lumen. These authors used intubation to collect the gastric secretions from the patient, who had previously received IV iodinated albumin. Sufficient protein-bound radioactivity was identified in the gastric secretions to explain the observed hypercatabolism of albumin. This technique has not been generally applicable to the quantitation of protein loss throughout the gastrointestinal tract because all intestinal secretions cannot be quantitatively collected. Also, there is rapid catabolism of the labeled proteins in the gastrointestinal lumen with reabsorption of the amino acids and the radioiodine label. The situation is further complicated by the fact that the salivary glands and gastric mucosa secrete the free radioiodine label.

These difficulties in the use of radioiodinated proteins led to the development by Gordon[34] of an indirect means of demonstrating excessive gastrointestinal protein loss by the use of IV administered radioiodinated polyvinylpyrrolidone (PVP). Radioiodinated PVP is a labeled synthetic polymer of high molecular weight in the range of smaller serum proteins that is unaffected by mammalian or bacterial enzymes and is poorly absorbed from the gastrointestinal tract. Hence, the fecal excretion of radioactivity following the IV administration of this material is a reflection of the loss of large molecules, such as serum proteins, from the blood into the gastrointestinal tract. Subsequently, new labeled macromolecules, including ^{51}Cr-labeled serum proteins,[77,93,97] ^{95}Nb-labeled albumin,[51] ^{59}Fe-labeled dextran,[4,49] and ^{67}Cu-labeled ceruloplasmin,[101] have been introduced and are superior to ^{131}I-PVP for the study of protein-losing gastroenteropathy.

The study of gastrointestinal protein loss with use of these agents has been of significance to the gastroenterologist in a number of ways. It has provided a better understanding of the pathogenesis of the hypoproteinemia seen in association with gastrointestinal disease. The use of techniques for demonstrating gastrointestinal protein loss may be the only way of pinpointing the intestinal tract as diseased, since many patients have hypoproteinemia and edema as the only clinical manifestations of their gastrointestinal disorder. The techniques for quantitation of gastrointestinal protein loss have also been of value in determining the site of the disease in the intestinal tract, in determining the activity of the gastrointestinal disease, and in following the efficacy of therapy of the intestinal disorder. Finally, as a result of such studies of protein metabolism, a number of new gastrointestinal diseases have been discovered.

Physiology and Pathophysiology

Study of the normal metabolism of serum proteins, especially albumin and the immunoglobulins, has led to concepts that assist in understanding the disturbances of protein metabolism found in patients with gastrointestinal disorders.[10,76,103,105] The protein that has been studied most extensively from this point of view is serum albumin. Albumin is synthesized by the liver and then delivered into the systemic circulation. Normally, the average synthetic rate for albumin is 130 to 230 mg/kg/day (approximately 10 to 14 g/day for a 70-kg man). Albumin is not restricted to the plasma compartment but is also distributed into the extracellular, extravascular spaces. From 36% to 53% of the body albumin pool is in the plasma compartment, with the remaining albumin in the extravascular pools. Normal individuals have a total circulating albumin pool (i.e., albumin in the plasma compartment) of 1.4 to 2.0 g/kg and a total exchangeable albumin pool (i.e., the albumin of all body pools) of 3.5 to 5.0 g/kg. The degradation of most serum proteins, including albumin, is a random process; i.e., a newly synthesized albumin molecule is as likely to be catabolized as one that has been in the circulation for some time. In addition, this random catabolic process has been shown to occur in the plasma compartment or in a body compartment in rapid equilibrium with the plasma.[16] For these reasons, albumin degradation rates are reported as the fraction of the plasma or intravascular pool of albumin catabolized per day (fractional catabolic rate). Normally, 7% to 11% of the intravascular pool of albumin is catabolized per day, corresponding to a half-time of albumin survival of 15 to 23 days.

The site of catabolism of the large serum proteins that have a long survival has not been adequately defined. Specifically, the role of the gastrointestinal tract in this process has been the subject of controversy. Albumin, gamma globulin, and other serum proteins have been demonstrated in the gastrointestinal secretions of normal individuals by electrophoretic and immunologic techniques.[35,42,71,84] Thus, the gastrointestinal tract has been shown to play a role in the physiologic degradation of serum proteins. A number of workers have suggested that such loss into the gastrointestinal tract is the major mode of disposal of the serum proteins in normal individuals.[3,111] They have estimated the magnitude of loss of albumin and gamma globulin into the gastrointestinal tract by determining the rate of loss of protein-bound radioactivity into the gastric and small intestinal secretions of normal animals that had received IV iodinated proteins. These workers estimated that from 38% to over 60% of the degradation of these proteins, in normals, could be explained by gastrointestinal protein loss.[3,111] It should be noted, however, that minor trauma to the intestinal mucosa during the intubation and surgical procedures involved in these studies, resulting in the loss of only 1 or 2 drops of plasma or lymph during the short study periods utilized, would have resulted in these high estimates for normal gastrointestinal catabolism of serum proteins.

Other workers, using different methods, have concluded that the normal gastrointestinal tract plays a less significant role in the catabolism of serum proteins. For example, removal of the subdiaphragmatic gastrointestinal tract of rodents results in only a 0% to 10% prolongation of the survival of iodinated albumin.[33,57] In addition, clearance studies performed using ^{51}Cr-albumin,[93,109] ^{67}Cu-ceruloplasmin,[101] ^{59}Fe-dextran,[49] ^{95}Nb-albumin,[51] or alpha-1-antitrypsin[9,20,30,89] showed that only 5% to 15% of the normal turnover of albumin and gamma globulin could be accounted for by enteric protein loss and that the contribution of the gastrointestinal tract to the catabolism of proteins with a shorter survival is even less. Thus, *bulk loss of serum into the gastrointestinal tract appears to be of only minor importance in the normal metabolism of serum proteins.*

Hypoproteinemia is an exceedingly common accompaniment of disease that may occur secondary to a variety of pathophysiologic mechanisms that affect the rate of synthesis, the patterns of distribution, or the rate of catabolism of serum proteins. The absence or extreme reduction in the serum concentration of a single plasma protein implies an inborn error of metabolism affecting the synthesis of that protein. Analbuminemia, analphalipoproteinemia, abetalipoproteinemia, and afibrinogenemia are examples of such disorders. In other patients one may see genetic or acquired defects in the ability to synthesize related proteins, such as the immunoglobulins, when the cell of origin of these proteins does not develop normally. Hypoproteinemia affecting several protein species caused by decreased protein synthesis may be found in malnutrition, liver disease, neoplastic disease, and many other chronic illnesses.

A second major mechanism resulting in hypoproteinemia is hypercatabolism of serum proteins. This may be restricted to a single protein, as in the isolated hypercatabolism of IgG in patients with myotonic dystrophy,[113] or may affect several proteins, as in patients with the Wiskott-Aldrich syndrome[11] or the syndrome of familial hypercatabolic hypoproteinemia.[100]

A third pathophysiologic mechanism resulting in hypoproteinemia is excessive loss of serum proteins into the urinary, respiratory, or gastrointestinal tract. Excessive loss of serum proteins into the gastrointestinal tract is a common disorder that plays a major role in the pathogenesis of the hypoproteinemia associated with many gastrointestinal diseases (Table 110–1). Excessive loss of serum proteins into the gastrointestinal tract may occur by a variety of mechanisms. One such mechanism is that of a disorder of gastrointestinal lymphatics leading to a loss of lymph fluid into the gastrointestinal lumen. A second mechanism is that of inflammation and ulceration of the mucosa of the gastrointestinal tract leading to exudation of plasma proteins. There are, in addition, a variety of diseases in which the mechanism of loss has not been defined.

In patients with protein-losing gastroenteropathy, the survival of albumin, IgG, IgA, IgM, and ceruloplasmin is markedly reduced.[87,101,103] The fraction of the intravascular pool catabolized per day over normal in a given patient is the same for each of these proteins. This is consistent with the concept that in patients with protein-losing gastroenteropathy there is bulk loss of serum proteins into the gastrointestinal lumen irrespective of the size of the molecules. This finding is in contrast with the urinary protein loss in patients with the nephrotic syndrome. In the latter disorder, low molecular weight proteins are lost preferentially because the sieving function of the glomerulus is partially retained. When serum proteins pass into the gastrointestinal tract, they are usually catabolized rapidly into their constituent amino acids. These are reabsorbed and made available to the body. However, *hypoproteinemia develops if the rate of loss of a protein exceeds the*

Table 110–1. DISORDERS ASSOCIATED WITH PROTEIN-LOSING ENTEROPATHY

I. *Diseases with disorders of intestinal lymphatics*
- Intestinal lymphangiectasia
- Intestinal lymphangiectasia with inflammatory disease
- Whipple's disease
- Retroperitoneal fibrosis
- Fistula between thoracic duct and small intestine
- Lymphangiectasia of colon
- Neoplasms involving mesenteric lymphatics
  - Lymphosarcoma
  - Hodgkin's disease
  - Mycosis fungoides
  - Mesenchymoma of mesentery
- Non-specific granuloma involving the small bowel and mesentery
- Angio-osteohypertrophy syndrome (cutaneous hemangioma, varicose veins, and hypertrophy of soft tissue and bone)
- Tuberculous peritonitis and mesenteric lymph node infection
- Congestive heart failure
  - Constrictive pericarditis
  - Interatrial septal defect
  - Tricuspid regurgitation
  - Familial myocardiopathy
  - Myocardiopathy with generalized myopathy
  - Congenital pulmonic stenosis
- Thrombosis of superior vena cava

II. *Diseases with ulceration of a region of the mucosa of the gastrointestinal tract*
- Esophageal carcinoma
- Gastric carcinoma
- Diffuse ulcerative gastritis
- Gastric carcinoid
- Generalized Kaposi's sarcoma
- Crohn's disease (regional enteritis)
- Acute infectious enteritis (staphylococcus, shigella, ameba)
- Chronic ulcerative (non-granulomatous) jejunitis
- Duodenal carcinoma
- Carcinoma of large bowel
- Ulcerative colitis

III. *Diseases with demonstrable pathology, but in which the mechanism of loss is not known*
- Stomach
  - Giant hypertrophy of the gastric mucosa (Menetrier's disease)
  - Hypertrophic gastropathy with hypersecretion
  - Atrophic gastritis
  - Gastric polyp
  - Postgastrectomy syndrome
  - Gastrocolic fistula
  - Gastric bezoar
- Intestines and related organs
  - Gluten-induced enteropathy, celiac disease, non-tropical sprue
  - Tropical sprue
  - Allergic protein-losing gastroenteropathy
  - Eosinophilic gastroenteritis
  - Jejunal stenosis
  - Jejunal diverticulosis
  - Blind loop syndrome
  - Tuberous sclerosis with congenital angiomatous malformation of small bowel
  - Hemangioma of small intestine

III. *Diseases with demonstrable pathology, but in which the mechanism of loss is not known (Continued)*
  - Acute transient gastrointestinal protein loss
  - Veno-occlusive disease of bowel
  - Arterio-occlusive disease of bowel
  - Incarcerated inguinal hernia
  - Kwashiorkor
  - Histoplasmosis of small bowel
  - Hookworm infection
  - Intestinal giardiasis
  - Intestinal capillariasis
  - Campylobacterosis
  - Diffuse colonic polyposis
  - Schistosomal polyposis of colon
  - Megacolon
  - Villous adenoma of rectum
  - Chronic pancreatitis
  - Zollinger-Ellison syndrome
  - Carcinoma of biliary tract
  - Cirrhosis of liver
- Generalized
  - Nephrotic syndrome
  - Cystic fibrosis
  - Dermatitis herpetiformis
  - Toxemia of pregnancy
  - Agammaglobulinemia
  - Dysgammaglobulinemia
  - Wiskott-Aldrich syndrome (eczema, thrombocytopenia, infections)
  - Scleroderma
  - Disseminated lupus erythematosus
  - Sjögren's syndrome
  - Rheumatoid arthritis
  - Sarcoidosis
  - Amyloidosis
  - Schönlein-Henoch purpura
  - Angioneurotic edema
  - Infectious mononucleosis
  - Paracoccidioidomycosis
  - Letterer-Siwe disease
  - Post-measles enteropathy
  - Mastocytosis
  - Metastatic malignant melanoma
  - Carcinoid syndrome
  - Waldenström's macroglobulinemia
  - Alpha chain disease
  - Cystic leiomyosarcoma
  - Cronkhite-Canada syndrome (diffuse gastrointestinal polyps with ectodermal changes)
  - Sjögren-Larsson syndrome (oligophrenia, ichthyosis, pyramidal tract disorder)
- Related to therapy
  - Factitious diarrhea with excessive laxative ingestion
  - Retained intestinal tube
  - Iodide ingestion in a patient allergic to iodides
  - Lactose ingestion in a patient with Crohn's disease
  - Pseudomembranous colitis secondary to antibiotic ingestion
  - Arsenic poisoning
  - Abdominal irradiation
  - Methotrexate therapy

body's capacity to synthesize that protein. Thus, hypoalbuminemia occurs in protein-losing gastroenteropathy since the albumin synthetic rate in such patients, estimated indirectly using radioiodinated albumin or directly using the ^{14}C-carbonate method, is normal or only increased to a maximum of twice normal.[114]

A similar limited capacity to accelerate albumin synthesis is noted in patients with the nephrotic syndrome and in normal individuals following plasmapheresis. A reduced level of serum protein likewise develops if the rate of synthesis of the excreted protein is not regulated by the concentration of that protein in the serum, as is the case with the immunoglobulins. Thus, synthesis of gamma globulin is usually normal and the serum concentration is reduced in patients with protein-losing gastroenteropathies that are not associated with an inflammatory disease process.[87] Immediately following the onset of protein-losing gastroenteropathy, the quantity of albumin or gamma globulin degraded exceeds that synthesized and the serum level falls. The serum level continues to decline until a new steady state is achieved at a lower protein level. At this new level the absolute quantity of the protein degraded daily (determined from the product of the lower than normal protein pool size and the higher than normal fraction of that pool catabolized or lost per day) again equals the daily synthetic rate of the protein.

The reduction in serum protein concentration is not the same for different proteins. The bulk process of gastrointestinal protein loss, in which a certain fraction of the intravascular pool of all proteins is lost into the gastrointestinal tract daily, has a much more profound effect on the serum concentration of a protein that normally has a low fractional catabolic rate than one with a high fractional catabolic rate.[102] If the plasma volume and rate of synthesis and endogenous catabolism of an immunoglobulin remain constant, the ratio of the serum concentration of a protein in a patient with bulk loss of proteins to the concentration of that protein in normal individuals can be predicted from the following formula:

Patient protein level (as fraction of the normal level of that specific protein) = normal fractional catabolic rate of that protein/normal fractional catabolic rate + fractional rate of bulk loss.

Thus, for example, in a patient with a bulk loss of 15% of the intravascular pool of serum proteins into the intestinal tract daily, the concentration of IgG with a normal fractional catabolic rate of 6%/day would be reduced to 26% of normal $\left(\text{i.e., } \frac{6}{6 + 15}\right)$. Through a similar analysis it can be shown that the concentration of IgE with a normal fractional catabolic rate of 92%/day would only be reduced to 86% of normal in the same patient $\left(\text{i.e., } \frac{92}{92 + 15}\right)$. With the very rapidly turning-over proteins and polypeptides (e.g., insulin) there would be no significant reduction in the serum level.

The loss of serum components in patients with protein-losing gastroenteropathy is not limited to the serum proteins. It has been shown that iron, copper[101] calcium,[63] and lipids[64] may be lost into the intestinal tract in these patients. Also, loss of lymphocytes into the intestinal tract, causing lymphocytopenia and abnormalities of cellular immunity, is a major feature in patients with disorders of lymphatic channels of the bowel.[87,110]

Methods for Demonstrating Protein-losing Gastroenteropathy

Because most proteins normally undergo complete degradation in the gastrointestinal lumen with subsequent absorption of the constituent amino acids, conventional nitrogen balance techniques cannot be used to detect protein-losing gastroenteropathy. Electrophoretic and immunochemical analyses of gastrointestinal secretions have been of value in detecting serum proteins in secretions but cannot be used to quantify gastrointestinal protein loss, since all the gastrointestinal secretions cannot be aspirated quantitatively. Measurement of enteric protein loss has therefore been performed by 2 different approaches. In the first approach, the magnitude of the loss of serum proteins into the gastrointestinal tract is estimated by determining the fecal excretion of the radioactive label following IV administration of radiolabeled macromolecules. In the second approach, gastrointestinal protein loss is quantitated by determining the fecal clearance of alpha-1-antitrypsin, a protein that is relatively resistant to catabolism by intestinal proteases.

Radiolabeled Macromolecules. The ideal radiolabel for this purpose should fulfill the following requirements: First, one should be able to attach the label to serum proteins without altering the metabolic behavior of the protein to which it is bound in terms of either survival or distribution. Second, there should be no absorption of the radioactive label from the gastrointestinal tract after catabolism of the protein, as this would result in an underestimation of the extent of the gastrointestinal protein loss. Third, there should be no excretion of the label into the gastrointestinal lumen except when the label is bound to protein. Such secretion in the salivary, gastric, or biliary fluids would result in an overestimation of the magnitude of the gastrointestinal loss. If these requirements are fulfilled, the labeled macromolecule could be used to determine the fraction of the protein pool lost into the gastrointestinal tract per day, as well as to determine the protein pool sizes and catabolic and synthetic rates. Although none of the radiolabeled macromolecules fulfill all these requirements,. the materials that are available do provide a great deal of useful information. In addition, a complete definition of the parameters of protein metabolism can be obtained with a combination of 2 techniques.

Radioiodinated Serum Proteins. The radioiodinated serum proteins were the first widely used radioactive macromolecules for the detection of gastrointestinal protein loss. They fulfill the first requirement; i.e., the serum proteins can be iodinated without altering their metabolism if great care is taken in the isolation, radiolabeling, and storage of the proteins. To perform a radioiodinated protein turnover, the iodinated protein is administered IV to a patient who is receiving oral iodide to block thyroidal uptake of the isotope. Following catabolism of the labeled protein, virtually all radioactivity is excreted into the urine and none is reincorporated into serum proteins. The radioactivity remaining in the serum is determined over the subsequent 2- to 3-week period. In some studies, the time course of decline of protein-bound radioactivity in the whole body is also determined. This latter can be obtained either by direct measurement, using a whole body counter, or may be determined by, the cumulative subtraction of daily urinary excretion of radioactivity from the initially injected dose.

The exact techniques used and the assumptions inherent in the various methods of analysis of iodinated protein turnover data have been reviewed.[27,105] The serum data alone can be analyzed to determine the size of the protein pools, rate of protein catabolism, and rate of protein synthesis as follows: the plasma protein radioactivity is plotted as a function of time on semilogarithmic paper as indicated in Figure 110–1. This plasma radioactivity curve is resolved into

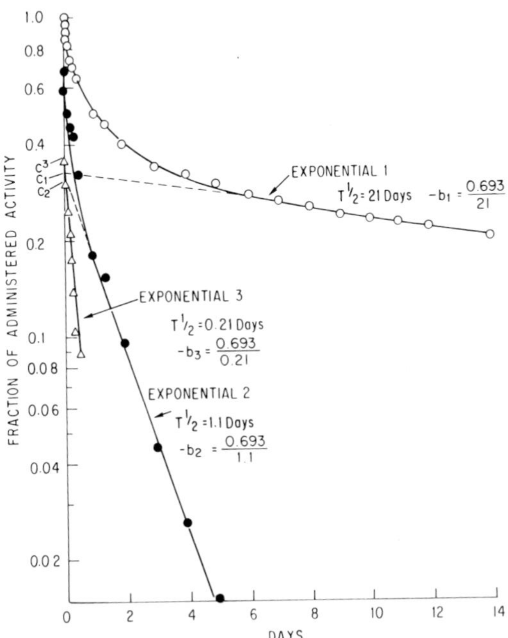

Figure 110–1. Graphic analysis of the plasma ^{125}I-albumin curve. The open circles represent actual measurements. The other points are graphically determined by "curve peeling." The original curve was plotted on semilogarithmic paper and its straight linear terminal portion was extrapolated to the ordinate to obtain the intercept c_1. The slope of this line is $-b_1$ (i.e., 1n 2/T½ in days). By subtracting the extrapolated line from the original curve, a new curve is obtained from which the slope and intercept value C_2 and $-b_2$ are obtained in the same manner as with the original curve. A third peeling yields C_3 and $-b_3$. Thus, the original curve may be described by three exponentials with slopes, $-b_1$, $-b_2$ and $-b_3$, and corresponding intercepts, c_1, c_2, and c_3. The metabolic parameters for albumin are determined from these slopes and intercepts using the formulas presented in the text.

2 or 3 exponential functions, each with an ordinate intercept c_i and a slope $-b_i$. The metabolic parameters are determined from these slopes and intercepts using the formulas shown at the bottom of the page.

Patients with protein-losing gastroenteropathy have reduced circulating pools of albumin, IgG, IgM, IgA, and ceruloplasmin. The synthetic rates for these proteins are normal or slightly increased. Their survival, however, is markedly reduced and the fractional catabolic rates (including endogenous catabolism and loss into the gastrointestinal tract) are markedly increased. For example, patients with protein-losing gastroenteropathy may catabolize over 70% of their plasma pool of albumin or IgG per day as compared with 6% to 10% of the plasma pool in normal individuals.

Although iodinated proteins have been very valuable in the study of the metabolic parameters of serum proteins in patients with protein-losing gastroenteropathy, they have certain limitations. There is rapid reabsorption of the radioiodide label following catabolism of the labeled protein in the intestinal lumen. There is also active secretion of radioiodide into the intestinal lumen in the salivary, gastric, and certain small intestinal secretions. The analysis of the data obtained from the serum and urinary radioactivity curves thus shows that hypercatabolism or loss, as opposed to decreased synthesis, is the cause of hypoproteinemia. The data, however, do not implicate the gastrointestinal tract as the site of this hypercatabolism. It should be noted that hypercatabolism resulting from disorders of endogenous catabolic mechanisms not involving loss of serum proteins can cause a very comparable pattern of protein metabolism. In an effort to overcome the problem of absorption of the radioiodine label, following catabolism of labeled protein lost into the intestinal tract, Citrin et al.[17] used intubation to collect the gastric secretions from a patient with giant gastric rugae who had previously received IV iodinated albumin. They were able to show significant protein-bound radioiodine in the gastric secretions of this patient. This technique has not had wide use, however, for the reason that all the gastrointestinal secretions cannot be collected. Another attempt to solve the problem of reabsorption of the iodide label by administering an ion exchange resin (Amberlite IRA 400) orally to trap the released radioiodine was also unsuccessful. This technique failed because significant secretion of non-protein-bound radioiodine into the intestinal tract persists. In addition, the resin does not trap most of the radioiodine liberated from proteins catabolized in the bowel lumen.[32] Thus, this technique does not provide any information that is not available using iodinated albumin turnover data alone and cannot be used to quantitate gastrointestinal protein loss.

^{51}Cr-labeled Proteins. A number of other labeled macromolecules have been proposed to circumvent the problems inherent in the use of iodinated serum proteins. The most widely used of these radiolabeled macromolecules for the detection of gastrointestinal protein loss are the ^{51}Cr-labeled serum proteins, including *^{51}Cr-labeled albumin,*[97,109] *^{51}Cr-labeled transferrin,* and serum proteins labeled in vivo by the IV administration of $^{51}CrCl_3$.[77,93] The ^{51}Cr label is neither significantly absorbed from nor secreted into the gastrointestinal tract. From 93% to 100% of the radioactivity of an orally administered dose of ^{51}Cr-albumin appears in the subsequent fecal collections. To use this radiolabeled macromolecule in a simple screening test, approximately 25 μCi of ^{51}Cr-albumin is administered IV. The stools over the subsequent 4 days are collected free of urine in 24-hour lots. They are then brought to a constant volume with water, homogenized, and counted with an appropriate standard in a gamma ray counter. The results are expressed as the percentage of the injected dose of radioactivity that is excreted in the stool in the 4 days following the IV administration of the isotope. Normal individuals excrete from 0.1% to 0.7% of the administered dose in the stool during this period, whereas patients with excessive gastrointestinal protein loss excrete from 2% to 40% of the dose.[97,109] Although the 4-day ^{51}Cr-albumin excretion study is a simple test that is of value in making the diagnosis of excessive gastrointestinal protein loss, it does not take full advantage of the relatively long survival of ^{51}Cr-albumin. It also does not provide data that can be meaningfully related to other parameters of protein metabolism determined with radioiodinated serum proteins.

A more meaningful measure of enteric protein loss, however, can be obtained if the clearance of ^{51}Cr-labeled serum protein is expressed as the fraction of the plasma pool or the milliliters of plasma lost into the gastrointestinal tract per day. This is accomplished by relating the fecal excretion of ^{51}Cr to the serum radioactivity curve in a fashion comparable to that of renal clearance techniques or to techniques used for quantitation of gastrointestinal red cell loss (Fig. 110–2). For these studies, stools are collected in daily lots for the 12-day period after IV administration of the ^{51}Cr-albumin and are processed and counted as just described. Serum samples are obtained 10 minutes after injection and daily thereafter and counted with an appropriate standard in a well-type gamma scintillation counter. Standards are used to correct for the differences in counting efficiency due to differences

$$\text{plasma volume (PV)} = \frac{\text{total activity injected intravenously}}{\text{activity/ml of plasma at zero time (extrapolated from samples taken during first few minutes of study)}} \tag{1}$$

$$\textbf{plasma pool of protein under study} = \textbf{plasma volume} \times \textbf{serum protein concentration} \tag{2}$$

$$\begin{array}{l}\textbf{Fraction of the total}\\ \textbf{body pool that is in}\\ \textbf{the intravascular space}\end{array} = \left(\sum_{i=1}^{n} \frac{c_i}{b_i}\right)^2 \Bigg/ \sum_{i=1}^{n} \frac{c_i}{(b_i)^2} \tag{3}$$

$$\begin{array}{l}\textbf{Fraction catabolic rate}\\ \textbf{(fraction of the intravascular}\\ \textbf{pool of protein catabolized per}\\ \textbf{day)}\end{array} = 1 \Bigg/ \left(\frac{c_1}{b_1} + \frac{c_2}{b_2} \cdots \frac{c_i}{b_i}\right) \tag{4}$$

$$\textbf{Absolute catabolic rate} = \textbf{fractional catabolic rate} \times \textbf{plasma protein pool} \tag{5}$$

If the patient is in the steady state, the synthetic rate is equal to the absolute catabolic rate for the protein.

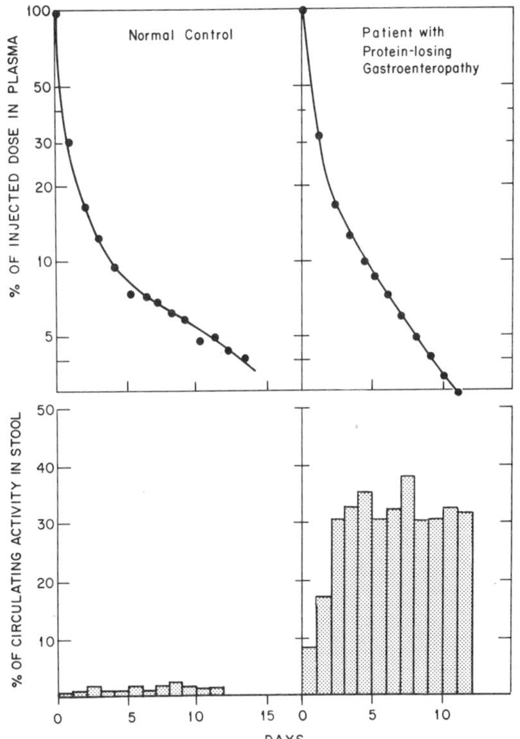

Figure 110–2. ^{51}Cr-albumin clearance studies in a normal control and in a patient with intestinal lymphangiectasia and protein-losing gastroenteropathy. Normal individuals clear from 0.2% to 1.6% of the plasma protein pool into the gastrointestinal tract daily, whereas the patient with intestinal lymphangiectasia and protein-losing gastroenteropathy cleared the protein from 30% of the circulating pool daily.

in geometry when counting serum and stool samples. The milliliters of plasma cleared into the gastrointestinal tract are then determined as follows:

$$\text{ml of plasma cleared of protein/day} = \frac{\text{counts in the stool in the 24-hr collection period}}{\text{counts/ml of serum 1 day before collection}}$$

This value assumes a transit time of 1 day between secretion of labeled protein into the gastrointestinal tract and its appearance in the stool. The mean value for milliliters of plasma cleared daily into the gastrointestinal tract over the period from the third to the twelfth day of study is determined. To calculate the fraction of the circulating protein pool cleared into the gastrointestinal tract per day, the milliliters of plasma cleared per day are divided by the plasma volume.

Another approach to obtain the clearance of plasma protein into the gastrointestinal tract that gives essentially identical results is to relate the total radioactivity excreted in the stools through the study period to the integral of the plasma radioactivity curve during this period. The clearance of plasma protein by this integral method may be expressed by the following equation:

$$Cl_{gi} = Q_f \Big/ \int_{to}^{tn} Q_p dt$$

where Q_f = cumulative fecal excretion of ^{51}Cr as a fraction of the injected dose and Q_p is the plasma radioactivity as a fraction of the injected dose. If the time is expressed in days, Cl_{gi} is equal to the fraction of the plasma pool cleared of protein into the intestinal tract daily. The integral $\int_{to}^{tn} Q_p\, dt$ represents the area under the plasma curve from the time of injection (to) until time at the completion of the study (tn). This area is usually determined by graphic resolution of a semilogarithmic plot of the plasma curve in a fashion comparable to that used for iodinated proteins. The curve is resolved into 2 or 3 exponential functions, each with an intercept c_i on the y axis and a slope $-b_i$. In this case,

$$Cl_{gi} = Q_f \Big/ \frac{c_{1to} - c_{1tn}}{b_1} + \frac{c_2}{b_2} \ldots \frac{c_i}{b_i}$$

where c_{ito} represents the intercept of the terminal slope $-b_1$ at the y axis and c_1t_n the value of the terminal slope at the conclusion of the study. Normal individuals clear the protein from 5 to 40 ml of plasma per day.[6,93,109] This is equal to a gastrointestinal clearance of 0.2% to 1.6% of the plasma pool of protein daily. In contrast, patients with excessive gastrointestinal protein loss clear from 50 to 1800 ml of plasma, representing from 2% to 60% of the intravascular pool of proteins into the intestinal tract daily.

Despite its advantages, ^{51}Cr-albumin has a significant limitation: a short apparent half-life of survival as compared with iodinated albumin. This half-life has been shown to be the result of elution of the chromium from the albumin with subsequent association of the label with other serum proteins, especially transferrin.[92] Although the elution of ^{51}Cr from the protein does not preclude its use in quantitating gastrointestinal protein loss by the clearance techniques (which assumes only that the specific activity of protein in the plasma is the same as that lost into the gastrointestinal tract), it does preclude the use of ^{51}Cr-albumin in the study of albumin catabolic and synthetic rates.

Intravenous administration of sterile $^{51}CrCl_3$ with in vivo labeling of a number of serum proteins has been advocated as an alternative technique for the detection of gastrointestinal protein loss.[77,92] Although a higher fraction of the administered radioactivity may be cleared by the kidney and reticuloendothelial system, the results of clearance studies using $^{51}CrCl_3$ are comparable to those using albumin labeled in vitro with ^{51}Cr.

^{131}I-Polyvinylpyrrolidone, ^{59}Fe-labeled Iron Dextran, ^{95}Nb-labeled Albumin, and ^{67}Cu-labeled Ceruloplasmin. A number of other radiolabeled macromolecules, including *^{131}I-polyvinylpyrrolidone,*[34] *^{59}Fe-dextran,*[4] *^{95}Nb-albumin,*[51] and *^{67}Cu-ceruloplasmin,*[101] which are not normally secreted or absorbed from the gastrointestinal tract, have been introduced for the evaluation of gastrointestinal protein loss. Each of these test substances is used in a fashion comparable to that used in ^{51}Cr-labeled serum protein studies; i.e., the fecal excretion of label is determined following the IV administration of the labeled macromolecules. These other test substances give results that are quite comparable to those obtained using ^{51}Cr-albumin. None of the other radiolabeled macromolecules appear to have major advantages over ^{51}Cr-labeled serum proteins for the routine detection of gastrointestinal protein loss.

Iodinated polyvinylpyrrolidone, a large polymer that is not metabolized by mammalian or bacterial enzymes, has proved to be a valuable material for use in a 4-day screening test for excessive gastrointestinal protein loss. However, the iodine-PVP bond is unstable on standing in vitro and in slightly alkaline solutions present in the small bowel in vivo. Also, variable amounts (10% to 68%) of the radioactive label that enters the gastrointestinal tract are absorbed.[34,46] Of greater significance, the PVP molecule is not a normal mammalian metabolite and differs from the serum proteins in size, structure, and charge. Unlike serum proteins administered IV, PVP disappears rapidly from the plasma and is either largely excreted into the urine or taken up by the reticuloendothelial system within 48 hours. It is thus only by inference that one gets information on serum protein metabolism with its use.

^{59}Fe-labeled dextran, another labeled non-protein macromolecule, has disadvantages similar to those of polyvinylpyrrolidone. A special advantage of this macromolecule, particularly in pediatric studies, is that there is little or no urinary excretion of the ^{59}Fe label during the study period in patients who do not have the nephrotic syndrome. Thus, one does not have to collect the stools free of urine. *^{95}Nb-labeled albumin* and especially *^{67}Cu-labeled ceruloplasmin* fulfill all the major requirements for techniques for the measurement of gastrointestinal protein loss. These radiolabeled macromolecules, however, are difficult and expensive to produce and are not commercially available. They are of special value in situations in which other techniques give conflicting results, as in the determination of the role of the normal gastrointestinal tract in plasma protein metabolism, whereas in the routine detection of gastrointestinal protein loss their expense precludes their use at this time.

Alpha-1-Antitrypsin Clearance. The measurement of fecal radioactivity after injection of the radiolabeled macromolecules is a valid approach for the quantitation of gastrointestinal protein loss. However, this test is not widely employed for routine patient care owing to the need to use radioactive products and to secure serial collections of feces free of urinary contamination. Furthermore, the radiolabeled macromolecules are no longer generally commercially available with the exception of $^{51}CrCl_3$ for in vivo labeling of serum proteins. In light of these problems, Crossly and Elliot[20] suggested an alternative approach that involves the quantitation of the fecal excretion of alpha-1-antitrypsin, a protein that is resistant to proteolysis. Alpha-1-antitrypsin has a molecular weight of 50,000 daltons and constitutes approximately 4% of the total serum protein content. In their initial studies, Crossly and Elliot[20] measured the alpha-1-antitrypsin concentration in saline extracts of random lyophilized fecal samples. In such studies, 250 mg of lyophilized feces is ground to a fine powder with a mortar and pestle, extracted with 5 ml of 0.9% saline by vigorous mixing with a vortex apparatus for 30 minutes, and centrifuged for 15 minutes at 4°C. The alpha-1-antitrypsin in a 5-μl aliquot of the supernatant is quantitated using commercially available immunodiffusion plates. These authors concluded that the measurement of alpha-1-antitrypsin provided a simple index of excessive loss of plasma proteins into the gastrointestinal tract.

Haeney and co-workers,[36] using a slightly different extraction procedure, did not obtain a correlation between fecal loss of alpha-1-antitrypsin and that of ^{51}Cr-albumin and questioned the validity of the fecal alpha-1-antitrypsin determination. However, in subsequent studies other workers have concluded that the determination of random fecal alpha-1-antitrypsin provides a reproducible method to screen for excessive intestinal protein loss.[89]

A more valid estimate for gastrointestinal protein loss was obtained by Florent and co-workers[30] and by other groups,[9,40,62] by quantitating the fecal clearance of alpha-1-antitrypsin. In these studies, the intestinal clearance expressed as milliliters (ml) of plasma cleared of alpha-1-antitrypsin into the intestinal tract per day was determined from the relationship:

$$\text{alpha-1-antitrypsin clearance (ml/d)} = \frac{V \times F}{P}$$

where V is the volume of the feces in ml/day, F is the alpha-1-antitrypsin concentration in the feces in mg/ml, and P is the serum alpha-1-antitrypsin concentration in mg/ml. In the studies of Florent et al.,[30] the upper limit of the normal antitrypsin clearance value was 13 ml/day. There was a highly significant correlation between the alpha-1-antitrypsin clearance and the ^{51}Cr protein clearance. There were no false-negative or false-positive determinations in the study of Hill and co-workers.[40] In the study of Florent et al.,[30] the positive predictive value of the test was 97.7% and the negative predictive value was 75%.

There are certain limitations in the use of this technique. The slope of the regression curve relating the alpha-1-antitrypsin fecal clearance to the $^{51}CrCl_3$ fecal clearance was 0.55, whereas theoretically it should be 1.0, considering that the 2 proteins are lost by passive diffusion and have similar molecular weights. One potential explanation for this discrepancy is that alpha-1-antitrypsin might be catabolized in the small intestine following its loss into the gastrointestinal tract. It is clear that such catabolism occurs for this protein when it is lost into the stomach inasmuch as alpha-1-antitrypsin is virtually completely destroyed by incubation with gastric juice ($pH<3$) at 37°C for 1 hour. In light of this latter observation, the use of alpha-1-antitrypsin clearance studies would not appear to be of value when gastric loss of serum proteins is suspected. However, the alpha-1-antitrypsin clearance appears to be a reliable clinical test for detecting excessive protein loss distal to the pylorus.

Critique of Methods. It is clear that there are many valuable techniques for the measurement of enteric protein loss. When considered in terms of the criteria for an ideal label, the information obtainable, and commercial availability, the techniques involving fecal clearance of IV administered $^{51}CrCl_3$ and those determining the intestinal clearance of alpha-1-antitrypsin are the most practical procedures for the diagnosis of protein-losing gastroenteropathy. If a complete analysis of protein metabolism is desired, ^{125}I serum proteins may be used simultaneously with ^{51}Cr-labeled serum proteins. The size of the protein pools and rates of protein catabolism and synthesis can be determined from the ^{125}I protein data and the rate of protein loss into the gastrointestinal tract quantitated with a ^{51}Cr-labeled protein clearance study. The site of loss of protein into the gastrointestinal tract may be determined in these studies by aspirating the gastrointestinal contents at different levels to determine the site of appearance of radioactivity following IV administration of ^{51}Cr-labeled serum proteins.

Diseases Associated with Protein-losing Gastroenteropathy

Protein-losing gastroenteropathy is a common phenomenon that has been demonstrated in association with a large number of disorders affecting the gastrointestinal tract (Table 110–1). It is not only noted with diseases restricted to the gastrointestinal tract, but may be a significant feature as well of a number of generalized disorders. Among these are congestive heart failure, immunodeficiency diseases, connective tissue disorders, the nephrotic syndrome, and metastatic malignancy. In many of these disorders a modest increase in the rate of enteric protein loss is but one of several abnormalities, and the primary gastrointestinal disorder is readily apparent from other more prominent gastrointestinal symptoms. In contrast to these patients, others with protein-losing gastroenteropathy are seen who have unexplained edema and hypoproteinemia as their only symptoms. If excessive gastrointestinal loss is demonstrated, the physician's diagnostic efforts must then be directed toward defining the specific disease affecting the gastrointestinal tract. In such cases the demonstration of protein-losing gastroenteropathy may be the only clue to a potentially fatal but treatable disorder.

Diseases with Disorders of Intestinal Lymphatics

Intestinal Lymphangiectasia

Clinical Manifestations. Intestinal lymphangiectasia is a disorder characterized by the early onset of edema, hypoproteinemia, and lymphocytopenia as a result of a generalized disorder of lymphatic channels, including dilated, telangiectatic lymphatic vessels of the small bowel.[104] This is a disease that primarily affects children and young adults, with a range in age of onset of symptoms from birth to 30 years in over 90% of cases.[8,42,64,73,79,94,104] The mean age of onset is 11 years. Males and females are affected equally. In the majority of cases (over 75%), the disease is sporadic. Intestinal lymphangiectasis has been associated with Noonan's syndrome in 3 cases,[39,91] congenital glaucoma in 3 cases, peliosis hepatis in 2 cases, Charcot-Marie-Tooth syndrome in 2 cases, and hypobetalipoproteinemia in 2 cases.[25] There have been at least 11 families with 2 to 4 affected siblings, suggesting a genetic etiology in some cases.

The major symptoms are *edema* and *diarrhea.* At the onset, the *edema* may be intermittent but later becomes a constant feature. The edema was clearly asymmetrical in 15% of the patients studied. Three of the patients presented with reversible blindness as a result of the development of macular edema. *Chylous effusions* developed during the course of their disease in 45% of the patients.

Gastrointestinal symptoms are usually mild but may on occasion be entirely absent or quite severe. Severe diarrhea and steatorrhea were present in 20%, mild diarrhea was present in 60%, and no gastrointestinal symptoms were present in the remaining 20% of the patients studied. Abdominal pain and vomiting were significant features in 15% of the patients. *Intestinal obstruction* due to adhesions may occur, especially in those patients with *chylous ascites. Hypocalcemic tetany* was present in 12% of the patients studied and was most common in those individuals with severe steatorrhea. *Growth retardation* (linear growth below the third percentile) is present in the majority of children with onset of edema and diarrhea within the first 10 years of life. Repeated episodes of lymphangitis of the extremity occur in some patients. In addition, there is an increased frequency of tuberculosis and reticuloendothelial malignancies,[106] possibly due to the lymphocytopenia and the inability to make a cellular immune response. Except for *edema,* physical examination is not remarkable. Inanition, malnutrition, and weight loss are not as prominent as in non-tropical sprue or celiac disease, except in the late stages of the disease in infants with severe intestinal lymphangiectasia and malabsorption.

The major laboratory findings are the *reduced concentration of the serum proteins* and *lymphocytopenia.* The mean total protein concentration of the 25 patients with intestinal lymphangiectasia seen at the National Institutes of Health was 3.5 g/dl with a mean albumin concentration of 1.8 g/dl. The IgG, IgA, and IgM concentrations were 4.5 ± 2.1, 1.15 ± 0.32, and 0.76 ± 0.26 mg/ml, respectively, in the patients, as compared with 12.1 ± 2.7, 2.6 ± 1, and 1.45 ± 0.6 mg/ml in control individuals. In addition, 50% of the patients had a *reduced serum transferrin* level and 30% had a *plasma fibrinogen* concentration below 200 mg/dl. In contrast, the serum concentrations of other proteins that ordinarily have a shorter survival were normal. Thus, the total alpha and beta globulin levels in patients with intestinal lymphangiectasia are nearly normal, and the serum concentration of the rapidly catabolized immunoglobulin IgE is within the normal range. The prothrombin time is normal in the majority of patients, but may be depressed in those with malabsorption.

The serum cholesterol level is normal or low in these patients, in contrast to the elevated levels seen in patients with hypoalbuminemia and the nephrotic syndrome. The mean cholesterol level in the patients with intestinal lymphangiectasia was 150 mg/dl. The total serum calcium, particularly the protein-bound fraction, may be slightly decreased. In those patients with steatorrhea the ionized serum calcium concentration, and in some cases the magnesium concentration, may be sufficiently reduced to produce tetany. The majority of patients with intestinal lymphangiectasia are not anemic and may even have a slightly elevated hematocrit level associated with a reduction in the plasma volume. Some patients are anemic, however, with a low serum iron and iron-binding protein. In these patients the peripheral red cells are mildly hypochromic. Extreme anemia is present in rare patients who have massive blood loss associated with an abnormal connection between the venous system and the intestinal lymphatic channels.[21]

Immunologic Studies. Although patients with intestinal lymphangiectasia have reduced serum concentrations of the major classes of immunoglobulin molecules, they make humoral immunologic antibody responses when challenged with antigens. Patients with intestinal lymphangiectasia show a more profound abnormality when the cellular immune system is evaluated. They are moderately to markedly lymphocytopenic, with a mean lymphocyte count of 710 ± 340/mm^3 as compared with 2500 ± 600/mm^3 in a control group of normal individuals.[87] This lymphocytopenia is due to the loss of lymphocyte-rich lymph fluid into the gastrointestinal tract secondary to the disorder of gastrointestinal lymphatic channels. *In vitro* studies of lymphocyte function have shown that patients with intestinal lymphangiectasia have relatively depleted populations of lymphocytes necessary for cell-mediated immunity; i.e., lymphocytes of patients with intestinal lymphangiectasia have impaired *in vitro* transformation to non-specific mitogens, specific antigens, and allogeneic cells when compared with equal numbers of lymphocytes from normal individuals.[110]

As a consequence of their lymphocytopenia and preferential depletion in long-lived thymus-dependent lymphocytes, patients with intestinal lymphangiectasia have *abnormalities of delayed hypersensitivity skin tests.*[87] Thus, less than 10% of patients with intestinal lymphangiectasia studied manifested positive skin reactions to mumps, trichophytin, *Candida albicans,* streptokinase-streptodornase, tetanus, or diphtheria antigens, whereas over 97% of the normal controls had a positive reaction to one or more of these agents. The presence of skin anergy should be kept in mind when patients with intestinal lymphangiectasia are evaluated for diseases such as tuberculosis, inasmuch as they cannot manifest a positive tuberculin test. None of the patients with intestinal lymphangiectasia studied could be sensitized to dinitrochlorobenzene (DNCB), whereas over 95% of the control population could be sensitized with this agent. In addition, patients with intestinal lymphangiectasia did not reject skin grafts from unrelated donors; such grafts have remained with no evidence of rejection in 5 patients studied during a 2-year period of observation. In addition, second-set grafts from the same donor have shown no evidence of rejection over a period of approximately 1 year.

Thus, *in summary* of the immunologic features, patients with intestinal lymphangiectasia have a primary abnormality in the development of lymphatic channels and secondarily lose lymphocytes and immunoglobulins into the gastrointestinal tract. The resultant lymphocytopenia and preferential depletion of long-lived recirculating lymphocytes lead to abnormalities of cellular immunity, with skin anergy and impaired homograft rejection.

Absorption Studies. *Steatorrhea* with increased chemical fecal fat has been found in over 75% of the patients; in about 50% the increase in fecal fat was minimal, being 7% to 10% of the ingested fat, while in another 25% it was greater than 10%. The vitamin A tolerance test may be abnormal. Fecal nitrogen may be normal or slightly increased. The carbohydrate absorption tests, including the glucose, D-xylose, and lactose tolerance tests, have usually been within normal limits in the limited number of patients who have been studied by these methods.

Roentgen Findings. The findings on barium meal study of the small bowel have been abnormal in over 75% of the patients. The most common findings are thickening and enlargement of the valvulae conniventes of the jejunum and ileum and increased secretions (Fig. 110–3). Slight jejunal dilatation with puddling and segmentation of contrast media is encountered to a lesser extent.[61,82]

Pedal lymphangiograms are abnormal in virtually all the patients, supporting the concept that this disease is a generalized lymphatic disorder.[70] Many patients have hypoplasia of the lymphatics of the lower extremity, with dermal backflow similar to that seen with primary lymphedema. No thoracic duct can be visualized in about one-fourth of the patients. In one case there was agenesis of the retroperitoneal lymph nodes. In a number of cases there was reflux of contrast medium into the mesenteric lymphatics with extravasation of contrast material into the proximal small bowel, or even into the peritoneum in a patient with chylous ascites.[13,64,95]

Jejunal Histology. Biopsy of the jejunal mucosa discloses the "hallmark" lesion of the disease, which is *dilatation of the lymph vessels of the mucosa and submucosa* (Figs. 110–4 and 110–5). In some areas the individual

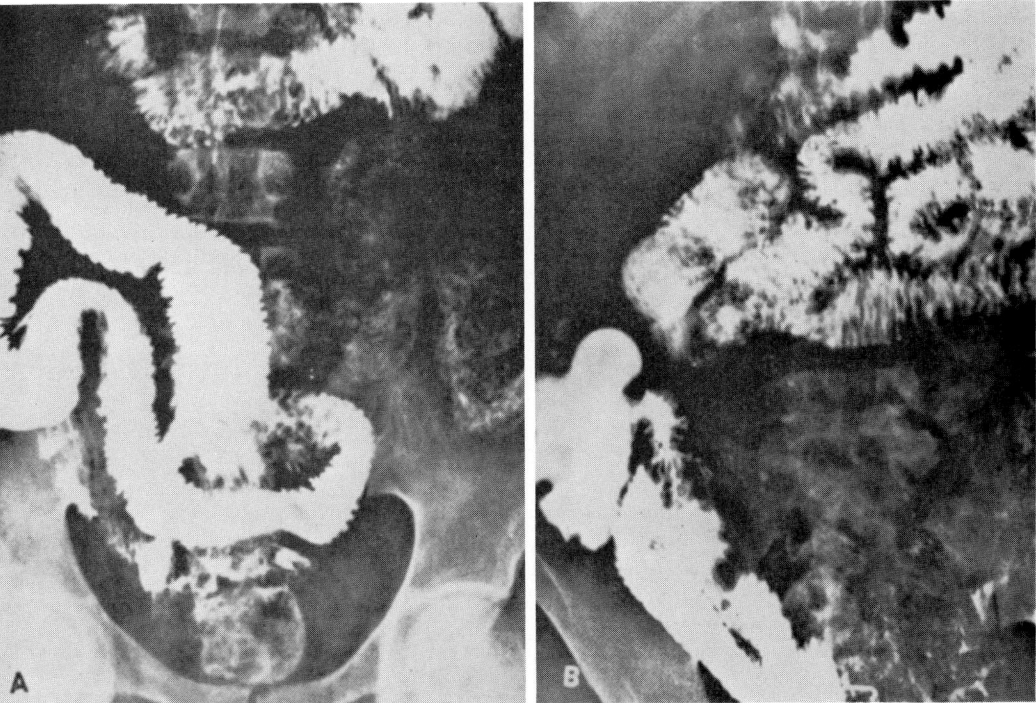

Figure 110–3. *A,* Slight dilatation of the proximal jejunum and moderate dilatation of the distal jejunum. This is associated with prominence of the folds and slight increase in secretions. *B,* The terminal ileum shows coarsening of the folds. There is no rigidity and no evidence of inflammatory change. (From Marshak RH et al. Radiology 1961; 77:893. Reproduced with permission.)

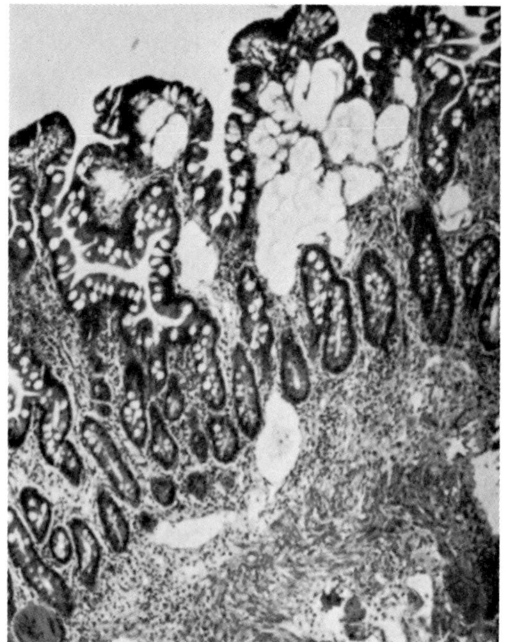

Figure 110–4. Peroral suction biopsy: villi distorted by several dilated lymph vessels. Note foamy lipophages in channel just above muscularis mucosae. (Hematoxylin and eosin, × 73.) (From Waldmann TA et al. Gastroenterology 1961; 41:197. © 1961, Williams & Wilkins. Reproduced with permission.)

villi containing dilated lymphatics have a normal architecture, but in others enlargement of many channels results in widening and distortion of the villi. The dilated lymphatic channels may contain foamy lipophages. These foamy macrophages do not contain the periodic acid–Schiff staining material present in Whipple's disease. In some patients, virtually every villus is involved and all peroral biopsy specimens show the classic features of this disease; in other patients, the lesions are more patchy in distribution and multiple biopsies are required before the diagnosis can be made.

Pathology. The gross appearance of the small intestine discloses edema of the affected areas. The serosal lymphatic vessels are dilated, and yellow nodules less than 5 mm in diameter can sometimes be seen along their course (Fig. 110–6). The mesenteric lymph nodes may contain similar yellow foci. The lumen of the bowel may be slightly dilated and the folds of Kerckring are prominent throughout. There is no atrophy of the mucosa as is found in sprue. In the affected areas, the villi are swollen and broader than normal. The villi may have enlarged bulblike tips, imparting a white pebbly appearance to the mucosal surface. A lipofuscin or seroid pigment may be seen in the external muscular layers.

The mesenteric lymphatics have a greatly thickened and fragmented elastica interna and there is hypertrophy of the muscular layers of the media. Fibrous tissue from the adventitia can penetrate and narrow the lumen of these vessels. The mesenteric lymph nodes show similar changes. The sinuses are usually dilated and relatively acellular.

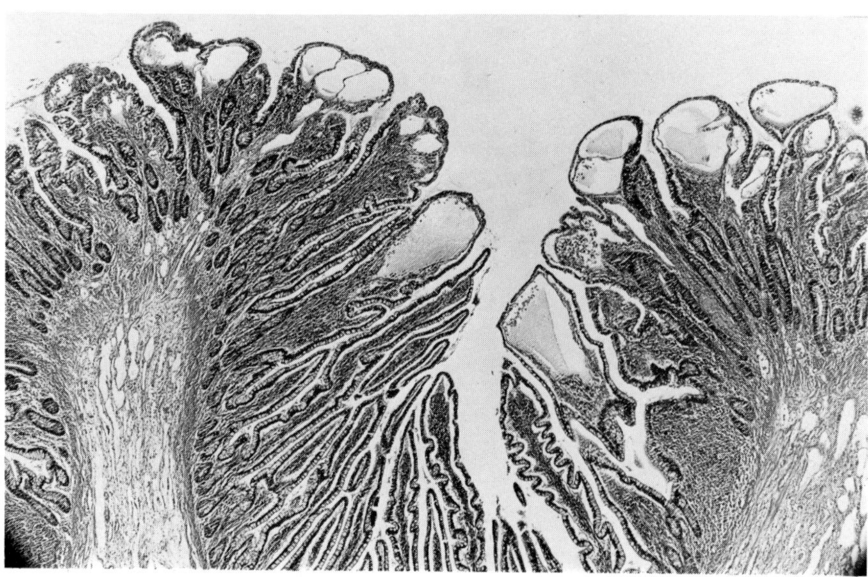

Figure 110–5. Intestinal biopsy from a patient with intestinal lymphangiectasia. Dilated lymphatic channels are present in mucosa and in submucosa. (Hematoxylin and eosin, × 27.) (From Strober W et al. J Clin Invest 1967; 46:1643. Reproduced with permission.)

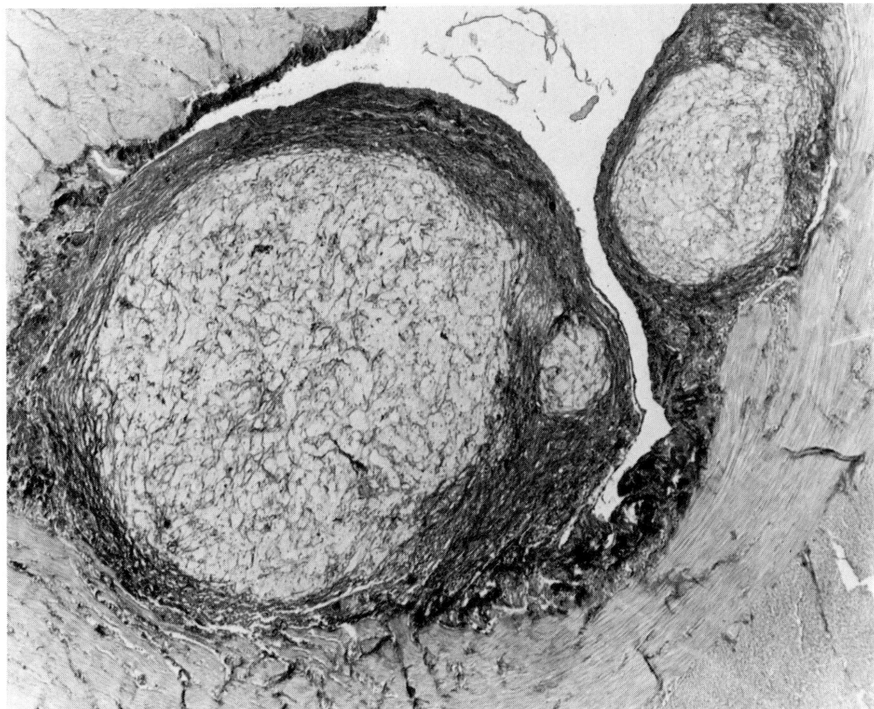

Figure 110–6. Laparotomy specimen. Serosal lymph vessels occluded by foamy lipophages. (Hematoxylin and eosin, × 48.) (From Waldmann TA et al. Gastroenterology 1961; 41:197. © 1961, Williams & Wilkins. Reproduced with permission.)

Foamy lipophages similar to those seen in the villi may be encountered. There is a marked reduction in the number of small lymphocytes of the mucosa and submucosa of the small bowel and the lymph nodes that may be secondary to the chronic gastrointestinal loss of long-lived recirculating lymphocytes.

Patients with intestinal lymphangiectasia thus appear to have a *generalized abnormality of lymphatic channel development* as their primary abnormality, with the loss of serum proteins and lymphocytes into the bowel as a secondary consequence of the disorder of gastrointestinal lymphatics. The pathogenesis of the lymphatic abnormalities in these patients remains obscure. A congenital malformation with a genetic etiology is most likely in those patients with an onset at birth and with a familial history of hypoproteinemia and chylous effusions. In other cases an acquired defect secondary to retroperitoneal fibrosis, pancreatitis, or other causes may be present.

Diagnosis and Differential Diagnosis. The diagnosis of intestinal lymphangiectasia should be suspected in patients, particularly of the younger age group, who have peripheral edema and a marked depression of the serum proteins that is not explained on the basis of proteinuria or hepatic disease. Both the serum albumin and gamma globulin are significantly reduced. The demonstration of a reduction in the serum concentration of these proteins with different sites of synthesis is of value in differentiating this syndrome from disorders of protein synthesis. Patients with intestinal lymphangiectasia have significant lymphocytopenia, a finding that is of major value in differentiating this disorder from diseases with protein loss into the intestinal tract due to mechanisms other than abnormalities of the intestinal lymphatic channels. There are 2 minimal essential features that must be demonstrated in order to make the diagnosis of intestinal lymphangiectasia. The first is the direct demonstration of excessive gastrointestinal protein loss by one of the techniques described earlier: an alpha-1-antitrypsin intestinal clearance test or a test with an IV administered radiolabeled macromolecule, such as ^{51}Cr-labeled serum proteins, ^{59}Fe-dextran, ^{95}Nb-albumin, ^{67}Cu-ceruloplasmin, or ^{131}I-PVP, to differentiate this syndrome from disorders in which the hypoproteinemia is secondary to decreased protein synthesis or accelerated endogenous protein catabolism. The second essential procedure for the diagnosis is the peroral gut biopsy; demonstration of dilated lymphatic channels of the small bowel is required for the diagnosis of intestinal lymphangiectasia.

LIVER DISEASE. Although hepatic disease is associated with hypoalbuminemia and edema with ascites, it can be differentiated from intestinal lymphangiectasia on clinical grounds and absence of hypogammaglobulinemia and lymphocytopenia. In addition, the hypoalbuminemia of liver disease can be shown to be the result of decreased albumin synthesis rather than excessive loss into the gastrointestinal tract.

IMMUNOLOGIC DEFICIENCY DISEASES. In infants, the differential diagnosis between primary immunodeficiency diseases and intestinal lymphangiectasia may be difficult. Over 50% of patients with congenital or acquired hypogammaglobulinemia have reduction in their serum albumin concentration in addition to reduction in gamma globulin concentration. Furthermore, 20% to 50% of these patients have significant gastrointestinal symptoms and many have lymphocytopenia. Patients with severe combined immunodeficiency disease present with many of the features seen in patients with intestinal lymphangiectasia, including hypoalbuminemia, hypogammaglobulinemia, diarrhea, lymphocytopenia, and skin anergy. The extreme reduction in immunoglobulin concentration, as well as the absence of severe gastrointestinal protein loss or dilated intestinal lymphatic channels in patients with the immunodeficiency syndromes, differentiates them from patients with intestinal lymphangiectasia.

CELIAC SYNDROME (Chapter 105). There are a number of similarities between patients with the celiac syndrome and those with intestinal lymphangiectasia. Patients with either disorder may have hypoalbuminemia and hypogammaglobulinemia associated with protein-losing gastroenteropathy. In addition, they may have steatorrhea and diarrhea as well as edema as major complaints. These 2 conditions, however, can be differentiated, by virtue of the fact that patients with the celiac syndrome have more severe steatorrhea and a greater impairment of various absorption tests, including those involving carbohydrate absorption. Patients with the celiac syndrome do not have the lymphocytopenia and abnormalities of delayed hypersensitivity that are present in patients with intestinal lymphangiectasia. In addition, patients with the celiac syndrome have an atrophic small intestinal mucosa with broad, thickened, blunted villi, whereas patients with intestinal lymphangiectasia have dilated lymphatic channels of the villi. Finally, remission with a gluten-free diet is seen in patients with the celiac syndrome, but not in patients with intestinal lymphangiectasia.

ALLERGIC GASTROENTEROPATHY. An abnormal response to dietary proteins (especially milk proteins) is a common cause of extreme gastrointestinal protein loss in infancy. Patients with allergic gastroenteropathy have hypoalbuminemia, hypogammaglobulinemia, and edema and may have diarrhea. In contrast to patients with intestinal lymphangiectasia, however, they do not have lymphocytopenia or skin anergy, and they have no dilated lymphatic channels demonstrable on peroral small intestinal biopsy.

WHIPPLE'S DISEASE (Chapter 109). Patients with Whipple's disease and those with intestinal lymphangiectasia have many features in common, including hypoalbuminemia, hypogammaglobulinemia, steatorrhea, edema, lymphocytopenia, and dilated lymphatic channels of the small bowel. However, the macrophages of the small intestine take the periodic acid–Schiff stain in patients with Whipple's disease but not in patients with intestinal lymphangiectasia. Furthermore, the gastrointestinal protein loss of patients with Whipple's disease responds to therapy with antibiotics and adrenal corticosteroids, whereas the patients with intestinal lymphangiectasia are not benefited by such therapy.

INTESTINAL LYMPHANGIECTASIA ASSOCIATED WITH AN INFLAMMATORY PROCESS. A group of patients have been identified by Fleisher and co-workers[29] who have dilated intestinal lymphatics and protein-losing enteropathy, but also have features that aid in distinguishing them from the majority of patients with intestinal lymphangiectasia. In contrast to patients with classic intestinal lymphangiectasia, these patients have a markedly elevated erythrocyte sedimentation rate and have normal or even elevated levels of serum immunoglobulins. Furthermore, in some cases there are transient abnormalities of the antinuclear antibody (ANA) and lupus erythematosus (LE) tests. It was suggested that the intestinal lymphangiectasia was secondary to an inflammatory process in these patients. Differing from the majority of patients with intestinal lymphangiectasia, these patients show partial or complete remission of all clinical features, including the protein-losing enteropathy, following corticosteroid therapy. In most cases, therapy with corticosteroids can be stopped after a period of months without recurrence of the protein-losing enteropathy.

CARDIAC DISEASE. The most important disease in the differential diagnosis of intestinal lymphangiectasia is the lymphopenic protein-losing enteropathy resulting from congestive heart failure. Of 60 patients seen at the National Institutes of Health with the tentative diagnosis of intestinal lymphangiectasia, 22 had had congestive failure, especially constrictive pericarditis. Patients with protein-losing gastroenteropathy due to congestive heart failure present with a clinical pattern that is very similar to that of intestinal lymphangiectasia; these patients have hypoproteinemia, edema, excessive gastrointestinal protein loss, lymphocytopenia, skin anergy, and dilated lymphatic channels of the small intestine. The patients with cardiac disease as their primary disease can be differentiated from those with primary intestinal lymphangiectasia because all of the former have an elevated venous pressure as well as other manifestations of right heart failure. Significant care should be taken to rule out cardiac disease in all patients with the tentative diagnosis of intestinal lymphangiectasia, considering that the disorders of lymphocyte and protein metabolism are completely reversible in such patients after surgical or medical therapy for the cardiac disease.

Treatment. There is no universally successful specific treatment for patients with intestinal lymphangiectasia. Rarely, only resection of a localized segment of affected bowel will relieve the clinical manifestations and disorders of protein metabolism.[42,50]

As noted, there may be a complete remission of the protein-losing enteropathy in patients with intestinal lymphangiectasia associated with an inflammatory disorder following corticosteroid therapy.[29] In over half the patients, a significant increase in serum protein concentration and reduction in edema have been reported when the patients were placed on a low fat diet or a diet in which long-chain triglycerides are replaced by medium-chain triglycerides.[43,52] There is a 2- to 3-fold increase in the thoracic duct flow following the administration of long-chain triglycerides. The use of a low fat diet or a diet using medium-chain triglycerides that are absorbed directly into the portal vein rather than through the lymphatics would be expected to have its effects through a reduction of lymph flow and pressure.

Prognosis. The usual course of intestinal lymphangiectasia shows relatively little or no progression. However, approximately 30% of the patients are unable to work because of extreme fatigue and weakness associated with the hypoproteinemia. In infants with associated severe diarrhea and malabsorption, the disease may be fatal. In these individuals, death may be related to extreme malabsorption, intestinal obstruction, or recurrent infections.

Congestive Heart Failure. Excessive gastrointestinal protein and lymphocyte loss has been demonstrated in patients with congestive failure secondary to a variety of cardiac diseases. [22,24,26,41,50,65,67,69,89,109] The majority of such patients have *constrictive pericarditis,* but isolated cases have been recorded with idiopathic cardiomyopathy, lupus erythematosus with pericarditis, Hodgkin's disease with chest irradiation causing constrictive pericarditis, congenital pulmonic stenosis, interatrial septal defect, rheumatic heart disease with tricuspid regurgitation, the carcinoid syndrome, and thrombosis of the superior vena cava. These diseases have diverse causes and different morphologic features, but the cardiac hemodynamics are similar in that they are characterized by *right heart failure* and an *elevation of the central venous pressure.*

Patients with cardiac disease and protein-losing gastroenteropathy present with *hypoproteinemia* and *edema* as the major clinical manifestations. Rare patients also develop hypocalcemic tetany. Despite an extreme rate of gastrointestinal protein loss, the symptoms referable to the intestinal tract are only moderate. *Diarrhea* is present in just over half of the patients, and approximately one-third have *steatorrhea.*

The major laboratory findings are comparable to those seen in intestinal lymphangiectasia, with marked *hypoalbuminemia* and *hypogammaglobulinemia*. Also seen are *lymphocytopenia* and an *immune deficiency state* characterized by an inability to manifest delayed hypersensitivity skin test responses and an inability to reject skin grafts from unrelated donors at a normal rate.[65,87] Thus, skin tests cannot be accurately interpreted in patients with congestive failure and protein-losing gastroenteropathy. This is especially important in the diagnostic evaluation of patients with constrictive pericarditis in whom tuberculosis is often a diagnostic possibility. This point is illustrated by the fact that some patients with constrictive pericarditis and a negative skin test for tuberculosis before therapy develop a positive skin test postoperatively, concomitant with a reversal of the protein-losing enteropathy and an elevation of the level of circulating lymphocytes.

Steatorrhea with increased chemical fecal fat may be found in some patients, but the D-xylose absorption test is normal. Roentgen examination of the gastrointestinal tract usually either is normal or shows edema of the small intestine. Dilatation of intestinal lymphatics comparable to that seen in intestinal lymphangiectasia has been demonstrated in patients with protein-losing enteropathy associated with constrictive pericarditis.[55,67,102]

The possible causes for hypoalbuminemia in patients with severe heart failure include: (1) hypervolemia with an increase in plasma volume and dilution of the serum proteins; (2) impaired synthesis of albumin owing to malnutrition or to hepatic fibrosis and cirrhosis associated with the cardiac failure; or (3) excessive loss of albumin into the gastrointestinal tract. Although hypervolemia and decreased albumin synthesis may contribute to the hypoalbuminemia in certain patients, the major pathophysiologic factor in patients with severe hypoalbuminemia appears to be protein-losing gastroenteropathy. The total exchangeable albumin of these patients may be less than 50% of normal, ruling out simple dilution as the cause. The rate of albumin synthesis is normal or slightly increased, eliminating the cause of impaired protein synthesis resulting from malnutrition or liver disease. However, the rate of albumin turnover is much more rapid than normal, with a high albumin fractional catabolic rate and a half-life of albumin survival of less than 4 days (normal 17 ± 2 days). Proteinuria is absent, but excessive protein loss into the gastrointestinal tract may be demonstrated by ^{131}I-PVP or ^{51}Cr-albumin tests.

The mechanism of the protein-losing enteropathy in congestive failure has not been conclusively elucidated. Davidson and coworkers[22] suggested that elevated systemic venous pressure in cardiac patients may lead to congestion of the lymphatics of the bowel wall with loss of protein-rich lymph into the gastrointestinal tract. This view is supported by a number of observations in animals and man that indicate that systemic venous hypertension leads to abnormal lymph drainage and lymph production. Blalock et al.[12] and Földi and associates[31] have demonstrated marked increases in thoracic duct pressure and have shown dilatation of the lymphatics of the bowel following ligation of the superior vena cava or experimental production of pericarditis in animals. Dumont et al.[28] carried out thoracic duct drainage in patients with intractable heart failure due to vascular disease. The thoracic duct was dilated in each case, and the lymph flow, as measured by cannulation, was increased. Similarly, Petersen and Ottosen[68] found increased thoracic duct flow (measured by cannulation) in patients with constrictive pericarditis. The foregoing studies suggest that venous hypertension causes an increase in lymph production as well as a functional obstruction to normal lymph drainage into the central veins. The suggestion that there is a functional disorder of gastrointestinal lymph drainage is supported by the observation that patients with protein-losing enteropathy and right heart failure have lymphocytopenia,[86] a feature that has been associated with the gastrointestinal loss of lymphocyte-rich lymph. In addition, some patients with congestive failure have markedly dilated lymphatic channels in the mediastinum and in the intestine.[55,67,112]

Treatment of the protein-losing enteropathy associated with congestive heart failure should be directed toward relieving the cardiac lesion. Complete or partial amelioration of the gastrointestinal protein and lymphocyte loss follows pericardectomy or repair of an interatrial septal defect. In patients without surgically correctable lesions, control of the congestive failure by medical means may also result in return to normal serum protein and lymphocyte levels. In adequately treated patients, the ability to manifest delayed hypersensitivity skin test responses returns to normal.

Granulomatous Disease of the Small Intestine and Mesentery. Holman et al.[42] and Schwartz and Jarnum[79] described patients with protein-losing gastroenteropathy and disorders of intestinal lymphatic channels who were found to have non-specific granulomatous lesions involving the jejunum (Chapter 111). Although the lesions are similar to other granulomatous disorders, they are apparently not sarcoidosis, tuberculosis, or Crohn's disease.

The major symptoms—diarrhea and peripheral edema—are similar to those of patients with intestinal lymphangiectasia. Malabsorption with steatorrhea may be present. Hypochromic anemia, hypoalbuminemia, and hypocalcemia are the major laboratory findings. Barium studies of the small bowel disclose an abnormal non-specific loss of the mucosal pattern. At laparotomy the major finding is diffuse dilatation of lymphatics of the mesentery and peritoneum. Dilated and stenotic loops of the small bowel may be encountered. In one patient, the lymph nodes showed greatly dilated lymphatics with acute and chronic inflammation. In another, there were reticuloendothelial hyperplasia, fibrosis, and giant cells containing crystals of unknown composition. One of the patients was asymptomatic following resection of the jejunal lesion.

Whipple's Disease (Intestinal Lipodystrophy). Hypoalbuminemia is present in over 80% of the patients with Whipple's disease in relapse (Chapter 109). Excessive loss of serum proteins into the gastrointestinal tract is the major factor causing this hypoalbuminemia.[59] Patients with Whipple's disease have lymphocytopenia, skin anergy, and dilatation of lymphatics of the intestinal mucosa. These findings suggest that an acquired abnormality of lymphatic channels may be involved in the pathogenesis of the protein-losing gastroenteropathy. Treatment with antibiotics alone, or with antibiotics and corticosteroids, results in a subsidence of diarrhea and malabsorption, disappearance of bacillary bodies from the intestinal mucosa, decrease in the periodic acid Schiff–positive macrophages in the lamina propria of the intestinal mucosa, and remission in the loss of proteins and lymphocytes into the intestinal tract.

Diseases with Ulceration of Mucosa of the Intestinal Tract

Inflammatory Diseases. Hypoproteinemia and hypoalbuminemia have been reported in from 20% to 75% of patients with Crohn's disease and ulcerative colitis (Chapters 126 and 127). Excessive loss of plasma proteins into the gastrointestinal tract has been shown to be the major factor in the hypoalbuminemia and reduction in total body protein pools observed.[84] The survival of radioiodinated albumin and gamma globulin was reduced and the fecal excretion of IV administered ^{131}I-PVP, ^{51}Cr-albumin, and ^{59}Fe-dextran was increased.[7,49,84] The magnitude of the gastrointestinal protein loss was shown to correlate with the extent and activity of the disease.[7] The mechanism of protein loss would appear to be the loss of blood and oozing of exudate containing plasma proteins from an inflamed ulcerating granular area.

Transient hypoproteinemia and edema associated with protein-losing gastroenteropathy have also been shown to complicate a prolonged episode of acute non-specific gastroenteritis or gastroenteritis associated with infection with staphylococcal, shigella, or salmonella organisms. In addition, excessive gastrointestinal protein loss has been described in association with infection with various parasites, including *Entamoeba histolytica, Giardia lamblia, Strongyloides,* and *Capillaria philippinensis.*

Malignant Diseases. Hypoalbuminemia is an exceedingly common accompaniment of malignancy. Decreased albumin synthesis appears to be the major pathophysiologic mechanism responsible for the hypoproteinemia, even in those patients who have normal liver function tests and who do not have malabsorption.[83,107] Protein-losing gastroenteropathy, however, has been shown to be a contributing factor in patients with esophageal, gastric, and colonic neoplasms, in patients with the carcinoid syndrome, and in a patient with alpha chain disease,[75] as well as in a small percentage of patients with lymphosarcoma, Hodgkin's disease, or mycosis fungoides.[48,88,109] In a series of patients with gastric carcinoma, excretion of ^{131}I-PVP was greater than normal in all patients, varying from 1.03% to 7.32% of the injected dose in a 5-day fecal collection, compared with the range in controls of 0.18% to 1.03%.[48] The patients with protein-losing gastroenteropathy associated with the carcinoid syndrome were either those with congestive heart failure and an elevated venous pressure or those with an unresected primary tumor of the stomach or small bowel.

Diseases Not Associated with Disorders of Intestinal Lymphatics or Ulceration of Gastrointestinal Mucosa

Giant Rugal Hypertrophy of the Stomach. Protein-losing gastroenteropathy was first demonstrated in patients with Menetrier's disease by Citrin and co-workers,[17] who used iodinated albumin turnover studies in conjunction with aspiration of the gastric secretions. Some patients with this disorder present with mild to severe postprandial indigestion, in some cases associated with vomiting and weight loss and in others with steatorrhea.[56] Other patients may present with severe hypoproteinemia and edema.

The patients with hypoalbuminemia have a shortened albumin survival and an increased fecal excretion of the radiolabeled macromolecules used for the detection of excessive gastrointestinal protein loss.[17,23,56,79] The abnormalities of plasma protein metabolism improve following subtotal gastrectomy. Although patients with the Menetrier's syndrome seldom, if ever, have hypersecretion of hydrochloric acid, a group of patients has been described who have hypertrophic gastropathy with hypersecretion and gastric protein loss[15,66,72] (Chapter 63). In one patient there was a reduction in the hypersecretion and excessive gastrointestinal protein loss following administration of atropine sulfate,[66] whereas in another the administration of propantheline (Pro-Banthine) had no beneficial effect.[72]

Allergic Gastroenteropathy. A significant cause of extreme protein-losing gastroenteropathy in infancy is a syndrome termed *"allergic gastroenteropathy."* This disorder is characterized by edema, iron deficiency anemia, eosinophilia, hypoalbuminemia, hypogammaglobulinemia, growth retardation, and features typical of allergy.[108] Patients present at an early age, usually within the first year of life, with edema as the major problem. The edema is most marked in the face, particularly in the periorbital area, but may become generalized. The gastrointestinal symptoms tend to be mild, in most cases limited to intermittent diarrhea. In some patients, vomiting following ingestion of certain foods and abdominal pain are associated features. In one patient, edema of the mouth and eyelids was noted immediately following ingestion of milk.[45] The patients frequently have asthma, eczema, allergic rhinitis, and other manifestations of allergy. Most of the patients are below the third percentile in height. There is a family history of asthma or eczema in most.

The laboratory findings include marked hypoalbuminemia and a reduction of the serum concentration of IgG, IgA, and IgM, but an elevated serum concentration of IgE. The patients have a normal or increased rate of albumin synthesis but an extremely shortened albumin survival half-time of 2.8 to 3.5 days and excessive fecal excretion of ^{131}I-PVP and ^{51}Cr-albumin following IV administration of these labeled macromolecules. The patients are significantly anemic, with a hemoglobin ranging from 6.6/dl to 9.9 g/dl. Their red cells are microcytic and hypochromic, with an associated low serum iron concentration. Most of the patients have a marked increase in the number of circulating eosinophils (over 2000 eosinophils/mm^3); none have had lymphocytopenia.

The patients do not have steatorrhea or abnormal glucose, lactose, or D-xylose tolerance tests. The stools are persistently positive for occult blood and are loaded with Charcot-Leyden crystals. No gastrointestinal parasites could be demonstrated in the patients studied. Roentgenography of the stomach and the gastrointestinal tract is either normal or may show mucosal edema of the small bowel. In the majority of patients, biopsies of the small bowel show a marked infiltration of the lamina propria by eosinophilic leukocytes as the only abnormality. There is no dilatation of the lymphatic channels of the bowel.

Therapy with a gluten-free diet has no effect on this syndrome. Following administration of oral iron, the hemoglobin returns to normal, but there is no effect on the eosinophilia or disorders of protein metabolism. Protein metabolism tends to return to or toward normal following corticosteroid administration.[81,108] In addition, in those patients studied there was a complete reversal or a significant amelioration of the disorders of protein metabolism and eosinophilia when the patients were placed on a hypoallergenic

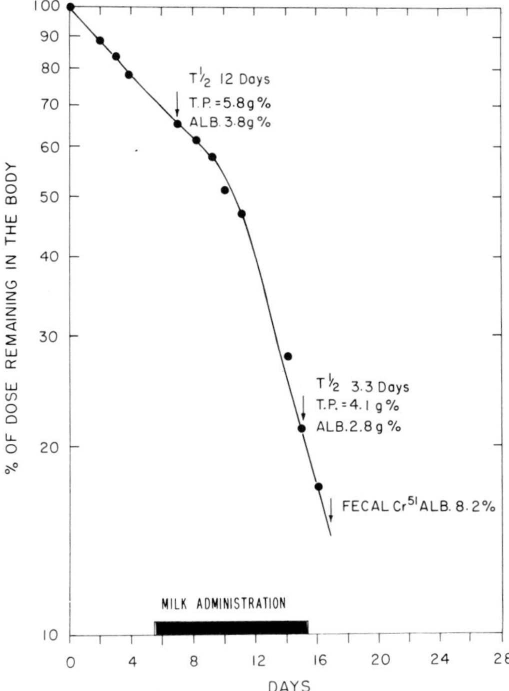

Figure 110–7. The effect of milk administration on the metabolism of ^{131}I-albumin in a patient with allergic gastroenteropathy. The survival ($T_{1/2}$ of albumin became markedly shortened ($T_{1/2}$ of 3.3 days on milk compared with $T_{1/2}$ of 12 days in control period) after addition of milk to diet. The 4-day fecal excretion of ^{51}Cr-albumin rose from the normal value of 0.24% during a control period on a hypoallergenic diet to 8.2% after 10 days of milk ingestion, indicating excessive gastrointestinal protein loss. (From Waldmann TA et al. N Engl J Med 1967; 276:762. Reproduced with permission.)

(specifically on a milk-free) diet. On reintroduction of milk, gastrointestinal protein loss (Fig. 110–7), hypoproteinemia, anemia, and, in many cases, asthma and rhinitis developed. In some patients, the offending antigen in milk has been shown to be beta lactoglobin.[60] It is felt that this syndrome is attributable to an abnormal response of the gastrointestinal tract to certain dietary constituents, especially milk, and that the condition is distinct from gluten-sensitive enteropathy.

Acute Transient Protein-losing Enteropathy. This form of protein-losing enteropathy often follows an infectious gastroenteritis. Clinical features are generalized edema and occasionally effusions in a child following a non-specific gastroenteritis.[98,115] The edema is associated with hypoproteinemia that may persist from 3 weeks to a few months. The laboratory picture is similar to that of an allergic gastroenteropathy and is characterized by hypoalbuminemia, hypogammaglobulinemia, anemia, and peripheral eosinophilia. In general, recovery occurs before gastrointestinal protein loss can be demonstrated. However, in those patients who have been examined during the acute phase, a shortened survival of albumin and excessive fecal excretion of macromolecules such as radioiodinated PVP and ^{51}Cr-albumin have been demonstrated.

Immunodeficiency Disease (Chapter 243). Since the initial description of X-linked agammaglobulinemia, over a score of immunodeficiency diseases have been described. Many of the patients with these primary disorders of the immune system have associated gastrointestinal disorders with hypoalbuminemia and protein-losing gastroenteropathy as secondary features.[2,5,18,19,37,42,44,74,96,99] Gastrointestinal disease is especially common in patients with common variable immunodeficiency disease. This appellation refers to a group of syndromes defined by the fact that immunologic deficiency and an increased rate of infection occur spontaneously following a period of apparently normal immunologic function. Immunologically, the patients lack plasma cells and have markedly decreased serum and secretory immunoglobulin levels as a result of decreased synthesis of these proteins. They manifest minimal or no antibody response to antigenic challenge. Some of the patients also have defective cellular immunity, with skin anergy and abnormalities of *in vitro* tests of delayed hypersensitivity. Patients with primary acquired hypogammaglobulinemia are susceptible to pyogenic infections leading to recurrent sinopulmonary infections, otitis media, conjunctivitis, and skin infections. Other complicating clinical features are splenomegaly, hepatomegaly, arthritis, Coombs-positive hemolytic anemia, amyloidosis, non-caseating granulomas, and a high occurrence rate of lymphoreticular and gastrointestinal neoplasms.

From 20% to 50% of these patients have diarrhea as a prominent symptom.[2,44,74,99] In the majority of patients, the diarrhea develops after the onset of recurrent respiratory infections. However, in some cases the diarrhea precedes the infections and may be the only clinical manifestation of the hypogammaglobulinemia. Most of the patients with gastrointestinal symptoms exhibit overt evidence of malabsorption, characterized by increased fecal fat; low serum, carotene, and vitamin E levels; and increased urinary excretion of 5-hydroxyindolacetic acid. Glucose, D-xylose, and vitamin B_{12} absorption tests are also abnormal in some patients. All the patients with common variable immunodeficiency disease and gastrointestinal disease studied by Waldmann and Laster[99] had hypoalbuminemia. The total body albumin pools were reduced in each of the patients studied by radiolabeled protein kinetic studies. In 4 of the patients there was defective albumin synthesis, whereas in 2 patients the albumin synthetic rate was within the normal range. In 3 patients excessive loss of albumin into the gastrointestinal tract was a significant factor in the hypoalbuminemia.

Two distinctive intestinal histologic patterns have been described in patients with common variable immunodeficiency disease. In the first, termed *"nodular lymphoid hyperplasia,"* there are lymphoid nodules evident as multiple small polyps within the mucosa. The architecture of the villi is relatively intact except for distortion by lymphoid nodules. The second histologic pattern, which may be found in patients with hypogammaglobulinemic sprue, is characterized by subtotal villous atrophy and lymphoid infiltration, but absence of plasma cells of the lamina propria.

A number of factors appear to be important in the pathogenesis of the diarrhea in hypogammaglobulinemia. Some patients have been shown to be chronically infected with shigella, salmonella, or staphylococcal organisms. Infection with *Giardia lamblia* is also very common in patients with this syndrome.[2] In some patients without known gastrointestinal bacterial pathogens or parasitic infection, significant intestinal intraluminal bacterial overgrowth is present.

The diarrhea, hypoalbuminemia, and protein-losing gastroenteropathy may respond to treatment. In some patients with hypogammaglobulinemic sprue, improvement was reported following institution of a gluten-free diet.[96,99] It should be noted that these patients were not challenged with gluten to confirm the association of gluten ingestion with the diarrhea. The diarrhea and protein-losing gastroenteropathy have also been successfully treated with antibiotics in some patients with gastrointestinal pathogens, as well as in some with an overgrowth of intraluminal intestinal bacteria. In addition, a course of metronidazole has been of value in eradicating *Giardia lamblia* infection, with an amelioration of the gastrointestinal symptoms and a return of the normal villous architecture.[2] Therapy with gamma globulin or with plasma infusions has been reported to be effective in controlling the diarrhea of some patients. It should be noted that, whereas there is a marked diminution or complete cessation of the gastrointestinal symptoms and abnormal enteric loss of albumin following effective therapy in these patients, the primary defect in gamma globulin synthesis is not affected. It is felt that the primary disorder in these patients is defective gamma globulin synthesis and an abnormality of cellular immunity. Protein-losing gastroenteropathy may be superimposed on this primary defect.

A similar pattern of immune deficiency, gastrointestinal disorder, and hypoalbuminemia associated with protein-losing enteropathy has been noted in association with a number of other immunodeficiency states. Thus, a number of patients with thymoma and hypogammaglobulinemia present with a pattern that is quite comparable to those with common variable immunodeficiency.[18] In addition, diarrhea, steatorrhea, infection with *Giardia lamblia,* and intestinal nodular lymphoid hyperplasia frequently accompany a dysgammaglobulinemia characterized by virtual absence of IgA and IgM and a moderately decreased level of IgG in the serum.[37] In addition, a spruelike syndrome with diarrhea, steatorrhea, and hypoalbuminemia has been noted in some patients with isolated IgA deficiency.[19] Patients with congenital X-linked agammaglobulinemia and an immune deficiency restricted to the circulating antibody system have a much lower rate of gastrointestinal disorders; protein-losing gastroenteropathy responsive to corticosteroid therapy has been described in patients with this form of immunodeficiency state.[99] Protein-losing gastroenteropathy has also been shown to be a common feature of patients with the Wiskott-Aldrich syndrome, an immunodeficiency syndrome characterized by thrombocytopenia, eczema, and a high rate of infections.[11] Patients with this syndrome appear to have a defect in the afferent limb of immunity and are unable to manifest either specific cellular or circulating immune responses to a number of antigens.

It seems clear from the foregoing considerations that involvement of the gastrointestinal tract and protein-losing gastroenteropathy are frequently associated features in patients with immunodeficiency syndromes.

Treatment of Protein-losing Gastroenteropathy

Since protein-losing gastroenteropathy is not a single disease entity, treatment depends on identification of the underlying disorder. With appropriate surgical, drug, or dietary therapy, over half the patients have a partial remission or complete amelioration of the hypoproteinemia and edema associated with protein-losing gastroenteropathy. Remission of gastrointestinal protein loss followed surgical resection of various localized lesions in the gastrointestinal tract, including gastric polyps, gastric carcinoids, gastric carcinomas, an eosinophilic granuloma of the stomach, giant hypertrophy of the gastric mucosa, congenital jejunal stenosis, localized granuloma of the ileum, colonic carcinomas, aganglionic segments of the bowel in patients with Hirschsprung's disease, and, in rare cases, localized segments of bowel with intestinal lymphangiectasia. Complete reversal of intestinal protein loss has followed successful repair of cardiac lesions in patients with an interatrial septal defect or with constrictive pericarditis.

Corticosteroids are effective in correcting gastrointestinal protein loss in some patients with ulcerative colitis, Crohn's disease, ileocolitis associated with agammaglobulinemia, allergic gastroenteropathy, and in some patients with intestinal lymphangiectasia who have an elevated sedimentation rate and normal or elevated immunoglobulin levels. Therapy with antibiotics is effective in reversing the gastrointestinal protein loss of patients with Whipple's disease and of some patients with immunodeficiency diseases. Cimetidine can be of value in the treatment of a patient with Menetrier's disease and protein-losing gastroenteropathy. Appropriate therapy with antiparasitic agents is effective in patients with hypogammaglobulinemia, giardiasis, and gastrointestinal protein loss. In addition, appropriate chemotherapeutic agents are of value in reversing the gastrointestinal protein loss associated with lymphomas affecting the intestinal tract.

Normal protein metabolism may return following a gluten-free diet in patients with non-tropical sprue or celiac disease and in individuals with agammaglobulinemia and an associated spruelike syndrome. A hypoallergenic diet, specifically a milk-free diet, has been effective in some patients with allergic protein-losing gastroenteropathy; in over half the patients with intestinal lymphangiectasia who are placed on a low fat diet there is an appreciable increase in the blood lymphocyte numbers and serum protein concentration, along with reduction of edema. An increase in the growth rate has been observed in treated children with this disorder. Jeffries and co-workers[52] and Holt[43] have shown that the albumin survival returned toward normal following institution of a low fat diet or a diet with medium-chain triglycerides replacing the long-chain triglycerides. The use of a low fat diet or a diet using medium-chain triglycerides, which are absorbed into the portal vein rather than through the intestinal lymphatics, would be expected to have its effect through a reduction in lymph flow and pressure in these patients with disordered lymphatic function.

References

1. Albright F, Bartter FC, Forbes AP. The fate of human serum albumin administered intravenously to a patient with idiopathic hypoalbuminemia and hypoglobulinemia. Trans Assoc Am Phys 1949; 62:204.
2. Ament ME, Rubin CE. Relation of giardiasis to abnormal intestinal structure and function in gastrointestinal immunodeficiency syndromes. Gastroenterology 1972; 62:216.
3. Andersen SB, Glenert J, Wallevik K. Gammaglobulin turnover and intestinal degradation of gammaglobulin in the dog. J Clin Invest 1963; 42:1873.
4. Andersen SB, Jarnum S. Gastrointestinal protein loss measured with ^{59}Fe-labelled iron-dextran. Lancet 1966; 1:1060.
5. Barandun S von, Aebersold J, Bianchi R, et al. "Proteindiarrhöe" zugleich ein Beitrag zur Frage der sogenannten essentiellen Hypoproteinämie. Schweiz Med Wochenschr 1960; 90:1458.
6. Beeken WL. Clearance of circulating radiochromated albumin and erythrocytes by the gastrointestinal tract of normal subjects. Gastroenterology 1967; 52:35.
7. Beeken WL, Busch HJ, Sylwester DL. Intestinal protein loss in Crohn's disease. Gastroenterology 1972; 62:207.
8. Ben Bouali A, Armand P, Barthe JP, et al. Lymphangiectasie intestinale primitive ou maladie de Waldmann. Sem Hop Paris 1979; 55:1935.
9. Bernier JJ, Florent C, Desmazures C, et al. Diagnosis of protein-losing enteropathy by gastrointestinal clearance of alpha 1-antitrypsin. Lancet 1978; 2:763.
10. Berson SA, Yalow RS, Schreiber SS, et al. Tracer experiments with I^{131} labelled human serum albumin: Distribution and degradation studies. J Clin Invest 1953; 32:746.
11. Blaese RM, Strober W, Levy AL, et al. Hypercatabolism of IgG, IgA, IgM and albumin in the Wiskott-Aldrich syndrome. A unique disorder of serum protein metabolism. J Clin Invest 1971; 50:2331.
12. Blalock A, Cunningham RS, Robinson CS. Experimental production of chylothorax by occlusion of the superior vena cava. Ann Surg 1936; 104:359.

13. Bookstein JJ, French AB, Pollard HM. Protein-losing gastroenteropathy: Concepts derived from lymphangiography. Am J Dig Dis 1965; 10:573.
14. Brambell FWR. The Transmission of Passive Immunity from Mother to Young. Vol 18, Frontiers of Biology. Amsterdam: North-Holland Publishing Co, 1970: 102.
15. Brooks AM, Isenberg J, Goldstein H. Giant thickening of the gastric mucosa with acid hypersecretion and protein-losing gastropathy. Gastroenterology 1970; 58:73.
16. Campbell RM, Cuthbertson DP, Matthews CM, et al. Behavior of ^{14}C- and ^{131}I-labelled plasma proteins in the rat. Int J Appl Radiat Isot 1956; 1:66.
17. Citrin Y, Sterling K, Halsted JA. Mechanism of hypoproteinemia associated with giant hypertrophy of gastric mucosa. N Engl J Med 1957; 257:906.
18. Conn HO, Quitiliani R. Severe diarrhea controlled by gamma globulin in a patient with agammaglobulinemia, amyloidosis, and thymoma. Ann Intern Med 1966; 65:528.
19. Crabbe PA, Heremans JF. Lack of gamma A-immunoglobulin in serum of patients with steatorrhoea. Gut 1966; 7:119.
20. Crossly JR, Elliot RB. Simple method for diagnosing protein-losing enteropathy. Br Med J 1977; 1:428.
21. Davidson JD, Flynn EP, Kirkpatrick JB. Protein-losing enteropathy and intestinal bleeding. The role of lymphatic venous connections. Ann Intern Med 1966; 64:628.
22. Davidson JD, Waldmann TA, Goodman DS. et al. Protein-losing gastroenteropathy in congestive heart failure. Lancet 1961; 1:899.
23. Dawson AM, Williams R, Williams, HS. Faecal PVP excretion in hypoalbuminaemia and gastrointestinal disease. Br Med J 1961; 2:667.
24. Díaz CJ, Linazasoro JM, López-García E, et al. Sobre la hipoalbuminemia en las pericarditis: Mecanismo y repercusiones. Estudios con proteinas marcadas de la rapidex de perdida y renovacion de la albumina del plasma. Rev Clin Esp 1960; 77:252.
25. Dobbins WO III. Hypo-β-lipoproteinemia and intestinal lymphangiectasia. Arch Intern Med 1968; 122:31.
26. Dolle W, Martini GA, Petersen F. Idiopathic familial cardiomegaly with intermittent loss of protein into the gastrointestinal tract. Ger Med Mon 1962; 7:300.
27. Donato L, Matthews CME, Nosslin B, et al. Applications of tracer theory to protein turnover studies. J Nucl Biol Med 1966; 10:3.
28. Dumont AE, Clauss RH, Reed GE, et al. Lymph drainage in patients with congestive heart failure. Comparison with findings in hepatic cirrhosis. N Engl J Med 1963; 269:949.
29. Fleisher TA, Strober W, Muchmore A, et al. Corticosteroid-responsive intestinal lymphangiectasia secondary to an inflammatory process. N Engl J Med 1979; 300:605.
30. Florent C, L'Hirondel C, Desmazures C, et al. Intestinal clearance of alpha 1-antitrypsin. A sensitive method for the detection of protein-losing enteropathy. Gastroenterology 1981; 81:777.
31. Földi M, Rusznyák I, Szabó GY. The role of lymph-circulation in the pathogenesis of edema. Acta Med Acad Sci Hung 1952; 3:259.
32. Freeman T, Gordon AH. The measurement of albumin leak into the gastrointestinal tract using ^{131}I-albumin and ion exchange resin by mouth. Gut 1964; 5:155.
33. Gitlin D, Klinenberg JR, Hughes WL. Site of catabolism of serum albumin. Nature (Lond) 1958; 181:1064.
34. Gordon RS Jr. Exudative enteropathy: Abnormal permeability of the gastrointestinal tract demonstrable with labelled polyvinylpyrrolidone. Lancet 1959; 1:325.
35. Gullberg R, Olhagen B. Electrophoresis of human gastric juice. Nature (Lond) 1959; 184:1848.
36. Haeney MR, Fields J, Carter RA, et al. Is faecal alpha 1-antitrypsin excretion a reliable screening test for protein-losing enteropathy? Lancet 1979; 2:1161.
37. Hermans PE, Huizenga KA, Hoffman HN, et al. Dysgammaglobulinemia associated with nodular lymphoid hyperplasia of the small intestine. Am J Med 1966; 40:78.
38. Herskovic T, Spiro HM, Gryboski JD. Acute transient gastroentestinal protein loss. Pediatrics 1968; 41:818.
39. Herzog DB, Logan R, Kooistra JB. The Noonan syndrome with intestinal lymphangiectasia. J Pediatr 1976; 88:270.
40. Hill RE, Hercz A, Corey ML, et al. Fecal clearance of alpha 1-antitrypsin: A reliable measure of enteric protein loss in children. J Pediatr 1981; 99:416.
41. Høedt K, Petersen VP, Schwartz M. Protein-losing gastroenteropathy in congestive heart failure. Lancet 1961; 1:1110.
42. Holman H, Nickel WF Jr, Sleisenger MH. Hypoproteinemia antedating intestinal lesions, and possibly due to excessive serum protein loss into the intestine. Am J Med 1959; 27:963.
43. Holt P: Dietary treatment of protein loss in intestinal lymphangiectasia. Pediatrics 1964; 34:629.
44. Hughes WS, Cerda JJ, Holtzapple P, et al. Primary hypogammaglobulinemia and malabsorption. Ann Intern Med 1971; 74:903.
45. Huntley CC, Bowers GW, Vann RL. Allergic protein-losing gastroenteropathy: Report of an unusual case. South Med J 1970; 63:917.
46. Jarnum S. The ^{131}I-polyvinylpyrrolidine (^{131}I-PVP) test in gastrointestinal protein loss. Scand J Clin Lab Invest 1961; 13:447.
47. Jarnum S. Protein-losing Gastroenteropathy. Oxford: Blackwell Scientific, 1963: 1.
48. Jarnum S, Schwartz M. Hypoalbuminemia in gastric carcinoma. Gastroenterology 1960; 38:769.
49. Jarnum S, Westergaard H, Yssing M, et al. Quantitation of gastrointestinal protein loss by means of Fe^{59}-labeled dextran. Gastroenterology 1968; 55:229.
50. Jeejeebhoy KN: Cause of hypoalbuminaemia in patients with gastrointestinal and cardiac disease. Lancet 1962; 1:343.
51. Jeejeebhoy KN, Jarnum S, Singh B, et al. ^{95}Nb-labelled albumin for the study of gastrointestinal albumin loss. Scand J Gastroenterol 1968; 3:449.
52. Jeffries GH, Chapman A, Sleisenger MH. Low-fat diet in intestinal lymphangiectasia: Its effect on albumin metabolism. N Engl J Med 1964; 270:761.
53. Jeffries GH, Holman HR, Sleisenger MH. Plasma proteins and the gastrointestinal tract. N Engl J Med 1962; 266:652.
54. Jones EA, Waldmann TA. The mechanism of intestinal uptake and transcellular transport of IgG in the neonatal rat. J Clin Invest 1972; 51:2916.
55. Kaihara S, Nishimura H, Aoyagi T, et al. Protein-losing gastroenteropathy as cause of hypoproteinemia in constrictive pericarditis. Jap Heart J 1963; 4:386.
56. Kalser MH: Protein-losing gastroenteropathy. *In:* Bockus HL, ed. Gastroenterology, Vol. 2, Ed. 2. Philadelphia: WB Saunders, 1964: 510.
57. Katz J, Rosenfeld S, Sellers AL. Sites of plasma albumin catabolism in the rat. Am J Physiol 1961; 200:1301.
58. Krag E, Frederiksen HJ, Olsen N, et al. Cimetidine treatment of protein-losing gastropathy (Menetrier's disease). A clinical and pathophysiological study. Scand J Gastroenterol 1978; 13:636.
59. Laster L, Waldmann TA, Fenster LF, et al. Albumin metabolism in patients with Whipple's disease. J Clin Invest 1966; 45:637.
60. Lebenthal E, Laor J, Lewitus Z, et al. Gastrointestinal protein loss in allergy to cow's milk betalactoglobin. Israel J Med Sci 1970; 6:506.
61. Marshak RH, Wolf BS, Cohen N, et al. Protein-losing disorders of the gastrointestinal tract: Roentgen features. Radiology 1961; 77:893.
62. Matuchansky C. Clairance intestinale de l' alpha-1-antitrypsine et entéropathie exsudative. Gastroenterol Clin Biol 1981; 5:183.
63. Milhaud G, Vesin P. Calcium metabolism in man with calcium^{45}: Malabsorption syndrome and exudative enteropathy. Nature (Lond) 1961; 191:872.
64. Mistilis SP, Skyring AP, Stephen DD. Intestinal lymphangiectasia: Mechanism of enteric loss of plasma-protein and fat. Lancet 1965; 1:77.
65. Nelson DL, Blaese RM, Strober W, et al. Constrictive pericarditis, intestinal lymphangiectasia, and immunologic deficiency. J Pediatr 1978; 86:548.
66. Overholt BF, Jeffries GH. Hypertrophic hypersecretory protein-losing gastropathy. Gastroenterology 1970; 58:80.

67. Petersen VP, Hastrup J. Protein-losing enteropathy in constrictive pericarditis. Acta Med Scand 1963; 173:401.
68. Petersen VP, Ottosen P. Albumin turnover and thoracic-duct lymph in constrictive pericarditis. Acta Med Scand 1964; 176:355.
69. Plaugh WH Jr, Waldmann TA, Wochner RD, et al. Protein-losing enteropathy secondary to constrictive pericarditis in childhood. Pediatrics 1964; 34:636.
70. Pomerantz M, Waldmann TA. Systemic lymphatic abnormalities associated with gastrointestinal protein loss secondary to intestinal lymphangiectasia. Gastroenterology 1963; 45:703.
71. Riva G, Barandun S, Koblet H, et al. Proteinverlierende gastroenteropathien: Klinik und Pathophysiologie. Protides Biol Fluids 1963; 11:168.
72. Roberts HJ. Hypertrophic gastropathy with hypersecretion and gastric protein loss. Aust NZ J Med 1971; 1:69.
73. Roberts SH, Douglas AP. Intestinal lymphangiectasia: The variability of presentation. A study of five cases. J Med 1976; 45:39.
74. Rosen FS, Janeway CA. The gammaglobulins. 3. The antibody deficiency syndromes. N Engl J Med 1966; 275:709.
75. Roth S, Havemann K, Kalbfleisch H, et al. Alpha-Ketten-Krankheit als malabsorptionssyndrom mit exsudativer enteropathie. Dtsch Med Wochenschr 1976; 101:1823.
76. Rothschild MA, Oratz M, Schreiber SS. Albumin synthesis. N Engl J Med 1972; 284:748.
77. Rubini ME, Sheehy TW. Exudative enteropathy. I. A comparative study of $Cr^{51}Cl$ and $I^{131}PVP$. J Lab Clin Med 1961; 58:892.
78. Schultze HE, Heremans JF. Molecular Biology of Human Proteins with Special Reference to Plasma Proteins. Vol. I. Amsterdam: Elsevier, 1966: 450.
79. Schwartz M, Jarnum S. Protein-losing gastroenteropathy. Danish Med Bull 1961; 8:1.
80. Schwartz M, Thomsen B. Idiopathic or hypercatabolic hypoproteinemia. Case examined by ^{131}I-labelled albumin. Br Med J 1957; 1:14.
81. Scudamoze HH, Phillips SF, Swedhund HA, et al. Food allergy manifested by eosinophilia, elevated immunoglobulin E level and protein-losing enteropathy: The syndrome of allergic gastroenteropathy. J Allergy Clin Immunol 1982; 70:129.
82. Shimkin PM, Waldmann TA, Krugman RL. Intestinal lymphangiectasia. Am J Roentgenol 1970; 110:827.
83. Steinfeld JL. I^{131} albumin degradation in patients with neoplastic diseases. Cancer 1960; 13:974.
84. Steinfeld JL, Davidson JD, Gordon RS Jr, et al. Mechanism of hypoproteinemia in patients with regional enteritis and ulcerative colitis. Am J Med 1960; 29:405.
85. Stoelinga GBA, Van Munster PJJ, Slooff JP. Chylous effusions into the intestine in a patient with protein-losing gastroenteropathy. Pediatrics 1963; 31:1011.
86. Strober W, Cohen LS, Waldmann TA, et al. Tricuspid regurgitation: A newly recognized cause of protein-losing enteropathy, lymphocytopenia and immunologic deficiency. Am J Med 1968; 44:842.
87. Strober W, Wochner RD, Carbone PP, et al. Intestinal lymphangiectasia: A protein-losing enteropathy with hypogammaglobulinemia, lymphocytopenia and impaired homograft rejection. J Clin Invest 1967; 46:1643.
88. Sum PT, Hoffman MM, Webster DR. Protein-losing gastroenteropathy in patients with gastrointestinal cancer. Can J Surg 1964; 7:1.
89. Thomas DW, Sinatra FR, Merritt RJ. Random fecal alpha 1-antitrypsin concentration in children with gastrointestinal disease. Gastroenterology 1981; 80:776.
90. Ulstrom RA, Smith NJ, Heimlich EM. Transient dysprotenemia in infants. A new syndrome. I. Clinical studies. Am J Dis Child 1956; 92:219.
91. Vallet HL, Holtzapple PG, Eberleen WR, et al. Noonan syndrome with intestinal lymphangiectasia. J Pediatr 1972; 80:269.
92. van Tongeren JHM, Majoor CLH. Demonstration of protein-losing gastro-enteropathy: The disappearance rate of ^{51}Cr from plasma and the binding of ^{51}Cr to different serum proteins. Clin Chim Acta 1966; 14:31.
93. van Tongeren JHM, Reichert WJ. Demonstration of protein-losing gastro-enteropathy: The quantitative estimation of gastrointestinal protein loss, using ^{51}-Cr-labelled plasma proteins. Clin Chim Acta 1966; 14:42.
94. Vardy P A, Lebenthal E, Schwachman H. Intestinal lymphangiectasia: A reappraisal. Pediatrics 1975; 55:842.
95. Vesin P, Roberti A, Bismuth V, et al. Protein and calcium-losing enteropathy with lymphatic fistula into the small intestine. *In:* Physiology and Pathophysiology of Plasma Protein Metabolism. Berne: Hans Huber, 1965: 179.
96. Vesin PS, Troupel JA, Renault H, et al. Enteropathie avec perte de proteines et steatorrhea. Etude par le PVP-I^{131} et la trioleine-I^{131} actcon du régine sans gluten. Bull Soc Med Hop (Paris) 1960; 76:261.
97. Waldmann TA. Gastrointestinal protein loss demonstrated by ^{51}Cr-labelled albumin. Lancet 1961; 2:121.
98. Waldmann TA. Protein-losing enteropathy. Gastroenterology 1966; 50:422.
99. Waldmann TA, Laster L. Abnormalities of albumin metabolism in patients with hypogammaglobulinemia. J Clin Invest 1964; 43:1025.
100. Waldmann TA, Miller EJ, Terry WD. Hypercatabolism of IgG and albumin: A new familial disorder. Clin Res 1968; 16:45.
101. Waldmann TA, Morel AG, Wochner RD, et al. Measurement of gastrointestinal protein loss using ceruloplasmin labeled with ^{67}copper. J Clin Invest 1967; 46:10.
102. Waldmann TA, Polmar SH, Balestra ST, et al. Immunoglobulin E in immunologic deficiency diseases. II. Serum IgE concentration of patients with acquired hypogammaglobulinemia, thymoma and hypogammaglobulinemia, myotonic dystrophy, intestinal lymphangiectasia and the Wiskott-Aldrich syndrome. J Immunol 1972; 109:304.
103. Waldmann TA, Schwab PJ. IgG (7S gamma globulin) metabolism in patients with defective gammaglobulin synthesis, gastrointestinal protein loss, or both. J Clin Invest 1965; 44:1523.
104. Waldmann TA, Steinfeld JL, Dutcher TF, et al. The role of the gastrointestinal system in "idiopathic hypoproteinemia." Gastroenterology 1961; 41:197.
105. Waldmann TA, Strober W. Metabolism of immunoglobulins. *In:* Progress in Allergy. Vol 13. Basel: S. Karger, 1969: 1.
106. Waldmann TA, Strober W, Blaese RM. Immunodeficiency disease and malignancy. Ann Intern Med 1972; 77:605.
107. Waldmann TA, Trier J, Fallon H. Albumin metabolism in patients with lymphoma. J Clin Invest 1963; 42:171.
108. Waldmann TA, Wochner RD, Laster L, et al. Allergic gastroenteropathy. A cause of excessive gastrointestinal protein loss. N Engl J Med 1967; 276:762.
109. Waldmann TA, Wochner RD, Strober W. The role of the gastrointestinal tract in plasma protein metabolism. Studies with ^{51}Cr-albumin. Am J Med 1969; 46:275.
110. Weiden PL, Blaese RM, Strober W, et al. Impaired lymphocyte transformation in intestinal lymphangiectasia: Evidence for at least two functionally distinct lymphocyte populations in man. J Clin Invest 1972; 51:1319.
111. Wetterfors J, Gullberg R, Liljedahl LO, et al. Role of the stomach and small intestine in albumin breakdown. Acta Med Scand 1960; 168:347.
112. Wilkinson P, Pinto B, Senior JR. Reversible protein-losing enteropathy with intestinal lymphangiectasia secondary to chronic constrictive pericarditis. N Engl J Med 1965; 273:1178.
113. Wochner RD, Drews G, Strober W, et al. Accelerated breakdown of immunoglobulin G (IgG) in myotonic dystrophy: A hereditary error of immunoglobulin catabolism. J Clin Invest 1966; 45:321.
114. Wochner RD, Weissman SM, Waldmann TA, et al. Direct measurement of the rates of synthesis of plasma proteins in control subjects and patients with gastrointestinal protein loss. J Clin Invest 1968; 47:3.
115. Wyngaarden JB, Crawford JD, Chamberlin HR, et al. Idiopathic hypoproteinenia: Report of a case with transient edema, depression of plasma, albumin and gammaglobulin and eosinophilia. Pediatrics 1952; 9:729.

Chapter 111

Miscellaneous Syndromes Associated with Malabsorption

Martin H. Kalser

Immunoproliferative Small Intestinal Disease (Alpha Heavy Chain Disease)

Immunoproliferative small intestinal disease (IPSID), a unique syndrome that begins as a benign disorder and progresses to a malignant state of intestinal lymphoma referred to as Mediterranean lymphoma, is discussed with small intestinal lymphoma in Chapter 112. It is considered here as well because malabsorption is a prominent feature of this disorder.

Etiology and Pathogenesis. Environment appears to be important in the unfolding of this syndrome. It is seen almost exclusively in lower socioeconomic populations among whom hygiene is poor and gastrointestinal parasitic infection and infectious diarrhea are prevalent.[1–3] Geographically, it occurs mostly in certain areas of the Middle East, the Mediterranean countries, South and Central Africa, Southeast Asia, and South and Central America.[2, 4–6, 15, 17] No specific enteric pathogen has been identified, but jejunal bacterial overgrowth may be found. Whether chronic bacterial infection and intestinal inflammation predispose to an abnormal immune response has not been established. The existence of an environmental factor is particularly evident in the lower frequency of IPSID in second as compared with first generation Israeli Jews of North African or Asian descent. This difference in frequency may reflect improved hygienic environment.[7]

There is also a strong association between this syndrome and certain HLA cell types (HLA–AW19, HLA–B12, and HLA–AG).[1] Chromosomal aberrations may represent a genetic marker for this entity.[8, 9]

The immunologic disturbance affects beta lymphocytes and results in production of a pathologic immunoglobulin with characteristics of alpha heavy chain antigen.[1] In addition to altered humoral immunity, alteration in cell-mediated immunity has been demonstrated in some patients.[2, 10]

Pathology. The jejunum appears to be affected first with extension into the duodenum. The mucosa is diffusely thickened and may display a cobblestone pattern resulting from thickened folds that assume a small nodular appearance. The characteristic microscopic pattern is of severe polymorphous or monomorphous cellular infiltration of the lamina propria and submucosa. The villi appear shortened and widened, and eventually complete villous atrophy may be present.

Epidemiology. The disease occurs predominantly in young men with the peak incidence in the third decade.[1] There is no racial predominance.[1] As has been noted, the disease is diffusely distributed in the lower socioeconomic groups of underdeveloped countries in many parts of the world. The major predisposing factors are poor sanitation and personal hygiene and high rates of infant and childhood infectious diarrhea and parasitic infections.

Clinical Aspects. *Diarrhea* is the major symptom. The diarrhea may spontaneously remit in the very early stages, but as the disease progresses it becomes chronic and persistent. Malabsorption becomes associated with consequent weight loss and symptoms of nutritional deficiency, such as anemia. The total course is one of slow progression as compared with the rather rapidly progressing intestinal lymphoma seen in Western countries. Initially the clinical course is more like tropical sprue (Chapter 106), but becomes more severe in its manifestations with time. Lactose intolerance is common, as with most intestinal malabsorption syndromes. Systemic toxicity with fever is unusual. Symptoms of obstruction or perforation, which are common in Western intestinal lymphoma, are decidedly unusual. Clubbing of the fingers and toenails occurs fairly often but ascites, hepatosplenomegaly, and peripheral lymphadenopathy are highly unusual.[1]

Laboratory evaluation discloses typical findings of malabsorption syndrome with anemia, hypoalbuminemia, hypocalcemia, and hypomagnesemia. The anemia may be associated with depressed serum iron, folate, or vitamin B_{12}. Intestinal parasites, particularly *Giardia lamblia,* are commonly encountered. Tests of malabsorption, including serum carotene, D-xylose, and fecal fat measurement, and tests for protein-losing enteropathy are abnormal (Chapter 27). Serum immunoglobulin levels are depressed more than can be explained on the basis of protein-losing enteropathy.[2, 11]

Diagnosis and Differential Diagnosis. The disorder would be suggested by the occurrence of persistent diarrhea and weight loss in a young individual, particularly a man in areas where the condition is endemic. Malabsorption would be suggested by evidence of nutritional deficiencies, and specific absorptive tests will confirm this. Small bowel barium radiographs disclose a "sprue-like" pattern of malabsorption (Chapter 102). In addition, thickening and nodularity of the mucosal folds may be seen. The demonstration of the specific alpha heavy chain peptide in serum provides support for the diagnosis (Chapter 112). Biopsy of the small bowel mucosa obtained perorally or enteroscopically (Chapter 103) can establish the diagnosis if the classic histologic changes are found.

Tropical sprue (Chapter 106) can clinically resemble IPSID in its early stages. Tropical sprue occurs in similar areas as IPSID but affects both native and long-term visitors to the area, whereas IPSID is reported only in the native population. All socioeconomic groups are affected in tropical sprue, but IPSID occurs mostly in the lower groups. Malabsorption and nutritional deficiencies are common in both, as are abnormalities in absorptive tests. The small bowel biopsy is abnormal in both with disturbed villus architecture and cellular infiltration of the lamina

Table 111–1. COMPARISON OF TROPICAL SPRUE AND IMMUNOPROLIFERATIVE SMALL INTESTINAL DISEASE (IPSID)

	Tropical Sprue	IPSID
Age	2nd to 4th decade	2nd to 3rd decade
Population	Native plus foreign long-time inhabitants	Native only
Sex	Men and women	Men predominantly
Geographic occurrence	Subtropical to tropical climates	Underdeveloped countries
Socioeconomic level	All	Lower groups
Bacteria in gut	Positive	Positive
Malabsorption	Positive	Positive
Protein-losing enteropathy	Late	Yes
Small bowel mucosa biopsy	Broad-clubbed villi; lamina propria infiltrate	Villous atrophy; marked cellular infiltrate
Nutritional deficiencies	Late	Early to late
Megaloblastic anemia	Late (common)	Intermittent
Folate deficiency	Late (common)	Intermittent
Abnormal serum protein	No	Alpha heavy chain peptide
Progression to lymphoma	No	Yes
Response to long-term antibiotics	Yes	Early only

propria, but an experienced observer may be able to recognize differences, particularly in the late stages. The abnormal alpha heavy chain peptide may be recovered in IPSID. Tropical sprue and early IPSID respond to bowel sterilization, but this is only of temporary duration in IPSID. IPSID progresses to primary intestinal lymphoma whereas tropical sprue remains a benign disease. The similarities and differences between these 2 disorders are summarized in Table 111–1.

Giardia lamblia infection (Chapter 232) can also be confusing, since this alone can result in intestinal malabsorption syndrome and is also a common finding in IPSID. When this parasite is found in a patient with malabsorption in an IPSID endemic area, a therapeutic trial of metronidazole (Chapter 232) would be appropriate.

Treatment. There is a definite response to tetracycline therapy in early stages of this disease[1, 11] (500 mg 4 times daily for about 1 month, and then twice daily for a total course of 6 to 12 months). The response rate decreases as the disease advances and exacerbations become progressively more frequent. Specific deficiencies, such as anemia, are treated with specific supplements.

Prognosis. The disease may spontaneously remit in the early stages, and tetracycline administration may induce remission for months or years. However, the disease is progressive and eventually fatal with development of intestinal lymphoma.

Malabsorption Syndrome with Intestinal Ulceration (Chronic Non-Granulomatous Ulcerative Jejunoileitis)

This syndrome is associated with high morbidity and mortality rates and with virulent small intestinal ulceration and malabsorption. Most cases are seen with celiac disease (Chapter 105) but other causes of malabsorption may be associated with this entity.

Etiology. In a detailed review of 40 cases, Baer at al.[12] classified 22 of the cases (55%) as celiac disease (gluten-induced enteropathy), 11 (27%) as "unclassified sprue," and 4 (10%) as other types of intestinal malabsorption, including one of adult alpha$_1$-antitrypsin deficiency and one of hypogammaglobulinemia. Three patients did not have significant blunting of the villi but rather an inflammatory reaction.[13] In addition, there were 7 cases of proven intestinal lymphoma, 4 with associated celiac disease. The ulcers are morphologically non-specific and without known cause.

Pathology. The ulcers are multiple in 90% to 95% of cases regardless of the causation. The overwhelming majority are in the jejunum, or both the jejunum and ileum, but have also been reported in the duodenum and colon (Table 111–2). Perforation occurs in about 50% of cases in jejunal or ileal ulcers. The intervening mucosa usually shows blunting of the villi. Granulomas are not seen. The walls of the involved segment and mesentery are thickened and the lymph nodes are enlarged. The histologic features are nonspecific and consist of an inflammatory infiltrate made up of lymphocytes, plasma cells, and granulocytes that extends variably to the muscularis or lamina propria but is concentrated mainly at the bases of the ulcers. Submucosal edema and fibrosis are also noted.

Clinical Features. Patients with underlying celiac disease display the typical symptoms of this disorder (Chapter 105) until the ulcerations and other changes develop. Non-celiac patients have villous blunting but do not

Table 111–2. MALABSORPTION SYNDROME WITH INTESTINAL ULCERATION*

		Complications			Ulcer Characteristics†								
Etiology	No.	*Bleeding No. (%)*	*Obstruction No. (%)*	*Perforation*	*S*	*M*	*J*	*I*	*J+I*	*C*	*Perforation*	Mortality No. (%)	Survival (5-year) No. (%)
Celiac	22	6 (27)	11 (50)	10	1	21	10	2	9	4	18 (81)	13 (59)	6 (27)
Unclassified sprue	11	6 (50)	2 (20)	5	1	10	4	1	6	0	5 (45)	10 (90)	1 (10)
Lymphoma	7	—	—	2	—	—	4	—	1	—	—	6 (86)	1 (14)
Miscellaneous‡	7	—	—	3	—	—	—	—	—	—	—	6 (86)	—

*Adapted from Baer et al.[12]
†S, single; M, multiple; J, jejunum; I, ileum; J+I, jejunum + ileum; C, colon.
‡Alpha$_1$-antitrypsin deficiency (1); hypogammaglobulinemia (1).

respond to a gluten-free diet or to corticosteroids. In general, they are older when the ulcerations develop as compared with celiac patients. Malabsorption in these patients is usually noted for only about 12 months before the appearance of the intestinal ulcers.

Symptoms of small intestinal ulcer development may be gradual or precipitous when perforation, bleeding, or obstruction occurs. Fever, abdominal pain, weight loss, and increased severity of diarrhea are the major clinical expressions. The character of the abdominal pain reflects the underlying lesion. If there is primarily an inflammatory reaction, the pain is localized. If ulceration has caused stricture formation, the symptoms are those of partial obstruction. Massive bleeding may also occur, as may free perforation with peritonitis.

Diagnosis and Differential Diagnosis. The diagnosis of this complication is strongly considered when a patient with intestinal malabsorption develops atypical symptoms of fever, abdominal pain, or hemorrhage, perforation, or obstruction. When there is no previous history of celiac disease or intestinal malabsorption, specific tests for intestinal absorption (Chapter 27) and small bowel biopsy (Chapter 101) may be abnormal and help establish the diagnosis of an underlying malabsorption syndrome. If the ulcers are chronic with cicatricial formation, barium radiographs of the small intestine may disclose areas of cicatricial narrowing with proximal dilatation.

The major entity requiring differentiation is *Crohn's disease* of the small intestine (Chapter 127). While certain aspects, such as chronic abdominal pain, fever, weight loss, and intermittent obstruction, are common to both syndromes, jejunal transport defects and abnormal jejunal biopsy with a flat villus pattern are seen in the malabsorption syndrome. Also, colonic involvement, while common in Crohn's disease, is highly unusual in malabsorption with ulceration.

Primary intestinal lymphoma (Chapter 107) may be difficult to distinguish from this syndrome. Both are clinically similar and differentiation may require careful histologic examination of the intestinal specimens by a pathologist experienced with these syndromes.

Complications. Severe complications are very frequent in this syndrome. Intestinal perforation with generalized peritonitis is probably the most lethal and occurs in over 40% of cases. Perforation may be the heralding expression of ulceration in 25% to 30% of cases. Intestinal obstruction is also common, occurring in one-third of patients, and may likewise be the initial mode of presentation. Gross gastrointestinal hemorrhage occurs in one-third of the cases.

Treatment. Surgical resection of the involved segment is the procedure of choice if the ulcer or ulcers are localized to one segment of the small bowel. Careful examination at the time of resection is required to exclude lymphoma. Resection is desirable because of the high occurrence rate of complications. If intestinal resection is not feasible because of the extent of the involved segment, or by the presence of multiple complicated ulcers, medical therapy can be tried. If abnormalities of the jejunal villi are present, the patient should be treated as for celiac disease with a strict gluten-free diet (Chapter 105). If there is failure to respond to a gluten-free diet, or if the patient is non-compliant, long-term steroid therapy with 20 mg of prednisone daily can be tried. Whereas prolonged remissions occur in about 10% of the patients receiving this treatment, perforation frequently recurs.[12] In the rare case in which new ulcers recur after one or more intestinal resections, it may be necessary, in my opinion, to resect almost all of the small intestine and then maintain the patient on chronic parenteral nutrition (Chapter 235).

Prognosis. The prognosis must be guarded. In patients with known celiac disease who develop this complication, the mortality rate may be as high as 60% and the 5-year survival no greater than 27%. In 40 cases of celiac disease, unclassified sprue, and miscellaneous malabsorption cases, the overall mortality rate was 72.5%.[13] In the unclassified sprue group (non-lymphoma), the mortality was 90% (10 of 11 cases) and only 10% had a 5-year survival. A similar high mortality was present in the lymphoma group with benign ulceration. Symptomatic ulcers commonly recur after surgery.

Mastocytosis (Urticaria Pigmentosa)

Systemic mastocytosis can be associated with secretory diarrhea (see later discussion and Chapter 8) or intestinal malabsorption.

The *etiology* of the malabsorption is not clear. Although serum histamine levels may be increased, gastric acid can be normal or low.[14] Hence, the sequence of events leading to malabsorption in the Zollinger-Ellison syndrome (Chapter 70) is not present. Furthermore, use of H_2 receptor blockers (cimetidine, ranitidine) is not effective in the treatment of the steatorrhea.[15]

The *clinical manifestations* of the disease include systemic as well as gastrointestinal expressions, with the latter occurring in about 23% of all patients with systemic mastocytosis.[16] Episodes of erythematous flushing, headache, tachycardia, and pruritus (urticaria pigmentosa) are features. The clinical symptoms resulting from malabsorption are similar to those seen with celiac sprue and include weight loss, tetany, and osteomalacia. *Physical examination* reveals the rash of urticaria pigmentosa (Chapter 18).

Laboratory studies may disclose a megaloblastic or iron deficiency anemia, low serum cholesterol, prolonged prothrombin time, low serum calcium, and low serum magnesium concentrations. In addition, serum phosphorus may be low and alkaline phosphatase may be elevated. Tests of absorption are abnormal and include low urinary excretion and low blood levels after oral administration of D-xylose, increased fecal fat, and increased fecal nitrogen. There may also be excessive loss of electrolytes in the stool.

In some cases, *small bowel roentgenograms* show submucosal nodularity[17] and may show segmental dilatation as well (Fig. 111–1). On endoscopic examination, nodular, urticaria-like submucosal lesions may be seen in the stomach. Radiographs of the bones disclose evidence of osteomalacia. Small bowel *biopsy* demonstrates edema and clubbing of the villi, but the villus pattern is essentially undisturbed; there usually is marked infiltration of the lamina propria with large numbers of eosinophils. In one reported case there was transient improvement on a gluten-free diet manifested by decrease in the number of stools and fecal loss of water, electrolytes, fat, and nitrogen; however, the response to the gluten-free diet was not complete.[18]

The *diagnosis* is to be suspected in a patient with typical cutaneous manifestations of urticaria pigmentosa and systemic manifestations of mastocytosis who has diarrhea and weight loss. The existence of intestinal malabsorption may be verified by appropriate

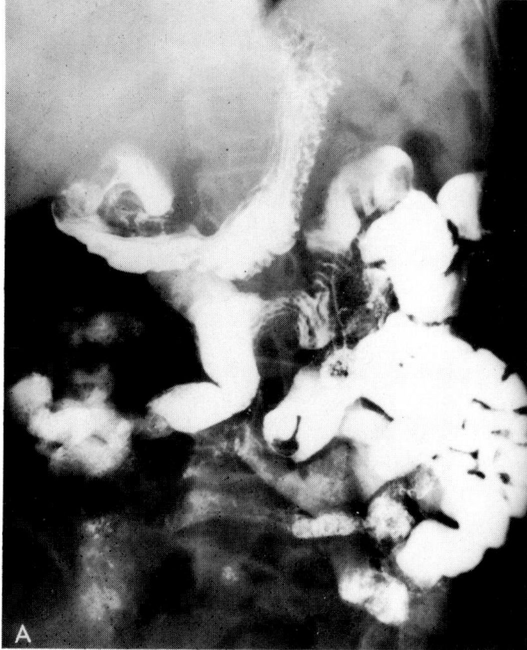

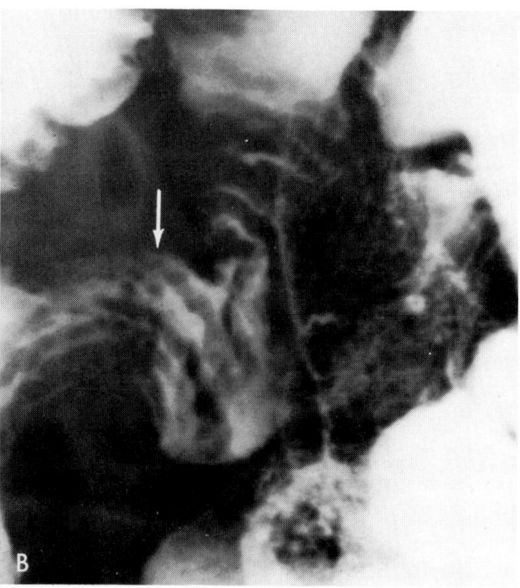

Figure 111–1. Patient S.S. *A,* This patient had systemic mastocytosis and urticaria pigmentosa of several years' duration with intermittent severe exacerbations of malabsorption characterized particularly by weight loss, watery diarrhea, and intractable tetany. The small bowel radiograph showed dilatation with segmentation of the jejunum. *B,* Enlargements in the jejunum were noted by arrow. This shows the nodularity of the jejunal mucosa.

tests (Chapter 27) and small bowel biopsy will disclose the changes that were earlier noted. The most specific test is that for urinary excretion of metabolites (N^+-methylhistamine and N^n-methylimidazolacetic acid), which is more specific than that of histamine itself. A level above 1 μmol/24 hours is abnormal. While the urine is being collected, it is important that the patient avoid microbially processed foods, such as cheese and sauerkraut, which may contain considerable histamine. Persistently high urinary levels of these metabolites are found also in chronic myelocytic leukemia and polycythemia vera. With these myeloproliferative syndromes, urinary excretion of the metabolites correlates with the number of basophil leukocytes. Paroxysmal increases of these substances in the urine may occur with anaphylactic drug reactions, wasp stings, or cold-induced urticaria.[16]

Treatment of malabsorption of system mastocytosis has not been impressively successful. General supportive measures and nutritional replacements are given as outlined for celiac disease in Chapter 102. H_2 receptor blockers, such as cimetidine and ranitidine, decrease some symptoms in some patients but rarely improve the malabsorption. Disodium cromoglycate has been shown to be effective in alleviating the gastrointestinal symptoms, including diarrhea and abdominal cramps, in a double-blind, cross-over study with placebo.[19] Only 1% of this drug is absorbed. The dose recommended is 100 mg 4 times a day. This drug acts by inhibiting the calcium-dependent, coupled, activation-secretion response of mast cells. Improvement is not present until the medication is given for 2 to 6 weeks and exacerbations after cessation of therapy occur in 2 to 3 weeks. While on the medication, alcohol can be ingested without precipitating symptoms. Despite amelioration of symptoms, the abnormal histaminuria and eosinophilia persist.[19]

Cronkhite-Canada Syndrome

This rare syndrome of ectodermal abnormalities with malabsorption and an exudative enteropathy is also considered in Chapter 138 from the standpoint of the intestinal polypoid lesions, which is one of its features. It primarily affects persons 40 to 70 years of age. The symptoms presented consist of severe intermittent watery diarrhea (occasionally containing blood), anorexia, weight loss, cramping abdominal pain, and peripheral edema. The *ectodermal abnormalities,* which may develop before the appearance of gastrointestinal symptoms,[20] include alopecia, hyperpigmentation and sclerodermatous changes of the skin, and atrophy of the finger- and toenails (onychodystrophy). Ophthalmologic alterations include cataracts and retinal detachment. Cerebellar ataxia has been reported,[20] and a case associated with multiple myeloma has been described.[21]

The *pathologic changes* consist of diffuse inflammatory mucosal reaction in the stomach, small bowel, and colon, with numerous inflammatory polyps throughout the length of the gut[22] (Chapter 138).

The *laboratory features* are those of severe malabsorption and of a protein-losing enteropathy (Chapters 27 and 110). D-xylose absorption is abnormal, serum folate and carotene concentrations are low, and fecal fat is increased. Serum albumin concentration also is very low and tests for intestinal protein loss are positive. Disaccharidase deficiencies exist and fecal losses of water and potassium are quite high, resembling a secretory diarrhea. The serum carcinoembryonic antigen (CEA) is elevated above 50 ng/ml.[20]

The *diagnosis* is suggested by the combination of skin lesions and alopecia combined with severe diarrhea, malabsorption, low serum albumin, and documented protein loss into the gut. The finding of multiple small polyps throughout the gastrointestinal tract on barium radiography and endoscopy confirms the diagnosis, particularly if histologic examination of these polyps shows an inflammatory reaction.

Remissions have been reported following dietary, steroid, and surgical *therapy.* However, the natural course of the disease is often characterized by spontaneous remissions, so that single case reports of improvement following specific therapy must be evaluated accordingly. A dramatic complete remission over a 2½-year follow-up period was reported following a 10-week course of enteral feeding through a nasogastric tube.[23] There was remarkable disappearance of the polyps, return of hair, and marked clinical improvement (Figs. 111–2 to 111–4). In other cases, remissions have been attributed to partial gastrectomy or partial colectomy[24, 25] even though the disease was in the remaining gut. Corticosteroids have been reported to be of benefit,[24] but this has not been confirmed.[20]

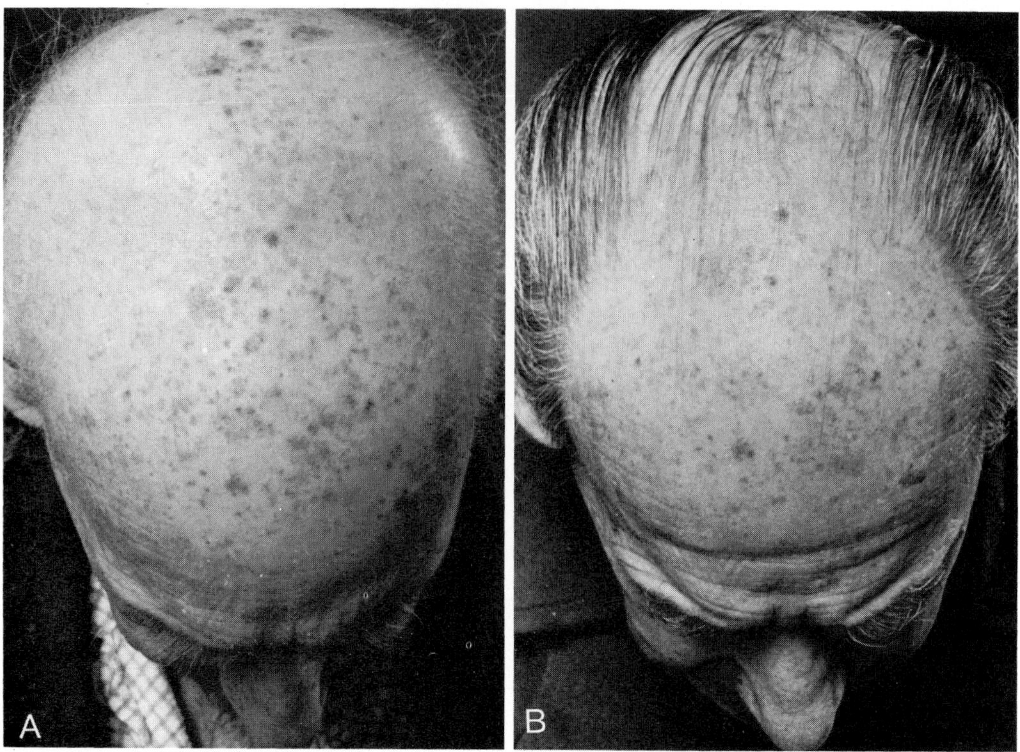

Figure 111–2. Appearance of the scalp in the Cronkhite-Canada syndrome. *A,* In August 1980, showing almost total alopecia. *B,* In January 1981, showing regrowth of hair. The patient had been balding for some years before the onset of the illness. (From Russel D, et al. Gastroenterology 1983; 85:180–5. Copyright 1983 by The American Gastroenterological Association. Reproduced with permission.)

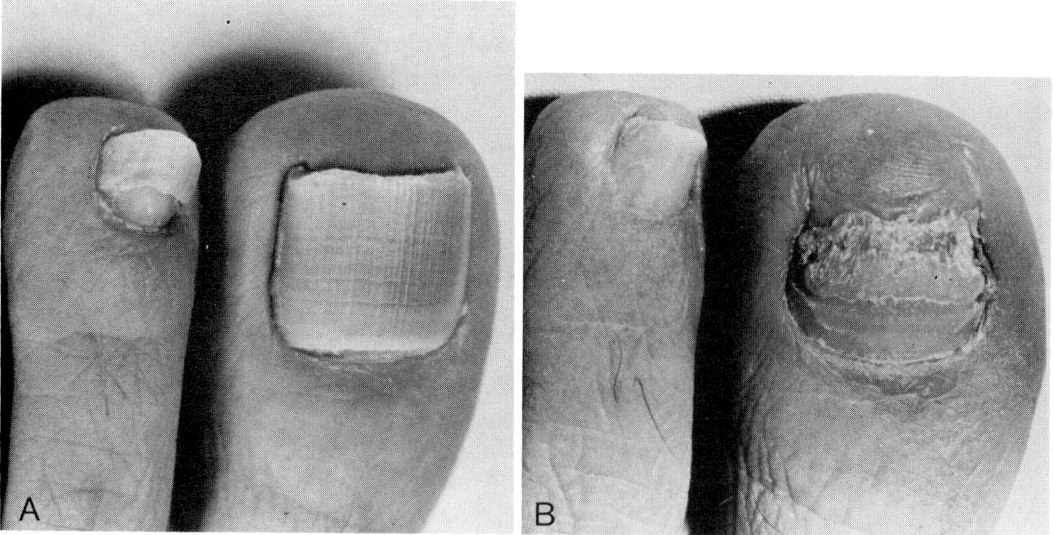

Figure 111–3. Appearance of toenails in the Cronkhite-Canada syndrome. *A,* In August 1980, showing onychodystrophy and lines of separation from the normal nail. *B,* In January 1981, showing regrowth of normal plate after separation. (From Russel D, et al. Gastroenterology 1983; 85:180–5. Copyright 1983 by The American Gastroenterological Association. Reproduced with permission.)

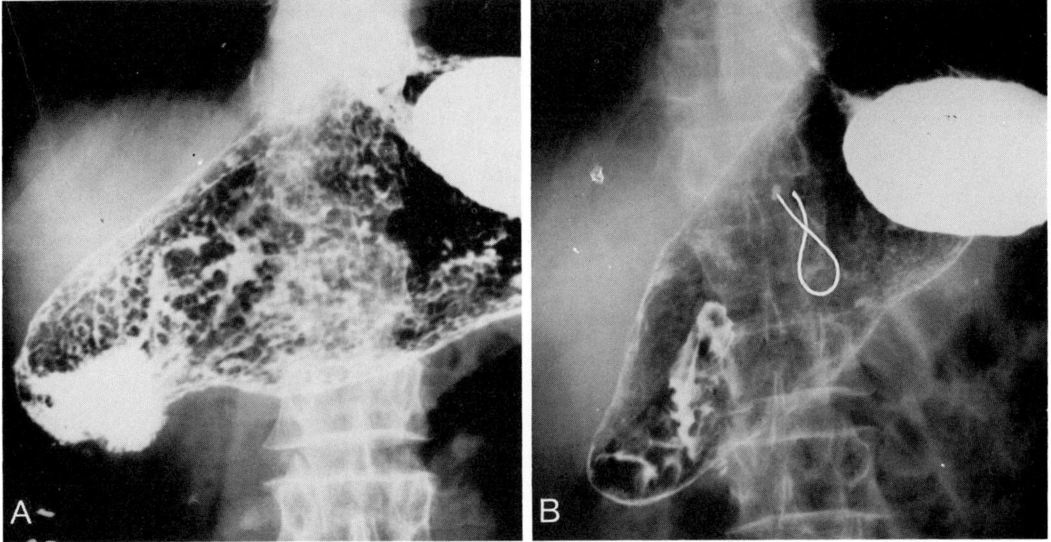

Figure 111–4. Upper gastrointestinal series in the Cronkhite-Canada syndrome. *A,* In August 1980, there were multiple filling defects in the stomach due to polyposis. *B,* In January 1981, the stomach appeared normal, with complete resolution of the gastric polyposis. (From Russel D, et al. Gastroenterology 1983; 85:180–5. Copyright 1983 by The American Gastroenterological Association. Reproduced with permission.)

Since the course of these seriously ill patients can be fatal, it would seem appropriate to use all medical agents considered to be possibly helpful in a trial of therapy. This would include nutritional supplemental therapy (enteral or parenteral) (Chapters 234 and 235) and corticosteroids, beginning with 60 to 80 mg/day of prednisone and then gradually decreasing after 2 weeks. Specific deficiencies, such as anemia, hypocalcemia, and hypoalbuminemia, should be treated with appropriate replacement therapy. Bowel sterilization with tetracycline, 500 mg 3 times a day for several weeks, may also be tried as in bacterial overgrowth situations (Chapter 107). If the patient does respond, the remission may be spontaneous rather than therapy-induced.

The *prognosis* varies markedly from an inexorable downhill course with inanition, anemia, and anasarca to spontaneous or therapy-induced remission. Death may be due to overwhelming infection. The overall mortality is about 43% with death in 6 to 18 months. Women generally have a more severe course than men.[26]

Abetalipoproteinemia

This is an inherited, autosomal recessive disorder of impaired fat assimilation due to a protein defect in lipoprotein synthesis by the intestinal mucosal cell. It occurs predominantly in Jews and people of Mediterranean background.

Pathophysiology. The basic defect in this syndrome resides in the synthesis of a specific apoprotein (apoprotein β), the protein moiety in lipoproteins. The apoproteins are designated by their carboxyl terminal amino acid; in this syndrome there is an apparent inability to synthesize the apoprotein with the amino acid serine on the carboxyl terminal (apoLP-ser). This is the major protein component of pre-beta lipoprotein (very low density lipoprotein, VLDL), beta lipoprotein (low density lipoprotein, LDL), and chylomicrons.[27] The concentration of high density lipoproteins (HDL) is also reduced by about 50%, since some HDL particles are derived normally from catabolism of chylomicrons.[28]

Infusion of lipoprotein IV has no effect on serum lipids. This confirms the theory that the defect in lipoprotein synthesis resides within the intestinal mucosal cells rather than being a defect in lipoprotein synthesis in another organ.[29]

The failure to synthesize chylomicrons and lipoprotein gives rise to disordered fat transport involving the delivery of triglycerides and cholesterol from the intestinal mucosa cells to the lymph. This results in defective release of fat from the mucosal cells with consequent increase of triglycerides within these cells. There is normal esterification of monoglycerides with free fatty acids by the mucosal cells to form triglycerides, but the concentration of intracellular triglycerides is 3 times normal. Similarly, triglyceride concentration is increased in the liver and there may be difficulty in the delivery of triglycerides and cholesterol from the liver to the blood.

Despite the failure of delivery of fat and cholesterol, most ingested fat in this syndrome is assimilated and only a fraction, 10% to 25%, is lost in the feces. The apparent alternate method of fat transport from the cell is not known. Total body synthesis of cholesterol is significantly higher than normal, but bile acid synthesis is normal. Cholesterol absorption is impaired. The increased sterol synthesis is secondary to increased loss that in turn is due to malabsorption of biliary cholesterol.[28]

The defect causing acanthocytosis of the red blood cells, as well as the cause of the changes in the central and peripheral nervous system and heart, is not known.

Pathology. The diagnostic finding in small bowel biopsy specimens is excessive fat droplets in the mucosal cells. The villus structure is normal and the cell and brush border are otherwise intact. The liver may show some degree of fatty infiltration.[30] The central nervous system shows demyelinization. The heart, in patients with congestive failure, discloses diffuse myocardial fibrosis without evidence of coronary artery disease.[31]

Clinical Features. The earliest manifestations are those of malabsorption, with the onset during the first few months of life. Diarrhea, steatorrhea, abdominal distention, and failure to thrive and grow are the major findings. Several years later, between the ages of 5 and 10 but before puberty, neurologic symptoms develop. These are indicative of cerebellar and basal ganglion involvement, although posterior column disease and peripheral nerve involvement may also be noted. Among the expressions of the neurologic changes are ataxia, intention tremors, nystagmus, absence of deep tendon reflexes, muscular weakness, particularly in the lower extremities, and athetoid movements.[32] Still later, the typical misshapen red cells, the acanthocytes, appear. Diminished peripheral vision due to retinitis pigmentosa also occurs. The last manifestation to appear is that of cardiac involvement with cardiomegaly and arrhythmias. Once involvement of the heart develops, death follows soon thereafter.[31] Although this syndrome is associated with a high mortality early in life, patients have been encountered in the fourth decade.[30]

Physical examination will reveal abdominal distention and evidence of emaciation in the more severe cases. Later in the course of the disease the signs of the neurologic involvement appear along with kyphoscoliosis, lordosis, and pes cavus.

Laboratory Findings. The major abnormalities are in the serum lipid components, which are depressed to a varying degree. The most severely depressed is the serum triglyceride concentration; this is frequently under 10 mg/dl as compared with a normal range of 50 to 150 mg/dl. Serum cholesterol is similarly markedly depressed, being under 50 mg/dl. These 2 components are usually absorbed from the intestine in chylomicrons into the lymph; in abetalipoproteinemia, postprandial chylomicrons are absent. Total serum fatty acids, free fatty acids, and phospholipids are also depressed. There is virtually complete absence of beta lipoprotein in the serum whether determined by ultracentrifugation, immunologically, or by lipoprotein electrophoresis. A characteristic finding in a peripheral blood smear is the presence of the crenated red cell with spines, the acanthocyte. The other usual biochemical studies are normal. There may be some degree of anemia.

Steatorrhea is a feature. Fecal fat excretion varies from 10% to 25% of fat intake[30, 32] and rarely is much greater. The serum carotene level is depressed. Prothrombin concentration may be depressed but bleeding due to prothrombin deficiency has not been reported. Similarly, there is no biochemical evidence of osteomalacia. Sugar absorption, as determined by the glucose tolerance and D-xylose tests, is normal.

Treatment. There is no known treatment for the extraintestinal manifestations and these are not reversible by any known therapy. Neurologic, retinal, and cardiac symptoms persist and progress once they develop.

Improvement in nutrition with amelioration of diarrhea and steatorrhea does occur with dietary therapy. Appreciable weight gain and improvement in overall status generally follow the consumption of a low long-chain triglyceride fat diet complemented by supplementary medium-chain triglycerides.

Increased fatty infiltration of the liver has been noted,[30] however, after 6 months of such therapy.

Collagen Vascular Diseases

The vasculitis syndromes as they affect the digestive system are discussed in Chapter 244. In this chapter, only the malabsorptive aspects of gastrointestinal involvement by some of the so-called collagen vascular diseases will be discussed.

Amyloidosis. Amyloid involvement of the small bowel resulting in malabsorption is quite unusual. Infiltration of the muscle layers, including the muscularis mucosa, by amyloid causes muscle atrophy and impaired motility. Malabsorption probably results from bacterial growth.[33] The major symptoms are those of diarrhea and steatorrhea. The results of laboratory tests, including those for malabsorption (Chapter 27), reflect impaired intestinal transport and increased fecal fat. Nutritional deficiencies are evidenced by low serum calcium, folate, and vitamin B_{12} levels. Small bowel barium radiography shows thickening of the mucosal pattern of the jejunum.

Scleroderma. Malabsorption is not unusual in scleroderma. It results from disturbed motility with stasis and bacterial overgrowth (Chapter 107). The diagnosis would be all the more suggested by the presence of scleroderma affecting the skin. Steatorrhea is present, with decreased absorption of D-xylose and vitamin B_{12}. Small bowel barium radiography shows dilatation of the gut with coarsening and thickening of the jejunal mucosa and very slow transit. Therapy consists of the use of wide-spectrum antibiotics and the dietary measures employed in malabsorption states, as discussed in the preceding chapters dealing with examples of this syndrome.

Systemic Lupus Erythematosus. Systemic lupus erythematosus has been reported in rare cases to be associated with malabsorption manifested by increased fecal fat and impaired D-xylose and vitamin B_{12} absorption. The small bowel mucosa shows abnormal morphologic patterns in the villi.[34]

Rheumatoid Arthritis. Malabsorption has been described in some cases of rheumatoid arthritis. In particular, D-xylose absorption is abnormal and there may be low serum folate levels. In one series of cases with malabsorption, small bowel biopsy was normal. The cause of the malabsorption is not known.[35]

Parasites

Parasites affecting the digestive tract are fully discussed in Chapter 232. Consideration is given here only to the element of malabsorption and to some parasitic infections in which malabsorption is a prominent feature. Giardiasis, coccidiosis, strongyloidiasis, and capillariasis can unequivocally result in malabsorption that is similar clinically to celiac or tropical sprue. In some parasitic infections, notably hookworm, malabsorption may be due to associated malnutrition[36, 37] or to tropical sprue in addition to the parasitic infection. This situation particularly obtains in disadvantaged socioeconomic groups.

Acquired Immune Deficiency Syndrome (AIDS). AIDS patients (Chapters 121 and 243) may have malabsorption secondary to chronic enteric infection with various parasites. Parasites involved include *Giardia lamblia* and coccidia (Cryptosporidium sp. and *Isospora belli*). These patients have typical findings of lymphopenia, inability to form recall antigens, and T cell defects characteristized by a marked decrease in T helper subset with inversion of the normal T helper to suppressor cell ratio (unpublished observations of Whiteside et al.[38]).

Giardiasis. Chronic infection with *Giardia lamblia* is not an infrequent cause of malabsorption in subjects with a normal immune system as well as in patients with immunodeficiency disease (Chapter 243). The clinical picture can be very similar to that of other causes of adult intestinal malabsorption syndrome as described in preceding chapters of this section. Diarrhea, abdominal cramps, distention, and weight loss may all be described, lasting from a few weeks or few months to many years. Tests of absorption are abnormal, including low serum carotene and folate levels, impaired D-xylose absorption, some impairment of vitamin B_{12} absorption, and an increase of fecal fat.[39] In general, malabsorption is only mild in degree and not all tests are abnormal in any given patient. Small bowel barium radiography in those with immunodeficiency disease may show nodular hyperplasia in addition to a malabsorption pattern; in some patients, only the malabsorption pattern is seen (Fig. 111–5). Small bowel biopsy is characterized by

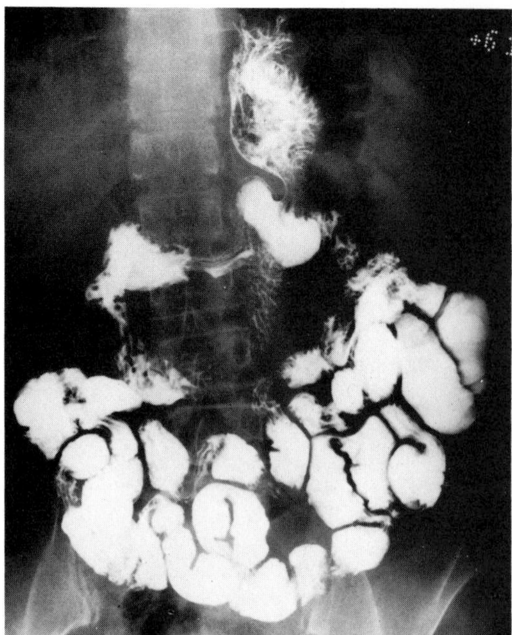

Figure 111–5. Patient H.Y. This patient had the diagnosis of malabsorption for 20 years; it was subsequently proved to be apparently due to giardiasis. Small bowel radiograph showed minimal dilation and segmentation compatible with malabsorption.

patchy involvement, with areas of abnormality interspersed among areas of normal structure. The structural changes vary from lymphoid hyperplasia to a flat mucosa with altered structure of the villi and infiltration of the lamina propria[39] (Fig. 111–6). Serum immunoelectrophoresis may show immunoglobulin deficiency, particularly of IgA; the pattern may also be normal. The best diagnostic test is the demonstration of giardia in the feces or in duodenal aspirate or a "touch preparation" of the mucosa of a small bowel biopsy. It must be emphasized that it takes an experienced histologist to recognize these organisms.

Marked clinical improvement follows therapy with metronidazole (Flagyl), 250 mg 3 times a day for 6 weeks. Improvement occurs within the first 2 to 3 weeks of treatment but the histologic and roentgen appearance do not revert to normal until later.[39] The following case description indicates how a correct diagnosis may be evasive.

H.Y. This patient was seen initially in 1973. Her symptoms had begun 29 years previously when the initial episode of watery diarrhea, anorexia, and weight loss occurred. This recurred intermittently throughout the years. In 1964, a small bowel biopsy was done and a diagnosis of tropical sprue was made. She was treated with supportive therapy and a low fat diet with apparent remission only to have periodic exacerbations. In January 1973, she again underwent intensive investigation and was found to have a megaloblastic anemia. Based on the small bowel biopsy, a diagnosis of gluten-induced enteroparthy was made. She was treated with folic acid and a gluten-free diet and symptoms cleared. Later in 1973, she had another severe exacerbation that led to her being seen by us.

Physical examination disclosed a thin white woman with minimal abdominal distention. Proctosigmoidoscopy was normal. Examination of the stool for ova and parasites on several occasions was negative. Hemoglobin was 11.5 g/dl. The white blood cell count and differential were normal. Laboratory studies, including a liver profile and serum electrolytes, were non-revealing; serum cholesterol was 136 mg/dl.

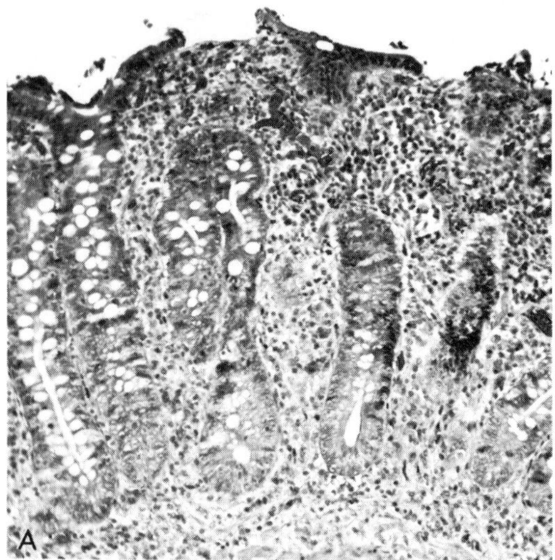

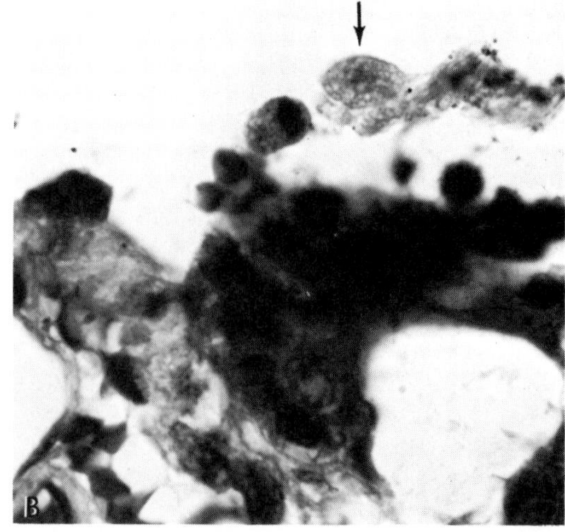

Figure 111–6. Patient H.Y. *A,* Peroral jejunal biopsy. (× 198.) This patient had giardiasis. There is total loss of villous pattern with heavy submucosal cellular infiltrate. *B,* Larger magnification (× 1584) of the surface showing a trophozoite of *Giardia lamblia* in the surface mucus (note arrow).

Malabsorption was evidenced by increased fat droplets in the stool on microscopic examination, a serum carotene of 19 μg/dl, and a D-xylose urinary excretion at 5 hours of 2 g following a 25-g oral dose. Serum protein electrophoresis disclosed a total protein value of 5.8 g/dl with albumin 2.9, alpha-1 globulin 0.2, alpha-2 globulin 0.46, beta 1.04, and gamma 1.19 g/dl, respectively. Serum immunoglobulin electrophoresis was definitely abnormal with an IgG level of 600 mg/dl (normal 700 to 1040 mg/dl). The IgM was 19 mg/dl with a normal of 37 to 104 mg/dl. The IgA was 136 mg/dl with a normal range of 60 to 490 mg/dl.

Small bowel radiographs showed segmental dilatation and other changes interpreted as consistent with the pattern of non-specific sprue pattern (Fig. 111–5).

The small bowel biopsy showed subtotal villous atrophy with the villi of the mucosa being flattened and atrophic. In the lamina propria there was dense infiltrate with plasma cells and eosinophils. Seen on the surface were scattered giardia, as noted in Figure 111–6.

The patient was given metronidazole (Flagyl), 750 mg/day in divided doses for 4 weeks. She became asymptomatic on this treatment and has remained so.

Coccidiosis. Chronic enteric infection with species of coccidia can result in both a severe secretory diarrhea[40] and malabsorption.[41] The clinical presentation of the malabsorption is the same as with other causes with diarrhea, steatorrhea, and nutritional deficiencies. Symptoms may be present for a number of years. Small bowel biopsy may show shortened villi, hypertrophied crypts, and infiltration of the lamina propria with eosinophils, polymorphonuclear leukocytes, and round cells. D-xylose absorption is abnormal and fecal fat is increased. The species involved are *Isospora belli* and *Cryptosporidium*. As has been noted, immunodeficient patients, including those with AIDS, are prone to this infection but it also occurs in immunologically normal individuals.[41] Response to treatment of the intestinal lesion (Chapter 232) is good and may be permanent in immunologically normal individuals; however, recurrences have been observed in immunodeficient patients after treatment (unpublished observations of Whiteside et al.[38]).

Hookworm. Impaired intestinal absorption has been noted with hookworm infection.[37] In many cases, however, other parasites and other causes for malabsorption may have been present as well. The malabsorption, particularly of protein, as well as the malnutrition may result from the intestinal reaction to the parasitic infection.[36] Small bowel biopsy does show mild mucosal atrophy and inflammatory involvement of the lamina propria, but the brush border is preserved. Tests of absorption show mild to moderate increases of fecal fat and impaired absorption of D-xylose. Small bowel barium radiograhs may show the malabsorption pattern. In some patients, treatment with diet can restore the malabsorption pattern to normal, whereas in others treatment of the parasitic infection as well as a nourishing diet is needed. No close correlation has been demonstrated between the degree of hookworm infection and the morphologic changes in the jejunum.[42]

Drugs

Various drugs can induce intestinal malabsorption in susceptible individuals. The reasons for this are not understood in all cases. With some it may be accentuation of folate deficiency, whereas with others, such as neomycin, specific changes occur that interfere with fat absorption.

Ethanol. Morphologic and functional changes in the small bowel occur with acute and chronic alcohol abuse in man[43, 44] (Chapter 156). Other causes of malassimilation in alcoholics include pancreatic insufficiency, liver disease with bile salt deficiency, and malnutrition. Prolonged administration of ethanol to chronic alcoholic patients as an isocaloric carbohydrate replacement can induce changes discernible only by electron microscopy. After 2 months of daily ethanol intake, changes may be seen in the mitochondria together with dilatation of the endoplasmic reticulum and cisternae of the Golgi apparatus.[44] Malabsorption of intestinal origin was present in over 60% of chronic alcoholics in one series of cases and was manifest by abnormal D-xylose test, impaired vitamin B_{12} absorption, and steatorrhea.[43]

Folate deficiency associated with chronic alcoholic ingestion may be the result of *decreased* small intestinal absorption rather than poor dietary habits alone. Indeed, folic acid malabsorption has been demonstrated in chronic alcoholic monkeys who were fed a nutritious diet together with alcohol for 24 months.[45] The liver also showed changes with steatosis and megamitochondria.

The mechanism of alcoholic injury to the small bowel mucosa appears to be at least partially due to accentuation of folate deficiency by ethanol ingestion. Combined ethanol ingestion and a folate-deficient diet in chronic alcoholic patients has been noted to result in decreased absorption of D-xylose, folic acid, glucose, water, and sodium.[46] Intestinal mucosal cell changes were noted by light microscopy in one chronic alcoholic person with severe folate deficiency; the duodenal mucosa demonstrated megaloblastic changes in the nucleus.[47]

Antibiotics. *Neomycin* is the antibiotic that classically has been shown to produce malabsorption. In small doses, 2 g/day, there is precipitation of bile salts with interruption of the micellar phase of lipid absorption. Mucosal damage occurs with larger doses of 3 to 12 g/day. This produces morphologic changes in the villi. A smaller dose also produces some lowering of serum cholesterol by inhibiting cholesterol absorption, secondary to its effect on the bile salts. With the larger doses there is malabsorption of glucose and D-xylose, as well as steatorrhea. The malabsorption is readily reversible[48, 49] (Fig. 111–7).

Steatorrhea has been reported following administration of tetracycline, chloramphenicol, and penicillin, but malabsorption resulting from these other antibiotics is less well documented.[50]

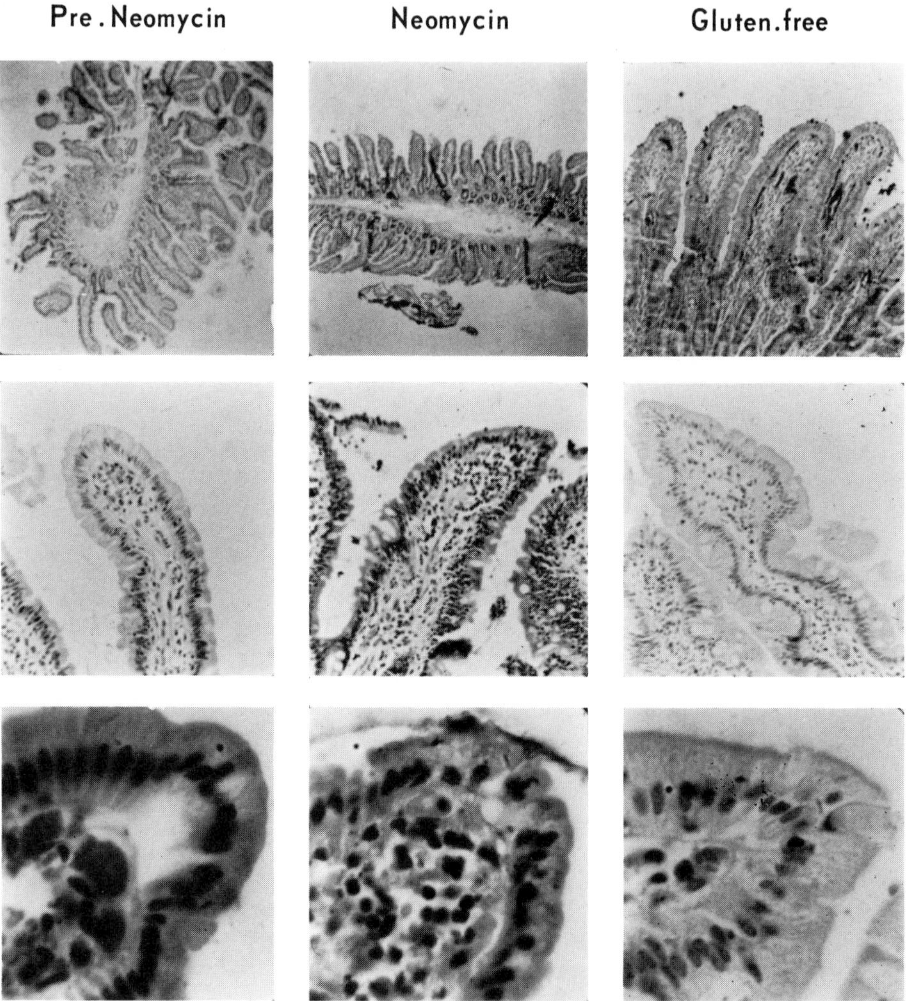

Figure 111–7. Peroral jejunal mucosal biopsy following ingestion of neomycin 4 to 8 g/day for 2 weeks, followed by a neomycin and gluten-free diet for a 2-week period. The changes to be noted in the neomycin period include (1) a decrease in total villous height associated with a clubbing tendency, (2) an increase in round cell infiltration and edema of the lamina propria, and (3) a reduction in height of epithelial cells lining the villous tips. Other changes noted less consistently are (1) vacuolization of the cytoplasm of the epithelial cells of the villous tips, and (2) the appearance of phagocytes with ingested cellular fragments in the basement membrane zone of the villi just below the villous tips. These changes are seen to be reduced during the neomycin-gluten–free period. (From Rogers AJ et al. JAMA *197*:117, 1966, Copyright, 1966, The American Medical Association. Reproduced with permission.)

Other Drugs. *Cholestyramine* can produce malabsorption of fat by precipitation of bile salts and also by interruption of micellar formation (Chapter 97). *Anticonvulsants,* such as phenytoin (Dilantin), inhibit absorption of folate as well as D-xylose[51] and megaloblastic anemia can result. Among other drugs capable of producing malabsorption of varying degree in isolated cases are colchicine and para-aminosalicylic acid.[48] *Colchicine* can produce a diffuse mucosal transport disorder with steatorrhea, azotorrhea, and increased fecal loss of water and electrolytes.[52] Serum carotene and cholesterol are depressed, and there is decreased absorption of D-xylose and vitamin B_{12}. Jejunal mucosal changes consist of edema and cellular infiltration in the lamina propria. Withdrawal of the drug results in complete recovery of intestinal function.

Triparanol has been reported to produce a malabsorption syndrome that clinically and by jejunal histologic features is indistinguishable from celiac disease. Patients respond to a gluten-free diet as well as to withdrawal of the drug.[48] Certain *cathartics,* particularly of vegetable origin, used in excess can cause hypokalemia as well as steatorrhea.[53]

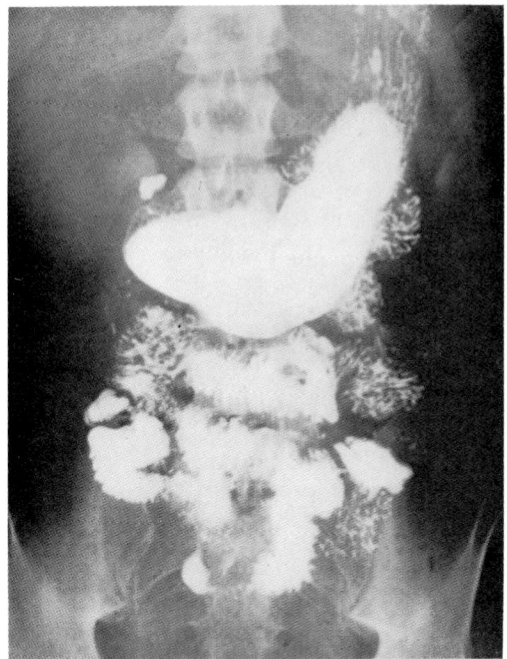

Figure 111–8. Patient M.W. with diabetic steatorrhea. The stomach appears to be enlarged and atonic. There is some dilatation of jejunal loops as well as thickening and coarsening of jejunal mucosa.

Endocrine Disorders

The interrelationship of endocrine and gastrointestinal disorders is described in Chapter 251. The discussion that follows is confined to certain endocrine disturbances that are associated with malabsorption and emphasizes the latter.

Diabetes Mellitus. Diabetes mellitus and intestinal malabsorption intertwine at several levels. This is in addition to diabetes mellitus associated with exocrine pancreatic disease. In children, the relation of diabetes mellitus to malabsorption is expressed in several ways. There is an increased frequency of diabetes in patients with celiac disease, approaching 10% in one series.[54] One group has also described malabsorption with steatorrhea in young children with severe diabetes who did not have associated celiac disease as evidenced by a relatively normal jejunal biopsy.[55] Diabetes and celiac sprue can also occur together in an adult but, overall, the prevalence of both together does not appear to be increased.

Diabetic steatorrhea is a distinct syndrome that occurs as a rare complication of diabetes mellitus.[56] It occurs predominantly in younger men several years after the onset of juvenile diabetes. Autonomic dysfunction is present and is evidenced by abnormal sweating patterns, impotence, and postural hypotension. There may be peripheral neuropathy, possibly autonomic neuropathy in the gut,[56a] and other manifestations of diabetic visceral involvement. The cause of the steatorrhea is not fully understood. It has been postulated that it is variably related to autonomic dysfunction, disturbed motility, pancreatic exocrine insufficiency, and bacterial overgrowth (Chapter 252) (Figs. 111–8 and 111–9). Therapy consists of control of the diabetes and the use of wide-spectrum antibiotic therapy, but results are not very encouraging. In most cases the prognosis is guarded, with death resulting from complications of the diabetes.

Hypoparathyrodism. Steatorrhea is not a universal finding in hypoparathyroidism. Indeed, fecal fat may be increased at one time and normal at another in a given patient on the same dietary intake. The cause of the steatorrhea is not known. Some cases clinically resemble celiac disease in that they may display anemia, tetany, clubbed fingers, and a flattened glucose tolerance test. Radio-

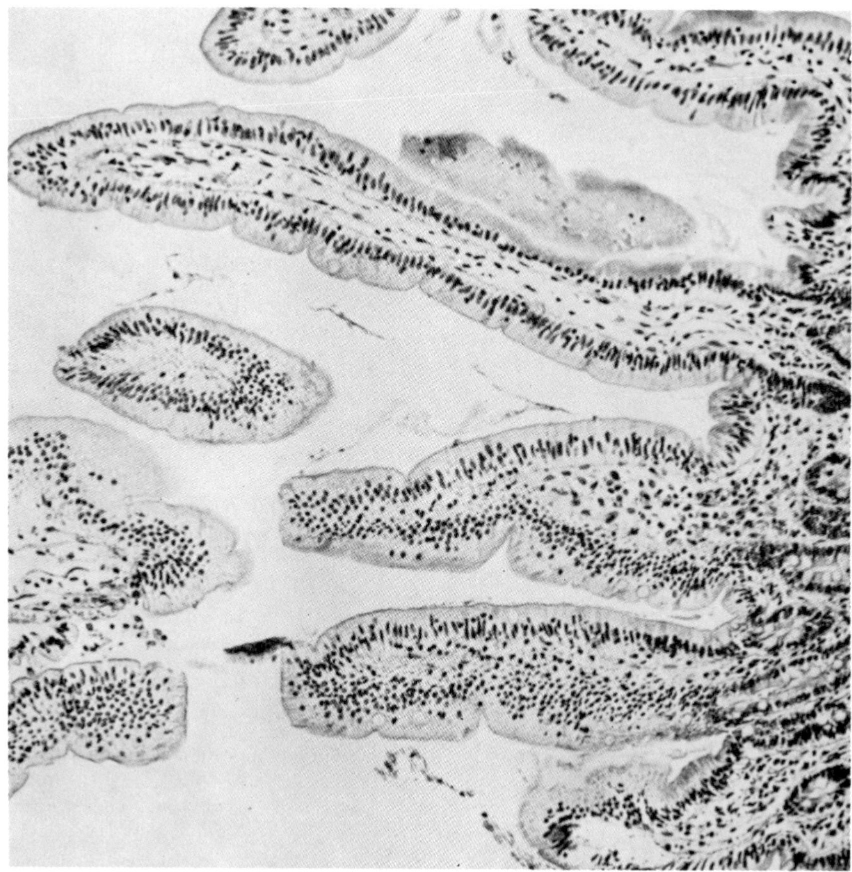

Figure 111–9. Patient M.W. with diabetic steatorrhea. The peroral jejunal biopsy discloses the normal, thin, "needle" villi. There is minimal jejunitis.

graphic abnormalities of the small bowel are also seen, including dilated loops, puddling, and flocculation of barium. These, however, can be seen in hypoparathyroidism in the absence of steatorrhea or other absorptive defects. Monilial infection has been thought to be a possible factor, but intestinal disturbances occur in the absence of this fungus.

The malabsorption manifestations are secondary to or occur concomitantly with hypoparathyroidism rather than hypoparathyroidism being secondary to the malabsorption.[57] The anemia results from impaired vitamin B_{12} assimilation. This is probably not the result of an intestinal defect, but more likely is secondary to histamine-resistant achlorhydria and failure to secrete intrinsic factor. In support of this is the ability to restore depressed absorption of vitamin B_{12} by the addition of intrinsic factor. There is also beneficial response of the malabsorption to parathyroid hormone and vitamin D therapy.

Thyrotoxicosis. Minimal steatorrhea may occur in patients with thyrotoxicosis on an ad libitum diet averaging about 250 g of dietary fat per day.[58] In only one reported case was the CA* less than 90%. In general, all other parameters of small bowel morphology and function are normal. Rapid small intestinal transit is viewed as the cause for minimal impairment of assimilation of a high dietary fat load. Propranolol (Inderal), a beta adrenergic blocking agent, when given to thyrotoxic patients, was found to decrease the degree of steatorrhea appreciably.[58]

Hypothyroidism. Hypothyroidism of various origins (spontaneous, postoperative, and thyroiditis-related) may be associated with intestinal malabsorption and mucosal histologic changes. Fecal fat is increased, serum vitamin A levels are depressed, and D-xylose absorption is abnormal. Histologi-

*CA = coefficient of fat absorption (normal $<$ 90%).

cally, a small bowel biopsy may show partial villous atrophy with plasma cell and lymphocyte infiltration of the lamina propria. Appropriate substitution therapy corrects the malabsorption and returns the histologic appearance of the jejunal mucosa to normal in 1 of 4 patients.[59]

Malignancy

Malabsorption and an abnormal jejunal mucosa have been demonstrated with malignancies of the gastrointestinal tract as well as other organs. There is a predisposition to malignancy in patients who have had celiac disease for over 10 years and have not been on a gluten-free diet. Not only are these patients liable to the development of lymphoma of the intestinal wall and mesenteric nodes (Chapter 112), but they have an increased occurrence rate of esophageal carcinoma as well[60] (Chapter 105). In extraintestinal lymphoma, a flat jejunal mucosa is present in the absence of lymphomatous involvement of the intestine and without apparent celiac disease. Functional and histologic changes of the small bowel have been reported as well in many other malignancies.[61]

A prospective study of small bowel morphology and function in patients with various types of neoplastic disease disclosed morphologic and absorptive changes.[61] Among the malignancies in which small bowel alterations were observed were primary cancers of the bronchus, stomach, colon, and urinary tract as well as malignancies of the reticuloendothelial system. Evidence of malabsorption, whether by decreased D-xylose or fat absorption, was present in over half the group. The degree of steatorrhea was minimal. Small bowel biopsy was abnormal in all the patients who had this procedure done. The dominant change was partial villous atrophy, but in one case a more severe form (subtotal villous atrophy) was seen.[61]

Little is known regarding the cause of the morphologic and functional changes that occur with malignancy, and the severity of the changes has not been correlated with the duration and stage of the malignancy. Possibly cachexia and malnutrition associated with malignant disease have a deleterious effect on the small intestinal mucosa. In this regard, however, it is of interest to note that a giant benign renal adenoma associated with intestinal malabsorption and atrophic jejunal mucosa has also been reported.[62]

Congestive Heart Failure

Minimal increase of fecal fat of unknown cause occurs in some patients with congestive heart failure (Chapter 247). However, the steatorrhea has not been correlated with the type of heart disease or with the duration of the congestive failure. In 2 of 3 patients studied,[63] the symptoms of congestive failure were of recent onset (about 1 month), whereas in the other patient the heart failure was chronic, requiring numerous hospital admissions for congestive failure. Digitalis therapy did not appear to be a factor, but some degree of mild hepatic dysfunction may also have been present and perhaps may have played a contributory role.

Folate malabsorption was noted in 28% and steatorrhea in 4% of one group of patients with congestive heart failure of various causes.[64] When the failure was reversed, absorption improved.

Congenital Short Small Intestine

A markedly shortened small bowel associated with congenital malrotation and malabsorption has been described.[65] Clinically the onset of symptoms is within a few days after birth. The major symptom is diarrhea that persists and is associated with failure to thrive and grow. In one case with this syndrome,[65] tests for malabsorption indicated a moderate steatorrhea with a CA of 45%, a flat glucose tolerance curve, decreased D-xylose excretion, and normal fecal pancreatic enzymes. Vitamin B_{12} absorption was normal, with normal serum levels and a negative Schilling test. Barium studies disclosed a markedly shortened small bowel with evidence of malrotation. At laparotomy the total small bowel beyond the ligament of Treitz measured 40 cm as compared with the normal 200 cm in a child of this age. Jejunal mucosal biopsy disclosed a normal villus pattern by light and electron microscopy. Adaptation apparently occurred in that the symptoms diminished markedly and malabsorption improved by age 7.

Collagenous Sprue

Some patients with what appears to be celiac disease do not respond as expected to a gluten-free diet. In some of these cases, collagen accumulation has been found in the affected bowel and has led to the suggestion that this alteration accounts for the poor therapeutic response (Chapter 105).

So-called collagenous sprue[66] is supposedly characterized by massive steatorrhea and azotorrhea, massive loss of water and electrolytes, severe hypokalemia, hypocalcemia, hypoalbuminemia, hypomagnesemia, dehydration, and an inexorable downhill course. The classic finding histologically is large masses of eosinophilic hyaline material in the lamina propria with the electron microscopic characteristics of collagen.[66]

Whether this is truly an independent entity or a variant of celiac disease is unsettled and debatable.

Voluntary Weight Reduction

Intestinal malabsorption with a flat jejunal mucosa on biopsy has been reported following severe voluntary weight reduction.[67] Such patients exhibit the typical syndrome of sprue with explosive diarrhea and laboratory evidence of hypocalcemia, hypomagnesemia, and hypokalemia. Tests disclose deficient D-xylose absorption, a flat glucose tolerance curve, a low serum carotene level, and increased fecal fat. Small bowel biopsy findings feature a flat mucosa with subtotal villous atrophy. Administration of a gluten-free diet is followed by complete amelioration of symptoms. In one case, improvement persisted even though the patient returned to a gluten-containing diet.[67]

The response to a gluten-free diet has been assumed to be non-specific, but the possibility remains that the voluntary weight reduction program exacerbated previously latent celiac disease.[67] While the observations remain valid that voluntary weight reduction can induce intestinal malabsorption, it is not known whether this is a distinct syndrome or whether it represents activated celiac disease.

Glucose-Galactose Malabsorption

Definition. Glucose-galactose malabsorption is a congenital disorder of transport of glucose and galactose resulting from a defect in the cell membrane carrier mechanism. The syndrome becomes apparent clinically soon after birth, with severe diarrhea following ingestion of glucose, glucose-containing disaccharides, oligosaccharides, or polysaccharides. It is associated with increased infant mortality, although some children do live to adult life following appropriate dietary therapy. There may be an associated defect of glucose transport in the renal tubules.

Genetics. The hexose transport defect is inherited as an autosomal recessive trait and asymptomatic heterozygotes may exist. It occurs as a single gene defect involving the carrier specific for active hexose uptake at the brush border. Cases have been reported from Sweden, Australia, France, and the United States, with one patient from the United States having Swedish ancestors.[68] It has been suggested that this disorder may be more prevalent in the Nordic ethnic group. There is an equal sex distribution in the limited number of reports to date and siblings commonly are affected. There is occasional evidence of heterozygosity in parents with slower uptake of glucose by the jejunal mucosa, but these parents are asymptomatic.[69]

Pathophysiology

Absorption Defect. The specific defect is in the uptake of glucose and galactose by the intestinal mucosal cell. There is no impairment of absorption of fructose or of the pentose D-xylose. Normally, glucose is absorbed at a faster rate than is fructose, but in this disease the reverse occurs. Following oral ingestion of glucose or galactose there is a flat tolerance curve with minimal elevation of blood levels. Perfusion studies show little absorption of glucose or galactose, even with extremely high concentrations of these sugars. Since the apparent absorption defect occurs at both high and low concentrations, both active and passive absorption appear to be affected. However, some glucose absorption in high concentrations does occur. Further evidence of brush border membrane carrier defect is the complete absence of uptake of radioactive ^{14}C-labeled glucose by mucosal biopsies from these afflicted patients. This is the same phenomenon noted in animals treated with phlorhizin, in which a specific defect is induced on the membrane carrier for glucose and galactose. Release of sugars from the intestinal mucosal cell is not affected, as demonstrated by radioactively labeled glucose studies. Absorption of the metabolically inactive analog of glucose, 3-O-methyl-D-glucose, which is actively absorbed but not metabolized, is also impaired.[70] Other aspects of normal active glucose absorption are not altered. These include ATP and a sodium-dependent energy pump. This was demonstrated by experiments with absorption of D-alanine, which is also actively absorbed and dependent upon the sodium pump. In patients with this disorder, the uptake and absorption of this amino acid are normal. Jejunal perfusion with a glucose and electrolyte solution of various concentrations was about 10% of normal controls. Impaired glucose absorption was also present at concentrations as high as 60 mM.[68–70]

Absorption of glucose following disaccharide administration is also markedly impaired, despite the fact that the brush border concentration of disaccharidase enzymes is normal (Chapter 104). The disaccharides are hydrolyzed normally at the brush border but absorption is markedly impaired. The histologic characteristics of the mucosa, by light and electron microscopy, are also well within normal limits.[71]

Fecal glucose and galactose are increased not only after ingestion of glucose and disaccharides but also after ingestion of starches. Normally these hexoses are completely absorbed in the duodenum, jejunum, and proximal ileum. No other absorptive defects other than transport of glucose and galactose are present. Fat, protein, minerals, and vitamins are absorbed normally.

There is a partial defect of renal tubular reabsorption of glucose. Glycosuria, with normal blood levels, does occur sporadically in these patients, but the maximum tubular reabsorption rate is normal.

Mechanism of Diarrhea. The diarrhea is primarily of osmotic type, with water and sodium secreted to dilute the hypertonic glucose solution within the intestinal lumen. Sodium fluxes are abnormal secondary to the defective glucose absorption; the inward flux is impaired. Glucose normally augments the potential difference (PD) of the jejunal mucosa when it is absorbed and this in turn facilitates sodium absorption.[68] In this disease, glucose does not influence the PD of the mucosa.

Sodium is absorbed in the jejunum by "solvent drag" secondary to glucose absorption (Chapter 95). Both mechanisms are negated in this disorder. At a concentration of 11 mM of glucose there normally is absorption of water and sodium from the perfusate fluid in the human jejunum. In these patients there is no secretion of water and sodium at this concentration.[68]

Bacterial fermentation leading to increased production of short-chain volatile fatty acids is not a cause of the diarrhea. Neomycin markedly reduced fecal flora in patients with this disorder, with the return of pH from acid to normal levels, but the diarrhea was not affected.[71]

Clinical Manifestations. The pathognomonic symptom is severe diarrhea appearing within a few days after birth when breast or formula feedings are first started in the infant. If unrecognized and untreated, persistent, unremitting diarrhea can lead to dehydration and death within a period of 6 months. The infant's appetite and general condition during the early stages remain good. An important clue is that the diarrhea rapidly ceases when all feedings are discontinued and parenteral fluids are given. Some patients with adequate fluid therapy can survive infancy, and there are case reports of the disease being uncovered in patients in the third and fourth decades of life.[68, 72] In the infant, serum hyperosmolality is a consequence of dehydration; despite losses of large amounts of water, there is no profound hyponatremia or hypocalcemia.

Development and growth in surviving children are normal. In later life they usually ingest a completely normal diet but have diarrhea of varying severity, cramping abdominal pain, and borborygmi. The usual diagnostic studies in these older individuals are completely normal and they frequently are given a diagnosis of irritable colon syndrome. The underlying basic congenital abnormality will not be recognized unless there is a high degree of suspicion.

Diagnosis. Severe *diarrhea* beginning within the first few days of life and persisting thereafter as long as the infant or child is feeding is the major clue to this disorder. It is important to remember that the diarrhea disappears with the cessation of oral feeding and institution of parenteral fluids. Examination of the stool shows *acid pH,* and bedside testing of the watery stools for glucose yields a strongly positive reaction. Intermittent glycosuria may also be present. Except for evidence of impaired glucose absorption, objective evaluation for systemic or gastrointestinal disease as the cause for the diarrhea is non-revealing in the adolescent or adult. The diagnosis may be established by comparing glucose absorption with fructose absorption. Flat blood curves occur after glucose administration but are normal after fructose. In contrast to malabsorption syndromes in which there also is a flat glucose tolerance, D-xylose absorption is normal in glucose-galactose malabsorption states. Stool glucose following glucose administration is quite high. However, in older individuals some absorption of glucose may occur.

Differential Diagnosis. Differential diagnosis in the infant embraces the exclusion of gastroenteritis, congenital disaccharidase deficiency, and celiac disease. The very early onset of severe diarrhea is not seen in celiac disease. Symptoms begin to appear when the diet is increased beyond breast milk or formula to include gluten-containing foods. Studies that include barium radiography of the small intestine, absorption tests, and small bowel biopsy give abnormal results in celiac disease and normal findings in glucose-galactose malabsorption. Congenital lactase deficiency in infants can be readily distinguished by substituting a non–milk-containing formula for the milk. This will alleviate the symptoms in cases of disaccharidase deficiency but not when there is glucose-galactose malabsorption. Glucose is not present in the stools in the former and is strongly positive in the latter, regardless of whether the source of carbohydrate is starch, disaccharides, or glucose. Lactose tolerance will give flat blood glucose levels in both, but glucose tolerance is normal in lactase deficiency.

Although only isolated reports of this syndrome beyond early childhood are available, it is possible that appropriate diagnostic measures may uncover less severe cases that have been attributed to the irritable bowel syndrome. Severe diarrhea early in infancy is not to be related simply to irritability of the bowel. Stool examination and tolerance tests can differentiate these syndromes. Lactase deficiency must be excluded; avoidance of milk provides clinical improvement in lactase deficiency but does not influence the clinical course of glucose-galactose malabsorption states. Stool examination for glucose, glucose or galactose tolerance tests, and brush border enzyme determinations afford laboratory help in differential diagnosis. In the adult, celiac disease can be readily differentiated from glucose-galactose malabsorption in that with celiac disease there is usually a latent adolescent period before re-exacerbation of symptoms in adulthood. Children with celiac disease fail to thrive and have impaired growth, whereas growth is normal in those with glucose-galactose malabsorption.

Treatment. During the acute phase of severe diarrhea with accompanying dehydration and electrolyte loss, the major form of therapy is replacement of fluids and minerals. Once the diagnosis is established in infants, special formulas are needed that exclude glucose or galactose in any form, either as free hexoses, disaccharides, or starches. In the early stages, diets may be employed consisting primarily of casein or soy bean flour as protein and corn oil as fat. Fructose can be added, 4% to 8%, with additional minerals and multivitamins. Later on a diet can be given of foods naturally high in protein and fat and low in carbohydrates. Such diets, given ad libitum, have been reported by these patients as they grow older.[71] Although sucrose is a disaccharide composed of fructose and glucose, some amount of this sugar can be tolerated by older patients.

Familial Enteropathy

This is a syndrome that occurs in infants from birth and is characterized by severe secretory diarrhea and malabsorption. It appears to have a familial incidence and the mortality rate is high.[73]

The *etiologic factor* is not known. Against any exogenous factor is the fact that symptoms begin at birth and persist when feeding is only from the mother's breast or when only parenteral nutrition is given for prolonged periods. The familial relation is evident in that siblings have the same illness. The family histories are consistent with an autosomal recessive mode of inheritance. Whereas the crypt cells at the base of the villus appear normal, the mucosal cells at the tip of the villus are abnormal with absence of microvilli and persistence of the secretory granules. This gives rise to the hypothesis that there is an inborn error of metabolism expressed as an inability of intestinal crypt cells to differentiate and mature normally into absorptive cells.

In *gross appearance,* the small intestine is dilated and its walls are paper thin. The main *histologic finding* is total villous atrophy with absent or irregular and shortened microvilli.

The *pathophysiology* of the syndrome is both an intestinal absorptive defect and abnormal secretion by the small intestinal mucosa. There is a net secretion of sodium and water in the basal state in the small intestine as determined from perfusion studies. This results in an increased volume of stool with a high concentration of sodium and potassium in the basal state. Stool volume may reach 100 to 200 ml/kg of body weight/24 hours. Malabsorption of fat, glucose, sodium, and water is present. Defective fat assimilation results from intestinal mucosal disease as well as from a decrease in conjugated bile salt concentration below the critical micellar concentration. Various disaccharidases in the mucosa are decreased, but pancreatic enzyme secretion is normal.

This disease is *clinically* expressed at birth with severe diarrhea, failure to thrive, and death usually before the age of 1 year. Parenteral hyperalimentation is needed to sustain fluid and electrolyte balance as well as an intake of adequate calories. The diarrhea persists even when nothing is given by mouth and the only reliable means of ensuring nutrient availability is by parenteral feedings. There is usually a history of early infant death in close relatives.

Diagnosis is suggested by the clinical history confirmed by tests of absorption and small bowel biopsy. Familial enteropathy differs from celiac disease and other causes of malabsorption in infants by its very early onset after birth, before gluten is introduced into the diet, and by the persistence of symptoms when nothing is given by mouth. No parasitic or other infectious agent capable of causing diarrhea and malabsorption has been found in these patients.

Treatment is limited to parenteral hyperalimentation (total parenteral nutrition, TPN). The diarrhea persists, but infants usually thrive on this regimen. Deterioration can occur when TPN is discontinued and oral feedings are restarted.

Prognosis must be severely guarded in view of the high mortality rate within the first year of life.

Fabry's Disease

This is a rare sex-linked familial disease of glycosphingolipid metabolism due to deficiency of lysosomal ceramide trihexosidase. Primarily involved are skin, cornea, kidney, heart, and nervous system. Symptomatic gastrointestinal involvement is unusual.[74]

The major *gastrointestinal complaints* are early satiety, episodic nausea, vomiting, cramping abdominal pain, and severe diarrhea. The basic pathologic lesion is believed to be impairment of the autonomic nervous system due to infiltration of the nerve ganglia (including Meissner's plexus) with ceramide trihexosidase. It is postulated that an autonomic neuropathy results, producing symptoms akin to those seen with the autonomic neuropathy of diabetes mellitus. Early satiety, nausea, and vomiting may all be noted when there is gastric stasis. Impaired jejunal motility with stasis also occurs as a consequence of the neuropathy. Bacterial overgrowth occurs and has been demonstrated to cause the severe diarrhea.[75] The ^{14}C glycocholate breath test is abnormal, confirming intestinal bacterial overgrowth.

Treatment consists of metoclopramide, 10 mg before each meal and at bedtime. This controls the early satiety and nausea and vomiting if present. Bowel sterilization with tetracycline, 250 mg 4 times a day for 10 days, will control the diarrhea; repeated courses may be needed if diarrhea recurs. The bile acid breath test returns to normal with the antibiotic therapy.[75]

Malabsorption in Normal Humans

Impaired absorption of carbohydrate and fat has been demonstrated in normal human subjects. The degree of malassimilation is dependent upon the source of the carbohydrate, whereas fat assimilation varies with the physical state of the food. This type of malassimilation has clinical relevance in 2 situations: (1) the total absorbed foodstuffs may be less than assumed or calculated, particularly in vegetarians; and (2) carbohydrate malassimilation may contribute to symptoms of distention, borborygmi, and abdominal discomfort.

Carbohydrate Malassimilation (Chapter 93). Carbohydrate malabsorption measured with the use of the hydrogen breath test (Chapter 27) has shown that assimilation varies with the source of the carbohydrate. Navy beans are poorly absorbed, with 18% being unassimilated. Baked potatoes have a 13% malabsorption rate. Carbohydrate malassimilation also varies with the type of flour used in making bread; 8% of the carbohydrate in oat bread and 6% in corn bread is malabsorbed. Bread or macaroni made from wheat flour is poorly absorbed (10% to 15%), while bread made from low gluten wheat or from rice flour is completely assimilated.[76, 77]

Fat Malassimilation. Assimilation of fat in peanuts varies with the physical state of the peanuts. Considerable malabsorption occurs when the whole peanut is ingested, 17.8% of the ingested fat being present in the feces.[78] Careful examination of the stools will show that portions of whole peanuts remain intact and therefore unavailable for lipid digestion. Grinding of the peanuts to form peanut butter resulted in enhanced fat assimilation; fecal fat was reduced from 17.8% to 7% of the ingested amount. The most complete assimilation occurs with the fat in the form of peanut oil; only 4.5% of the ingested fat is recoverable in the feces. The addition of high amounts of fiber substantially increases fecal fat following ingestion of peanut butter or peanut oil.[78]

Impaired Biotin Absorption (Juvenile Multiple Carboxylase Deficiency)

Juvenile multiple carboxylase deficiency is a syndrome in which metabolic biotin deficiency occurs consequent to biotin malabsorption or impaired biotin utilization because of biotin-responsive multiple carboxylase deficiency. The onset is in early childhood with acute symptoms of ataxia, alopecia, keratoconjunctivitis, erythematous rash, seizures, and lactic acidosis. A second phenotype with enzyme deficiency occurs in the neonatal period with life-threatening lactic acidosis, seizures, and rash.

Biotin absorption occurs from the proximal and distal small intestine. It has been postulated that there is a high affinity, low capacity ("low km") biotin transport system that enables the small amounts of biotin in the succus entericus to be taken up. This same cellular transport system may also be present in the renal tubule. Defect in this transport system as occurs with this syndrome in both the intestine and the renal tubules is expressed as a high renal clearance of biotin and rapid loss of biotin from the body pool. In the untreated patient, plasma and urinary concentrations of biotin are low.

Treatment in either the juvenile or neonatal type, whether due to metabolic enzyme deficiency or malabsorption of biotin, is by large dose biotin replacement, usually 10 mg/day, orally. The disease can become evident within 5 to 6 weeks of biotin deprivation.

The *prognosis* with treatment is excellent. All symptoms disappear and there is normal physical and mental growth.[79]

Secretory Diarrhea

Secretory diarrhea refers to watery diarrhea with marked increase in stool volume (above 750 ml/24 hours) associated with excess loss of electrolytes. It results either from excessive stimulation of secretion of water and ions or from inhibition of absorption. More commonly, this term is used to describe the watery diarrhea of high volume that persists when nothing is ingested. A classification of secretory diarrhea is presented in Table 111–3 with the various mediators.

Secretory diarrhea is discussed along with other types of diarrhea in Chapter 8. Its mention here is for completeness in the consideration of malabsorption syndromes and to emphasize that secretory diarrhea occurs with fatty acid malabsorption in the short bowel (Chapter 108) and with bacterial overgrowth syndromes (Chapter 107), as well as with impaired absorption of bile salts, such as occurs in ileal resection or disease (Chapters 97 and 108). Its management depends on its cause and the changes induced. For discussion of these the reader is referred to Chapter 8 and the other chapters where secretory diarrhea is a feature of the disorder under review.

Diverticula and Diverticular Disease of the Small Intestine

Martin H. Kalser and B. D. Pimparker

The first complete account of authentic diverticula in the mesenteric small intestine was given by Sir Astley Cooper in 1807.[90] Sir William Osler,[91] in an early contribution on this subject, counted 55 diverticula in the upper jejunum of a man 65 years of age on whom necropsy was done.

The jejunum and ileum share last place with the stomach in frequency of diverticula in the alimentary canal. The prevalence of these defects at necropsy varies between 0.006%[92] and 1.3%.[93] When searched for carefully, both at necropsy and on radiographs,[94, 95] the prevalence rate is at least doubled.

Table 111–3. SECRETORY DIARRHEA CLASSIFICATION*

Disease	Etiology	Mediator
Infections		
Cholera	Endotoxin	cAMP
E. coli	Endotoxin	cAMP
Hormonal (peptide)		
Gastric acid		
Gastrinoma	Gastrin	HCl
Mastocytosis	Histamine	HCl
Basophilic leukemia	Histamine	HCl
Intestinal-colon effect		
VIPoma (WDHA)	VIP	cAMP
Medullary carcinoma	Calcitonin	cAMP
Thyroid	Prostaglandin	
Ganglioneuroma	VIP	cAMP
Carcinoid	Serotonin	Motility
	Prostaglandin E_2	
Villous edema	Direct cell	Secretion
Mastocytoma	VIP	cAMP
Mastocytosis		
Familial enteropathy	Unknown	—
Other		
Ileectomy	Bile salts	cAMP
	Malabsorption	Motility
Short bowel	Hydroxy	cAMP
	Fatty acids	Motility
Laxative abuse	Castor oil	
	Phenolphthalein	
	Senna	
	Bisacodyl	
	Oxyphenisatin	

*Compiled from references 73 and 80 to 89.

Etiology. Klebs[96] was one of the first observers to mention that small intestinal diverticula occur often at the mesenteric border where the main blood vessels pierce the bowel wall. This was considered to be a weakened area in the bowel wall. Hansemann,[97] in 1896, made serial sections through bowel with its diverticulum and showed that the sac made use of the vascular channel to bulge through the muscle. Susceptibility to the formation of diverticula seems to decrease proportionately from the second portion of the duodenum to the terminal ileum, with possibly a slight increase in frequency in the terminal ileum. Most diverticula in the mesenteric portion of the small intestine are found in the upper part of the jejunum.[98] Frazer[99] attributed the relative frequency of diverticular formation in the jejunum to the facts that (1) the jejunum is 3 times the size of the ileum, resulting in a thinner longitudinal muscle coat, and (2) the individual arteries are larger in the jejunum. The lack of a peritoneal coat at the mesenteric border was also thought to make this a weaker area than the remaining circumference of the bowel. Edwards[100] expressed the belief that the diverticula start in a relaxed segment of small bowel between 2 segments in contraction by pushing a wedge of mucous membrane into the vascular gap. If this part of the intestinal wall contracts, the wedge may be driven back, but there will come a time when the impacted wedge is of such size that the contraction of the muscle about its base will consolidate its position by gripping it in the vascular gap. In time this may become permanent, and pressure will tend to increase its size.

Hansemann[97] produced diverticula by gas pressure and felt that this was the causative force. Rosedale,[101] using intraintestinal pressure of up to 1.5 pounds of mercury in 35 fresh postmortem specimens of jejunum, was unable to produce any definite outpouchings. Fraser[99] readily produced diverticula in postmortem gut with bismuth solution or oxygen, but with equal distention in the jejunum, ileum, and colon produced diverticula in the jejunum only. Butler[102] found arteriosclerosis of the mesenteric vessels in 4 of 5 patients with multiple jejunal diverticula. Because of this he carried out experiments in cadavers. Marked distention of the small intestine produced small pouches of the jejunal wall similar to the earliest stages of the multiple diverticula; they were best demonstrated in persons 65 or more years of age with generalized arteriosclerosis.

King,[103] on the other hand, doubted that blood vessels are a factor in the etiology of small intestinal diverticula, since some of the small diverticula have muscle; if the diverticula were simply mucous membrane hernias, there should be no muscle in their walls. The essential feature, according to King, is muscle weakness, probably due to hormonal, nervous, and chemical causes. Some observers have suggested, in addition, a myogenic deficiency such as fatty degeneration,[104] congenital hypoplasia,[105] senile atrophy or atony, and toxic myositis.[93]

Heterotopic pancreatic tissue may have some part to play in the development of sacs in the mesenteric small bowel.[106] Pancreatic heterotopia is found most often in persons in the fourth, fifth, and sixth decades of life, an age range coinciding with the greatest frequency of diverticulosis of the small intestine.[106] Nearly 70% of cases of pancreatic heterotopia are in the jejunum. Furthermore, of 77 cases of heterotopia in the jejunum, 3 (4%) were in the wall of a diverticulum. Among cases of heterotopia in the ileum, nearly 48% were in a Meckel's diverticulum while another 25% were in other types of ileal diverticula.

Pathology. Solitary diverticula of the jejunum or ileum usually occur in younger persons. They are congenital in type, and may be on the antimesenteric side of the bowel.[103] Some consider this type of diverticulum as a partial reduplication of the bowel.

Multiple diverticula are more common than single pouches, constituting between 54% and 100% of the total patients with diverticula of the mesenteric small intestine. Hansemann[97] reported patients with as many as 400 to 500 diverticula.

Multiple diverticula are usually on the mesenteric border, separating the leaves of the mesentery or bulging through one side of the mesentery. They often appear to be paired, one on each side of the bowel. Each diverticulum has its own opening. The openings into the bowel are usually large and the diverticula are able to drain well. At times, however, the openings are small or stenotic and may be obstructed by inflammatory changes, scar tissue, or fecaliths. The diverticula vary in size from minute projections to rounded sacs 10 cm or more in diameter.

If diverticula exist in the jejunum and ileum, there is at least a 25% chance that pouches will also be found elsewhere in the alimentary tract, particularly in the colon and duodenum.[98, 103, 107, 108]

Most jejunal and ileal diverticula are hernias of the mucous membrane that protrude through the muscular wall of the intestine at a point where there is a gap caused by the entrance of blood vessels near the mesenteric line. In effect, they are pulsion diverticula. A thin layer of muscular coat is carried with the mucosal bulge; this coat subsequently thins as the diverticulum increases in size. The walls may be quite thin and translucent, or they may be thickened by hypertrophy, fibrosis, or edema and inflammation.

On microscopic examination, the wall consists of serosa, mucosa, and submucosa with varying amounts of muscle. The fundus of the sac rarely contains a muscle layer, except for a few fibers of muscularis mucosae. The mucous membrane is usually intestinal in type but, as commented on earlier, may contain heterotopic gastric or pancreatic tissue.

Clinical Aspects. The condition occurs at any age, but is seen most often in elderly individuals; 80% to 90% of patients are above the age of 40 years. There is a preponderance of men, the rate of preponderance varying from 2:1 to 3:2. Of a total of nearly 500 patients reported, 39 were women. This is in contradistinction to duodenal diverticulosis, which occurs more often in women.[107]

In the great majority of patients, small intestinal diverticula are asymptomatic.[94] A very few patients have symptoms due to an interposed, usually acute complication. A few others present with a malabsorption syndrome with steatorrhea or megaloblastic anemia.[109] "Jejunal dyskinesia" has been used by Altemeier et al.[110] as a term to decribe a syndrome of varying degrees of acute and chronic non-mechanical ileus associated with jejunal diverticula. Colicky abdominal pain and borborygmi are the major manifestations.

Complications. Acute mechanical intestinal obstruction,[98] diverticulitis,[111] and hemorrhage[94] are the major acute complications (Table 111–4), with an overall occurrence rate of significant complications of 10%.[92, 98, 112]

The causes of mechanical *obstruction* include volvulus, stricture secondary to diverticular inflammation, and enteroliths extruded into the lumen. The severity of complicating diverticulitis may vary from edema to gangrene, abscess, and perforation with peritonitis or fistula formation. Blunt trauma may also cause rupture of a jejunal diverticulum.

Although *hemorrhage* is less commonly encountered as a complication of diverticulosis than are obstruction and inflammation, when it does occur it is frequently severe and potentially fatal.[113, 114] Hemorrhage from jejunal diverticula occurs in the later decades of life and usually presents with pronounced melena. Of 42 patients collected by Taylor,[113] 27 patients had sudden hemorrhage with shock, usually appearing without preceding abdominal complaints. In another report[114] of 35 patients with massive hemorrhage from jejunal diverticula, 7 died, a mortality rate of 20%. Although melena is the commonest manifestation of acute bleeding from these diverticula, hematemesis also occurs occasionally. There may be chronic bleeding or frequently recurring mild bleeding, but the

Table 111–4. COMPLICATIONS OF DIVERTICULA OF THE MESENTERIC SMALL INTESTINE

Acute mechanical intestinal obstruction caused by:
- Enteroliths extruded from diverticula
- Inflammatory mass associated with diverticulitis
- Volvulus of intestine
- Stricture of diverticular adhesions
- Pressure of filled diverticula on the intestine

Chronic intestinal obstruction due to:
- So-called jejunal dyskinesia
- Strictures or adhesions
- Inversion of diverticulum with intussusception
- Chronic volvulus

Inflammatory disturbances:
- Mild catarrhal inflammation leading to cyst formation due to closure of the neck of the sac
- Severe inflammation leading to gangrene and perforation resulting in:
  - Localized abscess formation
  - Generalized peritonitis
  - External or internal fistula formation

Hemorrhage

Rupture of diverticulum
- Spontaneous
- Traumatic
- Slow ooze leading to chronic asymptomatic pneumoperitoneum

Foreign bodies
- Food particles
- Bones
- Parasites

Blind loop syndrome
- Macrocytic megaloblastic anemia
- Steatorrhea

Neoplastic disease and formation of heterotopic tissue
- Benign
  - Heterotopic, gastric, or pancreatic tissue
  - Fibroma or lipoma
- Malignant
  - Carcinoid
  - Carcinoma
  - Sarcoma

frequency is not established; certainly, bleeding from small intestinal diverticula must be a rare cause of chronic gastrointestinal blood loss.

The occurrence of malabsorption with megaloblastic anemia is considered to be secondary to small bowel bacterial overgrowth. This condition, termed the bacterial overgrowth syndrome, is fully discussed in Chapter 107 and will be only briefly commented on here in relationship to small intestinal diverticula.

Montuschi,[115] in 1949, reported on a patient with diverticulosis of the small intestine with severe persistent hypoalbuminemia and steatorrhea. Zingg,[116] in 1950, after noting the association of megaloblastic anemia with intestinal diverticulosis, drew attention to the fact that the sprue syndrome might result from diverticulosis of the intestine. Badenoch and Bedford,[117] in 1954, described 2 patients with the triad of jejunal diverticulosis, steatorrhea, and megaloblastic anemia and suggested that stagnation within the narrow-mouthed diverticula might produce an effect similar to a blind loop of the gut. Prior to 1958, Scudamore et al.[118] could collect only 19 case reports of patients with this syndrome.

Cooke et al.[119] collected 31 patients from the literature who had intestinal diverticula together with steatorrhea and vitamin B_{12} malabsorption, and described a number of cases of their own. Of 21 patients with intestinal diverticulosis and macrocytic anemia, 13 had steatorrhea; another 2 had steatorrhea but without macrocytic anemia. It is interesting that intermittent partial small bowel obstruction was present in 11 of the 13 patients with steatorrhea, but in only 4 of 8 patients without quantitative evidence of steatorrhea. In their series of 33 patients with jejunal diverticula, Cooke et al. found steatorrhea in 9 of 27.

It should be emphasized that not all patients with blind loop syndrome from diverticulosis of the small intestine have both macrocytic anemia and steatorrhea. Patients have been described with diverticulosis and macrocytic anemia but without steatorrhea, as well as with diverticulosis and steatorrhea but without macrocytic anemia.

Radiologic Findings. A preliminary film of the abdomen is recommended; the sacs may contain air and be visible on an ordinary roentgenogram. In uncomplicated cases, the pouches are usually empty or contain fluid and chyme mixed with air. Occasionally, multiple fluid levels may be seen and may be mistaken for intestinal obstruction.[120, 121] On radiographs taken after ingestion of barium, the sacs appear as oval, circular, cup- or flask-shaped projections from the bowel lumen, best seen in tangential views. They are usually smooth in outline and show no distinct mucosal folds. They may appear as pedunculated collections of barium continuous with intestinal lumen or as residual round densities resembling bunches of grapes after emptying of the adjacent intestinal lumen. Occasionally they may be multiloculated. The intestinal loops are freely mobile, and this may account for a marked change in position of barium-filled diverticula on various films. Case[122] suggested that upright and lateral films are of more service and may occasionally demonstrate a level of opaque medium and a non-opaque fluid level capped with gas. Some diverticula are retentive. Enteroliths within them may simulate biliary or renal calculi. Diverticula may also produce marked distortion of the small intestinal outline, simulating the nutritional deficiency pattern.[123]

Diverticula in the region of the duodenojejunal junction present many diagnostic difficulties because of the stomach shadow. Those in the first few loops of the jejunum are usually easily visualized, whereas those occurring in the lower jejunum or ileum may be overlooked because of superimposed loops. The use of pressure devices, as well as frequent film exposures and perhaps serial filling of the small bowel by use of a tube inserted into the small gut, may be quite helpful in such cases. Fraser[99] suggested that intestinal diverticula may not visualize because they are in the mesentery and hence do not fill, or because they are so large that they hang down on the side of the bowel, kink their necks, and obstruct the entrance into them. Under these circumstances, filling may be obtained at times by placing the patient in the Trendelenburg position. Occasionally, because of partial or irregular filling, complicated diverticula are confused with intrinsic inflammatory disease of the small intestine. Rarely, a polyp-like neoplastic type of intraluminal defect may be visualized owing to an intraluminal diverticulum that is or has been inverted. Gross and colleagues[124] reported 3 unusual instances in which elongated diverticula originating from the small intestine pierced the right side of the diaphragm and extended into the thorax.

Diagnosis. The diagnosis of jejunal diverticulosis is established by barium study of the small intestine (Chapter 102), while the diagnosis of manifestations of disease resulting from this lesion is dependent upon the specific complication, whether malabsorption secondary to bacterial overgrowth (Chapters 27 and 107), gastrointestinal bleeding (Chapter 6), or obstruction (Chapter 122).

Treatment. Since the overwhelming majority of small intestinal diverticula are asymptomatic, no specific medical or surgical treatment is indicated when these are seen on barium radiographs. If the diverticula are believed to be the cause of bacterial overgrowth syndrome, appropriate bowel sterilization should be given (Chapter 107). Complications, such as diverticulitis, obstruction, perforation, or severe hemorrhage, require immediate supportive measures followed by appropriate surgical intervention.

Several surgical procedures are employed, depending on the nature of the complication. With a solitary, uninflamed diverticulum, excision of the pouch along with invagination of the stump by a pursestring suture is satisfactory. With multiple diverticula in a relatively short segment (under 12 inches), primary resection with end-to-end anastomosis can be done. With diffuse small bowel diverticulosis extending over a long segment, it is best to remove only that segment that is the cause of the complication. Side-to-side anastomosis, or bypass of a segment of gut with diverticula, or inversion of the whole diverticulum is best avoided.[92, 94]

References

1. Khojasteh A, Haghshenass M, Parrez H. Immunoproliferative small intestinal disease. A "Third-World lesion." N Engl J Med 1983; 308:1401–5.
2. Haghshenass M, Haghighi P, Abadi P, Kharazmi A, Gerami C, Nasr K. Alpha-heavy-chain disease in southern Iran. Am J Dig Dis 1977; 22:866–73.
3. Salem PA, Nassar HV, Shahid MJ. "Mediterranean abdominal lymphoma," or immunoproliferative small intestinal disease. I. Clinical aspects. Cancer 1977; 40:2941–7.
4. Selzer G, Sherman G, Callihan TR, Schwartz Y. Primary small intestinal lymphomas and alpha-heavy-chain disease: a study of 43 cases from a pathology department in Israel. Isr J Med Sci 1979; 15:111–23.
5. Gray GM, Rosenberg SA, Cooper AD, Gregory PB, Stein DT, Herzenberg H. Lymphomas involving the gastrointestinal tract. Gastroenterology 1982; 82:143–52.
6. Novis BH. Primary intestinal lymphoma in South Africa. Isr J Med Sci 1979; 15:386–9.
7. Selzer G, Sacks M, Sherman G, Naggan L. Primary malignancy lymphoma of the small intestine in Israel: changing incidence with time. Isr J Med Sci 1979; 15:390–6.

8. Nassar VH, Salem PA, Shahid MJ, et al. "Mediterranean abdominal lymphoma," or immunoproliferative small intestinal disease. II. Pathological aspects. Cancer 1978; 41:1340–54.
9. Gafter U, Kessler E, Shabtay F, Shaked P, Djaldetti M. Abnormal chromosomal marker (D14a+) in a patient with alpha-heavy-chain disease. J Clin Pathol 1980; 33:136–44.
10. Kharazmi A, Rezai MH, Abadi P, Nasr K, Haghighi P, Haghshenass M. T and B lymphocytes in alpha-chain disease. J Surg Oncol 1979; 11:365–74.
11. Doe WF. Alpha-chain disease: clinicopathological features and relationship to so-called Mediterranean lymphoma. Br J Cancer 1975; 22:866–73.
12. Baer AN, Bayless TM, Yardley JH. Intestinal ulceration and malabsorption syndromes. Gastroenterology 1980; 79: 754–65.
13. Jeffries GH, Steinberg H, Sleisinger MH. Chronic ulcerative (non-granulomatous) jejunitis. Am J Med 1968; 44:47–59.
14. Bank S, Marks IN. Malabsorption in systemic mast cell disease. Gastroenterology 1963; 46:535.
15. Roberts LJ, Sweetman BJ, Lewis RA, Austen F, Oates JA. Increased production of prostaglandin D_2 in patients with systemic mastocytosis. N Engl J Med 1980; 303:1400–4.
16. Keyzer JJ, DeMonchoy JGR, VanDoormaal JJ, Van Vorst Vader DC. Improved diagnosis of mastocytosis by measurement of urinary histamine metabolites. N Engl J Med 1983; 309:1603–5.
17. Clemmet AR, Fishbone G, Levine RJ. Gastrointestinal lesions in mastocytosis. Am J Roentgenol 1968; 103:405.
18. Broitman SA, McCray RS, May JC. Mastocytosis and intestinal malabsorption. Am J Med 1972; 48:382–91.
19. Soter NA, Austen F, Wasserman SI. Oral disodium cromoglycate in the treatment of systemic mastocytosis. N Engl J Med 1979; 301:465–9.
20. Ali M, Weinstein J, Biempica L, Halpern A, Das KM. Cronkhite-Canada syndrome: report of a case with bacteriologic, immunologic and electron microscope studies. Gastroenterology 1980; 79:731–6.
21. Rubin M, Tuthill RJ, Rosate EF, Cohen S. Cronkhite-Canada syndrome: report of an unusual case. Gastroenterology 1980; 79:737–41.
22. Shibuya C. An autopsy case of Cronkhite-Canada syndrome. Acta Pathol Jpn 1972; 22:171–83.
23. Russel DM, Bhathal PS, St. John DJB. Complete remission in Cronkhite-Canada syndrome. Gastroenterology 1983; 85:180–5.
24. Manousos O, Webster CV. Diffuse gastrointestinal polyposis with ectodermal changes. Gut 1966; 7:375–9.
25. Takalata J, Okubok K, Komepa T. Generalized gastrointestinal polyposis associated with ectodermal changes and protein-losing enteropathy with a dramatic response to prednisone. Digestion 1972; 5:153–61.
26. Johnson GK, Sorgell KH, Hensley GY. Cronkhite-Canada syndrome: gastrointestinal pathophysiology and morphology. Gastroenterology 1972; 63:140–52.
27. Gotto AM, Levy RI, John K. On the protein defect in abeta lipoproteinemia. N Engl J Med 1971; 284:813.
28. Illingworth DR, Conner WE, Lin DS, Diliberti J. Lipid metabolism in abeta lipoproteinema: a study of cholesterol absorption and sterol balance in two patients. Gastroenterology 1980; 78:68–75.
29. Lees RS, Ahrens EH. Fat transport in abeta lipoproteinemia. N Engl J Med 1969; 280:1261.
30. Law BH. Medium chain triglycerides in the treatment of pancreatic insufficiency and abeta lipoproteinemia. *In:* Senior J Jr. Medium Chain Triglycerides. Philadelphia: University of Pennsylvania Press, 1968:155.
31. Dische MR, Porro RS. The cardiac lesion in Bassen-Kornzweig syndrome. Am J Med 1970; 49:568.
32. Isselbacher KJ, Scheig R, Plotkin GR. Congenital beta lipoprotein deficiency: an hereditary disorder involving a defect in the absorption and transport of lipids. Medicine 1964; 43:347.
33. Kyle RA, Greipp PR. Amyloidosis (AL). Clinical and laboratory features in 229 cases. Mayo Clin Proc 1983; 58:665–83.
34. Bazinet P, Marin GA. Malabsorption in systemic lupus erythematosus. Am J Dig Dis 1971; 16:460.
35. Dryer NH, Kendall NJ, Hawkins CS. Malabsorption in rheumatoid arthritis. Ann Rheum Dis 1971; 30:626.
36. Mayoral LG, Carpathy K, Garcia FT. Intestinal malabsorption in parasitic disease. The role of protein malnutrition. Gastroenterology 1966; 50:856–7.
37. Sheehy TW, Meroley WH, Cox RS. Hookworm disease in malabsorption. Gastroenterology 1962; 42:148.
38. Whiteside ME, MacLoed CL, Barkin J, Pitchenick AE, Fischl MA. Chronic enteric coccidiosis in patients with the acquired immunodeficiency syndrome. (Submitted for publication.)
39. Ament ME, Rubin CE. Relation of giardiasis to abnormal intestinal structure and function in gastrointestinal immunodeficiency syndrome. Gastroenterology 1972; 65:216.
40. Leibman WM, Thaler MM, DeLorimer A, Brandenborg LL, Goodman J. Intractable diarrhea of infancy due to intestinal coccidiosis. Gastroenterology 1980; 78:579–84.
41. Trier JS, Mokey PC, Schimmel EM, Robles E. Chronic coccidiosis in man. Gastroenterology 1974; 66:923–35.
42. Aziz MA, Siddiqui AR. Morphologic and absorption studies of small intestine in hookworm disease (ancylostomiasis) in West Pakistan. Gastroenterology 1968; 55:242–50.
43. Roggin GM, Iber FL, Kater RMH, et al. Malabsorption in the chronic alcoholic. Johns Hopkins Med J 1961; 125:321.
44. Rubin E, Roybac BJ, Linderbaum J, et al. Ultra-structural changes in the small intestine induced by ethanol. Gastroenterology 1972; 63:801–14.
45. Romero JJ, Tamura T, Halsted CH. Intestinal absorption of (^{3}H) folic acid in the chronic alcoholic monkey. Gastroenterology 1981; 80:99–102.
46. Halsted ECH, Robles EA, Mezey E. Intestinal malabsorption in folate-deficient alcoholics. Gastroenterology 1973; 64:526–38.
47. Bianchi A, Chipman DQ, Breskin A, et al. Nutritional folic acid deficiency with megaloblastic changes in the small bowel epithelium. N Engl J Med 1970; 282:859.
48. Dobbins WO. Drug-induced steatorrhea. Gastroenterology 1968; 54:1193–5.
49. Rogers AI, Vloedman DA, Bloom EC, et al. Neomycin induced steatorrhea. JAMA 1966; 197:117.
50. Merliss RR, Hoffman A. Steatorrhea following the use of antibiotics. N Engl J Med 1951; 245:338.
51. Reynolds EH, Hallpike JF, Phillips RM. Reversible absorptive defects in anticonvulsive megaloblastic anemia. J Clin Pathol 1965; 18:593.
52. Race TF, Paes IC, Faloon WW. Intestinal malabsorption induced by oral colchicine. Comparison with neomycin and cathartic agents. Am J Med Sci 1970; 259:32.
53. Rawson MD. Cathartic colon. Lancet 1966; 1:1121.
54. Vrenick EJ, Simmons S, Murphy JS. Effect on hepatic morphology and treatment of obesity by fasting, reducing diets and small bowel bypass. N Engl J Med 1970; 282:829.
55. Hooft C, Devos E, Vanme JV. Celiac disease in a diabetic child. Lancet 1969; 2:161.
56. Wruble LD, Kalser MH. Diabetic steatorrhea: a distinct entity. Am J Med 1964; 37:118.
56a. Lincoln J, Bokor JT, Crowe R, Griffith SG, Haven AJ, Burnstock G. Myenteric plexus in streptozotocin-treated rats: neurochemical and histochemical evidence for diabetic neuropathy in the gut. Gastroenterology 1984; 86:654–61.
57. Jackson WPU. Steatorrhea in hypoparathyroidism. Lancet 1957; 272:1086.
58. Thomas FB, Caldwell JH, Greenberger NJ. Steatorrhea in thyrotoxicosis. Ann Intern Med 1973; 78:669.
59. Siurala M, Varis K, Labberg BA. Intestinal absorption and autoimmunity in endocrine disorders. Acta Med Scand 1968; 184:53–64.
60. Harris OD, Cooke WT, Thompson H. Malignancy in adult celiac disease and idiopathic steatorrhea. Am J Med 1967; 42:899.
61. Dymock IW, MacKay N, Miller V, et al. Small intestinal function in neoplastic disease. Br J Cancer 1967; 21:505.
62. McBrien MP, Hyde RD. Massive renal adenoma associated with intestinal malabsorption. Br J Surg 1970; 57:548.
63. Jones RD. Fat malabsorption in congestive cardiac failure. Br Med J 1961; 1:1276.
64. Hyde RD, Loehry CA. Folic acid malabsorption in cardiac failure. Gut 1968; 9:717.
65. Hamilton JR, Reilly BJ, Morecki R. Short small intestine associated with malrotation: a newly described congenital cause of intestinal malabsorption. Gastroenterology 1969; 56:124–36.
66. Weinstein WM, Saunders DR, Tygat GN, et al. Collagenous

sprue—an unrecognized type of malabsorption. N Engl J Med 1970; 283:1297.
67. Pittman FE. Primary malabsorption following extreme attempts to lose weight. Gut 1966: 7:154.
68. Phillips SF, McGill DB. Glucose-galactose malabsorption in an adult: perfusion studies with sugar, electrolyte and water transport. Am J Dig Dis 1973; 18:1017.
69. Mneuwisse GW, Dahlquist A. Glucose-galactose malabsorption. Acta Paediatr Scand 1968; 57:273.
70. Marks JF, Norton JR, Fordtran JS. Glucose-galactose malabsorption. J Pediatr 1966; 69:225.
71. Schneider AJ, Kinter WB, Stirling CE. Glucose-galactose malabsorption. N Engl J Med 1966; 274:305–12.
72. Mneuwisse GW, Dahlquist A. Glucose-galactose malabsorption. Lancet 1966; 1:858.
73. Davidson GP, Cutz E, Hamilton JR, Gall DG. Familial enteropathy: a syndrome of protracted diarrhea from birth, failure to thrive and hypoplastic villus atrophy. Gastroenterology 1978; 75:783–95.
74. Rowe JW, Gillian JI, Wartlin TA. Intestinal manifestations of Fabry's disease. Ann Intern Med 1974; 81:628–31.
75. O'Brien BD, Shintka TK, McDougall R, Walker K, Costopoulos L, Lentle B, Anhoct C, Freeman AT, Thomson ABR. Pathophysiologic and ultrastructural basis for intestinal symptoms in Fabry's disease. Gastroenterology 1982; 82:957–62.
76. Anderson H, Levine AS, Levitt MD. Incomplete absorption of the carbohydrate in all purpose wheat flour. N Engl J Med 1981; 304:891–2.
77. Levine AS, Levitt MD. Malabsorption of starch moiety of oats, corn and potatoes. Gastroenterology 1981; 80:1201.
78. Levine AS, Silvis SE. Absorption of whole peanuts, peanut oil and peanut butter. N Engl J Med 1980; 303:917–8.
79. Thoene JG, Lemons R, Baker H. Impaired intestinal absorption of biotin in juvenile multiple carboxylase deficiency. N Engl J Med 1983; 308:639–42.
80. Schwartz CJ, Kimberg DV, Sherrin HE, Field M, Said SI. Vasoactive intestinal peptide stimulation of adenylate cyclase and active electrolyte secretion in intestinal mucosa. J Clin Invest 1974; 54:536–44.
81. Kimberg DV, Field M, Johnson J, Henderson A, Gershon E. Stimulation of intestinal mucosal adenyl cyclase by cholera enterotoxin and prostaglandins. J Clin Invest 1971; 50:1218–30.
82. Gill DM, Evans DJ Jr, Evans DG. Mechanism of activation of adenylate cyclase in vitro by polymixin released, heat-labile enterotoxin of Escherichia coli. J Infect Dis 1976; 133[Suppl]:103–7.
83. Moss J, Vaughan M. Mechanism of activation of adenylate cyclase by cholecagen and E. coli heat-labile enterotoxin. *In:* Field M, Fordtran JS, Schultz SG, eds. Secretory Diarrhea. Bethesda, MD: American Physiological Society, 1980:107–23.
84. Kane MG, O'Dorisio TM, Krejs GJ. Production of secretory diarrhea by intravenous infusion of vasoactive intestinal polypeptide. N Engl J Med 1983; 309:1482–5.
85. Binder HJ. Pathophysiology of bile acid and fatty acid induced diarrhea. *In:* Field M, Fordtran JS, Schultz SG, eds. Secretory Diarrhea. Bethesda, MD: American Physiological Society, 1980:159–78.
86. Krejs GJ, Hendler RS, Fordtran JS.: Diagnostic and pathophysiologic studies in patients with chronic diarrhea. *In:* Field M, Fordtran JS, Schultz SG, eds. Secretory Diarrhea. Bethesda, MD: American Physiological Society, 1980:141–52.
87. Steven K, Lange P, Bukhone J, Rask-Madsen J. Prostaglandin E_2-mediated secretory diarrhea in villous adenoma of the rectum: effect of treatment with indomethacin. Gastroenterology 1981; 80:1562–6.
88. Harford WV, Krejs GJ, Santa Ana CA, Fordtran JS. Acute effects of diphenoxylate with atropine (Lomotil) in patients with chronic diarrhea and fecal incontinence. Gastroenterology 1980; 78:440–3.
89. Gardner J. Pathogenesis of secretory diarrhea. *In:* Field M, Fordtran JS, Schultz SG, eds. Secretory Diarrhea. Bethesda, MD: American Physiological Society, 1980:153–8.
90. Cooper A. Anatomy and Surgical Treatment of Crural and Umbilical Hernia. From 2nd Lond. 4d. by C. Aston Key. Philadelphia: Lea, 1807:87.
91. Osler W. Notes on intestinal diverticula. Ann Anat Surg 1881; 4:202.
92. Connolly PJ. Diverticula of the jejunum and ileum. J Mich Med Soc 1954; 53:868.
93. Spriggs EI, Marxer OA. Intestinal diverticula. Q J Med 1925; 19:1.
94. Orr IM, Russell JYW. Diverticulosis of the jejunum—a clinical entity. Br J Surg 1951; 39:139.
95. Ritvo M, Votta PJ. Diverticulosis of jejunum and ileum. Radiology 1946; 46:343.
96. Klebs TAE. Hanbuch der pathologischen Anatomie. Vol. I. Berlin: Hirschwald, 1869–1880:271.
97. Hansemann D. Ueber die Entstehung falscher Darmdivertike. Arch Pathol Anat 1896; 144:400.
98. Benson RE, Dixon EF, Waugh JM. Non-Meckelian diverticula of jejunum and ileum. Ann Surg 1943; 118:377.
99. Fraser I. Diverticula of the jejunum. Br J Surg 1933–34; 21:183.
100. Edwards HC. Diverticula and Diverticulitis of the Intestine. Bristol: John Wright & Sons, Ltd., 1939.
101. Rosedale RS, Lawrence HR. Jejunal diverticulosis. Am J Surg 1936; 34:369.
102. Butler RW. Traumatic rupture of intramesenteric diverticula of the jejunum. Br J Surg 1937; 25:277.
103. King ESJ. Diverticula of the small intestine. Aust NZ J Surg 1950; 19:301.
104. Edwards HC. Diverticula of the small intestine. Br J Radiol 1949; 22:437.
105. Cunliff WJ, Anderson J. Case of Cronkhite-Canada syndrome with associated jejunal diverticulosis. Br Med J 1967; 4:601.
106. Barbosa JJD, Dockerty MB, Waugh JM, et al. Pancreatic heterotopia: review of the literature and report of 41 authenticated surgical cases of which 25 were clinically significant. Surg. Gynecol Obstet 1946; 82:527.
107. Baskin RH Jr, Mayo CW. Jejunal diverticulosis. Surg Clin North Am 1952; 32:1185.
108. Lee RE, Finby N. Jejunal and ileal diverticulosis. Arch Intern Med 1958; 102:97.
109. Badenoch J, Bedford PD, Evans JR. Massive diverticulosis of small intestine with steatorrhoea and megaloblastic anemia. Q J Med 1955; 24:321.
110. Altemeier WA, Bryant CR, Wulsin JH. The surgical significance of jejunal diverticulosis. Arch Surg 1963; 86:732.
111. Milnes-Walker R. The complications of acquired diverticulosis of the jejunum and ileum. Br J Surg 1945; 32:457.
112. Nelson PA, Schmitz RL, Narsete EM. Jejunal diverticulosis complicated by "chronic non-mechanical" obstruction. Ill Med J 1954; 106:371.
113. Taylor MT. Massive hemorrhage from jejunal diverticulosis. Am J Surg 1969; 118:117.
114. Thomas CS Jr, Tinskly EA, Brockman SE. Jejunal diverticula as source of massive upper gastrointestinal bleeding. Arch Surg 1967; 95:89.
115. Montuschi E. Jejunal insufficiency with hypoproteinemic edema. Proc R Soc Med 1949; 42:868.
116. Zingg W. Schwere Diverticulosis Jejuni als Teilursache de Spruesyndromes. Gastroenterologia 1950; 75:353.
117. Badenoch J, Bedford PD. Massive diverticulosis of the upper intestine with steatorrhoea and megaloblastic anemia. Q J Med 1954; 23:464.
118. Scudamore HH, Hagedorn AB, Wollaeger EE, et al. Diverticulosis of the small intestine and macrocytic anemia with report of two cases and studies on absorption of radioactive vitamin B_{12}. Gastroenterology 1958; 34:66.
119. Cooke WT, Cox EV, Fone DJ. The clinical and metabolic significance of jejunal diverticula. Gut 1963; 4:115.
120. Rees JD. Diverticulosis of the jejunum. Am Surg 1956; 22:322.
121. Stromme A. Fluid levels in diverticula of the small intestine: radiological sign simulating obstruction. Br J Radiol 1956; 29:574.
122. Case JT. Diverticula of the small intestine other than Meckel's diverticulum. JAMA 1920; 75:1463.
123. Vogel F. Diverticulosis of jejunum. Gastroenterologia 1953; 80:377.
124. Gross RE, Edward MD, Neuhauser BD, et al. Thoracic diverticula which originated from the intestine. Ann Surg 1950; 131:363.

Chapter 112

Primary Small Intestinal Lymphoma

Daniel Rachmilewitz • Elimelech Okon

The small intestine may be affected by malignant lymphoma that is either localized or dispersed along its entire length. Several definitions are employed to characterize intestinal lymphomas. One defines lesions according to primary and secondary involvements. The extended definition[1] regards all lymphomas that have predominant small bowel lesions or that present initially with symptoms caused by intestinal involvement as *primary* lymphomas. A disseminated lymphomatous process originating elsewhere but affecting the small intestine in a localized or multifocal form is defined as a *secondary* lymphoma. This chapter, except for a passing comment at the end, deals with primary small intestinal lymphomas.

Primary small intestinal lymphoma (PSIL) is not a homogeneous group and can be further subdivided into "Western" type and alpha chain disease. Primary intestinal lymphoma of the "Western" type is characterized by discrete single or multiple lesions among which normal intestinal mucosa is preserved. Alpha chain disease is defined as a B lymphoid cell proliferation affecting the IgA secretory system and producing an abnormal immunoglobulin devoid of light chains. Khojasteh et al.[1a] have suggested that this form of PSIL, commonly referred to as "Mediterranean lymphoma," be termed "immunoproliferative small intestinal disease." The malignant proliferation in alpha chain disease involves large portions of the small intestine and normal mucosa does not intervene between affected regions. The epidemiology, pathologic findings, and clinical manifestations of PSIL are specific for each of the subtypes.

Etiology and Pathogenesis

The etiology and pathogenesis of PSIL are not known. However, the specific geographic distribution and the predilection of PSIL to appear among underprivileged populations suggest that environmental factors may have a role in its pathogenesis. A prolonged infection of the gastrointestinal tract and its resulting antigenic stimulation may lead to proliferation of lymphoid cells in the lamina propria. The lymphoid proliferation secondary to these environmental factors may also serve as the background for the oncogenic effect of a virus or any other unknown factor. The possibility of a predisposing genetic factor in the pathogenesis of alpha chain disease also has to be considered in view of the prevalence of this disorder among specific ethnic groups.

PSIL is also a recognized complication of celiac disease[2] and was reported in 9% of celiac disease patients.[3] In some instances the diagnosis of celiac disease is made prior to the diagnosis of the lymphoma, whereas in others the celiac disease is clinically occult and the diagnosis can easily be missed.[4] There is no evidence that patients with a suboptimal clinical response to a gluten-free diet or with persistent flat jejunal biopsy specimens are more prone to develop intestinal lymphoma.[3] *A gluten-free diet also does not seem to be effective in preventing the malignant complication* (Chapter 105).

Epidemiology

In the Western world, PSIL represents about 17% of all small bowel malignancies[5,6] and about 7.5% of all extranodal non-Hodgkins lymphomas.[7] In underdeveloped countries, PSIL accounts for more than two thirds of small bowel malignancies.[8] The "Western" type is usually observed in adults in the fifth and sixth decades[7] and in children under the age of 10 years.[1] The great majority of patients with alpha chain disease are between 10 and 30 years old.[9]

Primary Small Intestinal Lymphoma of the "Western" Type

Pathology. PSIL of the "Western" type involves the ileum in most patients. It may appear as a fungating mass (Fig. 112–1), as an ulcer with raised edges, or as plaquelike thickenings resembling mucosal nodules. An ulcerated and diffusely thickened segment of the bowel (Fig. 112–2), which causes narrowing of the lumen and sometimes simulates Crohn's disease, may also appear. A combination of these macroscopic forms may develop and be observed to exist simultaneously, especially in the advanced stages of the disease; a diffuse thickening of a segment in one area may be accompanied by a large lymphomatous mass extending into the mesentery and its lymph nodes in another area (Fig. 112–3).

Microscopically, all types of non-Hodgkin's lymphoma may be observed in the "Western" type of PSIL. However, certain histologic types tend to appear more commonly in specific macroscopic forms. PSIL appearing as a large fungating mass is usually of a more monomorphic histologic type, consisting of large lymphoid cells or immunoblasts. These correspond to the intermediate-grade malignant lymphoma (diffuse large cell type) and high-grade malignant lymphoma (large cell immunoblastic type).[11]

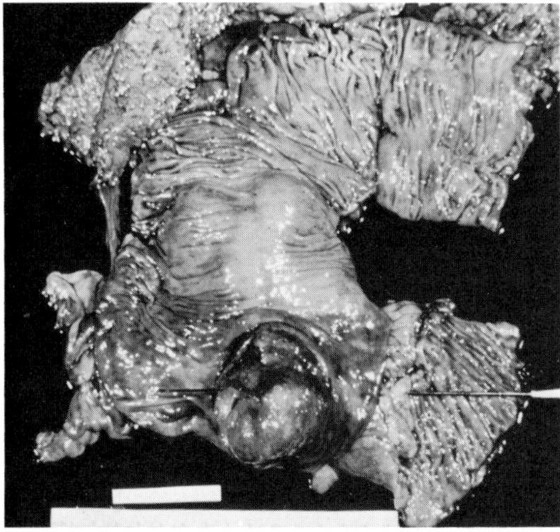

Figure 112–1. Primary small intestinal lymphoma presenting as a large fungating mass in the terminal ileum.

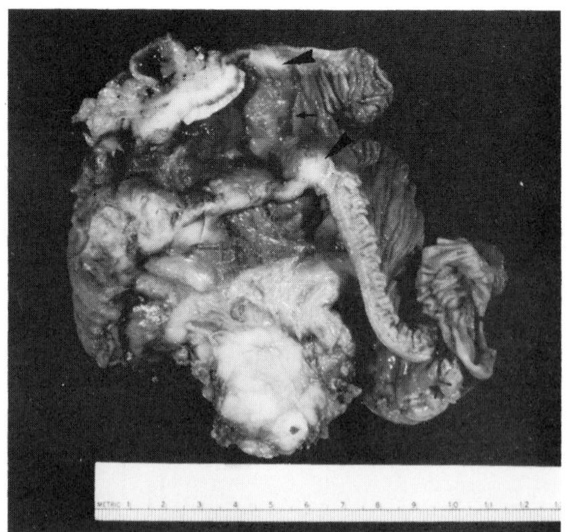

Figure 112–2. Primary small intestinal lymphoma presenting as a diffusely thickened segment of the jejunum. The large arrows mark the beginning of the thickened segment. Note that the lymphomatous infiltrate involves the entire wall, causing mucosal ulceration *(small arrow)*. The mesenteric lymph nodes are also involved.

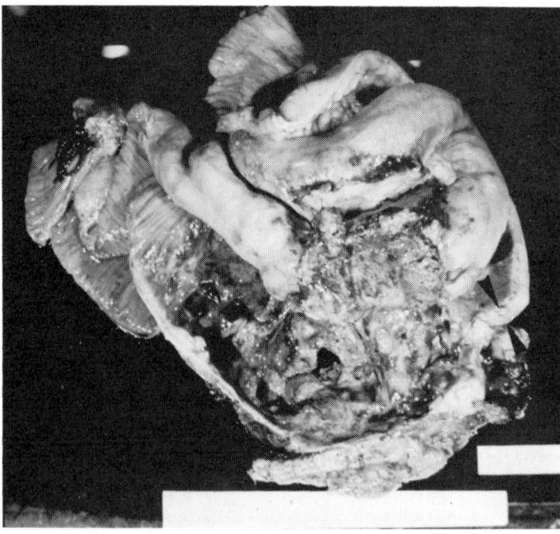

Figure 112–3. Primary small intestinal lymphoma presenting as a large abdominal mass. Note the conglomeration of several involved intestinal loops. The left lower loop is perforated. The arrows mark the infiltrated and thickened intestinal wall. The patient was a 22-year-old woman with Burkitt-type malignant lymphoma.

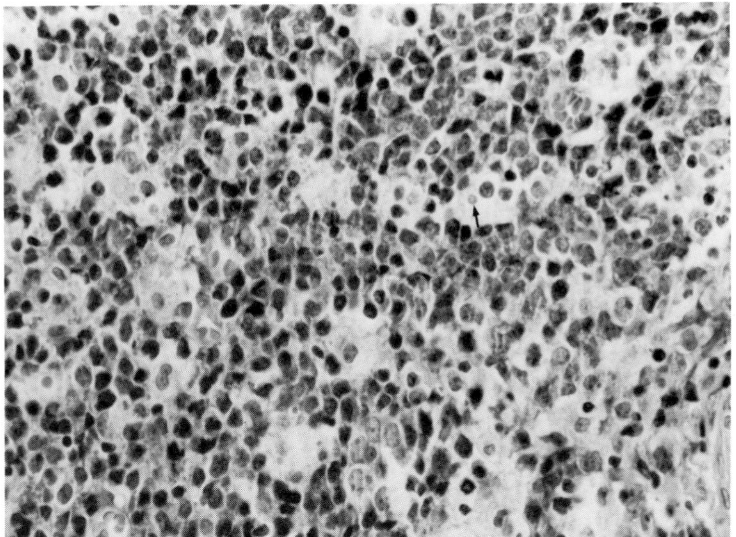

Figure 112–4. Primary small intestinal Burkitt-type lymphoma. This type of malignant lymphoma is composed of small noncleaved cells with a great number of macrophages showing pale cytoplasm containing tangible bodies *(arrow)*. (Hematoxylin and eosin, × 420.)

In children or adolescents, such a mass is usually composed of small noncleaved cells, at times showing Burkitt-type malignant lymphoma (Fig. 112–4). In older patients with segmental thickening or with multifocal involvement, the lymphomatous masses are of the small cleaved cell type, large lymphoid cell type, or, more frequently, appear as mixed small cleaved and large cell types. The diffuse pattern is histologically far more frequent than the follicular one. The high-grade malignant lymphomas (large cell immunoblastic type) often show plasmacytoid features (Fig. 112–5).

Clinical Features. The main clinical presentations are *obstruction, intussusception,* and *perforation.* In many patients the initial manifestation is such as to require management as a surgical emergency. Abdominal pain, usually crampy in nature, is frequently described. The pain is often associated with nausea and vomiting, reflecting partial obstruction. Malaise, fatigue, and slight weight loss may precede the other symptoms. Massive intestinal hemorrhage may occur, but occult intestinal bleeding is more common. Fever, when present, usually suggests either a complication or an extensive involvement of the malignant process. On physical examination, abdominal tenderness and the presence of an *abdominal mass* are the main findings. Hepatomegaly and splenomegaly

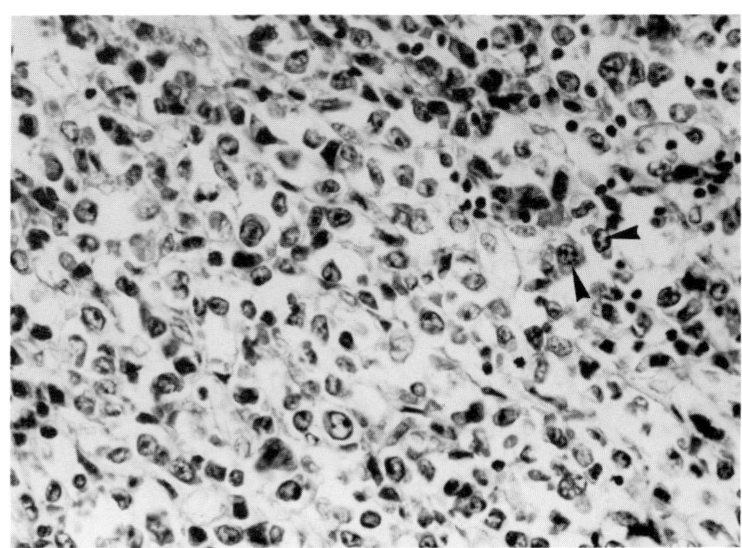

Figure 112–5. Primary small intestinal lymphoma appearing as high-grade large cell immunoblastic type. Note the lymphoplasmacytoid features in many of the cells *(arrows)*. (Hematoxylin and eosin, × 420.)

are generally found only in patients with extensive disease. The presence of intestinal obstruction (Chapter 122) or perforation is characterized by the respective typical findings.

Diagnosis. Routine hematologic and biochemical laboratory tests are of little value in diagnosis. Mild anemia is frequent, but abnormal cells are usually absent from the peripheral blood or bone marrow. Routine immunologic blood tests are usually within normal limits. Protein-losing enteropathy may be observed in patients with extensive disease.

Barium studies of the small intestine are helpful in defining the site, extent, and gross appearance of the lesions. Infiltration of the wall, distortion of mucosal folds, segmental constriction, and "aneurysmal" dilatation of the bowel may all occur (Fig. 112–6). The tumor may also appear as a polypoid mass projecting into the lumen. Mesenteric or extensive extraintestinal tumor spread may be manifested radiologically as extrinsic pressure defects.

Imaging procedures, such as computed tomography (Chapter 38) and magnetic resonance (Chapter 40), may provide useful diagnostic information by showing thickening of the wall (see Fig. 40–12), extension beyond the wall, and lymph node involvement.

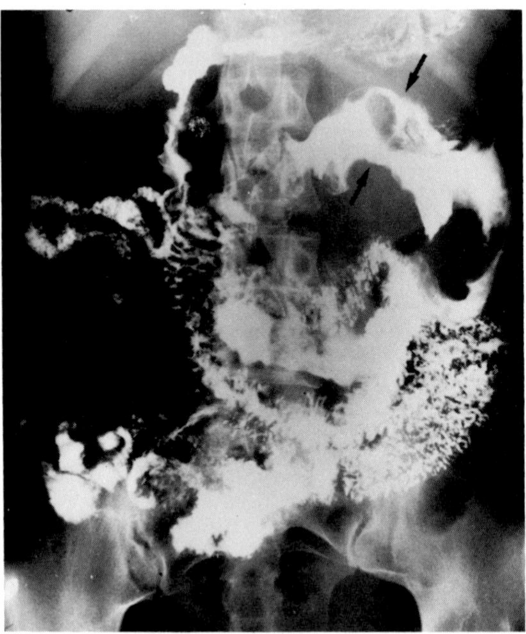

Figure 112–6. Barium contrast study of the small bowel from a patient with primary small intestinal lymphoma of the "Western" type. The mucosal folds in the duodenum are thickened, and there is an aneurysmal-like dilatation of a jejunal loop with irregular rigid margins and filling defects in the lumen *(arrows)*. There is also constriction of the involved segment, and the distance between adjacent loops is increased, suggesting mesenteric involvement. (Courtesy of Dr. Emerik Lax.)

Upper gastrointestinal endoscopy and ileal endoscopy performed with the colonoscope (see discussion of enteroscopy in Chapter 103) may help in the diagnosis of the disease when these respective regions of the small intestine are affected.

Differential Diagnosis. The "Western" type of primary intestinal lymphoma must be distinguished from other neoplasms, both benign (leiomyomas, adenomas, and lipomas) and malignant (carcinomas, sarcomas, and carcinoids)—all of which can present in the same way. Inflammatory diseases of the bowel (Crohn's disease, fungal infections, and tuberculosis) may also be considered in the differential diagnosis. Definitive diagnosis is established only by histologic examination of the tumor performed following laparotomy.

Treatment. The current trend in treating patients with PSIL of the "Western" type is to *surgically resect as much tumor mass as possible*. It is important that at the time of laparotomy the extent of involvement of the lymphomatous process be assessed by obtaining biopsy specimens from the liver and from mesenteric and para-aortic lymph nodes. Resection is followed by adjuvant radiotherapy and/or chemotherapy. In patients with disseminated tumors, chemotherapy may precede radiotherapy or surgical resection of residual lesions. When chemotherapy is administered to patients with lymphomas having high mitotic activity, such as Burkitt's lymphoma, massive cell lysis may lead to metabolic disturbances (hypocalcemia, hyperuricemia, and lactic acidosis). Allopurinol, careful correction of electrolyte and water imbalance, and sometimes even peritoneal dialysis or hemodialysis are needed in the final stages of treatment in these patients.

Prognosis. The histologic type, the extent of the intestinal disease, and the presence or absence of extraintestinal involvement are the important factors in prognosis. Recurrent disease following surgical resection ranges from 30% to 40%.[1, 7, 8, 12] When the disease involves extraintestinal sites, the 5 year survival is less than 10%.[1] Most deaths from PSIL occur within the first year after diagnosis. Patients alive after 10 years are considered to be cured.

Alpha Chain Disease (Mediterranean Lymphoma)

Alpha chain disease is a proliferative disorder of B lymphoid cells involving primarily the IgA secretory system. The plasma cells in this disorder produce a presumably homogeneous population of immunoglobulin (Ig) molecules that consist of incomplete alpha chains devoid of light chains. In rare instances, the abnormal protein secreted by the cellular infiltrate is polyclonal, consisting of a myeloma or lambda heavy chain protein.[13] Since the first description of alpha chain disease in 1968, more than 150 patients have been reported.

Two types of the disease have been recognized: a very rare respiratory form and a more common gastrointestinal form. The gastrointestinal form of the disease is extremely rare in Western developed countries. Most patients with this variety of the disorder originate from and live in countries where poor hygiene practices are common. Socioeconomically, they are in the lower classes.[13]

There is some confusion about the relationship of alpha chain disease to *Mediterranean lymphoma,* a disorder first reported from Israel in 1965.[14] Mediterranean lymphoma is also a primary diffuse intestinal lymphoma that affects underprivileged young adults and that has since been observed in other than Mediterranean countries. Like alpha chain disease, it may begin as an apparent benign plasma cell infiltration of the small intestine. In addition, alpha chain disease protein has been found in the sera of many patients with Mediterranean lymphoma, and the failure to detect it in all patients may be due to insensitivity of available techniques or to an advanced undifferentiated state of the malignant proliferating cells. Moreover, alpha chain disease protein can at times be detected in the jejunal secretion and a nonsecretory form of the disease has also been reported.[15] It seems, therefore, that *Mediterranean lymphoma and alpha chain disease are, in fact, the same entity.*

Pathology. In the alpha chain disease type of PSIL, there is diffuse lymphomatous infiltration of the mucosa and submucosa of a long segment of the small intestine, sometimes of its entire length. It usually affects the jejunum, with frequent extension into the duodenum and ileum. Mesenteric lymph nodes may be affected as well.

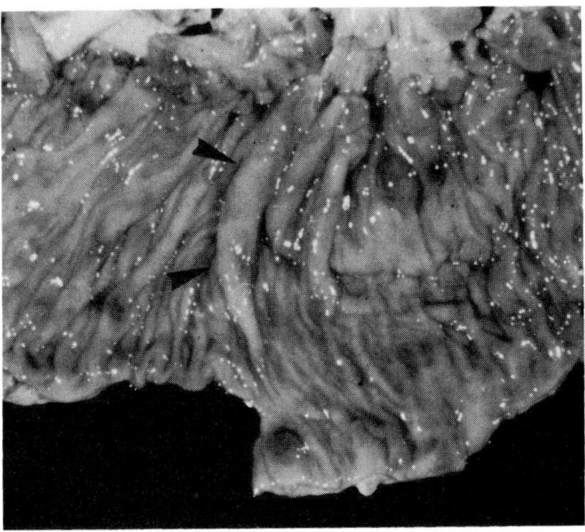

Figure 112–7. The jejunum of a patient with alpha chain disease. There is diffuse thickening and induration of the mucosa. Note the indurated and thickened mucosal folds in the center *(arrows)*.

Although most patients have diffuse thickening and induration of the affected segments of small intestine (Fig. 112–7), the macroscopic changes are sometimes very mild and the intestine and mesenteric lymph nodes may look normal at laparotomy. The most important histologic finding is extensive infiltration of the lamina propria and submucosa by a polymorphous or monomorphous cell infiltrate. The infiltrate leads to diminution in the number of crypts and can cause a reduction in the number of villi, some of which may appear shorter and wider; complete villous atrophy may even be found (Fig. 112–8). The surface epithelium may be altered and ulcerated. Most often, the polymorphous infiltrate is composed of small and large lymphoid cells, immunoblasts, plasma cells, eosinophils, neutrophils, and sometimes multinucleated giant cells. Many of the lymphoid cells have plasmacytoid features with an eccentrically placed nucleus and amphophilic cytoplasm (Fig. 112–9). The extent of the polymorphous infiltrate and the relative number of the various lymphoid cells change with progression of the disease. Indeed, the cells may differ in a given patient in various areas at the same time. When a monomorphous infiltrate predominates in the early stage of the disease, it is composed mainly of mature, bland-looking plasma cells; only a few atypical plasma cells and some large lymphoid cells can be traced within the infiltrate (Fig. 112–10).

In the more advanced stages, the lymphomatous infiltrate may penetrate deep into

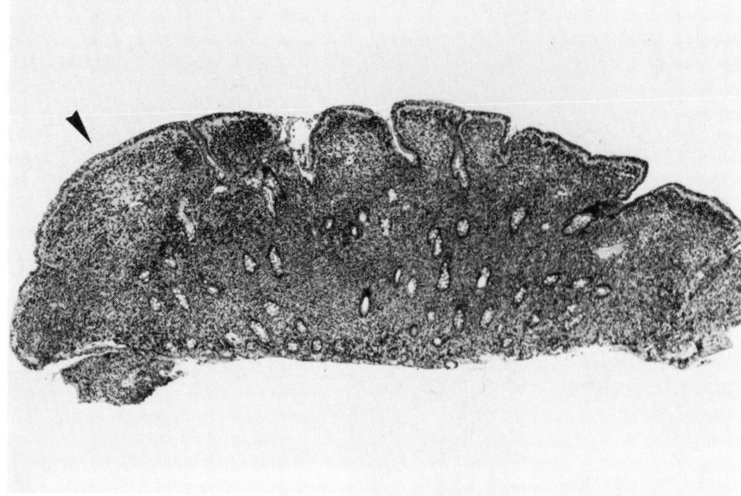

Figure 112–8. Jejunal biopsy specimen from a patient with alpha chain disease. The lamina propria is infiltrated extensively by a polymorphous infiltrate. There is diminution in the number of crypts and the villi are short and wide. On the left, the lymphomatous infiltrate caused complete villous atrophy *(arrow)*. (Hematoxylin and eosin, × 42.)

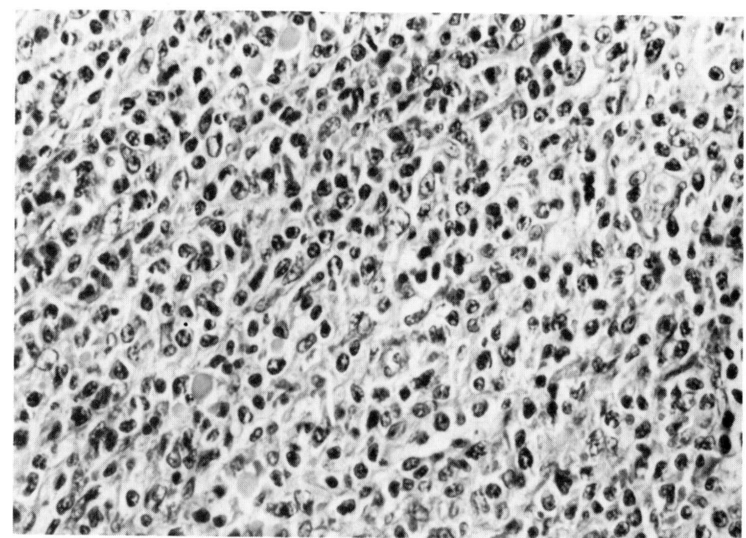

Figure 112–9. A polymorphous infiltrate in a jejunal biopsy specimen from a patient with alpha chain disease. The infiltrate includes small and large lymphoid cells, immunoblasts, and some neutrophils. Many of the lymphoid cells show lymphoplasmacytoid features. (Hematoxylin and eosin, × 420.)

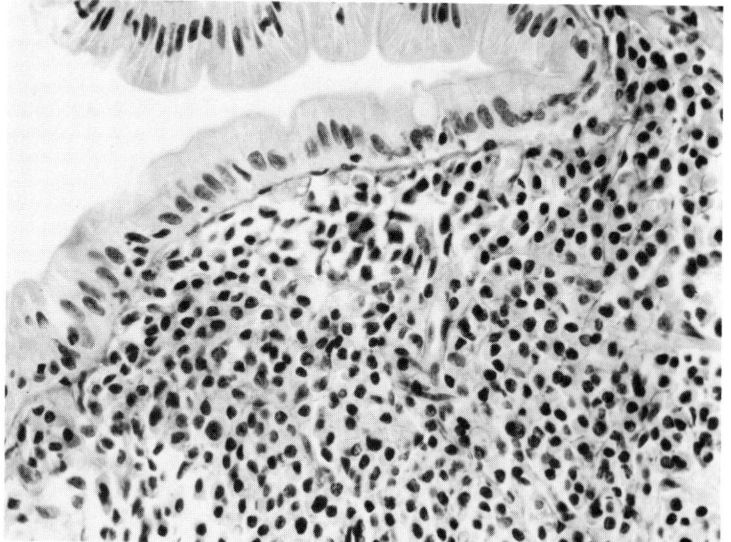

Figure 112–10. A jejunual biopsy specimen from a patient with alpha chain disease. The lamina propria is infiltrated by a dense monomorphous infiltrate composed mainly of mature bland-looking plasma cells. (Hematoxylin and eosin, × 420.)

the submucosa, destroy the muscularis propria, and even invade the mesenteric fat. Regional and mesenteric lymph nodes may already be involved early in the disease. In the early stage, the cells present in the lamina propria characteristically infiltrate the lymph nodes without affecting their normal architecture. In more advanced stages, there is effacement of the lymph node structure by the same infiltrate, but this is only rarely complete. The depth of penetration and the degree of cellular atypia may vary greatly from one region to another. Lymphoid cells invading deeper parts of the bowel are usually larger than those present in more superficial parts of the same segment.

With still further progression of the disease, a monomorphic proliferation of immunoblasts predominates in the intestine and lymph nodes, and the process manifests the typical features of immunoblastic lymphoma.[16] When the disease is widespread, it is indistinguishable from any other primary malignant lymphoma that secondarily involves various parenchymatous organs, such as the liver, lungs, kidneys, or spleen.

Immunofluorescence and immunoperoxidase studies reveal that the mature plasma cells contain alpha chains but lack the light chains. The large lymphoid cells usually do not show positive staining.

Clinical Features. The main clinical feature of alpha chain disease is *severe malabsorption,* and on many occasions this is the presenting symptom. Its onset can be either insidious or abrupt. *Abdominal pain* of variable intensity and localization, *vomiting,* and *loss of weight* are also frequent. The natural course of the disease is usually continuous, but at times partial spontaneous improvement is noted.

On physical examination, clubbing of the fingers is a very common finding. The abdomen is usually tender and distended. Edema and ascites can be found in advanced stages of the disease. Hepatosplenomegaly and lymphadenopathy are usually not evident when the patient is first seen. In later stages, "tumoral" symptoms of the nature of an abdominal mass, intestinal obstruction, or perforation can be observed.

Diagnosis. Anemia is usual but on most occasions is mild or moderate. Low serum albumin levels, hypocalcemia, and hypokalemia frequent. Dehydration and electrolyte imbalance may be so pronounced as to require emergency treatment. Hypokalemic nephropathy with polyuria may also occur.

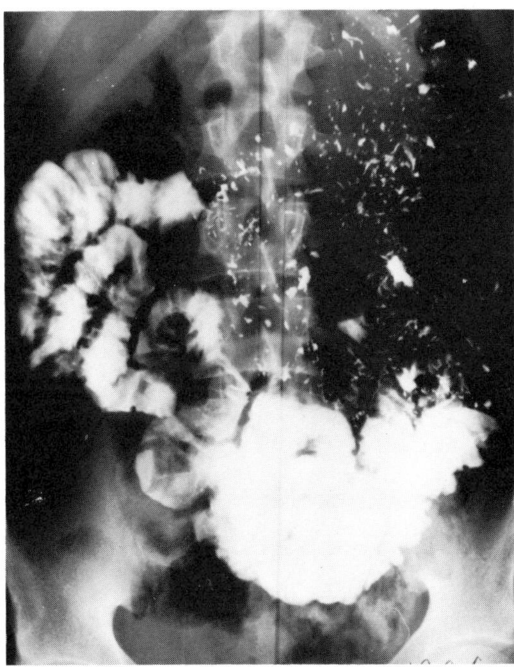

Figure 112–11. Barium contrast study of the small intestine from a patient with alpha chain disease. The small intestinal mucosa pattern is markedly abnormal. The mucosal folds are enlarged and there are polypoid filling defects. The bowel wall is edematous. Flocculation of the barium is also noted. (Courtesy of Dr. Emerik Lax.)

Frequently, increase in the intestinal isoenzyme of alkaline phosphatase is responsible for high serum activities of this enzyme. Serum lipid and cholesterol levels are low. Absorption tests such as D-xylose absorption and the Schilling test are usually abnormal. Protein-losing enteropathy and creatorrhea are almost constantly present.

Small intestinal barium meal roentgenograms usually show hypertrophic folds in the duodenum and jejunum; at times these have a pseudopolypoid pattern (Fig. 112–11). Strictures and filling defects secondary to enlarged mesenteric lymph nodes are also quite common. Imaging techniques of the nature of computed tomography (Chapter 38) and magnetic resonance (Chapter 40) may depict wall and adjacent changes, as noted earlier in the discussion of primary intestinal lymphoma. Multiple small bowel biopsies obtained either during endoscopy or by any other method are needed to establish the diagnosis. At times the diagnosis can be made only by examination of multiple full thickness intestinal biopsy specimens and mesenteric lymph nodes obtained at laparot-

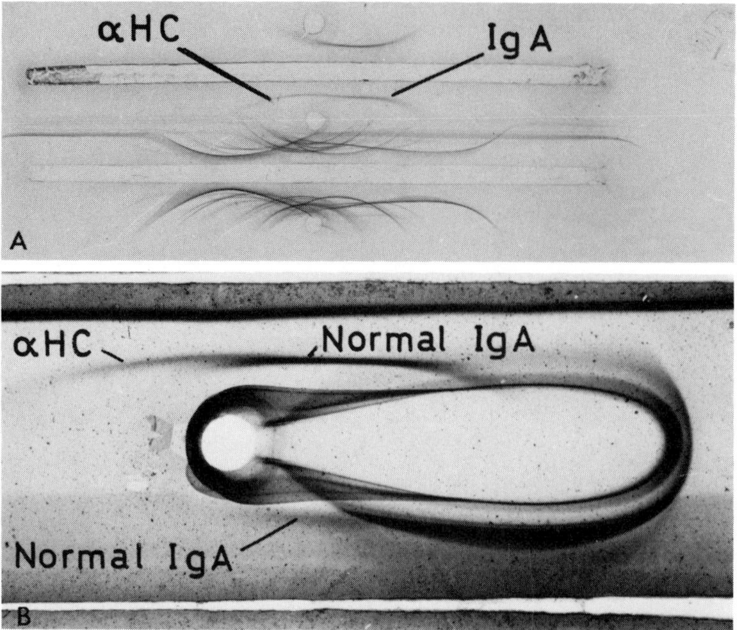

Figure 112–12. *A*, Immunoelectrophoresis of serum obtained from a patient with alpha chain disease (center well) and a control serum (outer wells). Lower trough contains anti–whole human serum and upper trough contains anti-IgA serum. The alpha chain (αHC) shows increased mobility toward the anode and forms a spur with the normal IgA globulin (IgA). *B*, Immunoselection immunoelectrophoresis of serum obtained from the same patient; 0.3 ml of anti-IgG antiserum was incorporated in the agar. The upper trough contains an anti-IgA serum and the lower one an anti-kappa or anti-lambda serum. Note that the normal IgA reacts with both antisera. The alpha heavy chain (αHC) does not react with antisera to the light chains (lower trough). (Courtesy of Dr. Avinoam Zlotnik.)

omy.[13] Bone marrow aspirate or biopsy is usually normal except for slight plasma cell infiltration. *Intestinal parasites, especially Giardia lamblia, are found in one third of the patients.*[17]

Immunologic Features. The alpha chain protein may be found on serum electrophoresis as a broad band in the α_2 and β_2 regions when present in sufficient concentration,[13] but in most instances the electrophoregram is normal. Immunoelectrophoresis with monospecific antisera to IgA is essential to disclose the diagnosis. An abnormal precipitin line extending from the α_1 to the slow β_2 regions, or showing a faster electrophoretic mobility than normal IgA, is usually observed (Fig. 112–12). However, several cases with normal mobility of the alpha chain protein have been described. Lack of precipitation with anti-kappa and anti-lambda antisera is not sufficient for the diagnosis of alpha chain disease, since several IgA myeloma proteins that contain light chains also fail to precipitate with such antisera. Immunoelectrophoresis with selected antisera to IgA-containing antibodies related to the conformational specificity of the Fab region is very specific and most sensitive for the diagnosis of alpha chain disease. In difficult cases, the protein has to be purified, reduced, and alkylated, and the lack of light chains should be demonstrated by gel electrophoresis.[13]

The serum levels of normal IgG and IgM are usually depressed. An exact quantitation of the alpha chain protein cannot be determined because of its small molecular weight, the consequent rapid diffusion, and the large rings formed by the immunodiffusion technique. Because of its tendency to polymerize and its lack of diffusion at times, the serum level of this protein may be falsely determined as zero. The concentration of the pathologic protein in the urine is also low because of its tendency to polymerize. However, the protein can be detected in concentrated urine. Bence Jones proteinuria is absent. The abnormal protein is also found in significant amount in jejunal fluid. When the protein is absent in the serum and jejunal fluid, immunofluorescence or biosynthetic methods can be used to prove its synthesis by the infiltrating cells.[13]

Differential Diagnosis. The clinical and radiologic picture of patients with alpha chain disease may closely resemble that of other intestinal mucosal diseases associated with malabsorption. Celiac disease (Chapter 105), Whipple's disease (Chapter 109), and amyloidosis (Chapter 111) especially have also to be considered in the differential diagnosis. Fever is not common with celiac disease and a gluten-free diet induces significant clinical improvement. The best way to distinguish among the various mucosal diseases is by multiple intestinal biopsy specimens taken from several levels of the small intestine to increase the chances of sampling involved mucosa.

Treatment. The various therapeutic indications and their time of application are still in dispute. Patients with disease limited to the intestine and manifested mainly by mature plasma cell infiltration may be treated first with *antibiotics* for several months. This treatment has to be followed by repeated intestinal biopsies and search for the disappearance of the alpha chain protein from the serum or jejunal juice. If there is no improvement within 3 months of therapy or if remission is not achieved within a reasonable time, *chemotherapy* should be given (Chapter 256). In patients with disseminated lymphomatous lesions, discrete tumors should be surgically resected when possible, followed by chemotherapy. Whether abdominal irradiation should precede the chemotherapy is still disputed. At all stages of the disease, supportive treatment with fluids, electrolytes, blood, and parenterally administered nutritive solutions is often essential.

Prognosis. The natural course of the disease is either one marked by *continuous* symptoms or one that is *interrupted* with spontaneous periods of clinical improvement. Remissions have been reported following antibiotic therapy.[18] Complete remission may be achieved with chemotherapy[19] but this occurs in only very few patients.

Secondary Small Intestinal Lymphomas

The small intestine may be secondarily involved in patients with malignant lymphoma. Clinically symptomatic secondary intestinal involvement, however, is not frequent. In most patients with lymphoma, intestinal symptoms occurring during treatment of the primary disease are not due to lymphomatous involvement of the gut. Moniliasis, ulcers, sepsis, and bleeding can all result from non-neoplastic lesions. Yet true tumor invasion of the gut can occur and usually is manifested as intestinal obstruction, perforation, or bleeding, necessitating emergency surgical intervention.

References

1. Herrmann R, Panahon AM, Barcos MP, Walsh D, Stutzman L. Gastrointestinal involvement in non-Hodgkin's lymphoma. Cancer 1980; 46:215–22.

1a. Khojasteh A, Haghshenass MD, Haghighi P. Immunoproliferative small bowel intestinal disease: A "third-world lesion." N Engl J Med 1983; 308:1401–5.

2. Stokes PL, Holmes GKT. Coeliac disease malignancy. Clin Gastroenterol 1974; 3:159–70.
3. Holmes GKT, Stokes PL, Sorahan TM, Prior P, Waterhouse JAH, Cooke WT. Coeliac disease, gluten free diet and malignancy. Gut 1976; 17:612–9.
4. Freeman HJ, Weinstein WH, Shnitka TK, Piercy JRA, Wensel RH. Primary abdominal lymphoma presenting manifestation of celiac sprue or complicating dermatitis herpetiformis. Am J Med 1977; 63:585–94.
5. Paetalunan RJG, Mayo CW, Dockerty MD. Primary malignant tumors of the small intestine. Am J Surg 1964; 108:13–8.
6. Fu YS, Perzin KH. Lymphosarcoma of the small intestine: A clinicopathologic study. Cancer 1972; 29:645–59.
7. Freeman C, Berg JW, Cutler SJ. Occurrence and prognosis of extranodal lymphomas. Cancer 1972; 29:252–60.
8. Chadli A, Lennert K. Les lymphomas malins non hodgkiniens du tube digestif. Ann Anat Pathol 1979; 24:231–50.
9. Seligmann M. Immunochemical, clinical and pathological features of α-chain disease. Arch Intern Med 1975; 135:78–82.
10. Lewin KJ, Kahn LB, Novis BH. Primary intestinal lymphoma of "western" and "Mediterranean" type alpha chain disease and massive plasma cell infiltration. Cancer 1976; 38:2511–28.
11. National Cancer Institute Sponsored Study of Classifications of Non-Hodgkin's Lymphomas: Summary and description of a working formulation for clinical usage. Cancer 1982, 49:2112–35.
12. Blackledge T, Bush H, Dodge OG, Crowther D. A study of gastrointestinal lymphoma. Clin Oncol 1979; 5:209–19.
13. Seligmann M, Rambaud JC. α-Chain disease: A possible model for the pathogenesis of human lymphomas. *In*: Good RA, Day SB, eds. Comprehensive Immunology, Vol. 4: Tomasy JJ, Good RA, eds. The Immunopathology of Lymphoreticular Neoplasms. New York and London: Plenum 1978: 425–47.
14. Ramot B, Sahin N, Bubis JJ. Malabsorption syndrome in lymphoma of small intestine. Isr J Med Sci 1965; 1:221–6.
15. Rambaud JC, Modigliani R, Nguyen Phouc BK. Non secretory alpha chain disease in intestinal lymphoma. N Engl J Med 1980; 303:53.
16. Selzer G, Sherman G, Callihan TR, Schwartz Y. Primary cell intestinal lymphomas and α heavy chain disease: A study of 43 cases from a pathology department in Israel. Isr J Med Sci 1979; 15:111–23.
17. Rambaud JC, Seligmann M. Alpha chain disease. Clin Gastroenterol 1976; 5:341–58.
18. WHO Meeting Report. Alpha chain disease and related small intestinal lymphoma. Arch Mal App Dig 1976; 65:591–607.
19. Zlotnik A, Levy M. α Heavy chain disease: A variant of Mediterranean lymphoma. Arch Intern Med 1971; 128:432–6.

Chapter 113

Carcinoid Tumor

Richard R. P. Warner

First clearly described in 1888,[1] the carcinoid tumor is a unique neoplasm, being neither completely malignant nor completely benign. It has been characterized as a "malignant neoplasm in slow motion" and a "missing link between benign neoplasm and carcinoma."[2] The name "Karcinoid" was applied to these tumors by Oberndorfer[3] in 1907 to indicate this intermediate status. Most carcinoids of fore- and midgut origin exhibit the histochemical ability to stain with silver salts. Hence they have also been labeled *argentaffinomas.*

Carcinoid tumors of the intestine arise from the argentaffin cells described by Kulchitsky in the mucosa near the base of the crypts of Lieberkühn. These enterochromaffin cells are now known to be part of the gut endocrine system and to have endocrinologic pluripotential. Their embryologic origin is from neuroectodermal cells of the neural crest.[4, 5] The argentaffin cell is included in the APUD cell concept of Pearce; hence the additional designation of carcinoid tumors as "carcinoid apudomas." APUD cells (amine precursor uptake and decarboxylation cells) are capable of producing multiple polypeptide hormones and bioamines.[6] Although functioning carcinoid tumors may elaborate one or several of these substances, serotonin is by far the most commonly elaborated pharmacologically active agent. Since 1954, when the clinical syndrome of flushing, diarrhea, wheezing, and heart disease resulting from humoral products of some carcinoid tumors was first described by Thorson et al.,[7] a number of cases of carcinoid tumors have been reported arising from enterochromaffin-like cells in a wide variety of extraintestinal sites. Many of these "ectopic" carcinoids have had histologic, histochemical, and endocrine features similar to those of the gut carcinoid.[8]

The majority of carcinoid tumors, regardless of their site of origin, do not cause clinical manifestations that are due to endocrine function. Most are also very slow growing, including those associated with the carcinoid syndrome. The often dramatic and bizarre clinical and chemical features of the rare carcinoid syndrome, the variant syndromes, and the milder incomplete syndrome constitute a "carcinoid spectrum."[9]

Pathology

Carcinoids in the small intestine appear grossly as submucosal nodules varying from pinhead size to several centimeters in diameter, but rarely are more than 5 cm in diameter. The majority are very small and are incidental findings. The minority that are associated with symptoms tend to be larger and in more than 90% of symptomatic cases are associated with metastases. Moertel et al.[2] observed metastases to be present in only 2% of lesions smaller than 1 cm in diameter, in approximately 50% of lesions 1 to 2 cm in diameter, and in about 80% of tumors larger than 2 cm in diameter.

The lesions are occasionally umbilicated or may be more clearly polypoid. Uncommonly, the mucosa that overlies them ulcerates. When sectioned, they are yellow to grayish white in color and ordinarily do not exhibit the necrosis often seen in adenocarcinomas. A primary carcinoid tumor rarely grows large enough to obstruct the lumen by its bulk.

However, when the tumor has invaded the muscular layer and extended beyond the gut wall, it often causes a marked local desmoplastic reaction as well as local smooth muscle hypertrophy. This fibrosis can lead to peritoneal adhesions, kinking of the bowel, and even intestinal obstruction.

Microscopically, carcinoid tumors are composed of rather small uniform epithelial cells separated by a delicate connective tissue framework. Their nuclei are also remarkably uniform, rarely showing mitosis or hyperchromatism. Anaplasia is uncommon. The cells almost always have abundant eosinophilic cytoplasmic granules that have many special staining and fluorescing properties. Of these, the most frequently utilized is the reaction with silver salts. After fixation in formalin, the direct reduction of silver salts by the granules to precipitate metallic silver is termed the *argentaffin* reaction. If prior exposure of the cells to an exogenous reducing agent is required before metallic silver will precipitate, the reaction is termed *argyrophil.* All argentaffin-positive cells are argyrophil-positive, but the reverse may not be true. In general, foregut carcinoids are either argyrophil or nonreacting, midgut tumors are argentaffin-positive, and hindgut carcinoids are mostly nonreactive to the usual silver staining techniques.[8, 10, 11] In addition to the classic histologic pattern, carcinoid tumors may display several other histologic features characteristic of their site of origin.[10] While the histologic appearance of a carcinoid tumor is usually easily identified, it may be difficult to determine whether the tumor is benign or malignant. It is generally accepted that the usual cytologic standards of tumor malignancy, such as mitosis and anaplasia, are not applicable to carcinoid.[12] *A diagnosis of malignancy must be based on gross and microscopic findings of invasiveness.*

In the small intestine, the ileum is the most common site of carcinoid (89%), followed by the jejunum (7%) and the duodenum (2%). Slightly over 2% of the small intestinal carcinoids occur in a Meckel's diverticulum. Besides the appendix and small intestine, other sites of carcinoid occurrence are (in order of decreasing frequency): the rectum and rectosigmoid, lung and bronchi, esophagus and stomach, pancreas, gallbladder, biliary tract, ovary and testis (argentaffin cell component of teratomas), right side of colon, and very rarely in various remote organs to which primordial neural crest cells have migrated.[8, 13–15] Particularly rare extraintestinal carcinoid sites are the thymus, urethra, prostate, urinary bladder, cerumen glands of the ear, breast, uterine cervix, and the parotid gland.

Associated Conditions. Carcinoids of the gut tend to be multicentric, with multiple primary tumors often appearing. This occurs particularly in the small intestine, where a second primary is present in approximately one third of the cases and sometimes even dozens of primaries occur.[2, 15] The tendency to multiplicity of carcinoids, however, is rare in the appendix.

Carcinoid tumors occur as part of the multiple endocrine neoplasia (MEN) syndrome, most usually type I, but occasionally type II.[5] This is considered part of a neuroectodermal dysplasia in which any of the endocrine neoplasia of neural crest origin may participate.[5,6] There is also an increased incidence of a second primary carcinoma of non-endocrine origin occurring in patients with carcinoid tumors. These metachronous or subsequent malignancies are usually in the gastrointestinal tract, particularly the colon.[2, 15, 16] Carcinoids of the intestine are also associated with a high incidence of benign renal cysts.[17]

With a few exceptions,[18] malignant carcinoids of the intestine follow a fairly predictable progressive pattern of invasiveness; they first invade the submucosa and underlying muscle coats and then the serosa and mesentery. Regional lymph nodes are usually invaded before a distant site, such as the liver, is involved as a consequence of blood vessel invasion. The malignancy of carcinoids of the small intestine, particularly the terminal ileum, is second only to that of carcinoids arising in the colon, where the primary tumor can grow larger before causing symptoms.[19] In one study, [12] about two thirds of all small intestinal carcinoids showed some degree of invasiveness, and almost 40% eventually spread to lymph nodes and beyond (16% distant metastases).

The liver is the most common site of distant metastasis.[2, 12, 18, 20] Other areas that may be involved are (in order of decreasing frequency): the mesentery and peritoneum, bone, lung, pancreas, skin, omentum, brain, spleen, mediastinum, adrenals, heart, kidney, thyroid, testis, and gallbladder. Although lytic lesions may occur, bone metastases are usually osteoblastic.

Pathophysiology

Although serotonin is not solely responsible for the humoral-related features of the carcinoid syndrome, as was originally thought, it does remain the most important contributor. Pathways of its synthesis and metabolism have been well delineated and frequently described[21] (Fig. 113–1). Blood levels can be measured and fluctuate considerably, depending on the influence of eating and many other factors.[22] Ithe major metabolite of serotonin is 5-hydroxyindolacetic acid (5-HIAA). In a normal adult, 5-HIAA is excreted in the urine over a 24-hour period in amounts ranging from 2 to 9 mg. Many foods and drugs and some disease states can alter the blood levels of serotonin and urinary 5-HIAA excretion or interfere with the urine assay.[(8,22)] The main foods that increase 5-HIAA are those that contain large amounts of serotonin: bananas, pineapple and its juice, red plums, eggplant, avocados, walnuts, and tomatoes. Glyceryl guaiacolate, acetanilid, mephenesin, methocarbamol, and phenothiazines can cause spurious measurements of 5-HIAA.[23,24] The most important of the non-carcinoid diseases that can increase blood serotonin, urinary 5-HIAA, and IAA are untreated malabsorption states (celiac disease, tropical sprue, Whipple's disease, stasis syndrome, cystic fibrosis) and chronic intestinal obstruction.[22] In these disorders the increased urinary excretion of tryptophan metabolites is not of the magnitude usually seen in the carcinoid syndrome and is rapidly corrected by antibiotics that alter the gut flora.

It should be noted that there are alternate routes for serotonin metabolism besides 5-HIAA, and this may explain the rare cases of carcinoid syndrome with elevated serotonin levels and normal 5-HIAA.[25]

Besides serotonin and its derivatives, the majority of functioning carcinoid tumors elaborate *bradykinin*.[26] Oates et al.[27] demonstrated the enzyme *kallikrein* in carcinoid tumors. Many catecholamines, particularly norepinephrine and epinephrine, as well as ethanol and other flush-provoking stimuli, release bradykinin and possibly other vasoactive products from carcinoid tumors.[27] *Kallikrein* converts kininogen (alpha$_2$-globulin) to the decapeptide lysyl-bradykinin, which in turn is rapidly changed to the nonapeptide bradykinin by plasma amino peptidase. Both

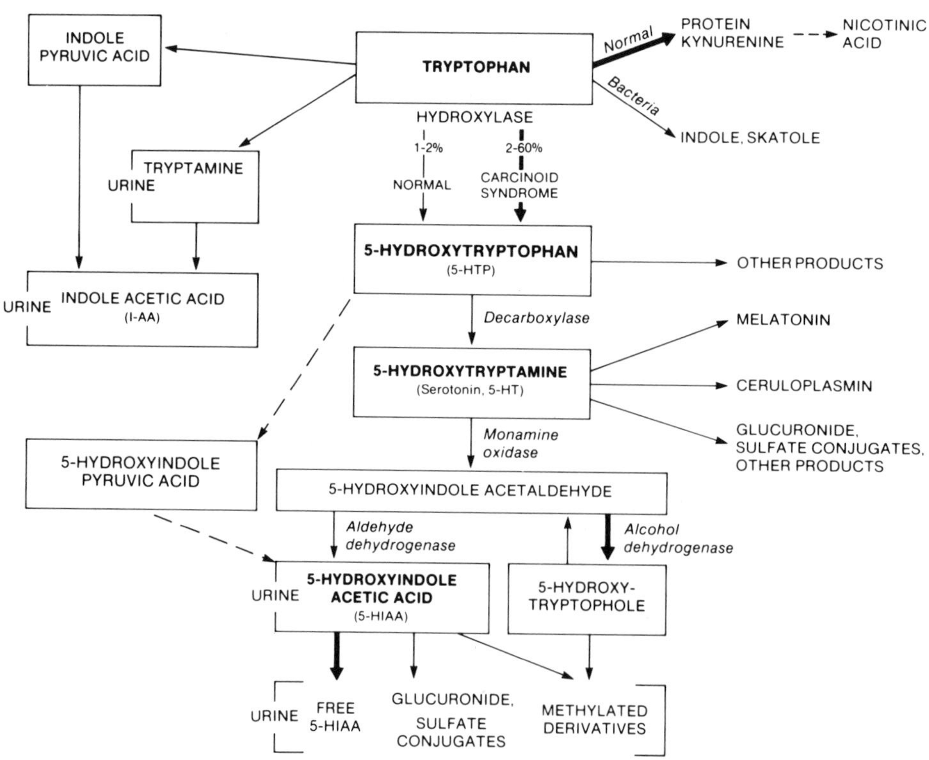

Figure 113–1. Principal metabolic pathways of tryptophan and serotonin.

the decapeptide and the nonapeptide have strong vasodilator and smooth muscle stimulating properties.

Prostaglandin E (PGE) blood levels have been found to be appreciably elevated in a majority of carcinoid syndrome patients.[28] Its role is unclear, since the PGE levels do not correlate with carcinoid syndrome symptoms, blood serotonin levels, or urinary 5-HIAA excretion. An uncertain role is also ascribed to *substance P* and *neurotensin,* which are also products of some carcinoid tumors.

On very rare occasions, midgut carcinoids secrete one or more of a host of *peptide hormones* in varying amounts, sometimes enough to cause a second endocrine syndrome superimposed on the carcinoid syndrome. Those peptide hormones documented to have been produced by midgut carcinoid tumors are: adrenocorticotropic hormone (ACTH), insulin, gastrin, vasoactive intestinal polypeptide (VIP), antidiuretic hormone (ADH), and calcitonin. Foregut carcinoids have also been known to produce these same substances, as well as others, with a slightly greater frequency than occurs in midgut carcinoids.[8]

Serotonin is probably mainly responsible for the diarrhea of the carcinoid syndrome and, perhaps along with other metabolic factors, causes the endocardial lesions. It may play a minor part in causing the flush and bronchospasm. Although, in general, there is a lack of correlation between the clinical severity of the carcinoid syndrome and the blood serotonin level and magnitude of the urinary 5-HIAA excreted,[13] serial measurements of these substances in each patient over a long period of time will reflect the progression of the disease in each individual. Increased serotonin and 5-HIAA may be seen in some cases of carcinoid without the clinical syndrome and in other instances the full syndrome may be present with only modest increases in these substances. However, as the disease worsens with the passage of time, the levels of serotonin and its metabolite usually increase progressively.

Plasma bradykinin levels rise abruptly in many, but not all, patients during provoked or spontaneous flushes. However, IV injected bradykinin does not cause the same quality of flush as that occurring spontaneously in many patients. Hence, complete understanding of the flush mechanism is still not clear.[27] The cherry-red patchy flush of some gastric carcinoids is due to the histamine that these tumors produce.[29]

The functioning carcinoid syndrome develops in one eighth to one third of invasive gut carcinoids and almost always requires the presence of liver metastases.[2, 12, 18] Moertel et al.[2] however, described the syndrome in 2 patients without hepatic metastases; one had only mesenteric node involvement, and the other had nodal and peritoneal implants. The prevailing concept is that a carcinoid discharging its products only into the portal venous system will not induce the syndrome because the liver rapidly inactivates serotonin and other pharmacologically active carcinoid tumor products. For the carcinoid syndrome to occur, functioning carcinoid tumors must be present in the liver, where they can grow large enough to have a significant humoral production with drainage of these substances directly into the hepatic veins and, thence, into the caval system. Infrequent exceptions occur when the functioning carcinoid arises in an extraintestinal site that has a venous drainage via the caval system, i.e., bronchus, ovary, testis, and, very rarely, mesenteric nodal metastases with abundant caval collaterals.

Although a carcinoid originating in any site can cause the functioning syndrome, in 75% to 80% of the cases the tumor arises in the small intestine, usually from the distal ileum.[14, 30] Appendiceal carcinoids rarely metastasize and almost never cause the functioning syndrome. Rectal carcinoids do have local and, infrequently, distal metastases, but also almost never cause the functioning syndrome. Approximately 10% of cases of the functioning syndrome stem from colon carcinoids. Another 10% come from bronchial carcinoids,[31] and, in rare instances, the syndrome is caused by a functioning carcinoid arising in some other extraintestinal site.

Epidemiology

Carcinoid tumors are common, with more than 4000 having been reported in the world's literature. The rate of occurrence of carcinoid tumor in necropsy studies has varied from 0.08% to 1.1%.[8] In a study from Malmö, Sweden, where the general hospital has an autopsy rate of 98%, the frequency of carcinoid found at all necropsy studies was 1.1%; none arose from the appendix. However, 6 appendiceal carcinoids were found operatively during the period of this study. MacDonald's report[12] indicates that a carcinoid will be found in 1 of every 200 to 300 appendices removed surgically. Various reports of carcinoid prevalence from both necropsy and clinical series have been collated and reviewed by Jaeger and Polk.[8] The appendix is the most frequent site of carcinoid tumors (35% to 40%), and carcinoid is the most common tumor of the appendix (77%). The small bowel is the next most common site for carcinoid tumor (33.7% of all carcinoids); carcinoids constitute 25% of all small intestinal tumors and 47% of all malignancies of the small intestine.[2]

Clinical Features

Carcinoid tumors occur in all age groups from infancy to the ninth decade. They are most common, however, in the age group from 50 to 60 years for non-appendiceal tumors and 30 to 40 years for appendiceal tumors. There is no overall sex difference in the frequency of carcinoids, although appendiceal carcinoids are more common in women and colonic carcinoids are more common in men. The frequency of carcinoid tumor also appears to be about the same in whites and blacks. Other than a few rare exceptions noted in the literature,[32] there is no familial tendency in the occurrence of these tumors.[14]

Non-specific Expressions. In the 25% of all small intestinal carcinoid cases that are symptomatic, *intermittent obstruction* is the most common presenting complaint.[2] This is usually due to kinking and fibrosis. Less common mechanisms associated with obstruction in these patients are constriction of the lumen, intussusception, and volvulus.

Second in frequency as the initial symptom is non-specific *abdominal pain.* This is seen in 41% of the cases. Less frequently occurring as a presenting symptom are melena, weight loss, change in bowel habits, and infarction of the small intestine due to either encroachment on the superior mesenteric artery or its more distal branches by metastatic carcinoid tumor or fibrosis associated with the tumor. Also contributing to this ischemic process may be the vasospastic effect of serotonin produced by the tumor. Other than evidence of intestinal obstruction, the most often noted clinical sign is a *palpable abdominal mass,* usually in the right upper quadrant.

In the very rare duodenal carcinoid, in addition to symptoms due to duodenal obstruction, ulceration, and bleeding, jaundice occurs infrequently. The functioning carcinoid syndrome is unlikely to arise from a duodenal carcinoid.

Carcinoid Syndrome. Since the first general acceptance of this rare dramatic constellation of signs and symptoms as a disease entity following its recognition and classic description in 1954,[7] many additional clinical and laboratory observations have underscored its variability and complexity.

Major Manifestations

CUTANEOUS FLUSHING. Episodic or paroxysmal flushing is the clinical hallmark of the syndrome. It consists typically of suddenly appearing erythema, which is deep red to violaceous or purple and involves the face and neck diffusely (Fig. 113–2). Less often it is patchy. Early in the disease, the flush is fleeting, 1 to 5 minutes, but later it may last hours and extend to involve the trunk and extremities. The flush is usually less apparent in black patients, who may simply complain of facial warmth or heat during attacks. It is usually accompanied by transient hypotension, and shock may occur in advanced cases.

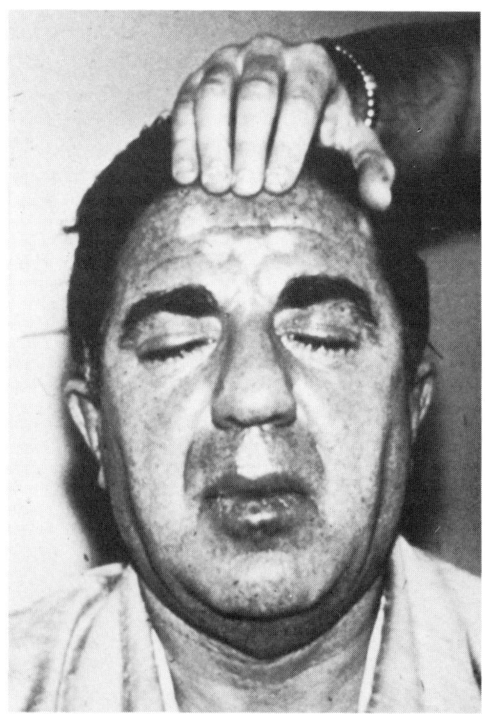

Figure 113–2. Carcinoid flush.

Cutaneous flushing occurs in about 75% of the cases and is second to diarrhea in frequency as a symptom of the syndrome.[33, 34]

DIARRHEA. This is generally considered the most frequent and disabling symptom of the carcinoid syndrome, occurring in more than 80% of patients.[34] Grahame-Smith,[13] however, reported it to be second to flushing in frequency. Chronic hypermotility of the gut with borborygmi and watery stools, which are sometimes explosive and accompanied by cramping, is the typical pattern. The diarrhea does not occur at the same time as the flushing episodes. Stools may vary from a few to more than 30 a day. The stools are nonbloody, unless bleeding results from peptic ulcer, ulceration of a primary tumor, gut infarction, or a coagulation defect. Steatorrhea and the features of malabsorption occur in a minority of patients. Transit time through the intestine may be extremely short, so that an upper gastrointestinal roentgen study may show that the first ingested barium has already reached the rectum and is distributed throughout the entire colon and small bowel while the patient is still drinking the initial barium.

VENOUS TELANGIECTASIA. These purplish lesions, which look like acne rosacea, appear late in the course of the disease in 50% of patients.[33] They occur on the skin of the face and neck, particularly the nose, upper lip, and malar area.

BRONCHOSPASM. These asthma-like episodes, which occur in only 10% to 20% of cases, are usually associated with paroxysmal flushing. It is exceedingly important that they not be mistaken for ordinary bronchial asthma attacks and not be treated with adrenergic agents, such as epinephrine. These drugs can precipitate bronchospastic and vasomotor attacks in patients with the carcinoid syndrome and may even cause death.

Cardiac Manifestations

VALVULAR LESIONS. Pathognomonic plaque-like deposits of a peculiar type of fibrous tissue develop in 25% to 50% of patients with carcinoid syndrome; these deposits occur on the endocardium of valvular cusps, the cardiac chambers, infrequently on the intima of the great veins, and sometimes on the intima of the great arteries.[34–37] Usually, this specific cardiac involvement develops late in the course of the disease. Patients with these lesions tend to have more highly functioning carcinoid tumors. This is evidenced by high blood levels of serotonin, very high urinary excretion of 5-HIAA, and exceptionally subnormal blood levels of tryptophan. The majority of these lesions develop on the right side of the heart, the most characteristic valvular lesions being tricuspid regurgitation and pulmonic stenosis. Considerably less often, the major valvular lesion may develop on the left side of the heart. In these instances there is almost always an atrial right-to-left shunt or a large highly functioning primary bronchial carcinoid. Cardiac arrhythmias occur frequently, and most of the patients with valvular lesions eventually develop heart failure.

HYPERKINEMIA. Some patients, both those with and without valvular lesions, develop heart failure due to excessively high cardiac output. This presumably results from continued chronic stimulation by the vasodilator substances released by the tumor.[38]

METASTATIC CARCINOID. Involvement of the pericardium or myocardium by metastatic carcinoid is an unusual but clinically important occurrence.[35, 39] I have observed it in 3 of 101 cases.

HEPATOMEGALY. Enlargement of the liver results from carcinoid metastases to this structure.

Minor Manifestations. There is a markedly increased frequency of *peptic ulcer* in association with metastatic carcinoid, both with and without the functioning syndrome.[12,29] Since dietary tryptophan is essential as a precursor for biosynthesis of protein and nicotinic acid, its diversion by a highly functioning carcinoid tumor to form large amounts of serotonin can result in the development of *hypoalbuminemia* and *pellagra*.[21] Poor dietary intake and diarrhea or malabsorption can augment this process. Besides weakness and edema, *profound muscle wasting* may occur as a reflection of poor protein synthesis. The rough, scaly skin lesions of pellagra may occur alone or along with mental changes. *Arthropathy* occurs in a small number of patients, who complain of stiffness and pain in the joints of their hands, particularly on releasing a tightly gripped object. This has been described as a specific arthropathy with characteristic radiologic findings.[40] A *myopathy* with distinct histologic features has been observed. It has been thought to be due to the effect of circulating serotonin on muscle fibers and has improved with cyproheptadine therapy.[41] There are a number of causes for muscle weakness and atrophy in carcinoid syndrome, but myopathy may be one that has not been sufficiently emphasized in the past. In addition to the fibrotic reaction locally associated with carcinoid tumors, extensive *fibrosis* can occur in the retroperitoneal area as well as in the mesentery and other sites. The fibrotic formation may obstruct viscera, such as the ureters,[42] or cause other bizarre manifestations, such as Peyronie's disease,[43] a plastic induration of the penis due to fibrosis.

Persistent *brawny edema* of the face, and to a lesser degree of the extremities, may appear as an advanced manifestation of the syndrome in some patients with severe flushing attacks. This is particularly true of those with a primary carcinoid of foregut origin.[44] Mild *hyperglycemia* due to the diabetogenic effect of serotonin may be noted in a minority of untreated patients. However, the glucose intolerance is usually mild and rarely of clinical significance.[45]

Variant Syndromes. In some functioning gastric and bronchial carcinoids, certain clinical and biochemical variations from the classic syndrome occur:

GASTRIC CARCINOID VARIANT SYNDROME. The flush with this very rare subset of gastric carcinoids is patchy, sharply demarcated, serpiginous, and cherry red rather than purplish. The tumors in these instances are ordinarily not associated with diarrhea or heart lesions. They usually are deficient in 5-HTP decarboxylase and hence secrete larger amounts of 5-HTP than 5-HT. Sometimes they form histamine, which may account for the particular flush exhibited as well as the increased prevalence of peptic ulcer. Patients with these tumors, as well as those with 5-HTP–secreting carcinoids from other sites, sometimes obtain significant benefit from treatment with methyldopa. By contrast, this decarboxylase inhibitor is usually of no help in typical cases of serotonin-secreting tumors.[29]

BRONCHIAL CARCINOID VARIANT SYNDROME. In this subset of patients, the flushes are very severe and long, lasting several hours to days. The flushes also tend to be preceded by disorientation, anxiety, and tremulousness. Associated with the flush are periorbital and facial edema, lacrimation, salivation, hypotension, tachycardia, diarrhea, dyspnea, asthma, oliguria, and sometimes nausea and vomiting. If left-sided cardiac lesions are also present, fatal pulmonary edema can occur. Corticosteroids and chlorpromazine are uniquely beneficial in this variant syndrome.[44]

Diagnosis

Non-functioning Tumors. Carcinoids of the small intestine, with or without metastases but not producing the functioning syndrome, are usually found at exploratory surgery undertaken because of undiagnosed symptoms. The latter consist of intermittent, slowly developing pain; obstruction; change in bowel habits; bleeding; and, in some cases of duodenal carcinoids, ulceration, duodenal obstruction, or biliary obstruction. A clinical suspicion of carcinoid tumor is sometimes supported by barium radiographic study of the gastrointestinal tract or by angiography. Metastatic involvement of the liver may be disclosed by a variety of scanning techniques.[46]

Some of the earlier studies of carcinoid tumors reported that most small primary carcinoids of the small intestine, even with medium-sized lymph node metastases, do not cause a significant increase in urinary excretion of 5-HIAA. However, I have found by measuring tumor serotonin content, as well as by carefully studying blood and urine, that some carcinoids with regional node involvement without liver metastases *do* produce enough serotonin to cause modest elevations in blood levels of this amine. They are also accompanied by a decrease in blood levels of tryptophan and small increases in urinary excretion of 5-HIAA. Therefore, accurate quantitative assays of each of these substances may occasionally be of diagnostic aid even in the absence of the carcinoid syndrome. Since these chemical abnormalities may be minor in degree, particular care must be taken to avoid the various factors noted earlier (food, drugs) that can alter these tests. In addition, interpretation of the test results must take into consideration the various noncarcinoid diseases noted earlier, which can cause similar minor chemical alterations. Whenever possible, a portion of any tumor removed at surgery that is suspected of being carcinoid should be retained. That fragment should not be fixed in formalin but should be kept frozen for possible future chemical assay.

Carcinoid Syndrome. The carcinoid syndrome is easily recognized when all of its major clinical manifestations are present. The diagnosis is confirmed by the finding (after appropriate dietary and drug precautions) of a 24-hour urinary excretion of 5-HIAA of more than 30 mg. It should be emphasized that *there is poor correlation between the 5-HIAA excretion and the clinical severity of the syndrome.* However, most patients with the complete syndrome who have moderate or severe flushing and diarrhea have a 24-hour urinary excretion of 5-HIAA of 100 to 1000 mg. The excretion of this metabolite may vary considerably from day to day so that reliance should not be placed on a single assay in a suspected case if a borderline or normal result is obtained. Since many patients neither present with nor subsequently develop all the manifestations of the carcinoid syndrome, it should be suspected in individuals with unexplained persistence of any 1 or 2 of the major features of the syndrome. In such cases, the *epinephrine provocative test* can be of considerable diagnostic assistance.

The observation that epinephrine and many other adrenergic agents provoke flushes in carcinoid syndrome led to the development of this bedside test.[47] A slow IV infusion of 5% dextrose in water is started, and the pulse and blood pressure are recorded every 30 seconds with the patient supine until a stable baseline is obtained. Epinephrine is then injected IV as a bolus in progressively increasing dosages at intervals of at least 5 minutes. The initial dose is 1 μg and the largest dose given is 10 μg. The patient is observed for flushing, hypotension, tachycardia, and other symptoms of carcinoid attacks. *The appearance of a flush alone or significant hypotension with or without a flush between 45 and 120 seconds after the injection and lasting for at least 1 minute is a positive response.* A positive test almost always occurs in patients who have spontaneous flushes.[48] Interestingly, the same effects occasionally occur in patients with carcinoid syndrome who have not yet had spontaneous flushing.[49] In patients with flushing due to other causes, the test gives negative results.[48] When a positive response occurs, the injection should not be repeated with larger doses of epinephrine. In some very active carcinoids, even the smallest dose of epinephrine or other catechols can precipitate a serious hypotensive episode. The latter may be reversed by the immediate IV injection of 5 mg of phentolamine. If this alpha adrenergic antagonist does not produce a paradoxical rise in the blood pressure, the only generally available vasopressor that will not exacerbate the attack and that can be used to treat it is methoxamine. Angiotensin, which is no longer commercially available, formerly was also used for this purpose.

Measurement of urinary 5-HIAA is the keystone of diagnosis in the carcinoid syndrome. This assay, which is almost universally available, is far preferable to the simple semiquantitative screening test that is positive only when 5-HIAA in the urine exceeds 30 mg/liter.[50] In patients with borderline urinary 5-HIAA elevation, I have found that quantitative assay of blood tryptophan, serotonin, and 5-HTP and measurement of urinary tryptamine and IAA excretion may be helpful in diagnosing a mild or variant carcinoid syndrome. Unfortunately, these uncommon tests are not generally available.

The most consistent abnormal finding I have seen in all cases of carcinoid syndrome is a reduction in the blood tryptophan level. This essential amino acid is the sole precursor of all the indole amines produced by carcinoid tumors. Greater than normal amounts of it will be metabolized by any tumors having indole metabolic function. Therefore, the finding of a subnormal blood tryptophan concentration in association with increased levels or increased excretion of any one or more of the indolic carcinoid products strongly supports the diagnosis of carcinoid syndrome.

A number of non-carcinoid tumors have rarely been found to produce serotonin, with and without the carcinoid syndrome; these include medullary carcinoma of the thyroid, oat cell carcinoma, bronchogenic carcinoma, hepatoma, some pancreatic islet cell tumors, and pheochromocytoma.[8] In the differential diagnosis of carcinoid syndrome, it is also sometimes necessary to consider other humoral causes of diarrhea. These include systemic mast cell disease, basophilic leukemia, Verner-Morrison syndrome, Zollinger-Ellison syndrome, ganglioneuroblastoma, and ganglioneuroma. Quantitative assays of histamine, VIP, gastrin, and catechols will help in differentiating these conditions from carcinoid syndrome. Furthermore, except for rare instances in the Zollinger-Ellison syndrome, serotonin and 5-HIAA are not increased in these diseases.

The final diagnosis of carcinoid tumor depends on histologic confirmation of either primary or metastatic tumor tissue obtained by surgical excision or biopsy (needle biopsy or endoscopic biopsy). Although routine histologic examination (hematoxylin and eosin stain) is often adequate, special silver staining techniques may be needed to be certain of the diagnosis. Occasionally, electron microscopy is necessary to demonstrate the neurosecretory carcinoid granules in order to confirm the diagnosis.

Treatment

Non-functioning Tumors. Carcinoid of the small intestine, whenever found and whether symptomatic or not, should be removed, particularly when the tumor is more than 2 cm in diameter. *The en bloc resection of these tumors should include 10 cm of bowel on either side of the lesion together with the regional lymph nodes.* Additional tumors should be sought and removed whenever one primary is found. However, because of their slow rate of growth and the problem of diarrhea if carcinoid syndrome develops later, surgery should be done with restraint to conserve as much small intestine as possible. Sometimes, simply bypassing an obstruction in a patient with either an inoperable primary tumor or with extensive metastases may provide palliation for years. Debulking the tumor may also help extend life.

In addition to standard histologic examination, unfixed tumor tissue should be saved (frozen) for serotonin and other assays. Even without the carcinoid syndrome, if carcinoid is suspected, urinary 5-HIAA should be measured before surgery, postoperatively, and at 6 month intervals if the tumor is found to have any invasiveness. If the tumor has any functioning quality, this may provide a marker to gauge progress.

In non-functioning tumors, vigorous cytotoxic chemotherapy is not advised except for situations in which huge metastatic carcinoid deposits cause symptoms because of their bulk. Because of their slow growth, these tumors are often better tolerated than are the chemotherapeutic agents to which they sometimes respond. Surgical resection of hepatic metastases is sometimes helpful in symptomatic patients.

Carcinoid Syndrome. Many treatment modalities are available for the carcinoid syndrome. However, the wide variations in severity of the syndrome and its complications make it necessary to exercise careful judgment in determining the degree of vigor and the type of treatment best for each individual patient.

General Supportive Measures. Nutritional factors include a high protein diet supplemented by niacin (50 mg twice a day) and multiple vitamins. In some cases, high protein elemental diet supplements and medium chain triglycerides are also of benefit. Adrenergic agonists should be avoided. These include all vasopressor agents except methoxamine and angiotensin, which should be used with caution and only for treatment of severe hypotension or shock. Use of sympathomimetic drugs, such as phenylephrine (Neo-Synephrine) used in decongestants, should be strictly limited. Also to be avoided are monoamine oxidase (MAO) inhibitors and ethanol. The patient should be shielded from abrupt endogenous catechol release by the avoidance of physical and emotional stress.

Anesthesia and surgery, even when minor, pose great risk for the carcinoid syndrome patient. Without specific preparation and precautions, serious complications (respiratory and cardiac) may occur. However, preparation with antiserotonin and antikinin agents and anesthesia using thiopental, pancuronium, and nitrous oxide significantly reduce the hazard.[51]

The diarrhea responds to various opiate preparations, diphenoxylate with atropine, or loperamide. Large doses of anticholinergics parenterally or by mouth are occasionally helpful. Pancreatic enzyme concentrates will occasionally improve steatorrhea and malabsorption, which in some cases result from a relative pancreatic insufficiency. Cholestyramine helps alleviate the diarrhea when a component is due to bile salt malabsorption. Potassium and magnesium supplements are often needed, along with other electrolytes depleted by the chronic diarrhea.

Surgery. The carcinoid syndrome cannot be completely cured except in those rare cases in which an extraintestinal primary tumor without metastasis is the cause and can be completely extirpated. There is a strong role for palliative surgery, however. When manifestations of the functioning syndrome are severe and poorly controlled medically, debulking the tumor mass may ameliorate the symptoms for long periods of time. This may involve shelling isolated tumor nodules from the liver, removing masses of involved mesenteric lymph nodes, or even performing partial hepatectomy. Occasionally, surgery will be required for relief of obstruction or bleeding associated with a primary intestinal tumor. In some instances, laparotomy may be done to ligate the hepatic artery and perhaps to insert a catheter into this vessel. In carefully selected patients with carcinoid heart valve involvement, prosthetic valve replacement can produce worthwhile palliation with reversal of right-sided cardiac failure.[52,53]

Radiotherapy. Except in instances of critical isolated lesions and painful bone metastases, external radiation therapy of carcinoid tumors is generally ineffectual. There is one report of favorable response to radiotherapy.[54] Effective palliation of the carcinoid syndrome has also been reported with hepatic artery injection of the beta emitter yttrium 90 attached to plastic microspheres.[55]

Chemotherapy. The indolent nature of nonfunctioning metastatic carcinoid tumors has limited the need for chemotherapy in these cases. Hence, experience with these agents in these situations is sparse. Moreover, available reports often do not distinguish well between patients with metastatic carcinoid with or without the functioning syndrome. In carcinoid disease without the syndrome, treatment with some agents or combinations may sometimes produce remission.[56] It is my impression that chemotherapy is more frequently helpful when coupled with other forms of treatment in ameliorating the symptoms of the carcinoid syndrome than it is in palliating carcinoid tumors without the syndrome. Conventional dosages may be used in non-functioning tumors.[56]

The subject of chemotherapy for the carcinoid syndrome has been well reviewed by Harris[57] (see also Chapter 256). The most helpful agents appear to be 5-fluorouracil, streptozotocin, BCNU, CCNU, adriamycin, methotrexate, cyclophosphamide, melphalan, and DTIC. Unfortunately, the more sensitive the tumor to chemotherapy, the greater the paradoxical exacerbation of the symptoms in response to treatment. This occurs because injury to the carcinoid tumor cell causes the cell to release its humoral products. Potent cytotoxic agents should not be administered in conventional dosage to any patient with active carcinoid syndrome because of the risk of provoking a severe, even fatal attack. An individualized prolonged schedule of treatment with reduced drug dosage should be made up for each patient and not initiated until the patient has been started and maintained on some effective combination of serotonin, alpha adrenergic, and bradykinin antagonist or blocking drugs. It is desirable to confirm the effectiveness of the protective drug regimen in each patient by demonstrating a weak or negative posttreatment response to the epinephrine provocative test in contrast to a positive pretreatment response.

Since lower than ordinary doses of chemotherapeutic agents are used in these patients, side effects are often mild. Therefore, once an effective drug regimen for suppression of carcinoid syndrome symptoms has been established and the initial chemotherapy has been administered in the hospital, subsequent chemotherapy can often be done on an ambulatory basis. The agents 5-fluorouracil and streptozotocin or 5-fluorouracil and CCNU have often been effective combinations that are well suited for prolonged ambulatory treatment.

Hepatic Artery Occlusion. Interruption of the hepatic arterial blood flow by operative ligation or percutaneous catheterization with Gelfoam embolus or another embolus injection has been reported to cause remissions in a number of carcinoid syndrome patients who have large deposits of functioning metastases in the liver.[58–61] Production of various vasoactive humoral substances by carcinoid tumors appears to decrease in response to ischemia. After an initial period of exacerbation, patients have marked improvement in flushing and diarrhea. Following simple occlusion of the hepatic artery, collateral vascular channels form quickly and revascularize the tumor.[62–64] To prevent this, some surgeons undertake complete dissection of the liver from all ligamentous and vascular connections except the portal vein, along with hepatic artery ligation.[61, 65] The carcinoid syndrome exacerbation provoked by hepatic artery ligation is sometimes very severe, and this treatment should not be undertaken without effective premedication and appropriate anesthesia. A schedule of treatment that I have used with good response in 17 patients with severe carcinoid syndrome has been: Chemotherapy for 3 to 9 months, followed by percutaneous hepatic artery catheterization with hepatic angiography, bolus chemotherapy injection, and Gelfoam embolus injection. The Gelfoam embolus migrates peripherally and blocks retrograde flow from collaterals in the hepatic arterial tree. Several weeks later, surgical hepatic artery ligation may be performed. Subsequently, the patient resumes systemic chemotherapy.

Pharmacologic Therapy. Alpha adrenergic blockers are often helpful in controlling flushing. Even though beta adrenergic agonists can precipitate flushing attacks, beta blockers are of no apparent benefit. Useful agents are phentolamine (Regitine), 25 to 50 mg orally 1 to 3 times a day; phenoxybenzamine (Dibenzyline), 10 mg orally, slowly increased to 30 mg daily; prochlorperazine (Compazine), 5 to 10 mg orally or IM every 4 hours; chlorpromazine (Thorazine), 10 to 25 mg orally or IM every 6 hours; and antiserotonin agents—methysergide (Sansert), 2 mg orally 1 to 3 times a day; cyproheptadine (Periactin), 2 to 8 mg orally every 4 to 6 hours; and the experimental tryptophan hydroxylase inhibitor *p*-chlorophenyl alanine (PCP). Although very effective in blocking synthesis of serotonin and improving diarrhea, PCP has too frequently caused severe allergic and central nervous system side effects to allow its unrestricted use.[66] Another antiserotonin agent that can be used parenterally for sedation and relief of pain in carcinoid syndrome is methotrimeprazine (Levoprome), 5 to 20 mg IM every 4 to 6 hours. *Morphine, a serotonin liberator, should be avoided in carcinoid syndrome patients.* For the initial pharmacologic treatment of a typical carcinoid syndrome patient, I prefer cyproheptadine, 2 to 4 mg orally 3 times a day, and phentolamine, 25 mg orally twice a day. Dosages can be subsequently adjusted, usually upward.

The observation that the carcinoid flush can be provoked by injection of pentagastrin[67] as well as by many gastrin stimuli (calcium, ethanol, and food intake), in addition to some catecholamines,[68] led to the suggestion that gastrin might be some sort of final common pathway for triggering the carcinoid flush. Therefore, *somatostatin,* which inhibits both release and action of gastrin, was tested in carcinoid patients and found to effectively inhibit spontaneous flushes as well as those provoked by these stimuli.[67, 68] However, measurement of plasma levels of gastrin and many other gut peptides before, during, and after flushes has not provided evidence of the involvement of these substances in the flush.[68] The secretory diarrhea of the carcinoid syndrome has also been effectively reversed by IV somatostatin.[69, 70]

I have observed that IV glucagon for a period of 48 hours (0.1 mg/hour) after hepatic dearterialization also has some effectiveness in suppressing carcinoid flushing and diarrhea.

In histamine-producing tumors, the flush may be inhibited by a combination of H_1 and H_2 antagonists, such as diphenhydramine (Benadryl) and cimetidine (Tagamet) in usual dosages.[71] Also, the flush associated with tumors that are deficient in 5-HTP decarboxylase and that elaborate large amounts of 5-HTP will often respond to alpha methyldopa (Aldomet).[29] The bronchospasm of carcinoid syndrome may respond to low doses of isoproterenol aerosol[8] and occasionally to corticosteroids. *Epinephrine and other adrenergic agonists must be withheld.* Perhaps by means of their antibradykinin and antiprostaglandin properties, corticosteroids exert a suppressant effect on carcinoid syndrome attacks and are therefore useful in carrying these patients through critical periods, such as surgery and chemotherapy.

There has been no evidence advanced that any of the known prostaglandin synthesis inhibitors are of help in carcinoid syndrome, except for anecdotal observations of the benefit of nutmeg.[72]

The protease inhibitor aprotinin (Trasylol), which is not available for human administration in the United States, has been used for several decades in Europe and several times has been reported to be successful in controlling carcinoid syndrome attacks during anesthesia.[73, 74] Likewise, leukocyte interferon treatment has been reported in a preliminary study to produce significant symptomatic and biochemical improvement in a small group of carcinoid syndrome patients.[74a]

Prognosis

Carcinoids of the small intestine usually have a very slow rate of growth and local and distant spread, and some even have periods of seemingly spontaneous arrest. Most of these tumors never extend beyond the region of their primary site and are incidental surgical or necropsy findings. Patients with metastases from these tumors, in the absence of the carcinoid syndrome, survive many years, even decades.[2] Even when the condition is very chronic and symptoms eventually lead to surgery, an operable lesion may still be found. Furthermore, when the lesion is unresectable, simple relief of the intestinal obstruction may be sufficient to allow the patient to live for many more months or years because of the slow growth of these tumors. In 28 patients with carcinoid of the small intestine followed by Moertel et al.,[2] the average survival was 8.1 years, with a range to 23 years from onset of symptoms to time of death. In Godwin's[15] series of over 500 patients with small intestinal carcinoid, the observed 5-year relative survival rates were 75% in tumors with no spread, 59% in tumors with regional metastases, 9% in tumors with distant metastases, and 54% overall. Van Sickle[75] reported a 5-year survival rate of 45% in a series of 61 patients with incompletely removed carcinoids of the small intestine.

The natural course and tempo of the disease are quite different in patients with the *carcinoid syndrome.* The majority of these individuals die much sooner, usually as a consequence of the pharmacologic effects of the hormonal products of their neoplasm. The few studies that have specifically evaluated survival indicate that it is usually much shorter than had previously been conceived. The range of survival, however, is quite wide. In a series of 91 cases, Davis et al.[34] observed a median survival of 38 months from the onset of flushing and a median survival of 23 months after the first finding of increased urinary 5-HIAA. Hajdu et al.,[18] in 9 cases, noted an average survival of less than 1 year after the diagnosis. These are older retrospective studies and the patients were either untreated or treated with earlier and less effective surgical and pharmacologic techniques than are now available.

Occasionally, large vascular metastatic carcinoid tumors in the liver will undergo infarction with autonecrosis and cystic degeneration. When this occurs, the vasoactive products of the tumor, as well as tissue breakdown products, flood the circulation and cause exacerbation of flushing, hypotension, diarrhea, and fever (carcinoid fever). Pain and tenderness over the liver will be present. These episodes may be followed by periods of improvement lasting many weeks or months.

Causes of Death. Even though only 25% of the patients with carcinoid syndrome develop heart valve lesions, the cardiac complications of arrhythmias and congestive heart failure account for 50% of their deaths.[33] The remainder succumb to various complications of carcinomatosis and the pharmacologic effects of their excessive circulating carcinoid products (cachexia, infection, hepatic failure, shock, electrolyte imbalance, gastrointestinal bleeding, renal failure, intestinal infarction, and intestinal obstruction).

References

1. Lubarsch O. Uber den primaren krebs des ileum, nebst beinerkungen ueber das gleichzeitige vorkammen van krebs und tuberculose. Virchows Arch [Pathol Anat] 1888; 111:280–317.
2. Moertel CJ, Sauer WG, Dockerty MB, Bagenstoss AH. Life history of the carcinoid tumor of the small intestine. Cancer 1961; 14:901–12.
3. Oberndorfer S. Uber die "kleinen dunndormcarcinome." Verh Dtsch Ges Pathol 1907; 11:113–6.
4. Pearse AGE. The cytochemistry and ultrastructure of polypeptide hormone-producing cells of the APUD series and the embryologic, physiologic and pathologic implications of the concept. J Histochem Cytochem 1969; 17:303–13.
5. Wichert RF, III. The neural ectodermal origin of the peptide secreting endocrine glands: A unifying concept for the etiology of multiple endocrine adenomatosis and the inappropriate secretion of peptide hormones by neuroendocrine tumors. Am J Med 1970; 49:232–41.
6. Pearse AGE. Neurocristopathy, neuroendocrine pathology and APUD concept. Z Krebsforsch 1975; 84:1–18.
7. Thorson A, Biorck G, Bjorkman G, Waldenstrom J. Malignant carcinoid of the small intestine with metastasis to liver, valvular disease of the right side of the heart (pulmonary stenosis) and tricuspid regurgitation without septal defects, peripheral vasomotor symptoms, bronchoconstriction, and an unusual type of cyanosis. Am Heart J 1954; 44:795–817.
8. Jaeger RM, Polk HC, Jr. Carcinoid apudomas. *In:* Hickey RC, ed. Current Problems in Cancer. Chicago: Year Book Medical Publishers, 1977. 1–53.
9. Sjoerdsma A, Melmon KL. The carcinoid spectrum. Gastroenterology 1964; 47:104–7.
10. Soga J, Tazawa K. Pathologic analysis of carcinoids: Histologic reevaluations of 62 cases. Cancer 1971; 28:990–8.
11. Lillie RD, Glenner CG. Histochemical reactions in carcinoid tumors of the human gastrointestinal tract. Am J Pathol 1960; 36:623–51.
12. MacDonald RA. A study of 356 carcinoids of the gastrointestinal tract: Report of four new cases of the carcinoid syndrome. Am J Med 1956; 21:867–78.
13. Grahame-Smith DG. The Carcinoid Syndrome. London: William Heinemann Medical Books Ltd, 1972.
14. Sanders RJ. Carcinoids of the Gastrointestinal Tract. Springfield, Ill: Charles C Thomas, 1973.
15. Godwin JD. Carcinoid tumors, an analysis of 2,837 cases. Cancer 1975; 36:560–9.
16. Brown NK, Smith MP. Neoplastic diathesis of patients with carcinoid: Report of a case with four other neoplasms. Cancer 1973; 32:216–22.
17. Hedinger C, Hardmeier T, Funk HU. Das argentaffine system des verdauungstraktes bei carcinoidsyndrom. Virchows Arch [Pathol Anat] 1966; 340/4:304–11.
18. Hajdu SI, Winawer SJ, Laird Myers WP. Carcinoid tumors. A study of 204 cases. Am J Clin Pathol 1974; 61:521–8.
19. Berardi RS. Carcinoid tumors of the colon (exclusive of the rectum): Review of the literature. Dis Colon Rectum 1972; 15:383–91.
20. Davis AJ. Carcinoid tumors (argentaffinomata). Ann R Coll Surg Engl 1960; 25:277–97.
21. Sjoerdsma A. Serotonin. N Engl J Med 1959; 261:181–8;231–7.
22. Warner RRP. Current status and implications of serotonin in clinical medicine. *In:* Dock W, Snapper I, eds. Advances in Internal Medicine. Chicago: Year Book Medical Publishers, 1967; 12:241–82.

23. Honet JC, Casey TV, Runyan JW, Jr. False-positive urinary test for 5-hydroxyindoleacetic acid due to methocarbamol and mephenesin carbamate. N Engl J Med 1959; 261:188–90.
24. Ross G, Weinstein B, Kabakow B. The influence of phenothiazine and some of its derivatives on the determinations of 5-hydroxyindoleacetic acid in urine. Clin Chem 1958; 4:66–76.
25. Davis RB, Rosenberg JC. Carcinoid syndrome with hyperserotoninemia and normal 5-hydroxyindoleacetic acid excretion. Am J Med 1961; 30:167–74.
26. Oates JA, Melmon K, Sjoerdsma A, Gillespie S, Mason DT. Release of a kinin peptide in the carcinoid syndrome. Lancet 1964; 1:514–7.
27. Oates JA, Butler TC. Pharmacologic and endocrine aspects of the carcinoid syndrome. Adv Pharmacol 1967; 5:109–28.
28. Jaffe BM, Condon C. Prostaglandin E and F in endocrine diarrheogenic syndromes. Ann Surg 1976; 84:516–24.
29. Oates JA, Sjoerdsma A.Unique syndrome associated with secretion of 5-hydroxytryptophan by metastatic gastric carcinoids. Am J Med 1962; 32:333–42.
30. Postlethwait RW. Gastrointestinal carcinoid tumors—a review. Postgrad Med 1966; 40:445–54.
31. Warner RRP, Southern AL. Carcinoid syndrome produced by metastasizing bronchial adenoma. Am J Med 1958; 24:903–14.
32. Moertel CG, Dockerty MG. Familial occurrence of metastasizing carcinoid tumors. Ann Intern Med 1973; 78:389–90.
33. Thorson A. Studies on carcinoid disease. Acta Med Scand 1958; 161(Suppl 334):1–132.
34. Davis Z, Moertel CG, McIllrath DC. The malignant carcinoid syndrome. Surg Gynecol Obstet 1973; 137:637–44.
35. Roberts WC, Sjoerdsma A. The cardiac disease associated with the carcinoid syndrome (carcinoid heart disease). Am J Med 1964; 36:5–34.
36. Lie JP. Carcinoid tumors, carcinoid syndrome, and carcinoid heart disease. Primary Cardiol 1982; 8:163–86.
37. Trell E, Rousing A, Ripa J, Torp A, Waldenstrom J. Carcinoid heart disease. Am J Med 1973; 54:433–44.
38. Schwaber JR, Lukas DS. Hyperkinemia and cardiac failure in the carcinoid syndrome. Am J Med 1962; 32:846–53.
39. Rich LL, Lisa CP, Nasser WK. Carcinoid pericarditis. Am J Med 1973; 54:522–7.
40. Plonk JW, Feldman JM. Carcinoid arthropathy. Arch Intern Med 1974; 134:651–4.
41. Swash M, Fox KP, Davidson AR. Carcinoid myopathy. Arch Neurol 1975; 32:572–4.
42. Morin LJ, Zuerner RT. Retroperitoneal fibrosis and carcinoid tumor. JAMA 1971; 216:1647–8.
43. Bivens CH, Marecek RL, Feldman JM. Peyronie's disease: Presenting complaint of carcinoid syndrome. N Engl J Med 1973; 289:844–5.
44. Melmon KL, Sjoerdsma A, Mason DT. Distinctive clinical and therapeutic aspects of the syndrome associated with bronchial carcinoid tumors. Am J Med 1965; 39:568–81.
45. Feldman JM, Plonk JW, Bivens CH, Lebovitz HE. Glucose intolerance in the carcinoid syndrome. Diabetes 1975; 24:664–71.
46. Weidner FA, Ziter FMH. Carcinoid tumors of the gastrointestinal tract. JAMA 1981; 245:1153–5.
47. Levine RJ, Sjoerdsma A. Pressor amines and the carcinoid flush. Ann Intern Med 1963; 58:818–28.
48. Vaidya AB, Wustrack KW, Levine RJ. Failure of epinephrine to provoke flushing in patients with systemic mastocytosis. Ann Intern Med 1971; 74:711–3.
49. Sjoerdsma A, Oates JA, Zaltzman P, Udenfriend S. Serotonin synthesis in carcinoid patients: Its inhibition by α-methyldopa, with measurement of increases in urinary 5-hydroxytryptophan. N Engl J Med 1960; 263:585–8.
50. Sjoerdsma A, Terry LL, Udenfriend S. Malignant carcinoid. A new metabolic disorder. Arch Intern Med 1957; 99:1009–12.
51. Miller R, Patel AU, Warner RRP, Parnes I. Anaesthesia for the carcinoid syndrome: A report of nine cases. Can Anaesth Soc J 1978; 25:240–4.
52. Okada RD, Ewy GA, Copeland JG. Echocardiography and surgery in tricuspid and pulmonary valve stenosis due to carcinoid syndrome. Cardiovasc Med 1979; 871–81.
53. Schoen FJ, Hausner RJ, Howell JF, Beazley HL, Titus JL. Porcine heterograft valve replacement in carcinoid heart disease. J Thorac Cardiovasc Surg 1981; 81:100–5.
54. Gaitan-Gaitan A, Rider WD, Bush RS. Carcinoid tumor—cure by irradiation. Int J Rad Oncol Biol Physic 1975; 1:9–13.
55. Simon N, Warner RRP, Baron M, Rudavsky AZ. Intra-arterial irradiation of carcinoid tumors of the liver. Am J Roentgenol Rad Ther Nuc Med 1968; 102:552–61.
56. Legha SS, Valdiviesco M, Nelson RS, Benjamin RS, Bodey P. Chemotherapy for metastatic carcinoid tumors: Experiences with 32 patients and a review of the literature. Cancer Treat Rep 1977; 61:1699–1703.
57. Harris AL. Chemotherapy for the carcinoid syndrome. Cancer Chemother Pharmacol 1981; 5:133–8.
58. Murray-Lyon IM, Parsons VA, Blendis LM, Dawson JL, Rake MO Laws JW, Williams R. Treatment of secondary hepatic tumors by ligation of hepatic artery and infusion of cytotoxic drugs. Lancet 1970; 2:172–5.
59. Jugdutt BL, Watanabe M, Turner FM. Hepatic artery ligation in treatment of carcinoid syndrome. Can Med Assoc J 1975; 112:325–7.
60. Allison DJ, Modlin IM, Jenkins WJ. Treatment of carcinoid liver metastasis by hepatic-artery embolization. Lancet 1977; 2:1323–5.
61. Berjian RA, Douglass HO, Jr, Nava HR, Karakousis C. The role of hepatic artery ligation and dearterialization with infusion chemotherapy in advanced malignancies in the liver. J Surg Oncol 1980; 14:379–87.
62. Plengvanit U, Chearanai O, Sindhvananda K, Damrongsak D, Tuchinda S, Viranuvatti V. Collateral arterial blood supply of the liver after hepatic artery ligation: Angiographic study of twenty patients. Ann Surg 1972; 175:105–10.
63. McDermott WV, Paris AL, Clause ME, Meissner WA. Dearterialization of the liver for metastatic cancer. Ann Surg 1978; 187:38–46.
64. Mays ET, Wheeler CS. Demonstration of collateral arterial flow after interruption of hepatic arteries in man. N Engl J Med 1974; 290:993–6.
65. Sparks FC, Mosher MB, Hallauer WC, Silverstein MJ, Roungel D, Passaro E Jr, Morton DL. Hepatic artery ligation and postoperative chemotherapy for hepatic metastases: Clinical and pathophysiological results. Cancer 1975; 35:1074–82.
66. Vaidya AB, Levine RJ. Hypothermia in a patient with carcinoid syndrome during treatment with para-chlorophenylalanine. N Engl J Med 1971; 284:255–7.
67. Frohlich JC, Bloomgarden ZT, Oates JA, McGuigan JE, Rabinowitz D. The carcinoid flush: Provocation by pentagastrin and inhibition by somatostatin. N Engl J Med 1978; 299:1055–7.
68. Long RG, Peters JR, Bloom SR, Brown MR, Vale W, Rivler JE, Grahame-Smith DG. Somatostatin, gastrointestinal peptides, and the carcinoid syndrome. Gut 1981; 22:549–53.
69. Davis GR, Camp RC, Raskin P, Kaejs GJ. Effect of somatostatin infusion on jejunal water and electrolyte transport in a patient with secretory diarrhea due to malignant carcinoid syndrome. Gastroenterology 1980; 78:346–9.
70. Dharmsathphorn K, Sherwin RS, Cataland S, Jaffe B, Dobbins J. Somatostatin inhibits diarrhea in the carcinoid syndrome. Ann Intern Med 1980; 92:68–9.
71. Roberts LJ II, Marney SR Jr, Oates JA. Blockade of the flush associated with metastatic gastric carcinoid by combined histamine H_1 and H_2 receptor antagonists. N Engl J Med 1979; 300:236–8.
72. Barrowman JA, Bennett A, Hillenbrand P, Rolles K, Pollock DJ, Wright JT. Diarrhea in thyroid medullary carcinoma: Role of prostaglandins and therapeutic effect of nutmeg. Br Med J 1975; 3:11–2.
73. Dery R. Theoretical and clinical consideration in anaesthesia for secretory carcinoid tumors. Can Anaesth Soc J 1971; 18:245–63.
74. Mason RA, Steane PA. Carcinoid syndrome: Its relevance to the anaesthetist. Anaesthesia 1976; 31:228–42.
74a. Oberg K, Funa K, Alm G. Effects of leukocyte interferon on clinical symptoms and hormone levels in patients with mid-gut carcinoid tumor and carcinoid syndrome. N. Engl J Med 1983; 309:129–33.
75. Van Sickle DG. Carcinoid tumors: Analysis of 61 cases, including 11 cases of carcinoid syndrome. Clev Clin Q 1972; 39:79–86.

Chapter 114

Small Intestinal Tumors (Other Than Lymphoma and Carcinoid)

Charles J. Lightdale • Paul Sherlock

The infrequent occurrence of small intestinal tumors is striking, considering the size of the small bowel and the prevalence of neoplasms in the stomach and colon. The first case report of a duodenal carcinoma was made by Hamburger in 1746, and Morgagni reported a case in 1761.[1, 2] A benign duodenal tumor was reported by Cruveilhier in 1835.[3] Raiford reviewed 88 cases of small intestinal tumors in 1932 and emphasized their relative rarity.[4]

Anatomy

The small intestine is a tube about 6 meters long extending from the pylorus to the ileocecal valve. It consists of 3 segments with no sharp divisions between them. The *duodenum,* which comprises the proximal 25 to 30 cm, adheres to the posterior abdominal wall and has submucosal glands (Brunner's glands). The remainder of the small bowel is on a mesentery and is divided into the *jejunum* (about 2.5 meters in length) and the *ileum.* The jejunum has abundant transverse circular folds (plicae circulares), whereas the ileum has fewer folds and more lymphoid tissue (Peyer's patches).[5]

Tumors of the small intestine may arise from any of its various cells. The innermost tissue layer, the mucosa, is composed of absorptive cells and intestinal glands. There are some smooth muscle cells comprising the muscularis mucosae just beneath the mucosa and a submucosa containing fibrocytes, endothelial cells, and lymphoid cells. The muscularis externa and fibrous serosa complete the intestinal wall.[6–9]

The most common tumors of the small bowel are *carcinoids,* arising from argentaffin cells in the intestinal glands. These tumors are described in Chapter 113, and small intestinal lymphoma is presented in Chapter 112. Consideration is given in this chapter, therefore, to the other forms of small bowel tumor.

Adenomas and adenocarcinomas arising from the intestinal glands and leiomyomas and leiomyosarcomas from the smooth muscle comprise the majority of these other small bowel tumors.[7–13] About half of all malignant tumors of the small intestine are adenocarcinomas, most of which occur in the proximal small intestine. Sarcomas, in contrast, are distributed more evenly throughout the length of the small bowel.[14–22]

Etiology and Pathogenesis

The factors that induce neoplastic changes in the small bowel may only be speculated upon, but it is likely that they differ for the various types of tumors. An area of great interest has been the identification of factors that may protect the small intestine from adenocarcinoma, which so much more often affects the stomach and colon.[23] Among these possible factors, the following command attention:

1. Transit time through the small bowel is rapid, and this may limit exposure of the

small bowel mucosa to carcinogens. In Raiford's early review,[4] most tumors were found in the ileum. This prompted him to postulate that relative stasis at the ileocecal valve might be a factor. Despite rapid transit, however, small bowel tumors have been produced in rats by feeding them nitrosourea compounds or bracken fern.[24,25]

2. Concentrations of carcinogenic substances may be lower in the more liquid small bowel contents than in the colon contents.

3. Enzyme systems may be more active in detoxifying carcinogens in the small intestine than in the stomach and colon. For example, benzpyrene is a known carcinogen, which is present in small quantities in a variety of foods.[26] Benzpyrene hydroxylase, present in the small intestine of man, converts benzpyrene into less active metabolites.[23] In rats, benzpyrene hydroxylase has been shown to be present in much greater concentration in the small intestine than in the stomach or colon.[27]

4. The bacterial population of the colon is much greater than that of the small intestine. The colon also has a large population of anaerobic bacteria, whereas these organisms are present in much lower percentage in the small intestine. The importance of anaerobic bacteria rests on the demonstration that they can convert natural bile acids into carcinogens.[28,29]

5. The immune system of the small intestine, both humoral and cellular, seems to be particularly effective. The small bowel is an active producer of IgA and has abundant T lymphocytes in the lymphoid nodules. Lowenfels[23] has suggested that small intestinal immunity may protect against oncogenic viruses. Calman[30] has similarly theorized that small bowel T cell immune systems may recognize neoplastic cells as foreign and eliminate them more efficiently than elsewhere in the gut. Experimentally, he showed that allogeneic tumors transplanted into normal mice survive much more readily if the recipient site is the stomach rather than the small intestine.

6. Several investigators have noted that the rapid proliferation of small intestinal mucosal cells may possibly have a protective effect against the growth of neoplasms. Bone and Wright[31] have referred to biomathematical models suggesting that neoplastic cell lines may replicate more slowly than normal mucosa and that when 2 cell lines grow competitively in close proximity, the more rapidly proliferating cells eventually dominate. Another theory developed by Lipkin and Quastler[32] holds that the small intestine has fewer retained proliferating cells than the stomach or colon. These are probably the cells involved in initial neoplastic transformation. Using tritiated thymidine and microautoradiographic techniques, it appears that fewer cells in the small intestine retain proliferative potential at the luminal surface of the glands. This characteristic of small intestinal mucosal kinetics may explain the lower rate of neoplastic change.

Epidemiology

Prevalence data relating to small bowel neoplasms are dominated by adenocarcinoma, the most common malignant tumor affecting the small intestine in most areas of the world (Fig. 114–1). Lowenfels[23] has shown that regional prevalence rates for small bowel cancer are significantly correlated with prevalence rates for colon cancer ($p<0.001$, $r=0.79$). A similar correlation in frequency rates was not evident between small bowel and stomach cancer.

The well known increased rate of colon cancer in Japanese migrating to Hawaii and the continental United States is also seen with small intestinal cancer. Interestingly, the prevalence rates for whites in Hawaii are likewise substantially higher than those for whites living elsewhere. In general, small bowel cancer is more common in developed Western countries than in underdeveloped countries.[33–36]

There are approximately 2000 new cases of small bowel cancer per year in the United States.[22] For the most part, surveys have shown a slight male preponderance, but there is no clear-cut predilection in the United States for racial groups or urban as compared with rural populations.[37, 38] Data from the Third National Cancer Survey showed a range in the age-adjusted prevalence rate of 0.6 to 1.9/100,000 American males and 0.4 to 0.9/100,000 American females.[39] Data from both Connecticut and Birmingham, England, showed a gradually increasing frequency of small bowel cancer in men with time.[25, 40] Symptomatic tumors tend to occur in individuals greater than 50 years old and the peak rate of occurrence of adenocarcinoma is in the sixth decade.[41]

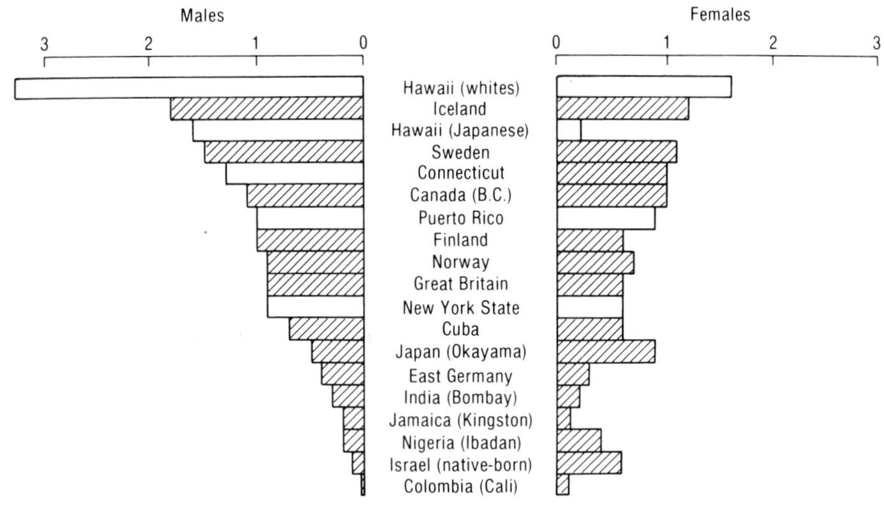

Figure 114–1. Age-adjusted (European) prevalence rates per 100,000 population for small intestinal cancer, by sex, for selected cancer registries: 1969–1971. (From Lightdale CJ et al. In Schottenfeld D, Fraumeni J Jr, eds. Cancer Epidemiology and Prevention. Philadelphia: WB Saunders, 1982. Reproduced with permission.)

Clinical Aspects

The symptoms produced by small bowel tumors will vary according to their size, location within the bowel wall, blood supply, and tendency to undergo necrosis and ulceration. The areas of the small bowel in which the tumor is located will also affect symptomatology.[22] For example, tumors arising from superficial mucosal surfaces, such as adenomas, tend to be polypoid and project into the bowel lumen. If sufficiently large, they may occlude the lumen and produce obstruction. They may also become the lead point in an intussusception, in which a length of bowel invaginates distally and causes obstruction. Adenomas may ulcerate and cause gastrointestinal bleeding, which is more likely to be occult than acute and gross.[42]

Most adenocarcinomas of the small intestine are annular in type, gradually narrowing the bowel lumen and producing *symptoms of obstruction*. Such symptoms include crampy abdominal pain, nausea, vomiting, and abdominal distention, which may be made worse by food intake. *Anorexia* and *weight loss* commonly accompany the obstructive symptoms. *Bleeding* is usually occult, but may be acute and obvious. *Perforation* is rare, usually producing a surgical abdomen. *Obstructive jaundice* may be a consequence of duodenal adenocarcinomas that involve the papilla of Vater. Adenocarcinomas in the duodenum are predominantly located in the periampullary region, and careful dissection of operative specimens is often required to differentiate primary duodenal from primary ampullary carcinomas. In some cases, it is impossible to define the site of origin.

Smooth muscle tumors arising from the muscularis externa may grow to large size before producing obstructive symptoms. Leiomyosarcomas tend to develop central ulcerations and, because of an abundant blood supply, may present with massive bleeding as a first symptom.

In general, malignant tumors of the small intestine are more likely to produce symptoms than benign tumors. Many benign tumors are incidental findings at surgery or necropsy and have never caused symptoms.[22] However, benign tumors are more likely to cause an intussusception than malignant tumors. In a study of symptomatic benign tumors of the duodenum, adbominal pain was present in 61% of patients and bleeding in 10%, whereas malignant tumors caused pain in 90% and bleeding in 15%.[43]

Disorders with an Increased Risk of Adenocarcinoma

Crohn's Disease (see also Chapter 127). There have been several reports indicating an increased incidence of small intestinal adenocarcinoma occurring in patients with Crohn's disease (regional enteritis). Darke et al.[44] estimated the prevalence of Crohn's disease in the United Kingdom and Sweden to be in the range of 9 to 33/10,000 population and the annual incidence of small bowel adenocarcinoma to be 0.3/10,000 persons per year. The expected incidence of small bowel carcinoma in a patient with Crohn's disease as calculated from these estimates would be about 1/billion/year. Since 40 cases were reported from 1957 to 1975 from the United States and Western Europe, the actual incidence appears to exceed the number of cases expected by chance. In a 1975 review, 15 of the 40 reported tumors were in surgically bypassed ileal segments, which may be a particular risk factor.[45] In addition, the great majority of reported adenocarcinomas occurred in the ileum, the most common site for Crohn's disease. This stands in contrast to de novo small bowel adenocarcinomas, which tend to cluster in the duodenum and proximal jejunum within 25 cm of the ligament of Treitz.

The cancers associated with Crohn's disease tend to occur in patients with longstanding disease and to present clinically mainly with symptoms of obstruction. The age at diagnosis of adenocarcinoma complicating Crohn's disease of the small intestine is younger by approximately 10 years than the corresponding age in de novo small intestinal adenocarcinoma.[46, 47] The overall risk factor for adenocarcinoma of the small bowel in patients with Crohn's disease has been estimated to be in the range of 100 times greater than the average risk for developing the disease.[33] Patients with Crohn's disease of the colon probably also have an increased risk for colonic adenocarcinoma, but of a much lower order of magnitude than the risk in ulcerative colitis.[48] There are a few reports of ileal adenocarcinoma developing in patients with ulcerative colitis and inflammatory changes in the ileum (backwash ileitis).[49]

Celiac Disease (see also Chapter 105). Celiac disease has been associated with an increased rate of development of malignancy, particularly lymphomas and carcinomas of the esophagus and pharynx.[49, 50] In the small intestine, lymphoma is the tumor most commonly associated with celiac disease.[51] However, at least 20 cases of adenocarcinoma of the small intestine in patients with celiac disease have been reported.[52–55] In several of these reports, the patients presented with the carcinoma, thereby raising questions as to tumor enteropathy or mucosal destruction due to the tumor. Most of the patients showed typically flat mucosa in areas remote from the cancer. In their report, Holmes et al.[55] described 3 patients with both biopsy-proven celiac disease and response to a gluten-free diet more than 5 years before the diagnosis of malignancy, leaving little room for controversy. Although most patients present with advanced disease, one of the patients reported by Holmes and Associates survived 8 years after surgical resection. It is not clear at this time whether strict adherence to a gluten-free diet lowers the rate of occurrence of malignancy in celiac disease. The development of symptoms such as malaise, anorexia, nausea, and diarrhea in patients adhering to a gluten-free regimen strongly suggests small bowel malignancy; anemia and occult gastrointestinal bleeding would further suggest adenocarcinoma.

Peutz-Jeghers Syndrome (see also Chapter 138). The Peutz-Jeghers syndrome features hamartomatous polyps throughout the small and large bowel and melanin spots on the oral mucosa, lips, and digits (Fig. 114–2). This is a rare disorder, first reported by Peutz[56] in 1921 and supported by a series of cases by Jeghers et al.[57] in 1949. As of 1969, a total of 321 cases had been reported, of which 29 occurred in the United States.[58] The condition appears to be transmitted as an autosomal dominant trait. The tumors are mostly hamartomas rather than adenomas (Fig. 114–3) and are characterized histologically by a peculiar branched tree arrangement of smooth muscle cells.[59] They are benign tumors for the most part, although malignant degeneration may occur.[60] In the 1969 series of Dozois et al.,[58] there were 11 malignant lesions in 321 patients, with 4 adenocarcinomas developing in the small intestine, 4 in the stomach, and 3 in the colon. Reid,[61] using strict criteria, calculated a lifetime incidence of small bowel adenocarcinomas of 2.4% in patients with Peutz-Jeghers syndrome.

The freckle-like lesions are typically found on the lips, but similar melanin spots have been described on the buccal mucosa, nose, and fingers. In some families, pigmentation occurs in the absence of gastrointestinal polyps. The hamartomas may be single, but are

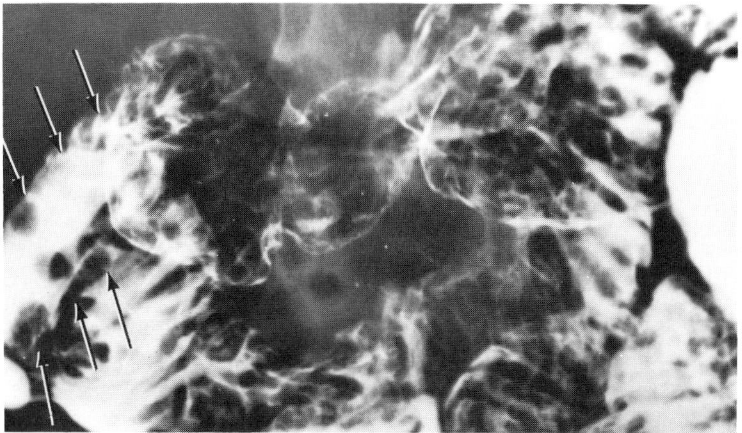

Figure 114–2. Barium radiograph showing multiple gastric and duodenal polyps (*arrows*) in patient with Peutz-Jeghers syndrome. (Courtesy of Dr. M. Edelman.)

usually multiple and most numerous in the jejunum and ileum. Intussusception is a frequent complication.

Familial Polyposis Syndromes (see also Chapter 138). Adenomas of the duodenum have been described in patients with familial polyposis coli. Although colon carcinoma develops in virtually all these patients not undergoing colectomy, they only rarely develop duodenal adenocarcinomas.[62–64] Familial polyposis of the entire gastrointestinal tract with adenomas of the jejunum and ileum has been reported, but, again, the potential for small intestinal cancer appears low.[65–67]

Gardner's syndrome appears to be a variant of familial polyposis. The syndrome was originally described as including osteomas, fibromas, and colonic adenomas, with a high incidence of colon cancer similar to that in familial polposis. A number of other soft tissue abnormalities have since been described, including gastric and small bowel adenomas. The small intestinal adenomas are most common in the duodenum. These lesions appear to have a greater tendency to undergo malignant change, particularly in the periampullary area than they do in other polyposis syndromes.[68–72]

In separate reports, Muir et al.[73] and Torre[74] have described patients with soft tissue tumors of the face, other soft tissue tumors, colon carcinomas, and duodenal carcinomas.

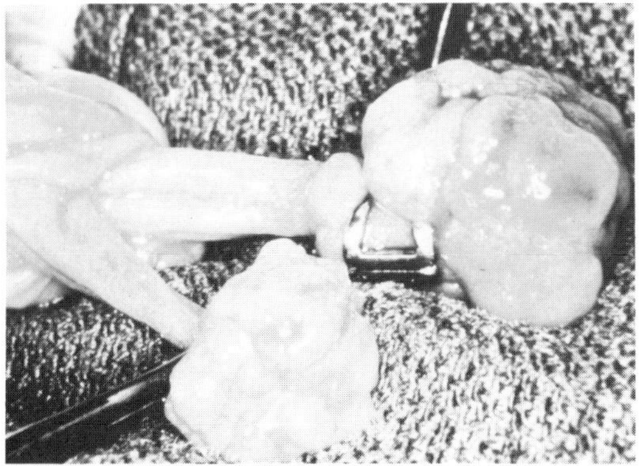

Figure 114–3. Surgical specimen showing pedunculated hamartomas resected from the jejunum of a patient with Peutz-Jeghers syndrome who developed an intussusception of the small bowel.

Diagnosis and Differential Diagnosis

There are no symptoms specific for small intestinal neoplasms of any type. Crampy abdominal pain, abdominal distention, nausea, vomiting, and gastrointestinal bleeding may arise from other obstructing or ulcerating bowel disease. For example, in patients with Crohn's disease, symptoms of a complicating carcinoma are indistinguishable from those produced by the inflammatory process.[45] Severe hemmorrhage would suggest the possibility of an ulcerated leiomyoma or leiomyosarcoma.[73–75]

Physical examination may provide additional information leading to a diagnosis of small intestinal tumor, but, again, findings are usually not definitive. An exception would be melanin spots typical of Peutz-Jeghers syndrome. A palpable abdominal mass is more suggestive of sarcoma than adenocarcinoma. Evidence of metastatic disease may be present, e.g., hepatomegaly, but these findings do not localize the malignancy to the small bowel.

The preoperative diagnosis of small intestinal tumors is generally made by barium contrast radiography.[76] A common error is to investigate a complaint of abdominal pain by performing a barium enema and barium meal series and to obtain roentgenograms showing the small intestine to a point only just beyond the ligament of Treitz; as a consequence, more distally situated neoplasms are missed (Fig. 114–4). There are no data regarding the detection of small intestinal malignancies at an early asymptomatic stage. The sensitivity of the barium meal roentgen examination of the small bowel may vary with the ability and interest of the radiologist. The more advanced the disease, the more likely it is to be detected.

Most adenocarcinomas produce a typical annular "apple core" or "napkin ring" deformity[77] (Fig. 114–5). Adenocarcinomas of the duodenum can be difficult to differentiate from advanced pancreatic carcinoma.[78] Leiomyosarcomas are more likely to present as a bulky mass, sometimes with a central ulceration.[73] Leiomyomas are the most common tumors found to arise from Meckel's diverticula.[79] Benign small bowel tumors, such as adenomas, are most prone to create a polypoid filling defect (Fig. 114–6) and are more likely to cause an intussusception than are malignant tumors, which stiffen the bowel wall.[8]

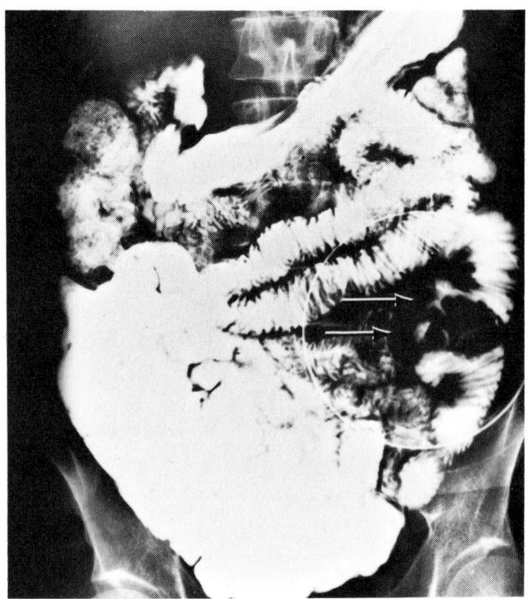

Figure 114–5. Barium radiograph showing a constricting adenocarcinoma of the jeunum *(arrows).* (Courtesy of Dr. M. Edelman.)

A useful technique in cases of small bowel tumors causing obstruction is to allow a mercury-weighted intestinal drainage tube to ad-

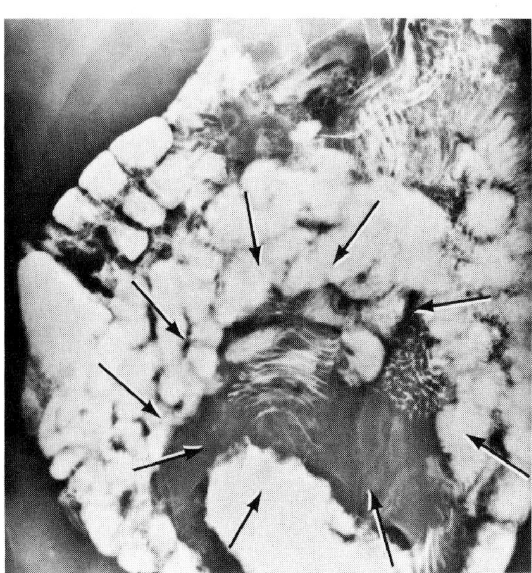

Figure 114–4. Barium radiograph showing the presence of a large mass displacing bowel loops *(arrows),* and an area of distention and extravasation of barium from the mid-small bowel due to an adenocarcinoma of the jejunum with a localized perforation. (Courtesy of Dr. M. Edelman.)

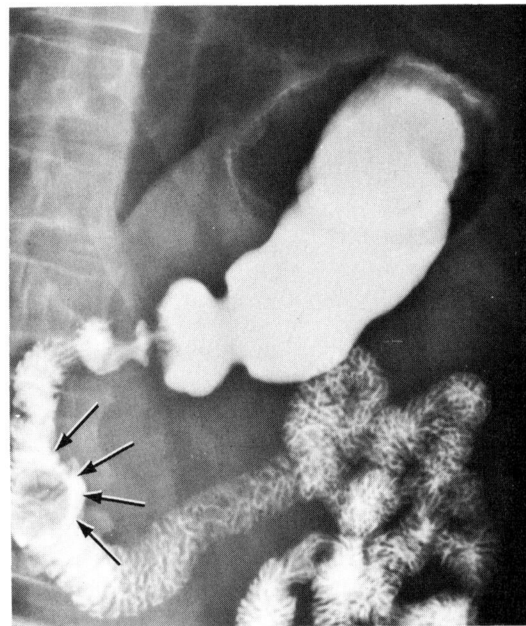

Figure 114–6. Barium radiograph showing smooth filling defect in the descending duodenum *(arrows)*: due to a leiomyoma. (Courtesy of Dr. M. Edelman.)

vance to the level of the obstruction and then to introduce barium or soluble contrast material through the tube. If there is continuous occult gastrointestinal bleeding and a small bowel lesion is suspected, a *tube aspiration test* may be performed. A long small-caliber tube with a mercury bag and aspiration holes at the tip is swallowed. As this tube progresses through the small intestine, material is periodically aspirated and tested for occult blood. If blood loss is detected, careful spot barium films are done of the area where the tip of the tube is located. Alternatively, a *string test* can be done. This involves swallowing a capsule with a long string and allowing the capsule to pass through the small bowel. The string is then retrieved and chemically tested for blood along its length to localize the bleeding. If there is more active bleeding from a possible small bowel source, *selective visceral angiography* may also be useful as a radiologic technique to identify bleeding sites and to localize a malignant lesion by finding typical neovascularity. *Radionuclide scanning* after administration of labeled red blood cells or technetium may also localize the site of a bleeding lesion in the small bowel, but will not provide a specific diagnosis.

Duodenal tumors may be detected and biopsied by upper gastrointestinal endoscopy. Modern fiberscopes routinely reach the third portion of the duodenum and newer, longer "enteroscopes" are under development (Chapter 41). Tumors of the terminal ileum may be reached in some patients by passing the ileocecal valve from the cecum with a colonoscope (Chapter 43).

There are, at present, no urine or blood tests that are of value in screening for small bowel neoplasms. The value of fecal occult blood testing in the detection of small intestinal tumors is unknown. As these tests become more widely used, data on small bowel tumors should become available.[81]

Post-bulbar peptic ulcer disease may produce symptoms more suggestive of bowel obstruction than of duodenal ulcer and may require differentiation from tumor. Barium roentgen studies show a markedly abnormal post-bulbar duodenum attributable to edema and spasm secondary to the benign ulceration. Duodenoscopy, biopsy, and cytologic studies will generally enable a correct distinction to be made between duodenal carcinoma and post-bulbar ulcer disease.

Adenomas may develop in the duodenal Brunner's glands and form polypoid growths

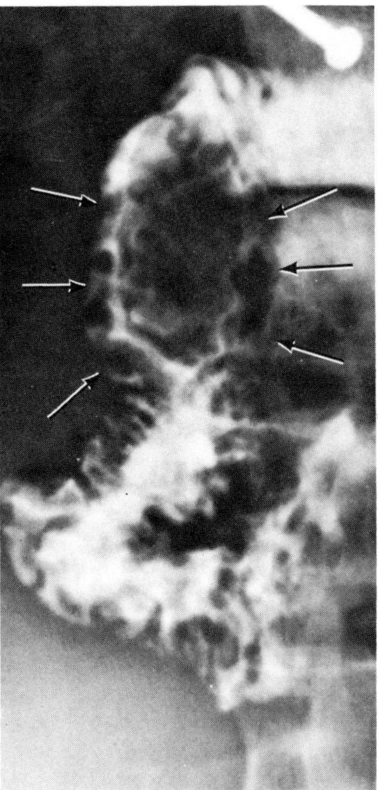

Figure 114–7. Barium radiograph showing a cystadenoma of a Brunner's gland *(arrows).* (Courtesy of Dr. M. Edelman.)

(Fig. 114–7). Endoscopy and biopsy may differentiate these from hyperplasia of Brunner's glands, which develops sometimes in the duodenal bulbs of patients with chronic hypersecretion of gastric acid. Brunner's gland hyperplasias are usually multiple, but single polypoid lesions sometimes occur.[81]

A preoperative diagnosis of complicating cancer in Crohn's disease or clear distinction between Crohn's disease and cancer may be difficult in the extreme. Both Crohn's disease and adenocarcinoma may produce weight loss, anorexia, an abdominal mass, obstruction, perforation, bleeding, and fistulization,[82] and the radiologic appearances of Crohn's disease and carcinoma may be indistinguishable.[83] Most cancers will eventually obstruct the small intestine. Changes in the appearance of or drainage from chronic fistulas in Crohn's disease may be an early sign of a complicating carcinoma.[45]

Miscellaneous Tumors

Simple tubular *adenomas* of the small intestine, most commonly found in the duodenum, have a very low malignant potential (Fig. 114–10), and carcinoma in Brunner's gland adenomas has not been reported.[81, 84] On the other hand, villous adenomas, again usually in the duodenum, appreciably often display carcinoma, both in situ and invasive.[84, 85] Indeed, about one third of villous adenomas found in the duodenum contain foci of adenocarcinoma, a rate approaching that of malignant change found in the colon when variations in interpretation are taken into account.[86] Villous adenomas are uncommon tumors in the duodenum, with only some 50 cases having been reported as of 1981.[85] They tend to grow larger in size than simple adenomas, the largest diameter at diagnosis usually exceeding 5.0 cm.[84] They are usually solitary, but a case of multiple duodenal villous adenomas has been reported.[87] Though they are soft and pliable, they may produce symptoms of obstruction because of their size. They may also be a source of blood loss. Diarrhea due to production of large amounts of mucus and electrolytes has not been reported with duodenal villous adenomas, probably because of the absorptive capacity of the small intestine. The development of obstructive jaundice in the presence of a duodenal villous adenoma suggests malignant infiltration.[87]

Villous adenomas have a typical appearance on roentgenograms taken after ingestion of barium. The so-called "mousse de savon" or "soap bubble" appearance they display is caused by their cauliflower-shaped, multilobulated nature with barium trapped in the interstices between the villous fronds (Fig. 114–8). Endoscopic biopsy usually confirms the diagnosis.[84,85] *Fibromas* and *fibrosarcomas* tend to produce syndromes similar to the leiomyomas and leiomyosarcomas, depending on whether they grow primarily into or outside the bowel lumen (Fig. 114–9). The intraluminal type may be a cause of intussusception, while the extraluminal type often becomes a palpable mass. As in the case of smooth muscle tumors, it may be difficult histologically to determine benign from malignant lesions in the absence of metastatic disease. The mitotic activity under light microscopic examination may sometimes predict malignant behavior.[8]

Lipomas are more common in the small intestine than in the stomach, but are seen less often than in the colon. They are usually small, rarely larger than 4 cm in diameter.

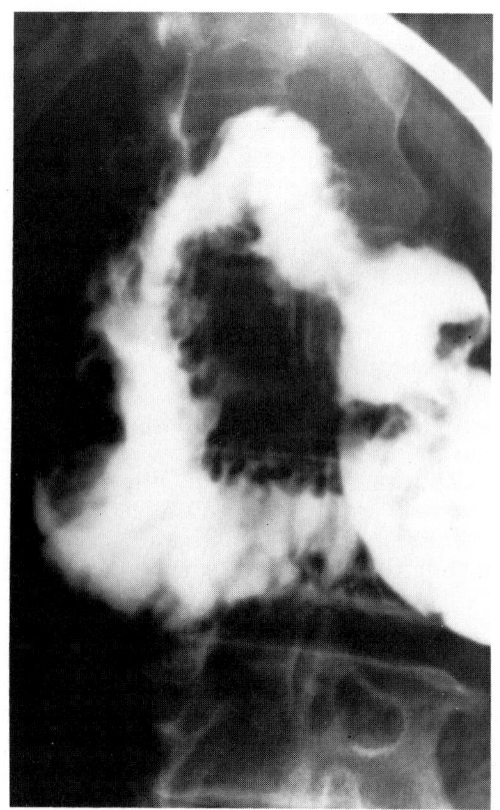

Figure 114–8. Barium radiograph showing a villous adenoma on the lateral wall of the duodenum measuring 3 to 4 cm in length. It projects as a large mass into the lumen. (Courtesy of Dr. E. Stewart.)

They may be single or multiple[88] and found incidentally at surgery or necropsy. Submucosal lipomas may produce an intussusception and on occasion may ulcerate and bleed. Rarely, lipomas are diffuse or grow to a large size from a subserosal origin, producing a palpable mass. Computed tomography, with the ability to make fine definition of density, may be helpful in the diagnosis of lipomas.[89]

Hemangiomas are more often multiple and may involve the gastrointestinal tract diffusely. They may vary in size from tiny pinpoint lesions to large cavernous hemangiomas several centimeters in size. Occasionally, they are polypoid and create intraluminal filling defects. Clinically, hemangiomas may be a source of gastrointestinal bleeding, either occult or massive. Angiography may allow nonsurgical diagnosis by identifying their characteristic vascular pattern.[90] Kaijser[91] classified hemangiomas of the gastrointestinal tract as follows:

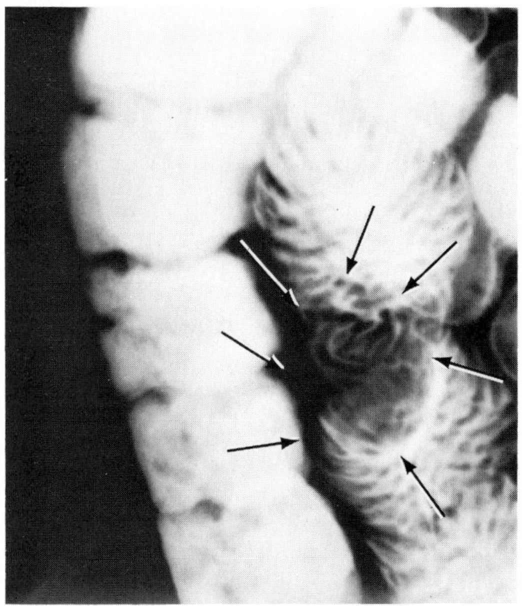

Figure 114–9. Barium radiograph showing fibrosarcoma of the jejunum creating a smooth filling defect *(arrows)* surrounded by normal mucosa. (Courtesy of Dr. M. Edelman.)

1. Multiple ectasias, considered to be hereditary and often involving the jejunum.
2. Cavernous hemangioma, affecting the colon more often than the small bowel.

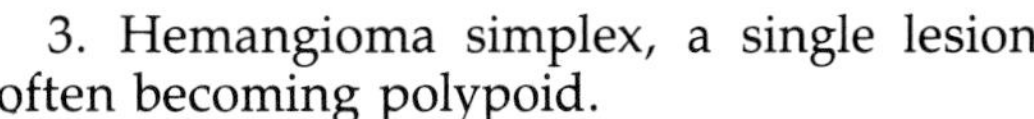

3. Hemangioma simplex, a single lesion often becoming polypoid.
4. Angiomatosis with gastrointestinal involvement (Osler-Weber-Rendu syndrome).

There are a number of even less common tumors occurring in the small intestine, with less than 100 cases reported in each category. These include *islet cell tumors, leiomyoblastoma, ganglioneuroma, neurofibroma* (usually as part of von Recklinghausen's disease), *lymphangioma, hemangiopericytoma, teratoma, choriocarcinoma, endometrioma, and osteoid and reticuloendothelial tumors.*

Metastatic Tumors

The relative infrequency of primary tumors in the small intestine does not hold equally for metastatic cancer. Possibly related to its greater surface area, the small bowel is the site of metastatic implants more frequently than are the stomach and colon.

Melanoma is the most common tumor giving rise to small bowel metastases.[92] In one third of the cases, no primary lesion can be identified, and in many other cases the primary tumor was removed from the skin or retina many years previously.[93] Frequently, after a quiescent period, the melanoma spreads explosively to involve organs such as the liver and lung as well as the gastrointestinal tract (Fig. 114–11). Melanoma metas-

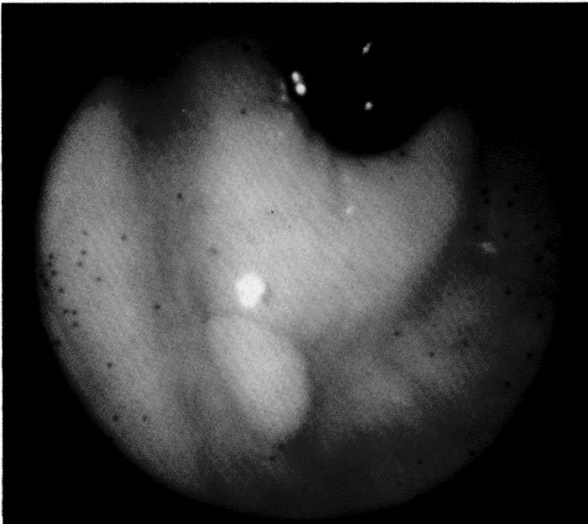

Figure 114–10. Endoscopic photograph showing retroflexed view of the base of the duodenal bulb. A small polyp is seen (bottom of the picture), which was found on biopsy to be an adenoma. The endoscope is seen coming through the pylorus (upper right corner). (Courtesy of the American Society for Gastrointestinal Endoscopy.)

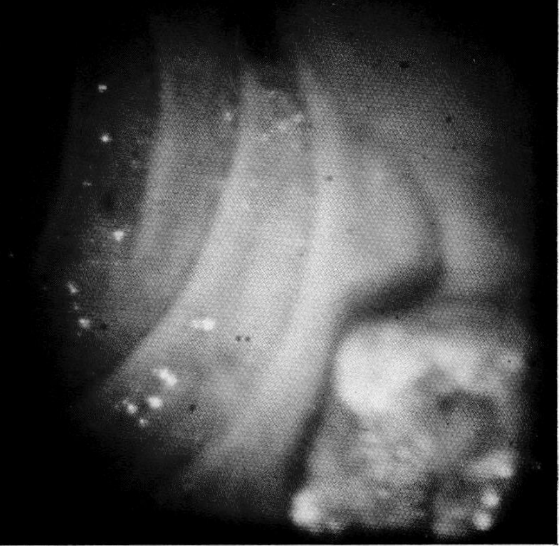

Figure 114–11. Endoscopic photograph showing a metastatic ulcerated melanoma located in the descending duodenum (lower right corner). This type of lesion produces a "target" or "bull's-eye" appearance on barium radiographs. (Courtesy of the American Society for Gastrointestinal Endoscopy.)

tases to the small bowel are usually multiple and may cause intussusception, obstruction, or bleeding (Fig. 114–12). Barium roentgenograms will usually show multiple intraluminal polypoid masses, sometimes with a central ulceration that produces a "bull's-eye" or "target" appearance[94] (Fig. 114–13).

Breast cancer is another primary neoplasm that commonly produces small bowel metastases. Patients treated with corticosteroids for breast cancer seem to develop a higher rate of gastrointestinal metastases.[95] These tumors may also involve the duodenum by direct spread from retroperitoneal lymph nodes. Cancers originating in the cervix, ovaries, colon, and kidneys may also involve the small intestine by direct extension.[92]

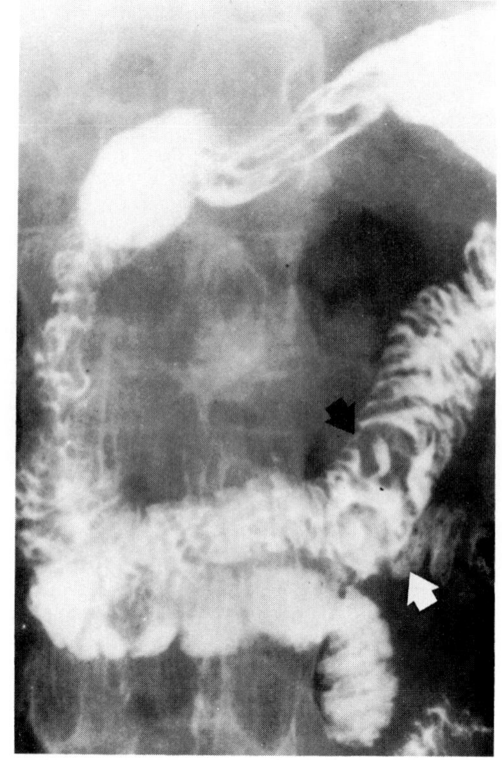

Figure 114–13. Barium radiograph of metastatic melanoma to the small bowel. Two lesions are seen in the third and fourth portions of the duodenum *(arrows).* These are about 1 cm in diameter and have central ulcerations within them ("target lesions"). (Courtesy of Dr. E. Stewart.)

Treatment and Prognosis

Benign symptomatic tumors are generally treated by simple surgical excision, removing as little small bowel as possible. The operative mortality is low and the prognosis is excellent.[48] Duodenal polyps and ileal polyps within reach, particularly when the polyps are pedunculated, may be removed endoscopically by cautery snare.[85]

Asymptomatic benign-appearing lesions found incidentally at surgery should also generally be excised to confirm their nature and to avoid future complications, such as intussusception or bleeding. When a benign-appearing small intestinal lesion is encountered as an incidental finding during a barium meal roentgen study done for other reasons, the decision as to what to do about it can be more difficult. Small (<2.0 cm), smooth polypoid or submucosal tumors may be observed by periodic radiologic studies for evidence of malignant change. Lesions within reach endoscopically may be snared and removed, if possible. If not, periodic repeat endoscopy with biopsy and cytologic study may be carried out. Factors such as the patient's age and general medical condition must be considered in each case when deciding whether to perform surgery on an asymptomatic patient with a benign-appearing lesion. When there are no contraindications and endoscopy is inconclusive, simple surgical excision is usually advised to confirm the diagnosis and prevent complications. Villous adenomas in the duodenum should be surgically excised because of the significant

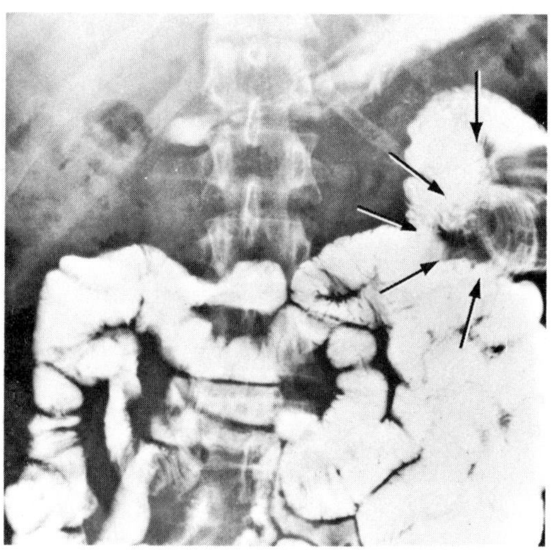

Figure 114–12. Barium radiograph showing melanoma metastatic to the small bowel with an area of intusussception *(arrows).* (Courtesy of Dr. M. Edelman.)

risk of malignant degeneration. These tend to be broad-based, sessile lesions that usually cannot be removed endoscopically.[97]

In syndromes involving diffuse multiple small bowel polyps, such as Peutz-Jeghers syndrome, surgery should be reserved for management of complications only. Duodenal polyps may be removed endoscopically if possible.[98] Prophylactic surgery for removal of all polyps is not indicated, as polyps tend to develop periodically in clusters throughout life.[99] When surgery is performed for symptomatic lesions, as many polyps as possible should be removed. Resection of the small bowel should be avoided, however, or kept to a minimum, since repeat operations may be required and short bowel syndrome is a risk.

Cancers of the small intestine are primarily managed surgically. With adenocarcinoma, surgery offers the only hope of cure. Adenocarcinomas metastasize early to regional lymph nodes and, hence, principles of wide resection are applicable.[48] Unfortunately, many lymph node metastases are located at the mesenteric root, where there is likely to be involvement of the superior mesenteric artery. Duodenal adenocarcinomas tend to spread by direct retroperitoneal extension. These require pancreatoduodenectomy, but are often unresectable.

Villous adenomas containing in-situ carcinoma can be managed safely by simple wide excision, but those with invasive cancer require a Whipple-type procedure.[97] The rare adenocarcinomas of the distal ileum are best managed by a resection including right hemicolectomy.

The overall resectability rate for small bowel adenocarcinoma is in the range of 50%, with 5-year survival in the range of 20%.[100, 101] If there is unresectable disease, a palliative resection of the main lesion is generally advised to relieve or prevent complications. Radiation therapy and chemotherapy have demonstrated minimal benefit. About 15% of patients with metastatic disease will have a brief beneficial response to 5-fluorouracil.[22]

Leiomyosarcomas are also managed surgically. In contrast to the adenocarcinomas, lymph node metastases are uncommon and spread is most often by direct peritoneal extension or hematogenously to the lungs and liver. Wide excision of the tumor mass is advised.[102] Leiomyosarcoma has a slower course than adenocarcinoma, and approximately half of the patients with resectable lesions will survive for 5 years after surgery.[22] Radiation therapy and chemotherapy have been essentially ineffective in the management of metastatic disease.

References

1. Hamburger GE. De ruptura intestini duodeni. *In:* Haller A, ed. Disputationes ad Morborium Historium et Curatiorum Facientes. Lausanne: MM Bausquet et Soc, 1757.
2. Keinerman J, Yardiumian K, Tarraki HT. Primary carcinoma of the duodenum. Ann Intern Med 1950; 32:451–65.
3. Cruveilhier J. Anatomie Pathologique du Corps Humain. Paris: JB Bailliere, 1835.
4. Raiford TS. Tumors of the small intestine. Arch Surg 1932; 25:122–77.
5. Grant, JCB. An Atlas of Anatomy by Regions. Baltimore: Williams and Wilkins, 1972.
6. Reith EJ, Ross MH. Atlas of Descriptive Histology. New York: Hoeber Medical Division, Harper and Row, 1967.
7. Morson BC, Dawson IMP. Tumors of the small intestine. *In:* Gastrointestinal Pathology. London: Blackwell Scientific Publications, 1972: 352–77.
8. Wood DA. Atlas of Tumor Pathology—Tumors of the Intestines. Sect VI, Fasc 22. Washington, DC: Armed Forces Institute of Pathology, 1967.
9. Dapena AV, Stein GN. Morphologic Pathology of the Alimentary Canal. Philadelphia: WB Saunders, 1970.
10. Lightdale CJ, Sherlock P. Tumors of the small and large intestine. *In:* Stein JH, ed. Internal Medicine: A Systematic Approach. New York: Elsevier North Holland, 1983: 147–55.
11. Silberman H, Crichlow RW, Caplan HS. Neoplasms of the small bowel. Ann Surg 1974; 180:157–61.
12. Southam JA. Primary tumors of the small intestine. Ann R Coll Surg Engl 1974; 55:129–33.
13. Treadwell TA, White RR. Primary tumors of the small bowel. Am J Surg 1975; 130:749–50.
14. Pagtalunan RJG, Mayo CW, Dockerty MB. Primary malignant tumors of the small intestine. Am J Surg 1964; 108:13–8.
15. Hampole MK, Jackson BA, Burkell CC. Primary malignant tumors of the jejunum and ileum. Can J Surg 1966; 9:159–65.
16. Brookes VS, Waterhouse JAH, Powell DJ. Malignant lesions of the small intestine. A ten-year survey. Br J Surg 1968; 55:405–10.
17. Haffner J, Semb L. Malignant tumors of the small intestine. Acta Chir Scand 1969; 135:543–8.
18. Vuori JV. Primary malignant tumors of the small intestine. Analysis of cases diagnosed in Finland 1953–1962. Acta Chir Scand 1971; 137:555–61.
19. Kyriakos M. Malignant tumors of the small intestine. JAMA 1974; 229:700–2.
20. Wilson JM, Melvin DB, Gray GF, Thorbjarnarson B. Primary malignancies of the small bowel: A report of 96 cases and a review of the literature. Ann Surg 1974; 180:175–9.
21. Ratner MH, Aust JC. Primary malignant neoplasms of the small intestine. Rev Surg 1975; 32:449–51.
22. Moertel CG. Small intestine. *In:* Holland JF, Frei E, eds Cancer Medicine, 3rd Ed. Philadelphia: Lea and Febiger, 1982: 1808–18.
23. Lowenfels AB. Why are small bowel tumors so rare? Lancet 1973; 1:24–6.
24. Evans I A, Mason J. Carcinogenic activity of bracken. Nature 1965; 208:913–4.
25. Takeuchi M, Ogiu T, Nakadate M, Odashima S. Induction of duodenal tumors in F344 rats by continuous oral administration of N-ethyl-N-nitrosourea. J Natl Cancer Inst 1980; 64:613–16.
26. Berg JW. Diet. *In:* Fraumeni JF Jr, ed. Persons at High Risk of Cancer: An Approach to Cancer Etiology and Control. New York: Academic Press, 1975: 201–24.

27. Wattenberg LW. Carcinogen-detoxifying mechanisms in the gastrointestinal tract. Gastroenterology 1966; 51:932–5.
28. Reddy BS, Martin CW, Wynder EL. Fecal bile acids and cholesterol metabolites of patients with ulcerative colitis, a high risk group for development of colon cancer. Cancer Res 1977; 37:1697–1701.
29. Hill MJ, Aries BC. Faecal steroid composition and its relationship to cancer of the large bowel. J Pathol 1971; 104:129–39.
30. Calman KC. Why are small bowel tumors rare? An experimental model. Gut 1974; 15:552–4.
31. Bone G, Wright NA. The rarity of small bowel tumors: An alternative hypothesis. Lancet 1973; 1:618.
32. Lipkin M, Quastler H. Cell retention and incidence of carcinoma in several portions of the gastrointestinal tract. Nature (Lond) 1962; 194:1198–9.
33. Lightdale CJ, Koepsell TD, Sherlock P. Small intestine. *In:* Schottenfeld D, Fraumeni J Jr, eds. Cancer Epidemiology and Prevention. Philadelphia: W B Saunders, 1982: 692–702.
34. WHO (World Health Organization). Cancer Incidence in Five Continents, Vol III. Lyon, France: International Agency for Research on Cancer, 1976.
35. Waterhouse JAH. Cancer Handbook of Epidemiology and Prognosis. London: Churchill Livingstone, 1974.
36. Lowe WC. Neoplasms of the Gastrointestinal Tract. Flushing, NY: Medical Examination Publishing Co, 1972.
37. Burbank F, ed. Patterns in Cancer Mortality in the United States: 1950–1967. Washington, DC: Natl Cancer Inst Monogr 1971; No 33.
38. Lilienfeld AM, Levine ML, Kessler II. Cancer in the United States. Cambridge, Mass: Harvard University Press, 1972: Appendix.
39. Cutler SJ, Young JR Jr. Demographic patterns of cancer incidence in the United States. *In:* Fraumeni JR Jr, ed. Persons at High Risk of Cancer: An Approach to Cancer Etiology and Control. New York: Academic Press: 307–42. 1975.
40. Eisenberg H, Campbell PC, Flannery JT. Cancer in Connecticut: Incidence Characteristics 1935–1962. Hartford, Conn: Connecticut State Department of Health, 1967.
41. Ingraham H. Cancer Control and Registry Report. Albany, NY: New York State Department of Health, 1974.
42. Darling RC, Welch CE. Tumors of the small intestine. N Engl J Med 1959; 260:397–408.
43. Kelsey JR Jr. Small bowel tumors. *In:* Bockus HL, ed. Gastreoenterology, Vol 2, 3rd Ed. Philadelphia: WB Saunders, 1976:459–72.
44. Darke SG, Parks AG, Grogono JL, Pollock DJ. Adenocarcinoma and Crohn's disease. A report of 2 cases and analysis of the literature. Br J Surg 1973; 60:169–75.
45. Lightdale CJ, Sternberg SS, Posner G, Sherlock P. Carcinoma complicating Crohn's disease. Report of seven cases and a review of the literature. Am J Med 1975; 59:262–8.
46. Fielding JR, Prior P, Waterhouse JAH, Cooke WT. Malignancy in Crohn's disease. Scand J Gastroenterol 1972; 7:3–7.
47. Nesbit RR Jr, Elbadawi NA, Morton JH, Cooper RA Jr. Carcinoma of the small bowel. A complication of regional enteritis. Cancer 1976; 37:2948–59.
48. Weedon DD, Shorter RG, Ilstrup DM, Huizenga KA, Taylor WF. Crohn's disease and cancer. N Engl J Med 1973; 289:1099–1103.
49. Schlippert W, Mitros F, Schulze K. Multiple adenocarcinomas and premalignant changes in "backwash" ileitis. Am J Med 1979; 66:879–82.
50. Harris OD. Malignancy in adult coeliac disease and idiopathic steatorrhea. Am J Med 1967; 42:899–912.
51. Holmes GKT, Stokes PL, Sorahan TM, Prior P, Waterhouse JAH, Cooke WT. Coeliac disease, gluten-free diet, and malignancy. Gut 1976; 17:612–9.
52. Ogilvie TA, Shaw HM. Primary tumors of the small bowel. Br Med J 1955; 1:142–5.
53. Petreshock EP, Pessah M, Menachemi E. Adenocarcinoma of the jejunum associated with nontropical sprue. Am J Dig Dis 1975; 20:796–802.
54. Javier J, Lukie B. Duodenal adenocarcinoma complicating celiac sprue. Dig Dis Sci 1980; 25:150–3.
55. Holmes GK, Dunn GI, Cockel R, Brookes VS. Adenocarcinoma of the upper small bowel complicating coeliac disease. Gut 1980; 21:1010–16.
56. Peutz JLA. A very remarkable case of familial polyposis of mucous membrane of intestinal tract and nasopharynx accompanied by peculiar pigmentations of skin and mucous membrane. Ned Moonschr Geneeskd 1921; 10:134–6.
57. Jeghers H, McKusick VA, Katz KH. Generalized intestinal polyposis and melanin spots of the oral mucosa, lips, and digits: A syndrome of diagnostic significance. N Engl J Med 1949; 241:993–1005.
58. Dozois RR, Judd ES, Dahlin DC, Bartholomew LG. The Peutz-Jeghers syndrome. Is there a predisposition to the development of intestinal malignancy? Arch Surg 1969; 98:509–15.
59. Bussey HJR, Veale AMO, Morson BC. Genetics of gastrointestinal polyposis. Gastroenterology 1978; 74:1325–30.
60. Matuchansky C, Babin P, Coutrot S, Druart F, Barbier J, Maire P. Peutz-Jeghers syndrome with metastasizing carcinoma arising from a jejunal hamartoma. Gastroenterology 1979; 77:1311–5.
61. Reid JD. Intestinal carcinoma in the Peutz-Jeghers syndrome. JAMA 1974; 229:833–4.
62. Qizilbash AH. Familial polyposis coli and periampullary carcinoma. Can J Surg 1976; 19:166–8.
63. Yao T, Iida M, Ohsato K, Watanabe H, Omae T. Duodenal lesions in familial polyposis of the colon. Gastroenterology 1977; 73:1086–92.
64. Ranzi T, Castagnone D, Velio P, Bianchi P, Polli EE. Gastric and duodenal polyps in familial polyposis coli. Gut 1981; 22:363–7.
65. Yonemoto RH, Slayback JB, Byron RL, Rosen RB. Familial polyposis of the entire gastrointestinal tract. Arch Surg 1969; 99:427–34.
66. Ranzi T, Castagone E, Velio P, Bianchi P, Polli EE. Gastric and duodenal polyps in familial polyposis coli. Gut 1981; 22:363–7.
67. Phillips LG Jr. Polyposis and carcinoma of the small bowel and familial colonic polyposis. Dis Colon Rectum 1981; 24:478–81.
68. MacDonald JM, Davis WC, Crago HR, Berk AD. Gardner's syndrome and periampullary malignancy. Am J Surg 1967; 113:425–30.
69. Melmed RN, Bouchier IAD. Duodenal involvement in Gardner's syndrome. Gut 1972; 13:524–7.
70. Schnur PL, David E, Brown PW Jr, Beahrs OH, ReMine WH, Harrison EG Jr. Adenocarcinoma of the duodenum and the Gardner syndrome. JAMA 1973; 223:1229–32.
71. Keshgegian AA, Enterline HT. Gardner's syndrome with duodenal adenomas, gastric adenomyoma and thyroid papillary-follicular adenocarcinoma. Dis Colon Rectum 1978; 21:255–60.
72. Hamilton SR, Bussey HJ, Mendelsohn G, Diamond MP, Pavlides G, Hutcheon D, Harbison M, Shermeta D, Morson BC, Yardley JH. Ileal adenomas after colectomy in nine patients with adenomatous polyposis coli/Gardner's syndrome. Gastroenterology 1979; 77:1252–7.
73. Muir EG, Bell AJY, Barlow KA. Multiple primary carcinomata of the colon, duodenum, and larynx associated with keratoacanthomata of the face. Br J Surg 1967; 54:191–5.
74. Torre D. Multiple sebaceous tumors. Arch Dermatol 1968; 98:549–52.
75. Cho KJ, Reuter SR. Angiography of duodenal leiomyomas and leiomyosarcomas. AJR 1980; 135:31-5.
76. Marshak RH, Lindner AE. Radiology of the Small Intestine, 2nd Ed. Philadelphia: WB Saunders, 1976. 77. Ekberg O, Ekholm S. Radiology in primary small bowel adenocarcinoma. Gastrointest Radiol 1980; 5:49–53.
78. Kato O, Kuno N, Kasugai T, Matsuyama M. Pancreatic carcinoma difficult to differentiate from duodenal carcinoma. Am J Gastroenterol 1979; 71:74–7.
79. Ewerth S, Hellers G, Holmstrom B, Nordenstam H. Carcinoma of Meckel's diverticulum. Acta Chir Scand 1979; 145:203–5.

80. Winawer SJ. Fecal occult blood testing. Am J Dig Dis 1976; 21:885–8.
81. Barnhart GR, Maull KI. Brunner's gland adenomas: Clinical presentation and surgical management. South Med J 1979; 72:1537–9.
82. Milman PJ, Gold BM, Bagla S, Thorn R. Primary ileal adenocarcinoma simulating Crohn's disease. Gastrointest Radiol 1980; 5:55–8.
83. Heathcote J, Knauer CM, Oakes D, Archibald WW. Perforation of an adenocarcinoma of the small bowel affected by regional enteritis. Gut 1980; 21:1093-6.
84. Gold BM. Duodenal filling defect. JAMA 1979; 241:2734–5.
85. Reddy RR, Schuman BM, Priest RJ. Duodenal polyps: Diagnosis and management. J Clin Gastroenterol 1981; 3:139–47.
86. Komorowski RA, Cohen EB. Villous tumors of the duodenum: A clinicopathologic study. Cancer 1981; 47:1377–86.
87. Hasleton PS, Shah S, Buckley CH, Tweedle DE. Ampullary carcinoma associated with multiple duodenal villous adenomas. Am J Gastroenterol 1980; 73:418–22.
88. Margolin FR, Lagois MD. Polypoid lipomatosis of the small bowel. Gastrointest Radiol 1980; 5:59–60.
89. Megibow AJ, Redmond PE, Bosniak MA, Horowitz L. Diagnosis of gastrointestinal lipomas by CT. AJR 1979; 133:743–5.
90. Sutton D, Murfitt J, Howarth F. Gastrointestinal bleeding from large angiomas. Clin Radiol 1981; 32:629–32.
91. Kaijser R. Hemangiomas of the gastrointestinal tract. Arch Klin Chir 1936; 187:351–65.
92. DeCastro CA, Dockerty MB, Mayo CW. Metastatic tumors of the small intestine. Surg Gynecol Obstet 1957; 105:159–65.
93. Richman A, Lipsey J. Melanoma of small intestine and stomach. J Mt Sinai Hosp 1951; 17:907-16.
94. Beirne MF. Malignant melanoma of the small intestine. Radiology 1955; 65:749–52.
95. Hartman WH, Sherlock P. Gastroduodenal metastases from carcinoma of the breast. An adrenal steroid-induced phenomenon. Cancer 1961; 14:426–31.
96. Chait MM, Kurtz RC, Hajdu SI. Gastrointestinal tract metastases in patients with germ-cell tumor of the testis. Am J Dig Dis 1978; 23:925–8.
97. Choctaw WT, Burbige EJ, McCandless CM. Duodenal villous adenoma. Am Surg 1980; 46:640–3.
98. Kurtz RC, Winawer SJ, Sherlock P. Endoscopy in the Peutz-Jeghers syndrome. Am J Gastroenterol 1974; 61:125-8.
99. Welch CE, Hedberg SE. Polypoid Lesions of the Gastrointestinal Tract, 2nd Ed. Philadelphia: W B Saunders, 1975: 194–9.
100. Rubin P. Cancer of the gastrointestinal tract. Small intestine: Diagnosis and treatment: Introduction. JAMA 1974; 229:699.
101. Garvin PJ, Herrman V, Kaminski DL, Willman VL. Benign and malignant tumors of the small intestine. Curr Probl Cancer 1979; 3(9):1–46.
102. Starr GF, Dockerty MB. Leiomyomas and leiomyosarcomas of the small intestine. Cancer 1955; 8:101–11.

Chapter 115

Intestinal Blood Flow

Robert H. Gallavan, Jr. • Eugene D. Jacobson

Anatomy

Arterial Supply. There are 5 arteries that provide blood to the small and large intestine: the superior mesenteric, inferior mesenteric, celiac, internal iliac, and pudendal. The superior mesenteric artery directs approximately 12% of cardiac output to the duodenum, jejunum, ileum, cecum, and ascending and tranverse colon (Fig. 115–1) and forms anastomoses with the celiac and inferior mesenteric arteries (Table 115–1 and Fig. 115–1). The inferior mesenteric artery carries approximately 6% of the cardiac output to the descending and sigmoid colon and the rectum and forms anastomoses with the superior mesenteric, internal iliac, and pudendal arteries (Table 115–1 and Fig. 115–2). The pancreaticoduodenal branch of the hepatic artery, which is the largest branch of the celiac artery, conveys blood to the duodenum and anastomoses with the superior mesenteric artery. The internal iliac and pudendal arteries provide a portion of the blood flow to the rectum and form anastomoses with the inferior mesenteric arteries (Table 115–1).[1]

The most significant aspect of this anatomic arrangement of the large arteries is the existence of extensive collateral circulations among the vascular beds of the small and large intestine. Thus, with one exception, the majority of the tissue in the intestines is perfused with blood from 2 major arteries. The notable exception, however, is the midportion of the small intestine, whose tissue is too far removed from the vascular imbrications of either the celiac or the inferior mesenteric artery to survive if superior mesenteric artery blood flow is compromised. It is not surprising, therefore, that the majority of patients reporting symptoms of intestinal ischemia are found to have lesions in this region, even though the underlying disease process may have attacked other regions of the intestinal vasculature as well. Furthermore, ischemia of the midgut usually proves fatal, whereas patients with ischemia of the colon usually survive the disease even if scarring of the organ develops at a later stage.

In general, the intestinal tract demonstrates an extensive collateral circulation at all levels. In addition to the anastomoses formed between the major arteries, the various branches of the superior and inferior mesenteric arteries divide and form a complex network of interconnecting vessels prior to entering the intestinal wall (Figs. 115–1 and 115–2). As will be discussed, collateralization is also evident in the microcirculation and venous drainage. This aids the intestines in compensating for catastrophic vascular insufficiency at all levels of the circulation.

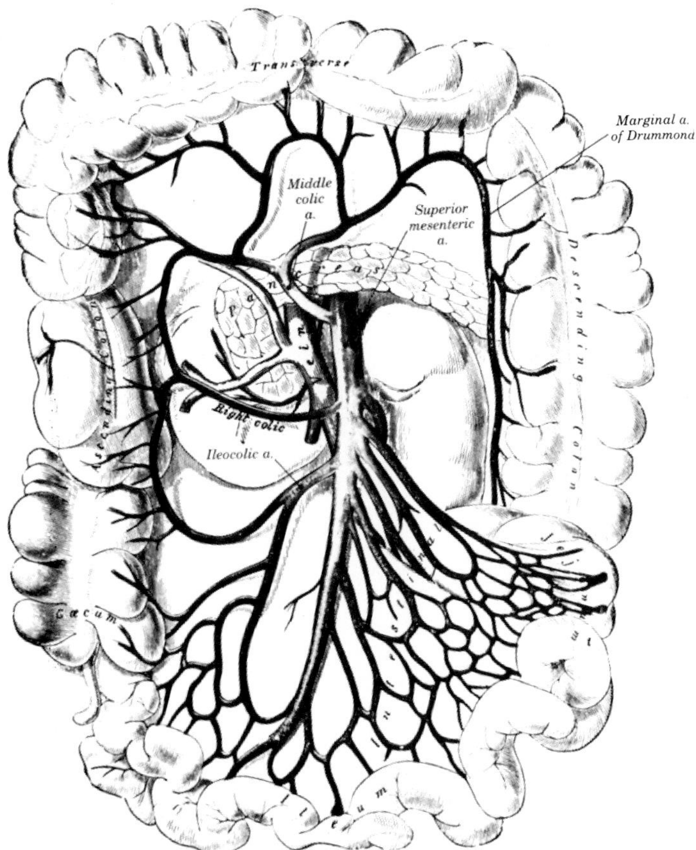

Figure 115–1. Major branches of the superior mesenteric artery in man. (From Mayo C, ed. Gray's Anatomy. Philadelphia: Lea and Febiger, 1973. Reproduced with permission.)

Intramural Vascular Anatomy. The small arteries of the intestinal vasculature arborize as they penetrate the serosa at the mesenteric border. Some of the branches extend around both sides of the intestinal wall and anastomose at the antimesenteric border, whereas others penetrate the muscularis and form the submucosal plexus. The vascular supply of the muscularis is derived from branches of both the submucosal plexus and the network of serosal arteries.[2]

In the small intestine, the vascular supply of the mucosa is derived from the submucosal plexus and consists of 2 groups of arteries. One group penetrates the muscularis mucosae and perfuses the capillaries surrounding the glands lining the crypts, whereas the second group enters the villi at

Table 115–1. MAJOR ANASTOMOSES OF THE SUPERIOR AND INFERIOR MESENTERIC ARTERIES

Artery	Branch	Portion of Intestine Perfused	Anastomoses with (arterial source)
Superior mesenteric artery	Inferior pancreaticoduodenal	Duodenum	Superior pancreaticoduodenal branch of the hepatic artery (celiac artery)
	Middle colic artery	Transverse colon	Left colic artery (inferior mesenteric artery)
Inferior mesenteric artery	Left colic artery	Descending colon	Middle colic artery (superior mesenteric artery)
	Superior hemorrhoidal	Upper rectum	Middle hemorrhoidal artery (internal iliac artery)
			Inferior hemorrhoidal artery (pudendal artery)

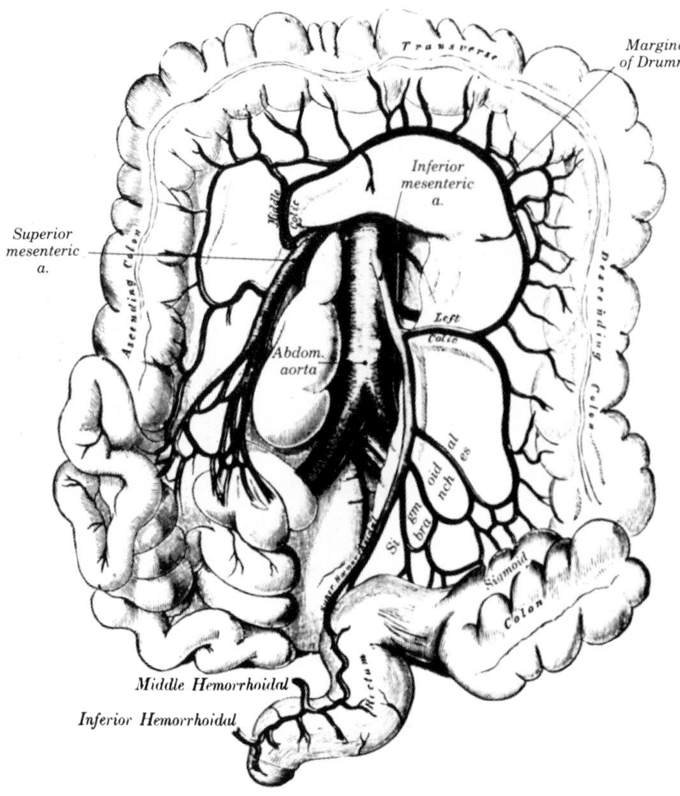

Figure 115–2. Major branches of the inferior mesenteric artery in man (From Mayo C, ed. Gray's Anatomy. Philadelphia: Lea and Febiger, 1973. Reproduced with permission.)

their bases and arborizes into a dense network of capillaries (Fig. 115–3).[2] In the large intestine, the arteries that provide blood to the mucosa are distributed along the undersurface of the mucosa and give off arteriolar and capillary branches that pass to the mucosal surface between the colonic glands. This forms a "honeycomb" plexus of capillaries at the mucosal surface (Fig. 115–4).[3]

Generally, 1 or 2 veins drain each villus of the small intestine and join the venous network of the glandular region. In both the small and large intestine, the venous drainage of the glandular region merges sequentially with the venous effluent from the submucosal plexus, the muscularis, and the serosal network before exiting from the serosa at the mesenteric border.[2]

There are several consequences of this anatomic arrangement of the intestinal vasculature. The first is that all the arteries and veins that deliver blood to and drain blood from the submucosa and mucosa must pass through the muscularis and be subject to compression during forceful contractions of the intestinal wall. Similarly, the muscularis

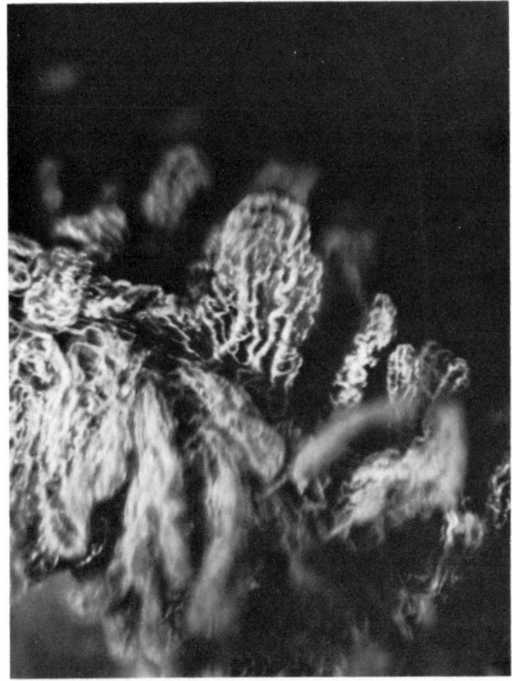

Figure 115–3. Human jejunal villus (× 60). The arteriole is on the left and the venule is on the right. (U.S. Army photograph.)

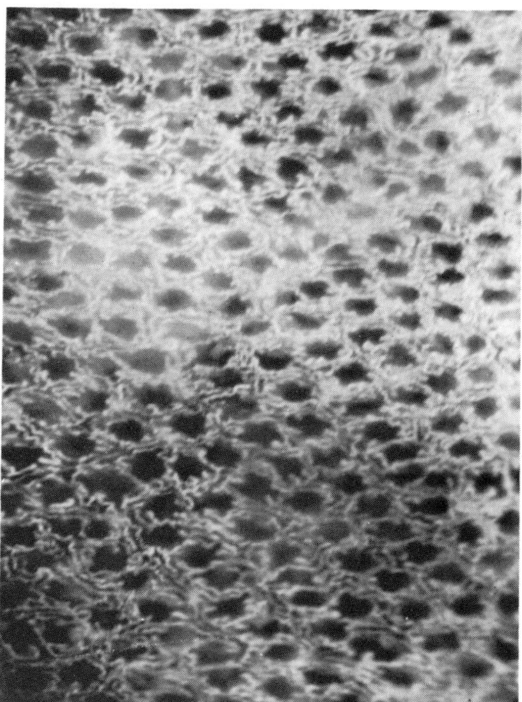

Figure 115–4. Luminal surface of the colonic mucosa in man (× 80). (U.S. Army photograph.)

is a fairly rigid tissue in comparison to the mucosa. Hence, when pressure in the lumen increases during distention of the bowel, the vessels of the mucosal layer are subjected to the greatest compressive force. Since the submucosal and mucosal layers of the intestinal wall receive approximately 75% of total intestinal blood flow and are metabolically the most active components of the wall, compensatory mechanisms must offset the compressive effects of normal intestinal motility and mild distention on mucosal blood flow. These mechanisms will be discussed in the section on the relationship between blood flow and motility.

Another important aspect of the microcirculatory anatomy of the small intestine is the arrangement of arteries, capillaries, and veins in the villi. As seen in Figure 115–3, the artery and vein of the villus are in sufficiently close approximation to allow a *countercurrent exchange* of lipid-soluble substances between the 2 vessels. Investigators have proposed that there is a movement of physically dissolved oxygen from the arteriole (or perhaps the capillaries, where its concentration is higher) into the vein that drains blood in a countercurrent direction. Effectively, this short circuits some of the oxygen being delivered and leads to a gradient of PO_2 from the base to the tip of the villus. Indeed, Bohlen[4] has measured a PO_2 gradient from the base of the villus (PO_2 = 24 mm Hg) to the tip (PO_2 = 13 mm Hg) in rats. In addition, Svanvik and Lundgren[5] and Bond et al.[6] have shown that ^{85}Kr is absorbed slowly from the lumen, whereas other less diffusible substances are absorbed relatively quickly. This would suggest that absorbed ^{85}Kr in the venous drainage of the villus is moving down its concentration gradient to the artery.

Two additional possible consequences of a countercurrent exchange in the villus are: (1) simple absorption of lipid-soluble substances from the lumen of the small intestine would be hindered, and (2) the epithelial cells at the tip of the villus would be subject to chronically low PO_2.

Following absorption into the epithelial cell, most dietary fats are packaged intracellularly into chylomicrons and are delivered to the systemic circulation via the lymphatics and not via the veins of the villi. Hence, it does not seem likely that countercurrent exchange would appreciably impede lipid absorption.

The most significant effect of countercurrent exchange in the small intestine appears to be the reduction of oxygen delivery to the villus tip. This has been suggested as one reason for the high rate of epithelial cell turnover under normal conditions. It is even more likely that the countercurrent exchange of oxygen contributes to the rapid development of lesions on the tip of the villi during periods of intestinal ischemia. It should be noted, however, that the high rate of epithelial cell turnover is essential for the maintenance of body iron levels, since the amount of iron that can be absorbed from the gut depends upon the concentration of iron within the epithelial cells. The iron content of the latter is fixed at the time the cell is formed[7] so that a constant turnover of epithelial cells is necessary for adjustment to sudden changes in iron metabolism.

In addition to its role as a *countercurrent exchanger,* the microcirculation of the villus may act as a *countercurrent multiplier.* It has been proposed that absorption of solutes at the surface of the villus creates an osmotic gradient between the centrally located arteriole and the peripheral capillaries.[5] The gradient would cause water to move from the artery to the capillaries and be carried away in the venous system, whereas the osmolality in the arterial blood would increase progressively as the blood flowed through the tip of the villus. This cycle would repeat itself until a steady state was achieved in which the osmolality at the tip of the villus was considerably greater than 300 mOsm/kg. Based upon a cryoscopic technique, osmolalities for the absorbing villus in man of 800 to 1000 mOsm/kg water have been calculated.[5]

In the rat intestine, comparisons were made of the sodium concentration in the distal half of the villus and in the submucosa, both at rest and during coupled absorption of sodium and glucose from the lumen.[8] At rest, the sodium concentration was 200 to 225 mM in the villus, but only 140 to 150 mM in the submucosa. The villous concentration increased during absorption to 250 to 400 mM within 1 minute following superfusion with glucose in saline. Because of differences in the anatomy of these species,[9] it is likely that the human villus is a more efficient countercurrent multiplier than that of the rat. The ability of the intestine to increase the osmolality of the tip of the villus so dramatically could explain its ability to absorb water from hyperosmotic solutions. This increase in osmolality may also contribute to the absorptive hyperemia, as a hyperosmotic environment can produce a decrease in vascular smooth muscle tone.

Venous Drainage. As the veins of the small and large intestine exit the serosal wall, they begin to coalesce into a number of major veins running parallel to the branches of the superior and inferior mesenteric arteries. The veins of the small intestine and the ascending and transverse colon combine to form the superior mesenteric vein, which joins the splenic vein to form the portal vein. The venous drainage from the descending and sigmoid colon and the upper rectum enters the inferior mesenteric vein, which then empties into the splenic vein. Part of the venous drainage from the rectal venous plexus is directed through the middle and inferior hemorrhoidal veins to the internal iliac veins.[1] The rectal venous plexus thus serves as an anastomosis between the portal and systemic venous circulations, as do the esophageal veins. Consequently, hemorrhoidal and esophageal varices may appear in portal hypertension.

The portal vein conveys the venous drainage of the splanchnic region to the liver. Although a reciprocity of flow between the portal venous and the hepatic arterial circulations has been reported, it usually consists of changes in arterial blood flow in response to changes in portal venous flow, rather than the opposite.[10] As will be discussed, diseases of the liver can have profound effects on the intestinal circulation if associated with either portal hypertension or hypoproteinemia.

Summary. The 3 important functional aspects of vascular anatomy that relate to the regulation of intestinal blood flow are: (1) The intestinal vasculature is characterized by a well developed collateral circulation at all levels of the gut except the midportion of the small intestine. This explains why ischemic necrosis of this area occurs when superior mesenteric artery blood flow is compromised. (2) Although the veins draining the intestine also have a large number of anastomoses, vascular anomalies at the level of the superior or inferior mesenteric veins, the portal vein, or the liver can produce profound disturbances in intestinal blood flow and function. (3) The close approximation of arteries and veins in the villi of the small intestine makes it possible for the villus to be the site of countercurrent exchange. This would contribute to a lower P_{O_2} at the tip of the villi and make the small intestine particularly vulnerable to intestinal ischemia (especially since the efficiency of oxygen countercurrent exchange would increase as the velocity of flow decreases).

Regulation of Blood Flow

The forces that govern the movement of blood through the vasculature can be classified as either propulsive or resistive. The *propulsive force* is the pressure gradient $(P_1 - P_2)$ from the arterial to the venous side of the vascular bed. The *resistive forces* include, but are not limited to, the length of the blood vessel (l), its internal radius (r), and the viscosity of the blood (η). A variation of the law of Poiseuille is often used to express the relationship between blood flow (Q), the pressure gradient $(P_1 - P_2)$, and resistance (R):

$$Q = \frac{P_1 - P_2}{R} \qquad \text{(Equation 1)}$$

$$\text{where: } R = \frac{8l\eta}{\pi r^4} \qquad \text{(Equation 2)}$$

Although this relationship was derived for homogeneous fluids moving through rigid tubes and ignores factors such as pulsatile pressure and turbulence, it is a useful approximation of the behavior of blood as it moves through blood vessels.[11]

According to Equation 1, blood flow may be altered by varying either the pressure gradient ($P_1 - P_2$) or the resistance (R) (Fig. 115–5). Although mean systemic arterial pressure (P_1) and portal venous pressure (P_2) do vary under conditions such as shock or systemic or portal hypertension, the moment to moment regulation of intestinal blood flow is mediated by changes in resistance. This is true of all systemic vascular beds and allows each organ to adjust its blood flow independently and to compensate for variations in the pressure gradient.

As mentioned earlier, the 3 major factors that contribute to vascular resistance are vessel length (l), vessel radius (r), and the viscosity (η) of blood (Equation 2). Although vessel length can change when the intestines are distended and although the viscosity of blood does change as it passes through the vascular bed, both are relatively constant and neither plays a significant role in the regulation of intestinal blood flow. Furthermore, according to Equation 2, resistance is inversely related to the fourth power of the radius, i.e., a small change in the radius will have a large impact on the resistance. Hence, the major regulation of peripheral blood flow involves the alteration of internal vessel diameter by means of changes in vascular smooth muscle tone. The major anatomic site for resistance to flow in a vascular bed occurs at the level of the arterioles. The wall of the arteriole is relatively thick in comparison with total vessel diameter and is composed of a relatively large proportion of vascular smooth muscle. In such a vessel, only a small change in muscle tone is required to alter the internal radius appreciably and, thereby, the blood flow.[11]

Although the arterioles provide the greatest resistance to flow, changes in the diameter of large and small arteries and the veins can also substantially affect intestinal blood flow. Therefore, it is convenient to consider the intestinal circulation as a series of vascular beds, each with its own contribution to total vascular resistance. In such a system, total resistance is equal to the sum of the resistances of each component. The following sections consider the contribution of each compartment to total resistance and the conditions under which it is likely to change.

Intestinal Blood Vessels and Vascular Resistance

Large and Small Arteries. This category includes all arterial vessels from the major branches of the aorta down to but not including the arterioles, i.e., vessels whose outside diameter exceeds 25 μ. The total drop in pressure as blood flows from the aorta to the mesenteric arterioles is approximately 13 mm Hg, representing 15% of the total resistance to blood flow across the intestinal vasculature.

The small and large arteries do not participate in the moment to moment regulation of intestinal blood flow because their inner diameter is fairly constant. This is a consequence of the relatively small amount of vascular smooth muscle in the vessel wall, as well as the anatomic arrangement of the smooth muscle and a less extensive sympathetic innervation.[11] There are, however, a number of conditions that can produce a significant reduction in the diameter of these vessels and thereby reduce intestinal blood

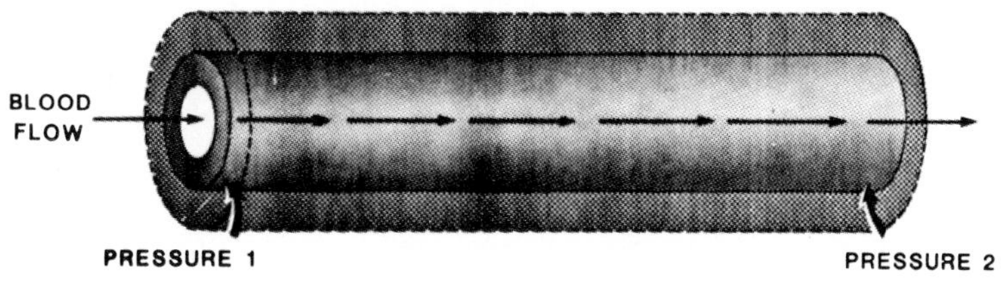

$$\text{BLOOD FLOW} = \frac{\text{PRESSURE 1 - PRESSURE 2}}{\text{RESISTANCE}} = \frac{\text{PRESSURE GRADIENT}}{\text{RESISTANCE}}$$

Figure 115–5. The relationship between blood flow, blood pressure, and resistance in a blood vessel.

flow. These include compression of the small arteries during intestinal contractions, distention of the gut, and partial or total occlusion of the arterial lumen due to atherosclerotic plaques, thrombi, and emboli or as a result of the vasospasm found in peripheral vascular disease. The effect of any of these conditions on intestinal blood flow will depend on the site of occurrence, the degree of occlusion, and the efficiency of compensatory mechanisms.

There are 2 ways in which the intestine can compensate for reductions in large or small artery diameter. The first, as discussed previously, is to bypass the occluded vessel by means of the extensive collateral network within the intestinal vasculature. This is an effective response only as long as the number of vessels occluded is small and the sites of occlusion are not centrally located. Occlusions of the large intestinal arteries, especially the superior mesenteric artery, are more serious and severely tax the ability of the collateral circulation to maintain tissue perfusion.[12]

The second compensatory mechanism involves a decrease in vascular resistance at the level of the arterioles. As noted earlier, total resistance across the vascular bed is equal to the sum of the resistances of each component. Therefore, it is possible, within limits, to maintain vascular resistance and intestinal blood flow at a constant level by decreasing arteriolar resistance as large and small artery resistances increase. Since the large and small arteries normally generate only 15% of total intestinal vascular resistance and the arterioles account for 55% of resistance, a substantial decrease in large or small artery diameter would be required to overwhelm the compensatory capacity of the arteriolar bed. Thus, intestinal blood flow has been found to be within the normal range in patients with reductions of superior mesenteric artery diameter in excess of 50%.

Although resting intestinal blood flow may be maintained in the face of such extreme reductions in arterial diameter, this does not mean that such reductions are without consequences. It may be that extreme reductions in large vessel diameter would require nearly maximal dilation of the arteriolar bed to maintain resting blood flow at normal levels. Under these conditions, the intestinal vasculature may be unable to respond to a demand for additional blood flow, e.g., as would occur at mealtime. Symptoms of intestinal angina occur at such times in the *"small meal syndrome."*

Arterioles. The arterioles are the major resistance vessels of the small intestine. Mean arterial pressure decreases 45 mm Hg as blood flows through these vessels, which generate 55% of total intestinal vascular resistance. Regulation of intestinal blood flow is mediated almost exclusively by changes in arteriolar diameter. Arteriolar vascular smooth muscle tone is controlled by a dynamic interplay among a variety of local and systemic regulatory pathways. These pathways and their role in the regulation of intestinal blood flow will be discussed later.

Precapillary Sphincter and Capillaries. Mean arterial pressure decreases approximately 18 mm Hg across the capillary bed, which accounts for 22% of total vascular resistance. The capillaries are essentially rigid tubes and have no vascular regulatory role. The precapillary sphincters are individual smooth muscle cells that surround the arteriolar-capillary juncture and serve to regulate the number of perfused capillaries (Fig. 115–6). Although these sphincters open and close in response to local and systemic influences, they contribute very little to the regulation of intestinal resistance and do not play a significant role in the regulation of total intestinal blood flow.

Veins. Under normal circumstances, there is little resistance to flow through the venous network (8% to 10% of total intestinal vascular resistance). This is due to the large diameter of the veins, which is considerably greater than that of corresponding arteries. The walls of the veins are thinner and contain proportionally less smooth muscle than is found in the arterial walls.[11] Venous smooth muscle serves mainly to mobilize pooled venous blood in response to systemic needs and does not contribute to the regulation of intestinal blood flow. However, increases in mesenteric venous resistance under obstructive conditions, such as cirrhosis of the liver, carcinoma of the liver, portal vein thrombosis, or systemic venous hypertension as a result of congestive heart failure, are far more serious than obstruction of large arterial inflow and cannot be compensated for by arteriolar dilation.

Unlike the arterial network of the intestinal tract, which draws blood from several sources, nearly all intestinal venous blood

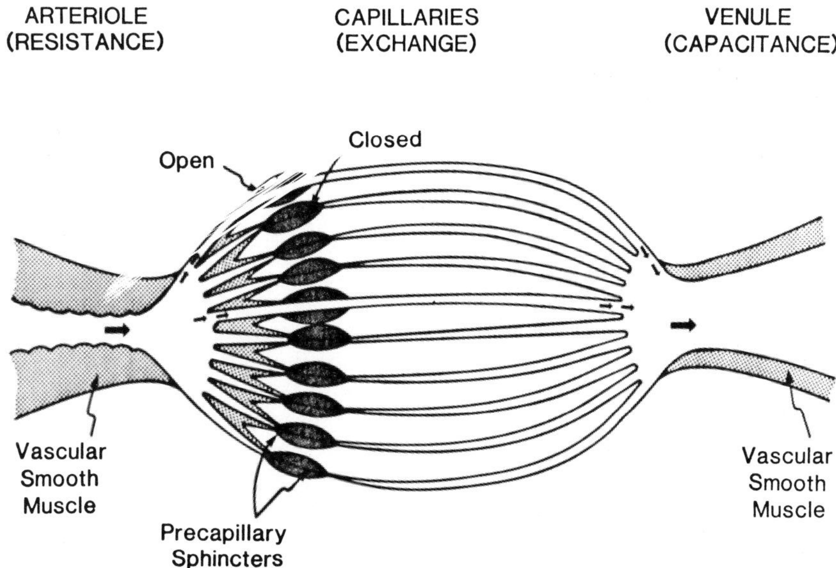

Figure 115–6. Anatomy of the intestinal microcirculation. Note that at any given time, the majority of capillaries are not perfused with blood.

must pass through the portal vein and the liver. Therefore, any increase in resistance at either of these sites will significantly increase portal venous pressure and reduce flow to the entire gastrointestinal tract. This reduction is due to both the decrease in the arterial-venous pressure gradient and a vascular response unique to the intestinal vasculature—the venous-arteriolar response.

It would be expected that normally as venous resistance increased, arteriolar resistance would decrease in order to maintain intestinal blood flow, similar to arterial obstruction. However, one consequence of such a response would be an increase in capillary hydrostatic pressure, which would lead to filtration of fluid out of the capillaries and into the intestinal lumen and tissues. The body could not long tolerate such a loss of fluid, and it appears that this is prevented by the venous-arteriolar response.

The *venous-arteriolar response* is characterized by an increase in arteriolar resistance whenever venous pressure increases.[2] It is believed to be a myogenic response, i.e., it is characteristic of vascular smooth muscle itself and is not mediated by intercellular control mechanisms even though it may be modulated by them. The venous-arteriolar response is part of the compensatory process elicited during the development of portal hypertension. This process involves both a decrease in mesenteric arterial inflow and, if the condition evolves slowly, the development of collateral circulation to increase venous outflow. However, the ability of the intestinal vasculature to compensate for this condition is limited, and the advanced stages of liver disease are characterized by loss of fluid into the peritoneal cavity with the formation of ascites.

Control of Intestinal Vascular Resistance

General. The foregoing discussion of the different components of the intestinal vasculature indicated that the ability of the intestine to regulate blood flow under both normal and pathogenic circumstances depends almost entirely upon its ability to regulate arteriolar vascular smooth muscle tone. The deep embedment of the arterioles in the tissue that they perfuse is ideally suited to permit a rapid response to both local and systemic regulatory pathways. Surprisingly, very little specific information is available about these regulatory pathways. Before discussing individual pathways, however, it may be useful to review the general regulatory principles involved.

In the intestine, as in the stomach, skeletal muscle, heart, and brain, regulation of blood flow appears to be directed toward the maintenance of oxygen delivery at a level adequate to meet the metabolic demands of the tissue. Thus, an increase in systemic arterial pressure is met by an increase in intestinal vascular resistance to prevent excessive intestinal blood flow, and a decrease in arterial pressure prompts a decrease in vascular resistance to prevent a decrease in blood flow. This ability of the intestine to maintain a relatively constant blood flow in the face of changes in perfusion pressure is termed *pressure autoregulation* (or more simply *autoregulation*).

Autoregulation is mediated by local or intrinsic regulatory pathways. On the other hand, there are circumstances in which the body must sacrifice intestinal blood flow to satisfy other demands, such as increased skeletal muscle blood flow during exercise or maintenance of systemic blood pressure during circulatory shock. Under these conditions, extrinsic regulatory pathways are activated. These are pathways that originate outside the intestinal tract and serve the needs of the body as a whole. There is a constant interaction between the intrinsic and extrinsic regulatory pathways, the final effect on arteriolar vascular smooth muscle tone representing the algebraic sum of these opposing influences.

Extrinsic Regulatory Pathways

NEURAL. The intestine is innervated by both the sympathetic and the parasympathetic branches of the autonomic nervous system. In general, the parasympathetic nerves have very little direct effect on intestinal blood flow, their main purpose being to regulate intestinal secretion and motility. The sympathetic nervous system appears to act primarily on intestinal blood vessels and to have very little effect on intestinal function.[13]

The major neurotransmitter of the sympathetic nervous system is *norepinephrine,* a potent intestinal vasoconstrictor. Therefore, intestinal blood flow decreases initially under conditions that elicit sympathetic discharge, such as fear, exercise, or shock. The control of the sympathetic nervous system over intestinal blood flow is not absolute, however, and the intestinal vasculature exhibits a phenomenon referred to as *autoregulatory escape.*

As the name implies, autoregulatory escape involves the activation of local mechanisms that offset the effects of sympathetic nervous activity. Thus, if the fibers of the sympathetic nervous system are stimulated, the initial response is a decrease in intestinal blood flow. As noted earlier, intrinsic mechanisms operate to maintain a constant blood flow; despite continuous stimulation by sympathetic nerves, blood flow begins to return to the control level and the intestinal tract escapes the vasoconstrictive effects of sympathetic discharge. In an extreme condition, such as shock, the intestinal vasculature loses its ability to escape the effects of sympathetic discharge, perhaps because of the activation of humoral regulatory mechanisms in addition to the neural activation.

HUMORAL. Blood-borne agents that appear to alter intestinal resistance include circulating catecholamines (epinephrine and norepinephrine), angiotensin II, and vasopresin. Gastrointestinal hormones, such as glucagon, vasoactive intestinal polypeptide (VIP), and cholecystokinin (CCK), are dilator agents but probably never achieve concentrations in the systemic circulation sufficient to dilate mesenteric vessels directly. The circulating catecholamines, angiotensin II, and vasopressin are all vasoconstrictors and under resting conditions are not released in sufficient quantities to affect blood flow. However, under extreme conditions, such as hemorrhagic shock, they circulate in concentrations sufficient to decrease intestinal blood flow and reinforce the effects of sympathetic activation.

Intrinsic Regulatory Pathways

NEURAL. In addition to the fibers of the autonomic nervous system, both the small and large intestine have 2 discrete networks of intramural nerves: (1) the myenteric (Auerbach's) plexus, which lies between the circular and longitudinal muscle layers, and (2) the submucosal (Meissner's) plexus, which is in the submucosal layer.[1] A number of substances that have been proposed as intramural nerve fiber transmitters have also been shown to dilate the intestinal vasculature, including VIP, substance P, the enkephalins, and adenosine triphosphate (ATP).

Although it is quite possible that alterations in intestinal blood flow or function would result in intramural nerve fiber stimulation and the release of neurotransmitters, it is difficult to see how this would constitute an effective regulatory mechanism. The fact that these fibers are confined to the neural plexuses, which are anatomically separated from the mass of intestinal tissue, requires the neurotransmitter to diffuse a considerable distance across many membranes before acting on enough blood vessels to alter intestinal blood flow appreciably. This is especially true of the fibers of the myenteric plexus. The fibers of the submucosal plexus, however, could release their neurotransmitters into the submucosal vessels, which are in an in-series relationship with the mucosal vessels. At present, it is uncertain whether intramural nerve fibers and their neurotransmitters help regulate intestinal blood flow.

HORMONAL. Three gastrointestinal hormones that are synthesized and released in the walls of the gastrointestinal tract may play a role in the regulation of intestinal blood flow (Chapter 241). Secretin, gastrin, and CCK have been claimed to be intestinal vasodilators and are released into the circulation following a meal. Of the 3 hormones, CCK is the most likely candidate as a mediator of postprandial hyperemia. CCK is a potent intestinal dilator and preferentially dilates the mucosal blood vessels in a manner similar to the postprandial response. Furthermore, it may be vasoactive at the levels reached in the systemic circulation following a meal,[2] although this is disputed.[14]

Both secretin and gastrin dilate the intestinal vasculature but are not vasoactive at the levels reached following a meal. Furthermore, synthetic secretin, which is not contaminated with CCK and VIP (as is extracted secretin), is not vasoactive.[14] It is possible that the tissue concentrations of these hormones are significantly higher than their blood levels. If so, this would allow CCK, and perhaps other hormones, to mediate at least the postprandial intestinal hyperemia and possibly other aspects of intestinal blood flow.

PARACRINE SUBSTANCES. In addition to the classic gastrointestinal hormones, there are a variety of vasoactive paracrine substances that are synthesized and released within the small and large intestine, including serotonin (5HT), histamine, bradykinin, and the prostaglandins. Histamine, bradykinin, and the prostaglandins PGE_2, PGD_2, and PGI_2 are all intestinal vasodilators. The thromboxanes (TxA_2 and TxB_2) and PGF_2 are vasoconstrictors, and the response to serotonin varies.[2]

Histamine dilates the mesenteric circulation through both its H_1 and H_2 receptors.[15] There is evidence that histamine may play an important role in the postprandial intestinal hyperemia. Blockade of H_1 histamine receptors has been shown to reduce considerably both the increase in blood flow and the increase in metabolism induced by food.[16] On the other hand, prostaglandins, which appear to be important in the maintenance of resting intestinal blood flow, apparently act to inhibit postprandial intestinal hyperemia.[17]

Serotonin does not appear to play a direct role in the regulation of postprandial intestinal hyperemia.[2] It has been proposed, however, as a possible mediator of the vasodilator response to mucosal irritation. In addition, serotonin may be involved in the vasodilator response to the infusion of secretin or CCK and so may play an indirect role in the regulation of intestinal blood flow.[2] Although bradykinin is a potent intestinal vasodilator, there is no current evidence to indicate that it is a physiologic regulator of intestinal blood flow.

METABOLIC REGULATION. Metabolic factors have long been recognized as one of the major pathways in the regulation of intestinal blood flow. It has been assumed that some metabolic by-products are vasoactive owing to their direct effects on arteriolar vascular smooth muscle. As tissue metabolism increases, the amount of dilator metabolites produced increases, and if these metabolites are not carried away in the venous effluent, their tissue concentrations increase. By definition, this increase in the concentration of dilator metabolites would result in a decrease in arteriolar vascular smooth muscle tone. The resulting increase in blood flow would wash out the dilator metabolites until a new steady state was achieved. The concentration of dilator metabolites in the tissue in this situation would be the same as that at rest. However, both metabolism and blood flow would be increased, the latter at least transiently, and would lead to phasic changes in local blood flow. Similarly, if the metabolic rate decreased, the concentration of dilator metabolites would decrease and arteriolar vascular smooth muscle tone would increase. Again, blood flow would decrease until resting dilator tissue concentrations of metabolites were restored.[13]

There is no question that metabolic regulation of intestinal blood flow plays a major role in autoregulation and autoregulatory escape and that it acts to moderate the deleterious effects of the venous-arteriolar response on intestinal blood flow. However, at present there is no clear evidence to indicate which metabolite or metabolites mediate these responses. Some possible mediators are K^+, H^+, P_{CO_2}, lactate, prostaglandins, histamine, adenosine, and adenine nucleotides, as well as tissue osmolality and P_{O_2}, but none has been demonstrated to be closely linked with metabolically induced changes in blood flow. It may be that alterations in the entire metabolic environment mediate the circulatory response rather than changes in just 1 or 2 particular metabolites.

MECHANICAL INFLUENCES. This category includes compression of the small arteries during intestinal contractions or distention and the myogenic response. The effects of external compression will be discussed more fully later, but in general they do not have a regulatory role per se. Mention has already been made of the myogenic response in relation to the venous-arteriolar reflex, and it may also play a role in autoregulation. The myogenic response is an inherent property of vascular smooth muscle and involves a reflex contraction whenever the muscle is stretched. Conversely, a decrease in stretch evokes a decrease in muscle tone.

The controlling factor in the myogenic response is the transmural pressure, i.e., the difference between intravascular pressure and tissue pressure. Either systemic or portal hypertension will increase the transmural pressure and stretch the vascular smooth muscle, resulting in a reflex vasoconstriction. Conversely, a decrease in transmural pressure due to systemic hypotension or external compression will decrease vascular smooth muscle stretch and result in vasodilation. Although this mechanism can be invoked to explain autoregulation, the actual contribution of the myogenic response to autoregulation in the intestine is controversial.[2] There is no doubt, however, that the myogenic response mediates the intestinal venous-arteriolar response.

Summary. Intestinal blood flow is determined by the pressure gradient through the vascular bed and by vascular resistance. The major determinant of vascular resistance is the internal radius of the arterioles, which is inversely proportional to vascular smooth muscle tone. Although the pressure gradient may change under extreme conditions, the moment to moment regulation of intestinal blood flow is mediated by changes in arteriolar resistance.

The level of resistance in the intestinal vasculature is determined by the constant interplay of a number of regulatory mechanisms. In general, extrinsic systems act to reduce intestinal blood flow in order to maintain systemic arterial pressure and to divert blood to other organs. Intrinsic mechanisms maintain tissue perfusion at levels that are sufficient to meet metabolic demand and to mediate functional vascular responses such as the postprandial intestinal hyperemia.

Extrinsic control is exercised mainly by the sympathoadrenal complex, with additional input from angiotensin II and vasopressin under extreme conditions, such as shock or heart failure. Intrinsic control is a complex phenomenon that may be mediated by neural, hormonal, paracrine, metabolic, or myogenic mechanisms. Normally, the metabolic regulation of intestinal blood flow dominates resting blood flow and probably mediates autoregulatory responses. In addition, metabolic influences may counteract the effects of the venous-arteriolar response on intestinal blood flow and probably play a significant role in postprandial intestinal hyperemia. Paracrine substances may be important in maintaining intestinal blood flow and appear to play a role in postprandial intestinal hyperemia, as do the gastrointestinal hormones. The myogenic response mediates the venous-arteriolar response and may contribute to autoregulation.

Blood Flow and Intestinal Function

The 2 principal functions of the gastrointestinal tract, absorption and secretion, are dependent upon an adequate supply of blood. In the intestine, the active transport of nutrients and solutes, either out of or into the intestinal lumen, requires a continuous delivery of oxygen and metabolic substrates to the cells of the villi and crypts. Similarly, passive absorption of nutrients depends upon the removal of absorbed nutrients from the mucosa in order to sustain the diffusion gradients across the mucosal epithelia. The intestinal vascular smooth muscle receives a considerably smaller fraction of total intestinal blood flow than does the mucosa. Yet it is essential that perfusion of the muscularis is adequate, since normal intestinal motility is necessary for other intestinal functions. Paradoxically, the direct effect of intestinal visceral muscle contraction is to impede the flow of blood both to itself and to the mucosa. The following sections will consider the relationship between blood flow and absorption/secretion and the effects of motility and luminal distention on intestinal blood flow.

Absorption and Secretion

Water. Water moves passively across membranes in response to osmotic or hydrostatic gradients in all tissues of the body. In the absorbing intestine, the osmotic gradient is maintained by 2 mechanisms: (1) the continuous active transport of sodium and other solutes from the lumen into the interstitial space, and (2) the continuous removal of absorbed water and solutes by the venous and lymphatic circulations.

The movement of fluids between the capillary and interstitial spaces is described by the following equation:

$$J_{v,c} = K_{f,c}\,[(P_c - P_t) - \sigma_d(\pi_p - \pi_t)] \quad \text{(Equation 3)}$$

where $J_{v,c}$ is the capillary filtration rate, the rate at which fluid moves across the capillary wall; $K_{f,c}$ is the capillary filtration coefficient, an index of the exchange capacity of the blood vessels; σ_d is the osmotic reflection coefficient, an index of the permeability of the capillary to large molecular weight molecules such as proteins; P_c and P_t (referred to along with π_p and π_t as the *Starling forces*) are, respectively, the capillary and tissue hydrostatic pressures; and π_p and π_t are, respectively, the plasma and tissue colloid oncotic pressures, which are related to the protein concentration in each compartment.[15]

This equation is a precise representation of *Starling's hypothesis* that the rate at which fluid moves across the capillary wall is determined by the balance of those forces that favor the movement of water out of the capillary (P_c and π_t) and those favoring its movement into the capillary (P_t and π_p). Because capillary hydrostatic pressure is far greater than tissue hydrostatic pressure, the hydrostatic pressure gradient ($P_c - P_t$) favors filtration of fluid out of the capillary. Conversely, plasma colloid oncotic pressure gradient ($\pi_p - \pi_t$) favors absorption of fluid into the capillary. If ($P_c - P_t$) exceeds $\sigma_d(\pi_p - \pi_t)$, then $J_{v,c}$ is positive and filtration occurs. If ($P_c - P_t$) is less than $\sigma_d(\pi_p - \pi_t)$, then $J_{v,c}$ is negative and absorption occurs. Under resting conditions, filtration is favored and the filtered fluid is returned to the systemic circulation by means of the lymphatic circulation.

During absorption of fluid and solutes from the lumen of the gut, the movement of water into the mucosal interstitial space has 2 effects on the Starling forces. The first is an increase in tissue hydrostatic pressure (P_t) by increasing the volume of fluid in the interstitial space. The second effect is a reduction in tissue colloid oncotic pressure (π_t) by dilution of the interstitial fluid, thereby reducing the concentration of protein in the interstitial space. As seen in Equation 3, an increase in P_t will reduce the hydrostatic pressure gradient ($P_c - P_t$), which normally favors filtration, and a decrease in π_t will increase the colloid oncotic pressure gradient ($\pi_p - \pi_t$), which normally favors absorption. The net result is a reversal of the net fluid flux ($J_{v,c}$) in the capillaries from filtration to absorption. Additionally, the increase in tissue hydrostatic pressure increases the rate of movement of interstitial fluid into the lymphatics. Both mechanisms serve to remove absorbed water from the intestinal tissues.

Intestinal secretion under normal circumstances and in response to agents such as cholera toxin is not a passive process. Secretion involves the active transport of ions into the intestinal lumen and the subsequent passive movement of water down its osmotic gradient. This, in turn, reduces the amount of water in the interstitial space, thereby reducing tissue hydrostatic pressure (P_t) and increasing tissue colloid oncotic pressure (π_t). The net result is enhancement of the movement of water out of the capillaries and into the interstitial space. As regards intestinal fluid absorption and secretion, therefore, alterations in capillary fluid dynamics are normally secondary events; the primary mechanism for absorption and secretion is the active transport of ions and other solutes across the mucosal epithelium.[16]

One condition, however, can produce intestinal secretion by means of a direct effect on the balance of the Starling forces, i.e., portal venous hypertension. Any increase in venous blood pressure is reflected back into the capillaries and produces an increase in the capillary hydrostatic pressure. This, in turn, increases the rate of fluid filtration into the interstitium and thence into the intestinal lumen and lymphatic circulation simply as a result of the increased hydrostatic pressure gradient. If this condition is also accompanied by a decrease in the plasma protein concentration, as is the case in advanced stages of liver disease, the rate of fluid filtration is even greater. This ensues because of the decrease in plasma colloid oncotic pressure, the principal Starling force favoring movement of fluid back into the capillary.[17]

Two physiologic mechanisms act to compensate for the effects of venous hypertension on fluid filtration. The first is an increase in lymph flow due to the increase in tissue hydrostatic pressure; although this does not alter the rate of fluid filtration, it does preserve total body fluid volume. The second compensatory mechanism is the venous-arteriolar reflex or response. As mentioned previously, any increase in mesenteric venous pressure produces a reflex increase in arteriolar resistance and this acts to reduce capillary hydrostatic pressure. However, increased arteriolar resistance would diminish intestinal blood flow and could lead to malabsorption of nutrients.

The capacity of these 2 mechanisms to compensate for the effects of portal venous hypertension appears to depend upon the etiology of the disease process. In cases of acute portal venous hypertension, such as that produced by partial or total occlusion of the portal vein, the compensatory mechanisms are ineffectual and fluid loss is considerable. If untreated, the condition results in death within a few hours. If the venous hypertension develops slowly, as in the case of cirrhosis of the liver, ascites and watery diarrhea do not develop until the final stages of the disease.[17]

Nutrients. Superior mesenteric artery blood flow is considerably increased following a meal. The increased flow is directed to those portions of the intestine that have been exposed to chyme, implying a functional relationship between intestinal blood flow and nutrient absorption. The small intestine is exposed to a wide variety of nutrients that are generally classified according to their mechanism of absorption as active or passive. The latter category is further divided into those nutrients that are lipid soluble and those that are water soluble.

In general, there appears to be a positive linear correlation between intestinal blood flow and the passive absorption of lipid-soluble substances.[5, 16] Although the exact relationship varies according to the individual nutrients, intestinal absorption of lipid-soluble substances appears to be flow-limited. On the other hand, passive absorption of water-soluble substances with a molecular weight greater than 100 is flow-independent. This is due to the relative impermeability of the intestinal epithelium to these nutrients so that absorption is diffusion-limited. The absorption of actively transported nutrients is generally flow-independent as well, provided that flow is at a level sufficient to meet the metabolic demands of the active transport processes.

While the relationship between blood flow and the absorption of individual nutrients in isolated intestinal segments appears to be fairly clear, the integrated response of the intact small intestine to chyme is considerably more complex. The presence of bile in the lumen appears to enhance the hyperemic effect of food considerably, without altering intestinal metabolism or the rate of nutrient absorption and despite the lack of any direct effect of bile on intestinal blood flow.[18] There is additional evidence that the intermediates of protein digestion may have vasodilatory effects in the small intestine even though the absorbed end products do not. Thus, the presence of chyme in the intestinal lumen apparently activates a variety of local regulatory mechanisms (neural reflexes or the release of paracrine substances) that alter blood flow independent of the process of nutrient absorption.

The absorption of nutrients from the intestinal lumen is associated on the whole with at least a moderate increase in intestinal blood flow, an effect that appears to facilitate the absorptive process. Furthermore, intestinal ischemia may inhibit nutrient absorption, even though it would probably require a severe ischemic condition to result in malnutrition due to malabsorption. The malabsorption syndrome has rarely been reported in patients with congestive heart failure, a disease associated with intestinal ischemia as well as portal hypertension. The infrequency of the malabsorption syndrome with intestinal ischemia may be due to the capacity of the small bowel to absorb nearly all nutrients in the proximal part of the organ, leaving the distal small intestine to act as an absorptive "reserve."[19] Although it is true that patients with the "small meal syndrome" (abdominal angina) are often malnourished, this is due to the behavioral response to pain and not to ischemic malabsorption.

Motility and Distention

THE EFFECTS OF BLOOD FLOW ON MOTILITY. Increases in intestinal blood flow apparently have no effect on either colonic or small bowel motor activity. Similarly, reductions in muscularis blood flow of 50% to 70% do not appear to damage intestinal smooth muscle.[20] This is probably related to the lower metabolic rate of smooth muscle relative to the mucosal tissues and the ability of smooth muscle to meet these demands during periods of ischemia by means of anaerobic glycolysis.

Total occlusion of the mesenteric artery or extreme hypoxia (75% reduction in arterial PO_2) has been shown to elicit an immediate but transient increase in intestinal motility. This period of increased activity lasts from 1 to 5 minutes and appears to be neurally mediated. Following this initial response to ischemia or anoxia, intestinal motility decreases and smooth muscle contractions are abolished within 15 minutes. Intestinal motility has been shown to return quickly to control levels, even after 3 hours of ischemia. More prolonged ischemia, however, results in permanent damage.[20]

THE EFFECTS OF MOTILITY ON BLOOD FLOW. As noted previously, all arteries and veins that perfuse the intestinal wall must pass through the muscularis and are subject to total or partial occlusion during intestinal smooth muscle contractions. Of the 3 layers of the intestinal wall, the mucosa and submucosa receive the greatest share of total intestinal blood flow and are the most likely to suffer the adverse effects of intestinal motility.

The consequences of intestinal smooth muscle contractions in relation to mucosal blood flow depend on the nature of the contraction (rhythmic versus tonic), the strength of the contraction, and the length of intestine involved. Ordinarily, only tonic contractions of considerable strength and involving a considerable portion of the intestinal wall, such as those seen in the colon during bulk movement following a meal, result in a sustained decrease in local mucosal blood flow. The lack of change in blood flow during less strenuous motor events is due to 2 efficient compensatory mechanisms of the gut that offset the effects of motility on intestinal blood flow.[21]

The most important compensatory mechanism is the autoregulatory ability of the intestinal circulation. As noted earlier, any increase in intestinal arterial resistance can be compensated for by a corresponding decrease in arteriolar resistance, which preserves normal tissue perfusion. The second compensatory mechanism is the extensive network of collateral vessels within the intestinal wall. Most intestinal contractions involve only 1 to 2 cm of the intestinal wall. Therefore, reductions in mucosal blood flow due to the compression of arteries passing through the active portion of the wall are compensated for by increased blood flow through the arteries of adjacent, quiescent portions of the intestine. Together these 2 compensatory mechanisms alleviate the deleterious effects of intestinal motility on mucosal blood flow in all but the most severe and extensive intestinal visceral muscle contractions.[20,21]

THE EFFECTS OF DISTENTION ON BLOOD FLOW. An increase in intestinal luminal pressure acts on the intestinal vasculature in a manner similar to intestinal visceral muscle contractions, i.e., increased pressure in the lumen compresses the relatively compliant mucosal layer and its blood vessels against the more rigid muscularis layers. Distention tends to compromise mucosal blood flow but, as in the response to motor events, there are several compensatory mechanisms that stabilize mucosal blood flow. Autoregulation of intestinal blood flow and an unidentified neural reflex act to maintain mucosal blood flow. In addition to these 2 direct compensatory mechanisms, receptive relaxation of intestinal visceral muscle acts indirectly to maintain mucosal blood flow by reducing pressure in the lumen.

Pressure within the lumen generally does not exceed 20 mm Hg in cases of intestinal blockage, whereas blood flow is not compromised until pressure reaches 30 mm Hg. In rare cases, pathologic conditions can produce a luminal pressure of 50 mm Hg, but even at these levels the reduction in mucosal blood flow is not great.[20, 21]

References

1. Michels NA. Blood Supply and Anatomy of Upper Abdominal Organs with Descriptive Atlas. Philadelphia: JB Lippincott, 1955.
2. Granger DN, Richardson PDI, Kvietys PR, Mortillaro NA. Intestinal blood flow. Gastroenterology 1980; 78:837–63.
3. Reynolds DG, Kardon RH. Methods of studying the splanchnic microvascular architecture. *In:* Granger DN, Bulkley GB, eds. Measurement of Blood Flow, Applications to the Splanchnic Circulation. Baltimore: Williams and Wilkins, 1981: 69–88.
4. Bohlen HG. Intestinal tissue PO_2 and microvascular responses during glucose exposure. Am J Physiol 1980; 238:H164–71.
5. Svanvik J, Lundgren O. Gastrointestinal circulation. *In:*

Crane RK ed. International Review of Physiology, Vol. 12. Baltimore: University Park Press, 1977: 1–34.
6. Bond JH, Levitt DG, Levitt MD. Quantitation of countercurrent exchange during passive absorption from the dog small intestine. J Clin Invest 1977; 59:308–18.
7. Crosby WH. The control of iron balance by the intestinal mucosa. Blood 1963; 22:441–9.
8. Bohlen HG. Na + -induced intestinal interstitial hyperosmolality and vascular responses during absorptive hyperemia. Am J Physiol 1982; 242:H785–9.
9. Winne D. The vasculature of the jejunal villus. *In*: Kramer M, Lauterbach F, eds. Intestinal Permeation. Amsterdam: Excerpta Medica, 1975: 56–7.
10. Richardson PDI, Withrington PG. Physiological regulation of the hepatic circulation. Ann Rev Physiol 1982; 44:57–69.
11. Folkow B, Neil E. Circulation. London: Oxford University Press, 1971.
12. Boley SJ, Brandt LJ, Veith FJ. Ischemic disorders of the intestine. Curr Probl Surg 1978; 15:1–85.
13. Tepperman BL, Jacobson ED. Mesenteric circulation. *In:* Johnson LR, ed. Physiology of the Gastrointestinal Tract. New York: Raven Press, 1981: 1317–36.
14. Bowen JC, Pawlik WW, Fang WF, Jacobson ED. Pharmacological effects of gastrointestinal hormones on intestinal oxygen consumption and blood flow. Surgery 1975; 78:515–9.
15. Richardson PDI, Granger DN. Capillary filtration coefficient as a measure of perfused capillary density. *In:* Granger DN, Bulkley GB, eds. Measurement of Blood Flow, Applications to the Splanchnic Circulation. Baltimore: Williams and Wilkins, 1981: 319–36.
16. Mailman D. Relationships between intestinal absorption and hemodynamics. Ann Rev Physiol 1982; 44:43–55.
17. Bynum TE. Hepatic mechanisms. *In:* Frohlich ED, ed. Pathophysiology. Altered Regulatory Mechanisms in Disease. 3rd Ed. Philadelphia: JB Lippincott, 1984.
18. Tepperman BL, Jacobson ED. The gastric and intestinal vasculatures. *In:* Duthie HL, Wormsley KG, eds. Scientific Basis of Gastroenterology. 2nd Ed. Edinburgh: Churchill Livingstone (in press).
19. Borgstrom B, Dahlqvist A, Ludh G, Sjovall J. Studies of intestinal digestion and absorption in the human. J Clin Invest 1958; 36:1521–36.
20. Chou CC. Relationship between intestinal blood flow and motility. Ann Rev Physiol 1982; 44:29–42.
21. Walus KM, Jacobson ED. Relation between small intestinal motility and circulation. Am J Physiol 1981; 241:G1–15.

Chapter 116

Ischemic Bowel Disease

Arvey I. Rogers • Jay L. Cohen

Ischemic bowel disease results when hypoxic injury to the small and/or large intestine complicates varying degrees of occlusion of the mesenteric arterial or venous circulation.[10, 48] Clinical manifestations depend primarily on the anatomic site of injury, the nature of the occlusive process, and the degree and duration of the ischemic insult. A high index of clinical suspicion is essential to ensure early recognition. Advances in understanding of the complex anatomic and physiologic factors regulating gut blood flow (Chapter 115) and refinements in radiologic diagnostic techniques and in radiologic and surgical therapeutic procedures, along with improved life support systems, have reduced the high rates of morbidity and mortality consequent to delayed diagnosis, intestinal gangrene, perforation with peritonitis, and non-viable intestine. It is the intent of this chapter to highlight these advances.

An appreciation of the relevant functional anatomy and physiology of the mesenteric circulation is basic to understanding the underlying mechanisms and the clinical consequences of the intestinal hypoxia. This understanding, in turn, should facilitate the rational selection and confident application of diagnostic studies and assure earlier and increasingly effective management.

Mesenteric Vasculature

Anatomy

The vascular anatomy of the gut is well described in the preceding chapter (Chapter 115). Some of this is highlighted here as well, however, because of the pertinence of the mesenteric vasculature and its anatomic characteristics to ischemic disease of the bowel.

Arterial. With the exception of the esophagus and distal rectum, the gastrointestinal tract is oxygenated by arterial blood delivered by 3 unpaired branches of the aorta: the celiac axis, the superior mesenteric artery, and the inferior mesenteric artery. An extensive collateral circulation depends upon the development and patency of numerous anastomotic channels linking these major arterial trunks (Fig. 116–1). Whatever the cause, a reduction in oxygen delivered to the gut wall by way of these arteries or their collateral channels is the inciting event and critical determinant of hypoxic injury of the bowel. Understanding the arterial and parallel venous anatomy constituting the mesenteric circulation provides a basis for appreciating the clinical consequences of reduced flow involving one or several major vessels and the organs they supply.[10, 33, 48, 57, 83, 111] Chapter 115 provides important information relevant to mesenteric vascular anatomy. Further details are provided here.

Celiac Axis. The celiac axis, a large vessel arising at almost right angles to the aorta at the level of the T12 to L1 vertebrae, rapidly divides into its 3 major branches: hepatic, left gastric, and splenic arteries. The stomach receives arterial blood from all 3 branches. The lesser curvature is supplied by the left gastric artery, which occasionally anastomoses with the right gastric branch of the hepatic artery. The gastroduodenal branch of the hepatic artery gives origin to the right gastroepiploic and superior (posterior and anterior) pancreaticoduodenal arteries. The splenic artery divides into the short gastric and left gastroepiploic arteries, which provide circulation to the greater curvature of the stomach and anastomose with the right gastroepiploic artery.

Important interconnections exist between branches of the celiac and superior mesenteric arteries. The

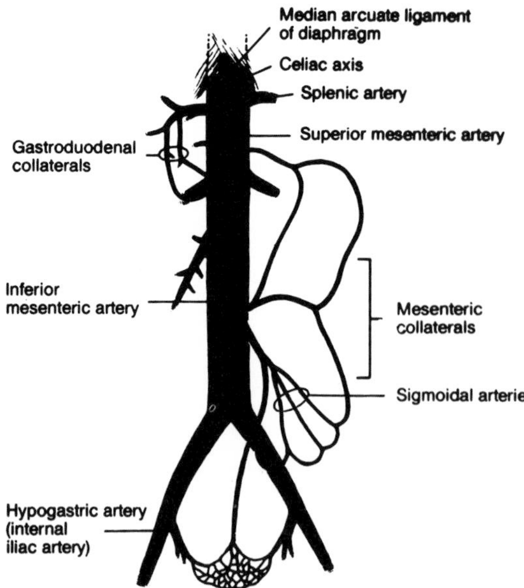

Figure 116–1. Mesenteric arterial circulation and major collateral and anastomotic channels.

superior pancreaticoduodenal branches of the gastroduodenal artery anastomose with the inferior (posterior and anterior) pancreaticoduodenal branches of the superior mesenteric artery to form the pancreaticoduodenal arcades. The latter provide a rich blood supply to the duodenum and neighboring head of the pancreas as well as an important communication between 2 of the 3 major mesenteric arterial trunks. The generous circulation to and anastomotic channels about the stomach account for the rarity of isolated gastric infarction.[48]

Superior Mesenteric Artery. Arising just beneath the celiac axis, the superior mesenteric artery originates from the anterior surface of the aorta posterior to the body of the pancreas at the level of the L1 vertebra. Its downward and forward course takes it over the uncinate process of the pancreas and anterior to the third portion of the duodenum. The inferior pancreaticoduodenal branch arising early from this artery has already been discussed as a major collateral channel that assures adequacy of the arterial circulation through the pancreaticoduodenal arcades when flow by way of the celiac axis is compromised. Three major branches of the superior mesenteric artery, the middle colic, right colic, and ileocolic arteries and up to 20 intestinal branches, provide arterial blood to the entire small intestine, the cecum, and the ascending, hepatic flexure, and proximal transverse colon regions. The intestinal branches arising from the superior mesenteric artery just proximal and distal to the origin of the ileocolic branch form a series of 3 or 4 arcades before penetrating the intestinal wall as end arteries *(arteriae rectae).* The main trunk of the superior mesenteric artery continues as the ileocolic artery, supplying the terminal ileum, cecum, and proximal ascending colon. The right colic artery, which may arise from a common middle colic–right colic trunk (50% of the population) or the superior mesenteric artery directly (40%), supplies blood to the ascending colon and hepatic flexure. The middle colic artery supplies the proximal portion of the transverse colon and anastomoses with right and left colic (branch of the inferior mesenteric artery) arteries.[10, 83, 111]

Inferior Mesenteric Artery. The smallest in caliber of the 3 main mesenteric arteries, the inferior mesenteric branch, arises from the aorta at the level of the L3 vertebra; divides into the left colic and sigmoid arteries, which provide blood to the distal transverse, descending, and sigmoid colon; and terminates as the superior rectal artery, which supplies the proximal rectum. The distal rectum is supplied by the middle and inferior rectal branches of the internal iliac artery by way of its hypogastric branch.[82]

Anastomotic Considerations (Fig. 116–1).[111]. The left colic branch of the inferior mesenteric artery and the middle branch of the superior mesenteric artery form an anastomotic connection known as the *arc of Riolan* or the *meandering mesenteric artery.* Injection of the ileocolic artery results in filling of the right, middle, left, and sigmoid arteries through a central anastomotic artery known as the *marginal artery of Drummond.* This artery parallels the entire colon, giving rise to its own arteriae rectae. It must be adequate enough to compensate for reduced arterial flow to the colon in circumstances of compromised flow through the middle or left colic arteries. In some patients, however, this artery is an unimportant channel.

It is theoretically possible, hence, for 1 of the 3 major mesenteric arteries to supply all of the intra-abdominal viscera if sufficient collateral flow has had time to develop through 1 of the 3 major collateral channels described, i.e., pancreaticoduodenal arcade (celiac axis–superior mesenteric artery); arc of Riolan (superior mesenteric artery–inferior mesenteric artery), and marginal artery of Drummond (superior mesenteric artery–inferior mesenteric artery–iliac artery). Acute occlusive disease developing on a background of previously normal mesenteric arterial flow (superior mesenteric artery embolus) or involving end arteriae rectae (vasculitis) cannot undergo compensation by collateral channels, and segmental or diffuse gut ischemia thus results.

Finally, it is important to recall that regions of the colon and rectum supplied through anastomotic connections, e.g., the distal transverse colon and splenic flexure (superior mesenteric artery–inferior mesenteric artery) and the rectum (inferior mesenteric hypogastric arteries), are relatively underperfused. They are designated "watershed" areas and are therefore more susceptible to ischemic injury complicating inferior mesenteric artery occlusion or underperfusion.[76, 77, 100]

Venous. For the most part, veins parallel arteries in the mesenteric circulation. The superior mesenteric and splenic veins join to form the portal vein, which enters the liver. The inferior mesenteric vein drains into the splenic vein. Collaterals between the splanchnic and systemic circulations function importantly when portal hypertension or occlusion of the inferior vena cava develops. Superior mesenteric vein thrombosis is the major cause of mesenteric venous thrombosis.[47, 48]

Table 116–1. ACUTE MESENTERIC ISCHEMIA: PATHOPHYSIOLOGY

Arterial spasm Inadequate collateral flow Reduced perfusion pressure	Secondary occlusion	ARTERIAL (spasm, embolus, thrombus) VENOUS (thrombus)	May result in:
Ischemia → Infarction → Gangrene → Perforation → PERITONITIS			

→ = May lead to.

Acute Ischemic Syndromes

Temporary or permanent reductions of mesenteric arterial or venous flow are the primary factors in the development of gut wall ischemia.[10, 15] Inadequate collateral flow, arterial spasm, and a reduction in perfusion pressure may initiate or aggravate the ischemic insult to the small intestine and/or colon (Table 116–1). The most serious consequence is tissue infarction, which can eventuate in gangrene, perforation, and peritonitis. Failure to diagnose ischemia accurately prior to development of gangrene, the progression of bowel infarction even after the inciting or aggravating factors are corrected, the high frequency of non-occlusive mesenteric ischemia, and the fact that acute mesenteric ischemia primarily affects older persons already afflicted with cardiovascular, renal, or other systemic disorders together account for the high mortality rates of 50% to 70%.[13] Half of the cases of acute mesenteric infarction are caused by embolic or thrombotic occlusion of the superior mesenteric artery. Of the remaining 50%, half are due to non-occlusive infarction and half result from occlusion of the inferior mesenteric artery, mesenteric venous thrombosis, or arteritis.[87] Some investigators attribute a greater proportion of instances of vascular insufficiency to non-occlusive disease.[8]

Superior Mesenteric Artery Ischemia

Etiology. Acute mesenteric artery insufficiency results from occlusion or from non-occlusive vasoconstriction of the major mesenteric arteries or their branches.[55,84–87,96,99,104] The superior mesenteric artery is virtually always involved (Fig. 116–2). Causes vary, but most patients have associated cardiovascular and/or generalized atherosclerotic disease.

Arterial atherosclerosis, embolism, dissection of an aortic aneurysm, fibromuscular hyperplasia, and oral contraceptive–associated thromboembolic disease are the major causes of acute occlusion of one or more of the major mesenteric arteries. Small arterial branches, including intramural arteriae rectae, may become involved in systemic disorders associated with vasculitis (Chapter 244).

The most common of the foregoing causes is *atherosclerotic disease,* usually involving and occluding 2 of the 3 mesenteric arteries. The luminal occlusion as a rule is at or proximal to the aortic origin of the vessel,[48, 58] but the atherosclerotic process may involve any portion of the artery or its branches. Emboli generally lodge at bifurcations of branches of major vessels and therefore can be easily distinguished from thrombi at the time of surgery, should this be undertaken.[86]

Conditions leading to systemic *hypoperfusion* predispose to the occurrence of mesenteric artery insufficiency on the basis of reflex vasoconstriction.[13, 15, 54, 85, 89] Non-occlusive ischemia, congestive heart failure, cardiac chamber dilatation or arrhythmias, hypotension, and hypovolemia are common antece-

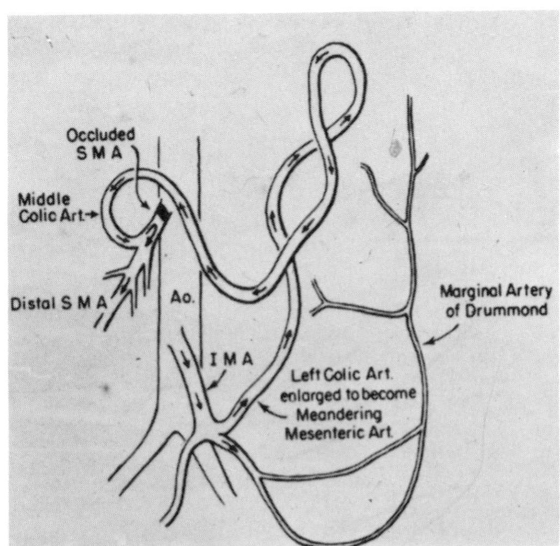

Figure 116–2. Stenosis of the superior mesenteric artery (SMA) associated with a large marginal artery of Drummond.

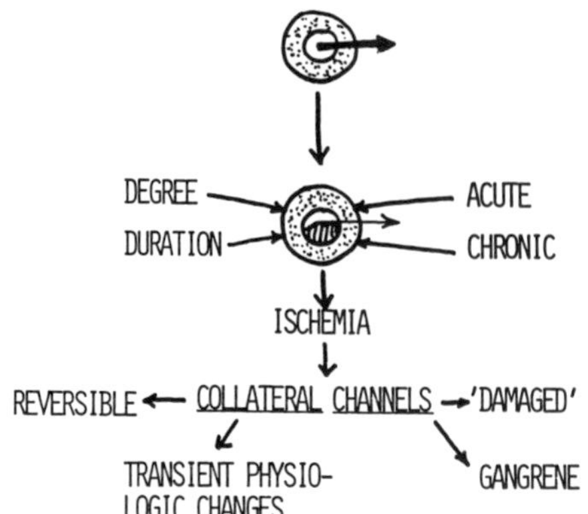

Figure 116–3. Schema illustrating pathophysiology of mesenteric ischemia and emphasizing factors that influence severity and outcome.

dents. Hypoxemia and drug-induced arterial vasoconstriction (e.g., digoxin, adrenergic agents, and vasopressin) are additional factors that may initiate or aggravate non-occlusive intestinal ischemia.

Pathophysiology.[15] When arterial occlusion is abrupt, complete, prolonged, or occurs in the absence of adequate compensatory collateral vascular channels, it is likely that irreversible ischemia of the intestinal wall will result. On the other hand, when the occlusive process is gradual, incomplete, or transient and well-developed collateral channels exist, reversible ischemia is likely (Fig. 116–3). The anatomic and physiologic responses to mesenteric occlusion that results in a reduction in arterial perfusion pressure are reviewed in Chapter 115. Essentially, it has been determined that a critical time interval of several hours exists during which local and humoral factors can maintain adequate intestinal blood flow distal to a major vessel occlusion. Prolongation of the occlusive process may result in a sustained reduction in arterial perfusion pressure and progressive ischemia secondary to reflex vasoconstriction, even if the initial occlusive insult is reversed[15] (Fig. 116–4).

Edema, hemorrhage, and sloughing of the sensitive oxygen-deprived intestinal mucosa and submucosa are the predictable sequential pathologic responses to ischemic injury, whatever its etiology. Clinical and radiologic manifestations can be explained on their basis and may predict severity of the ischemic insult. Spasm of the muscularis mucosae, the earliest response to hypoxia, is replaced within hours by ileus. This varies with the severity of intestinal wall injury and is followed by gangrene and perforation. Fibrosis and scarring of the intestinal wall may complicate severe deep injury that did not lead to perforation at the time of the acute insult.[48]

Clinical Features.[8, 10, 26, 28, 29, 48, 54, 55, 61, 87, 99, 105, 123, 124] Occlusive or non-occlusive mesenteric ischemia is most likely to develop in individuals over age 50 with any of the following conditions: (1) valvular or atherosclerotic cardiac disease; (2) chronic congestive heart failure, poorly responsive to digitalis and/or diuretic therapy; (3) cardiac arrhythmias, irrespective of etiology; (4) hypovolemia or hypotension complicating traumatic or pathologic conditions such as burns, gastrointestinal or surgically associated hemorrhage, pancreatitis, protracted vomiting, fulminant diarrhea, intestinal obstruction, or vigorous diuresis; (5) recent myocardial infarction; and (6) previous history of arterial emboli to the extremities.[8, 15, 55]

The clinical features of occlusive and non-occlusive disease are too indistinct to consider separately. Abdominal pain, the most common symptom, is encountered in 78% to 100% of conscious patients. It varies in duration, severity, character, and location but is usually abrupt in onset, diffuse, mid-abdominal, colicky, and severe enough to prompt the patient to seek medical assistance. Less than 15% of patients experiencing acute occlusion of the superior mesenteric artery have had antecedent abdominal angina. Other complaints, seen in less than 50% of patients with proven gut wall ischemia or infarction, include "collapse" (fainting, weakness, stupor), vomiting or diarrhea (either of which may be bloody),

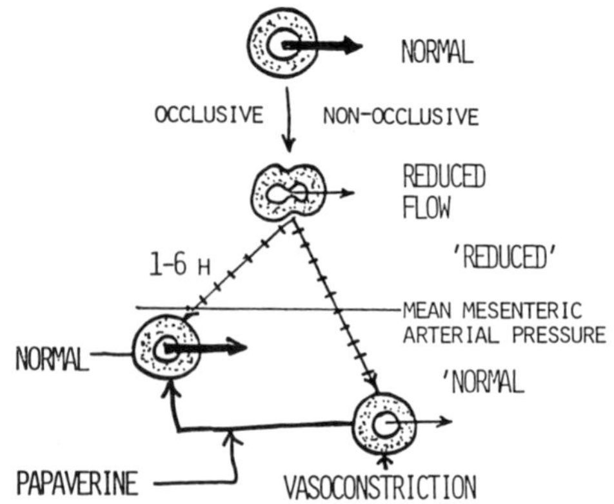

Figure 116–4. Schema illustrating effect of arterial occlusion, critical time interval for "reversibility" to occur, and persistence of spasm despite relief of major occlusive process.

dyspnea, and confusion. The simultaneous onset of spontaneous evacuation of the bowel is a classic symptom of acute occlusive mesenteric ischemia. Non-occlusive ischemia is less likely to be associated with a defecation urge or actual defecation.

Unexplained abdominal distention of gastrointestinal bleeding may be the only manifestations of non-occlusive or occlusive mesenteric ischemia in 15% to 25% of patients who experience pain.[10, 15, 48] Initially, gastrointestinal bleeding is usually evident only as occult blood. Physical findings vary with the severity of the ischemic insult. Early in the presentation, the patient's complaint of pain is disproportionate to the physical findings on abdominal examination. Bowel sounds may be normal or hyperactive, and there may be little or no abdominal tenderness. With progression of the ischemic process, intermittent mid-abdominal pain may become constant and poorly localized. Abdominal distention develops and bowel sounds diminish in frequency and intensity. Transmural necrosis is associated with involuntary guarding and rebound tenderness, features consistent with serositis or perforation with peritonitis. With progression of the ischemic process to frank infarction, systemic manifestations become more prominent and the patient experiences tachycardia, hypotension, fever, hemoconcentration, and pronounced leukocytosis with a left shift. Nausea, vomiting, back pain, hematemesis and/or rectal bleeding, and findings suggesting intestinal obstruction may be observed. These findings indicate advanced disease with an extremely poor prognosis.[10,15,48,55,61,69] One of the most important points to remember about the clinical presentation of ischemic bowel disease is that the clearest sign of early preinfarction ischemia is the presence of severe abdominal pain with an absence of objective abdominal findings in a patient at high risk for the development of ischemic bowel disease.[8]

Diagnosis. No single or set of physical or laboratory findings is specific or pathognomonic for the diagnosis of gut ischemia or ischemic injury, nor can these findings accurately differentiate occlusive from non-occlusive varieties of mesenteric arterial disease. In addition to stress of inflammation-related leukocytosis and hypovolemia induced by fluid loss with resultant hemoconcentration, few other consistently abnormal laboratory findings have been described. Elevated serum amylase activity (rarely more than 2-fold), elevated serum phosphate and intestinal alkaline phosphatase activity, increased excretion of phosphate in the urine, and raised peritoneal fluid phosphate levels usually indicate more severe gut wall injury.[5, 60, 102] Metabolic acidosis is a late and non-specific finding. Based on data from experimental studies in canine models, Barnett et al.[5] demonstrated that a base deficit was an ineffective aid in differentiating mesenteric occlusion from other intra-abdominal catastrophes. Cooke and Sande[26] confirmed that metabolic acidosis cannot be used to differentiate ischemia from an infarcted gut in humans with mesenteric vascular disease. Vomitus and/or stool may contain blood; this finding varies with the site and severity of ischemic injury to the gastrointestinal tract.

Radioisotope techniques utilizing ^{99m}Tc-pyrophosphate or diphosphonate and ^{99m}Tc-colloid sulfur–labeled leukocytes have been evaluated in experimental settings with animals for their ability to diagnosis ischemic injury; they have not yet proved sufficiently reliable or reproducible for human use. Laparoscopy, by making it possible to see the serosal surface of the bowel, enables the possible existence of transmural infarction to be assessed. It is not recommended as a routine procedure in this setting, however.[48]

Abdominal pain films may reveal: (1) dilated small intestinal loops with air-fluid levels consistent with mechanical obstruction or pseudo-obstruction; (2) bowel wall thickening and "thumbprinting" or scalloping; (3) loop separation and thickening of the valvulae conniventes (Fig. 116–5), and (4) intramural or portal air (late findings suggesting clostridial infection). None of these findings is specific enough to be relied upon exclusively for diagnostic purposes.[8, 10, 15]

Contrast studies should *not* be undertaken early in these patients. Barium will move slowly through the atonic small intestine and will also obscure angiographic findings.

Boley and his colleagues[13] have advocated early mesenteric angiography when mesenteric vascular disease is clinically suspected. In addition to identifying major vessel occlusion by embolus or thrombus, it is possible to recognize vasoconstriction as a consequence of non-occlusive ischemia. Four reliable angiographic criteria facilitate recognition of vasoconstriction: (1) narrowing at the origins of branches of the superior mesenteric artery; (2) spasm or other irregularities in the

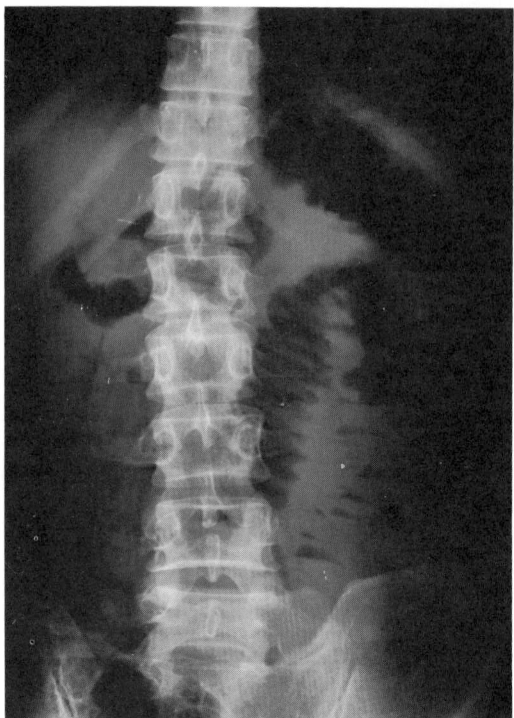

Figure 116–5. Plain abdominal film demonstrating ileus, edema of valvulae, and loop separation by edema in patient with acute ischemic injury of small intestine.

branches of this artery, (3) spasm of the arcade, and (4) impaired filling of intramural vessels. These findings, seen in up to 50% of such patients, have greatest diagnostic validity for non-occlusive ischemia when volume status is normal and the patient is not in shock or receiving vasopressors.[13] Thus, mesenteric angiography may identify splanchnic vasoconstriction and superior mesenteric artery occlusion by embolus or thrombosis. It may also provide anatomic evidence concerning collateralization, the condition of other arterial channels, and the feasibility of subsequent angioplasty or revascularization[52] (Fig. 116–6).

The diagnosis of an infarcted gut may be delayed, or its presence may not be recognized until surgery is undertaken or the patient has died and necropsy is performed. With today's technology and the advances in understanding of the clinical presentation of mesenteric vascular ischemic disease, the frequency of early diagnosis should progressively increase.[8]

Management (Fig. 116–6). Resuscitation, cardiopulmonary support, correction of conditions that predispose to mesenteric artery hypoperfusion, and avoidance of potent vasoconstrictors are general principles that govern the first few hours of management of patients with suspected acute mesenteric artery insufficiency (AMI). If a pressor agent is necessary to maintain blood pressure, *dopamine* (Dopastat) should be utilized. Every effort should be made to prepare the patient for possible surgical intervention before serious complications of congestive heart failure or shock arise. Operative intervention must be considered imminent when peritoneal signs are present and persistent.[26, 29, 48, 55, 96, 99]

Because of (1) mortality figures of 70% to 90% for acute mesenteric ischemic disease, (2) progressive bowel infarction despite correction of the vascular or systemic causes, and (3) recognition of the increasing frequency of occurrence of non-occlusive mesenteric ischemia, Boley and his colleagues[8, 10, 13] developed an aggressive roentgenologic (angiographic) and surgical approach in patients with suspected acute mesenteric ischemia due to occlusion or underperfusion through the superior mesenteric artery. A flush aortogram is first performed to detect aneurysm, dissection, and emboli, as well as to assess collateralization. This is followed by selective angiography of the superior mesenteric artery. Using strict criteria for patient selection, accurately interpreting non-occlusive angiographic findings, applying selective intra-arterial infusion of vasodilating agents, and making earlier decisions about corrective surgery and "second look" operations allowed Boley et al.[13] to reduce the mortality rate to 54% in their initial group of 50 patients. A subsequent controlled trial in 45 other patients with emboli to the superior mesenteric artery compared the outcome utilizing traditional management methods (25 patients) against a strict program employing *intra-arterial papaverine* as a vasodilating agent (20 patients).[11] There was a 20% survival in the control group compared with 55% for patients on the vasodilator protocol, and 4 patients required no surgery. With respect to those recovering, it should be noted that spontaneous reversal of ischemia in some patients was described by Vyden[117] in 1973.

Boley et al.[13] have emphasized that the successful management of patients with acute mesenteric ischemia placed on their

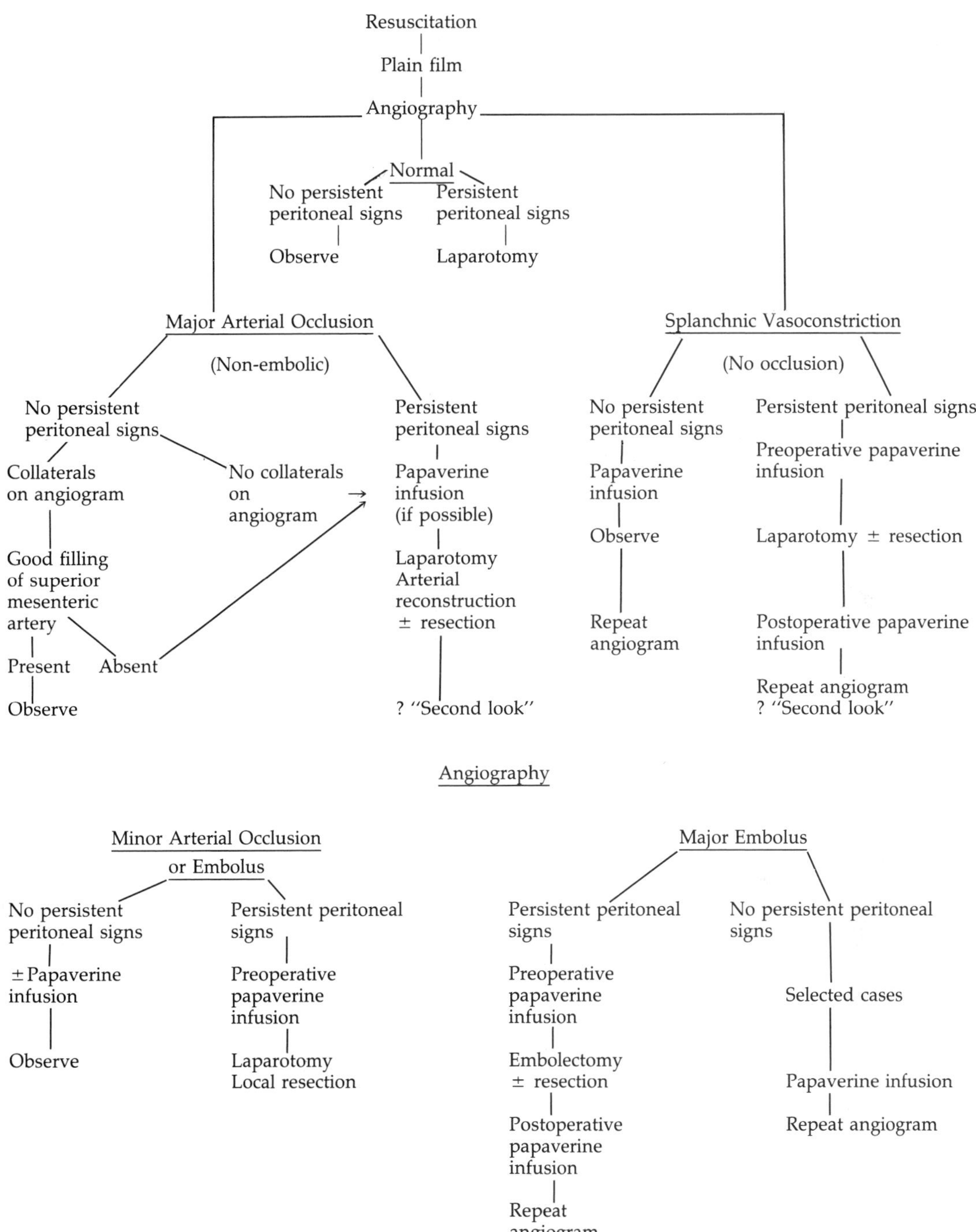

Figure 116–6. Management of superior mesenteric artery ischemia. (From Boley SJ, Borden EB. Acute mesenteric ischemia. *In:* Najarian JS, Delaney JP, eds. Advances in Gastrointestinal Surgery. Copyright © 1984 by Year Book Medical Publishers, Inc., Chicago. Reproduced with permission.)

protocol (Fig. 116–6) requires a high index of suspicion that acute mesenteric ischemia exists, early (less than 12 to 24 hours) mobilization of the angiographer and surgeon, and prompt institution of intra-arterial papaverine infusion. The papaverine infusion is often continued postoperatively following intestinal resection or extraction of an arterial clot.

A variety of vasodilating substances (histamine, phenoxybenzamine, glucagon, papaverine, dopamine, PGE_1)[1, 31, 116] have been utilized or considered to reverse vasoconstriction. The largest clinical experience, however, has been with papaverine in both occlusive and non-occlusive varieties of acute mesenteric ischemia.[8, 15] When initial angiography reveals a major vessel occlusion or non-occlusive vasoconstriction, a bolus intra-arterial injection of 25 mg of tolazoline is employed to facilitate complete visualization of the postobstructive or terminal vasculature. If there is no suspicion of peritonitis, a continuous papaverine infusion of 30 to 60 mg/hour (1 mg/ml) is begun through a catheter secured in the superior mesenteric artery. Repeat angiograms are performed to assess benefit. If a vasodilatory response is observed, the papaverine infusion is continued. At a predetermined time interval, follow-up angiography is performed to assure that the vasoconstrictive features are reversed, and papaverine-free perfusate is substituted. When vasoconstriction remains controlled, papaverine is discontinued. Persistence of vasoconstriction or development of peritoneal signs during infusion of papaverine provides a clear indication for laparotomy and possibly embolectomy, thrombectomy, and/or resection of infarcted bowel.

More than 90% of papaverine is inactivated during passes through the liver, allowing large doses to be given continuously over long periods of time. It is unusual for catheters to clot during continuous infusions. Angiocatheters may be utilized for infusing thrombolytic substances when major or minor vessel occlusion is encountered. Use of anticoagulants is controversial.[8, 13]

Surgical intervention is required when peritoneal signs persist or develop during infusion. Surgery is ideal when acute embolization to the superior mesenteric artery occurs in a young individual without pre-existing extensive arterial disease and should also be undertaken when chances for anatomic success and survival are felt to be good in an elderly, often infirm individual with multisystem disease.[11, 13, 54, 55, 86]

A poor outcome is correlated directly with the extent of infarcted intestine discovered at surgery. Every effort should be made to diagnose non-occlusive mesenteric infarction in order to avoid unnecessary early surgery.[8, 10, 13, 97] The discovery of substantial narrowing of the superior mesenteric artery or other vessels on angiography indicates need for operative or non-operative correction on an elective basis when the patient is more stabilized. There is no exact method for determining the viability of ischemic, non-infarcted bowel at the time of surgery.[17, 27, 65] Visual inspection, palpation of vessels, Doppler ultrasonography, electromyography, injection of radiolabeled microspheres, and intraoperative fluorescein angiography have all been utilized with varying degrees of success.[48, 72] "Second look" operations should be performed if doubt or concern exists about the viability of initially resected intestine. Intra- and postoperative intra-arterial papaverine infusion may reduce the requirement for "second look" surgery.[13] Katz and Williams[66] advocate steroid delivery by the retrograde venous route as a unique therapy for ischemic disease, but this approach has yet to be evaluated widely.

Patients surviving resective surgery usually fare quite well. Short bowel syndromes or malabsorption complicating resection or mucosal injury to bowel left *in situ* can be adapted to by the patient[114] (Chapter 108). Short- or long-term parenteral hyperalimentation has improved survival figures for patients who have undergone extensive resection or who have permanent impairment of small bowel function.

Ischemic Colitis

Boley and colleagues[12] described reversible vascular occlusion of the colon in 1963. Marston et al[77] characterized the syndrome further in 1966 when they described stages and outcomes. Lesions that resulted were ulcerative and hemorrhagic in nature, transitory, and limited to the mucosa and submucosa, or they were more severe, progressing rapidly to necrosis and gangrene. In many patients, the clinical picture was one of mucosal inflammation.

Table 116–2. ISCHEMIC COLITIS: CAUSES*

Impaired left ventricular function
Hypovolemia (hemorrhage, dehyration)
Major artery damage or occlusion:
Aortoiliac reconstruction
Abdominoperineal resection of the rectum
Occlusion of the inferior mesenteric artery:
Thrombosis
Therapeutic embolization
Inadvertent surgical ligation
Miscellaneous:
Hypercoagulable states
Vasculitis
Amyloid
Ruptured aortic aneurysm
Obstructing colorectal cancer
Drugs:
Oral contraceptive agents
Ergot
Vasopressin
Bilateral nephrectomy/transplant

*References 10, 15, 33, 38, 46, 48, 57, 68, 70, 74, and 109.

Etiology (Table 116–2).[48] Occlusion or underperfusion of large and/or small arteries supplying the colon wall predisposes to ischemic injury.[3] Generalized atherosclerosis and impaired left ventricular output secondary to myocardial dysfunction are the leading causes. Sustained hypovolemia complicating hemorrhage, diarrhea, diuresis, or plasma loss, as in pancreatitis, may be implicated. Hyperviscous states predispose to ischemia by reducing the rate of arterial blood flow. Digitalis use during states of hypoperfusion and/or passive congestion may provoke segmental arterial spasm, yet should not be withheld when indicated. The common denominator producing ischemia in all of these circumstances is *hypoxia*.

Pathophysiology.[3, 100, 101] Colonic vascular and circulatory characteristics, splanchnic hemodynamics, intraluminal pressure, and colonic flora interplay to effect or aggravate hypoxic injury to the colonic wall.[100] A major vascular channel providing arterial flow to the colon is the marginal artery of Drummond, which receives its blood volume and pressure from the superior and inferior mesenteric arteries and the hypogastric branch of the iliac artery.[83] Critical points of anastomosis exist in 2 separate areas of the colon: (1) at the junction between the superior and inferior mesenteric arteries near the splenic flexure (Griffith's point), and (2) between the inferior mesenteric artery and the hypogastric vessels (critical point of Sudeck) near the rectosigmoid region. When splanchnic flow is reduced, these regions are most sensitive to ischemic injury. Any region of the colon, however, is subject to focal ischemia. Williams and Wittenberg[125] found ischemic colitis to be located in the left colon in 73% of patients, in the transverse colon in 14%, in the right colon in 8%, and in the rectum and rectosigmoid in 5%. The vast potential for collateral flow mandates that at least 2 of the 3 major arterial channels be occluded before ischemic symptoms occur. A major reduction in splanchnic flow, albeit transient, leads to constriction of intramural arterioles and subjects to ischemic injury those regions of the colon at anastomotic sites that are relatively underperfused. This phenomenon explains the development of ischemia of the colon in the absence of major arterial or venous obstruction.[3, 100, 101] The actual role of spasm, however, has been challenged.[125]

Distention of the colon lumen secondary to mechanical obstruction or paralytic ileus may produce local hemodynamic disturbances and focal circulatory insufficiency in distended regions of the colon.[9, 100] Since the tension in the colon wall is directly proportional to luminal diameter and intraluminal pressure (law of Laplace), the cecum is especially sensitive. This is especially true in individuals with already compromised blood flow. Experimental studies by Boley, et al.[9] have clearly demonstrated the effects of bowel distention on raising intraluminal pressure, reducing total blood flow, and reducing arterial-venous oxygen differences by impairing oxygen extraction in the distended colon wall.

Finally, the "virulence" of colonic microbial flora must be considered in the pathogenesis of inflammation, necrosis, and gangrene complicating ischemic injury to the mucosa.[100]

Clinical Features (Table 116–3).[10] Ischemic colitis affects both sexes at an average age of 70 years but is becoming increasingly recognized as a frequent cause of "inflammatory" colon disease in patients over age 50.[16, 125] The entity may occur in much younger individuals as a presumed complication of oral contraceptive use or without plausible explanation.[4, 34, 43] Irrespective of the age of onset or the cause, classic symptoms include the abrupt onset of crampy lower left or midline abdominal pain, occasional nausea and vomiting, and bloody diarrhea, the last feature clearly dominating the clinical picture. As a

Table 116–3. ISCHEMIC COLITIS: CLINICAL FEATURES

Age:
70 or older
Cause:
Idiopathic
Hypotension
Hypoperfusion
Symptoms:
Abdominal pain
Diarrhea
Rectal bleeding
Diagnosis:
Endoscopy (with or without biopsy)
Barium enema examination
Exclusion
Course:
Severe
Peritonitis
Mild
Resolution in less than 2 weeks
Stricture

rule, patients do not appear acutely ill and only rarely have associated hypotension or features of acute peritonitis, inasmuch as the gangrenous form of ischemic colitis occurs in only an estimated 10% of ischemic episodes. The patients are usually afebrile, have normal or slightly raised pulse rates, and present with mild abdominal distention and diffuse or left lower quadrant abdominal tenderness. A "mass" attributed to edematous thickening of the sigmoid colon wall may be palpated in the left iliac fossa.[48] Digital rectal examination is normal or reveals only mild left wall tenderness with bright blood on the examining finger. Kaminski et al.[64] and Margolis et al.[75] described toxic megacolon resulting from ischemic injury complicated by left colon strictures and deep gangrenous ulcers of the wall of the colon. Their elderly patients presented with acute generalized abdominal pain, massive colonic distention, and signs of systemic toxicity (fever, tachycardia). In the series of Margolis et al.,[75] all 3 patients described milder symptoms of abdominal pain and distention that preceded the onset of the more acute presenting symptom complex by several weeks. Devroede and his associates[32] described 36 patients ranging in age from 40 to 79 years with fecal incontinence, rectal pain, or both, which were thought to be secondary to chronic rectal ischemia. This diagnosis was based on the histologic evidence of atrophy and fibrosis of the lamina propria of rectal mucosa, findings absent in asymptomatic healthy controls.

Diagnosis. *Differential diagnosis* should include infectious and idiopathic inflammatory colitis, pseudomembranous colitis, acute diverticulitis, colon neoplasia, sigmoid volvulus complicated by strangulation obstruction, and pancreatitis.[82] Very infrequent involvement of the rectum or right colon and the absence of multiple skip areas of involvement as well as of deep transmural fissuring, abscesses, cobblestoning, and sinus tracts all mitigate against the roentgenologic diagnosis of idiopathic or granulomatous inflammatory bowel disease.

Laboratory findings are non-specific and reveal changes consistent with mild inflammation. Anemia may be present, especially if the patient experienced significant blood loss from recent surgery or if the colonic bleeding recurred frequently over several weeks prior to establishing the diagnosis. Microscopic examination of the stool or rectal discharge reveals both red and white blood cells. Cultures are negative.

Proctosigmoidoscopy may reveal a grossly normal rectum, non-specific changes of edema or hyperemia, or granular or friable mucosa beginning in the anus and extending proximally in a continuous fashion, consistent with idiopathic ulcerative colitis.[67, 82] Endoscopy may be carried out with a flexible proctosigmoidoscope or a colonoscope so that the rectosigmoid and left colon regions may be inspected.[40, 48, 58, 67, 82, 103] Colonoscopy, however, should be performed with great care or not done at all in a patient with "active" colitis because of the realistic danger of inducing a perforation or diminishing further the already compromised blood flow by increasing intraluminal pressure.[9, 40, 58, 103]

When the rectum is spared, the sigmoid colon may show striking changes of edematous mucosa with associated submucosal hemorrhages, scattered areas of mucosal ulceration, and bluish-black nodules representing mucosal gangrene. The findings of bluish-black nodules and a sharp line of demarcation between involved and uninvolved mucosa and the rapid resolution of these findings on repeated examination are the endoscopic features felt to be most consistent with the diagnosis of ischemic colitis. Mucosal biopsy findings include mucosal necrosis with varying degrees of submucosal necrosis and hemorrhage, submucosal granulation tissue, fibrosis or hyalinization with-

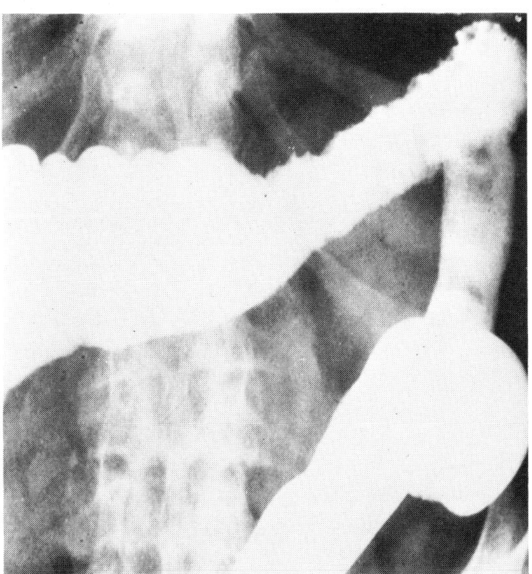

Figure 116–7. Ischemic colitis showing spasm, edema, and "thumbprinting" of splenic flexure.

out granuloma formation, hemosiderin-laden macrophages in the mucosa and submucosa, and intravascular fibrin platelet thrombi.[40, 58]

The *radiologic* diagnosis of ischemic colitis may be suggested by the presence of "thumbprinting" abnormalities in the wall of a mildly dilated air-filled segment of colon observed on abdominal plain films.[45, 67, 76] If a barium enema examination is performed early, the classic sign of ischemic colitis is that of thumbprinting or scalloping of the barium column caused by localized elevation of the mucosa consequent to submucosal hemorrhage and edema (Fig. 116–7). Associated spasm in the involved segment is usual. Both findings may disappear in several days or persist for several weeks. Mucosal ulcerations may develop several weeks following the initial ischemic event. Intramural barium may be identified but is a finding that may also be encountered in patients with Crohn's disease and diverticulitis. Stricture formation may begin within 3 weeks of the ischemic episode; the strictures are long and benign in appearance. If fibrosis occurs asymmetrically, sacculations or pseudodiverticula may develop on the opposite wall.

All of the changes that have been described are reversible up to the point of stricture formation.[7] Annular carcinoma must be considered in the differential diagnosis of stricturing, particularly because carcinoma has been found in up to 10% of patients with ischemic colitis.[45, 67, 76]

Angiography is generally felt to be of limited diagnostic value because spontaneously occurring ischemic colitis is usually not a consequence of large vessel occlusion. Furthermore, the significance of discovering large vessel occlusion must be established in each case. While a more severe clinical course of ischemic colitis can be predicted to some extent by angiographic findings revealing major vessel occlusion, this is not always true.[125] Johnson and Nabseth[62] found that 44% of 99 cases of ischemic colitis complicating aortic surgery had only mucosal involvement or stricture. Williams and Wittenberg[125] reported an equal prevalence rate of mild disease in 46 patients with occlusive and nonocclusive ischemic colitis; survival figures were also comparable. The decision to perform angiography in patients with presumed ischemic colitis should be based, therefore, on determining if there is major vessel occlusion in order to facilitate diagnosis, even though proof of arterial occlusion does not establish with absolute certainty the diagnosis of ischemic colitis.[125]

In the series reported by Brandt and his colleagues,[16] it was possible to diagnose ischemic colitis in 75% of 81 patients whose symptoms of colitis began after age 50; in 85% of those given this diagnosis, confirmation was based on definite clinical and pathologic criteria. Failure to utilize specific criteria, however, was responsible for initially incorrect discharge diagnoses in 50% of this same group.

Management. Management initially consists of general supportive measures, including maintenance of adequate blood volume and red blood cell mass, Po_2, and cardiac output. Antibiotics are usually included (Table 116–4), and analgesics may be necessary for pain control. Severe abdominal pain that

Table 116–4. ISCHEMIC COLITIS: RECOMMENDATIONS FOR ANTIBIOTIC COVERAGE*

Cefoxitin, 1 to 2 g q 4 h (does not cover *Enterococcus* and some *Bacteroides fragilis* spp.)
OR
Clindamycin, 600 mg q 6 h *plus* an aminoglycoside, 80 mg q 8 h (adjust with altered renal function)
OR
Metronidazole, 750 mg q 6 h *plus* ampicillin, 6 to 12 g/day, *plus* an aminoglycoside

*Greenman R, personal communication.

persists, intensifies, or becomes generalized, especially when associated with abdominal distention, rebound, guarding, fever, and leukocytosis, should suggest actual or impending colonic infarction, gangrene, pronounced serositis, perforation, and, possibly, peritonitis. Radiographic distention of the segment of colon involved in the ischemic process is highly suggestive of full-thickness gangrene.[77] Under these circumstances, early exploratory surgery is recommended.

Resection of severely ischemic or infarcted colon with reanastomosis or temporary diverting ileostomy or colostomy is the preferred surgical approach.[125] When resection is undertaken, it is essential that the surgeon be able to assess accurately the adequacy of the circulation to the remaining bowel; use of intra-operative Doppler-detected serosal pulsations is becoming an almost indispensable technique for this purpose.[27] Colonic decompression by endoscopy and surgical cecostomy are attractive alternatives to resection, but neither has been evaluated systematically.[3]

Fibrotic stricturing, usually of the left colon and rectosigmoid region, may complicate ischemic colitis. Colonic narrowing associated with ischemic injury and spasm is usually reversible. As noted earlier, long (8 to 10 cm), smooth, tapered, benign strictures begin to form 3 weeks following the ischemic episode.[45, 67, 76] It is essential that a colon carcinoma be excluded in such instances,[120] as also remarked earlier. Diagnostic colonoscopy, brushings, washings, and biopsy are required to exclude colon carcinoma presenting as an ischemic insult. Symptoms related to stricture development are few, and the need for corrective surgery is extremely infrequent.

Mesenteric Venous Thrombosis

Frequency. First described as a distinct entity in 1935, mesenteric venous thrombosis accounts for only 0.01% to 0.06% of hospital admissions and in-hospital diagnoses and is responsible for an estimated 5% to 15% of cases of intestinal ischemia occurring in the absence of mechanical small bowel obstruction. Early reports attributing a frequency of 30% to 40% of ischemic episodes to venous thrombosis reflected the assumption that this entity was the etiologic factor in cases of gut ischemia when arterial occlusion could not be identified. A great majority of these cases, however, probably represented arterial nonocclusive ischemia.[47]

Pathophysiology. Experimental ligature occlusion of the superior mesenteric vein in dogs results in a reproducible pathophysiologic sequence: venous dilatation, bleeding into the mesentery, bowel wall cyanosis and congestion, arterial spasm, paralytic ileus, and weeping of culture-negative serosanguineous fluid from the bowel wall and mesentery into the peritoneal cavity.[90] The experimental studies of Polk[90] and Friedenberg et al.[41] showed associated marked hypovolemia and hemoconcentration, reduced superior mesenteric arterial flow, tachycardia, hypotension, leukocytosis, and acidosis. The thrombosis developing proximal to the venous occlusion extended into peripheral tributaries. Bowel wall hemorrhage was associated with separation of mucosa and submucosa, but there was no progression to wall necrosis or perforation. Death resulted from cardiovascular collapse. In some animals, arterial spasm resulted in associated arterial thrombosis. When Friedenberg and his colleagues[41] occluded the venous drainage of isolated loops of small intestine, irreversible necrosis developed within 14 hours. Mesenteric arteriographic sequences have been described that include arterial spasm, prolonged arterial phase, opacification of the thickened bowel wall, and non-visualization of the mesenteric portal venous system.

Not all of these observations are strictly applicable to the patient who develops spontaneous occlusion of the mesenteric venous system, because there are frequently associated systemic or local intra-abdominal disorders.

Etiology. Mesenteric venous thrombosis may be a primary event ("agnogenic"),[81] or it may occur secondary to a wide variety of disorders altering blood coagulation, blood flow, or venous endothelium.[19, 41, 61, 78, 121] Table 116–5 lists the disorders associated with mesenteric venous thrombosis categorized as primary or secondary to hypercoagulable states, inflammation, stasis, or abdominal trauma. Agnogenic thrombo-occlusion may be on a basis of altered coagulability. The superior mesenteric vein is affected primarily, with the inferior mesenteric vein involved less than 6% of the time.[47]

Clinical Features.[44, 61] As in arterial occlusion, the predominant presenting complaint

Table 116–5. DISORDERS ASSOCIATED WITH MESENTERIC VENOUS THROMBOSIS

Primary ("agnogenic")

Hypercoagulable states:
- Neoplasms
- Antithrombin deficiency
- Thrombocytosis
- Polycythemia vera
- Oral contraceptive use

Inflamation:
- Abscess (pelvic, intra-abdominal)
- Peritonitis
- Inflammatory bowel disease
- Diverticulitis

Stasis:
- Portal hypertension
- Congestive heart failure
- Congestive splenomegaly

Abdominal trauma:
- Surgery (splenectomy)
- Blunt trauma

in mesenteric venous thrombosis is acute, intense, diffuse, crampy abdominal pain. Unlike arterial occlusion, however, the pain may be present to some degree for a month or more before its more acute onset. Initially, the pain is disproportionate to the minimal abdominal physical findings. Nausea and vomiting are encountered in up to 50% of patients, who also have low-grade fever, mild hypovolemia, and abdominal distention with normal or reduced bowel sounds. Tympany to percussion may be absent because of fluid-filled small intestinal loops. Abdominal tenderness develops rapidly, but features of peritonitis are late in onset. Ascites is detectable only rarely, unless pre-existing. Stools are positive for gross or occult blood in 30% to 100% of reported cases.[61] Gross bleeding is more likely when the inferior mesenteric vein is involved in the thrombo-occlusive process.

Hemoconcentration and leukocytosis are the only consistent, non-specific laboratory findings. An elevation of phosphate in serum and peritoneal fluid has been reported in animals with experimentally induced mesenteric venous occlusion and in humans in whom the disorder developed spontaneously. Elevations in activity of intestinal alkaline phosphatase have been noted when ischemia and infarction complicate primary or associated arterial occlusion. The finding of serosanguineous peritoneal fluid, sometimes with elevated amylase activity, is common.[47]

Diagnosis. Radiographic findings on plain abdominal radiographs and the results of CT scanning or angiography may be helpful.[20, 80] Demonstration of small intestinal ileus with air-fluid levels together with striking bowel wall thickening and mucosal irregularity strongly suggests the diagnosis.[20] Ascites is a late finding. Arterial occlusion, intramural hemorrhage on the basis of trauma or anticoagulants, vasculitis, infiltrative pathology, and angioneurotic edema may produce similar findings. Air in the bowel wall or portal vein is a late finding.

Air-fluid levels and contrast enhancement of the bowel wall on CT studies have been described in patients with mesenteric venous thrombosis.[47] CT and ultrasonography may also diagnose neoplastic thrombosis of the superior mesenteric vein.[79]

Barium contrast studies confirm the abdominal plain film findings of dilatation, intestinal wall thickening, and submucosal hemorrhage. Angiographic reports are few but are purported to show arterial spasm, reduced blood flow to the affected intestinal wall, and absence of venous drainage.[47] Technetium scintiscanning has been used to diagnose mesenteric venous thrombosis, but there is no broad clinical experience with this method.[87]

Diagnosis may be delayed for days to weeks and is established only infrequently prior to surgery or death.

Management. Volume replacement to compensate for fluid losses into the gut is essential to stabilize cardiovascular status and to prevent hypoperfusion and complicating arterial occlusive or non-occlusive infarction. Antibiotic coverage and heparin are not recommended for routine use, although there are some data to support their use. For example, heparin pretreatment, volume restoration, correction of acidosis, and intraperitoneal antibiotic administration improved certain parameters without prolonging life in experimental animals.

Definitive treatment requires surgery. The findings of venous thrombosis, persistent arterial pulsations, and extrusion of thrombus from cut mesenteric veins provide confirmatory evidence for the diagnosis. All bowel affected by the thrombotic process should be removed along with all thrombosed mesenteric veins. The extent of bowel wall and venous tributary involvement is difficult to determine. Intraoperative Doppler ultrasonography may be useful in this regard.[27] Because postoperative recurrence is usually at the anastomotic site, wide excision to assure venous patency is essential. Thrombectomy alone is undertaken cautiously and only when a large central vein is occluded. "Second look" operations are advocated when there is any clinical suspicion of progressive disease, since smaller thrombi may be overlooked. From 1 to 3 of 4 patients are expected to survive following successful surgical intervention with resection of involved bowel and thrombus-containing veins. Patients who do not have surgery or who are unable to undergo resection have a 100% mortality.

Postoperative recurrent thrombosis has been reported in up to 29% of patients. The thrombosis usually develops within 11 days but may not appear until 40 days following initial surgery.[63] Recurrence is usually at the anastomosis. The frequency of occurrence is higher in patients with previous thrombophlebitis and is associated with a mortality of up to 37%.[63] To offset risks of postoperative recurrence, predominantly in idiopathic or agnogenic forms of thrombosis, anticoagulation is recommended. This is effected initially with heparin (for 7 to 10 days) and for up to 10 additional weeks with warfarin (Coumadin). Indications for anticoagulation are less clear in secondary varieties of mesenteric venous thrombosis. The discovery of depressed antithrombin III levels following resolution of the venous thrombotic process and discontinuance of heparin therapy is an indication for prolonged anticoagulation.[88] The risk of anticoagulant-induced hemorrhage may outweigh that of thrombosis, especially when there is coexistent cirrhosis or malignancy.

Chronic Ischemic Syndromes

Abdominal Angina

Chronic ischemic syndromes are considerably less common than those resulting from acute ischemic insults to the small and large intestine. In part, this difference in frequency can be attributed to the potential for developing extensive collateral flow in the mesenteric circulation. While accounting for the low prevalence of documented cases of chronic mesenteric ischemia, the existence of extensive collateral circulation adds to the difficulty of firmly diagnosing this frequently reversible disease entity.

Most cases of chronic visceral ischemia are secondary to intrinsic disease of the mesenteric vessels, with atherosclerosis accounting for over 90% of known causes. Aortic aneurysms, fibromuscular hyperplasia, thromboangiitis obliterans, and congenital anomalies are extremely rare causes.[15, 22] Extrinsic compression of mesenteric vessels, specifically the celiac axis, by neural or ligamentous tissue has been implicated as a cause of chronic ischemic disease.[35, 51, 113]

Postprandial abdominal pain is the major symptom resulting from chronic mesenteric vascular insufficiency. Its occurrence is somewhat analogous to exercise-induced angina pectoris on the basis of coronary artery insufficiency. The pain is viewed as arising from muscular spasm of the gut wall induced by reduction in the level of tissue oxygen secondary to insufficient arterial perfusion during periods of increased metabolic demand. Figure 116–8 illustrates that trunk patency, PO_2, arteriolar resistance, capillary perfusion pressure, and tissue O_2 demands are all determinants of the development of abdominal angina.

The term *"abdominal angina"* was first used by Baccelli[2] in 1918 to describe a syndrome of postprandial abdominal cramping pain associated with chronic intestinal ischemia. In the 1930s, Dunphy[36] theorized that there was a link between intestinal angina and chronic splanchnic arterial occlusion. Increased inter-

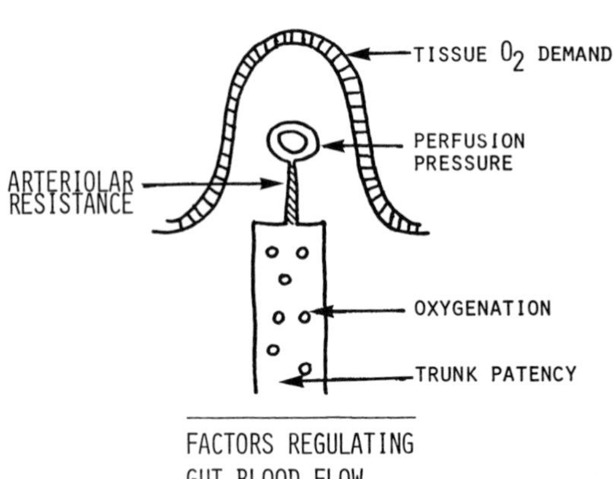

Figure 116–8. Schema illustrating determinants of abdominal angina resulting in spasm of muscularis mucosae and/or mucosal injury of a "villus."

Table 116–6. CHRONIC MESENTERIC ISCHEMIA: CLINICAL FEATURES

Predisposing factors:
- Advanced age
- Diabetes mellitus
- Hypertension

Causes:
- Intrinsic
  - Atherosclerosis (> 90% of cases)
  - Aortic aneurysms
  - Fibrointimal hyperplasia
  - Arteritis
  - Congenital anomalies
- Extrinsic
  - Celiac axis compression

Symptoms:
- Postprandial abdominal pain (most common)
- Weight loss
- Diarrhea
- Malabsorption
- Non-specific gastrointestinal complaints

Diagnosis:
- Consistent history
- Exclusion of disorders simulating gastrointestinal disease
  - Pancreatic carcinoma
  - Retroperitoneal tumor
  - Penetrating ulcer
- Angiography

est was sparked by Mikkelson[36a] in 1957, when he proposed a possible surgical approach to mesenteric vascular disease. One year later, Shaw and Maynard[106] reported that endarterectomies had relieved symptoms in 2 patients with significant stenosis of the superior mesenteric artery.

Clinical Features (Table 116–6). Advanced age, diabetes mellitus, and hypertension are cited as the most frequent predisposing factors in the development of chronic mesenteric ischemia. Cigarette smoking also appears to play a role. Interestingly, in contrast to other forms of atherosclerotic disease, symptomatic mesenteric vascular disease seems to occur more frequently in women than in men.[22, 29, 92, 112, 126] This predisposition in women has not been uniformly noted, however, although most reported series are small.

Abdominal pain or discomfort is the most consistent symptom, being reported in up to 100% of patients.[29, 53, 56, 92, 112, 126] The pain, most often located in the upper abdomen or periumbilical region, typically begins 15 minutes to 1 hour after meals and usually subsides within 1 to 4 hours. Described initially as a dull ache, the pain may become severe and colicky with progression of the disease. Various positions, such as squatting or lying in the prone position, have been claimed by patients to alleviate symptoms. The severity of the pain correlates with the amount of food ingested, and this commonly instigates voluntary decrease in meal size. Total caloric intake frequently diminishes as a consequence, and frank sitophobia may ensue.

The self-imposed decrease in food intake results in progressive and often significant *weight loss,* another important feature of the disease. Other less consistent symptoms include flatulence, bloating, nausea, vomiting, and non-specific alterations in bowel habits. Diarrhea may be observed in up to 50% of cases, and although malabsorption has been described,[30] it is rarely severe enough to account for the significant loss of weight.[15, 29, 53, 56]

Important *physical findings* are limited and non-specific. Signs of inanition predominate. The abdominal examination is often unremarkable, even during episodes of meal-induced pain, but mild distention may be encountered. Evidence of atherosclerosis is commonly seen. Abdominal bruits, while frequent, are not pathognomonic.[29, 53, 56] It has been suggested that phonoangiographic detection of a diastolic component to a bruit may correlate with angiographically significant disease.[98] The diagnostic value of this finding, however, has not been adequately assessed.

Laboratory findings are likewise non-specific and, in general, are not helpful except to exclude other causes of abdominal pain and weight loss. Steatorrhea, up to 20 g of fat/24 hours, may be present and may not always resolve after successful revascularization.[106, 114, 119] Other tests for malabsorption (e.g., D-xylose) (Chapter 27) yield variable results but are generally normal.

Diagnosis. The diagnosis of chronic mesenteric ischemia remains a challenge for a number of reasons. Elderly patients commonly present with vague, often non-specific abdominal complaints. Initial standard laboratory and radiologic evaluation may yield completely normal findings. Because of possible reactions to contrast media and the possible presence of renal insufficiency, local thrombosis, and hemorrhage, physicians are often reluctant to order angiography, particularly when symptoms are vague and the initial evaluation produces negative findings. This reluctance may be manifested further by the usual lengthy lag between the onset of symptoms and definitive diagnosis, reported in one series to average 12 months.[92] In addition, the finding of severe atherosclerotic disease of the splanchnic vessels does not by itself establish the diagnosis of chronic mesenteric insufficiency.

The importance of a careful history cannot be overemphasized. The existence of consistent postprandial abdominal pain should be confirmed and sitophobia differentiated from anorexia. It has been advised that patients with atypical pain be observed closely, inasmuch as the typical pattern of pain will ultimately ensue if mesenteric ischemia is responsible.[15]

Care must also be exercised to exclude other gastrointestinal disorders that may simulate mesenteric ischemia. Chronic pancreatic or peptic ulcer disease and a variety of gastrointestinal neoplasms may present with abdominal pain, weight loss, and alteration in bowel function. Mesenteric insufficiency commonly resembles and brings to mind pancreatic carcinoma. Thorough serologic evaluation, contrast studies, endoscopy, and ultrasonography or CT should help exclude these several conditions. When a patient presents with typical postprandial abdominal pain and weight loss and causes other than chronic mesenteric ischemia have been excluded, angiography should be performed.

Angiographic examination should include biplane flush aortography as well as selective celiac, superior mesenteric, and inferior mesenteric artery injections when possible.[83, 93] It is important to obtain both lateral and anteroposterior views. The former are needed to visualize in profile the origins of the mesenteric vessels as they arise anteriorly from the aorta. Atherosclerotic lesions will usually be found within the proximal 1 to 2 cm of the origin of the vessels,[91, 111] allowing for the development of collateral flow in distal segments (Fig. 116–9). Severe disease is most often found involving the celiac and superior mesenteric arteries. While the inferior mesenteric artery may be involved, it more often serves as the major source of collateral circulation by way of the meandering mesenteric artery of Drummond. Anteroposterior views on angiography are necessary to assess collateral circulation and the pattern of blood flow. The finding of prominent collateral vessels indicates both significant stenosis of a major vessel and chronicity of the disease process.[6, 21] Connolly and Kwaan[22] state that the finding of a large meandering mesenteric artery is pathognomonic of severe stenotic disease of 2 of the 3 major mesenteric vessels.

The major limitation of angiography, other than the morbidity associated with an invasive procedure, is that important information derived from it pertains only to anatomy and not to blood flow. Digital subtraction angiography may produce results comparable to conventional angiography in studies of the aorta.[18] While arterio-occlusive disease is a major limiting factor to blood flow, the extensive collateral potential of the mesenteric circulation can allow adequate oxygen delivery in the presence of complete occlusion of 2 major vessels. This fact becomes evident from numerous angiographic and necropsy studies demonstrating the frequent occurrence of severe occlusive disease of the mesenteric circulation in asymptomatic patients. Furthermore, despite the frequent finding of occlusion of the major mesenteric arteries, the number of documented cases of chronic intestinal ischemia remains relatively small.

The potential for collateral flow is so great that despite reported cases of single-vessel disease causing ischemic symptoms, most physicians are reluctant to make a diagnosis without greater than 50% occlusion of at least 2 vessels.[53, 56, 92, 124, 126] Even then, the significance of occlusion of one or all of the major vessels is controversial and cannot alone be accepted as proof of the existence of chronic mesenteric ischemia.

Methods to assess splanchnic blood flow indirectly are currently being investigated. Hansen et al.,[49] determining hepatic blood flow through the use of indocyanine green, demonstrated inability of patients with intestinal ischemic disease to increase splanchnic blood flow following a test meal. After reconstructive surgery, the postprandial rise in blood flow paralleled that of a control group. The technique, while difficult to perform, provides hope of being able to assess blood flow, the critical parameter in mesenteric ischemic disease, more accurately.

Management

Arterial Reconstruction. Arterial reconstruction remains the mainstay of therapy for chronic mesenteric insufficiency. The deci-

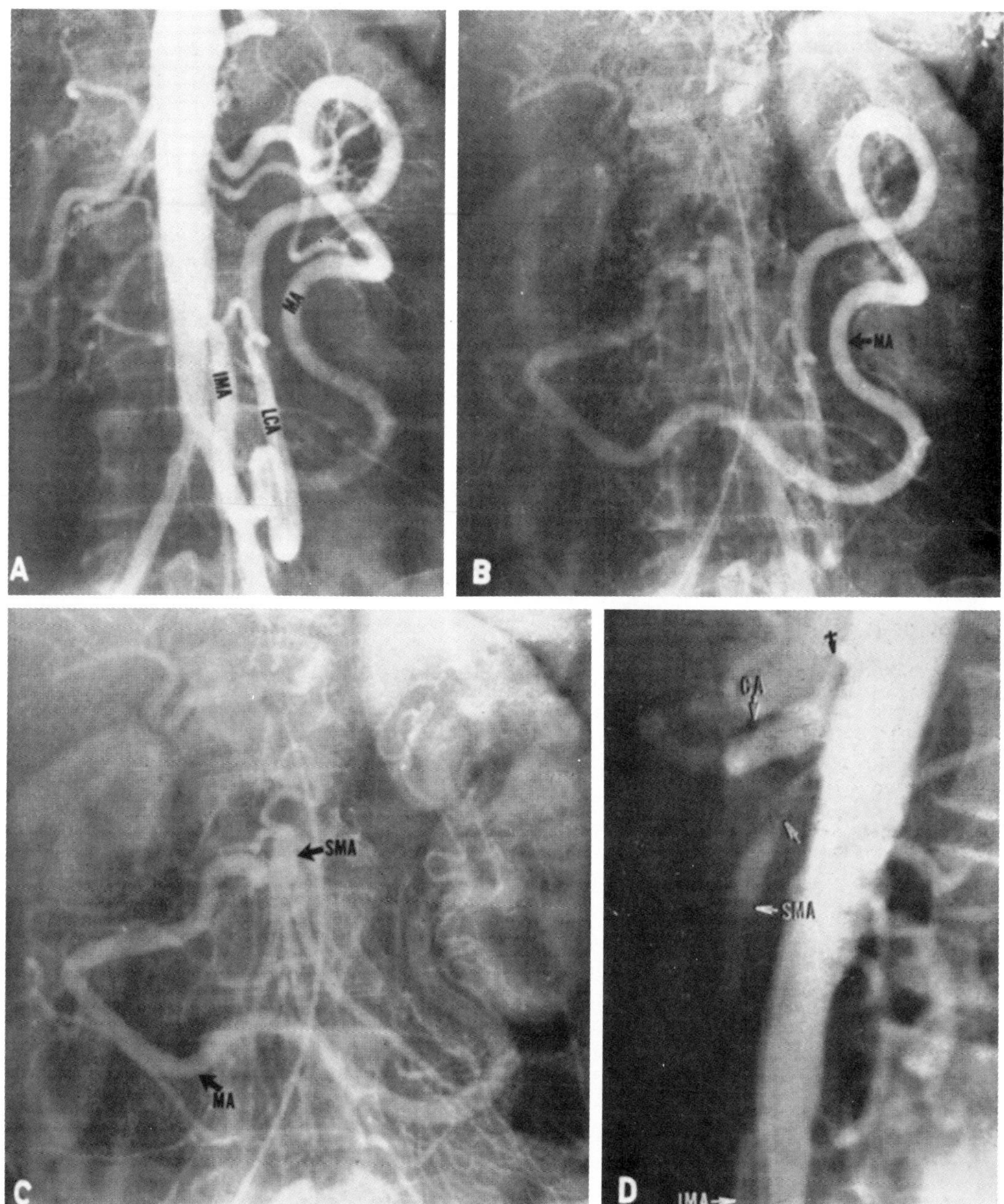

Figure 116–9. Superior mesenteric artery occlusion associated with large marginal artery as seen by angiography. *A*, Flush aortogram revealing dilated inferior mesenteric artery (IMA) and its left colic (LCA) branch continuing as a marginal artery (MA). *B*, Marginal artery continues to join with middle colic branch of superior mesenteric artery to provide blood to right transverse colon. *C*, MA fills (SMA). *D*, Lateral view of aorta showing stenosis of the celiac artery (CA) and SMA. The inferior mesenteric artery (IMA) is not occluded. (From Kahn P, Abrams HL. Radiology 1964; 82:429–41. Reproduced with permission.)

sion to operate should be based on a careful consideration of the severity of symptoms, a reasonable degree of certainty concerning the relationship of the symptoms to the objective evidence of substantial vascular disease, and, finally, the overall operative risk. Cardiovascular status should be adequately compensated and nutritional deficits, anemia, hypovolemia, and hypoxia corrected preoperatively.

Corrective surgical techniques include endarterectomy, prosthetic or saphenous vein bypass grafting, and reimplantation.[22, 23, 25, 29] Because of the relative infrequency of chronic mesenteric ischemia, there are no large prospective comparative trials of the various available techniques; as a result, there is continuing controversy concerning the ideal surgical approach. *Endarterectomy*,[106] the first and at one time a very popular reconstruction technique, no longer is considered the preferred method.[15] Because the procedure is technically difficult and requires greater operative exposure, simultaneous correction of aneurysmal disease or infrarenal aortic obstruction may not be possible.[29] Utilizing a "trapdoor" transaortic approach that allows accessibility to both celiac and superior mesenteric arterial ostia, Stoney et al.[110, 112] obtained good results with endarterectomy.

The most commonly employed method of arterial reconstruction of the splanchnic vessels is that of *bypass grafting*. Perioperative mortality rates range from 5% to 17%[53, 56, 96, 110, 126] and overall results are encouraging, regardless of variations in technique. Stoney and his colleagues[110, 112] advocate the use of antegrade grafts because their experience with retrograde grafting was disappointing. Ultimately, it is likely that the decision concerning a specific surgical procedure will depend upon the patient's general clinical status, the anatomic considerations, and the surgeon's personal experience and preferences.

A question frequently raised concerns the number of vessels that should or must be bypassed when more than one mesenteric artery is significantly obstructed. While single-vessel reconstruction is usually sufficient to re-establish adequacy of mesenteric arterial flow, Hollier et al.[56] suggest that long-term surgical successes correlate better with more complete revascularization. In this connection, their review of the surgical management of 56 patients with chronic mesenteric ischemia is of interest. Of 51 survivors of a variety of surgical procedures, 96% experienced immediate relief of abdominal pain and other related symptoms. However, 26.5% of this group experienced recurrent symptoms during a mean follow-up period of 38 months (5 months to 21 years). The authors demonstrated an inverse relationship between the recurrence of symptoms and the number of obstructed arteries bypassed, citing a 50% recurrence rate when only 1 of 2 or 3 occluded vessels was revascularized. Recurrent symptoms developed in only 11% of those patients in whom all occluded vessels were revascularized. No correlation could be shown to exist between recurrence rate and techniques of revascularization or type of graft employed.

Prophylactic Revascularization. Several reports suggest that chronic mesenteric ischemia may be a harbinger of acute ischemic insults in up to 50% of patients.[124] However, in most documented cases of acute occlusion of a mesenteric vessel, the history was notable for its lack of antecedent symptoms. Presently, the majority of instances of acute ischemic events are caused by embolic or non-occlusive arterial disease. Furthermore, the finding of asymptomatic and unsuspected mesenteric arterial occlusive disease during angiographic studies performed for other reasons or at the time of postmortem examination is not uncommon. These observations have resulted in controversy concerning prophylactic revascularization in patients with asymptomatic but anatomically appreciable mesenteric arterial occlusion.[15, 22–24] It would seem advisable presently to consider revascularization when contemplating unrelated vascular surgery that could further compromise the marginal flow and its dependence upon collateral channels (e.g., aortoiliofemoral, renal arterial, or aortic aneurysm reconstructive surgery).

Balloon Angioplasty. Advances in interventional radiography have resulted in the developemnt of a non-operative approach to the management of chronic mesenteric ischemia. There are now a number of reports of the successful management of mesenteric arterial disease by means of percutaneous transluminal angioplasty using Grunzig balloons.[42, 44, 95, 115] Experience is still too limited, however, to allow an adequate assessment of this procedure. It is likely that it will enjoy an important place in the management of high-risk surgical candidates and as a temporizing measure before definitive surgical revascularization.

Celiac Compression Syndrome

Recurrent abdominal pain attributed to compression of the celiac axis by surrounding anatomic structures has been termed the "*celiac compression syndrome*."[37, 73, 108, 112, 113, 118, 122] Compression is usually contributed to by the inferior portion of the median arcuate ligament or the celiac ganglion. Great controversy has been generated regarding the nature, pathophysiology, and even the existence of this syndrome since it was first described by Harjola,[50] Rob,[94] and Dunbar et al.[35]

Clinical Features.[14] Unlike patients with chronic mesenteric ischemia secondary to intrinsic vascular pathology, patients with celiac compression syndrome are younger and in general good health. Abdominal pain, the most consistent symptom, is usually epigastric in location and not of the predominantly postprandial nature described by patients with chronic mesenteric ischemia. Other symptoms, including weight loss, nausea, and diarrhea, have been variably described. Physical findings are usually of no assistance. A high midline abdominal systolic bruit, which frequently decreases with deep inspiration, is considered by some to be the most common associated physical finding.[96] Unfortunately, it is not encountered with great frequency.

Diagnosis. Diagnosis rests on the exclusion of other important causes of epigastric pain in a young individual, such as gastroesophageal reflux, gastritis, peptic ulcer disease, duodenitis, or pancreatitis. Mesenteric angiography typically reveals compression of the celiac axis reflected by an asymmetric smooth tapering of the axis,[126] often associated with poststenotic dilatation. The degree of compression may vary with respiration. It must be emphasized, however, that even with the characteristic compressive changes, caution must be exercised in making a firm diagnosis of celiac compression syndrome since similar findings may be demonstrated in asymptomatic subjects.

Management.[71, 113] When surgical management is deemed advisable clinically, the corrective methods employed include revascularization of the celiac axis by division of the median arcuate ligament, bypass, or reconstruction with or without associated ganglionectomy. Non-systematic patient selection, differing operative approaches, and incomplete follow-up are felt to account for the variability in reported results. In one large series,[39] while 83% of the patients were relieved initially of abdominal pain, only 41% remained symptom-free when followed for a period of 3 to 11 years. It has not been possible to predict long-term results on the basis of either presenting complaints or type of surgery.

Unanswered Questions. Many questions must be addressed if the celiac compression syndrome is to gain general acceptance as a legitimate basis for abdominal pain or even if it is to be included in classifications of mesenteric ischemic disorders.[107] This issue has been addressed by Brandt and Boley.[14] One aspect of the syndrome that makes considering it an important cause of mesenteric ischemia especially difficult is the fact that only a single vessel is involved. It was pointed out in the earlier discussion on chronic mesenteric ischemia that at least 2 of the major vessels must be partially or completely occluded for the syndrome of chronic abdominal pain to be present. An alternative mechanism proposed to explain the ischemia that may result from compression of the celiac axis is the phenomenon of "arterial steal."[14] This mechanism postulates that increased flow from the superior mesenteric artery to the celiac axis to accommodate for the reduction in flow imposed by compression of the celiac axis results in decreased blood flow to the small bowel, particularly during digestion. Conversely, increased flow to the small bowel postprandially by way of the superior mesenteric artery has been theorized to result in a reduction in flow to the distribution of the celiac axis, with resulting ischemia. Neither theory has been substantiated and there is contrary, albeit inconclusive, evidence.[14] Finally, it has been suggested that the mechanism for pain associated with celiac compression is neurogenic in origin. This theory suggests that the pain arises from the celiac ganglion, which has impinged on the celiac artery.[73]

In my opinion, celiac axis compression remains a poorly defined syndrome with insufficient evidence to either confirm or exclude it as a cause of abdominal pain. Considerable caution must be exercised in recommending surgery for patients suspected of having this disorder. Indeed, surgery should probably be reserved only for those cases in which exploratory surgery is contemplated to establish a definitive diagnosis.

References

1. Athanasoulis CA, Wittenberg J, Bernstein R, Williams F. Vasodilatory drugs in the management of nonocclusive bowel ischemia. Gastroenterology 1975; 68:146–50.
2. Baccelli F. Cited by Goodman EH: Angina abdominis. Am J Med Sci 1918; 155:524.
3. Barcewicz PA, Welch JP. Ischemic colitis: current trends. Conn Med 1979; 43:695–8.

4. Barcewicz PA, Welch JP. Ischemic colitis in young adult patients. Dis Colon Rectum 1980; 23:109–14.
5. Barnett SM, Davidson ED, Bradley EL III. Intestinal alkaline phosphatase and base deficit in mesenteric occlusion. J Surg Res 1976; 20:243–6.
6. Barth KH, Scott WW, Harrington DP, Siegelman SS. Abnormalities in the sequence of filling and emptying of mesenteric arteries. Gastrointest Radiol 1978; 3:85–9.
7. Bell RH, Creaghe SB, Goldberger LE. Reverisble ischemic pancolitis. Am J Surg 1981; 141:279–81.
8. Boley SJ. Early diagnosis of acuute mesenteric ischemia. Hosp Prac 1981; 16:63–71.
9. Boley SJ, Agrawal GP, Warren AR, et al. Pathophysiological effects of bowel distention on intestinal blood blow. Am J Surg 1969; 117:228–34.
10. Boley SJ, Brandt LJ, Veith FJ. Ischemic diseases of the intestines. *In* Current Problems in Surgery. Chicago: Year Book Medical Publishers, 1978: 1–5.
11. Boley SJ, Sammartano R, Brandt LJ, Sprayregan S. New concepts in the management of emboli of the superior mesenteric artery. Surg Gynecol Obstet 1981; 153:561–9.
12. Boley SJ, Schwartz S, Lash L, et al. Reversible vascular occlusion of the colon. Surg Gynecol Obstet 1963; 116:53–60.
13. Boley SJ, Sprayregan S, Seigelman SS, Veith FJ. Initial results from an aggressive roentgenological and surgical approach to acute mesenteric ischemia. Surgery 1977; 82:848–55.
14. Brandt LJ, Boley SJ. Celiac axis compression syndrome. A critical review. Am J Dig Dis 1978; 23:63–40.
15. Brandt LJ, Boley SJ. Ischemic intestinal syndromes. *In* Najarian JS, Delancy JP, eds. Advances in Surgery. Chicago: Year Book Medical Publishers, 1981: 1–45.
16. Brandt L, Boley S, Goldberg L, et al. Colitis in the elderly. Am J Gastroenterol 1981; 76:239–45.
17. Bulkley GB, Zuidema GD, Hamilton SR, et al. Intraoperative determination of small intestinal viability following ischemic injury. Ann Surg 1981; 193:628–37.
18. Buonocore E, Meaney TF, Borkowski GP, et al. Digital subtraction angiography of the abdominal aorta and renal arteries: Comparison with conventional angiography. Radiology 1981; 139:281–6.
19. Carnahlo ACA, Vaillancourt RA, Cabral RB, et al. Coagulation abnormalities in women taking oral contraceptives. JAMA 1977; 237:875–8.
20. Clement AR, Chang J. The radiologic diagnosis of spontaneous mesenteric venous thrombosi. Am J Gastroenterol 1975; 63:209–15.
21. Connolly JE, Abrahms HL.Kieraldo JH. Observation on the diagnosis and treatment of obliterative disease of the visceral branches of the abdominal aorta. Arch Surg 1965; 90:596–606.
22. Connolly JE, Kwaan JHM. Management of chronic visceral ischemia. Surg Clin North Am 1982; 62:345–56.
23. Connolly JE, Kwaan JHM. Prophylactic revascularization of the gut. Ann Surg 1979; 190:514–22.
24. Connolly JE, Stemmer EA. Intestinal gangrene as the result of mesenteric arterial steal. Am J Surg 1973; 126:197–204.
25. Connelly TL, Perdue GD, Smith RB III, Anslem JD, McKinnon WM. Elective mesenteric revascularization. Am Surg 1981; 47:19–25.
26. Cooke M, Sande MA. Diagnosis and outcome of bowel infarction on an acute medical service. Am J Med 1983; 75:984–92.
27. Cooperman M, Martin EW Jr, Carey LC. Determination of intestinal viability by Doppler ultrasonography in venous infarction. Ann Surg 1980; 191:57–8.
28. Corday E, Gold H, Vyden JK. Gastrointestinal vascular syndromes. Hosp Pract 1970; 5:57–65.
29. Crawford ES, Morris GC, Myhre HO, Roehy JOF Jr. Celiac axis, superior mesenteric artery and inferior mesenteric artery occlusion: surgical considerations. Surgery 1977; 82:856–66.
30. Dardik H, Seidenberg B, Parker J. Intestinal angina with malabsorption treated by elective revascularization. JAMA 1967; 194:1206.
31. Davis LJ, Anderson J, Wallace J, Jacobson ED. Experimental use of prostaglandin E_1 nonocclusive mesenteric ischemia. AJR 1975; 125:99–110.
32. Devroede G, Vobecky S, Massé S, et al. Ischemic fecal incontinence and rectal angina. Gastroenterology 1982; 83:970–80.
33. Dick AP, Graff R, Gregg MCC, et al. An arteriographic study of mesenteric arterial disease. Gut 1967; 8:206–20.
34. Duffy T. Reversible ischaemic colitis in young adults. Br J Surg 1981; 68:34–7.
35. Dunbar JD, Molnar W, Berman F, Marable SA. Compression of the celiac trunk and abdominal angina: preliminary report of 15 cases. AJR 1969; 95:731–44.
36. Dunphy JE. Abdominal pain of vascular origin. Am J Med Sci 1936; 192:102.
36a. Mikkelson WP. Intestinal angina—its surgical significance. Am J Surg 1953; 94:262.
37. Edwards AJ, Hamilton JD, Nichol WD, Taylor GW, Dawson A. Experience with coelic axis compression syndrome. Br Med J 1970; 1:342–5.
38. Ernst CB, Hagihara PF, Daugherty ME, et al. Ischemic colitis incidence following abdominal aortic reconstruction. Surgery 1976; 80:417–21.
39. Evans WE. Long-term evaluation of the celiac band syndrome. Surgery 1974; 76:867–71.
40. Forde KA, Lebwohl O, Wolff M, Voorhees A. The endoscopy corner: reversible ischemic collitis—correlation of colonoscopic and pathologic changes. Am J Gastroenterol 1979; 72:182–5.
41. Friedenberg MJ, Polk HC Jr, McAlister WH, Shochat SJ. Superior mesenteric arteriography in experimental mesenteric venous thrombosis. Radiology 1965; 85:38–45.
42. Furrer J, Gruntzig A, Kugelmeier J, et al. Treatment of abdominal angina with percutaneous dilation of an arteria mesenterica superior stenosis. Cardiovasc Intervent Radiol 1980; 3:43–4.
43. Ghahremani GC, Meyers MM, Farman J, Port RB. Ischemic disease of the small bowel and colon associated with oral contraceptives. Gastrointest Radiol 1977; 2:221–8.
44. Golden DA, Ring EJ, McLean GK, et al. Percutaneous transluminal angioplasty in the treatment of abdominal angina. Am J Radiol 1982; 139:247–9.
45. Gore RM. Calenoff L, Rogers LF. Roentgenographic manifestations of ischemic colitis. JAMA 1979; 241:1171–3.
46. Gore RM, Marn CS, Vjiki GT, et al. Ischemic colitis associated with systemic lupus erythematosus. Dis Colon Rectum 1983; 26:449–51.
47. Grendell JH, Ockner RK. Mesenteric venous thrombosis. Gastroenterology. 1982; 82:358–72.
48. Grendell JH, Ockner RK. Vascular diseases of the bowel. *In* Fordtran JS, Sleisenger MH, eds. Gastrointestinal Disease. 3rd Ed. Vol 1. Philadelphia: WB Saunders, 1983: 1543–68.
49. Hansen HJB,Engell HC, Ring-Larsen H, et al. Splanchnic blood flow in patients with abdominal angina before and after arterial reconstruction. Ann Surg 1977; 186:216–20.
50. Harjola PT. A rare obstruction of the celiac artery. Ann Chir Gynaecol Fenn 1963; 52:547–50.
51. Harjola PT, Lantiharju A. Celiac axis syndrome: abdominal angina caused by external compression of the celiac artery. Am J Surg 1968; 115:864–9.
52. Harper DR, Buist TAS. Selective angiography in acute midgut ischemia. Gut 1978; 19:132–6.
53. Hertzer NR, Beven EG, Humphries AW. Chronic intestinal ischemia. Surg Gynecol Obstet 1977; 145:321–8.
54. Hertzer NR, Beven EG, Humphries AW. Acute intestinal ischemia. Am Surg 1978; 44:744–9.
55. Hildebrand HD, Zierler RE. Mesenteric vascular disease. Am J Surg 1980; 139:188–92.
56. Hollier LH, Bernat PE, Pairolero PC, Payne WS, Osmundson PJ. Surgical management of chronic intestinal ischemia: a reappraisal. Surgery 1981; 90:940–6.

57. Horsburgh AG. Vascular surgery of the gut. Br J Hosp Med 1980; August, 113–8.
58. Hunt RH, Buchanan JD. Transient ischemic colitis—colonoscopy and biopsy in diagnosis. J Roy Nav Med Svc 1979; 65:15–9.
59. Jamieson WG, Lozon A, Durand D, Wall W. Changes in serum phosphate levels associated with intestinal infarction and necrosis. Surg Gynecol Obstet 1975; 140:19–21.
60. Jamison WG, Taylor MB, Troster M, Durand D. The significance of urine phosphate measurements in the early diagnosis of intestinal infarction. Surg Gynecol Obstet 1979; 148:374–88.
61. Jenson CB, Smith GA: A clinical study of 51 cases of mesenteric infarction. Surgery 1956; 40:930–7.
62. Johnson WC, Nabseth DC. Visceral infarction following aortic surgery. Ann Surg 1974; 180:312–8.
63. Jona J, Cummins GM Jr, Head HB, Govostis MC. Recurrent primary mesenteric venous thrombosis. JAMA 1974; 227:1033–5.
64. Kaminski DL, Keltner RM, Willman VL. Ischemic colitis. Arch Surg 1973; 106:558–63.
65. Katz S, Wahab A, Murray W, Williams LF. New parameters of viability in ischemic bowel disease. Am J Surg 1974; 127:136–41.
66. Katz S, Williams F. A new treatment for ischemic bowel disease: Steroid delivery via retrograde venous route. Am J Surg 1978; 135:791–4.
67. Kilpatrick ZM, Farman J, Yesner R, Spiro HM. Ischemic proctitis. JAMA 1968; 205:64–70.
68. Lambert M, dePeyer R, Muller AF. Reversible ischemic colitis after intravenous vasopressin therapy. JAMA 1982; 247:666–7.
69. Laufman H, Scheinberg S. Arterial and venous mesenterial occlusion. Analysis of forty-four cases. Am J Surg 1942; 58:84–92.
70. Lescher TJ, Bombeck T. Mesenteric vascular occlusion associated with oral contraceptive use. Arch Surg 1977; 112:1231–2.
71. Levin DC, Baltaxe HA. High incidence of celiac axis narrowing in asymptomatic individuals. AJR 1972; 116:426–9.
72. Mann A, Fazio VW. A comparative study of the use of fluorescein and the Doppler device in the determination of intestinal viability. Surg Gynecol Obstet 1982; 154:53–5.
73. Marable SA, Kaplan MF, Berman FM, Molnar W. Celiac compression syndrome. Am J Surg 1968; 115:97–102.
74. Margolis DM, Etheredge EE, Garza-Garza R, et al. Ischemic bowel disease following bilateral nephrectomy or renal transplant. Surgery 1977; 82:667–73.
75. Margolis IB, Faro RS, Howells EM, Organ CH. Megacolon in the elderly. Ischemic or inflammatory? Ann Surg 1979; 190:40–4.
76. Marshak RH, Lindner AE, Maklansky D. Ischemia of the colon. Mt Sinai J Med 1981; 4:180–90.
77. Marston A, Pheils MT, Thomas ML. Morson BC. Ischaemic colitis. Gut 1966; 7:1–15.
78. Matthews JE, White RR. Primary mesenteric venous occlusive disease. Am J Surg 1971; 122:579–83.
79. Merritt CRB. Ultrasonic demonstration of portal vein thrombosis. Radiology 1979; 133:425–7.
80. Moncada R, Reynes C, Churchill R, Love L. Normal vascular anatomy of the abdomen on computed tomography. Radiol Clin North Am 1979; 17:25–37.
81. Naitove A, Weismann RE. Primary mesenteric venous thrombosis. Ann Surg 1965; 161:516–23.
82. Nelson RL, Schuler JJ. Ischemic proctitis. Surg Gynecol Obstet 1982; 154:27–33.
83. Novelline RA, Waltman AC, Athanasoulis CA, Baum S. Recent advances in abdominal angiography. Adv Intern Med, 1976; 21:417–49.
84. Olearchyk AS, Cogbill CL. Acute intestinal ischemia. Milit Med, 1979; April, 245–8.
85. Ottinger LW. Nonocclusive mesenteric infarction. Surg Clin North Am 1974; 54:689–98.
86. Ottinger LW. The surgical management of acute occlusion of the superior mesenteric artery. Ann Surg 1978; 188:721–31.
87. Ottinger LW. Mesenteric ischemia. N Engl J Med 1982; 307:535–7.
88. Peters TG, Lewis JD, Filip DJ, Morris L. Antithrombin III deficiency causing postsplenectomy mesenteric venous thrombosis coincident with thrombocytopenia. Ann Surg 1977; 185:229–31.
89. Polansky BJ, Berger RL, Byrne JJ. Massive non-occlusive intestinal infarction associated with digitalis toxicity. Circulation 1964; 30(Suppl):141–5.
90. Polk HC Jr. Experimental mesenteric venous occlusion. III. Diagnosis and treatment of induced mesenteric venous thrombosis. Ann Surg 1966; 163:432–44.
91. Reiner L, Jimenez FA, Rodriquez FL. Atherosclerosis in the mesenteric circulation; observations and correlations with aortic and coronary atherosclerosis. Am Heart J 1963; 66:200–9.
92. Reul GJ, Wulasch DC, Sandiford FM, et al. Surgical treatment of abdominal angina: review of 25 patients. Surgery 1974; 75:682–9.
93. Reuter SR, Olin T. Stenosis of the celiac artery. Radiology 1965; 85:617–27.
94. Rob C. Diseases of the abdominal aorta. Manit Med Rev 1965; 45:552–7.
95. Roberts L, Wertman DA, Mills SR, et al. Transluminal angioplasty of the superior mesenteric artery: an alternative to surgical revascularization. Am J Radiol 1983; 141:1039–42.
96. Rogers DM. Thompson JE, Garrett WV, et al. Mesenteric vascular problems: a 26 year experience. Ann Surg 1982; 195:554–63.
97. Russ JE, Haid SP, Yao JST, Bergan JJ. Surgical treatment of nonocclusive mesenteric infarction. Am J Surg 1977; 134:638–42.
98. Saar MG, Dickson ER, Newcomer AD. Diagnostic bruit in chronic intestinal ischemia: recognition by abdominal phonoangiography. Dig Dis Sci 1980; 25:761–2.
99. Sachs SM, Morton JH, Schwartz SI. Acute mesenteric ischemia. Surgery 1982; 92:646–53.
100. Saegesser F, Loosli H, Robinson JWL, Roenspies U. Ischemic diseases of the large intestine. Int Surg 1981; 66:103–17.
101. Sakal L, Keltner RM, Kaminski D. Spontaneous and shock-associated ischemic colitis. Am J Surg 1980; 140:755–60.
102. Sawer BA, Jamieson WG, Durand D. The significance of elevated peritoneal fluid phosphate level in intestinal infarction. Surg Gynecol Obstet 1978; 146:43–45.
103. Scowcroft CW, Sanowksi RA, Kozarek RA. Colonoscopy in ischemic colitis. Gastrointest Endosc 1981; 27:156–61.
104. Seltzer MH, Roberts B. Acute superior mesenteric artery occlusion with a case report. Ann Surg 1969; 169:498–501.
105. Semb BKH, Halvorsen JF, Fossdai JE, Eide J. Visceral ischaemia following coeliac and superior mesenteric artery occlusion. Acta Chir Scand. 1977; 143:185–90.
106. Shaw RS, Maynard EP III. Acute and chronic thrombosis of the mesenteric arteries associated with malabsorption. N Engl J Med 1958; 228:874–8.
107. Sleisenger MH. The celiac artery syndrome—again? Ann Intern Med, 1977; 86:355–6.
108. Stanley JC, Fry WJ. Median arcuate ligament syndrome. Arch Surg 1971; 103:252–8.
109. Stillman AE, Weinberg M, Mast WC, Palpant S. Ischemic bowel disease attributable to ergot. Gastroenterology 1977; 72:1336–7.
110. Stoney RJ, Ehrenfeld WK, Wylie EJ. Revascularization methods in chronic visceral ischemia caused by atherosclerosis. Ann Surg 1977; 186:468–76.
111. Stoney RJ, Reilly LM. Chronic visceral ischemia. An often overlooked cause of abdominal pain. Postgrad Med 1983; 74:111–8.
112. Stoney RJ, Wylie EJ. Recognition and surgical management of visceral ischemic syndromes. Ann Surg 1966; 164:714–22.

113. Szilagyi DE, Rian RL, Elliot JP, Smith RF. The celiac artery compression syndrome: Does it exist? Surgery 1972; 72:849–63.
114. Tilson MD, Stansel HC. Abdominal angina: intestinal absorption eight years after successful mesenteric revascularization. Am J Surg 1976; 131:366–8.
115. Uflacker R, Goldany MA, Constant S. Resolution of mesenteric angina with percutaneous transluminal angioplasty of a superior mesenteric artery—studies using a balloon catheter. Gastrointest Radiol 1980; 5:367–9.
116. Ulano H, Treat E, Shanbour LL, Jacobson ED. Selective dilation of the constricted superior mesenteric artery. Gastroenterology 1972; 62:39–47.
117. Vyden JK. Recovery from acute intestinal ischemia without bowel resection. JAMA 1973; 226:776–7.
118. Watson WC, Sadikali F. Celiac axis compression. Experience with 20 patients and a critical appraisal of the syndrome. Ann Intern Med 1977; 86:278–84.
119. Watt JK, Watson WC, Haase S. Chronic intestinal ischemia. Br Med J 1967; 2:199–202.
120. West BR, Ray JE, Gathright JB. Comparison of transient ischemic colitis with that requiring surgical treatment. Surg Gynecol Obstet 1980; 151:366–8.
121. Whelan MA, Kain P. Mesenteric complications in a patient with polycythemia vera. Am J Gastroenterol 1982; 77:526–8.
122. Wihas AA, Laws HL, Jander HP. Surgical treatment of the celiac axis compression syndrome. Am J Surg 1977; 133:688–91.
123. Williams LF Jr. Vascular insufficiency of the bowels. DM 1970; August, 1–38.
124. Williams LF. Vascular insufficiency of the intestines. Gastroenterology 1971; 61:757–77.
125. Williams LF, Wittenberg J. Ischemic colitis: A useful clinical diagnosis, but it is ischemic? Ann Surg 1975; 182:439–48.
126. Zelenock GB, Grahm LM, Whitehouse WM. Splanchnic arteriosclerotic disease and intestinal angina. Arch Surg 1980; 115:497.

Chapter 117

Angiography in Vascular Disorders of the Gut

Stanley Baum • Hugh A. Jordan

In the little more than 2 decades since its introduction,[1–3] mesenteric angiography has developed into a valuable diagnostic as well as therapeutic technique. In the 1960s and early 1970s, angiographers learned how to selectively catheterize most major arteries in the body and gained experience in the transcatheter infusion of various drugs that pharmacologically manipulate splanchnic blood flow.[4] The past decade saw the expansion of transvascular therapy to include the use of: (1) deliberate embolization to stop refractory bleeding and infarct tumors,[5, 6] (2) percutaneous transluminal dilatation as an alternative to surgical reconstruction of arterial stenoses and occlusions,[7] and (3) the application of intravascular techniques to other tubular systems in the body, notably the biliary and urinary tracts.[8–13]

It is likely that with the further development and application of computer assisted techniques, such as computed tomography (CT), magnetic resonance imaging (MRI), and digital subtraction angiography (DSA), the diagnostic applications of selective mesenteric angiography will become less important. There probably will be increased emphasis, however, on transvascular therapeutic procedures. This chapter is an account of the current place of angiography in both diagnosis and transvascular therapy in the management of vascular diseases of the gastrointestinal tract or alimentary tract lesions with a vascular component.

Angiographic Anatomy

Familiarity with the vascular anatomy of the alimentary tract and its variants is vital, of course, to the angiographer and to the interpretation of angiographic findings. The arterial supply to the gut, the intramural vascular arrangement, and the venous drainage from the alimentary tract are reviewed in Chapters 35, 115, and 116. Figures 117–1 to 117–4 summarize these features as they appear to the angiographer and as they serve as guides in the interpretation of the angiography findings. Figures 117–1 and 117–4 also appear in Chapter 35, and an illustration resembling Figure 117–4 appears in Chapter 116. Nevertheless, both figures are shown here again to facilitate understanding of the angiographic aspects of vascular disease of the gut.

The fact that the vasculature of the gut is characterized by variants and unusual patterns emphasizes the need to know the intricacies of the vascular anatomy.[14–16] For example, the right colic artery varies in its origin, arising from the superior mesenteric artery in 40% of cases, the middle colic artery in 30%, or the ileocolic artery in 12%; in 18% it may be absent, being replaced by the descending branch of the middle colic artery.[14]

Another important variation from the angiographic standpoint is the origin of the middle colic artery from the dorsal pancreatic

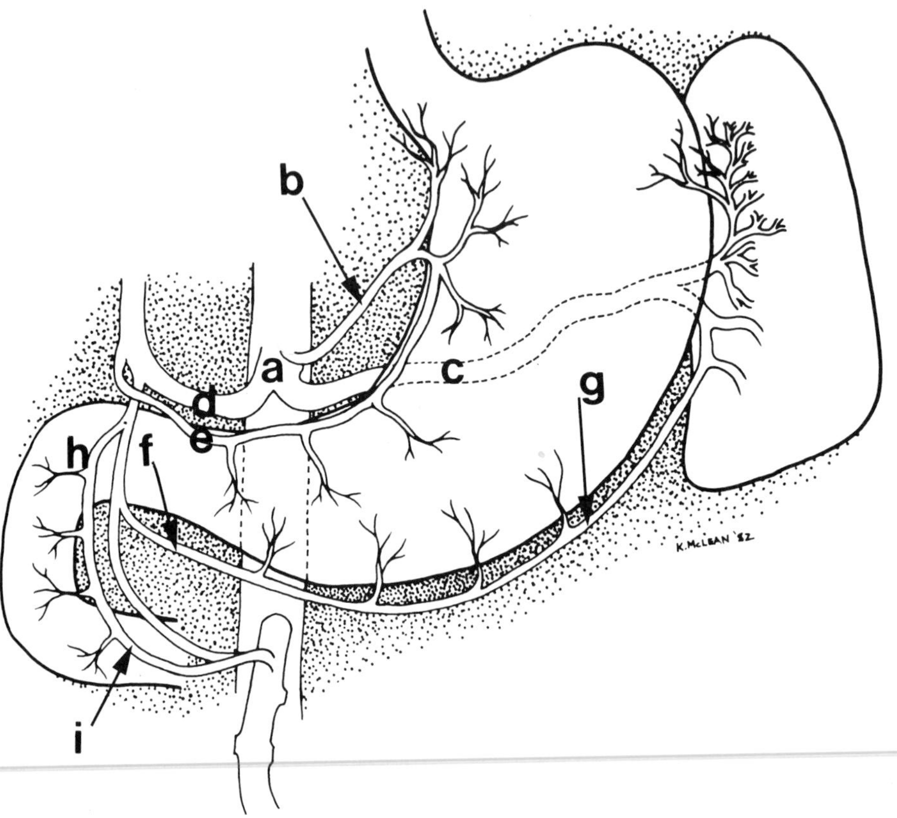

Figure 117–1. Arterial anatomy of the stomach and duodenum. *a,* Celiac axis. *b,* Left gastric artery. *c,* Splenic artery. *d,* Common hepatic artery. *e,* Right gastric artery. *f,* Right gastroepiploic artery. *g,* Left gastroepiploic artery. *h,* Superior pancreaticoduodenal artery. *i,* Inferior pancreaticoduodenal artery. (From Marshak RH et al. Radiology of the Stomach. Philadelphia: WB Saunders 1983. Reproduced with permission.)

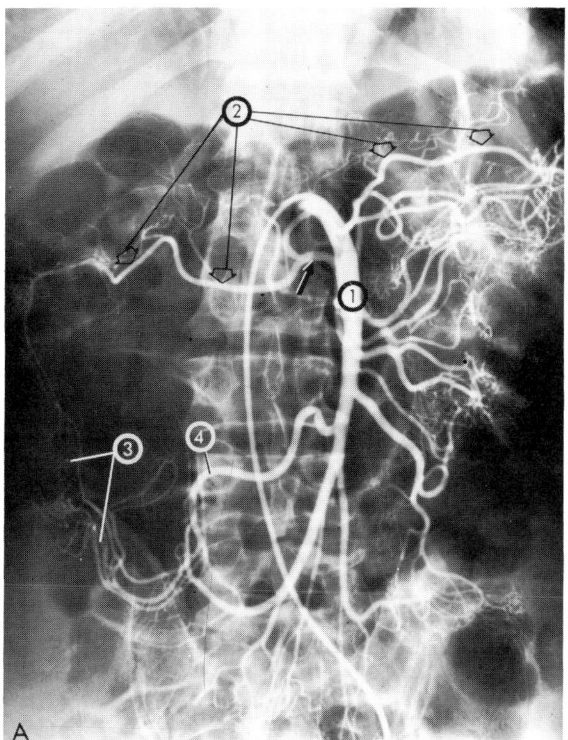

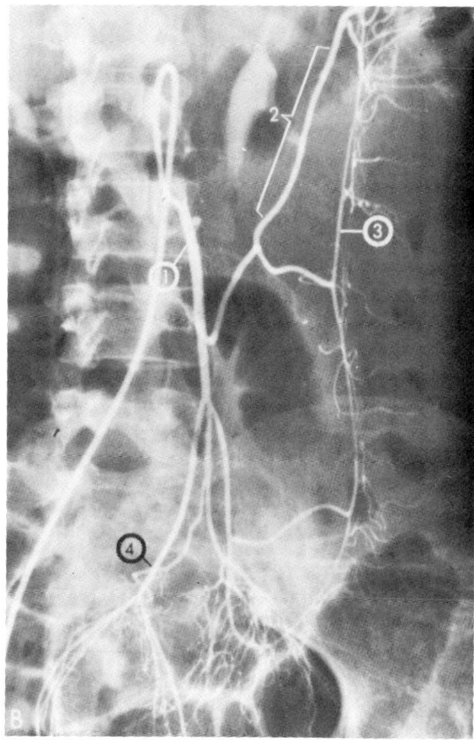

Figure 117–2. *A,* Selective superior mesenteric arteriogram during the arterial phase demonstrates the contribution of the superior mesenteric artery to the ascending and transverse portions of the colon. The middle colic artery (1) arises directly from the superior mesenteric artery and supplies the branches to the transverse colon (2), anastomosing with the right colic branch (3) of the ileocecal artery (4). *B,* Normal inferior mesenteric artery (1) gives rise to the ascending left colic artery (2) that will anastomose with the middle colic artery of the superior mesenteric artery. This anastomosis is very effective in supplying collateral flow in occlusive disease. The marginal artery of Drummond (3) runs along the mesenteric border of the colon. One of the descending branches of the inferior mesenteric artery is the superior hemorrhoidal artery (4), which is another important anastomosis for collateral flow.

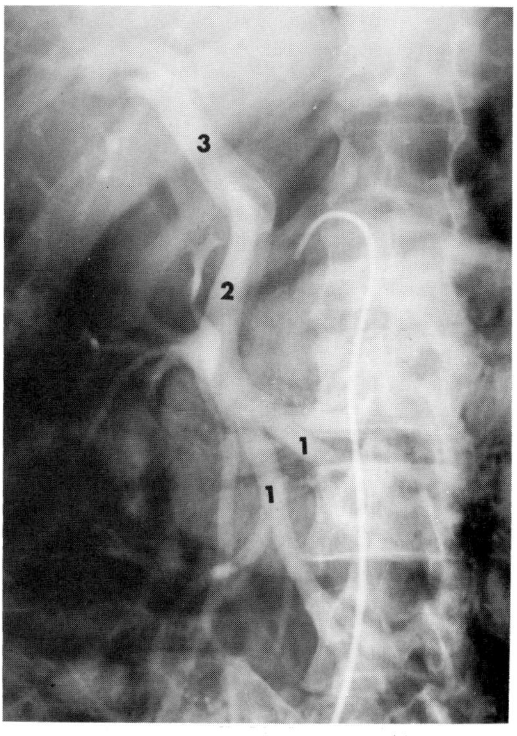

Figure 117–3. The venous phase of a superior mesenteric arteriogram performed immediately after the injection of 25 mg of tolazoline in the superior mesenteric artery shows excellent opacification of jejunal vein (1), the superior mesenteric vein (2), and the portal vein (3).

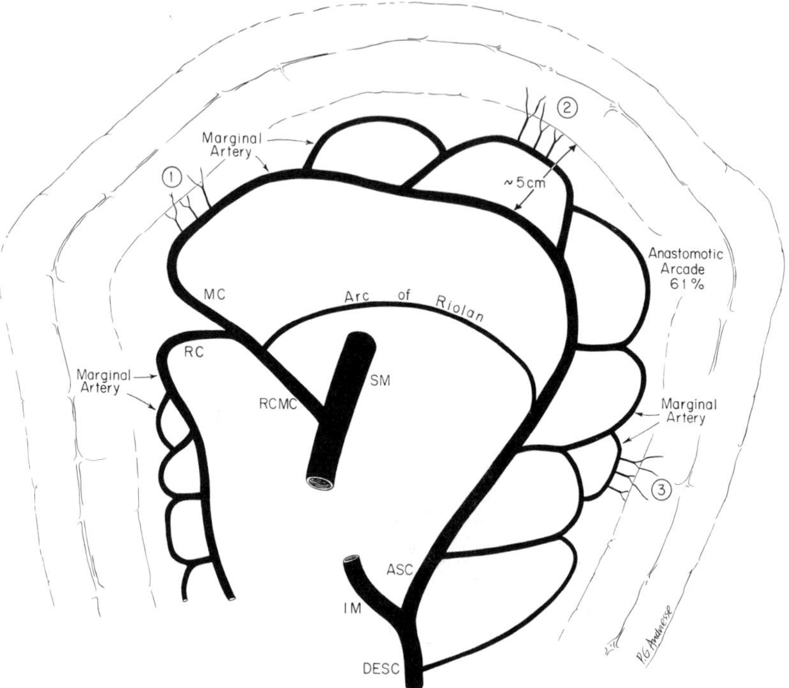

Figure 117–4. Marginal artery of Drummond, arc of Riolan, and Griffith's point. The marginal artery is that continuous artery that is closest to and parallel with the wall of the colon. It is the only artery that gives rise to the vasa recta, which are short, straight arteries supplying the bowel wall. Although a continuous artery, its components may represent several different arteries ranging from the right colic, middle colic, or ascending and descending branches of the left colic arteries themselves to primary, secondary, or even higher order arcades. The vasa recta arise from the entire length of the marginal artery, but schematically they are shown arising in only 3 groups. Group 1 arises from the middle colic artery itself; group 2 arises from a primary arcade; and group 3 arises from a secondary arcade. (From Nebessal et al., Kornblith, Pollard, and Michaels. Superior Mesenteric Arteries: A Correlation of Angiograms and Dissections. Boston: Little, Brown, 1969. Reproduced with permission.)

artery, a branch of the celiac axis. An accessory second middle colic artery may be present (10% of cases), arising from the normal middle colic artery and anastomosing with a branch of the inferior mesenteric artery to form the arc of Riolan[14] (Fig. 117–4).

Opacification of veins by following the contrast material well into the venous phase of the study should be a part of every selective superior or inferior mesenteric arteriogram. The information that may be obtained can play a vital role in evaluating diseases of the gastrointestinal tract. By way of illustration, jejunal and ileal veins draining blood from the small bowel into the superior mesenteric vein may form varices in patients with portal hypertension and, on occasion, give rise to acute gastrointestinal hemorrhage.[17]

Developmental Anomalies

By demonstrating vascular changes or bleeding, mesenteric angiography may contribute valuable information in certain developmental anomalies of the bowel.

Mid-Gut Volvulus. Congenital anomalies of rotation and fixation of the intestinal tract may cause intestinal obstruction in newborns and infants. In adults, mid-gut volvulus may be asymptomatic or it may present with intermittent attacks of abdominal pain, occasionally accompanied by nausea, vomiting, and diarrhea. The angiographic diagnosis of potential vascular compromise rests on the demonstration of twisting of branches of the superior mesenteric artery around the root of the mesentery[18] (Fig. 117–5). Computed tomographic examination of such patients shows the abnormal relationships of the superior mesenteric artery and vein as they enter the root of the mesentery, and this study may give the first clue to the diagnosis.[19]

Volvulus of the cecum, a limited form of mid-gut volvulus due to failure of descent and fixation of the cecum and ascending colon, also presents with intermittent attacks of abdominal pain. Because of the difficulty in making a clinical diagnosis, mesenteric angiography has been performed and attention drawn to the characteristic angiographic "coiled spring" appearance that the branches of the ileocolic artery assume as a result of volvulus of this part of the large bowel.

Duplications. Localized duplications of the intestine, most common in the ileum, may compromise blood supply to the bowel if they become very large or are associated with volvulus. Mesenteric angiography documents the vascular compromise and the displacement of arteries and veins. Hemorrhage due to the presence of gastric mucosa and peptic ulceration may also be demonstrated in this way.

Congenital Diverticula. Mesenteric angiography may contribute importantly when these lesions are complicated by bleeding (see discussion on Bleeding that follows).

Bleeding

(See also Chapter 6)

Upper Intestinal Bleeding. It is now accepted that *barium studies* are inappropriate in the investigation of acute upper intestinal bleeding. Not only may the results be equivocal or misleading, but the presence of barium in the bowel precludes the effective subsequent use of angiography.

Endoscopy today is generally regarded as the primary investigative procedure in upper intestinal hemorrhage[20, 21] but has important limitations,[22] particularly when the bleeding emanates from a lesion in the upper gut. Identification of the source of bleeding is circumscribed by the limited portion of the gut that can be examined with present endoscopes (see Chapter 103 for discussion of enteroscopy). Moreover, laser and other coagulation methods to arrest bleeding are not widely available and may not be applicable even when the site is visualized. Hence, angiographic diagnosis and transcatheter therapy have come to play increasingly important and even crucial roles in the diagnosis and management of upper intestinal hemorrhage (see Chapter 35 for a description of the basic diagnostic procedure).

In 1963, experimental animal studies demonstrated the ability of angiography to show arterial or capillary bleeding at rates as low as 0.5 ml/minute.[23] In addition, bleeding can be controlled in many cases by infusing vasoconstrictor drugs or particulate emboli through the same angiographic catheter.[24–28] Because of this potential for therapy, selective arteriography is carried out in many bleeding patients even when the cause of bleeding has been established by other techniques.

Vasopressin is commonly administered to produce vasoconstriction. It was originally infused IV in doses of 20 to 30 units over a period of 15 to 20 minutes,[29, 30] but this rela-

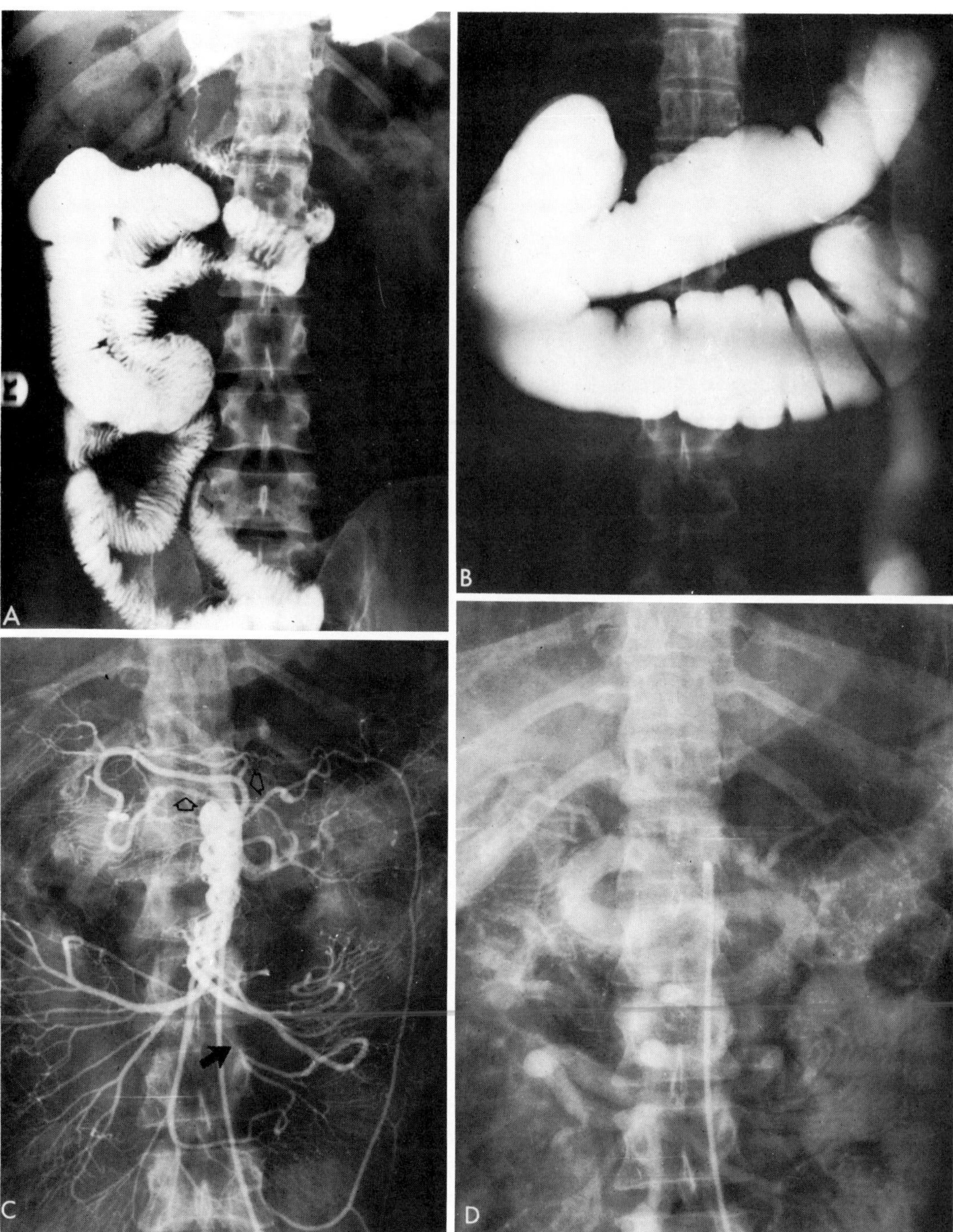

Figure 117–5. Angiographic findings in midgut malrotation with volvulus. *A,* Barium meal examination of the stomach, duodenum, and small intestines demonstrates malrotation with an abnormal location of the ligament of Treitz. *B,* Barium enema demonstrates most of the colon in the left half of the abdomen with an abnormal position of the cecum and ascending colon. *C,* Arterial phase of a selective superior mesenteric arteriogram shows marked twisting of the jejunal and ileal branches around the ileocolic branch, producing a "barber pole sign." The narrowing of the proximal portion of the midjejunal artery *(solid black arrow)* is probably caused by the midgut volvulus. The middle and right colic arteries *(open arrows)* are in the upper and left portions of the abdomen. *D,* The venous phase of the superior mesenteric arteriogram demonstrates dilatation of the jejunal, ileal, and superior mesenteric veins, which are twisted around the root of the mesentery, presumably as a result of the volvulus. The angiographic findings in both the arterial and venous phases suggest malattachment of the mesentery.

Illustration continued on opposite page

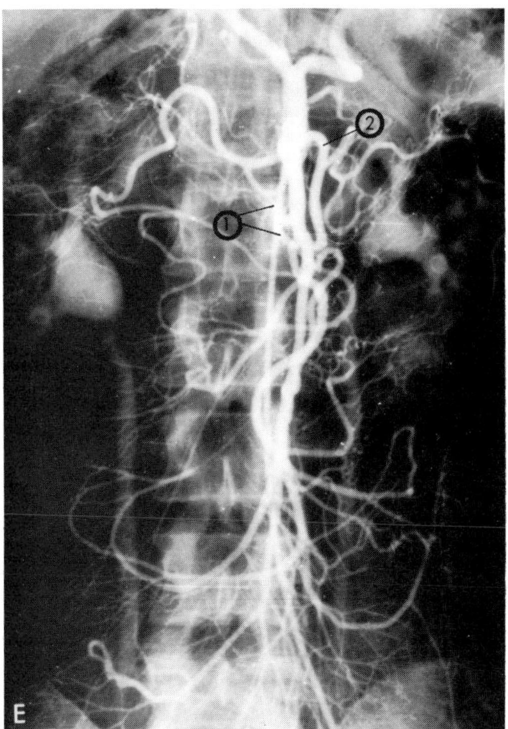

Figure 117–5 *Continued. E,* Following corrective surgery, the postoperative superior mesenteric arteriogram demonstrates the jejunal branches (1) arising from the right side of the superior mesenteric artery while the middle colic artery (2) arises from the left side. Only one jejunal branch remains loosely twisted around the main mesenteric trunk.

tively high dose was associated with serious side effects, such as a decrease in cardiac output secondary to a reduction in coronary artery blood flow.[31] These shortcomings can be avoided by infusing the vasoconstrictor in low doses at a rate in the range of 0.1 unit/minute[32] through an angiographic catheter inserted into the principal artery supplying the area of bleeding. Cardiac output is not affected by this method of administration and prolonged or repeated infusion over periods of days is not attended by bowel ischemia or infarction or by tachyphylaxis. A small but definite antidiuretic effect does occur, however, and care must be taken to avoid fluid overload.

Similar low doses of vasopressin infused IV have been found to have an equal effect in lowering portal venous pressure; since this route avoids the hazards associated with intra-arterial catheters, it is now the approach of choice.[33–35] The vasopressin should be delivered through a centrally placed catheter, as extravasation of the drug may lead to ischemic necrosis of tissue.

When pharmaceutical vasoconstriction does not arrest bleeding and the arterial supply to the bleeding site has been clearly delineated, occlusion of the feeding vessel may be attempted. The most commonly used material to effect such embolization is Gelfoam, cut and rolled into pledgets and soaked in a sclerosing agent. Stainless steel coils are also used to provide a more permanent occlusion. Tissue adhesives, such as 2-isobutyl cyanoacrylate (bucrylate), have been advocated as well, and absolute alcohol has given some encouraging results.[36–39]

Duodenum. Pyloroduodenal bleeding due to chronic peptic ulceration may respond to intra-arterial vasopressin alone (Figs. 117–6 and 117–7), but this occurs in less than 50% of cases[40] (Fig. 117–8). Suggested reasons for this high failure rate include: (1) The dual blood supply of the duodenum from branches of the celiac and superior mesenteric arteries. Injection of contrast material into the inferior pancreaticoduodenal artery during vasopressin infusion of the gastroduodenal artery may show continuing extravasation at the ulcer site. This problem has been surmounted by infusing both limbs of the vascular arcade simultaneously with vasopressin through separate arterial catheters. (2) Inability of an artery encased in a chronic inflammatory mass at the base of an ulcer to constrict in response to vasopressin. (3) Erosion by the ulcer of a large vessel, such as the gastroduodenal artery. A small proportion of these patients will respond to Gelfoam or steel coil embolization of the gastroduodenal artery[40] (Fig. 117–9). As a general rule, surgical intervention is necessary for such patients if they are judged fit to withstand the procedure, inasmuch as the surgical ligation of the bleeding vessel can be accompanied by a vagotomy or other appropriate procedure to prevent recurrence of bleeding.

Small Bowel. Hemorrhage into the small intestine, apart from the duodenum, is uncommon. The most frequent causes are tumors, arteriovenous malformations, or Crohn's disease. Because abnormal vessels are present in these lesions, vasopressin infusion often fails to control the bleeding. If the patient is unfit for surgery, embolization with Gelfoam may achieve hemostasis, although there is a real danger of bowel infarction due to the end-arterial nature of the vasa recta of the small bowel.

Angiography has a place in both the diagnosis of bleeding lesions of the small bowel

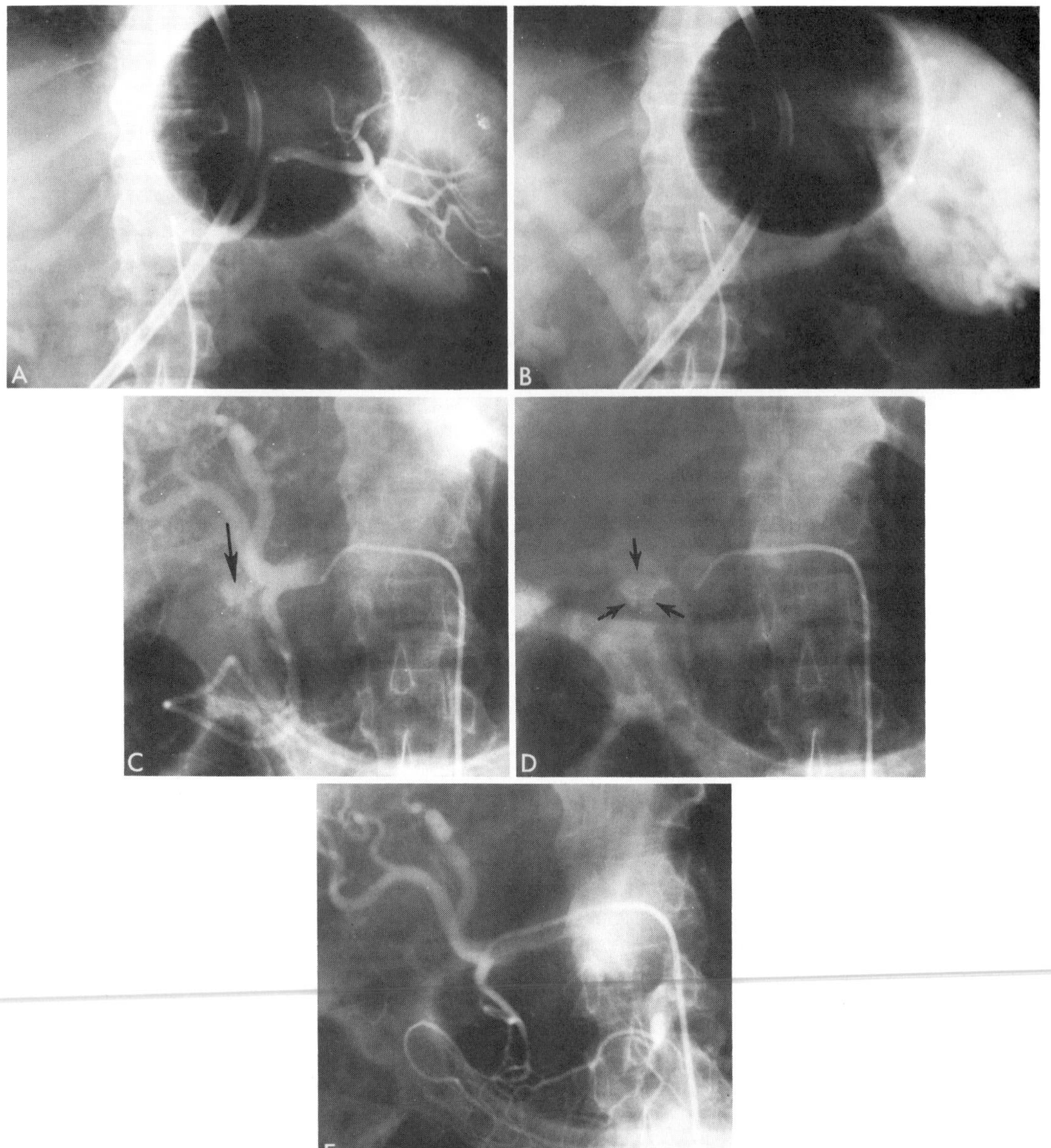

Figure 117–6. Bleeding duodenal ulcer in a patient with known cirrhosis, portal hypertension, and varices. *A,* Selective splenic arteriogram, arterial phase, demonstrates an enlarged spleen. *B,* The venous phase of the selective splenic arteriogram shows patency of the splenic and the portal vein with hepatopetal flow. The gastric balloon of the Litton tube compresses the gastric varices. *C,* Selective hepatic artery injection demonstrates extravasation of contrast material from a branch of the gastroduodenal artery in a bleeding duodenal ulcer *(arrow)*. *D,* Increasing extravasation is noted at the end of the venous phase of the hepatic artery injection *(arrows)*. *E,* Arteriogram during the infusion of 0.15 unit/minute of surgical Pituitrin into the gastroduodenal artery demonstrates cessation of bleeding. The patient was infused for 36 hours. He did not rebleed after the catheter was removed, and he was discharged from the hospital 5 days later.

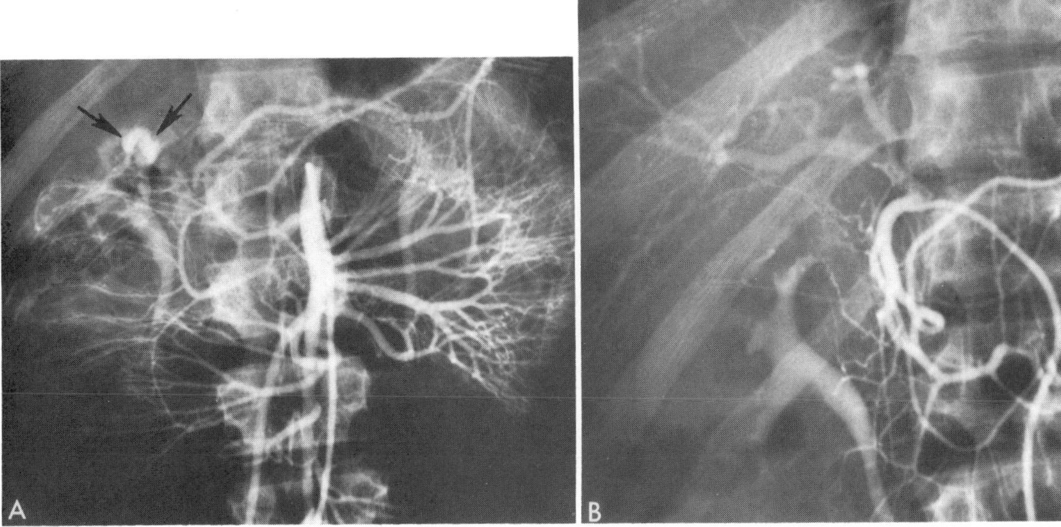

Figure 117–7. A 15-year-old boy with a bleeding duodenal ulcer controlled by the intra-arterial infusion of Pituitrin. *A,* Superior mesenteric arteriogram demonstrates extravasation in the duodenal cap *(arrow)* from a branch of the inferior pancreaticoduodenal artery. *B,* The gastroduodenal artery has been selectively catheterized and infused with 0.1 unit/minute of surgical Pituitrin. An arteriogram performed during the infusion fails to demonstrate any further bleeding. Clinically there was also cessation of hemorrhage.

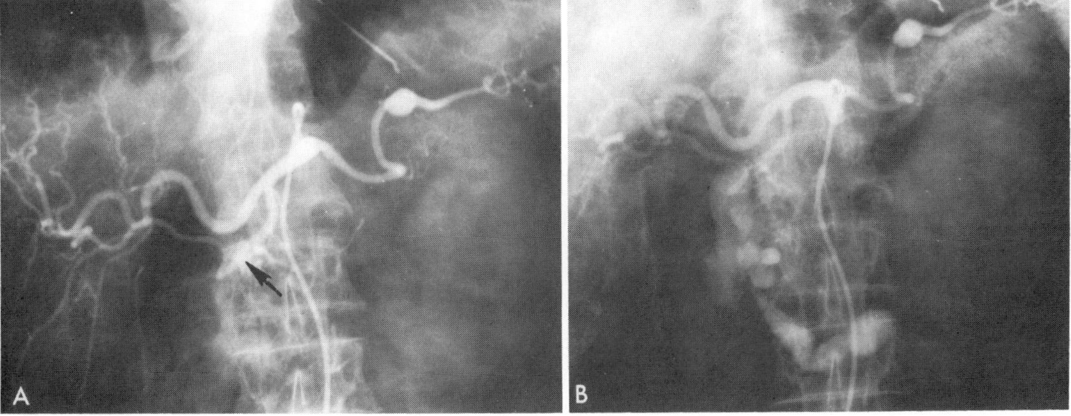

Figure 117–8. Erosion into the gastroduodenal artery by a duodenal ulcer. *A,* Celiac arteriogram shows extravasation from the gastroduodenal artery *(arrow)*. *B,* During the late phase of the celiac arteriogram, there is massive extravasation into the second and third portions of the duodenum. Attempts to control the bleeding by infusing surgical Pituitrin were unsuccessful.

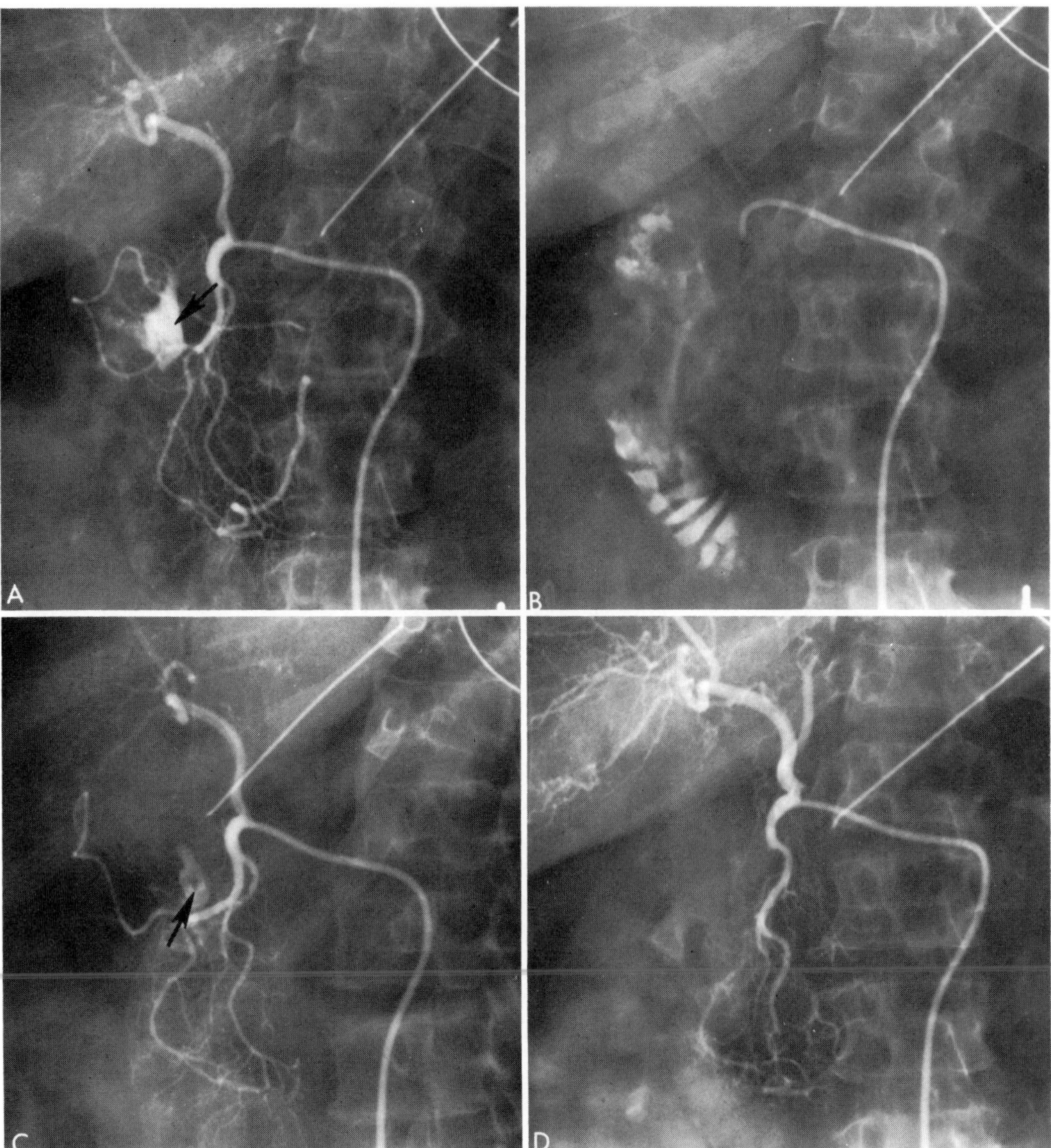

Figure 117–9. Massively bleeding duodenal ulcer controlled by the selective embolization of a small amount of autologous clots. *A* and *B,* Selective gastroduodenal arteriography demonstrates massive extravasation of a contrast material *(arrow)* from a branch of the superior pancreaticoduodenal artery into the duodenum. *C,* The infusion of 0.3 unit/minute of surgical Pituitrin directly into the gastroduodenal artery was unsuccessful in controlling the bleeding, and a repeat arteriogram shows continued extravasation *(arrow)*. *D,* Several strands of autologous clots were injected through the catheter directly into the superior pancreaticoduodenal artery. A repeat arteriogram showed that the bleeding was controlled by embolization technique.

and their localization for subsequent surgical removal. Owing to the mobility and overlapping coils of the small bowel, the exact location of the lesion at the time of the diagnostic study is frequently not sufficiently clarified to allow the surgeon to limit resection to the small segment of intestine containing the lesion. To overcome this problem, the angiogram may be repeated on the morning of surgery and a catheter placed selectively in the superior mesenteric artery. A coaxial 3F catheter is then passed through the original angiographic catheter into the branch of the superior mesenteric artery supplying the segment of bowel containing the lesion. The catheters are then secured in place and the patient is taken to the operating room. When the small bowel is displayed at surgery, injection of methylene blue through the 3F inner catheter discolors the segment of bowel containing the lesion, which is then resected. Immediate specimen radiography with the vessels injected with radiopaque silicon rubber confirms that the lesion has been resected before the surgeon closes the abdomen.[41]

Mesenteric Varices. Fine venous anastomoses exist between small portal tributaries of the mesenteric veins on the parietal surface of the viscera and the systemic venous channels in the retroperitoneum and abdominal wall. Although most of the varices in portal hypertension occur in the esophagus, rectum, and around the umbilicus, some patients as noted earlier, exhibit intestinal varices as a result of dilatation of these preexisting intestinal collaterals. This is especially true in patients who have had previous abdominal surgery and who develop adhesions between loops of bowel and the abdominal wall (Fig. 117–10). In portal hypertension, these varices may become huge and are capable of bleeding in a manner similar to esophageal varices.

Localized varices involving the superior mesenteric vein and its tributaries can be secondary to either pancreatic malignancy invading the mesenteric vein as it crosses the head of the pancreas or neoplasms of the gastrointestinal tract secondarily involving the mesentery. Carcinoid tumors may also produce extensive desmoplastic reaction in the mesentery, thereby occluding multiple tributaries of the superior mesenteric vein. In all these instances the venous dilatation may cause bleeding as a result of erosions of the overlying mucosa and rupture of the dilated venous channels.[42, 43] The value of angiography in these patients is to document the venous obstruction and the presence of varices and to exclude other sources of hemorrhage.[42]

Upper Intestinal Bleeding in Children. The 3 most common causes of acute bleeding into the bowel in children are peptic ulceration, portal hypertension, and Meckel's diverticulum. Ectopic gastric mucosa, an invariable associated change when bleeding occurs in Meckel's diverticulum, can usually be demonstrated with a ^{99}technetium pertechnetate scan,[44–46] and, if necessary, angiography may reveal extravasation in the diverticulum[47, 48] (Fig. 117–11).

Lower Intestinal Bleeding. Accumulated experience provides a basis for the following general conclusions: (1) Massive large bowel bleeding is usually due to diverticular disease[49–51] (Chapter 135) (Figs. 117–12 and 117–13), but may also arise from ischemic and inflammatory bowel disease (Fig. 117–14), vascular malformations, and rarely from carcinoma. (2) Chronic intermittent blood loss is commonly due to angiodysplasia.[52–54] (3) An appreciable proportion of lower intestinal hemorrhage encountered in hospital practice is iatrogenic, associated especially with chemotherapy and anticoagulants.[55] Patients with leukemia also frequently bleed into the lower intestinal tract.[56] (4) Radionuclide scans, which demonstrate extravasation with a high degree of sensitivity and may indicate the site of bleeding, have an established place in the investigation of lower intestinal tract hemorrhage[57–59] (Chapter 36).

Acute Bleeding. A ^{99}technetium sulfur colloid scan is performed first to confirm active bleeding, to define which patients are likely to benefit from visceral angiography, and to indicate which mesenteric vessels should primarily be studied at angiography[57–59] (Chapter 36).

^{99}Technetium sulfur colloid circulates in the intravascular space after peripheral IV injection. If bleeding is occurring at the time, a small fraction of the injected activity extravasates into the bowel from the point of bleeding. With each recirculation a smaller amount of activity enters the bowel as the reticuloendothelial system progressively removes the radiopharmaceutical from the circulation. As the intravascular space is cleared of activity, contrast develops between the

Text continued on page 1952

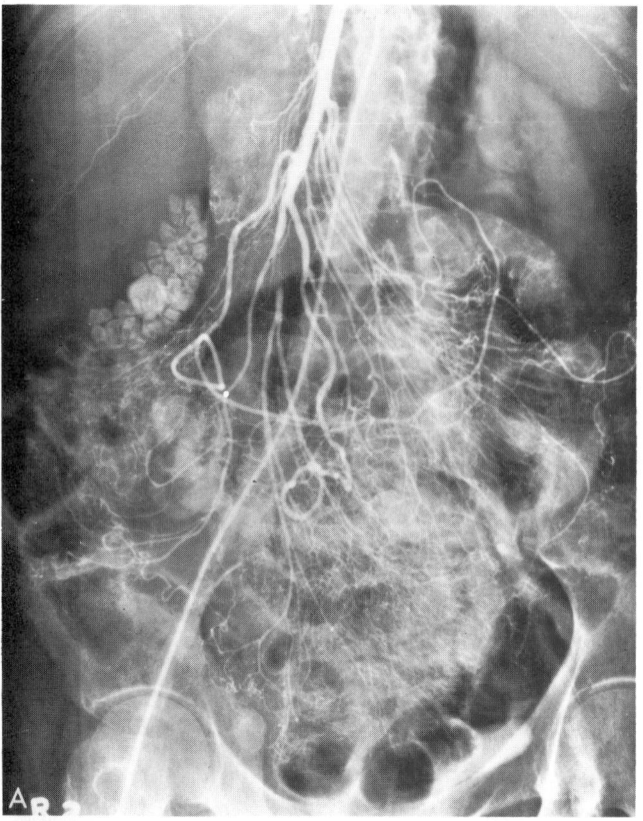

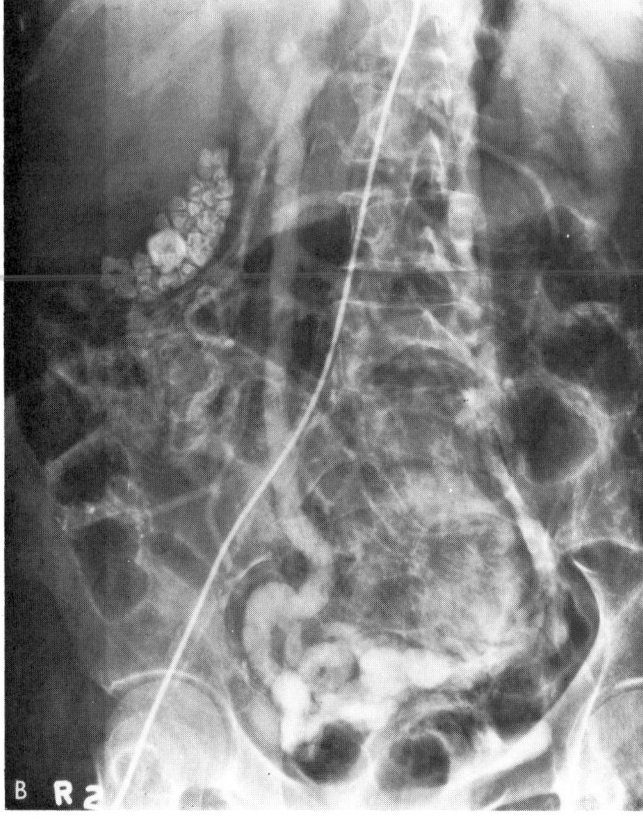

Figure 117–10. Bleeding mesenteric varices. A 68-year-old woman known to be cirrhotic presenting with lower gastrointestinal bleeding. *A*, Selective superior mesenteric arteriogram failed to demonstrate any evidence of a site of arterial bleeding. *B*, During the venous phase of the superior mesenteric arteriogram, retrograde flow is seen down the superior mesenteric vein into large varicosities in the pelvis. On later films in the serial study the contrast material was seen draining by way of the left ovarian vein. This patient had had pelvic surgery many years before. The pelvic varices decompressed the mesenteric vein via the gonadal venous system. At surgery adhesions containing large varicosities were seen between the pelvic organs and ileal loop of small bowel. In the resected specimen of the ileum one of the large veins in the wall of the ileum was bleeding as the result of an overlying area of mucosal ulceration. (From Baum S. *In*: Marshak RH, Lindner AE. Radiology of the Small Intestine. 2nd Ed. Philadelphia: WB Saunders, 1976. Reproduced with permission.)

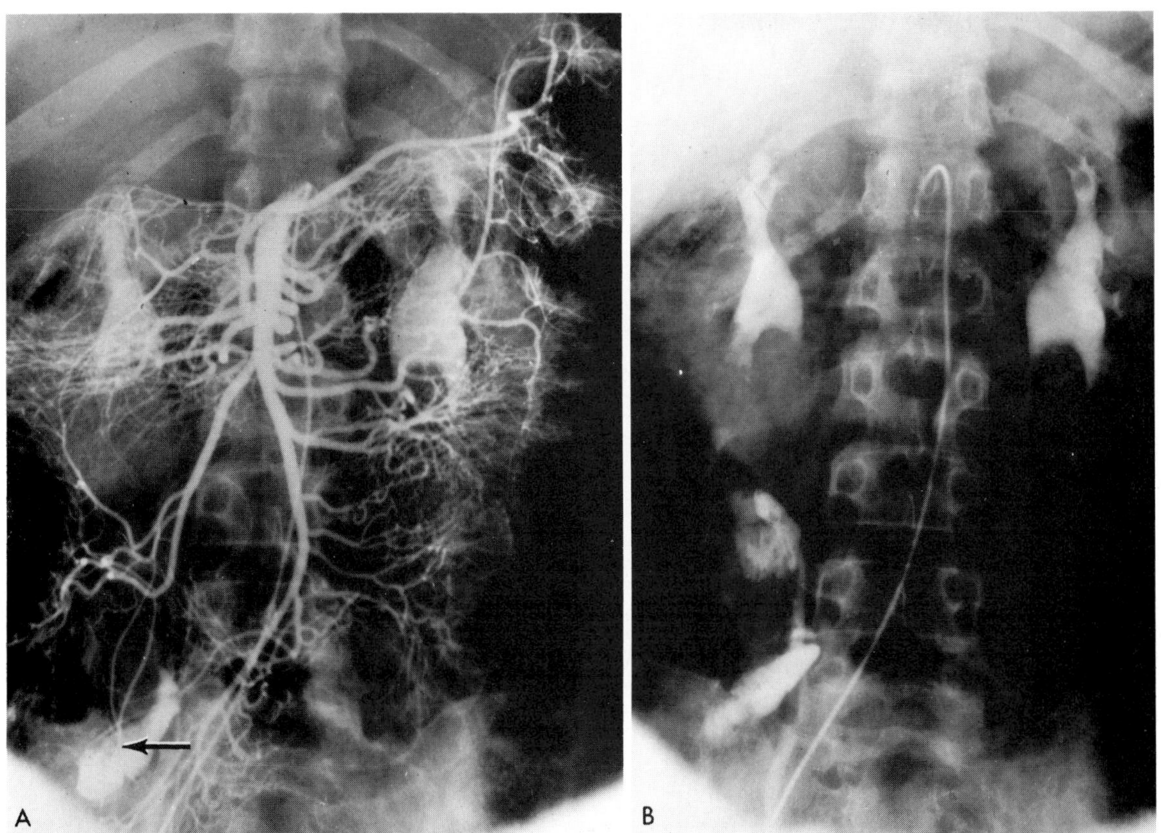

Figure 117–11. Angiographic demonstration of a bleeding Meckel's diverticulum. *A,* During the arterial phase of a selective superior mesenteric arteriogram, extravasation is seen originating from a branch of the ileocolic artery *(arrow)*. *B,* Fifteen seconds after the injection, contrast material remains within the bleeding Meckel's diverticulum. (From Baum S. *In*: Marshak RH, Lindner, AE. Radiology of the Small Intestine. 2nd Ed. Philadelphia: WB Saunders, 1976. Reproduced with permission.)

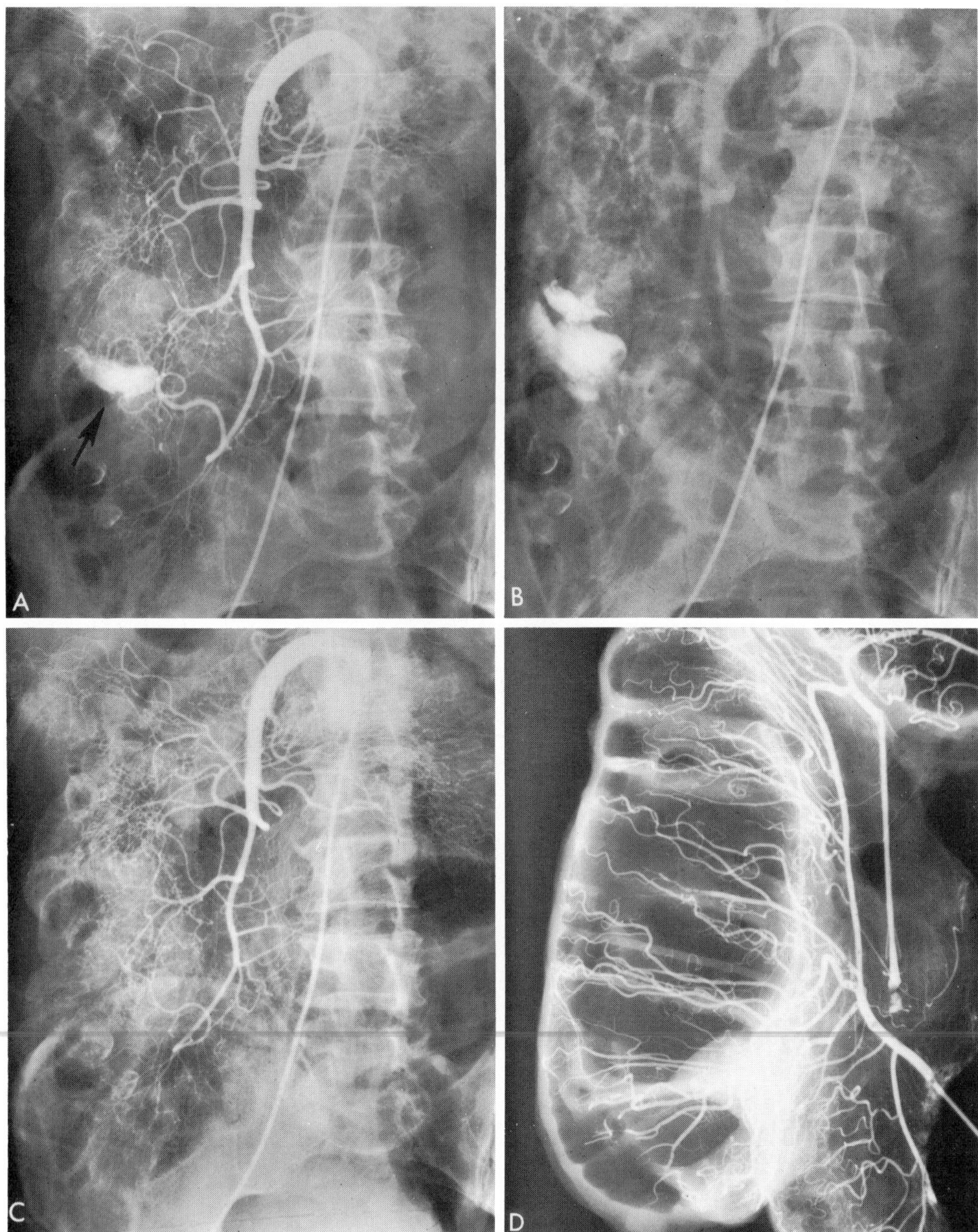

Figure 117–12. Massively bleeding right-sided diverticulum in a 55-year-old man controlled with intra-arterial infusion of vasopressin. *A,* Massive extravasation of contrast material from a branch of the ileocolic artery *(arrow). B,* Persistent contrast material within the colon during the late venous phase of the examination. *C,* Repeat superior mesenteric arteriogram during the infusion of 0.2 unit/minute of vasopressin demonstrates constriction of the peripheral branches of the mesenteric artery without any evidence of extravasation. The infusion was maintained at a rate of 0.2 unit/minute for 24 hours, then decreased to 0.1 unit/minute for another 18 hours, at which time the catheter was removed. *D,* An elective right-sided colectomy was performed 10 days later and the right colic artery was injected with a barium-gelatin mixture. Multiple diverticula were present in the right colon and could be seen on the injected specimen by the bowing that they produced on the adjacent arteries *(arrows).*

Illustration continued on opposite page

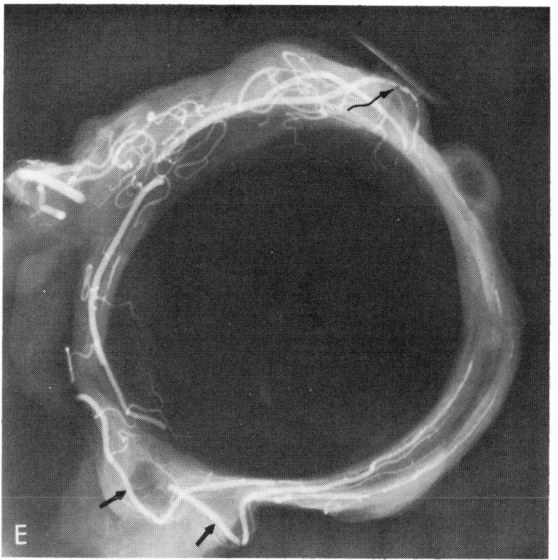

Figure 117–12 *Continued. E,* Cross section of the colon of the level of the diverticulum that was bleeding demonstrates multiple diverticula in that area with characteristic bowing of the adjacent arteries. The artery overlying the diverticulum that was bleeding exhibits marginal irrregularity, presumably due to thrombosis (curved arrow). (From Waltman AC et al. Geriatrics 1974; 29:48. Reproduced with permission.)

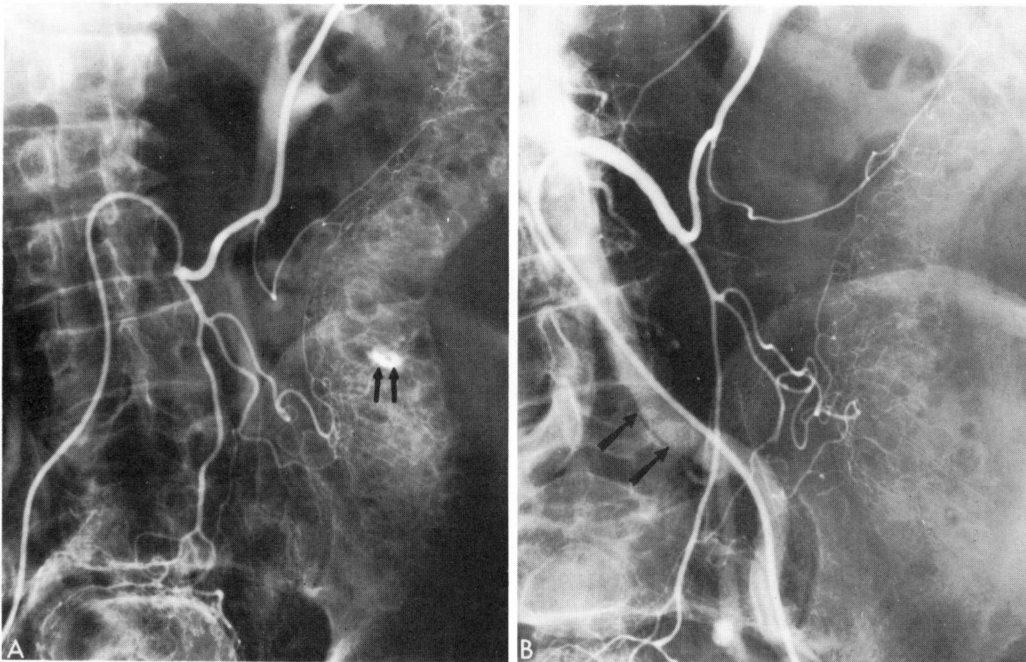

Figure 117–13. Inferior mesenteric arteriogram of a 73-year-old man with a bleeding diverticulum in the sigmoid colon. *A,* Arterial phase of the examination showed extravasation of contrast material within the diverticulum *(arrows). B,* During the infusion of vasopressin at 0.2 unit/minute a repeat arteriogram shows constriction of the peripheral branches of the inferior mesenteric artery without extravasation. Reflux into the aortoiliac vessels *(arrows)* confirms the increase in peripheral resistance within the inferior mesenteric bed, resulting in reflux of contrast material into the abdominal aorta.

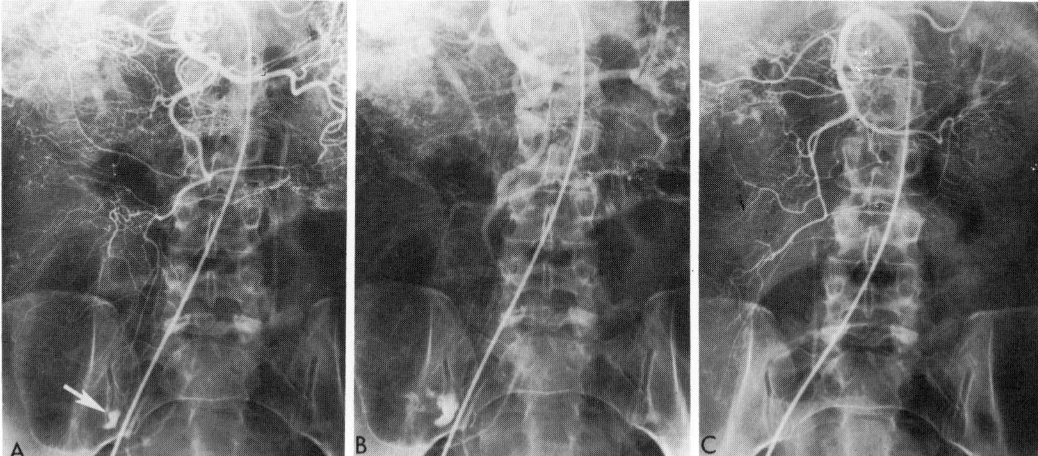

Figure 117–14. Right-sided ulcerative colitis bleeding controlled with the intra-arterial infusion of vasopressin. *A,* Superior mesenteric arteriogram demonstrates bleeding from a cecal branch of the ileocecal artery *(arrow)*. *B,* Extravasated contrast material persists within the cecum during the venous phase of the arteriogram. *C,* In order to avoid emergency surgical intervention, vasopressin was infused into the superior mesenteric artery. Superior mesenteric arteriogram during the infusion of vasopressin at a rate of 0.2 unit/minute for 15 minutes shows constriction of the peripheral branches of the artery with cessation of further bleeding.

extravasated activity and the diminishing intravascular background[57, 58] (Fig. 117–15).

The actual site of extravasation can usually be inferred from (1) the location and configuration of the extravasated activity, and (2) the change in appearance on serial images as the intraluminal activity is propelled onward by peristalsis. This usually allows differentiation between activity in the small and large bowel (Figs. 117–16 and 117–17).

The sensitivity of this investigation is such that bleeding rates as low as 0.1 ml/minute can be detected, as compared with a minimum of 0.5 ml/minute for angiographic visualization.

As the half-life of ^{99}technetium sulfur colloid in the circulation is 2 minutes, only bleeding occurring within the first 10 to 15 minutes after injection will appear on the image, but this simple, inexpensive, and non-invasive test can be readily repeated as soon as there is clinical evidence of rebleeding.

Scintigraphy demonstrates extravasation and may suggest its site but gives no information about the nature of the bleeding lesion. In the often elderly arteriosclerotic patient in whom acute colorectal hemorrhage typically occurs, it may be deemed reasonable to institute a trial of IV vasopressin and defer further investigation of the abnormality responsible for the bleeding to a later date. Postoperative large bowel hemorrhage also responds readily to vasopressin alone in many cases[60, 61] (Figs. 117–18 to 117–20).

Patients treated with IV vasopressin can be monitored during therapy by clinical parameters and by further technetium sulfur colloid scans to identify those continuing to bleed or who rebleed and will require surgical intervention. In such cases, angiography is required to confirm the location of the bleeding site as well as to indicate the nature of the bleeding lesion. This information will enable the surgeon to limit the procedure in many cases to directed segmental colonic resection, and thereby lower operative morbidity and mortality.

Intense activity in the liver and spleen largely restricts the usefulness of technetium sulfur colloid scintigraphy to the lower gastrointestinal tract. Blood pool imaging using technetium-labeled red blood cells avoids this problem and, in addition, has the theoretical advantage of a greatly increased half-life in the circulation. This allows visualization of extravasation up to 24 hours after injection of the isotope.[59, 62] Its benefits, however, are largely offset by the greatly reduced sensitivity of the labeled red blood cell technique as a result of increased background activity from labeled red blood cells in the intravascular space. As a consequence, a bleeding rate of 3 to 6 ml/minute is required before extrava-

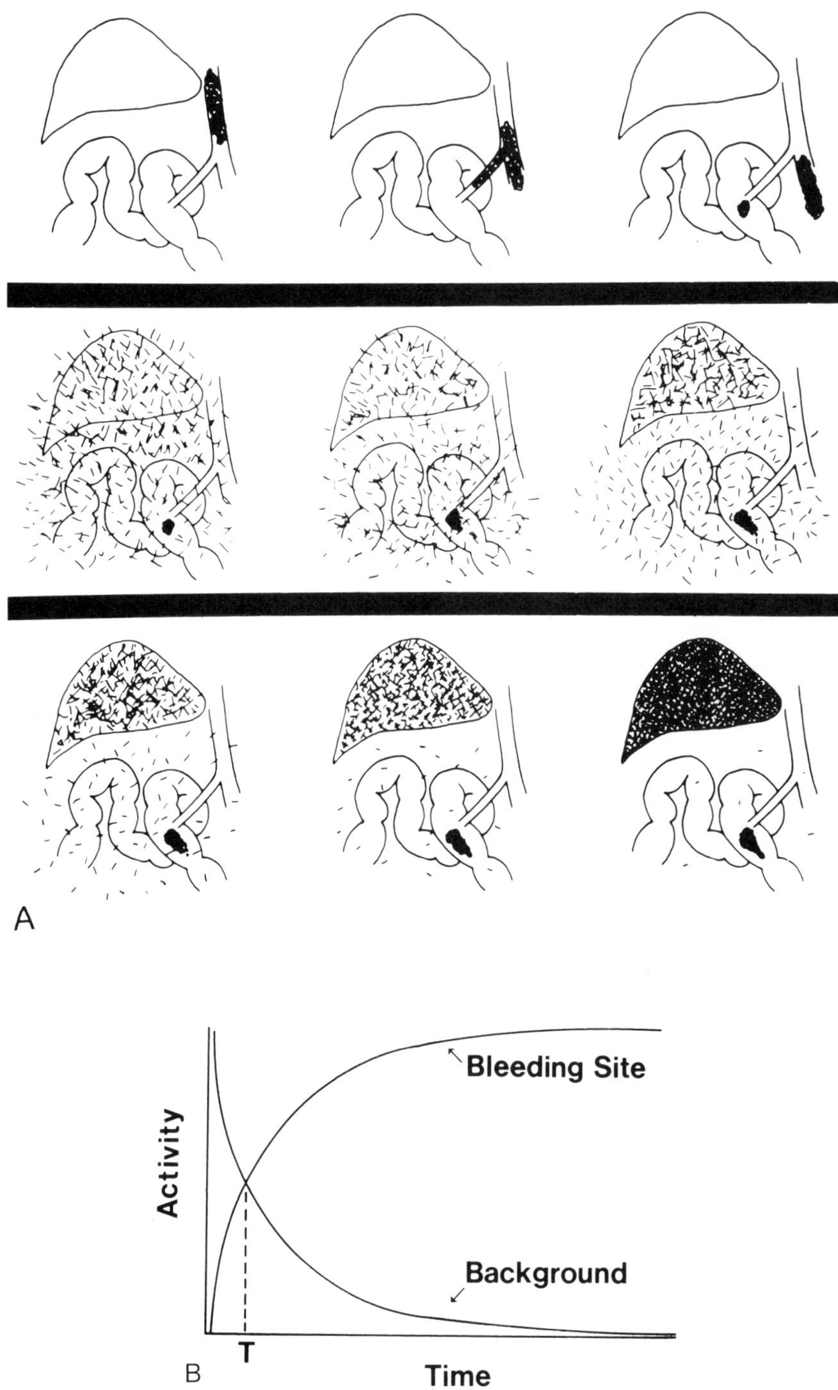

Figure 117–15. Demonstration of gastrointestinal bleeding with ^{99m}technetium sulfur colloid—basic concept. *A,* The radionuclide has been injected IV. At the bleeding site a fraction of the injected activity extravasates and is eliminated from the circulation. This phenomenon is repeated each time the blood recirculates. Because of rapid clearance of the radionuclide by the reticuloendothelial system, a contrast is eventually reached between the extravasated activity and the surrounding background, allowing visualization of the bleeding site. *B,* Graph depicting the events in *A.* The background activity decreases exponentially immediately after IV administration of the agent. The activity at the bleeding site increases exponentially in the opposite direction. A contrast is reached between the bleeding site and the surrounding background activity when the 2 curves cross (Point T).

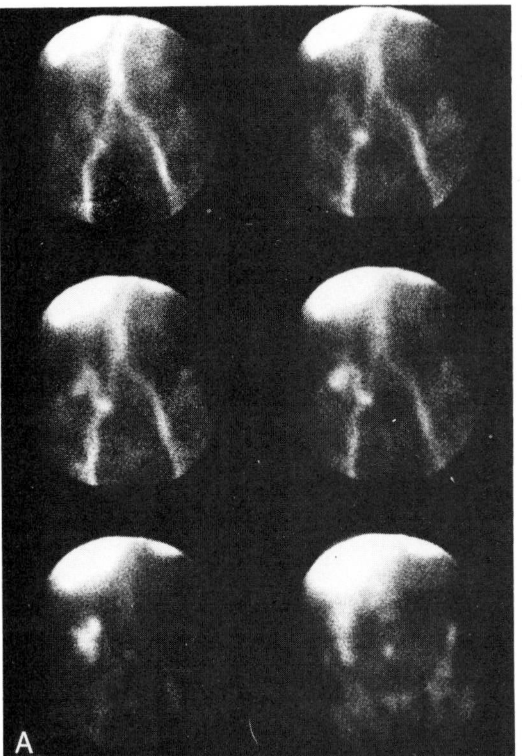

Figure 117–16. Bleeding from the terminal ileum. *A,* Shortly after the injection of ^{99m}Tc sulfur colloid a point of extravasation is noted in the right lower quadrant overlying the iliac vessel *(left top).* The activity gradually moves upward and laterally into a wider lumen *(top right, middle left and right).* Finally, the extravasated blood moves upward toward the liver *(lower left and right).* The findings were interpreted as showing a bleeding site in the terminal ileum, very close to the ileocecal vale. *B* and *C,* Superior mesenteric artery angiogram in the same patient shortly after the scan shows extravasation of the contrast medium in the terminal ileum exactly at the site shown on the scan. *B* is early phase, and *C* is late phase of the angiogram.

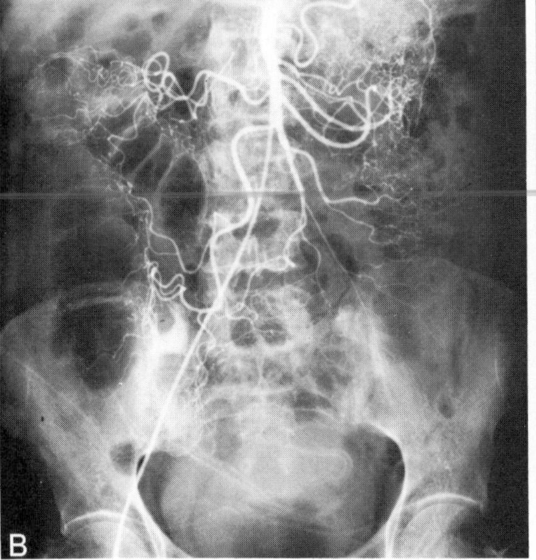

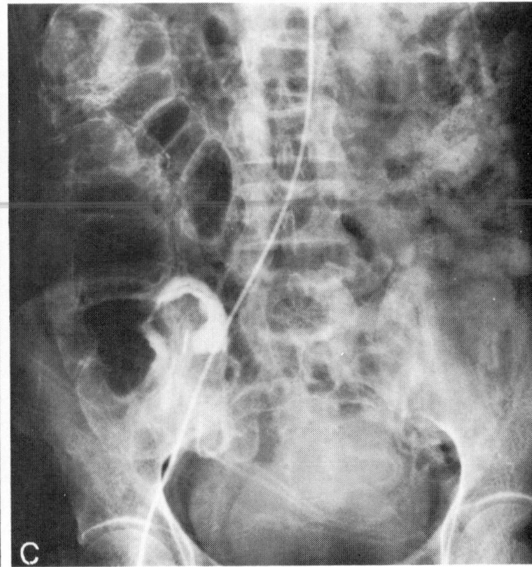

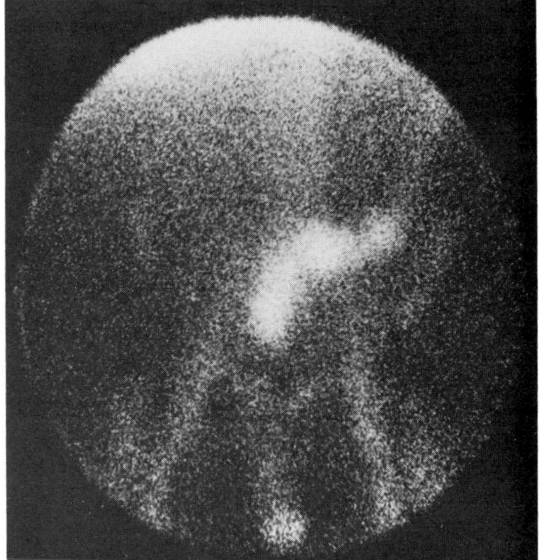

Figure 117–17. Bleeding sigmoid lesion. Scintigram showing extravasated activity in the pelvis with a configuration corresponding to that of the sigmoid colon. The activity subsequently moved into the rectum and disappeared with bowel evacuation, confirming the location of the lesion. This patient was treated successfully with IV vasopressin without further investigation.

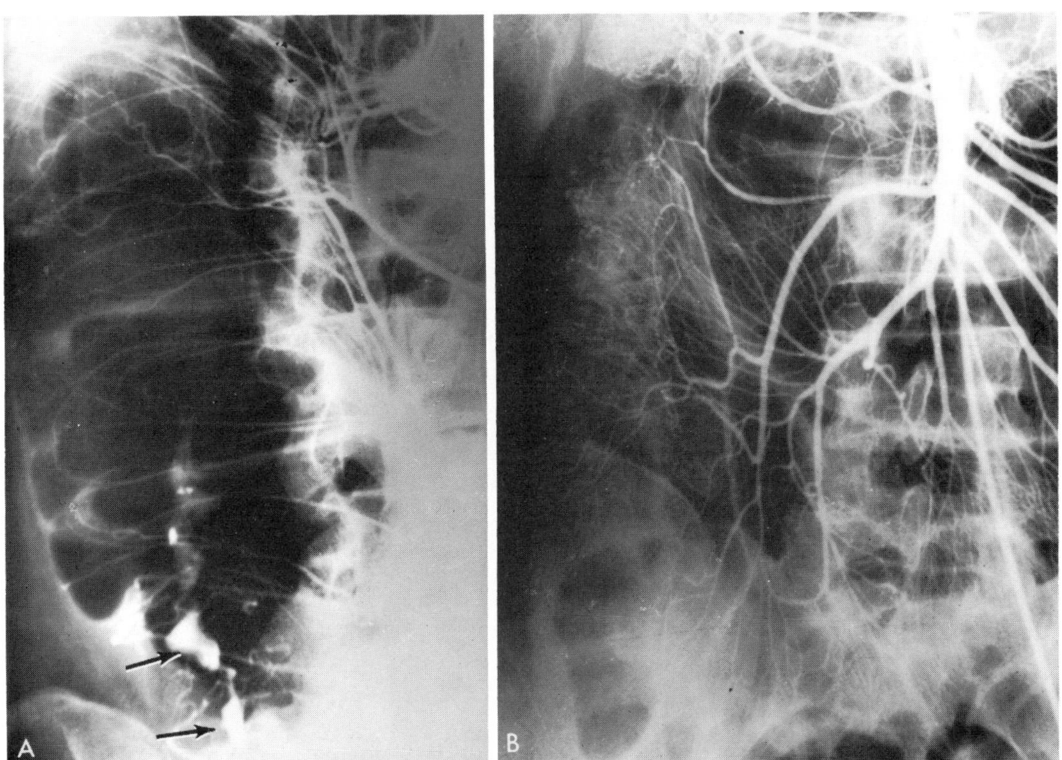

Figure 117–18. Hemorrhage from an appendiceal stump. This 28-year-old man had bright red rectal bleeding 2 weeks after an appendectomy. *A,* Superior mesenteric arteriogram demonstrates massive extravasation originating from the ileocolic artery at the tip of the cecum *(arrow)*. *B,* During the infusion of 0.2 unit/minute of vasopressin, no further evidnce of extravasation was seen. The patient was discharged 3 days later and has had no recurent bleeding.

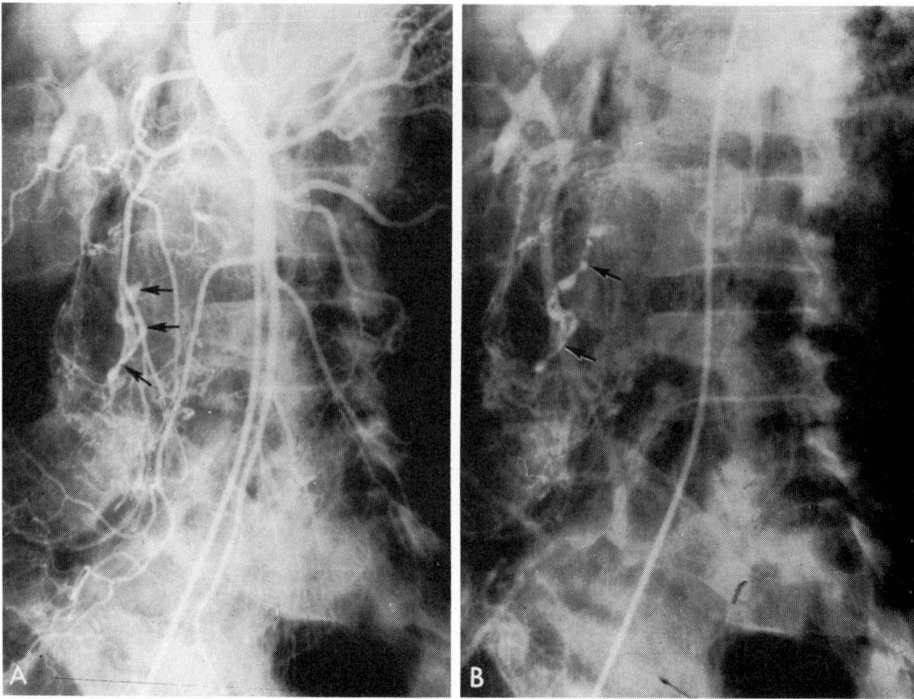

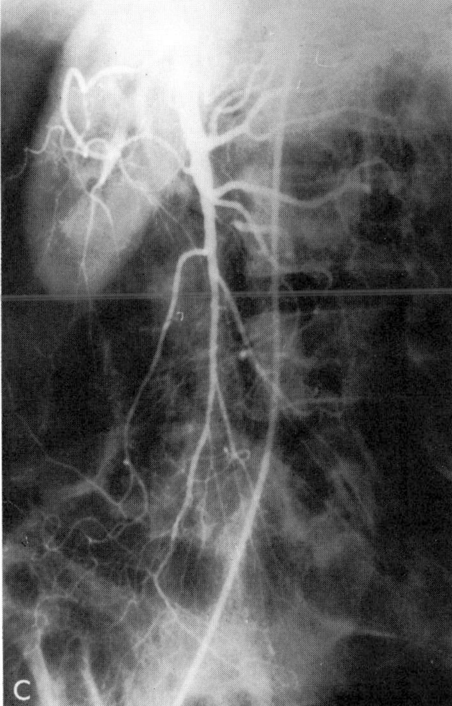

Figure 117–19. Gastrointestinal bleeding following closure of a transverse colostomy as part of a 3-stage procedure for carcinoma of the sigmoid. *A,* Arterial phase of the superior mesenteric arteriogram shows extravasation of contrast material from a branch of the right colic artery *(arrows). B,* The extravasated contrast material persists during the late venous phase of the study *(arrows). C,* During the infusion of vasopressin into the superior mesenteric artery for 15 minutes, the angiogram was repeated and there is no longer evidence of extravasation. The patient was treated with vasopressin infusion for 2 days and no recurrent bleeding occurred after termination of the infusion. (From Athanasoulis CA et al. Radiology 1974; 113:37. Reproduced with permission.)

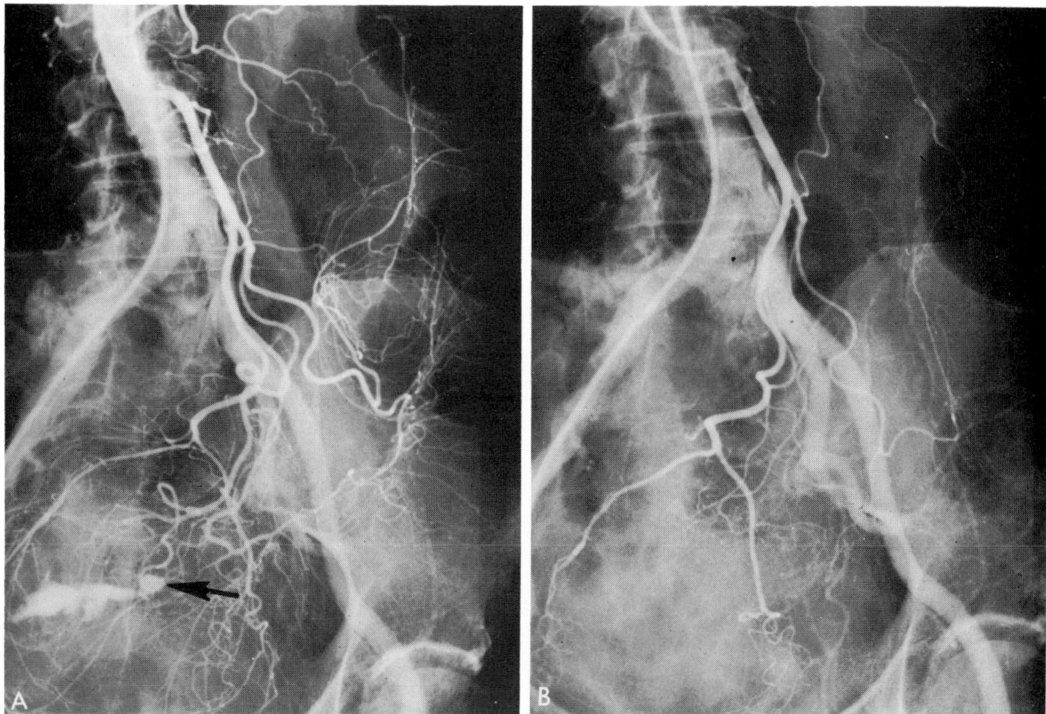

Figure 117–20. Massive lower gastrointestinal bleeding after colonoscopic removal of a polyp. *A,* Inferior mesenteric arteriogram during the arterial phase shows bleeding from a sigmoidal branch of the inferior mesenteric artery *(arrow)*. *B,* Repeat inferior mesenteric arteriogram during the infusion of 0.2 unit of vasopressin for 20 minutes showed no further bleeding. The infusion was continued at the same rate for 12 hours and then decreased to 0.1 unit/minute for another 12 hours, with clinical control of the bleeding.

sation can be identified.[63] In addition, continuous imaging of the patient over 24 hours after injection is impractical in a busy department, and anything less is likely to lead to misrepresentation of the actual site of bleeding. Furthermore, increased peristalsis associated with gastrointestinal hemorrhage may move the extravasated activity a long way in either direction from the bleeding point by the time the delayed image is obtained.[63]

Chronic Intermittent Bleeding. Arteriovenous malformations of various kinds may be associated with both acute hemorrhage and chronic intermittent bleeding. Those in the upper gastrointestinal tract and in the small bowel are most often congenital in origin, occur mainly in young patients, and may be associated with inherited conditions such as hemorrhagic telangiectasia.[64] Large bowel vascular malformations, on the other hand, occur mainly on the right side of the colon in elderly patients. They are commonly known as *"angiodysplasia."* This term is a bit unfortunate, as it suggests a developmental origin, whereas the bulk of evidence indicates that the malformations are acquired lesions. The lesions are considered by many to be a form of ischemic large bowel disease associated with chronically raised intraluminal pressure, resulting in poor mucosal perfusion and submucosal arteriovenous shunting[52] (Chapter 116).

An association between angiodysplasia and aortic stenosis has been well documented.[50, 64–69] Inasmuch as aortic stenosis is associated with reduced cardiac output and chronic tissue ischemia as a result of decreased perfusion, its association with angiodysplasia may be further evidence of the acquired nature of the latter.

The prevalence rate of angiodysplasia in resected and necropsy "normal" colon specimens from elderly subjects appears to be related to the diligence with which the lesion is sought by the pathologist. Rates as high as 50% have been recorded.[65] The question then arises as to whether these lesions are only incidentally present and not the true source of bleeding. The low rate of rebleeding after segmental colonic resection for angiographically demonstrated angiodysplasia, however, suggests that these lesions are indeed responsible for the hemorrhage.[53, 54] Such apparently contradictory findings may be reconciled if only those angiodysplastic lesions large enough to be visualized at angiography actually cause blood loss of sufficient degree to be recognized clinically.

The ^{99}technetium sulfur colloid scan is usually negative in patients with angiodysplasia, as bleeding rarely occurs during the examination. The angiographic appearance of the vascular abnormality consists of dilated, tortuous small branches of the mesenteric artery, usually in the cecum or ascending colon, with a dense capillary blush of the involved segment and early opacification of a prominent draining vein (Fig. 117–21). Angiography in these patients is usually performed on an elective or semielective basis because of the chronic nature of the blood loss; for that reason, contrast extravasation in the lumen of the colon is rarely seen.

Identification of these vascular abnormalities is very difficult at surgery. The serosal aspect of the bowel may look perfectly normal; even transillumination at the operating-

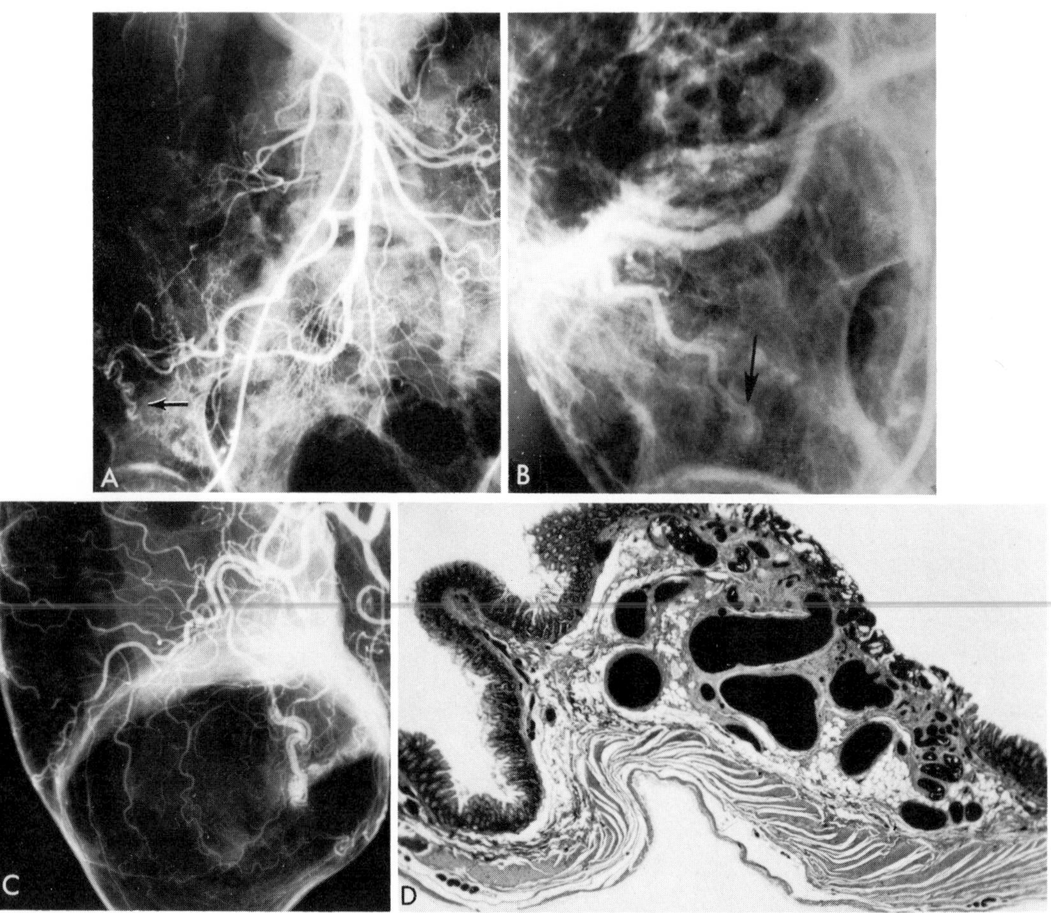

Figure 117–21. Angiodysplasia of the cecum in an elderly man wih chronic gastrointestinal bleeding. *A,* Arterial phase of a superior mesenteric arteriogram demonstrates a dilated and tortuous artery in the cecum *(arrow). B,* Magnification angiogram during the venous phase of the study demonstrates an early draining vein coming from the same areas as the abnormal artery *(arrow). C,* Radiograph of the injected surgical specimen shows dilated arterial and venous structures of the angiodysplasia corresponding to the findings on the arteriogram. *D,* Photomicrograph of the area of the angiodysplaia in the wall of the cecum shows the grossly dilated submucosal vascular channels. The vascular channels are distended because of the vascular injection technique employed.

room table may not prove helpful. The pathologist also has difficulty in finding these lesions unless many serial sections are made. We have found that it is useful to inject the arteries of the resected specimen with either a gelatin barium solution or silicon rubber material, which prevents collapse of the vessels prior to histologic section. Radiographs can be taken of the specimen and the attention of the pathologist drawn to the specific area of abnormality (Fig. 117–21). Pathologically, the lesions are not true arteriovenous malformations but rather seem to be a cluster of submucosal ectatic vascular lakes consisting of both arteries and veins. Apparently, bleeding occurs as a result of small erosions and ulcerations of the overlying mucosa.

Vascular Disorders

Vascular gastrointestinal disease may occur as a result of disorders affecting either the large or the small vessels of the gut. With modern angiographic techniques, large vessel disease is easy to diagnose. Small vessel disease, on the other hand, can be exceedingly difficult to detect despite magnification techniques and improved radiographic resolution.[70–72] Functional disorders of the small vessels (such as vasoconstriction in low flow states) or the superimposition of functional on organic abnormalities (e.g., constriction of vessels adjacent to an artery occluded by an embolus) further complicate the issue. It is also certain that an overlap exists with disorders affecting both large and small vessels.[71]

Without entering into a detailed discussion of all the disorders affecting the large and small vessels of the gut, this section will deal with the applications of angiography in the following conditions: atheromatous occlusions, embolic occlusions, low flow states, aneurysms, vasculitis, degenerative vascular disease, and structural vascular changes. The first 3 of these entities are the most common causes of bowel ischemia and are discussed along with the other causes for ischemic bowel disease in the preceding chapter (Chapter 116).

Acute Mesenteric Ischemia

Occlusive. It takes approximately 6 hours from the onset of complete ischemia until bowel infarction occurs.[73, 76] Early diagnosis, therefore, is essential. If clinical suspicion is high, a plain film of the abdomen should be obtained, followed by mesenteric angiography.[75]

Midstream abdominal aortography in both the anteroposterior and lateral planes should be performed. The value of the lateral aortogram cannot be overemphasized, because it is in the lateral view only that the origins of the mesenteric arteries can be appreciated[75, 76] (Fig. 117–22). Selective superior mesenteric arteriography is necessary to establish the level of occlusion, to demonstrate the presence of additional distal arterial occlusions, and to document the degree and extent of collateral vessel development and the patency of the mesenteric veins (Fig. 117–23). Occlusion of the superior mesenteric artery secondary to aortic dissection can also be diagnosed with abdominal aortography (Fig. 117–24).

Obstruction of the superior mesenteric artery resulting in bowel ischemia results principally from acute thrombosis due to atheroma and embolic disease, with the 2 being about equally divided in frequency. Thrombosis more often involves the origin or the proximal segment of the superior mesenteric artery, whereas emboli usually lodge at bifurcations, such as the origin of the middle colic artery[76] (Figs. 117–22 and 117–25).

Administration of thrombolytic agents may reverse superior mesenteric arterial thrombotic or embolic occlusions.[77] The enzyme streptokinase is a plasminogen activator and as such accelerates fibrinolytic breakdown of thrombus. Unfortunately, systemic therapy with the drug carries a risk of serious bleeding. This led to the development of local streptokinase therapy in which lower doses of the enzyme are delivered over a period of up to 48 hours through an angiographic catheter placed as close to the thrombus as possible.

An ideal thrombolytic agent would act only on plasminogen intimately related to fibrin within a thrombus and so avoid bleeding complications due to systemic activation of plasminogen. Such an agent, known as human extrinsic (tissue type) plasminogen activator, has been developed[78, 79] and should be available for clinical use in the future. Its expense, however, may limit its application.

Streptokinase has been delivered through an angiographic catheter placed selectively in the mouth of the superior mesenteric artery in cases of thromboembolic occlusion of

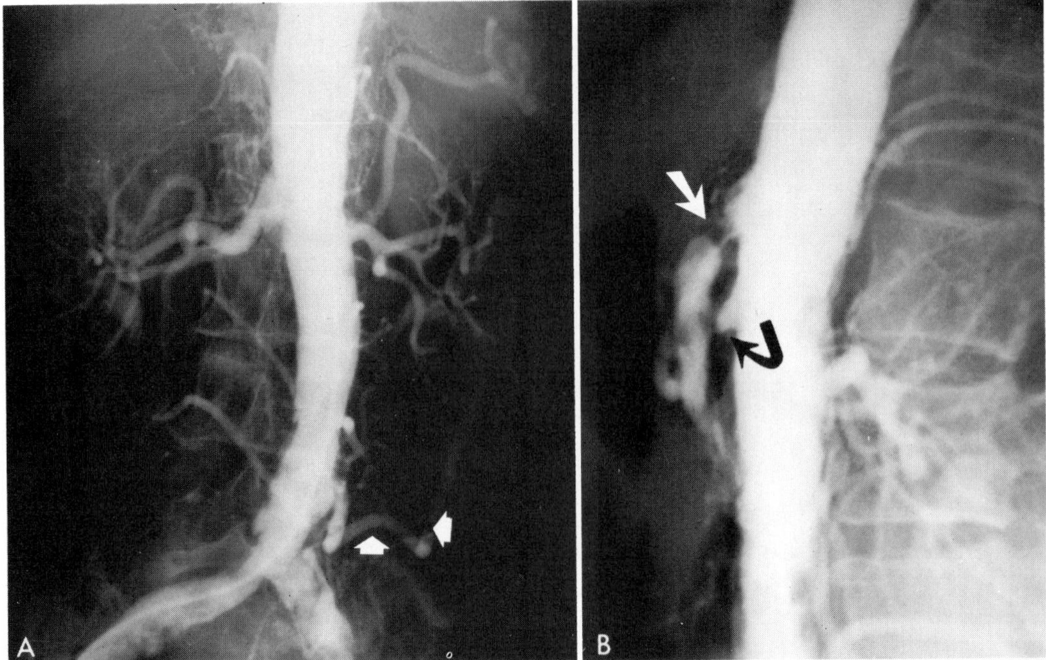

Figure 117–22. Value of the lateral aortogram in evaluation of the mesenteric arteries. Aortography was performed in this 72-year-old woman because of postprandial epigastric pain. A bruit was heard over the epigastrium. Barium studies of the gastrointestinal tract were negative. *A*, Midstream abdominal aortogram, anteroposterior view, shows an enlarged left colic artery from the inferior mesenteric artery *(arrows)*. The celiac axis and the superior mesenteric artery cannot be evaluated with this projection. *B*, Lateral view; there is severe stenosis of the celiac axis *(straight white arrow)* and complete occlusion of the superior mesenteric artery *(curved black arrow)*.

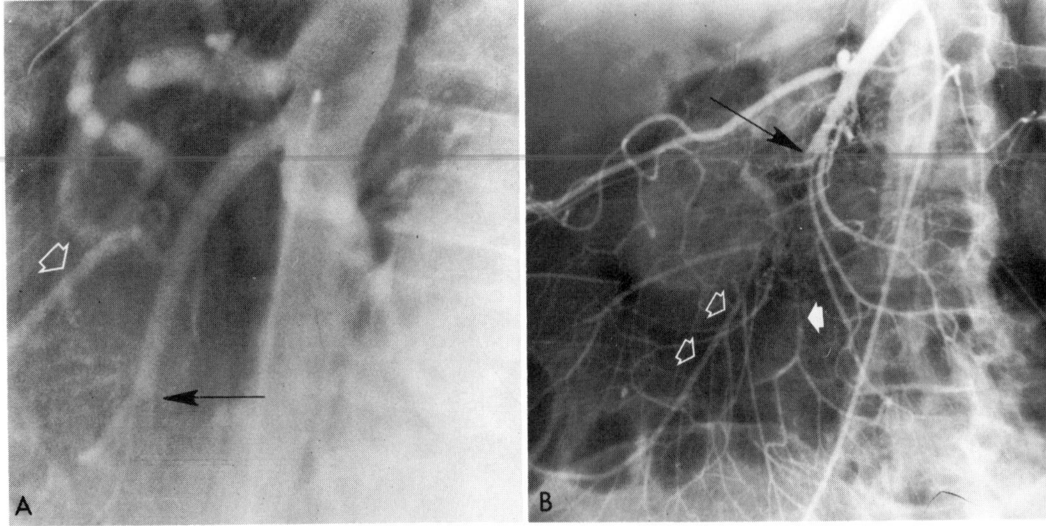

Figure 117–23. Embolic occlusion of the superior mesenteric artery in a 48-year-old woman with atrial fibrillation. *A*, There is occlusion of the superior mesenteric artery *(black arrow)* beyond the origin of the middle colic artery *(white open arrow)*. *B*, The selective superior mesenteric arteriogram shows to better advantage the level of the occlusion *(black arrow)*. With the selective injection, reconstitution of the distal superior mesenteric artery is demonstrated *(open white arrows)* and occlusion of additional jejunal branches *(small white arrow)* can be appreciated.

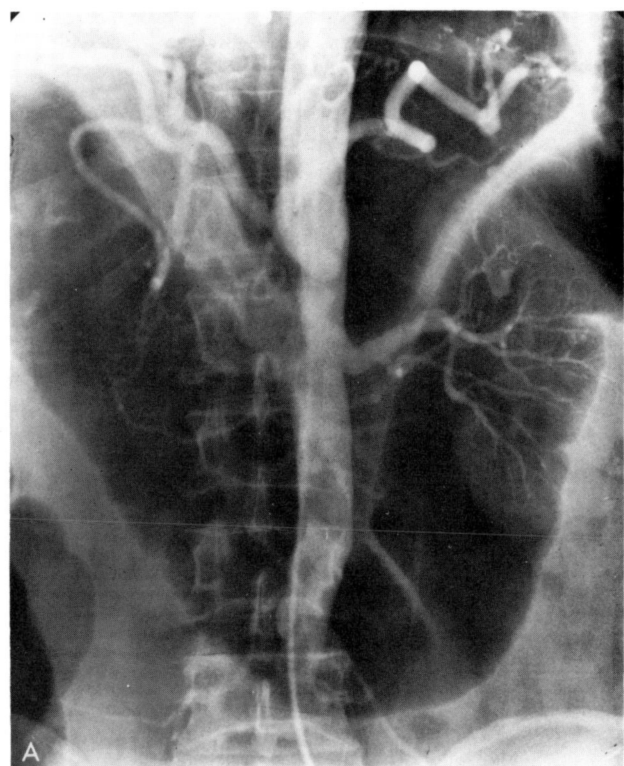

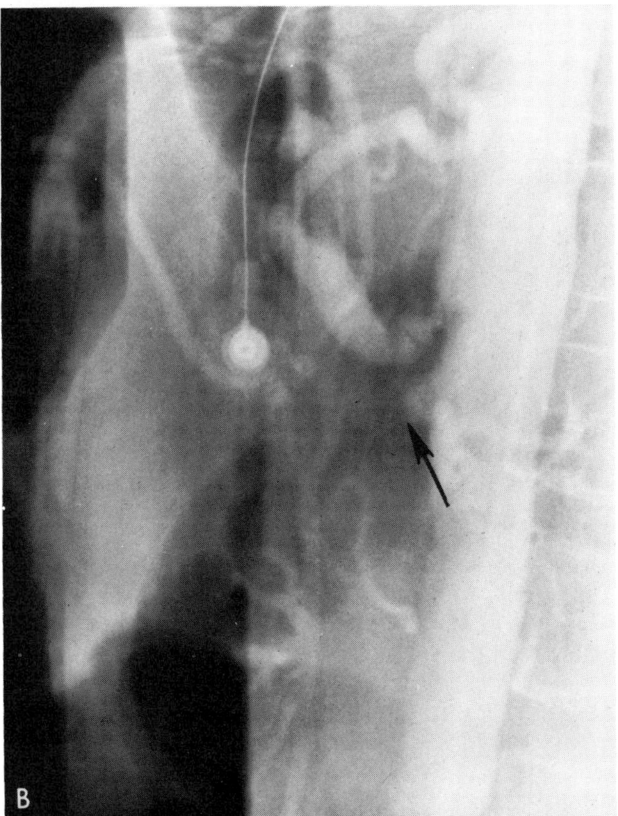

Figure 117–24. Dissecting aneurysm of the thoracic aorta extending into the abdomen and occluding the right renal and superior mesenteric artery. This 55-year-old man was brought to the hospital after being found unconscious. On physical examination the abdomen was distended and no bowel sounds could be heard. *A,* Abdominal aortography demonstrates a dissection of the abdominal aorta with occlusion of the right renal and superior mesenteric arteries. *B,* A lateral film of the abdomen shows with better definition the complete occlusion of the superior mesenteric artery immediately distal to its origin *(arrow).* (From Baum S. *In*: Marshak RH, Lindner AE: Radiology of the Small Intestine. 2nd Ed. Philadelphia: WB Saunders, 1976. Reproduced with permission.)

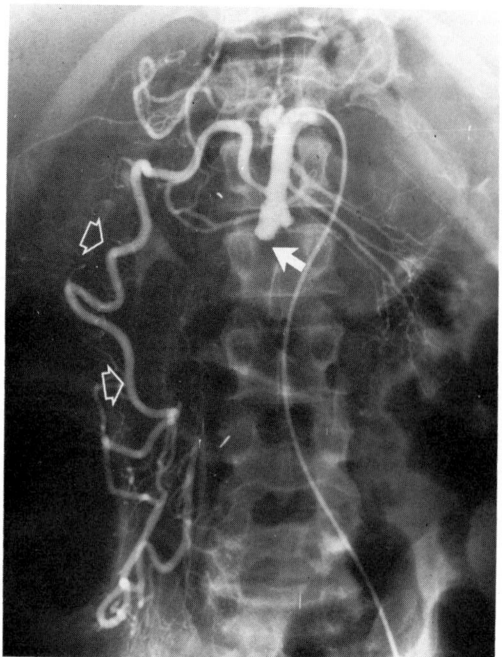

Figure 117–25. Embolic occlusion of the superior mesenteric artery from a thrombus in an akinetic segment of the left ventricle. There is complete occlusion of the superior mesenteric artery *(solid arrow)* distal to the origin of the middle colic artery. Some collateral flow exists to the bowel by way of the middle colic–right colic anastomosis *(open white arrows).*

that vessel,[77] with resultant lysis of thrombus and re-establishment of the circulation in the involved bowel. It is obviously essential that such therapy be instituted before necrosis of bowel occurs, i.e., in the first 6 hours after onset of symptoms in a patient with no signs of peritoneal irritation; otherwise, hemorrhage into the bowel would seem almost inevitable.

Atheromatous lesions at the origin of the mesenteric arteries are extremely common in patients without symptoms of bowel ischemia. The clinical setting and the presence or absence of large collateral vessels help determine the significance of superior mesenteric artery stenosis or occlusion.[76, 80, 81]

In the presence of hemodynamically significant stenosis or occlusion at the origin of the superior mesenteric artery, collateral flow develops through the pancreaticoduodenal arcades and the marginal anastomotic artery of the colon (Fig. 117–26). If the superior mesenteric artery is occluded distal to the origin of the middle colic artery, neither the marginal nor the pancreaticoduodenal arcades are functional. In these instances, small mesenteric collateral vessels form in an attempt to bridge the occlusion, but they are generally not adequate to maintain viability of the bowel.[14, 15, 71, 72]

The inferior mesenteric artery is frequently occluded by atherosclerosis or in the course of development of abdominal aortic aneurysms. In these usually asymptomatic patients, the marginal vessel can be seen at angiography extending from the middle colic to the left and distal inferior mesenteric arteries.[14–16, 71, 82]

Low Flow State. Angiographically, at surgery, and at necropsy, the intestinal arteries and veins are not found to be occluded in this form of intestinal ischemia (Chapter 116). The evidence suggests that vasoconstriction is the prominent factor in the development of ischemic symptoms in these patients. Clinically, the entity is seen most commonly in patients following myocardial infarction or congestive heart failure, in those who have undergone major thoracic or abdominal surgery, and in patients ingesting digitalis, a potent mesenteric vasoconstrictor.[70, 71, 76, 82, 83]

The fact that no arterial occlusions are found may only reflect the present limitation of angiographic resolution of small-sized vessels. However, with the data available today, it seems logical to replace the concept "nonocclusive ischemia" with the term "low flow state," which better denotes the underlying pathophysiology.[84]

The diagnosis can be made only with mesenteric angiography, and the angiographic features are mainly those of intense mesenteric vasoconstriction[85–87] (Fig. 117–27*A*). The most peripheral branches of the superior mesenteric artery are very slow to fill, and some areas of the gut do not appear to be perfused. Because of the intense peripheral vasoconstriction, concentric areas of narrowing are seen in many of the major branches of the mesenteric artery, especially at their origins. This may be associated as well with irregularity of the intestinal branches and abnormal tapering patterns. The angiographic changes may reverse with infusions of vasodilator drugs directly into the superior mesenteric artery (Fig. 117–27*B*). If they do not, it is assumed that the vascular changes are fixed and are not functional.[70, 71, 75, 85–87]

In veiw of the extremely high mortality of bowel ischemia secondary to low flow states, an aggressive diagnostic and therapeutic approach has been developed. Mesenteric

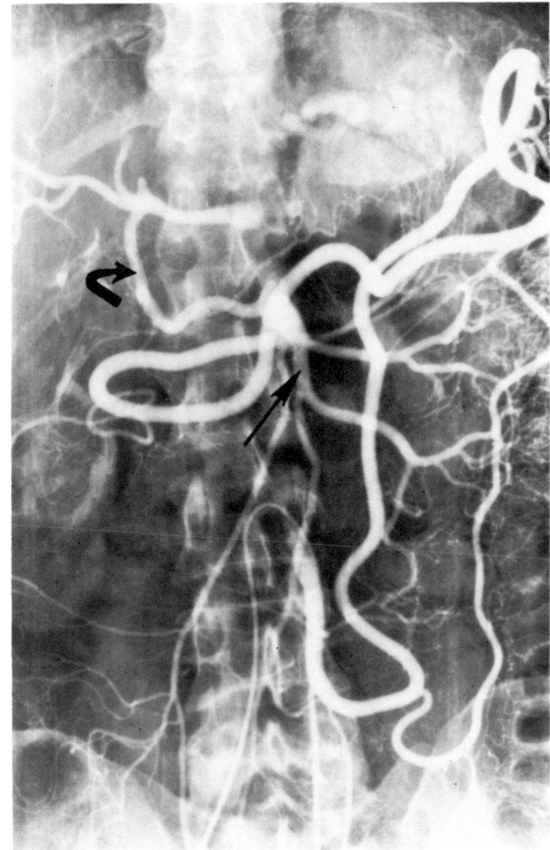

Figure 117–26. Asymptomatic, complete occlusion of the celiac and superior mesenteric arteries with excellent collateral filling via the inferior mesenteric artery. Selective inferior mesenteric arteriography demonstrates collateral filling of the superior mesenteric artery *(straight arrow)* by way of the marginal anastomotic artery of the colon extending from the left colic to middle colic arteries. The celiac axis fills via the inferior pancreaticoduodenal artery *(curved arrow)*. (From Baum S. *In*: Marshak RH, Lindner AE. Radiology of the Small Intestine. 2nd Ed. Philadelphia: WB Saunders, 1976. Reproduced with permission.)

angiography is performed as soon as the diagnosis of acute bowel ischemia is suspected.[83, 88] In the absence of organic large vessel occlusion and in the presence of local or generalized mesenteric vasoconstriction, papaverine is infused directly into the mesenteric artery in an attempt to reverse vasoconstriction, promote bowel perfusion, and prevent further extension of the ischemic process or progression to infarction. During the infusion, measures should be taken to provide adequate volume support, improve cardiac function, and control sepsis. An exploratory laparotomy may be performed, depending on the clinical signs at the end of 10 to 12 hours of infusion.[76, 84]

The recommended sequence of radiologic procedures and therapeutic approaches in bowel ischemia secondary to occlusion or low flow states is summarized in Figure 117–28.[75]

Ischemic Colitis. The colitis of ischemic bowel disease probably results from mucosal devitalization caused by decreased arterial perfusion of the bowel wall. This may be due to actual arterial occlusive disease or, as is more often the case, to low perfusion states (Chapter 116). Angiography has little to offer in this group of patients. Selective inferior mesenteric arteriography usually does not show arterial or venous occlusions; what is found rather is hypervascularity of the bowel wall with intense opacification of the draining veins (Fig. 117–29). These findings are considered non-specific and are the result of hyperemia associated with the inflammatory response in the ischemic segments of the bowel.

Preoperative aortography can be helpful in preventing colonic ischemia in patients requiring abdominal aortic reconstruction. If the inferior mesenteric artery is the main or the only vessel supplying the bowel, as in patients with stenosis or occlusion of the celiac or superior mesenteric artery, preoperative knowledge of this abnormality would alert the surgeon and prevent colonic infarc-

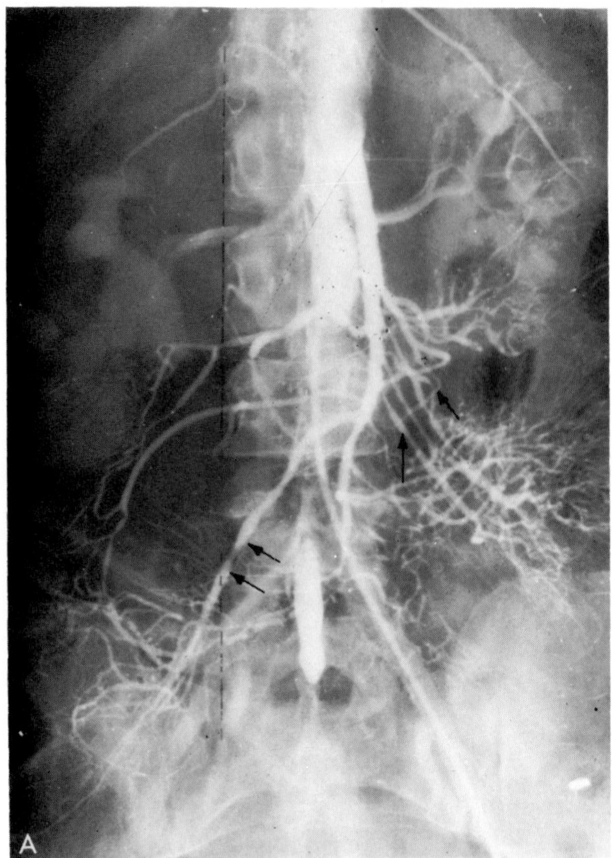

Figure 117–27. Treatment of non-occlusive mesenteric ischemic disease by the selective arterial infusion of vasodilating agents. *A,* Selective superior mesenteric arteriography demonstrates multiple narrowed segments of both the small and medium-sized vessels *(arrows),* as well as a marked decrease in the peripheral filling of the small mesenteric branches.

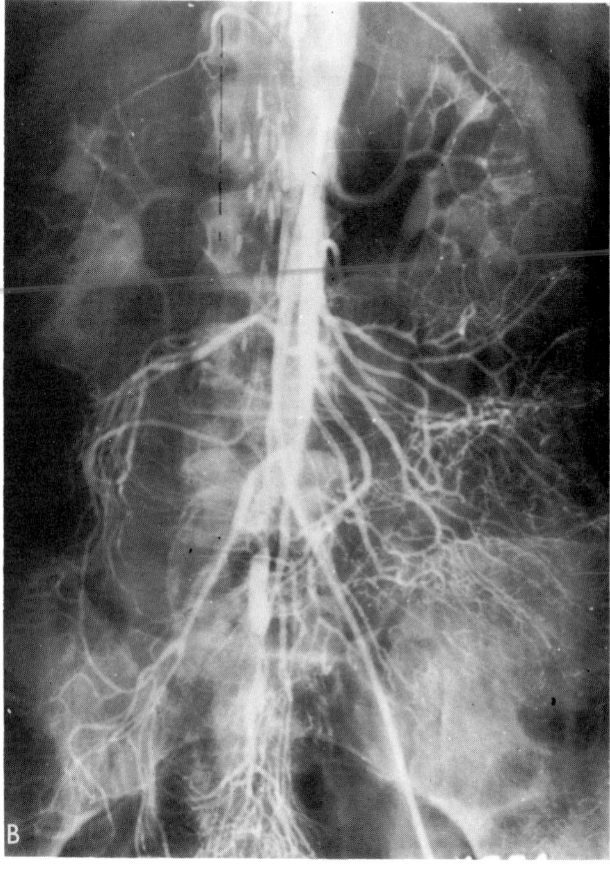

Figure 117–27 *Continued. B,* Repeat superior mesenteric arteriography after the injection of 25 mg of Priscoline demonstrates an increase in the amount of peripheral arterial filling, less reflux in the abdominal aorta indicating a decrease in peripheral resistance, and dilatation in many of the segments of narrowing noted on the pre-Priscoline arteriogram. (From Baum S. *In*: Marshak RH, Lindner AE: Radiology of the Small Intestine. 2nd Ed. Philadelphia: WB Saunders, 1976. Reproduced with permission.)

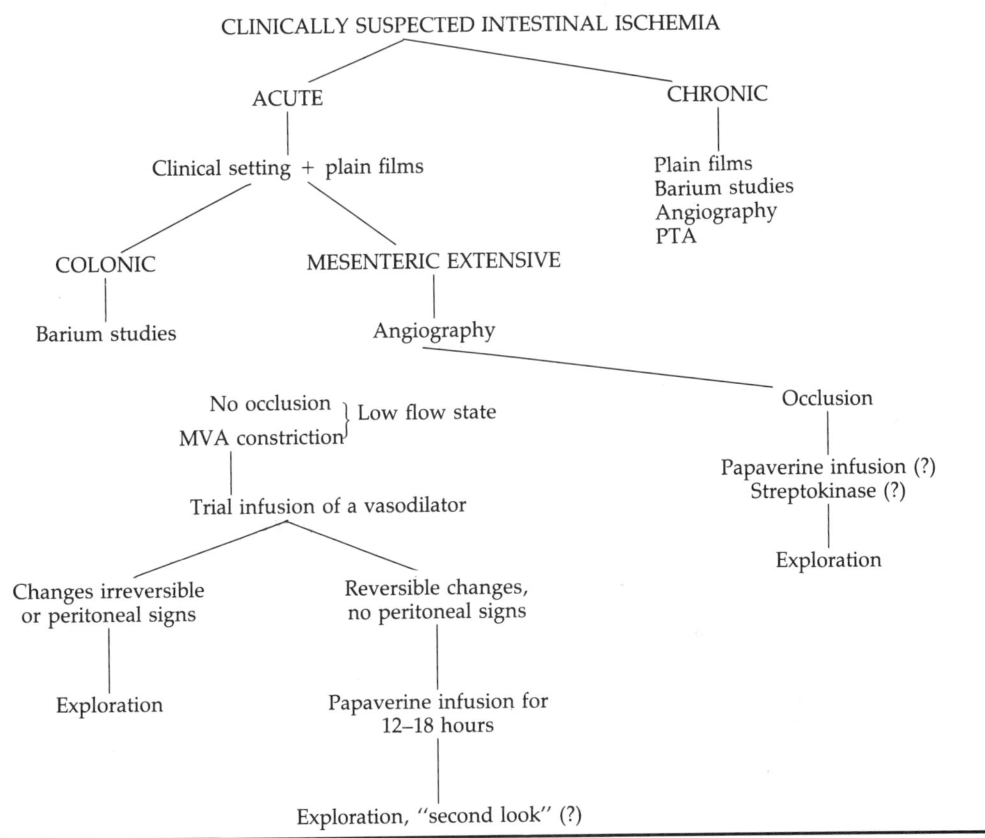

Figure 117–28. Sequence of radiologic procedures in intestinal ischemia. MVA = mesenteric vascular arterial; PTA = percutaneous transluminal angioplasty.

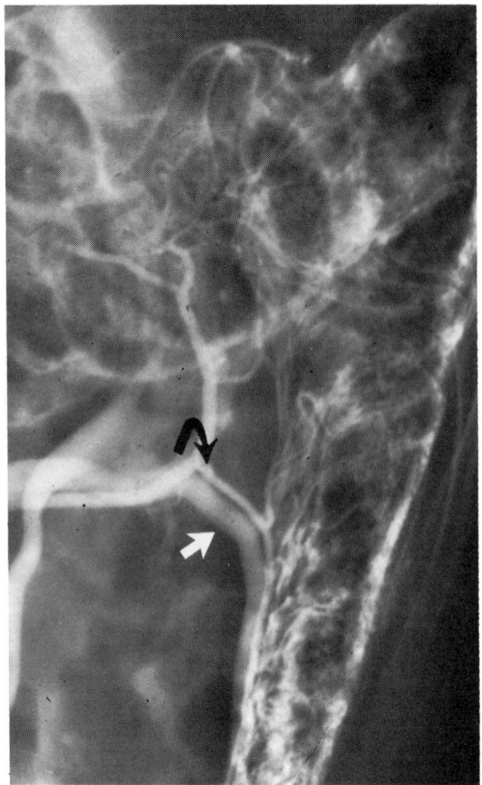

Figure 117–29. Colonic ischemia in a man with diarrhea and crampy abdominal pain. Inferior mesenteric arteriogram shows patent arteries *(curved arrow)*, veins *(straight arrow)*, and hypervascularity of the bowel wall.

tion that otherwise occurs in about 2% of patients undergoing reconstruction of the abdominal aorta.[75, 89]

Chronic Mesenteric Ischemia. Severe stenosis or complete occlusion of the mesenteric arteries due to atherosclerosis is usually the cause of chronic intestinal ischemia or so-called intestinal angina (Chapter 116). A firm angiographic diagnosis of chronic intestinal ischemia is beset with difficulty because 75% of the adult population have angiographic evidence of artherosclerosis of the mesenteric vessels, and anatomic defects found angiographically do not always correlate with the clinical symptoms[76, 83, 90] (Fig. 117–30). The generous collateral pathways make it hard to evaluate the significance of a demonstrable angiographic abnormality. It is reasonable, however, to assume that a patient with abdominal pain and weight loss not otherwise explained has chronic intestinal ischemia when arteriographic studies show narrowing of more than 50% of the lumen of 2 of the 3 mesenteric vessels.[83] Aortography and mesenteric arteriography remain the only methods by which atherosclerosis or other vascular abnormalities involving the mesenteric arteries can be demonstrated. These procedures, therefore, should be performed in patients in whom abdominal symptoms cannot be explained by other clinical, radiologic, or laboratory tests.

From the standpoint of management, percutaneous transluminal angioplasty has been shown to be a safe and effective alternative to surgical bypass grafting or endarterectomy in the treatment of stenosis at the origin of the superior mesenteric and/or celiac artery productive of abdominal angina[91] (Fig. 117–31).

In addition to vessel stenosis or occlusion from atherosclerosis, angiography may demonstrate other abnormalities such as fibromuscular hyperplasia of the visceral arteries,[92] encasement of the mesenteric vessel by tumor or fibrosis, atherosclerotic or mycotic aneurysms of the superior mesenteric artery, and occasionally extrinsic compression of the celiac axis by the median arcuate ligament, the so-called celiac axis syndrome[93] (Figs. 117–32 to 117–34).

Aneurysms

Aortic Aneurysms. Approximately 5% of atherosclerotic aneurysms of the abdominal aorta extend above the renal arteries and involve the superior mesenteric artery and the celiac axis.[94] The inferior mesenteric artery is practically always occluded by an abdominal aneurysm. Aortic dissections, although rarely originating in the abdomen, frequently extend from the thoracic aorta to involve the abdominal aorta and compromise arterial blood flow to the kidneys and/or the viscera.[95] An acute abdomen secondary to mesenteric arterial occlusion may occasionally be the presenting symptom in a patient with aortic dissection. The importance of establishing this diagnosis preoperatively is obvious.

Aneurysms of the Visceral Arteries. With the exception of the splenic artery, atheromatous aneurysms of the celiac and superior mesenteric arterial branches are rare. In the majority of cases, such aneurysms are traumatic or mycotic in nature or the result of digestion of the arterial wall by leaking pancreatic enzymes in patients with pancreatitis (Fig. 117–35). In patients with fibromuscular arterial disease, aneurysms resulting from

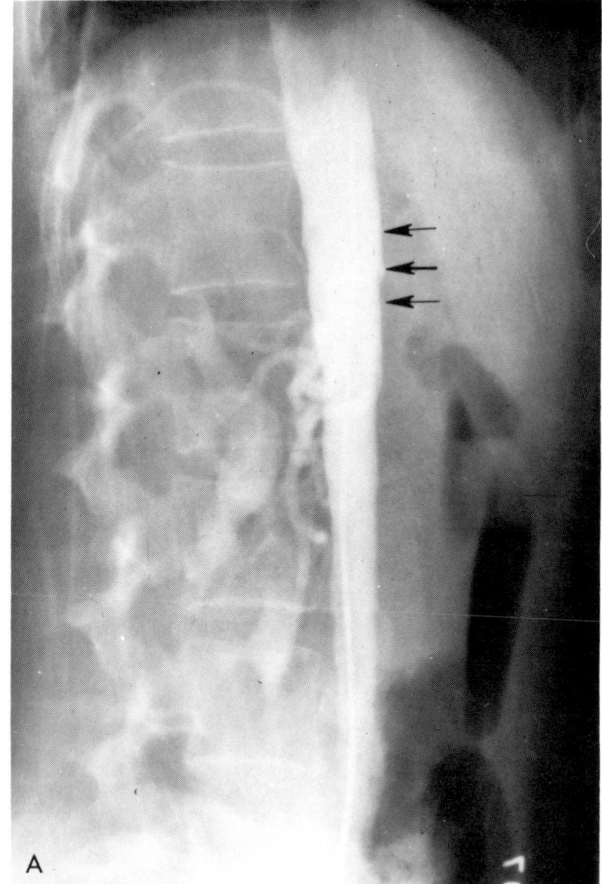

Figure 117–30. A 56-year-old woman with abdominal pain secondary to atherosclerotic occlusions at the origins of the celiac and superior mesenteric arteries. *A,* A lateral abdominal aortogram fails to demonstrate filling of either the celiac or superior mesenteric arteries *(arrows).*

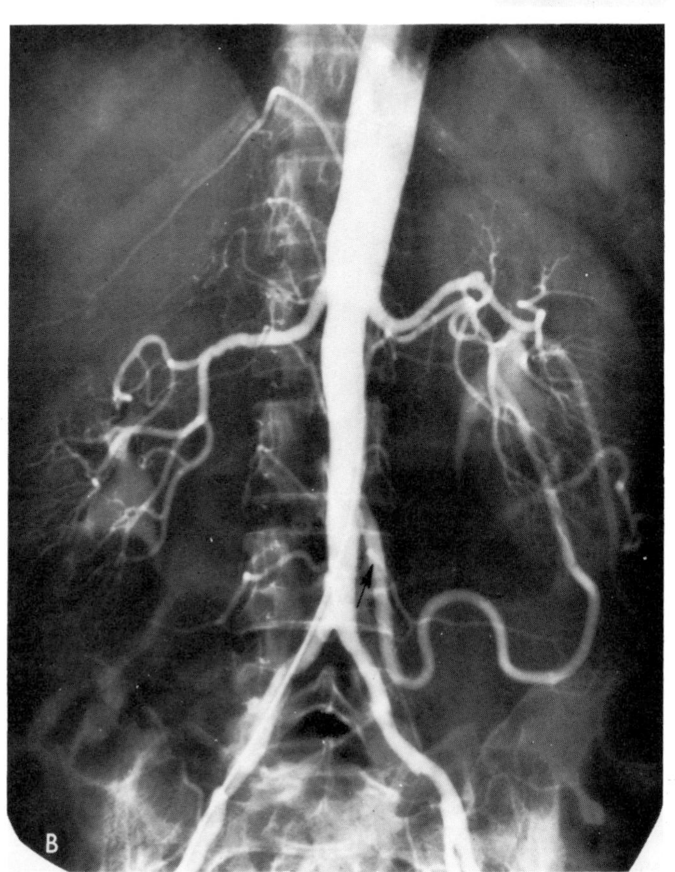

Figure 117–30 *Continued. B,* In the A-P projection both renal arteries are filled without any evidence of either the celiac or the superior mesenteric artery. The inferior mesenteric artery *(arrows)* is large and serves as the major collateral vessel.

Illustration continued on following page

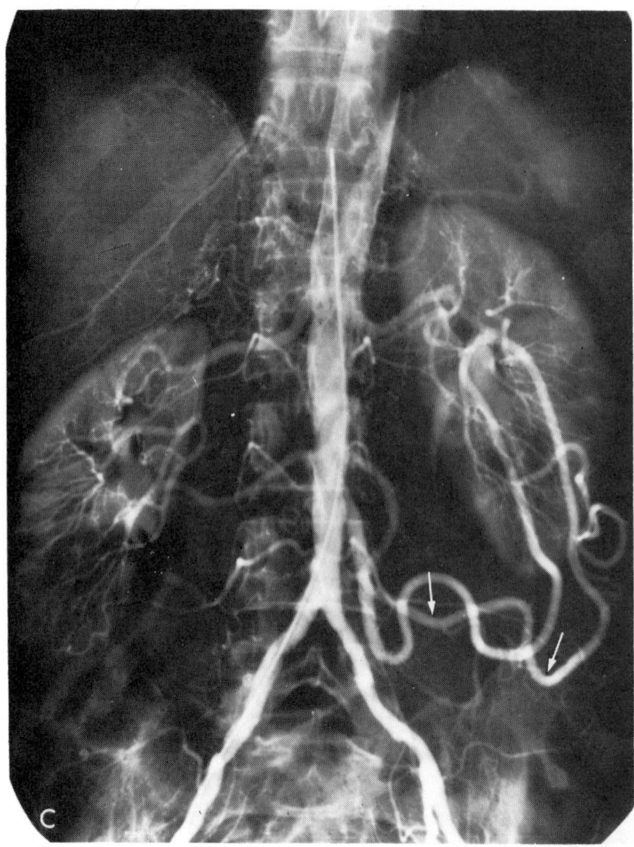

Figure 117–30 *Continued. C,* Several seconds after the injection of contrast material into the abdominal aorta, the marginal anastomotic artery of the colon is identified *(arrows)* coursing in a retrograde direction from the inferior mesenteric artery.

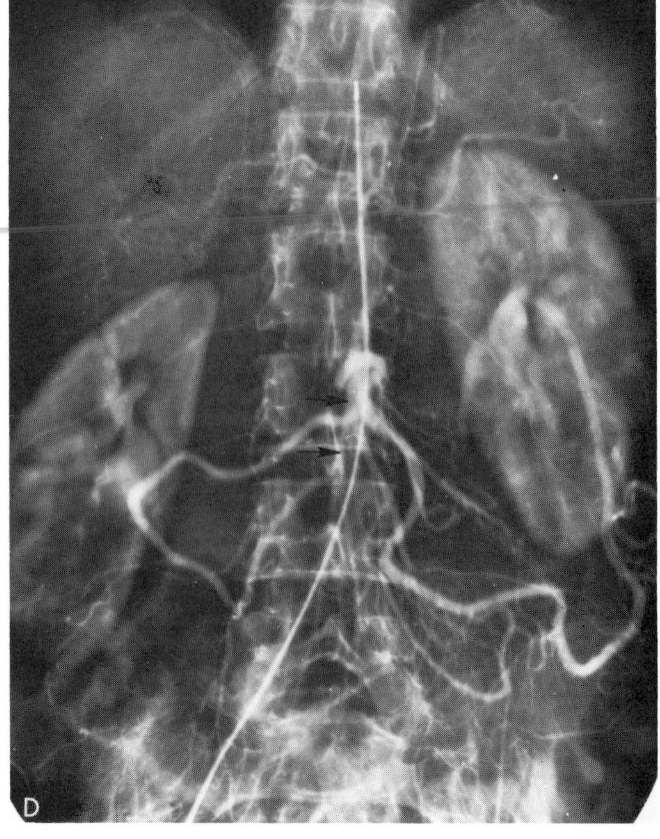

Figure 117–30 *Continued. D,* Ten seconds after the injection of contrast material, the superior mesenteric artery *(arrows)* reconstitutes by way of the marginal anastomotic artery. The celiac axis has reconstituted through collaterals from the lumbar, intercostal and inferior phrenic arteries. (From Baum S. *In*: Marshak RH, Lindner AE. Radiology of the Small Intestine. 2nd Ed. Philadelphia: WB Saunders, 1976. Reproduced with permission.)

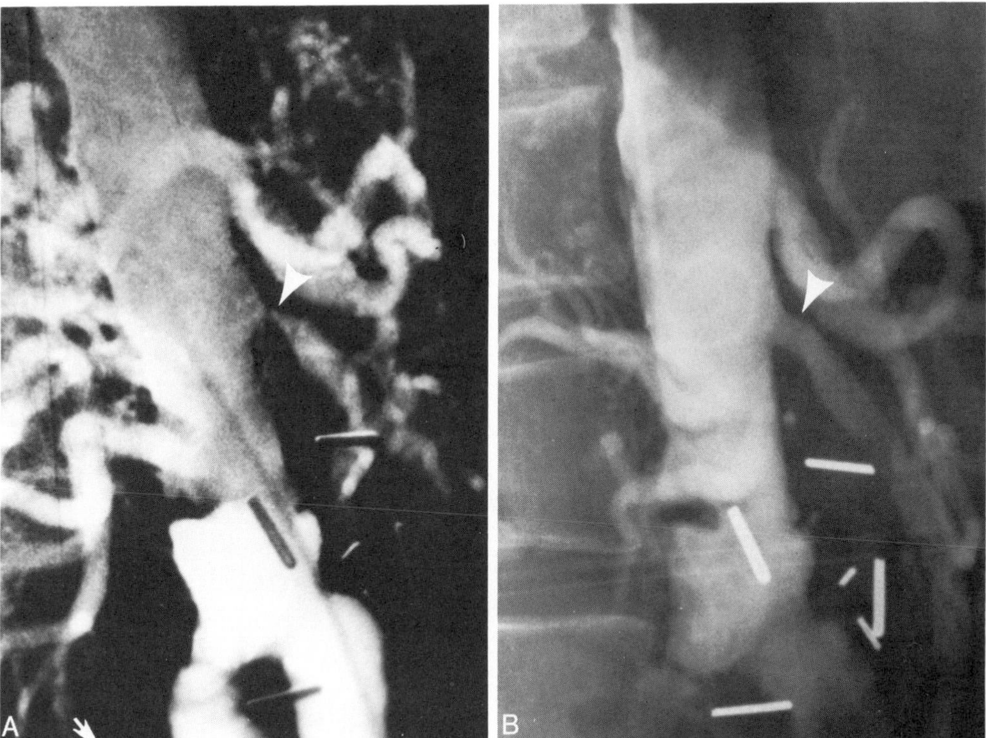

Figure 117–31. Percutaneous transluminal angioplasty of superior mesenteric artery stenosis. *A,* Preliminary lateral aortogram in this patient with intestinal angina shows a tight stenosis of the origin of the superior mesenteric artery *(arrowhead)*. *B,* After balloon dilatation the vessel is widely patent *(arrowhead)*. The patient's symptoms resolved after dilatation.

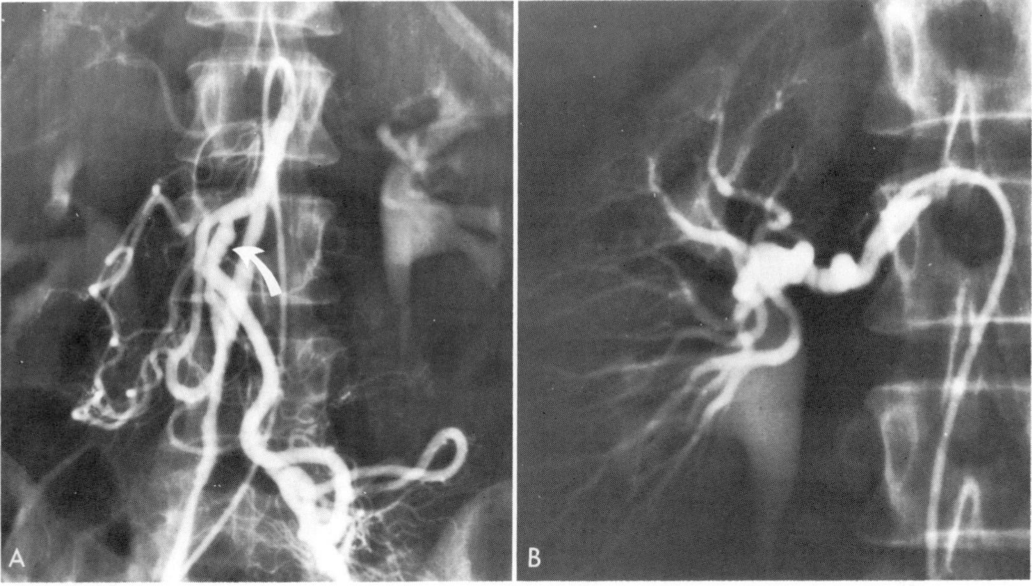

Figure 117–32. Fibromuscular dysplasia of the superior mesenteric artery (SMA) in a patient with chronic epigastric pain. *A,* Superior mesenteric arteriogram reveals a corrugated appearance of the SMA *(arrow)*. Multiple branches are occluded. *B,* Renal arteriogram in the same patient shows the typical "string of pearls" appearance of medial fibroplasia.

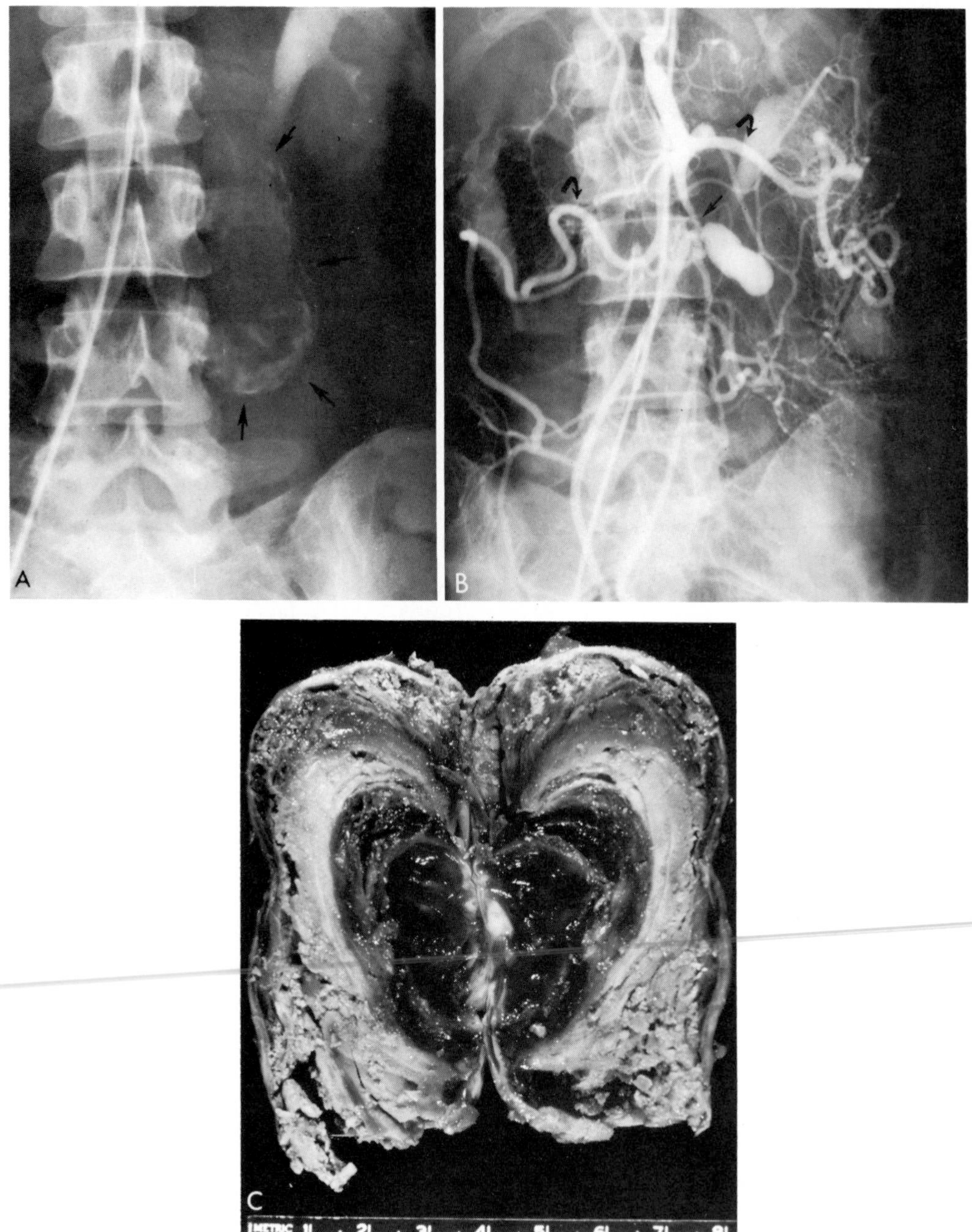

Figure 117–33. Mycotic aneurysm of the superior mesenteric artery (SMA) in a woman with a history of rheumatic heart disease. *A,* A mass lesion with a calcified rim *(arrows)* is noted on the radiograph of the abdomen. *B,* Superior mesenteric arteriogram shows a false aneurysm contained within the calcific density seen in *A.* The aneurysm has retracted the superior mesenteric artery, reducing its lumen *(straight arrow).* Flow to the distal SMA is predominantly by way of the middle colic artery *(curved arrows). C,* Photograph of the resected specimen showing the false aneurysm with surrounding clot.

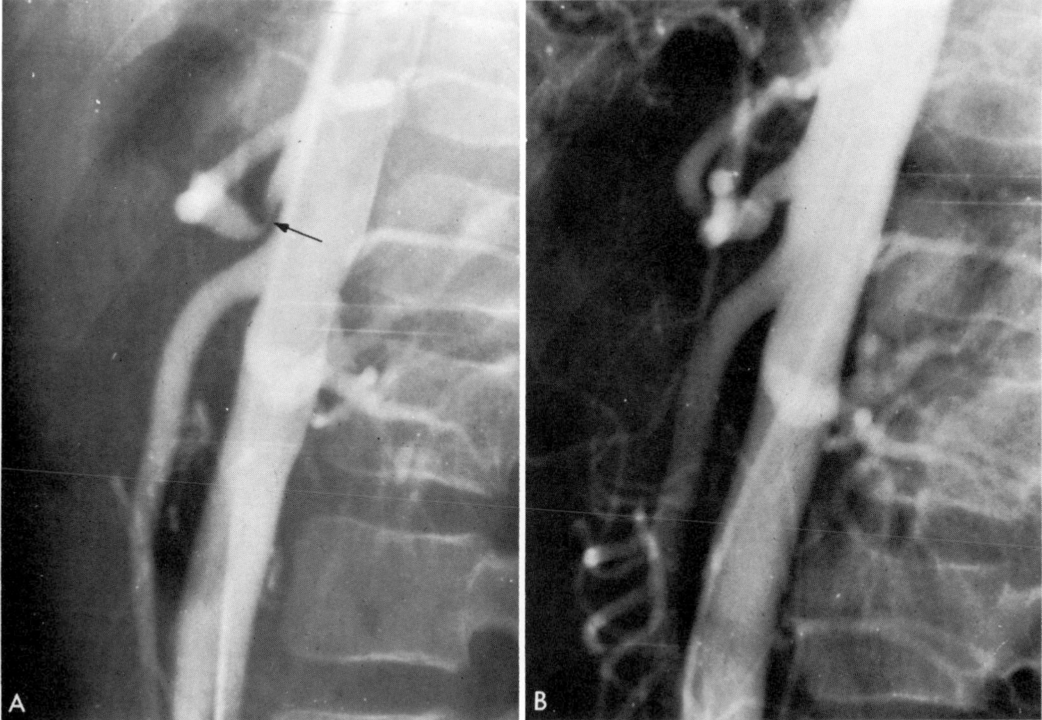

Figure 117–34. Celiac artery syndrome in a 12-year-old boy with epigastric pain. A bruit could be heard over the epigastrium. *A,* Lateral abdominal aortogram shows compression of the celiac axis by the median arcuate ligament *(arrow)*. *B,* Repeat aortogram following surgical division of the constricting ligament shows restoration of the celiac artery lumen. The child became asymptomatic following the operative procedure.

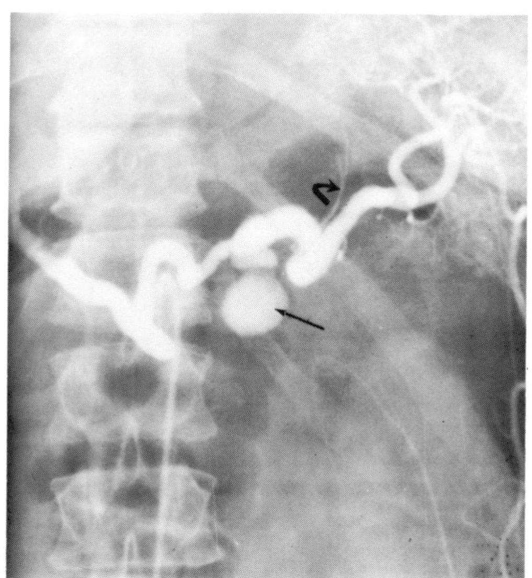

Figure 117–35. Rupture of a non-calcified splenic artery aneurysm secondary to pancreatitis. Selective celiac arteriogram shows a splenic artery aneurysm with opacification of a false sac *(straight arrow)*. There is displacement of pancreatic branches *(curved arrow)* due to the presence of a large hematoma around the aneurysm.

intramural dissections may be the dominant arteriographic finding.

In cases of celiac artery occlusion, increased flow and turbulence in the pancreaticoduodenal arcades may lead to aneurysm formation (Fig. 117–36). Gastrointestinal or intra-abdominal bleeding and/or occlusion of major arterial branches are potential complications of visceral artery aneurysms.[96–98]

Vasculitis. Vasculitis of the mesenteric vessels may be primary, part of a systemic disease, or local (secondary to inflammation of the tissues surrounding the vessels).

Polyarteritis nodosa, lupus erythematosus, scleroderma, rheumatoid arthritis, and dermatomyositis have all been known to produce a necrotizing arteritis of the small or medium-sized vessels with perivascular inflammation and fibrinoid necrosis (Chapter 244). The arterial involvement may be segmental with only a small portion of the wall being involved. This is especially true in polyarteritis nodosa. The end result of the arterial injury may be rupture, aneurysm formation, fibrosis, or thrombosis.[70, 71, 99]

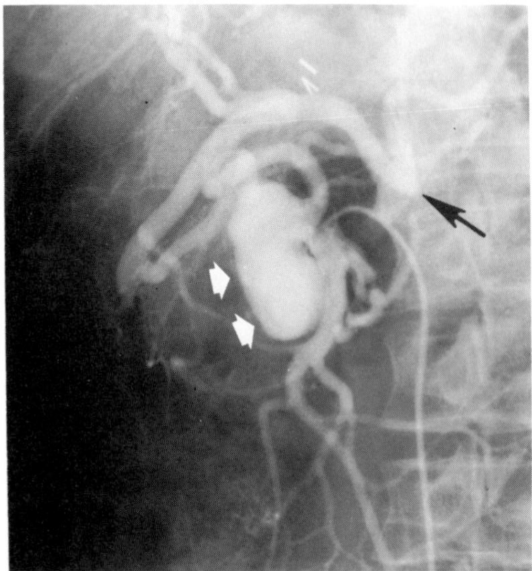

Figure 117–36. Aneurysm of the pancreaticoduodenal artery in a patient with celiac artery occlusion. The presenting symptom was obstructive jaundice. Superior mesenteric arteriogram shows an aneurysm of the inferior pancreaticoduodenal artery *(white arrows)*. There is retrograde filling of the celiac axis *(black arrow)*. Jaundice was the result of hemorrhage from the aneurysm and compression of the common bile duct.

Magnification arteriography is essential for the diagnosis of these lesions when small vessels are involved (Fig. 117–37). Conventional angiography should be sufficient to diagnose lesions involving larger-sized vessels, such as the colic arteries.[70, 71]

An interesting feature of polyarteritis nodosa has been the involvement of the middle and the left colic arteries. Necrosis of the wall of the vessel produces aneurysmal dilatation associated with areas of intramural dissection, giving a very characteristic nodularity and beaded appearance (Fig. 117–38). This can lead to intra-abdominal and/or retroperitoneal hemorrhage, mesenteric infarction, and, occasionally, intestinal perforation.[86, 100]

Local vasculitis secondary to inflammation surrounding the vessels may be the result of peptic ulceration, pancreatitis, ileocolitis, or the desmoplastic reaction resulting from external radiation or intra-abdominal malignancies.[71, 99]

Degenerative Disease. Degenerative disease may produce narrowing of the small visceral arteries owing to thickening and fibrosis of the media. These lesions are not related to atherosclerosis.[99]

Structural Diseases of the Small Vessels. Included in this category are pseudoxanthoma elasticum and hereditary hemorrhagic telangiectasia.[99]

Tumors

Angiography has played only a minor part in the study of bowel tumors inasmuch as adenocarcinomas are not highly vascular[16, 101, 102] and simpler examinations, such as barium radiography, endoscopy, and biopsy, usually provide sufficient information for diagnosis.

Some of the more unusual tumors do show increased vascularity and some specific angiographic features. These are worthy of mention because they must be recognized when fortuitously discovered or deliberately sought at angiography. Leiomyomas, leiomyosarcomas, hemangiopericytomas, and villous adenomas are an otherwise dissimilar group of tumors that have in common the angiographic features of sharply circumscribed hypervascularity and neovascularity and early venous filling (Fig. 117–39).

The angiographic diagnosis of carcinoid tumor of the small bowel may be made on the basis of the vascular distortion due to the extreme thickening, fibrosis, and shortening of the mesentery that occurs in association with this tumor, rather than the non-specific angiographic features of the tumor itself (Chapter 113). The hypervascular appearance may actually represent crowding of the mesenteric arcades due to retraction of the mesentery as well as the development of collateral vessels distal to areas of occlusion (Fig. 117–40). The veins coursing within the mesentery may also be encased and, on occasion, patients present with signs of intestinal ischemia due to vascular compromise. This may progress to complete occlusion of the superior mesenteric vein with resulting small bowel infarction[16, 95, 103] (Fig. 117–41). Other lesions that may simulate the mesenteric changes of carcinoid are lymphomatous involvement of the mesentery and certain forms of mesenteric panniculitis (Chapter 230).

Inflammatory Bowel Disease

Crohn's Disease (Regional Enteritis). In the acute phase of this condition, selective arteriography usually demonstrates a marked

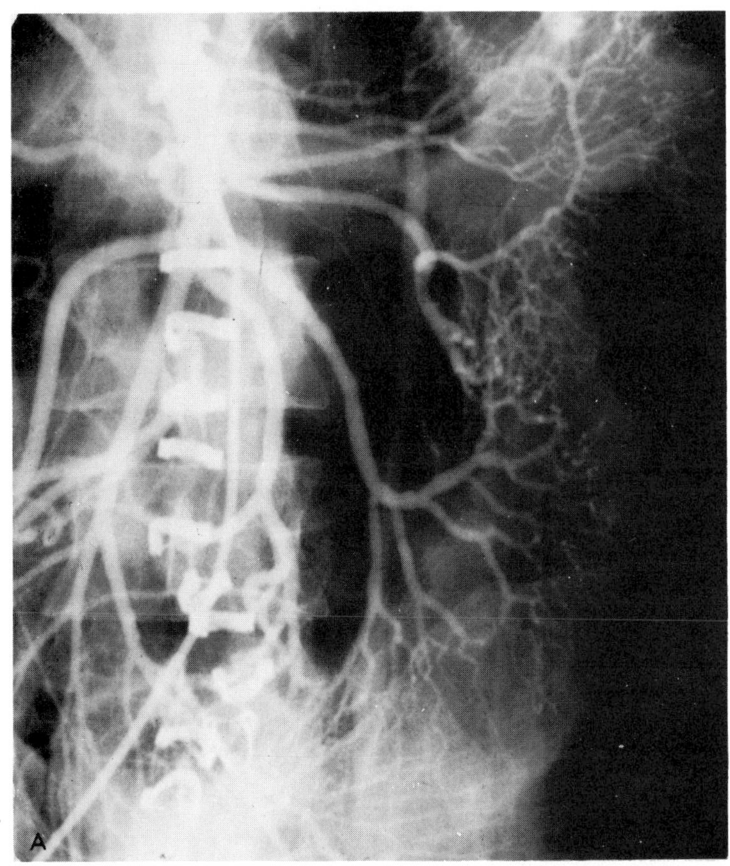

Figure 117–37. Periarteritis of the midjejunal arterial branches resulting in infarction of 4 feet of small bowel. *A*, Selective superior mesenteric arteriography demonstrates marginal irregularity of the vessels going to the midjejunum.

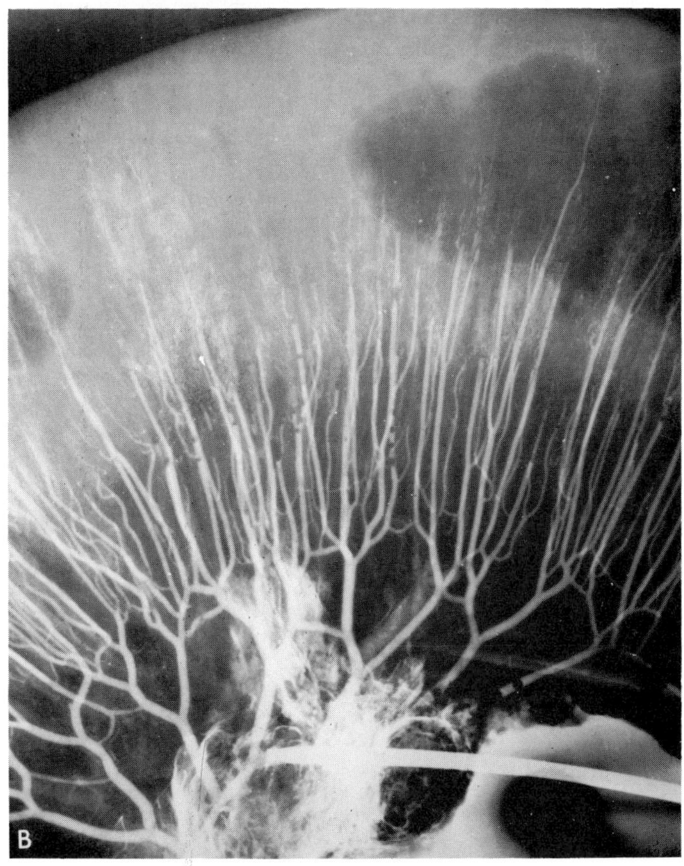

Figure 117–37 *Continued. B,* Injection specimen using 0.05 mm focal spot demonstrates occlusion of almost all the intramural peripheral arterial branches in the involved segment of bowel. The occlusions themselves are probably in branches measuring less than 100 μ in diameter. (From Baum S. *In*: Marshak RH, Lindner AE. Radiology of the Small Intestine. 2nd Ed. Philadelphia: WB Saunders, 1976. Reproduced with permission.)

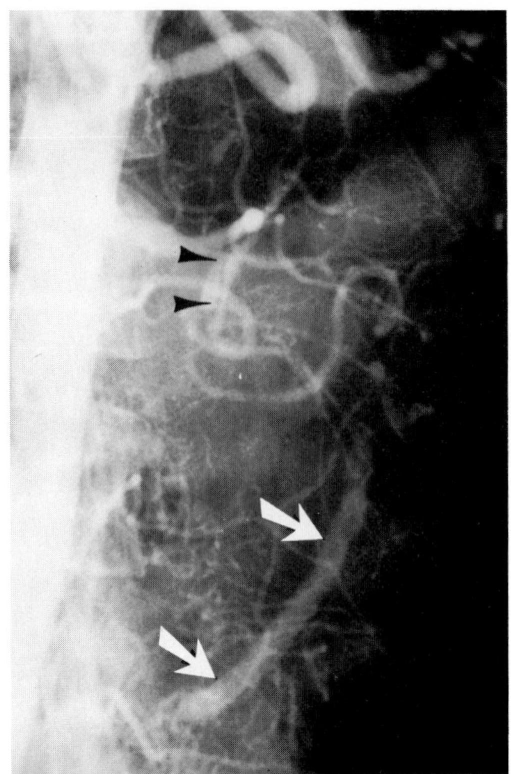

Figure 117–38. Periarteritis of the colic artery. This elderly woman presented with intra-abdominal bleeding. Midstream aortogram shows a sausage-like structure *(white arrows)* representing dissection of the left colic artery. The black arrowheads point to dissection of the renal artery. At operation, rupture of the left colic artery was found with bleeding into the sigmoid mesocolon.

increase in blood supply to the affected area of the bowel. The peripheral segmental arteries to the involved intestine are dilated, tortuous, and markedly disorganized as they enter the bowel wall. During the capillary phase, the thickened bowel wall exhibits an intense parenchymal blush (Fig. 117–42). When the acute phase subsides, the mesenteic vessels may return to a normal appearance. However, because of the marked mesenteric thickening and fibrosis in patients with this progressive disease, small bowel arterial branches within the mesentery become irregular, stenotic, and occasionally occluded.

Ulcerative Colitis. The normal arteriographic appearance of the colon is relatively hypovascular compared with the vascular pattern of the stomach and small bowel; very few arterial branches can be identified on the antimesenteric surface (Fig. 117–2*A* and *B*), and the bowel wall is only faintly opacified in the capillary phase. The arteriographic findings of acute ulcerative colitis are: (1) dilatation of the proximal as well as the distal arterial branches, and (2) a characteristic nontapering appearance of the vasa recta that course through the colon from the mesenteric to the antimesenteric surface.[3, 104, 105] The appearance resembles that of a stepladder, with the vessels remaining uniform in caliber as they penetrate the bowel wall. During the capillary phase of the study, there is an intense blush of the wall corresponding to the area of maximal inflammation, and dilated, tortuous veins can be seen coming from the diseased colon (Figs. 117–43 and 117–44). These are, in fact, the angiographic appearances of any acute colitis, regardless of cause, and they contrast with the vascular distortion and tortuosity noted in Crohn's disease of the small intestine. When the process is less acute, angiographic findings are correspondingly less striking, and when patients are in remission, the arteriogram is often normal.

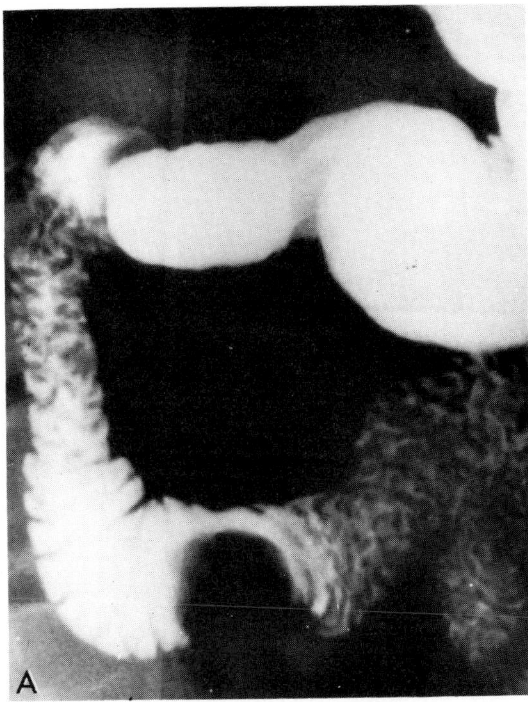

Figure 117–39. Leiomyoma of the third portion of the duodenum. *A,* Spot film of an upper gastrointestinal series shows a mass in the third portion of the duodenum. The patient presented with low-grade gastrointestinal bleeding. *B,* Selective direct serial magnification arteriography of the gastroduodenal artery shows abundant tumor vessels arising from the inferior pancreaticoduodenal artery, supplying a mass corresponding to the defect noted on the barium examination.

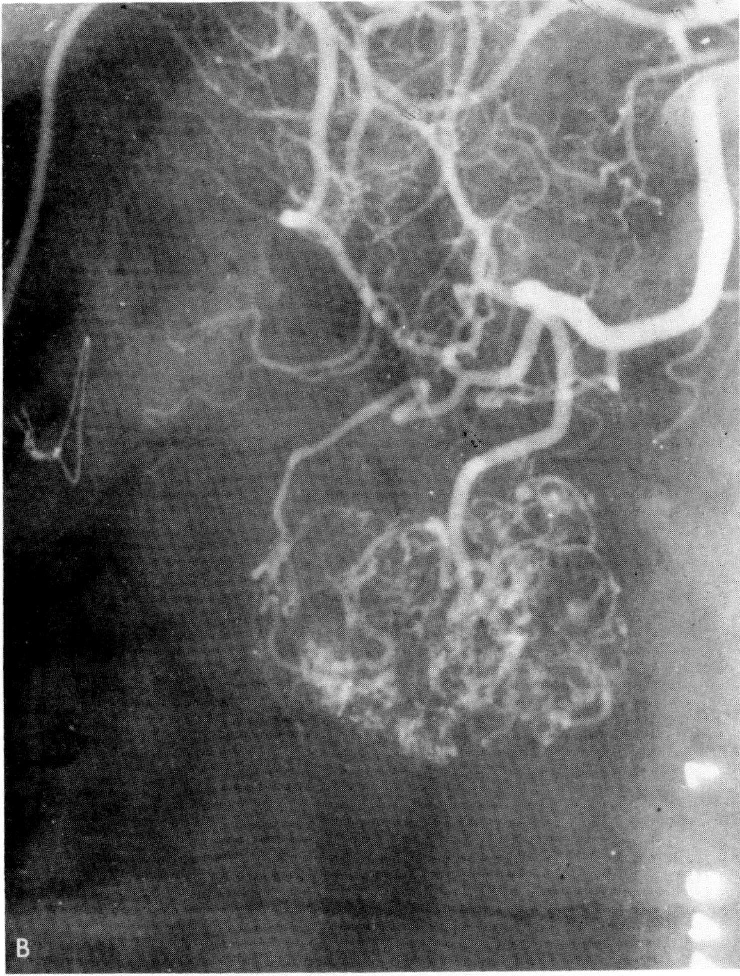

Illustration continued on following page

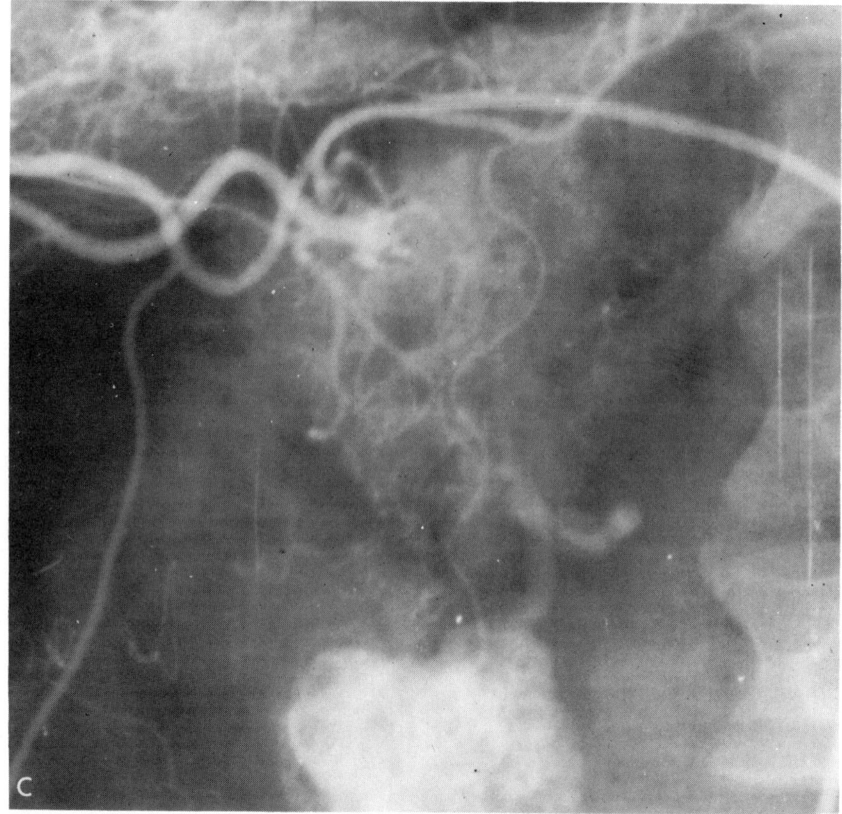

Figure 117–39 *Continued.* *C,* During the late phase of the same injection there is an intense blush of the tumor. A duodenal leiomyoma was confirmed at surgery. (From Baum S. *In*: Marshak RH, Lindner AE. Radiology of the Small Intestine. 2nd Ed. Philadelphia: WB Saunders, 1976. Reproduced with permission.)

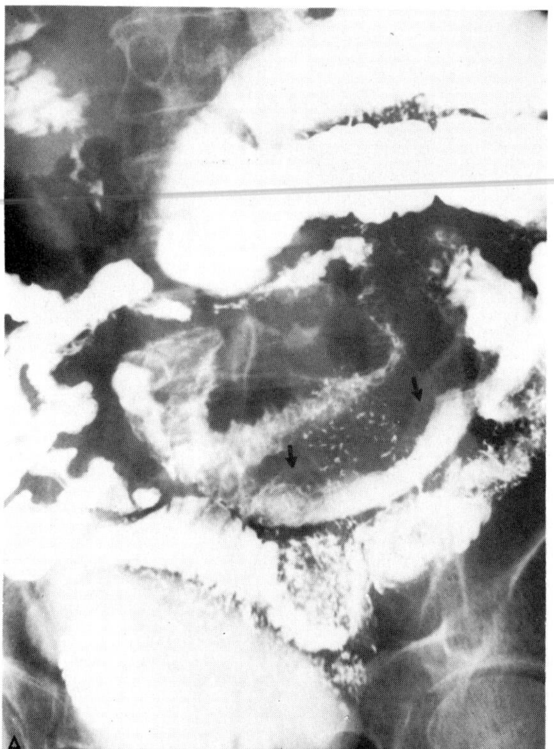

Figure 117–40. Ileal carcinoid tumor with metastases and fibrosis in the root of the mesentery presenting as ischemic enteritis. *A,* Barium meal examination showing a rigid loop of jejunum in the left lower quadrant of the abdomen *(arrows).*

Illustration continued on opposite page

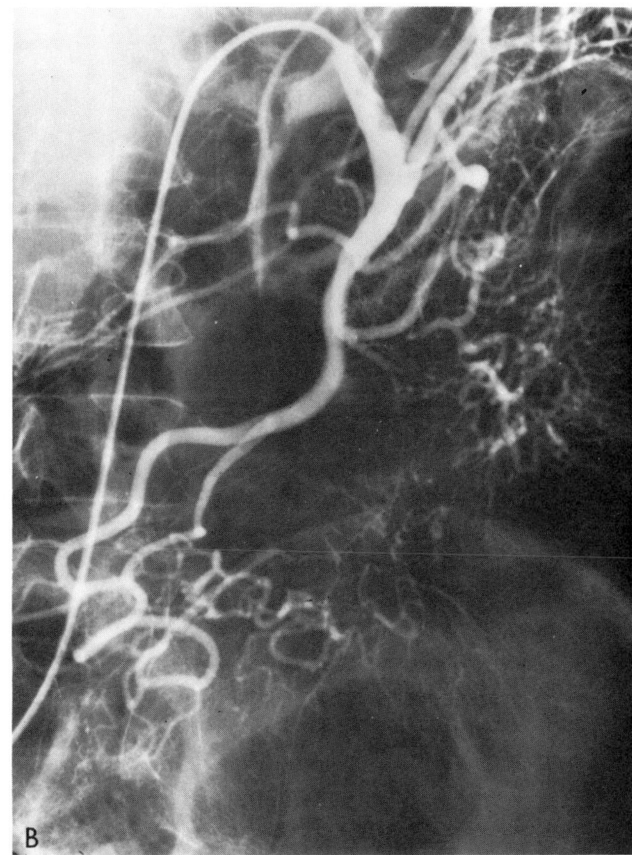

Figure 117–40 *Continued. B,* Selective superior mesenteric arteriography demonstrates a lack of filling of many of the jejunal branches in the area of abnormality noted on the barium study. *C,* A magnified view of the abnormal area demonstrates encasement resulting in marked narrowing and occlusion of many of the jejunal arteries *(upper arrows)* as well as attempts at collateral filling of the abnormal jejunal segments *(lower arrow)*. At surgery a carcinoid of the ileum was found with metastases and fibrosis in the mesenteric lymph nodes and mesentery, resulting in encasement of the mesenteric arteries. (From Baum S. *In*: Marshak RH, Lindner AE. Radiology of the Small Intestine. 2nd Ed. Philadelphia: WB Saunders, 1976. Reproduced wih permission.)

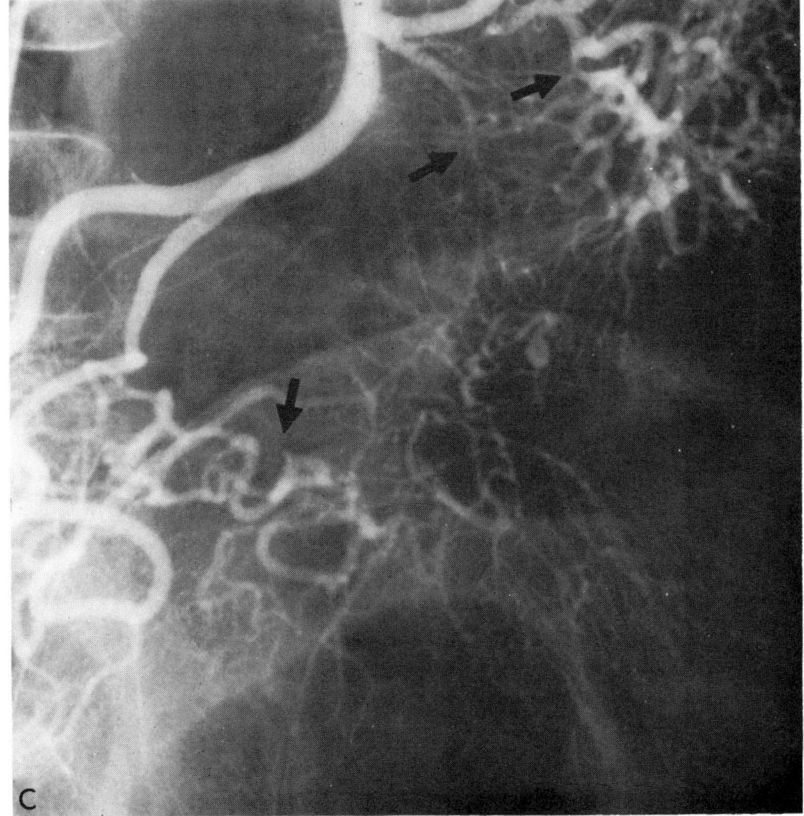

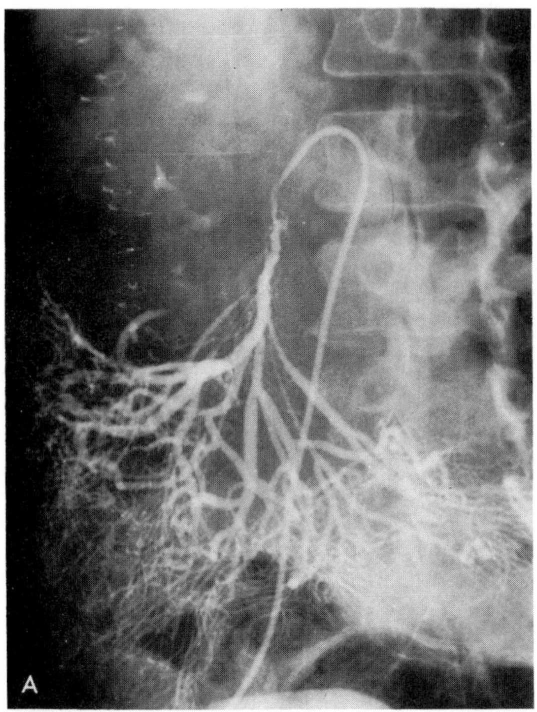

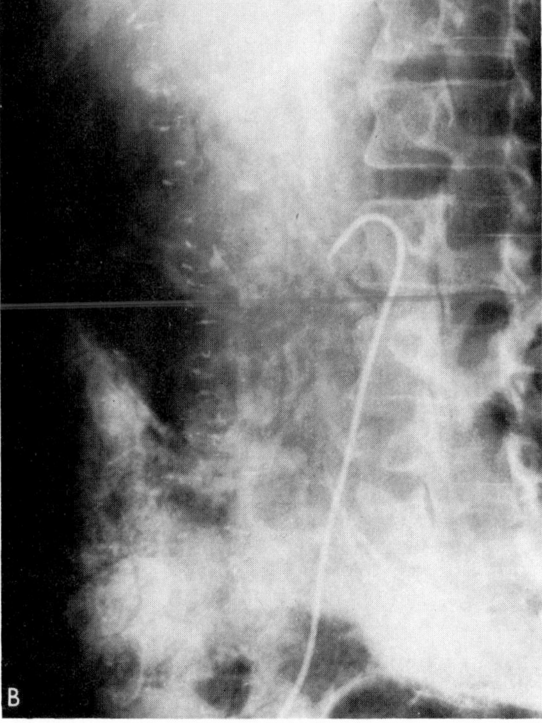

Figure 117–41. Desmoplastic reaction in the root of the mesentery from an ileal carcinoid, resulting in gangrene of the small bowel. *A,* Selective superior mesenteric arteriography demonstrates marked narrowing of the proximal 5 cm of the superior mesenteric artery in a patient complaining of severe abdominal pain. *B,* The venous phase of the study demonstrates the superior mesenteric vein completely occluded with intrahepatic branches of the portal vein filling via collaterals. This patient died of mesenteric infarction, and at postmortem examination the changes in the root of the mesentery were seen to be caused by an extreme desmoplastic reaction. There was no evidence of metastatic tumor. (From Baum S. *In*: Marshak RH, Lindner AE. Radiology of the Small Intestine. 2nd Ed. Philadelphia: WB Saunders, 1976. Reproduced with permission.)

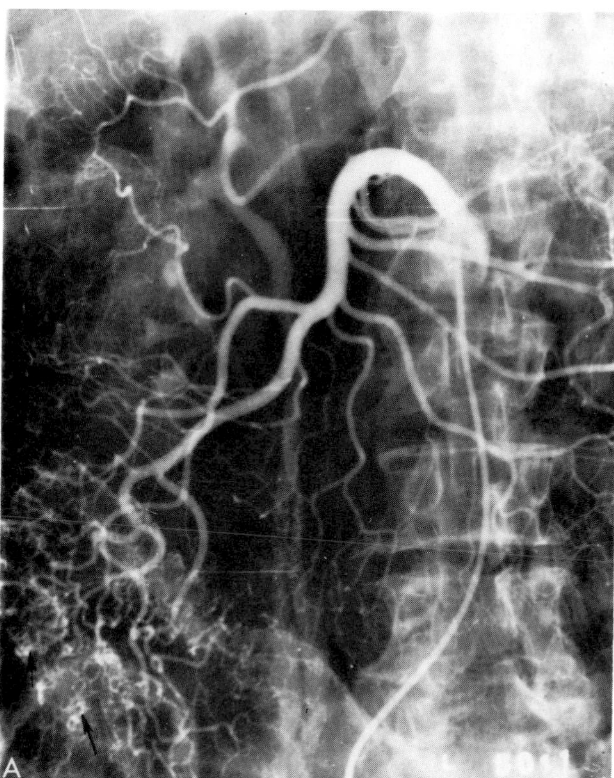

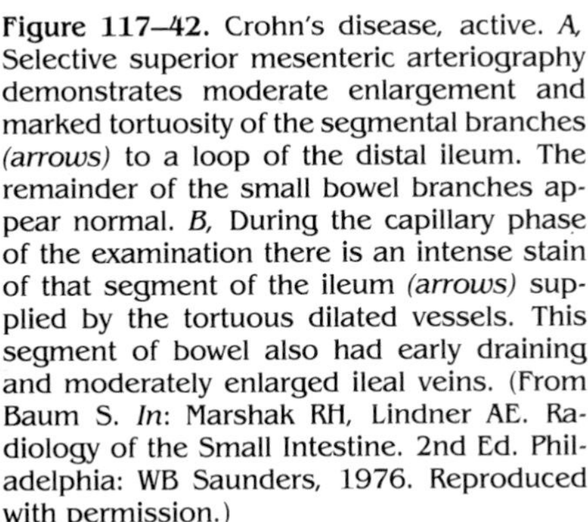

Figure 117–42. Crohn's disease, active. *A,* Selective superior mesenteric arteriography demonstrates moderate enlargement and marked tortuosity of the segmental branches *(arrows)* to a loop of the distal ileum. The remainder of the small bowel branches appear normal. *B,* During the capillary phase of the examination there is an intense stain of that segment of the ileum *(arrows)* supplied by the tortuous dilated vessels. This segment of bowel also had early draining and moderately enlarged ileal veins. (From Baum S. *In*: Marshak RH, Lindner AE. Radiology of the Small Intestine. 2nd Ed. Philadelphia: WB Saunders, 1976. Reproduced with permission.)

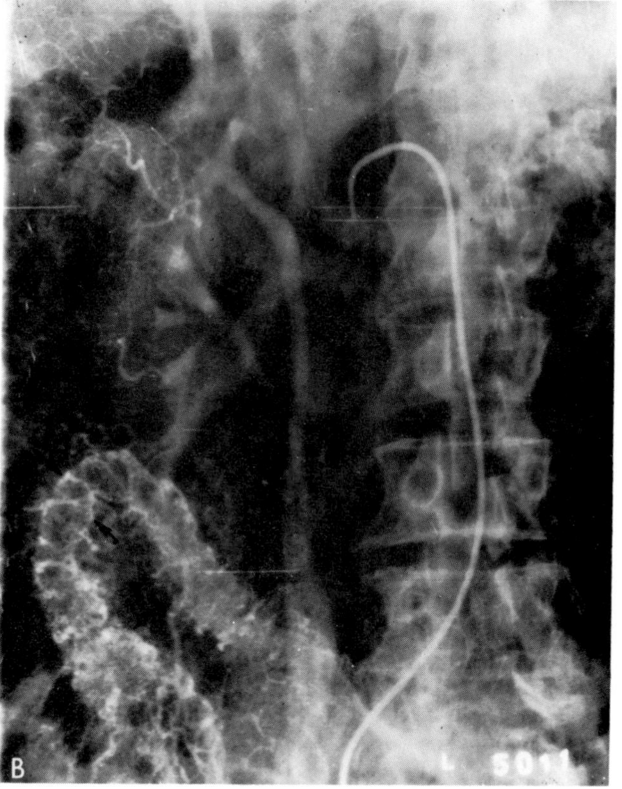

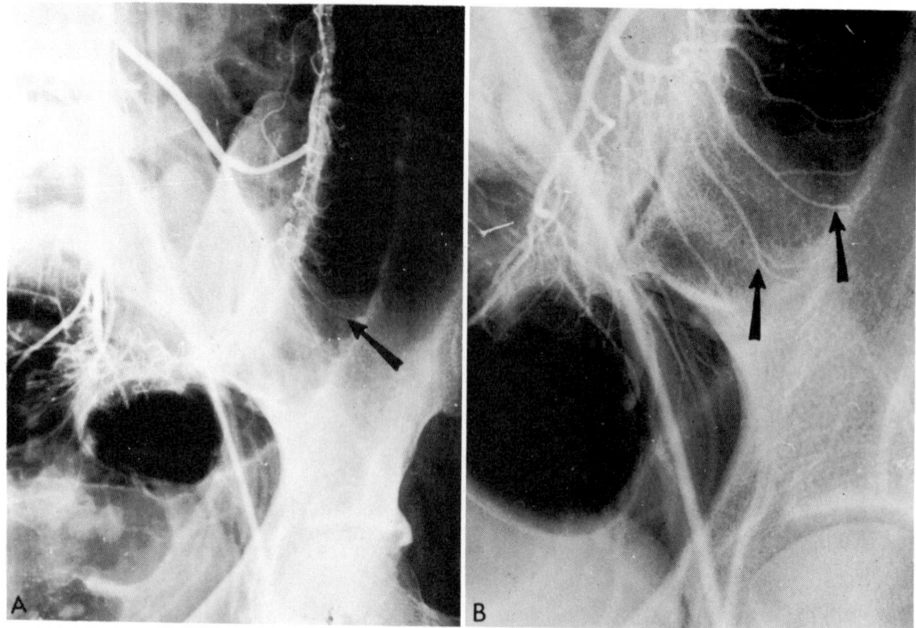

Figure 117–43. Acute ulcerative colitis involving the sigmoid and descending colon. *A,* Selective inferior mesenteric arteriogram demonstrates moderately dilated vasa recta going to the descending colon exhibiting a non-tapered appearance as they approach the antimesenteric surface of the bowel wall *(arrow)*. *B,* Direct serial magnification examination of the same patient demonstrates the non-tapered appearance of the vessels to better advantage *(arrows)*.

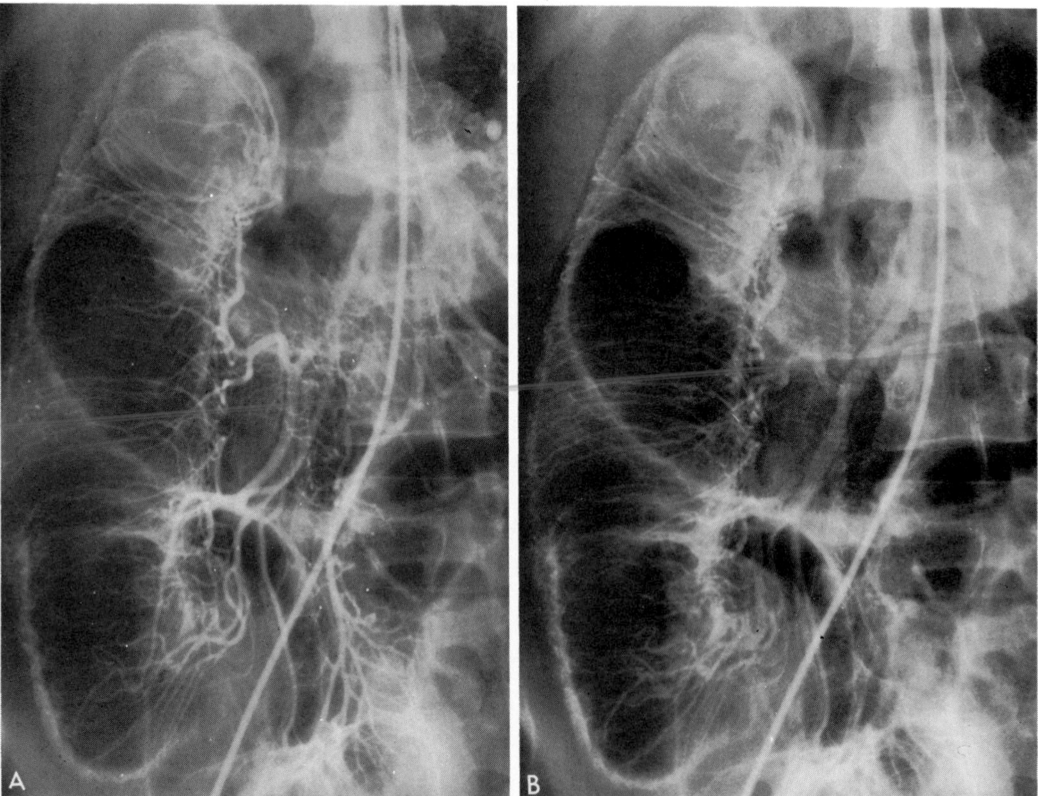

Figure 117–44. Right-sided colitis. *A,* Arterial phase of a selective superior mesenteric arteriogram demonstrates the characteristic non-tapered "stepladder" appearance of the vasa recta in the ascending colon. Since ulcerative colitis is primarily a mucosal inflammatory process, the non-tapered appearance of the vessels going to the bowel is completely consistent with the pathologic changes. A transmural colitis such as that seen in Crohn's disease exhibits a different angiographic pattern because of the marked tortuosity and distortion of the vessels as they penetrate the bowel wall. *B,* During the late capillary phase of the examination, there is an intense blush of the bowel wall and early draining veins, indicative of the hyperemia that is present.

References

1. Baum S, Roy R, Finkelstein AK, Blakemore WS. Clinical application of selective celiac and superior mesenteric arteriography. Radiology 1965; 84:279–95.
2. McAlister WH, Margulis AR, Heinbecker P, Spjud H. Arteriography and microangiography of gastric and colonic lesions. Radiology 1962; 79:769–82.
3. Odman P. Percutaneous selective angiography of the superior mesenteric artery. Acta Radiol 1959; 51:24–30.
4. Baum S. Arteriography in the diagnosis of gastrointestinal bleeding. *In:* Abrams HL, ed. Angiography. Vol 2. Boston: Little Brown, 1971:1121.
5. White RI, Stranberg JD, Gross, GS, Barth KH. Therapeutic embolization with long-term occluding agents and their effects on embolized tissues. Radiology 1977; 125:677–87.
6. Gianturco C, Anderson JH, Wallace S. Mechanical devices for arterial occlusion. AJR 1975; 124:428–35.
7. Gruntzig A, Kumpe DA. Technique of percutaneous transluminal angioplasty with the Gruntzig balloon catheter. AJR 1979; 132:547–52.
8. Hoevels J, Lunderquist A, Ihse I. Percutaneous transhepatic intubation of bile duct for combined internal-external drainage in pre-operative and palliative treatment of obstructive jaundice. Gastrointest Radiol 1978; 3:23–31.
9. Ring EJ, Oleaga JA, Freiman DB, Husted JW, Lunderquist A. Therapeutic applications of catheter cholangiography. Radiology 1978; 128:333–8.
10. Burhenne HJ. Non-operative retained biliary tract stone extraction: a new roentgenologic technique. AJR 1973; 117:388.
11. Pereiras RV, Regingold OJ, Hutson D, Mejie J, Viamonte N, Chiprut RO, Schiff ER. Relief of malignant obstructive jaundice by percutaneous insertion of a permanent prosthesis in the biliary tree. Ann Intern Med 1978; 89:589–93.
12. Stables DP, Holt SA, Sheridan HN, Donohue RE. Permanent nephrostomy via percutaneous puncture. J Urol 1975; 114:684–7.
13. Pfister RC, Newhouse JH. Intervention of percutaneous pyeloureteral techniques. II. Percutaneous nephrostomies and other procedures. Radiol Clin North Am 1979; 17:351–63.
14. Michels NA. Blood Supply and Anatomy of the Upper Abdominal Organs. Philadelphia: JB Lippincott, 1955.
15. Nebesar RA, Kornblith PL, Pollard JJ. Celiac and Superior Mesenteric Arteries: A Correlation of Angiograms and Dissections. Boston: Little Brown, 1969.
16. Reuter SR, Redman HC. Gastrointestinal Angiography. Philadelphia: WB Saunders, 1972.
17. Gray RK, Grollman JH. Acute lower gastrointestinal bleeding secondary to varices of the superior mesenteric venous system. Radiology 1974; 111:559–61.
18. Buranasiri S, Baum S, Nusbaum M, Tumen H. The angiographic diagnosis of mid-gut malrotation with volvulus in adults. Radiology 1973; 109:555–63.
19. Nichols DM, Li DK. Superior mesenteric vein rotation: a computed tomography sign of midgut malrotation. AJR 1983; 141:707–10.
20. Dagradi AE, Ruiz RA, Weingarten ZG. Influence of emergency endoscopy on the management and outcome of patients with upper gastrointestinal hemorrhage. Am J Gastroenterol 1979; 72:403–15.
21. Webb WA, McDaniel L, Johnson RC, Doyle Haynes C. Endoscopic evaluation of 125 cases of upper gastrointestinal bleeding. Ann Surg 1981; 193:624–7.
22. Graham DY. Limited value of early endoscopy in the management of acute upper gastrointestinal bleeding. Am J Surg 1980; 140:284–90.
23. Nusbaum M, Baum S. Radiographic demonstration of unknown sites of gastrointestinal bleeding. Surg Forum 1963; 14:374–5.
24. Athanasoulis CA, Waltman AC, Courcy WR, Baum S. Control of hemorrhagic gastritis by the interarterial infusion of vasopressin. Gastroenterology 1973; 64:693 (Abstract).
25. Baum S, Nusbaum M. The control of gastrointestinal hemorrhage by selective mesenteric arterial infusion of vasopressin. Radiology 1971; 98:497–505.
26. Baum S, Nusbaum M, Tumen H. The control of gastrointestinal hemorrhage by selective mesenteric arterial infusions of Pitressin. Gastroenterology 1970; 58:926 (Abstract).
27. Conn HO, Ransby GR, Storer EK. Selective interarterial vasopressin in the treatment of upper gastrointestinal hemorrhage. Gastroenterology 1972; 63:634–45.
28. Nusbaum M, Baum S, Kuroda K, Blakemore WS. Control of portal hypertension by selective mesenteric arterial drug infusion. Arch Surg 1968; 97:1005–13.
29. Schwartz SI., Bales HW, Emerson GL. The use of intravenous Pituitrin in the treatment of bleeding esophageal varices. Surgery 1959; 45:72–81.
30. Shaldon S, Sherlock S. The use of vasopressin (Pitressin) in the control of bleeding from the oesophageal varices. Lancet 1960; 2:222.
31. Drapanas T, Crowe CP, Shim WKT, Shente WG. The effect of Pitressin on cardiac output and coronary, hepatic and intestinal blood flow. Surg Gynecol Obstet 1961; 113:438.
32. Nusbaum M, Baum S, Sakiyalak P. Pharmacological control of portal hypertension. Surgery 1967; 62:299–310.
33. Barr JW, Lakin RC, Rosch J. Similarity of arterial and intravenous vasopressin on portal and systemic hemodynamics. Gastroenterology 1975; 69:13–9.
34. Johnson WC, Widrid WC, Ansell JE. Control of bleeding varices by vasopressin: a perspective randomized study. Ann Surg 1977; 186:369–76.
35. Chojkier M, Groszmann RJ, Atterbury CE, Bar-Meir S, Blei AT, Frankel J, Glickman MG, Schade G, Taggart GJ, Conn HO. A controlled comparison of continuous interarterial and intravenous infusions of vasopressin in hemorrhages from esophageal varices. Gastroenterology 1979; 77:540–6.
36. Lunderquist A, Barjesson B, Owman T, Bengmark S. Isobutyl 2-cyanoacrylate (Bucrylate) in the obliteration of gastric coronary vein and esophageal varices. AJR 1978; 130:1–6.
37. Yune HY, Klattee C, Richmond BD, Rabe FE. Absolute ethanol in thrombotherapy of bleeding of esophageal varices. AJR 1982; 138:1137–42.
38. Uflacker R. Percutaneous transhepatic obliteration of gastroesophageal varices using absolute alcohol. Radiology 1983; 146:621–5.
39. Keller FS, Rosch J, Dotter CT. Transhepatic obliteration of gastroesophageal varices with absolute alcohol. Radiology 1983; 146:615–20.
40. Waltman AC, Greenfield AJ, Novelline RA, Athanasoulis CA. Pyloroduodenal bleeding and interarterial vasopressin: clinical results. AJR 1979; 133:643–6.
41. Dodson TF. Intraoperative localization of small bowel bleeding sites with combined use of angiographic methods and methylene blue injection. Surgery 1980; 87:77–84.
42. Feldman M, Smith VM, Warner CG. Varcies of the colon. Report of three cases JAMA 1962; 179:729–35.
43. Gray R, Grollman JH, Acute lower gastrointestinal bleeding secondary to varices of the superior mesenteric venous system: Angiographic demonstration. Radiology 1974; 111:559–61.
44. Jewett TC, Duszynski DQ, Allen JE. The visualization of Meckel's diverticulum with technetium 99Tc pertechnetate. Surgery 1970; 68:567–70.
45. Fletcher P, Andrews TJ. Abdominal scanning for bleeding Meckel's diverticulum using 99Tc pertechnetate. Aust Paediatr J 1978; 14:246–7.
46. Petrokubi RJ, Baum S, Rohrer GV. Cimetidine administration resulting in improved pertechnetate imaging of Meckel's diverticullum. Clin Nucl Med 1978; 3:385–8.
47. Hall TJ. Meckel's bleeding diverticulum diagnosed by mesenteric angiography. Br J Surg 1975; 62:882–4.
48. Faris JG, Whitley JE. Angiographic demonstration of Meckel's diverticulum: case report and review of the literature. Radiology 1973; 108:255–6.
49. Barr AH, DeLaurentis DA, Parry CE, Keohane RB. Angiography in the management of massive lower gastrointestinal tract hemorrhage. Surg Gynecol Obstet 1980; 150:226–8.
50. Talman EA, Dixon DS, Gutierrez FE. Role of arteriography in rectal hemorrhage due to arterial venous malformations and diverticulosis. Ann Surg 1979; 190:203–13.
51. Behringer GE, Albright NL. Diverticular disease of the colon, a frequent cause of massive rectal bleeding. Am J Surg 1973; 125:419–23.

52. Baum S, Athanasoulis C, Waltman A, Galdabini J, Schapiro R, Warshaw A, Ottinger L. Angiodysplasia of the right colon; a cause of gastrointestinal bleeding. AJR 1977; 129:789–94.
53. Welch CE, Athanasoulis CA, Galdabini JJ. Hemorrhage from the large bowel with special reference to angiodysplasia and diverticular disease. World J Surg 1978; 2:73–83.
54. Boley SJ, Sammartano R, Adams A, DiBiasea-Kleinhaus S, Sprayregan S. On the nature and etiology of vascular ectasias of the colon. Gastroenterology 1977; 72:650–60.
55. Giacchino JL, Geis WP, Pickleman JR, Dado DV, Freeark RJ. Changing perspective in massive lower intestinal hemorrhage. Surgery 1979; 86:368–76.
56. Kawamura S, Sawada Y, Fujiwara S, Kawatsu S, Chiba Y, Yoshida Y. Clinical and pathologic studies of gastrointestinal hemorrhage in acute leukemia. Tohoku J Exp Med 1979; 127:342–52.
57. Alavi A, Dann RW, Baum S, Biery DN. Scintigraphic detection of acute gastrointestinal bleeding. Radiology 1977; 124:753–6.
58. Alavi A, Ring EJ. Localization of gastrointestinal bleeding; superiority of 99-technetium sulfur colloid compared with angiography. AJR 1981; 137:741–8.
59. McKusick KA, Froelich J, Callahan RJ, Winzelberg G, Strauss HW. 99-Tc red blood cells for detection of gastrointestinal bleeding: experience with 80 patients. AJR 1981; 137:1113–8.
60. Athanasoulis CA, Waltman AC, Ring EJ, Smith JC, Baum S. Angiographic management of post-operative bleeding. Radiology 1974; 113:37–42.
61. Baum S, Athanasoulis CA, Waltman AC. Gastrointestinal hemorrhage. Part II. Angiographic diagnosis in control. Adv Surg 1973; 7:149.
62. Winzelberg GG, Froelich JW, McKusick KA, Waltman AC, Greenfield AJ, Athanasoulis CA, Strauss HW. Radionuclide localization of lower gastrointestinal hemorrhage. Radiology 1981; 139:465–9.
63. Alavi A. Letter to the editor. Radiology 1982; 142:801.
64. Richardson JD, Max MH, Flint LM, Schweisinger W, Howard M, Aust JB. Bleeding vascular malformations of the intestine. Surgery 1978; 3:430–6.
65. Meyer CT, Troncale FJ, Galloway AS, Sheahan DG. Arterial venous malformations of the bowel. Medicine 1981; 1:36–48.
66. Schoenfeld Y, Eldar M, Bedazovsky B, Levy MJ, Pinkhas J. Aortic stenosis associated with gastrointestinal bleeding: a survery of 612 patients. Am Heart J 1980; 7:178–82.
67. Bogokowsky H, Slutzki S, Alon H. Angiodysplasia as a cause of colonic bleeding in the elderly. Br J Surg 1979; 5:315–6.
68. Bourdette D, Greenberg B. Twelve year history of gastrointestinal bleeding in a patient with calcific aortic stenosis and hemorrhagic telangiectasia. Am J Dig Dis 1978; 1:777–9.
69. Gelfand ML, Cohen T, Ackert JJ, Ambos M, Mayadag M. Gastrointestinal bleeding in aortic stenosis. Am J Gastroenterol 1979; 71:30–8.
70. Baum S. Small vessel angiography of the gut. *In:* Hilal SK, ed. Small Vessel Angiography. Imaging, Morphology, Physiology and Clinical Applications. St. Louis: CV Mosby, 1973; 454–78.
71. Baum S. Small bowel angiography. *In:* Marshak RM, Linder AE, eds. Radiology of the Small Intestine. Philadelphia: WB Saunders, 1976.
72. Bosniak MA. In vivo magnification arteriography of the bowel wall. Am J Surg 1967; 114:39–62.
73. Galloway J, Walker PA, Mavor TE. Mesenteric arterial occlusions as a vascular emergency. Br J Surg 1969; 56:431–4.
74. Mavor GE. Acute occlusion of the superior mesenteric artery. Clin Gastroenterol 1972; 1:639–45.
75. Athanasoulis CA, Novelline RA, Waltman AC. Intestinal ischemia. *In:* Clearfield H, Dinosa A, eds. The Role of Angiography in Diagnosis and Therapy. New York: Grune & Stratton, 1976.
76. Williams LF. Vascular insufficiency of the intestines. Gastroenterology 1971; 61:757–71.
77. Flickinger EG, Johnsrude IS, Ogburn NL, Weaver MD, Pories Wj. Local streptokinase infusion for superior mesenteric artery thromboembolism. AJR 1983; 140:771–2.
78. Riijken DC, Collen D. Purification and characterization of the plasminogen activator secreted by human melanoma cells in culture. J Biol Chem 1981; 256:7035–41.
79. Weimar W, Stibbe J, Van Seyen AJ, Billiau A, DeSomer P, Collen D. Specific lysis of an iliofemoral thrombus by administration of extrinsic (tissue type) plasminogen activator. Lancet 1981; 2:1018–20.
80. DeMuth WE, Fitts WT, Patterson LT. Mesenteric vascular occlusion. Surg Gynecol Obstet 1959; 108:209–18.
81. Derrick JR, Pollard HS, Moore RM. The pattern of arterial sclerotic narrowing the celiac and superior mesenteric arteries. Ann Surg 1959; 1409:684–74.
82. Kahn P, Abrams HL. Inferior mesenteric arterial patterns; angiographic study. Radiology 1974; 82:429.
83. Williams LF, Kim JP. Non-occlusive mesenteric ischemia. *In:* Boley SJ, ed. Vascular Disorders of the Intestine. New York: Appleton-Century-Crofts, 1971: 519.
84. Boley SJ, Sprayregen S, Veith FJ. An aggressive roentgenologic and surgical approach to acute mesenteric ischemia. Ann Surg 1973; 5:355–67.
85. Athanasoulis CA, Wittenberg J, Berstein R, Williams LF. Vasodilatory drugs in the management of non-occlusive bowel ischemia. Gastroenterology 1975; 68:146–50.
86. Habboush EF, Wallace HW, Nusbaum M, Baum S, Drtch P., Blakemoore WS. Non-occlusive mesenteric vascular insufficiency. Ann Surg 1974; 180:819–22.
87. Siegelman SS, Sprayregen S, Boley SJ. Angiographic diagnosis of mesenteric arterial vasoconstriction. Radiology 1974; 112:533–42.
88. Wittenberg J, Athanasoulis CA, Schapiro JH, Williams LF. A radiological approach to patients with acute extensive bowel ischemia. Radiology 1974; 106:13–24.
89. Ottinger LW, Darling RC, Nathan MJ, Linton RR. Left colon ischemia complicating aortoiliac reconstruction. Arch Surg 1972; 105:841–6.
90. Dick AP, Graft R, Gregg D. An arteriographic study of mesenteric arterial disease. Gut 1967; 8:206–20.
91. Golden DA, Ring EJ, McLean GK, Freiman DB. Percutaneous transluminal angioplasty in the treatment of abdominal angina. AJR 1982; 139:247–9.
92. Palubinskas AJ, Ripley HR. Fibromuscular hyperplasia in extrarenal arteries. Radiology 1964; 82:451–5.
93. Rob C. Celiac axis syndrome. *In:* Boley SJ, ed. Vascular Disorders of the Intestine. New York: Appleton-Century-Crofts, 1971: 543.
94. Brewster DC, Retana A, Wortman AC, Darling RC. Angiography in the management of abdominal aortic aneurysms: its value and safety. N Engl J Med 1975; 292:822–5.
95. Case records of the Massachusetts General Hospital (case 1-1973. N Engl J Med 1973; 288:36–43.
96. Case records of the Massachusetts General Hospital (case 19-1975). N Engl J Med 1975; 292:1068–73.
97. Sethi GK, Nelson RM. Gastroduodenal arterial aneurysms: report of a case in review of the literature. Surgery 1976; 79:233–5.
98. Smith GW, Hill CH. Aneurysms of the branches of the abdominal aorta: diagnosis, management and results. Surgery 1967; 61:505–15.
99. Feller E, Ricket R, Spirro NM. Small vessel disease of the gut. *In:* Boley SJ, ed. Vascular Disorders of the Intestine. New York: Appleton-Century-Crofts, 1971: 483.
100. Buranasiri S, Baum S, Nusbaum M, Finkelstein D. Periarteritis of the middle colic artery: arteriographic, surgical and pathological correlation. Am J Gastroenterol 1973; 59:73–6.
101. Baum S. Selective arteriography. *In:* Stein GN, Finkelstein AK, eds. An Atlas of Tumor Radiology: The Duodenum, Small Intestine and Colon. Chicago: Year Book Medical Publishers, 1973:308.
102. Boijsen E. Superior mesenteric arteriography. *In:* Abrams HL, ed. Angiography. Vol II, 2d Ed. Boston: Little Brown, 1971:1091.
103. Reuter SR, Boijsen E. Angiographic findings in two ileal carcinoid tumors. Radiology 1966; 87:836–40.
104. Boijsen E, Reuter SR. Mesenteric angiography in the evaluation of inflammatory and neoplastic disease of the intestine. Radiology 1966; 87:1028–38.
105. Lunderquist A. Angiography in ulcerative colitis. AJR 1967; 99:18.

Chapter 118

Acute Non-parasitic Diarrhea

Herbert L. DuPont

Acute diarrhea is the second most common clinical illness in our society. It is an even more important problem among certain populations: infants in day care centers, mentally retarded persons in custodial institutions, male homosexuals, and persons traveling from industrialized to developing countries. For a rational approach to this pervasive disorder, its nature must first be clearly delineated. Definitions of diarrhea, however, differ (Chapter 8). Probably the best definition, and the one to be used here, is "the passage of a greater number of stools with decreased form than usual."

Previously, we were able to show the cause of acute diarrhea in only 10% to 15% of cases. With the availability now of electron microscopy, tissue culture, and serologic techniques, as well as refined bacteriologic procedures, we can detect an agent in 50% to 80% of cases, depending upon age of the host and the severity and duration of illness when studied. An etiologic agent commonly cannot be found in very young infants with diarrhea. In most severe cases of diarrhea in older children and adults, an agent usually can be detected. For most cases of acute diarrhea in which symptoms are mild, it is not important to make an etiologic diagnosis. On the other hand, for those with severe illness or in patients with a highly communicable pathogen, such as a strain of *Shigella*, etiologic assessment may lead to appropriate and important antimicrobial therapy.

Pathogenesis

Acute diarrhea results when along with enteric infection there is a change in the balance between input and output of solute in the intestinal tract. Of the 3 general mechanisms that lead to the passage of increased numbers of unformed stools (active intestinal secretion, decreased absorption, and motility alterations) (Chapter 8), the first is the most important in infectious diarrhea.[1] Increase in intestinal secretion is stimulated by a host of bacterial enterotoxins and enteric hormones. Table 118–1 shows how a variety of bacterial enterotoxins influence cyclic nucleotide levels in the gut. When elaborated, each results in intestinal secretion. With diffuse damage to the small bowel mucosa or its brush border, absorption is impaired, leading to an osmotic diarrhea.[2]

Bacterial enterotoxins stimulate motility changes analogous to mass peristalsis.[3] Invasive agents may also variably alter motility

Table 118–1. EFFECT OF BACTERIAL EXOTOXINS ON CYCLIC NUCLEOTIDE METABOLISM

Exotoxin	Cyclic Nucleotide	
	Adenylate Cyclase	*Guanylate Cyclase*
Enterotoxigenic *E. coli*		
Heat-labile toxin (LT)	Stimulation	
Heat-stable toxin (ST)		Stimulation
Shigella (Shiga) toxin	Probably stimulation	
Yersinia enterocolitica		
Heat-stable toxin		Stimulation
Clostridium difficile		
Cytotoxin	Inhibition	Stimulation

patterns.[4] Intestinal hypomotility or stasis alters intestinal absorption by increasing the contact time of solute with the absorbing surface and by producing an increase in the "unstirred layer" effect.[5] The high flow velocity associated with increased secretion may additionally decrease absorption of solutes and water, contributing to osmotic diarrhea.[6] Viral agents are characteristically associated with vomiting, which is best explained by a virus-induced delay in gastric emptying.[8] When distention of the gut reaches a maximum, which occurs in cholera-like illness, the gut will not distend further and acts as a rigid conduit.[7]

Table 118–2 outlines the virulence characteristics of the non-parasitic diarrhea-producing enteropathogens. Some of these properties will be discussed in this section, while others that deal more with the evolution of the clinical syndrome produced will be discussed later in this chapter.

A great deal of confusion exists about *Escherichia coli* as an enteric pathogen. During the 1940s and 1950s, *E. coli* organisms belonging to certain serotypes were implicated in hospital nursery outbreaks of diarrhea. These strains were termed "enteropathogenic *E. coli* (EPEC)," a term restricted today to these serotype-identified strains. The general serotypes currently identified as potential EPEC strains are 026, 044, 055, 086, 0111, 0114, 0119, 0125, 0127, 0128ac, 0142, and 0158. EPEC strains have now been implicated as causative agents in protracted diarrhea of infancy,[9] and virulence characteristics have been at least partially defined. EPEC strains have been shown to elaborate enterotoxic substances active in the perfused rat intestine,[10] and a preliminary study further indicated that these strains may produce a toxin immunologically related to that elaborated by *Shigella dysenteriae 1* (the Shiga bacillus).[11] However, the most constant pathogenic mechanism of the EPEC strains is enteroadherence (Fig. 118–1). Approximately 80% of EPEC strains (as determined by serotype) will be positive for adherence[12] in Hep II tissue culture cells, the standard assay of adhesion for these strains.[13]

Isolates of *E. coli* 0157:H7 have been identified in diarrheal stools of patients with an illness clinically designated as "hemorrhagic colitis." Infection was traced to contaminated hamburgers obtained from a variety of sources, including a large national chain restaurant.[14]

The second form of *E. coli* diarrhea is due to enterotoxigenic strains. These organisms possess a variety of pathogenic properties that are characteristically under plasmid control.[15] Most strains implicated in human illness possess surface (capsular) antigens of fimbriate structure, which render the organisms adherent to the small bowel epithelial lining of the host. Strains also elaborate one or more secretory toxins that are active in animal or tissue culture assays (Fig. 118–2 and 118–3). A protein of 80,000 to 90,000 molecular weight, antigenically and biologically related to cholera toxin, is characteristically produced. This toxin is customarily referred to as heat-labile toxin (LT) because it is susceptible to heat. LT induces intestinal

Table 118–2. VIRULENCE CHARACTERISTICS OF THE NON-PARASITIC ENTERIC PATHOGENS

Microbial Agent	Host/Parasite Interaction
Rotavirus, Norwalk agent	Penetration of small bowel mucosa, inflammation, malabsorption, delayed gastric emptying
Vibrio cholerae	Adherence, secretion: adenylate cyclase secondary to heat-labile toxin
Enteropathogenic *E. coli* (EPEC)	Adherence with characteristic intestinal damage, release of enterotoxins?
Enterotoxigenic *E. coli* (ETEC)	Virulence plasmids: colonization fimbriae, heat-labile and heat-stable enterotoxins (LT and ST)
Shigella and invasive *E. coli*	Invasiveness and release of a Shiga-like toxin, small bowel infection followed by colonic phase of infection with variable degrees of inflammation
Salmonella	Attachment (fimbrial surface antigens) and invasiveness, nature of mucosal inflammation determines host response
Campylobacter	Invasiveness and release of heat-stable enterotoxins

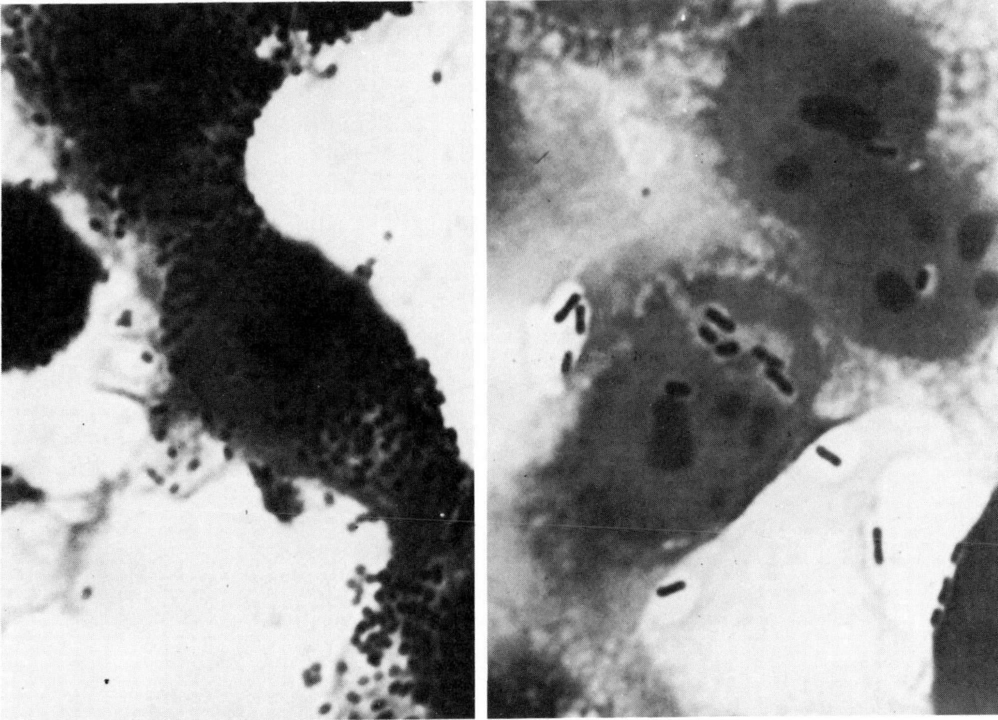

Figure 118–1. Adherence test for *E. coli* using HEP-II cell line enteropathogenic *E. coli* strain JCP-88. *Left,* 4+ adherence; *right,* ACTC control *E. coli* strain showing non-adherence (× 1000; carbol fuchsin stain).

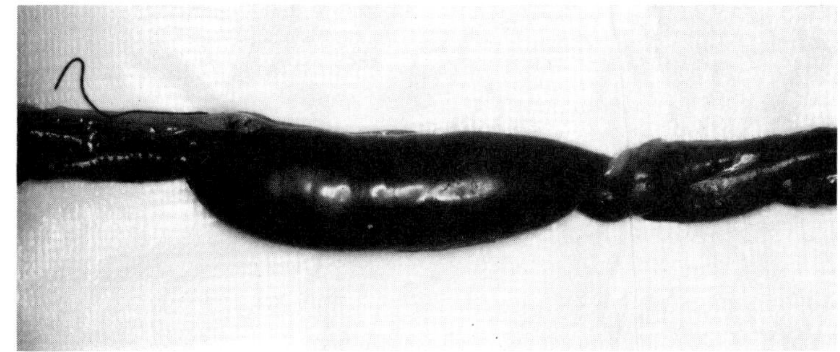

Figure 118–2. Rabbit intestinal loop test for heat-labile *E. coli* enterotoxin. Dilated loop of rabbit ileum 18 hours after injection of filtrates containing the toxin. (From DuPont HL, Pickering LK. Infections of the Gastrointestinal Tract: Microbiology, Pathophysiology and Clinical Features. New York: Plenum Publishing Co., 1980. Reproduced with permission.)

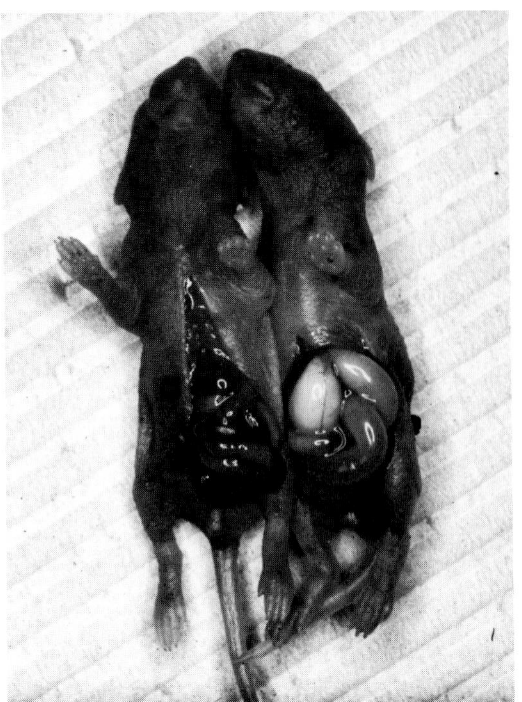

Figure 118–3. Suckling mouse assay for heat stable *E. coli* toxin. Dilated intestine (*right*) 2 to 4 hours after intragastric inoculation of filtrates containing the toxin. (From DuPont HL. Med Clin North Am 1978; 62:945–60. Reproduced with permission.)

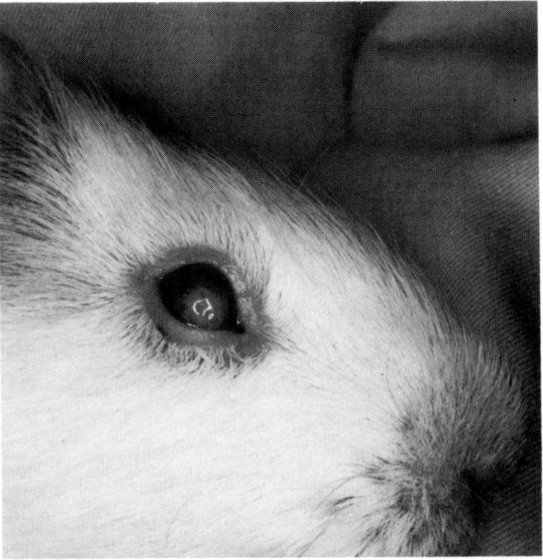

Figure 118–4. Guinea pig eye model of invasiveness (Sereny test). An invasive *E. coli* or Shigella strain placed earlier in the conjunctival sac produces purulent keratoconjunctivitis.

secretion by stimulating adenylate cyclase. Heat-stable toxin (ST) is also commonly produced. Two or more STs may be produced by *E. coli* differing in terms of methanol solubility and activity in animal models.[16] Enterotoxigenic *E. coli* (ETEC) may produce LT or ST (commonly both). Strains producing only LT may cause diarrhea and may be responsible for outbreaks of illness. However, there is a clearer association with diarrhea for strains producing only ST or LT plus ST. Occasionally, *E. coli* strains not belonging to EPEC serotypes and not producing conventional LT or ST are implicated in cases of diarrhea.

A third form of diarrheogenic *E. coli* has been characterized. These *E. coli* are invasive for the intestinal tract, producing an illness indistinguishable from shigellosis.[17] To verify an *E. coli* strain as invasive, a heavy suspension of the strain is dropped into the conjunctival sac of a guinea pig soon after the strain is isolated. Invasive strains induce purulent keratoconjunctivitis (Fig. 118–4).

Shigella and Salmonella are the prototypes of invasive enteric pathogens. In shigellosis, the organisms invade superficially, showing progressively fewer bacteria deeper into the mucosa. Superficial intestinal inflammation is intense, with ulceration and local hemorrhage. In salmonellosis, the epithelial lining is largely left intact and the bacteria commonly reach the lamina propria. Strains of Shigella and Salmonella produce enterotoxins that probably contribute to the occurrence of diarrhea through secretory pathways.[18,19] In Salmonella infection, the nature of the host leukocytic inflammatory response determines the clinical expression of disease to a large degree. With Salmonella gastroenteritis, there is a polymorphonuclear leukocytic response and the organisms are locally contained in most cases. In the systemic forms of salmonellosis, a mononuclear leukocytic infiltrate is seen, which appears to correlate with transit through the portal tributaries to the systemic circulation.

Campylobacter strains invade the colonic mucosa, producing inflammatory infiltrates in the lamina propria, crypt abscesses, and epithelial ulcerations,[20] features that are similar histologically to the colitis seen in idiopathic inflammatory bowel disease.[21] The invasive nature of the organism undoubtedly explains the rapid development of humoral antibody to the infecting strain and the occasional recovery of the organism from peripheral blood early in the infection. Rarely, patients with Campylobacter infection may present with massive lower intestinal hemorrhage.[22] Campylobacter strains have been studied in the laboratory for pathogenic mechanisms, and conflicting data have been generated. In certain studies, heat-stable toxins have been produced,[23] whereas in others, production of conventional toxins has not been documented.[24] The invasive nature of one Campylobacter strain was well demonstrated in a model of infection in 3-day-old chickens.[25]

Epidemiology

Modes of Spread. The infectious agents responsible for non-parasitic diarrhea are spread to those destined to become ill through a number of different pathways. Among these are food or water contaminated by persons, animals, or the environment and person-to-person or person-to-environment-to-person spread. Although the concept of dose response of man to enteric pathogens applies in the majority of situations, it assumes that the host is healthy in all respects. Table 118–3 offers a brief perspective on several bacterial enteropathogens about which sufficient data exist to allow speculation as to dose response and expected route of transmission. Cholera and ETEC diarrhea characteristically occur after ingestion of a large inoculum that has multiplied in a food or water vehicle.

A small inoculum of Shigella (100 to 200 cells) will produce illness in up to one-fourth of those exposed. This dose response information helps us understand how Shigella can be spread from person to person and why secondary spread is so common in families and in day care centers and other settings where people are living in close proximity with one another. In developing regions, shigellosis is usually a food-borne enteric disease. While a food or water vehicle is occasionally seen in the United States, the expected route of transmission is person-to-person. Non-typhoid Salmonella and Campylobacter strains are characteristically spread from animals to man through a food vehicle. Person-to-person spread of Salmonella does occur. This is characteristically seen in the hospital setting among those with disability, in homes for the elderly or retarded, and among infants.

While low doses of Salmonella ($< 10^3$) can result in infection,[26] the relative rarity of person-to-person spread when compared with the situation for Shigella suggests a difference in dose for the 2 enteric pathogens. While growth of Salmonella occurs when food is left at room temperature, this may not be the case for Campylobacter. However, a lower dose of Campylobacter probably is sufficient to produce illness.

The transmission dynamics of *viral gastroenteritis* have not been fully worked out. It appears that rotaviruses and Norwalk-like agents are generally spread through a water vehicle. The Norwalk-like agents cause explosive outbreaks affecting whole segments of the community, regardless of age, when water contamination occurs.

Rotavirus infection typically occurs in children less than 3 years of age, and non-

Table 118–3. DOSE OF ORGANISMS REQUIRED FOR INFECTION AND EXPECTED MODE OF SPREAD FOR SELECTED BACTERIAL ENTEROPATHOGENS

		Mode of Transmission		
Microbial Agent	**Dose Implicated***	***Person-to-Person***	***Food***	***Water***
Vibrio cholerae	High	Rare	Common	Common
ETEC	High	Rare	Common	Probable
Shigella	Low	Common	Common in developing countries	Occurs
Salmonella	Moderate	Occurs in infants and elderly and debilitated persons	Common	Occurs
Campylobacter	Low	Unknown	Common	Occurs

*High = $>10^5$ viable cells; moderate = 10^3 to 10^5; low = $<10^3$.

typhoid salmonellosis is most common in infants less than 1 year of age. In developing countries, ETEC strains are important in the age group affected by rotavirus. Campylobacter is a cause of diarrhea in all age groups, but half of the patients are between the ages of 16 and 35 years.[27] EPEC strains have been clearly shown to be important only in hospital nurseries where newborn children are housed. These strains have also been shown to be important causes of endemic diarrhea in young children, producing protracted diarrhea associated with dehydration and poor growth.[9,13]

Importance of Various Agents. The various enteric pathogens may show regional differences in importance (Table 118–4). Cholera endemic areas are largely characterized, although spread outside of known regions does occur. Rotavirus is a common cause of diarrhea in children under the age of 3 years in all regions of the world. Rotavirus diarrhea characteristically occurs in the cooler months of the year, especially in regions with temperate climates. The other major causes of pediatric diarrhea in all regions are Shigella, Campylobacter, and EPEC strains. ETEC and Giardia are particularly important in diarrhea occurring in developing regions. Shigella infections show regional patterns of importance, differences for which there are no obvious explanations. Campylobacter diarrhea is important in all regions of the world and may show an inverse proportion of cases when compared with Shigella prevalence. In selected areas where Shigella accounts for as many as 15% of cases (Houston, Mexico), Campylobacter is seen in 3% to 5% of cases, while in regions where Campylobacter is implicated in 10% to 20% of cases (Denver, Toronto, Scandinavia), Shigella isolates are far less common. *Yersinia enterocolitica* may be a cause of acute diarrhea in any region of the world. It shows a striking association with colder climates, however. *Y. enterocolitica* is commonly associated with diarrhea in Scandinavia and in Canada,[28] where it is characteristically seen in the summer. *Aeromonas hydrophila* has been associated with diarrhea in certain regions of the world including Canada, Thailand, and Western Australia.

Food-borne disease is discussed in Chapter 119.

Special Considerations.

Traveler's Diarrhea. When persons from industrialized regions travel to developing areas, the occurrence rate of acute diarrhea among them is approximately 40%. Illness is most common in young children, but all age groups are susceptible. The causative agents (Table 118–4) reflect the organisms prevalent in the area being visited. ETEC can be found in just under 50% of cases. The frequency of this group of organisms in these circumstances is probably a reflection of local prevalence as well as the relative lack of occurrence of ETEC infection in developed countries. Immunity to ETEC occurs rapidly as persons remain in endemic areas,[29, 30] presumably as a result of repeated exposure to the organism. Food is an important vehicle of transmission of bacterial agents in all areas,[31] while water probably remains an important source of bacterial enteropathogens in rural areas and in selected areas for Giardia and viruses.

Infants in Day Care Centers. It is becoming increasingly clear that day care centers represent important settings for the transmission

Table 118–4. ESTIMATED RELATIVE IMPORTANCE OF ENTEROPATHOGENS

Microbial Agent	Endemic Pediatric Diarrhea: *United States*	Endemic Pediatric Diarrhea: *Developing Country*	Food-borne Diarrhea in the United States*	Diarrhea of Travelers
Rotavirus	20%–40%	20%–40%	Unknown	10%
Enterotoxigenic *E. coli*	1%–4%	20%–40%	Rare	40%
Enteropathogenic *E. coli*	10%	10%	?	Unknown
Shigella	3%–15%	3%–15%	7%	15%
Salmonella	4%	3%–7%	40%	7%
Campylobacter	3%–15%	3%–15%	?	3%
Giardia	4%	4%–20%	Rare	3%
Unknown	40%	30%–40%	0	22%
Clostridium perfringens	?	?	11%	?
Staphylococcus aureus	?	?	26%	?

*Percentages given are based on outbreaks with an identified agent. (From Sours HE, Smith DG. Outbreaks of foodborne disease in the United States. 1972–1978. J Infect Dis 1980; 142:122–5. Reproduced with permission.)

of enteric agents among young infants who are exposed for the first time to other children who are also not toilet-trained.[32] These centers may constitute in a community an important reservoir of many enteric pathogens, including hepatitis A, Giardia, rotavirus, Shigella, and *Clostridium difficile*.[33]

Male Homosexuals and Immunocompromised Persons. Male homosexuals commonly experience a wide variety of infectious diseases, with the enteric pathogens being the most important cause of morbidity in this setting. Table 118–5 lists the agents most commonly involved. Usually, the agents important in diarrheal disease are spread by the fecal-oral route through oral-anal contact. This concept is supported by a study of patients seen at a venereal disease clinic where sexual transmission of enteric parasites was evaluated.[34] Women and heterosexual men were free of parasites, while the prevalence of *Entamoeba histolytica* or *Giardia lamblia* was 6% in bisexual men and 22% in homosexual men. A history of oral-anal sexual contact correlated with higher rates of infection.

Organisms probably can be transmitted through direct rectal inoculation into an area of mucosal damage (*Neisseria gonorrhoeae, Chlamydia trachomatis),* but this mode of spread is largely unproved.

Male homosexuals may develop severe deficits in immunologic capabilities and experience a wide array of infections caused by organisms of normally low virulence. *Acquired immune deficiency syndrome (AIDS)* is a partially characterized disorder of immune responsiveness that may be associated with enteric infection due to cytomegalovirus, herpes simplex, and cryptosporidia.[35, 36] Patients severely immunocompromised from any cause also show increased susceptibility to enteric pathogens. Classically, Salmonella infection with spread to the systemic circulation is seen in cancer patients.[37] The same agents seen in AIDS, including cytomegalovirus, can be found as well in those with compromised immunity. Yersinia, *Clostridium difficile,* and viral agents, including enteric adenoviruses, rotavirus and Coxsackie virus, also are encountered fairly commonly.[38]

Table 118–5. ENTERIC INFECTIOUS DISEASES IN MALE HOMOSEXUALS

Epidemiologic Setting	Enteric Infection
Fecal oral spread largely through oral-anal contact	Shigellosis, salmonellosis, campylobacteriosis, giardiasis, amebiasis
Direct rectal inoculation	Gonococcal and chlamydial proctitis
Altered immunocompetence	Cytomegalovirus, herpes simplex, and cryptosporidial colitis

Clinical Aspects

Clinical manifestations of enteric infection may reflect the virulence characteristics of the involved pathogen. Rotavirus and Norwalk-like agents lead to vomiting in most cases. In cholera and ETEC, profuse watery diarrhea classically occurs. Patients with cholera have no fever, while those with illness due to ETEC may have low-grade fever. Protracted diarrhea in an infant suggests disaccharidase deficiency following rotavirus infection, giardiasis, or EPEC illness. In half of the patients with shigellosis, a progressive descending intestinal tract infection occurs. This begins with fever and is followed by watery diarrhea with voluminous stools. One to 3 days later, the stools decrease in volume ("fractional" stools), a greater number are passed, and blood and mucus are seen in the stool. The early phase of infection relates to small bowel infection and perhaps to release of Shigella enterotoxin as well; the second dysenteric phase corresponds to the presence of the organisms in the colonic mucosa, the target organ in shigellosis. During the second phase, lower abdominal pain may be severe and fecal urgency and tenesmus are common. A history suggesting a descending intestinal tract infection, progressing from a small bowel to primarily a colonic type of disease, suggests shigellosis. Patients with Campylobacter diarrhea often have fever, and dysenteric stools (blood and mucus) frequently are passed. Campylobacter infection resembles shigellosis, although most cases of the former are clinically milder and illness may not last as long. In Salmonella gastroenteritis, patients usually present with low-grade fever and watery diarrhea. The stools often contain mucus; gross blood is present in slightly less than 10% of the cases.

Table 118–6 lists the agents to consider in patients with a given clinical finding. Despite differences in virulence characteristics of the enteric pathogens, most patients with intestinal infection do not have a characteristic clinical picture. In the majority of patients,

Table 118–6. CORRELATION OF ENTERIC PATHOGENS WITH CLINICAL FINDINGS IN CLASSIC CASES OF INFECTIOUS DIARRHEA

Clinical Finding	Microbial Agents
Profuse "cholera-like" diarrhea	*Vibrio cholerae*, ETEC, Shigella (early), Salmonella (in those with altered gastric physiology)
Vomiting (intense)	*Staphylococcus aureus* food poisoning, viral gastroenteritis
High fever	Shigella, Salmonella, Campylobacter, Yersinia, *Clostridium difficile*
Dysentery (bloody stools)	Shigella, Campylobacter, Salmonella, Yersinia, *Vibrio parahemolyticus, Clostridium difficile*
Protracted diarrhea (>3 weeks)	Disaccharidase deficiency from viral gastroenteritis, diarrhea due to EPEC or Giardia, or small bowel bacterial overgrowth

selected laboratory studies must be relied upon to help make a diagnosis and/or empiric therapy for diarrhea must be initiated without previous establishment of the cause.

Diagnosis

In approaching the patient with non-parasitic diarrhea, a working etiologic categorization can be structured from such data as the presence or absence of associated cases, profuse diarrhea, fever, vomiting, dysentery, or a protracted course. Most patients with mild diarrhea need not be evaluated beyond clinical assessment, since the cost of laboratory studies cannot be justified when illness in most instances lasts only a few days. On the other hand, there are indications for laboratory tests that may lead to specific antimicrobial therapy with shortening of the clinical illness and reduction in secondary transmission.

When associated cases of diarrhea occur among family members, a group of friends, or multiple patrons of an eating establishment, a common exposure would be suspected and an incubation period constructed. In the setting of an outbreak of enteric disease when the incubation period is less than 4 hours and vomiting is the most common symptom, a diagnosis of staphylococcal food poisoning can be made. With other agents, infection characteristically is associated with symptoms and the incubation period is 8 hours or longer. Watery diarrhea without fever suggests *Clostridium perfringens* or *Bacillus cereus.* Afebrile watery diarrhea associated with abdominal cramps or pain and appearing 7 to 22 hours after eating a meat product, especially in the spring or fall, is probably due to *C. perfringens. B. cereus* food-borne disease has 2 forms. One is expressed by upper gastrointestinal symptoms developing within 1 to 6 hours (resembling staphylococcal food poisoning); the other is indistinguishable from *C. perfringens* illness with quite similar incubation periods and symptoms.[39] The presence of fever in a proportion of the cases is more compatible with Salmonella, Campylobacter, or Shigella infection. When a community-wide outbreak occurs, especially when vomiting is an important feature, a Norwalk-like viral agent is probably the cause.

Considering the low cost of the test and the value of the information given, the *fecal leukocyte test* is a good starting point for the laboratory evaluation of acute diarrhea. It should be obtained in any patient with moderate to severe diarrhea. For practical purposes, this would be any hospitalized patient, those with profuse diarrhea, and those with fever or dysentery. The optimal stain for most cases is methylene blue. Either a wet mount preparation[40] or a dried heat-fixed fecal smear can be examined with dilute methylene blue under oil (Fig. 118–5). When a male homosexual is being evaluated, a Gram stain is preferable to look for intracellular gram-negative diplococci indicative of gonococcal proctitis. Mucus should be selected for study whenever present in a stool sample, using a wooden applicator stick to secure a mucus strand.

Numerous leukocytes in a fecal smear indicate the presence of diffuse inflammation of the colonic mucosa; they do not betoken or connote the presence of a specific microorganism. Early in the course of shigellosis, during the small bowel phase, stools are characteristically negative for leukocytes, as is the case for diarrhea due to Salmonella

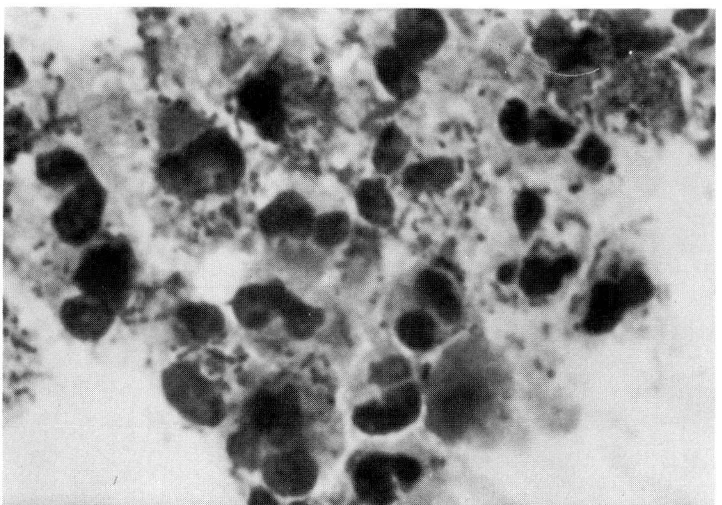

Figure 118–5. Methylene blue stain of heat fixed stool. The numerous polymorphonuclear leukocytes seen microscopically indicate the presence of a diffuse colitis.

and Shigella during the recovery phase. Patients with small bowel inflammation, focal colitis, or those bleeding into the gastrointestinal tract usually do not have numerous leukocytes, presumably because of dilution. The major causes of fecal leukocyte–positive stools (diffuse colitis) are listed in Table 118–7.

A stool culture is reserved for those patients admitted to the hospital, those with dehydration or protracted forms of diarrhea (lasting ≥1 week), and those with fever (≥40°C), dysentery, or fecal leukocyte–positive stools. Virtually all diagnostic laboratories have the expertise to isolate Shigella, Salmonella, and Campylobacter when a stool culture is ordered. These agents together account for 20% to 25% of cases of acute nonparasitic diarrhea.

Proctosigmoidoscopy is a useful procedure in selected cases of diarrhea. For most cases of infectious diarrhea it usually gives much the same information as the fecal leukocyte test (presence or absence of colonic or rectal inflammation). However, endoscopy can be additionally valuable in helping to diagnose antibiotic-associated colitis, amebiasis (selective sampling of ulcers), villous adenoma, or early idiopathic inflammatory colitis.

Additional tests are available in certain areas. A commercially available immunoassay for rotavirus (Rotazyme test) can be utilized to diagnose rotavirus gastroenteritis. Serotyping of *E. coli* (to identify EPEC strains), toxin testing, studies of invasiveness (guinea pig eye test), and radioimmunoassay for Norwalk virus can be done at present in only a limited number of research centers.

Table 118–7. ROUTINE LABORATORY TESTS: WHEN TO PERFORM AND AGENTS SOUGHT

Tests or Procedures	Indications	Microbial Agent
Fecal leukocyte test	Any case of moderate to severe diarrhea	Shigella, Salmonella, Campylobacter; occasionally Yersinia, *Vibrio parahemolyticus, Clostridium difficile,* and gonococcal proctitis
Stool culture	Hospital admission; dehydration with diarrhea; profuse diarrhea; temperature >40°C; diarrhea >1 week in duration; positive fecal leukocytes; passage of bloody stools	Shigella, Salmonella, Campylobacter (upon special request, Yersinia, Aeromonas, Vibrio, EPEC strains)
Parasitic examination	Diarrhea >1 week in duration; recent travel to developing region, Soviet Union, Rocky Mountains; bloody stools with few leukocytes	*Giardia lamblia, Entamoeba histolytica*

Treatment

In the initial evaluation of a patient with diarrhea, the first consideration is a determination of the need for hospitalization. Indications for admission to a hospital include: (1) the presence of significant (10%) dehydration manifested by tachycardia, extreme dryness of the mucous membranes, lack of tears, oliguria approaching anuria, ability to palpably depress the fontanel if open, loss of skin elasticity and turgor, skin mottling, cool extremities, apathy, and mild somnolence; (2) intractable vomiting; (3) extremes of age; (4) serious underlying disorder; and (5) severe systemic toxicity.

The cornerstone of therapy for all forms of diarrhea is fluid and electrolyte replacement. In most forms of acute diarrhea, active intestinal secretion probably occurs with impairment of sodium transport across the intestinal wall. Glucose transport, however, is largely left intact. Also, glucose absorption carries sodium and water with it.[41] An oral solution has been recommended by the World Health Organization for the therapy of diarrhea; the solution has 90 mEq/liter of sodium and 20 mEq/liter of potassium (Table 118–8). It has been used extensively in the field and under supervision can replace the losses associated with intense (cholera-like) diarrhea.[42] This solution can be produced by combining with 1 liter of water the following ingredients: sodium chloride, 3.5 g; sodium bicarbonate, 2.5 g; potassium chloride, 1.5 g; and glucose, 20 g. Free fluid should be given with this high sodium solution to prevent the development of hypernatremia.[43] In the United States, lower amounts of sodium are sufficient to replace losses in cases of mild to moderately severe diarrhea. Pedialyte, Lytren, and Gatorade are good solutions for oral therapy. Soft drinks plus salted crackers can also be used to replace fluid and salt losses. In Table 118–8 the sodium and potassium contents of a few of the readily available solutions are compared.

Table 118–9. NONSPECIFIC THERAPY FOR ACUTE DIARRHEA

Agent	Mechanisms	Comment
Bismuth subsalicylate	Antisecretory	Salicylate absorption; black stools
Loperamide or diphenoxylate	Antimotility, antisecretory	Rapid onset of action; rarely will worsen invasive forms; overdose liability in children
Kaopectate	Adsorbent	Makes stools more bulky; safe

Drugs are often used for symptomatic relief of diarrhea. Table 118–9 offers a brief perspective on the more commonly used preparations. *Bismuth subsalicylate* is an effective agent for treating secretory diarrhea.[44] The amount of salicylate absorbed is significant when one 8-ounce bottle is taken over 3½ hours (the recommended dose) and is equivalent to taking 8 aspirin tablets.[45] *Loperamide* (Imodium) and *diphenoxylate* (Lomotil) are the most rapidly active of the agents listed and are the most effective in relieving cramps and pain. The opiate-like agents have classically been considered to have primarily antimotility effects, but their effect on fluid movement may be of more importance.[46] Patients with high fever or bloody stools should not receive these preparations because of the possibility of worsening of the illness as a consequence.[47] *Kaopectate* increases the form of the

Table 118–8. ORAL FLUID THERAPY OF ACUTE DIARRHEA

Preparation	Indication	Electrolyte Content (mEq/liter)	
		Sodium	*Potassium*
WHO formula*	Dehydration or cholera-like diarrhea	90	20
Pedialyte	Mild to moderate diarrhea	30	20
Lytren		30	25
Gatorade		23	3
Pepsi-Cola		6.5	0.8
7-Up		4.6	0.1
Coca-Cola		0.4	1–13
Apple juice, canned		1.7	26

*Available in packets to add to water.

stool, perhaps allowing some conscious control of the timing of evacuation. However, fluid losses probably are not prevented by adsorbent compounds such as Kaopectate.

For more severe diarrhea, antimicrobial agents are useful (Table 118–10). The microbial agents that may produce diarrhea and are responsive to appropriate specific drug therapy include enterotoxigenic *E. coli*, enteropathogenic *E. coli*, Shigella, and Campylobacter. *Trimethoprim/sulfamethoxazole* (TMP/SMX) currently is the drug of choice for severe illness due to ETEC, EPEC, and Shigella.[48,49] *Furazolidone* also is effective against these forms of diarrhea.[50] For Campylobacter, *erythromycin* or furazolidone probably is the drug of choice, although their use late in the course of the disease is only minimally effective.[51] While Salmonella gastroenteritis should not be treated with antibiotics for reason of prolongation of fecal shedding of organisms[52] or conversion into more severe illness,[53] Salmonella bacteremia must be treated with antimicrobial agents. Since 6% to 8% of patients with Salmonella gastroenteritis develop bacteremia, patients with high fever, profuse diarrhea, or, in fact, any patient ill enough to justify hospitalization, probably should be treated with ampicillin, chloramphenicol, or TMP/SMX.

Newer agents are being developed for treating acute bacterial diarrhea. One such agent, *bicozamycin*, a poorly absorbable antibiotic, was found to be an effective form of therapy for traveler's diarrhea due to strains of ETEC, Shigella, and possibly Salmonella and for illness unassociated with an identifiable agent.[54]

Prevention of Traveler's Diarrhea. Knowing that diarrhea occurs in nearly half of all persons traveling from industrialized to developing regions and that most of the cases of diarrhea are caused by bacterial agents has led to attempts to prevent the illness by prophylactic administration of drugs. Kean and associates[55] initially established, even before the important causes were known, that antibiotics could prevent much of the illness during short-term exposure. Subsequently, *doxycycline*[56] and then *trimethoprim/sulfamethoxazole*[57] have been shown to prevent traveler's diarrhea, primarily through their effect on ETEC strains.[58] TMP/SMX has an advantage over other available compounds in that it is also active against most strains of Shigella. *Bismuth subsalicylate* protects rabbit intestinal loops from the effects of cholera and ETEC enterotoxins.[59] This action led to field studies evaluating the effectiveness of this anti-inflammatory agent in the preven-

Table 118–10. ANTIMICROBIAL THERAPY FOR BACTERIAL DIARRHEA

Microbial Agent	Drug	Dose: *Children*	Dose: *Adults*
ETEC (traveler's diarrhea)	Trimethoprim (TMP) + Sulfamethoxazole (SMX)	TMP 10 mg/kg/day + SMX 50 mg/kg/day (po) in 2 equally divided doses for 3–5 days	TMP 160 mg + SMX 800 mg (po) bid for 3–5 days
	or Furazolidone (FX)	FX 5 mg/kg/day (po) individual doses qid for 5 days	FX 100 mg qid (po) for 5 days
EPEC or enteroadherent *E. coli*	TMP + SMX	As for ETEC	As for ETEC
Shigella	TMP + SMX	As for ETEC	As for ETEC
Campylobacter	Erythromycin (ER)	ER 25–50 mg/kg/day (po) in 4 equally divided doses for 7 days	ER 500 mg qid (po) for 7 days
	or Furazolidone (FX)	FX 5 mg/kg/day (po) in divided doses qid for 5–7 days	FX 100 mg qid (po) for 5–7 days
Salmonella* (bacteremic)	Ampicillin	200 mg/kg/day (IV) in 6 equally divided doses for 10–14 days	Ampicillin 6 g/day (IV) in 6 equally divided doses for 10–14 days

Non-bacteremic disease is not treated with antibiotics (see text).

tion of traveler's diarrhea.[60] When taken in a dose of 60 ml 4 times a day, bismuth subsalicylate prevented illness for 3 weeks while subjects remained at risk. Doses of this magnitude are probably impractical for most travelers. Nevertheless, the demonstration that a nonantibiotic compound can prevent the illness is exciting.

Not all travelers at risk should be encouraged to take drugs prophylactically. Side effects of the drugs are real, including the development of gastrointestinal symptoms and skin rashes. Also, intestinal flora will commonly develop resistance during drug administration,[61] which could present problems. It is our recommendation that antibiotic prophylaxis be reserved for certain business persons on critical short-term assignment and for those with other underlying disease. Doxycycline is given in a dose of 100 mg twice a day on the day of travel, then 100 mg daily for the period at risk. TMP/SMX is given in a dose of one double strength tablet (TMP 160 mg/SMX 800 mg) each day, beginning on the day of travel and continuing for 1 to 2 days after returning home. For those away from home for more than 2 weeks, antibiotic prophylaxis is probably inappropriate. All travelers should be aware that where they eat and what they eat will to a large degree determine whether diarrhea occurs.[62]

References

1. Field M. Intestinal secretion. Gastroenterology 1974; 66:1063–84.
2. Lifshitz F, Coello-Ramirez R, Gutierrez-Topete G, Cornado-Cornet, MC. Carbohydrate intolerance in infants with diarrhea. J Pediatr 1971; 79:760–7.
3. Borgström B, Dahlqvist A, Lundh G, Sjövall J. Studies of intestinal digestion and absorption in the human. J Clin Invest 1957; 36:1521–36.
4. Weisberg PB, Carlson GM, Cohen S. Effect of *Salmonella typhimurium* on myoelectrical activity in the rabbit ileum. Gastroenterology 1978; 74:47–51.
5. Dietschy JM, Sallee VL, Wilson FA. Unstirred water layers and absorption across the intestinal mucosa. Gastroenterology 1971; 61:932–4.
6. Matuchansky C, Huet PM, Mary JY, Rambaud JC, Bernier JJ. Effects of cholecystokinin and metoclopromide on jejunal movements of water and electrolytes and on transit time of luminal fluid in man. Eur J Clin Invest 1972; 2:169–75.
7. Dillard RL, Eastman H, Fordtran JS. Volume-flow relationships during the transport of fluid through the human small intestine. Gastroenterology 1965; 49:58–66.
8. Meeroff JC, Schreiber DS, Trier JS, Blacklow NR. Abnormal gastric motor function in viral gastroenteritis. Ann Intern Med 1980; 92:370–3.
9. Rothbaum R, McAdams AJ, Giannella R, Partin JC. A clinicopathologic study of enterocyte-adherent *Escherichia coli:* A cause of protracted diarrhea in infants. Gastroenterology 1982; 83:441–54.
10. Klipstein FA, Rowe B, Engert RF, Short HB, Gross RJ. Enterotoxicity of enteropathogenic serotypes of *Escherichia coli* isolated from infants with epidemic diarrhea. Infect Immun 1978; 21:171–8.
11. O'Brien AD, LaVeck GD, Thompson MR, Formal SB. Production of *Shigella dysenteriae* type 1-like cytotoxin by *Escherichia coli.* J Infect Dis 1982; 146:763–9.
12. Rowe B. Enteropathogenic *Escherichia coli* (EPEC)—Importance and pathophysiology *In:* Holme T, Holmgren J, Merson MH, Möllby R, eds.: Acute Enteric Infections in Children. New Prospects for Treatment and Prevention. Amsterdam: Elsevier/North Holland Biomedical Press, 1981: 101–6.
13. Clausen CR, Christie DL. Chronic diarrhea in infants caused by adherent enteropathogenic *Escherichia coli.* J Pediatr 1982; 100:358–61.
14. US Dept Health and Human Resources, PHS, MMWR, November 5, 1982, Vol 31, No 43, pp 580 and 585.
15. Evans DG, Evans DJ Jr, DuPont HL. Virulence factors of enterotoxigenic *Escherichia coli.* J Infect Dis 1977; 136:S118–23.
16. Burgess MN, Bywater RJ, Cowley CM, Mullan NA, Newsome PM. Biological evaluation of a methanol-soluble, heat stable *Escherichia coli* enterotoxin in infant mice, pigs, rabbits, and calves. Infect Immun 1978; 21:526–31.
17. DuPont HL, Formal SB, Hornick RB, Snyder MJ, Libonati JP, Sheahan DG, LaBrec EH, Kalas JP: Pathogenesis of *Escherichia coli* diarrhea. N Engl J Med 1971; 285:1–9.
18. Keusch GT, Grady GF, Mata LJ, McIver J. The pathogenesis of Shigella diarrhea. I. Enterotoxin production by *Shigella* dysenteriae 1. J Clin Invest 1972; 51:1212–8.
19. Koupal LR, Deibel RH. Assay, characterization, and localization of an enterotoxin produced by *Salmonella.* Infect Immun 1975; 11:14–22.
20. Blaser MJ, Parson RB, Wang WL. Acute colitis caused by *Campylobacter fetus* ss. *jejuni.* Gastroenterology 1980; 78:448–53.
21. McKendrick MW, Geddes AM, Gearty J. Campylobacter enteritis: A study of clinical features and rectal mucosal changes. Scand J Infect Dis 1982; 14:35–8.
22. Michalak DM, Perrault J, Gilchrist MJ, Dozois RR, Carney JA, Sheedy PF II. *Campylobacter fetus* ss *jejuni:* A cause of massive lower gastrointestinal hemorrhage. Gastroenterology 1980; 79:742–5.
23. Butzler JP, Skirrow MB. Campylobacter enteritis. Clin Gastroenterol 1979; 8:737–63.
24. Manninen KI, Prescott JF, Dohoo IR. Pathogenicity of *Campylobacter jejuni* isolates from animals and humans. Infect Immun 1982; 38:46–52.
25. Ruiz-Palacios GM, Escamilla E, Torres N. Experimental *Campylobacter* diarrhea in chickens. Infect Immun 1981; 34:250–5.
26. Blaser MJ, Newman LS: A review of human salmonellosis. I. Infective dose. Rev Inf Dis 1982; 4:1096–106.
27. Walder M. Epidemiology of Campylobacter enteritis. Scand J Infect Dis 1982; 14:27–33.
28. Marks MI, Pai CH, LaFleur L, Lackman L, Hammerbera O. Yersinia enterocolitica gastroenteritis: A prospective study of clinical, bacteriologic, and epidemiologic features. J Pediatr 1980; 96:26–31.
29. DuPont HL, Olarte J, Evans DG, Pickering LK, Galindo E, Evans DJ Jr. Comparative susceptibility of Latin American and United States students to enteric pathogens. N Engl J Med 1976; 295:1520–1.
30. Brown MR, DuPont HL, Sullivan PS. Effect of duration of exposure on diarrhea due to enterotoxigenic *Escherichia coli* in travelers from the United States to Mexico. J Infect Dis 1982; 145:582.
31. Tjoa W, DuPont HL, Sullivan PS, Pickering LK, Holguin AH, Olarte J, Evans DG, Evans DJ Jr. Location of food consumption and travelers' diarrhea. Am J Epidemiol 1977; 106:61–6.
32. Pickering LK, Evans DG, DuPont HL, Vollet JJ III, Evans DJ Jr. Diarrhea caused by Shigella, rotavirus, and giardia in day care centers: Prospective study. J Pediatr 1981; 99:51–6.
33. Kim KH, DuPont HL, Pickering LK. Outbreaks of diarrhea associated with *Clostridium difficile* and its toxin in day care centers: Evidence of person-to-person spread. J Pediatr 1983; 102:376–82.

34. Phillips SC, Mildvan D, William DC, Gelb AM, White MC. Sexual transmission of enteric protozoa and helminths in a venereal-disease-clinic population. N Engl J Med 1981; 305:603–6.
35. Weinstein L, Edelstein SM, Madara JL, Falchuk KR, McManus BM, Trier JS. Intestinal cryptosporidiosis complicated by disseminated cytomegalovirus infection. Gastroenterology 1981; 81:584–91.
36. US Dept Health and Human Services, PHS, MMWR, November 12, 1982, Vol 31, No 44, pp 589–92.
37. Han T, Sokal JE, Neter E. Salmonellosis in disseminated malignant diseases: A seven-year review (1959–1965). N Engl J Med 1967; 276:1045–52.
38. Yolken RH, Bishop CA, Townsend TR, Bolyard EA, Bartlett J, Santos GW, Saral R. Infectious gastroenteritis in bone-marrow-transplant recipients. N Engl J Med 1982; 306:1009–112.
39. Terranova W, Blake PA. *Bacillus cereus* food poisoning. N Engl J Med 1978; 298:143–4.
40. Harris JC, DuPont HL, Hornick RB. Fecal leukocytes in diarrheal illness. Ann Intern Med 1972; 76:697–703.
41. Schultz SG, Curran PF. Coupled transport of sodium and organic solutes. Physiol Rev 1970; 50:637–718.
42. Sack RB, Cassels J, Mitra R, Merritt C, Butler T, Thomas J, Jacobs B, Chaudhur A, Mondal A. The use of oral replacement solutions in the treatment of cholera and other severe diarrheal disorders. Bull WHO 1970; 43:351–60.
43. Cleary TG, Cleary KR, DuPont HL, El-Malih GS, Kordy MI, Mohieldin MS, Shoukry K, Shukry S, Wyatt RG, Woodward WE. The relationship of oral rehydration to hypernatremia in infantile diarrhea. J Pediatr 1981; 99:739–41.
44. DuPont HL, Sullivan PS, Pickering LK, Haynes G, Ackerman PB. Symptomatic treatment of diarrhea with bismuth subsalicylate among students attending a Mexican university. Gastroenterology 1977; 73:715–8.
45. Pickering LK, Feldman S, Ericsson, CD, Cleary TG. Absorption of salicylate and bismuth from bismuth subsalicylate-containing compound (Pepto-Bismol). J Pediatr 1981; 99:654–6.
46. Schiller LR, Davis GR, Santa Ana CA, Morawski SG, Fordtran JS. Studies of the mechanism of the antidiarrheal effect of codeine. J Clin Invest 1982; 70:999–1008.
47. DuPont HL, Hornick RB. Adverse effect of lomotil therapy in shigellosis. JAMA 1973; 226:1525–8.
48. DuPont HL, Reves RR, Galindo E, Sullivan PS, Wood LV, Mendiola JG. Treatment of travelers' diarrhea with trimethoprim/sulfamethoxazole and with trimethoprim alone. N Engl J Med. 1982 ; 307:841–44.
49. Thorén A, Wolde-Mariam T, Stintzing G, Wadström T, Habte D. Antibiotics in the treatment of gastroenteritis caused by enteropathogenic *Escherichia coli*. J Infect Dis 1980; 141:27–31.
50. DuPont HL, Ericsson CD, Galindo E, Mendiola J. Furazolidone therapy of travelers' diarrhea. (in press).
51. Anders BJ, Lauer BA, Paisley JW, Reller LB. Double-blind placebo controlled trial of erythromycin for treatment of campylobacter enteritis. Lancet 1982; 1:131–2.
52. Aserkoff B, Bennett JV. Effect of antibiotic therapy in acute salmonellosis on the fecal excretion of salmonellae. N Engl J Med 1969; 281:636–40.
53. Rosenthal SL. Exacerbation of salmonella enteritis due to ampicillin. N Engl J Med 1969; 280:147–8.
54. Ericsson CD, DuPont HL, Sullivan PS, Galindo E, Evans DG, Evans DJ Jr. Bicozamycin, a poorly absorbable antibiotic, effectively treats travelers' diarrhea. Ann Intern Med 1983; 98:20–5.
55. Kean BH, Schaffner W, Brennan RW, Waters SR. The diarrhea of travelers. V. Prophylaxis with phthalylsulfathiazole and neomycin sulphate. JAMA 1962; 180:367–71.
56. Sack DA, Kaminsky DC, Sack RB, Itotia JN, Arthur RR, Kapikian AZ, Ørskov F, Ørskov I. Prophylactic doxycycline for travelers' diarrhea. Results of a prospective double-blind study of Peace Corps volunteers in Kenya. N Engl J Med 1978; 298:758–63.
57. DuPont HL, Galindo E, Evans DG, Cabada FJ, Sullivan PS, Evans DJ Jr. Prevention of travelers' diarrhea with trimethoprim-sulfamethoxazole and trimethoprim alone. Gastroenterology 1983; 84:75–80.
58. DuPont HL, West H, Evans DG, Olarte J, Evans DJ Jr. Antimicrobial susceptibility of enterotoxigenic *Escherichia coli*. J Antimicrobial Chemother 1978; 4:100–2.
59. Ericsson CD, Evans DG, DuPont HL, Evans DJ Jr, Pickering LK. Bismuth subsalicylate inhibits activity of crude toxins of *Escherichia coli* and *Vibrio cholerae*. J Infect Dis 1977; 136:693–6.
60. DuPont HL, Sullivan PS, Evans DG, Pickering LK, Evans DJ Jr, Vollet JJ, Ericsson CD, Ackerman PB, Tjoa WS. Prevention of travelers' diarrhea (emporiatric enteritis)—prophylactic administration of subsalicylate bismuth. JAMA 1980; 243:237–41.
61. Murray BE, Rensimer ER, DuPont HL. Emergence of high-level trimethoprim resistance in fecal *Escherichia coli* during oral administration of trimethoprim or trimethoprim-sulfamethoxazole. N Engl J Med 1982; 306:130–5.
62. DuPont HL, DuPont MW. Travel with Health. New York: Appleton-Century-Crofts, 1981.

Chapter 119

Food Poisoning

Cedric Garland • Elizabeth Barrett-Connor

Definition

In its broadest sense, food poisoning encompasses any illness that has as a necessary causal factor ingestion of a foodstuff. Such a definition would include diverse parasitic (e.g., trichinosis), viral (e.g., hepatitis), and rickettsial (e.g., Q fever) diseases, as well as diseases caused by the contamination of food with sundry toxic substances (e.g., pesticides or heavy metals). In this chapter only bacterial food poisoning, toxic or invasive, and illness caused by the presence of natural food toxins, i.e., those not introduced by man, will be considered.

Food poisoning is most easily recognized when there is an outbreak in which 2 or more persons experience a similar illness after ingestion of the same food. Isolated cases are rarely identified unless there is an unusual etiologic agent recovered from the patient (e.g., an unusual *Salmonella* organism known to be present in a brand of commercial chocolate), an obvious association with a particular food (e.g., sickness following ingestion of wild mushrooms), or a distinctive clinical syndrome (e.g., botulism).

In many food poisoning outbreaks, no specific agent is found. This may reflect inadequate culture techniques for fastidious bacteria, lack of representative samples of suspect foods by the time the investigation is undertaken, or limitations of test models for toxins. Comparison of food histories in ill and well persons who attended the same banquet, for example, may provide different attack rates in sick and well persons for a particular food item. In this case the food, if not the specific agent, can be identified. The nature of the suspect food, coupled with the incubation period and the clinical picture, often supports a specific diagnosis although the agent or its toxin cannot be recovered. Several excellent reviews of differential diagnosis have been published.[1–5] A summary of differential diagnosis and a guide to the workup of a food poisoning outbreak are given at the end of this chapter.

Bacterial Food Poisoning

Over 80% of food poisoning outbreaks of known etiology are caused by bacterial contamination of food. Bacterial food poisoning can occur only when the food is contaminated, able to support the growth of bacteria, and maintained at the right temperature for sufficient time to permit growth of organisms to yield either an infectious dose or a preformed toxin. It follows that most bacterial food poisoning outbreaks result from improper cooking, storage, or handling of food and are preventable.

Bacterial food poisoning usually is manifested as a neurologic disease (botulism) or gastroenteritis. Gastroenteritis is due either to invasion of the gut epithelium or to the action of an enterotoxin. In general, invasive agents cause a loss of intestinal mucosal integrity and an illness with a longer incubation period, more systemic signs, including fever, and blood and leukocytes in the stool. In contrast, enterotoxins are emetic or cause a secretory diarrhea with no change in villous architecture; the clinical picture is characterized by a shorter incubation period, little or no fever, and no fecal leukocytes or blood.

Clostridium botulinum

Botulism. Botulism, perhaps the oldest recognized form of food poisoning, was attributed to sausage during the first century AD and derived its name from the Latin word for sausage. In 1897, Van Ermengem clearly showed that the disease was caused by a toxic substance in food. In the early 20th century, a number of epidemics in the United States associated with commercial canned products led to an understanding of the canning procedures necessary for safe foods[6]; over 80% of subsequent cases have been attributed to improperly prepared home-canned products.[7] The largest outbreak ever reported in the United States occurred in 1977, when 59 cases followed ingestion of a hot sauce prepared from home-canned jalapeño peppers served in a Mexican restaurant.[8] Occasional outbreaks attributed to commercially prepared foods, most notably smoked fish and canned salmon and vegetables, continue to occur.

Clostridium botulinum is a gram-positive anaerobic bacillus present throughout the environment that produces heat-resistant spores under suitable conditions. The spores germinate, grow, and produce a heat-labile neurotoxin, but only under anaerobic conditions and only with a pH of 4.0 or greater. The ability to produce some types of toxin is dependent on the infection of the bacillus with a bacteriophage; different phages appear to be responsible for different toxins. Four (A, B, E, and F) of the 8 antigenic types of botulinal toxin have been responsible for food-borne human illness. In the United States, type A toxin is most commonly associated with food poisoning; this form is most frequently reported from states west of the Mississippi. In Europe, most botulism is type B; in the United States, this form is most commonly reported east of the Mississippi. Type E botulism, reported most commonly from Japan, Canada, Alaska, and Scandinavia, is usually associated with uncooked fish or other marine products. Type F botulism is rare.

Food-borne toxigenic botulism is caused by the ingestion of a preformed botulinal neurotoxin.[9,10] These toxins are among the most potent known poisons; nanogram doses may be lethal. On a weight basis, type A toxin is more potent than type B, and type B in turn, is more potent than type E. Partial proteolysis of some toxins in the gastrointestinal tract may potentiate their toxicity. Absorbed toxin binds to the external surface of peripheral nerve membranes; type A toxin is most tightly bound to neural tissue, type E next, and type B least well bound. The toxin interacts in terminal axons with a nerve cell receptor and alters the ability of intracellular calcium to trigger exocytosis of acetylcholine granules.[11] The result is a characteristic neuroparalytic syndrome involving peripheral cholinergic synapses. The pathogenesis of the gastrointestinal symptoms is unknown.

Clinical Features. As with most preformed toxin food poisonings, there is no fever and the incubation period is short, usually 12 to 36 hours, but may be as long as 8 days. In general, the earlier the onset, the more severe the illness. Signs and symptoms are gastrointestinal and neurologic. Gastrointestinal symptoms usually appear first and include nausea, vomiting, abdominal pain, and diarrhea. Although occasionally severe, gastrointestinal symptoms in most cases are mild or absent.

Neurologic abnormalities reflect toxin-induced blockade of cholinergic transmission in ganglionic synapses, postganglionic parasympathomimetic synapses, and neuromuscular junctions. The earliest neurologic findings typically are diplopia, dysarthria, dysphagia, dysphonia, and a dry, painful mouth, sometimes leading to a misdiagnosis of pharyngitis. Ophthalmoplegia, with or without ptosis and pupillary abnormalities, almost always precedes lower cranial and peripheral nerve impairment. The descending weakness or paralysis is usually bilateral, but not necessarily symmetrical, and occurs in the absence of numbness and paresthesias in most cases.[12] Postural hypotension is common. Constipation may be a serious problem. Although patients are occasionally somnolent, the mental status remains normal. The case-fatality rate is presently about 15%, but rates as high as 70% have been reported, usually due to complications of respiratory muscle paralysis.[12] Improved survival is probably primarily due to advances in intensive respiratory care.

Survivors recover completely but slowly; recovery is dependent on ultraterminal sprouting of the nerve to form a new motor endplate on the postsynaptic muscle.[13] Classically, recovery begins first in the muscles of respiration, speech, and swallowing. Constipation, ocular paresis, exercise intolerance, and generalized weakness may persist for months.[14]

Diagnosis. Botulism is most readily diagnosed when there is an outbreak. A clinical diagnosis can usually be made based on the cardinal features of botulism: (1) ophthalmoplegia followed by descending bilateral paresis; (2) no sensory deficits; (3) normal mental status; and (4) absence of fever.

Specific diagnosis rests on the demonstration of botulinal toxin and/or *C. botulinum* in serum, vomitus, gastric contents, or suspect foods. Since *C. botulinum* is rarely found in normal stool, demonstration of the organism or its toxin in stool establishes the diagnosis. Both serum and feces obtained before antitoxin is administered should be frozen and sent to a reference laboratory where mice and antisera are available for toxicity studies and neutralization tests. However, laboratory analysis fails to confirm the diagnosis in one-third of probable cases, possibly because the toxin is bound to nerve tissue and is not in the specimens submitted for analysis.[15]

Electromyography is useful in distinguishing botulism from the Guillain-Barré syndrome: in botulism, muscle action potential is usually diminished in response to a single supramaximal stimulus, but paired or repetitive supramaximal stimuli cause facilitation of the action potential.

Treatment. The specific treatment of neurologic botulism is administration of equine antitoxin. This should be given early, inasmuch as antitoxin is effective only before and during the binding of toxin to neural receptors.[16] The benefit of antitoxin is most clearly established for type E botulism, in which reversal of paralysis is often prompt; in contrast, patients with type A or B disease do not show dramatic improvement.

Both trivalent (ABE) and bivalent (AB) antitoxins are available commercially in the United States. A polyvalent antitoxin for types C, D, F, and G is manufactured by the Serum Institute of Denmark. When, as is usually the case, the toxin is unknown, trivalent (ABE) antitoxin should be administered. Antitoxin and information about treatment are available on a 24-hour basis from the Centers for Disease Control in Atlanta. Skin testing for allergic reaction should precede the use of antitoxin. Approximately 10% of patients show allergy to horse serum and must be desensitized. Approximately 20% of recipients have an adverse reaction.[17]

Supportive therapy includes close attention to vital capacity. Severe respiratory insufficiency may develop rapidly, in which case intubation or tracheostomy and intensive respiratory care may be life-saving. Cathartics, high enemas, and gastric lavage are recommended to eliminate residual toxin in early illness, but should be used with care in patients with ileus. The value of penicillin in the treatment of botulism is unproved; aminoglycosides may worsen the paralysis[18]; and guanidine hydrochloride is of no benefit.[19]

Prevention. Careful attention to appropriate heating and cooling procedures during home canning would prevent most outbreaks. Because the toxin is heat-labile, usual cooking (either boiling for 10 minutes or heating to 80°C for 30 minutes) will also prevent disease associated with improperly canned or smoked foods.

A single case of botulism is considered to be an outbreak and should be reported to the appropriate health authorities so that other exposed persons can be identified and additional cases prevented. When exposed asymptomatic persons are identified in conjunction with a food-borne outbreak of botulism, induced vomiting, gastric lavage, and purgatives are recommended to remove unabsorbed toxin. Watchful waiting rather than prophylactic antitoxin is generally recommended because of the risk of serum sickness or anaphylaxis associated with horse serum.

Infant Botulism. Infant botulism was first reported in 1976,[20] although in retrospect the first case (proved by laboratory tests) was encountered in California in 1931.[21] Arnon and co-workers[22] were the first to elucidate the epidemiology and have provided an excellent review.[23] As of January 1981, a total of 189 cases had been recognized worldwide, 181 of which were in the United States. Illness is almost entirely limited to infants less than 6 months of age. Of the several hundred items fed to California infants with botulism, only honey was found to contain *C. botulinum* spores. However, only one-third of cases are associated with the ingestion of raw honey; in the remainder, the source is unknown. Breast feeding may offer some protection against the acute fatal form of infant botulism, but does not preclude the more common subacute type of illness.[23] Typically, the infant is the only family member who is ill, and feces of family members contain neither *C. botulinum* nor its toxin.

Etiology. The responsible clostridia are the same as those described in adults. The distribution of toxin types associated with illness is likewise similar, with cases caused by type B toxin predominantly east of the Mississippi and cases caused by type A toxin predominantly west of it. Unlike botulism in older children and adults, however, infant botulism is caused by the ingestion of spores, not preformed toxin. Clostridium spores can multiply and produce toxin in the intestine of some infants. Studies in animal models suggest that the restricted age distribution reflects the lack of postnatally acquired gut flora that act as competitors of clostridial multiplication.[24]

Clinical Features. Illness may be abrupt in onset and lead to sudden death without a recognized prodrome. In these circumstances, the syndrome is indistinguishable historically and pathologically from typical infant crib death. The majority of recognized cases have a gradual onset, manifested initially as constipation followed by hypotonia and descending symmetrical flaccid paralysis. Early findings include less vigorous sucking, weak crying, and loss of neck and limb muscle strength. Examination discloses ptosis, ophthalmoplegia, reduced facial expression, dysphagia, pooled oral secretions, decreased gag reflex, and poor anal sphincter tone. Fever is not seen in the absence of suppurative complications. Weakness is maximum by 2 weeks, persists for another 2 to 3 weeks, and then very slowly resolves to complete recovery. Although relapses are sometimes seen, most infants recover without detectable sequelae.

Diagnosis. Rapid diagnostic support may be obtained by electromyography when the characteristic pattern known as Brief, Small, Abundant motor-unit action Potentials (BSAP) is seen; the absence of BSAP, however, does not exclude the diagnosis of infant botulism. Diagnosis is confirmed by identification of botulinal toxin and/or *C. botulinum* organisms in the stool. Both toxin and organisms may be present in fecal specimens up to 8 weeks after clinical recovery. Circulating toxin is rarely demonstrated.

Treatment. Because of the possibility of progressive paralysis or sudden apnea, hospitalization with access to an intensive care unit is indicated. Treatment is supportive, with particular attention to pulmonary hygiene and nutrition. Evaluation of head control is the most sensitive physical finding indicative of adequate neuromuscular function and signifies that oral feedings can be resumed.[25] No benefit from antitoxin therapy has been established in infant botulism. Most infants have recovered without antitoxin, the use of which entails a risk of severe anaphylaxis, even in the neonate. Antibiotics are not associated with a more rapid clearance of *C. botulinum* from stool or with a more favorable clinical course. Since infant botulism is a prolonged intestinal infection with continued release and absorption of toxin, high colonic saline enemas may enhance fecal excretion of toxin.

Prevention. Raw honey should not be fed to infants less than 12 months of age.

Staphylococcus

Staphylococcal food poisoning had been well described previously, but Dack and coworkers in the 1930s[26] were the first to draw attention to its importance, to distinguish staphylococcal enterotoxin from other staphylococcal toxins, and to reproduce the illness in human volunteers. Today, staphylococcal food poisoning is one of the most common reported causes of food-borne disease in the United States. It accounts for one-fifth to one-fourth of all confirmed cases and is probably greatly underreported.[27] Occasional outbreaks are attributed to unpasteurized milk or other dairy products from animals with infected udders. The great majority of cases, however, derive from foods contaminated by food handlers who are nasal or skin carriers, only 20% of whom have clinically obvious staphylococcal hand lesions.[28] Typically high-protein moist foods such as custards, creams, and meat (particularly ham and pork products) are contaminated during preparation. Contaminated unrefrigerated food allows bacterial multiplication and toxin production prior to ingestion.

Agents. Staphylococci are gram-positive aerobic cocci; most do not produce an enterotoxin. Staphylococcal food poisoning is usually due to enterotoxin-producing, penicillinase-positive *Staphylococcus aureus* of phage group III or IV. Some outbreaks have been associated with enterotoxin-producing *Staphylococcus epidermidis*.[29] Of the 5 or more antigenically distinct enterotoxins (exotoxins), types A and D are most often associated with food poisoning. Individual cultures of *S. aureus* may produce more than one type of toxin. Staphylococcal toxin is extremely potent, as little as 1 μg/100 g of food causing disease.[30] It is also resistant to temperature extremes, such as prolonged refrigeration or boiling for 30 minutes.

Disease is caused by ingestion of preformed toxin. The ingested enterotoxin is rapidly absorbed from the gut and appears to exert its emetic effect by stimulation of the central nervous system. Gastroscopic examination of patients with staphylococcal food poisoning shows gross abnormalities[30]; it is not clear whether these are the result of pernicious vomiting or causally related to the gastroenteritis.

Clinical Features. The usual incubation period is 2 hours, with a range of 30 minutes to 7 hours. The onset typically is abrupt, with nausea, abdominal cramps, vomiting, and prostration as predominant findings. Diarrhea is much less common and fever is absent. Shock and death occur rarely, usually in infants or debilitated adults. The duration of illness is ordinarily less than 24 hours.

Diagnosis. The clinical picture is very characteristic and often suffices for diagnosis, particularly in an outbreak. Because *S. aureus* is present in 2% to 30% of routine stool cultures, recovery of the organism from the stool is insufficient for diagnosis. Specific diagnosis requires the demonstration of large numbers of staphylococci ($>10^6$ organisms/g) in food or vomitus or the demonstration of enterotoxin. Failure to recover organisms from an incriminated food is not unusual when the food has been cooked or cured long enough to kill staphylococci after their toxin has been formed. When staphylococci are recovered, phage typing is helpful for epidemiologic investigation. Enterotoxin bioassay and seroassay studies are available only in specialized research laboratories. Because it is rarely possible to detect toxin in vomitus, feces, and serum, only suspect foods and cultural filtrates are assayed.

Treatment. No treatment is required for most patients. Very young or very old patients may require fluid and electrolyte replacement. Antibiotics are not indicated.

Prevention. Proper food handling would prevent this disease. Once toxin has formed, usual cooking will not destroy the heat-stable toxin.

Clostridium perfringens

Clostridium perfringens, formerly *C. welchii*, was first recognized as a common cause of food poisoning in 1953.[31] Precooked or reheated meat and meat products, such as gravies or stews, are most often incriminated.[32] During processing, foods of animal origin become contaminated with *C. perfringens* from animal intestinal contents. Inadequate cooking or holding temperatures allow the heat-resistant spores to multiply in large numbers. Human feeding studies show that 10^8 organisms are required to produce disease, so that illness only follows ingestion of heavily contaminated food.[33]

C. perfringens is a ubiquitous non-motile, spore-forming, anaerobic, gram-positive bacillus found in soil, raw meat, and the intestinal tract of many animals and man. Of the 5 major toxigenic types, only type A is frequently associated with food poisoning. Spores of *C. perfringens* type A can be either heat-resistant or heat-sensitive; most outbreaks are associated with the heat-resistant strains, which can survive boiling up to 6 hours. Both lecithinase-positive and lecithinase-negative strains have been associated with food poisoning outbreaks and shown to produce enterotoxins.[34] Symptoms are caused by a heat-labile enterotoxin (CPE), which is released by lysis of sporangia after ingestion of large numbers of vegetative type A *C. perfringens*.[35] Like most other enterotoxins, CPE appears to act by blocking fluid and electrolyte resorption from the gut.[36]

Clinical Features. The average incubation period is 8 hours, with a range of 5 to 24 hours. Major symptoms are abdominal cramps and watery diarrhea. Nausea is relatively common, vomiting is less often seen, and fever is absent. Stools do not contain mucus and rarely contain blood or leukocytes. Recovery within 24 hours is the rule. Death is very rare.

Diagnosis. Because *C. perfringens* is frequently found in food and human feces, isolation of the organism alone is insufficient for diagnosis. Quantitative cultures of stool or incriminated food showing at least 10^5 spores/g are compatible with *C. perfringens* food poisoning. Correct interpretation of quantitative cultures requires anaerobic culture of fresh or refrigerated material. The detection of enterotoxin from fecal samples obtained early in the illness has been shown to be diagnostic.[37] Because there are over 90 serotypes of *C. perfringens*, serotyping is useful to demonstrate that food and stool contain the same organism.[38] Inasmuch as patients may have other serotypes in their stool, at least 3 isolates should be serotyped for comparison with the food isolate.

Treatment. Most patients require no treatment. Very young or debilitated patients may require IV fluids. Antibiotics are not indicated.

Prevention. Disease control relies primarily on the prevention of multiplication of the organism in cooked food. Frozen beef or poultry should be thawed in the refrigerator, cooked to a core temperature of 75°C, and eaten or refrigerated immediately after cooking. Leftovers should be reheated to at least 60°C to destroy vegetative cells.

Pig-bel. Pig-bel, or enteritis necroticans, a rare type of food poisoning seen primarily in Papua, New Guinea, is caused by type C *C. perfringens*.[39] The organism is usually transmitted by contaminated pig meat. Typically, there is an acute onset of severe abdominal pain, vomiting, diarrhea, prostration, and shock. Case-fatality rates may be 50% or higher. At necropsy there is a diffuse necrotizing enteritis of the jejunum, ileum, and colon. Antitoxin appears to be of no benefit in treatment,[40] but a beta toxoid has been shown to prevent pig-bel in New Guinea.[41]

Bacillus cereus

The association of *Bacillus cereus* with food-borne disease was first recognized in Europe in the 1950s,[42] The first United States outbreak was reported in 1970.[43] Between 1971 and 1974, 18 outbreaks of *B. cereus* infection in England were associated with consumption of fried rice.[44] Recognized outbreaks have been attributed about equally to improperly handled cooked rice and to diverse other ingestants.[45] In one survey, 52% of 1500 food ingredients were positive for *B. cereus*.[46]

Organism. B. cereus is an aerobic, motile, spore-forming, gram-positive rod. Spores are ubiquitous in soil, vegetation, and many raw and processed foods. They survive boiling and steaming and germinate and multiply at ambient temperatures. Strains of *B. cereus* elaborate at least 2 enterotoxins. Emetic illness is associated with strains that cause vomiting in monkeys and produce no fluid secretion in the rabbit ileal loop system; isolates from outbreaks manifesting primarily diarrhea cause diarrhea in monkeys and produce a heat-labile toxin that stimulates the adenyl cyclase–cyclic AMP system.[47–49]

Clinical Features. There appear to be 2 distinct clinical syndromes related to the strain differences just noted. Fever does not occur with either form. The emetic form usually but not always is associated with ingestion of fried rice.[50] It is characterized by an incubation period of 1 to 6 hours, nausea, vomiting, abdominal cramps, and relatively little diarrhea and simulates staphylococcal food poisoning. The diarrheal form is attended by lower abdominal pain and tenesmus, usually has a longer incubation period (6 to 16 hours), and simulates clostridial food poisoning.

Diagnosis. Specific diagnosis rests on recovery of the organism from the stool or suspected food. Inasmuch as *B. cereus* can sometimes be found in the stools of well persons, isolation of this microorganism from the stool is not in itself sufficient to identify the cause of the outbreak. Its recovery would assume significance, however, if negative stools were obtained from an appropriate control group. Approximately 50% of food ingredients may contain *B. cereus*. Hence, only heavy contamination (10^5 or more organisms/g of food) is confirmatory. Because *B. cereus* grows better on non-selective than on enteric media, many laboratories will fail to identify the organism unless this possibility is specifically noted with the culture request.

Treatment. Recovery is usually complete in less than 48 hours and antibiotics are not recommended.

Prevention. Disease can be prevented by proper food handling. For example, *B. cereus* heat-resistant spores on rice survive boiling. If the rice is then left at room temperature, vegetative forms can multiply and produce toxin that will not be inactivated during stir frying or rewarming. Prompt refrigeration of boiled rice prevents this sequence of events.

Salmonella

Non-typhoidal salmonellosis is the leading cause of bacterial food poisoning in the United States and other Western cultures. Between 1972 and 1978, salmonellae accounted for more than one-third of reported food-borne outbreaks and nearly one-half of all reported cases of confirmed bacteria-caused food poisoning in the United States.[27] More recently, nearly one-third of salmonella outbreaks have been reported from hospitals and institutions.[51] Virtually all outbreaks are traced to a food of animal origin, such as contaminated milk, eggs, poultry, shellfish, or red meat. The largest reported outbreak occurred in 1974, when over 3000 persons who ate potato salad at a Navaho barbeque were affected.[52] Nationwide outbreaks have been attributed to commercial products.

Most salmonellosis reflects the wide distribution of non-typhoidal salmonellae in domestic animals used as food, particularly poultry and poultry products. Following the establishment of *Salmonella hadar* in the stock of a large turkey breeder in England, this serotype rose from relative obscurity to become the second most prevalent serotype isolated from patients in England and Wales during the period between 1971 and 1979.[53] Food-borne outbreaks caused by infected food handlers are uncommon, as are secondary cases in noninstitutional settings.

Most *Salmonella* food poisoning is caused by the species *S. enteritidis*. The infectious dose varies with the serotype and with host characteristics, such as reduced gastric acid. Salmonellae that are not destroyed by gastric acid penetrate and multiply in the lamina propria and epithelial cells of the lower intestine, where they stimulate a polymorphonuclear leukocyte exudate. Accordingly, leukocytes are seen on microscopic examination of the stool. Despite the lack of invasion of the upper gut mucosa, enterotoxin-mediated alterations in fluid and electrolyte transport probably occur in both the large and small intestine. Diarrhea is produced by one or more of several toxins identified in animal model systems.[54–56]

Clinical Features. The incubation period usually is 6 to 72 hours, but may be as long as 2 weeks. In a typical case, headache, nausea, and vomiting are followed by abdominal cramps and diarrhea. Stools may contain mucus or small amounts of blood and vary in number from 3 to more than 40/day. Most patients are febrile (38° to 40°C). Although diarrhea and fever may persist as long as 2 weeks, most patients recover within 5 days.

Diagnosis. Salmonellae are readily recovered from stool or food on most enteric media. Rarely, lactose-fermenting strains may be missed by cultural procedures in common use.[57] The chance of recovering salmonellae from stool is enhanced if a swab containing a generous amount of stool is incubated overnight in an enrichment broth, such as selenite F or tetrathionate, prior to plating on enteric media. At least 2 enteric media, such as eosin–methylene blue (EMB), Salmonella-Shigella (SS), MacConkey, Tergitol F, or xylose-lysine-deoxycholate (XLD), should be employed. In 50% of cases, the stool culture remains positive for at least 2 weeks after the onset of illness. Serotyping or phage typing is useful in the evaluation of outbreaks.

Treatment. Antibiotics do not alter the clinical course of *Salmonella* enterocolitis. Indeed, they may actually prolong the duration of fecal excretion of salmonellae.[58] However, when the patient is ill enough to be hospitalized or when there is septicemia or localized extraintestinal infection, treatment with ampicillin or trimethoprim/sulfamethoxazole is recommended.

Prevention. Since foods of animal origin are the most frequent source of human salmonellosis, most disease in man can be prevented by adequate refrigeration, thorough cooking of food, and avoidance of cross-contamination in the kitchen, e.g., not returning the cooked chicken to the same unwashed cutting board. Although most infected food handlers are the victims rather than the cause of outbreaks, handwashing after defecation and before food preparation is also recommended.

Shigella

From 1961 through 1978, 84 outbreaks of common source food-borne shigellosis were reported in the United States.[59] Infected food handlers have been responsible for most food-borne outbreaks; the vehicle is often a food item, such as a salad, that requires extensive handling in preparation.[60]

Shigellae are non-motile gram-negative bacteria for which man is the natural host and reservoir. The 4 species of *Shigella* comprise 39 recognized serotypes, any of which can cause disease. *Shigella sonnei* is the most common species in the United States, Western Europe, and Japan, and *S. flexneri* is most common in developing countries. *S. dysenteriae* and *S. boydii* are less common; the former is noteworthy for the greater severity of disease and for the propensity to induce bacteremia, otherwise uncommon in shigellosis. Some serotypes can be further subdivided by colicin and phage typing for epidemiologic investigation. Shigellae also produce an enterotoxin (exotoxin), the most potent of which is produced by *S. dysenteriae*. Other details and characteristics of *Shigella* are described in Chapter 118, where the role of these bacteria in nonparasitic diarrhea is considered.

Clinical Features. The incubation period is 1 to 7 days. Onset is typically abrupt with fever, cramping abdominal pain, and diarrhea without gross blood; red blood cells and leukocytes can be seen microscopically, however. The majority of infections are manifested only as this early phase, which lasts 1 to 3 days. In a proportion of patients, varying with age, inoculum, and infecting serotype, *Shigella* infection manifests itself at the very outset as classic bacillary dysentery or progresses to this condition. Such patients have an increasing number of scanty stools containing blood and mucus; tenesmus is common, but fever is often absent. Dysentery may persist for a week or longer and may be fatal if untreated. Patients demonstrating the entire clinical spectrum from mild watery diarrhea to severe dysentery may be seen during an outbreak. Convulsions complicate shigellosis in a significant proportion of children, often in the absence of high fever or evidence of pre-existing idiopathic epilepsy.

Diagnosis. Definitive diagnosis is based on the isolation of shigellae from freshly passed stool or from a rectal swab. In outbreaks, positive stool cultures are found in about two-thirds of cases. Usual enteric media are inhibitory for some strains; therefore, at least 2 different media, such as SS, EMB, MacConkey, or XLD agar, should be used concurrently. The sooner after passage the stool is processed and the more media used, the greater the likelihood of isolation of shigellae. Serotyping, colicin typing, phage typing, and fluorescent antibody techniques can be used to ascertain that isolates are epidemiologically related, although multiple colicin types have been observed in some outbreaks.

Treatment. Antimicrobials decrease the duration of illness and fecal excretion of shigellae in both mild and severe cases. Unfortunately, multiply resistant shigellae are common, and the choice of therapy, as well as the need for it in mild cases, must be determined based on local considerations of cost and antibiotic sensitivity patterns.[61] At present, trimethoprim/sulfamethoxazole appears to be the treatment of choice. Fluid and electrolyte replacement is required in some cases. Antidiarrheal drugs that inhibit gut motility should be avoided, since they occasionally increase the severity or duration of illness.[62]

Prevention. Careful handwashing prior to food handling should prevent food-borne shigellosis.

Escherichia coli

Food has been incriminated as a source of enterotoxic *Escherichia coli* (ETEC)–associated traveler's diarrhea in Mexico[63] and in common source outbreaks of ETEC-associated gastroenteritis in Japan.[64] The first convincing demonstration that food was the vehicle for transmission of ETEC diarrhea in the United States was reported in 1982; in this common source outbreak, 83% of over 500 cases were associated with ingestion of Mexican food in a restaurant.[65] Enteroinvasive *E. coli* are a less common cause of gastroenteritis. In the United States, a large outbreak was related to contaminated cheeses imported from France.[66] The usual source of food contamination with *E. coli* is an infected food handler with poor personal hygiene. A large dose, on the order of 10^8 *E. coli*, is required to cause illness.[67]

A detailed description of *E. coli* and its characteristics will be found in Chapter 118, where the contribution of this organism to nonparasitic diarrhea is discussed.

Clinical Features. After an incubation period of 1 to 3 days, most patients experience diarrhea and abdominal cramps. Nausea, vomiting, and fever are less common. Recovery is usually complete within 3 days, although it takes a week or longer for some patients to feel completely well.

Diagnosis. A specific diagnosis of *E. coli* gastroenteritis presently requires an enormous amount of time and effort. It is, therefore, rarely attempted in the absence of an outbreak. In an outbreak, a presumptive diagnosis of *E. coli* gastroenteritis is made when a known pathogenic serotype is isolated from the stools of most patients and is absent in the stools of controls. Many outbreak-associated isolates—and enterotoxin-producing food isolates—are nonserotypeable strains or strains not previously recognized as pathogenic.[68,69] Therefore, laboratory tests for invasive or toxigenic properties are usually required. The diagnosis of ETEC is based on finding toxin-producing *E. coli* in the stool or demonstrating a 4-fold rise in serum antitoxic antibodies; invasive *E. coli* can also be demonstrated by specific tests (Chapter 118). The responsible food handler is usually culture-negative by the time the epidemiologic investigation is carried out, because fecal carriage is usually transient.

Treatment. Oral or occasionally IV rehydration is required in some cases. No studies document antimicrobial benefit even though neomycin, colistin (Coly-Mycin), and gentamicin shorten the duration of fecal carriage of enteropathogenic *E. coli.*

Prevention. Good personal hygiene by food handlers should prevent *E. coli* food poisoning.

Cholera

Food-borne outbreaks of cholera have been reported associated with raw or partially cooked seafood, such as shrimp (Philippines, 1962), mussels (Naples, 1973), fish (Guam, 1974), cockles (Portugal, 1974),[70] and marine bivalves (Sardinia, 1973 and 1979).[71] In the United States, a 1978 outbreak was associated with the ingestion of cooked crabs.[72] Both of the recognized biotypes, classic *Vibrio cholerae* and the El Tor variant, can cause food poisoning; the latter hardier biotype has been the cause of most recent outbreaks. Persons who develop clinical cholera in endemic areas or during outbreaks frequently have hypochlorhydria or achlorhydria. Emphasizing the importance of this are studies in volunteers in whom neutralization of gastric acid reduced the infectious dose to less than 10^6 organisms.[73]

Organism. *V. cholerae* is an actively motile, gram-negative, curved bacterium with a single polar flagellum. Man is the only natural host. Both of the major serotypes of *V. cholerae,* Inaba and Ogawa, whether of classic or El Tor biotype, produce an immunologically identical thermolabile exotoxin. This toxin stimulates adenyl cyclase activity of intestinal epithelial cells, causing increased levels of adenosine monophosphatase and hypersecretion of fluids and electrolytes.[74] There is little inflammatory response and few leukocytes on stool examination. *V. cholerae* adheres to but does not invade the intestinal mucosa, which remains intact.

Clinical Features. The incubation period ranges from several hours to 3 days. The clinical picture varies from mild, simple diarrhea to profuse watery diarrhea of abrupt onset. In the latter case, stools are gray, have a slightly "fishy" odor, and contain mucus, which imparts the characteristic "rice-water" appearance. Vomiting often follows the onset of diarrhea. Massive diarrhea and vomiting may cause a 10% to 15% fluid loss, resulting in profound dehydration and shock. In such cases, pulse and blood pressure may be unmeasurable, the skin assumes a marked wrinkled appearance, and body temperature is normal or subnormal. Muscle cramps and oliguria are common. Even in extremis most patients remain lucid and complain of severe thirst. In severe untreated cases, the case-fatality rate may exceed 50%.

Diagnosis. Severe cholera is a clinical diagnosis; laboratory confirmation is important mainly for epidemiologic and control purposes. *V. cholerae* grows readily in a variety of routine laboratory media but is inhibited by most selective media used in enteric bacteriology. Therefore, the laboratory must be advised that cholera is suspected in order to recover the organism. Thiosulfate–citrate–bile salt (TCBS) agar is the preferred medium. Phage typing is useful in the workup of an outbreak.

Treatment. Treatment should be initiated immediately and not await the 1- to 2-day period required to recover the organism. Large volumes of IV fluids and electrolytes are required for patients in shock; milder cases can be treated with an oral electrolyte solution containing glucose. Antibiotics, such as tetracycline, shorten the course of diarrhea and thereby reduce fluid replacement needs.[75] With appropriate therapy, mortality should be less than 1% and complete recovery the rule.

Prevention. Good personal hygiene by food handlers and adequate cooking of potentially contaminated food can prevent this disease. Killed vibrio vaccines are relatively ineffective but toxins, toxoids, and somatic antigens show promise as immunizing agents.

Non-O Group 1 *Vibrio cholerae*. *V. cholerae* strains that do not agglutinate in *V. cholerae* O-1 antiserum (formerly called *noncholera vibrios*) have been associated with food-borne gastroenteritis. Five cases associated with the eating of raw oysters were reported in 1979 in the United States.[76] Some non–O-1 *V. cholerae* strains produce a toxin similar to cholera toxin. Illness is similar to cholera except that some affected persons have dysentery, the mechanism of which is unknown.

Vibrio parahaemolyticus

Vibrio parahaemolyticus was first recognized as a cause of human gastroenteritis in 1950 in Japan, where it now accounts for more than 50% of bacterial food poisoning in the summer months. First confirmed as a cause of food poisoning in the United States when a large outbreak followed the consumption of steamed crabs in 1971,[77] 13 outbreaks had been reported by the end of 1972.[78] *V. parahaemolyticus* has been isolated from a variety of marine fish and shellfish and from coastal and estuarine waters of the world during the warm summer months; outbreaks are similarly seasonal. In Japan, most outbreaks are attributed to raw fish; in the United States, cooked shellfish is the most common vehicle. Inadequate cooking or refrigeration, contamination of cooked seafood with uncooked seafood, or use of sea water in food preparation has been incriminated.[79] Contamination of food by infected food handlers and person-to-person spread have not been demonstrated.

Organism. *V. parahaemolyticus* is a halophilic, motile, facultatively anaerobic, gram-negative rod. Strains are separated into 2 groups (Kanagawa-positive and Kanagawa-negative) based on their ability to lyse human red blood cells. Both Kanagawa-negative and Kanagawa-positive strains produce enterotoxin, but only Kanagawa-positive strains are recovered from ill persons and cause diarrhea in human volunteers with an infectious dose of 2×10^5 organisms. Pathogenic mechanisms have been studied in a number of animal models with conflicting results.[80] Most investigators have failed to demonstrate an enterotoxin in the rabbit ileal loop system; Yet cell-free filtrates produce diarrhea in kittens and monkeys. *V. parahaemolyticus* also has invasive properties, but dysentery occurs in the minority of human cases.

Clinical Features. The incubation period is usually 12 to 15 hours but may be as short as 3 or as long as 96 hours. By far the most common clinical syndrome is an abrupt onset of abdominal pain and explosive watery diarrhea, with or without fever and vomiting, simulating salmonellosis. Less commonly there is a dysenteric illness; the stools contain gross blood and mucus and proctosigmoidoscopy reveals discrete ulcers. This syndrome simulates shigellosis or amebic dysentery. Recovery is usually complete in 2 to 5 days, although some deaths have been reported.

Diagnosis. Recovery of this organism from the stool requires deviation from the usual enteric bacteriology protocols. *V. parahaemolyticus* does not grow well on SS or EMB agar; it grows best on TCBS agar, which has a high salt concentration and an alkaline pH. Recovery of organisms from seafood, but not feces, is enhanced by prior enrichment in a salt-containing broth.[80] During an outbreak, there is little similarity between strains isolated from patients and food; strains from patients are nearly always Kanagawa-positive, but strains recovered from food are usually Kanagawa-negative. Further, there are often multiple serotypes isolated from patients and from food.

Treatment. Antibiotic therapy is not of proven value. However, antibiotics do reduce the duration of fecal excretion of organisms. Most strains are sensitive to tetracycline and resistant to ampicillin.

Prevention. *V. parahaemolyticus* can survive freezing and heating to 80°C for 15 minutes. Raw seafood should be avoided, and cooked or processed seafood must not be left unrefrigerated. Cross-contamination between raw and cooked marine food should be avoided.

Campylobacter

Campylobacter gastroenteritis, first reported in 1957,[81] was not recognized as one of the most common enteric infections of man until the 1970s. The development at that time of selective culture techniques permitted the organism (previously called *Vibrio fetus*) to be isolated from stools. Many animal species are infected, but most human infections are sporadic and unrelated to animal exposure. Foods implicated in *Campylobacter* outbreaks include raw milk, raw meat (including raw liver used as alternative cancer therapy), and processed poultry products.[82,83] In one survey, *Campylobacter jejuni* was isolated from the rectums of over 80% of broiler poultry in a city market.[84] The infectious dose is unknown, but may be relatively small; one volunteer became ill after ingesting 500 organisms.

Organism. *Campylobacter* organisms are small, motile, curved, gram-negative bacilli that are microaerophilic. Two species of *Campylobacter* (*C. jejuni* and *C. fetus* ss. *fetus* [formerly *intestinalis*]) cause disease in man. The former is usually manifested by diarrhea in previously healthy individuals; the latter as septicemia in immunocompromised or debilitated hosts. Although it was previously thought that bacteremia was uncommon with *C. jejuni* infections, an outbreak associated with eating processed turkey showed that *C. jejuni* bacteremia may also be a sequel to food-borne infection due to this organism.[83] The disease appears to be due to invasion of the intestinal epithelium, as evidenced by the frequent presence of leukocytes and blood in the stool and the findings in a limited number of proctosigmoidoscopic examinations.

Clinical Features. The incubation period is not well established but is probably between 2 and 11 days. The clinical picture usually includes diarrhea, abdominal pain, and fever. Headache, myalgia, and vomiting may precede diarrhea by 24 hours or more. Frank dysentery, simulating shigellosis or inflammatory bowel disease, is seen in approximately half the cases; much higher or lower frequencies of dysentery have been reported in some series. The striking abdominal pain in some cases suggests appendicitis. The duration of illness is usually less than 1 week, but relapses occur in up to 25% of cases.

Diagnosis. Direct examination of stool by phase contrast microscopy often reveals the characteristic "seagull" appearance of the organisms. Definitive diagnosis by stool culture is made only when the laboratory is specifically advised to look for this agent. A selective medium composed of a blood agar to which antibiotics have been added (usually vancomycin, polymyxin B, and trimethoprim), a temperature of 43°C, and reduced (5% to 8%) oxygen are usually required. The combined yield of 2 commercial media (campy-BAP and campy-Thio) is superior to either medium used alone.[82] Serologic tests are also available and are positive in a high proportion of cases. In some cases, organisms can be recovered from the stool as long as 3 weeks after illness.

Treatment. Most infections are self-limited. Erythromycin rapidly eradicates fecal carriage and is recommended for patients with prolonged or severe illness.[83] *Campylobacter* is generally not susceptible to such commonly used drugs as ampicillin or trimethoprim/sulfamethoxazole.

Prevention. Knowledge of the epidemiology of *Campylobacter* food poisoning is in its infancy. Thorough cooking of poultry and meat and avoidance of unpasteurized milk are recommended. *Campylobacter* can survive freezing for at least 3 weeks, so frozen products are not necessarily safe.

Yersinia

Although *Yersinia enterocolitica* infection of animals is relatively common, its importance in man has come to be appreciated only in recent years owing to the development of better techniques for culture of the organism from fecal specimens.[85] The largest reported outbreak in the United States occurred in New York State in 1976, when ingestion of contaminated chocolate milk resulted in the hospitalization of 36 children, 16 of whom had appendectomies for symptoms.[86]

Y. enterocolitica is a gram-negative coccobacillary organism that produces a heat-stable enterotoxin and is also invasive in some models.[85,87,88] However, enterotoxin production in vivo occurs only at temperatures lower than those found in the human intestinal tract so that its role in the pathogenesis of diarrhea is uncertain. Fecal leukocytes and red blood cells compatible with invasive colitis are seen in some cases. The infectious dose is unknown. Person-to-person transmission has been documented.

Clinical Features. The usual incubation period is 5 to 7 days, following which acute abdominal pain and fever occur. A mild form with fever, watery diarrhea, vomiting, and abdominal pain usually affects children less than 5 years of age and subsides spontaneously in 1 to 2 days. In older children and adults, a longer illness often begins with fever, abdominal cramps and vomiting; diarrhea may also be present but in only about half the cases. Mesenteric adenitis or ileitis is relatively frequent, leading in some cases to appendectomy. A myriad of other features may also be seen from time to time, including rash, erythema nodosum, and arthritis resembling Reiter's syndrome or acute rheumatic fever.

Diagnosis. Diagnosis can be made by stool culture in only half the cases. The stool sample should be collected as early in the illness as possible. It is important that the stool specimens be cultured on enteric media after refrigeration at 4°C for at least 2 weeks (cold enrichment) or incubated at 25°C. Serologic agglutinin tests are positive in at least 80% of cases; either a single elevated titer (≥1:128) or a 4-fold rise is considered diagnostic. Serotyping and biotyping of isolates are important to exclude non-pathogenic *Yersinia* and to document the same *Yersinia* type in ill persons and suspect foods.

Treatment. Antimicrobial therapy does not appear to alter the course of the gastroenteritis. Nevertheless, antibiotics are used in patients with a more severe clinical syndrome.[89] The drug of choice has not been established; most isolates are resistant to ampicillin but sensitive to a wide variety of other antibiotics.

Prevention. Other than proper food handling, no specific preventive modalities are known. Refrigeration of contaminated food does not prevent bacterial multiplication, since this organism grows well at refrigerator temperatures.

Miscellaneous Bacteria

Assorted other bacteria have been implicated in food poisoning outbreaks, including group A streptococci, enterococci, *Klebsiella* spp., and *Pseudomonas* spp. Of these, group A β-hemolytic streptococci are the most important. Typically, a nasopharyngeal carrier contaminates a high-protein moist food, which is then inadequately refrigerated before serving. An outbreak of streptococcal sore throat follows in 1 to 3 days.

Non-bacterial Food Poisoning

Non-bacterial food poisoning is much less common than bacterial food poisoning, but includes serious diseases with high case-fatality rates. Most non-bacterial food poisonings are characterized by a short incubation period and an afebrile extra-gastrointestinal illness, with or without associated gastroenteritis. Mushroom and marine toxins are by far the most important causes of nonbacterial food poisoning in terms of both numbers of cases and severity of illness. Excellent reference sources are available.[90,91] Regional poison control centers provide regularly updated information on the diagnosis and management of non-bacterial poisonings. An example is the Rocky Mountain Poison Center *Poisindex.*[92]

Mushrooms

Mushroom poisoning usually results from eating poisonous species of mushrooms that are mistaken for harmless types. About 100 of the more than 2000 species of mushrooms are poisonous to humans. Persons harvesting wild mushrooms may collect more than one poisonous species, and the resulting natural history of response to the different toxins present may be complicated by the different latency periods and symptoms associated with each.

Mushrooms of the genera *Amanita* and *Galerina* account for the largest number of deaths in the United States and Western Europe, but the frequency of poisoning due to *Russula* may be increasing, especially in refugees to the United States from Southeast Asia.[93] It has been estimated that 90% of deaths from mushroom poisoning in the United States and Western Europe are due to consumption of *Amanita phalloides* ("death-cap") mushrooms. Fatal poisoning due to mushrooms of the genus *Gyromitra,* especially *Gyromitra esculenta,* is common in Eastern Europe but rare in the United States and Western Europe.[92] Oral ingestion of mushrooms of the genus *Gyromitra* and related types is not essential for poisoning to occur, since inhalation of vapors produced while cooking has induced toxicity.

Most of the toxins of the common poisonous mushrooms are thermostable, and many can persist after desiccation and storage for several years. The mechanism of action of the mushroom toxins, still incompletely understood, has been the subject of several reviews.[94–96] At least 8 amatoxins and 7 phallotoxins have been isolated from *Amanita* spp. The amatoxins are cytotoxic, interfering with the transcription of DNA and RNA, and most of the symptoms and pathologic changes that they produce reflect cellular necrosis. The phallotoxins probably are not absorbed from the gut and contribute little to the symptoms of mushroom poisoning. Some *Amanita* spp. produce isoxazoles that act on the central nervous system to compete with the gamma-aminobutyric acid (GABA) transmitter and cause psychotropic symptoms. False morels, mushrooms of the genus *Gyromitra,* produce a toxin (gyromitrin) that acts as a pyridoxine antagonist and causes hemolysis and gastrointestinal irritation. *Amanita muscaria* and other mushrooms contain L-(+)-muscarine and other thermostable cholinergic compounds that produce a peripheral cholinergic effect.

Clinical Features. Two types of mushroom poisoning have been identified: one with an incubation period of usually less than 4 hours and manifested primarily by confusion, delirium, and visual disturbances or by symptoms suggestive of cholinergic poisoning; the other has a usual incubation period of 10 to 14 hours and is expressed as gastroenteritis. The first type is usually caused by *Russula* and related genera; the second is most often caused by *Amanita* (amatoxin), *Gyromitra* (gyromitrin), and related genera. Late manifestations of amatoxin poisoning are hepatic and/or renal failure and cardiomyopathy. Late manifestations of gyromitrin poisoning include jaundice and seizures. Case-fatality rates vary widely, with average rates as high as 50% for *Amanita, Galerina,* and related mushrooms and as low as 1% for *Russula.*[92]

Diagnosis. Clinical diagnosis is usually based on a history of consumption of wild mushrooms. The diagnosis should particularly be suspected in refugees and other foreigners, for whom the services of a translator may be necessary. The presentation of harmless species by the patient, relatives, or friends may be misleading, since the patient may have eaten other species that are poisonous. Whenever possible, mushrooms should be identified by a mycologist. Mushroom specimens, gastric contents, and stool can be assayed for toxins by thin-layer chromatography and radioimmunoassay.[97]

Treatment. Aggressive treatment of mushroom poisoning should be initiated promptly, even if the species involved cannot be immediately identified. Poisoning by any species of mushrooms should be treated with induction of vomiting if the patient is conscious and has an intact gag reflex or with endotracheal intubation and immediate gastric lavage with a large-bore tube if the patient is unconscious. Emesis or gastric lavage should be performed regardless of when the patient is first seen, although in cases of poisoning due to *Amanita, Galerina,* and related genera little benefit appears to result if the removal of gastric contents is initiated 6 or more hours after ingestion or after vomiting and diarrhea have spontaneously occurred. All patients with mushroom poisoning should be given a slurry of activated charcoal by mouth (adults: 60 to 100 g; children: 30 to 60 g). Cyclic enterohepatic circulation of toxins may be blocked by repeated administration of the charcoal slurry every 4 hours for 2 days. Catharsis with magnesium sulfate (adults: 30 g; children: 250 mg/kg) is also recommended.

Poisoning by mushroom toxins may result in a need for intensive supportive treatment, including mechanical respiratory assistance, correction of fluid and electrolyte imbalances, and possible administration of specific antidotes. All patients should be carefully monitored with appropriate laboratory tests for changes in hepatic and renal function. These often require major supportive measures, such as hemodialysis. Activated charcoal hemoperfusion may remove mushroom toxins and has been recommended.[98]

Several specific therapies have been recommended for particular types of mushroom poisoning: thioctic acid for *Amanita* and *Galerina* mushroom poisoning, pyridoxine hydrochloride for *Gyromitra* poisoning, methylene blue for methemoglobinemia, and atropine for cholinergic symptoms. Only the last 2 treatment modalities, however, have demonstrated benefit. Massive doses of corticosteroids have also been recommended but proof of their efficacy is wanting.

Prevention. Mushroom poisoning can be prevented only by avoiding consumption of all wild mushrooms. Poisonous species of mushrooms cannot be reliably identified using existing taxonomic keys, and there is no test available to the consumer that can accurately identify toxic species.

Ciguatera Fish

Ciguatera fish poisoning is the most commonly reported illness associated with eating finned fish in the United States.[99] It is common in southern Florida, Hawaii, the South Pacific Islands, and the Caribbean.[100,101] Ciguatera poisoning accounts for about 7% of all reported food-borne disease outbreaks of known cause.[27] About 50 cases/year are reported to the Centers for Disease Control (90% from Hawaii and Florida). It may occur after consumption of moray eels, barracuda, grouper, snapper, and bottom-dwelling fish ecologically associated with coral reefs in tropical and temperate climates and is most common in late spring and early summer.

The cause of the illness is a toxin or mixture of toxic agents produced by the dinoflagellate *Gambierdiscus toxicus* that accumulates in finned fish through the marine food chain.[102] The mechanism of action of ciguatera toxin in man is unknown.

Clinical Features. The usual incubation period is 1 to 6 hours, but may be shorter or longer. Gastrointestinal symptoms usually appear first and neurologic symptoms later. About 9 of 10 patients develop *diarrhea*; 7 of 10 experience *vomiting*; 4 of 10 complain of *abdominal pain*; and 6 of 10 have *paresthesias* (including circumoral paresthesias), weakness, and arthralgias, especially marked in the knees and ankles. Acutely ill patients may experience *bradycardia* and *hypotension*, and many patients have generalized *myalgias* and *pruritus*. The most characteristic finding is *circumoral paresthesias*, although the frequency reported in various series ranges from 36% to 89%. The median duration of the acute illness is 4 hours. The case-fatality rate is less than 1/1000, but neurologic symptoms may persist for months or years.[109]

Diagnosis. The diagnosis of ciguatera fish poisoning is based on the characteristic clinical picture combined with a recent history of consumption of the appropriate species of fish or eels. Specimens of suspect seafood can be sent to reference laboratories, where bioassay procedures or enzyme-linked immunosorbent (ELISA) techniques can be used to identify toxicity.[91,103,104]

Treatment. Treatment is supportive. If hypotension develops (usually following the occurrence of bradycardia), fluids and atropine have been recommended. *Pralidoxime*, a cholinesterase reactivator, has been widely used without notable success, as have calcium gluconate, corticosteroids, vitamin B complex, and ascorbic acid. The pharmacologic basis for use of pralidoxime is unclear, since ciguatera toxin does not appear to be a direct cholinesterase inhibitor.

Prevention. The toxins that cause ciguatera poisoning are heat-stable, so that even prolonged cooking does not provide protection against poisoning. Control of ciguatera poisoning may require monitoring of blooms of *Gambierdiscus toxicus* and other toxic microorganisms or bioassay surveillance of potentially ciguatoxic fish, especially bottom-dwelling shore fish caught in the vicinity of reefs in a belt extending from 35°N to 35°S latitude. An effective centralized system for timely reporting of fish poisoning is also of value in preventing subsequent cases. An energetic health education effort should be an integral part of such a system.

Scombroid Fish

Scombroid fish poisoning results from eating fish, mostly from the suborder Scombroidea, that have been handled with inadequate refrigeration.[105] The suborder Scombroidea includes tuna, mackerel, and bonito. Mahimahi (*Coryphaena hippurus*) have also caused this disease. Sashimi (raw tuna) was implicated in an outbreak of the disease in 15 persons who ate at Japanese restaurants in San Francisco, California.[106] Disease is caused by scombrotoxin, a mixture of histamine and related substances, produced when *Proteus morganii, Klebsiella pneumoniae,* and other bacteria (most of which are endogenous) decarboxylate the free histidine normally present in scombroid fish, converting it to histamine. Isoniazid is a potent inhibitor of diamine oxidase, an enzyme that is active in the metabolism of histamine. Scombroid fish poisoning has been observed in patients taking isoniazid who ate poorly refrigerated tuna, but not in others who ate the same fish but were not receiving isoniazid.[107] Fresh tuna contains 1 mg/100g scombrotoxin; decomposed tuna contains 1000 mg/100 g. Scombrotoxin is heat-stable and not destroyed by the regular procedures used in cooking and canning tuna.[108]

Clinical Features. Symptoms usually begin within 15 to 45 minutes after ingestion and include many features characteristic of a histamine reaction: prominent flushing, headache, vertigo, abdominal cramps, and, in some cases, nausea, vomiting, diarrhea, and a generalized burning sensation.[108] The median duration of illness is 4 hours, and the case-fatality rate is virtually zero. Persons sharing a single meal of scombroid fish may have a range of symptoms varying from none to severe discomfort, since scombrotoxins are unevenly distributed in fish flesh, and sections only a few centimeters apart may have widely different concentrations.

Diagnosis. The diagnosis is based on the characteristic signs and symptoms occurring less than 1 hour after consumption of tuna, mahimahi, mackerel, bonito, skipjack, or other scombroid fish. It can often be determined that the fish was poorly refrigerated or had a "peppery" taste. Laboratory determination of the histamine content of samples of the suspect fish may help to establish the diagnosis, but control samples should also be tested from scombroid fish known to be nontoxic. Raw samples of fish can additionally be cultured for *Proteus morganii, Salmonella, Clostridium, Shigella, E. coli,* and *Enterobacter,* all of which can convert histidine to histamine.

Treatment. Symptoms are usually relieved promptly by parenteral antihistamine therapy. Bronchospasm may be relieved by sympathomimetics.

Prevention. Inasmuch as the toxin that produces scombroid fish poisoning is heat-stable, cooking will not provide protection against the disease. Scombroid fish must be eaten soon after they are caught or must be frozen or canned immediately. Fish left in the sun for more than 2 hours should not be eaten.

Paralytic Shellfish

Paralytic shellfish poisoning results from eating mussels, clams, oysters, or other bivalve molluscs—raw, cooked, or canned—which have ingested marine dinoflagellates of the genus *Gonyaulax.*[109] Crab and shrimp do not concentrate toxins from *Gonyaulax.* Dinoflagellates multiply during the warm season and impart a red to brown discoloration ("red tide") to the water in which they grow.[110] Red tides occur throughout the world, and human outbreaks of poisoning have been described from Nova Scotia to Malaysia. In the Northern Hemisphere, many jurisdictions prohibit the collection of shellfish during the period from May 1 to October 31 and closely monitor commercial shellfish for toxin during this period. The Washington clam (*Saxidomus nuttalli*) can retain toxin year-round and may produce paralytic shellfish poisoning in some areas at any time of the year.

The *Gonyaulax* toxin, saxitoxin, is not denatured by extended cooking in neutral or acid solutions or by commercial canning. Saxitoxin inhibits neuromuscular conduction by a reversible blockade of sodium channels in nerve and skeletal muscle. At high doses, inhibition can also occur in cardiac and smooth muscles.

Clinical Features. Paralytic shellfish poisoning has a median incubation period of 30 minutes. Early symptoms include paresthesias or numbness of the lips, mouth, tongue, or face, followed by paresthesias of the extremities. Dysphagia, a choking sensation and difficulty in speaking, as well as dizziness and severe frontal headache, may occur. Gastrointestinal symptoms are uncommon. Respiratory failure and death may occur within the first 12 hours. The reported case-fatality rate ranges from 0% to 9%.[103]

Diagnosis. The diagnosis is based on the characteristic clinical picture occurring during or immediately following consumption of fresh or canned bivalve shellfish or broth. Toxin levels can be determined in fresh shellfish by mouse bioassay or spectrofluorometry.

Other diseases due to consumption of shellfish can be differentiated by symptoms and latency periods. *Erythematous shellfish reactions* (rash, headache, occasional death) occur in allergic individuals after a latency period of several hours. *Gastrointestinal shellfish poisoning,* with nausea, vomiting, and diarrhea, but no paresthesias or neurologic symptoms, develops 10 to 12 hours after ingestion of shellfish contaminated with any of a variety of bacterial pathogens.

Treatment. If the patient is conscious and has an intact gag reflex, *vomiting should be induced.* If the patient is unconscious or has an absent or equivocal gag reflex, *endotracheal intubation* and *gastric lavage* (large-bore tube) should be performed. An oral slurry of *activated charcoal* (adults: 60 to 100 g; children: 30 to 60 g) should be given, and a *magnesium sulfate cathartic* (adults: 30 g; children: 250 mg/kg) should be administered. Dehydration should be prevented with IV normal saline. Respiratory failure is a major hazard in paralytic shellfish poisoning, and the patient must therefore be closely monitored. If adequate tidal volume or oxygenation cannot be maintained, *mechanical assistance to respiration* and creation of an artificial airway may be necessary. Hypotension may require administration of fluids and, if unsuccessful, vasopressors. *Activated charcoal hemoperfusion* to assist in removal of the toxin should be performed if improvement has not occurred with standard care.

Prevention. Toxic shellfish cannot be identified by any testing method readily available to the potential consumer. The toxins that cause paralytic shellfish poisoning are heat-stable, so even extended cooking will not prevent the disease. Consumption of bivalve molluscs should be avoided during the warm months, especially those collected in the zone from 30°N to 30°S latitude. Certain molluscs, such as the Washington clam, must be avoided at all times.

Neurotoxic Shellfish

This form of bivalve shellfish poisoning is milder than paralytic shellfish poisoning. It results from eating shellfish contaminated with a heat-stable toxin from the red tide dinoflagellate *Gymnodinium breve*, a microorganism found off the Gulf and Atlantic coasts of Florida, Spain, France, Morocco, England, the Cape West Coast of South Africa and other coastal areas. However, human disease is rare[111]; only 5 cases were reported in the United States between 1972 and 1978.[27] Two heat-stable neurotoxins have been isolated from *Gy. breve*, at least one of which acts by stimulation of postganglionic nerve fibers.

Clinical Features. Symptoms begin within 3 hours of consumption of bivalve shellfish and include paresthesias, nausea, vomiting, diarrhea, and reversal of temperature sensation. Ataxia may follow, but paralysis has not been reported.[103] The illness is self-limited and the case-fatality rate is virtually zero.

Diagnosis. The diagnosis of neurotoxic shellfish poisoning is based on the clinical picture and a history of recent consumption of bivalve shellfish during the warm months. If the suspect shellfish is available, laboratory tests can differentiate the toxin of *Gy. breve* from that of *Gonyaulax* microorganisms.

Treatment. An oral slurry of *activated charcoal* (adults: 60 to 100 g; children: 30 to 60 g) and a cathartic should be administered. No other treatment is necessary for this self-limited disease.

Prevention. Extended cooking provides no protection against neurotoxic shellfish poisoning. The only effective protection is avoidance of bivalve shellfish during the warm months.

Puffer Fish

This neurotoxic poisoning is caused by eating any of 50 species of puffer fish (family Tetrodontidae) found in the Atlantic, Pacific, and Indian Oceans.[91,112] About 50 cases and 30 deaths occur each year in Japan where "fugu," a species of puffer fish, is considered a delicacy. The viscera and other parts of these fish contain tetrodotoxin, the most potent nonprotein toxin found in nature. Tetrodotoxin is a neurotoxin that produces effects similar to those of saxitoxin and in large doses causes defects in cardiac conduction and contractility.

Clinical Features. Neurologic and gastrointestinal symptoms usually begin within 10 to 40 minutes following ingestion of the fish but may be delayed for 3 or more hours. Symptoms include paresthesias, especially of the lips and tongue, dizziness, ataxia, excessive salivation, nausea, vomiting, diarrhea, epigastric pain, twitching, dysphagia, aphonia, convulsions, and paralysis, most prominent in the respiratory muscles. The pupils constrict at an early stage of the illness, but become dilated later and the light reflex disappears. Cyanosis, hypotension, convulsions, and cardiac arrhythmias follow. Most victims remain conscious until shortly before death, which usually occurs within the first 6 hours. Death occurs in 60% of cases, usually as a result of respiratory paralysis.[91] The prognosis improves dramatically if the patient survives the first 6 hours.

Diagnosis. The diagnosis of puffer fish poisoning is based on the characteristic clinical picture and a history of recent consumption of fish or fish stock from the family Tetrodontidae. Tetrodotoxin can be detected in the fish by reference laboratories.

Treatment. *Gastric emptying* by induced vomiting or gastric lavage with a cuffed endotracheal tube should be initiated as soon as poisoning by Tetrodontidae is suspected. Tetrodotoxins slow the rate of gastric emptying, so removal of toxic gastric contents may be possible for several hours after ingestion. If there is difficulty swallowing, oral fluids must be withheld to reduce the possibility of aspiration. In any event, IV fluids may be necessary to prevent or treat hypotension caused by toxin-induced vasodilation. If hypotension is present, use of a plasma expander has been recommended (at least until urinary output exceeds 40 ml/hr), but if the central venous pressures rises with restoration of urinary output, inotropic agents may be needed. *Endotracheal intubation* should be performed if the patient experiences difficulty with saliva or respiratory secretions. Patients with respiratory paralysis require assistive respiratory devices. The electrocardiogram should be continuously monitored, since arrhythmia and bradycardia are common; complete atrioventricular dissociation may require insertion of a temporary pacemaker. Anticholinesterases may be helpful in restoring muscle function.[112]

Prevention. Tetrodotoxin is not destroyed by cooking, and the only effective prevention is avoidance of puffer fish as food. Tetrodontidae are served legally only in specially licensed restaurants in Japan.

Mycotoxins

Various microfungi have been associated with food poisoning. Entire textbooks have been devoted to mycotoxins,[113,114] although human illness due to these agents is relatively rare today. A classic example is ergot poisoning. The only other form of mycotoxicosis recognized to have seriously affected entire populations, i.e., alimentary toxic aleukia due to T-2 toxin from *Fusarium* spp., is also primarily of historical interest. A large number of fatal cases occurred in the Soviet Union during World War II after consumption of bread made from moldy overwintered grain.[115]

Aflatoxins from *Aspergillus flavus* have attracted considerable interest because of their possible role in the induction of primary liver cancer. Much larger doses of aflatoxin (2 to 6 mg/day over several weeks) have been associated with an acute hepatitis characterized by jaundice, ascites, and portal hypertension.[116] Aflatoxin-reated disease can be prevented by eliminating food storage conditions that favor growth of *A. flavus* and discarding seriously contaminated supplies of nuts, grains, or dried fruits.

Plant Alkaloids

Plants containing toxic or pharmacologically active alkaloids grow throughout the world.[117] Some varieties, such as the foxglove (*Digitalis purpurea*), are dried and purified for orthodox clinical uses. Acute or chronic poisoning can result from ingestion of plant alkaloids used as teas, spices, folk remedies, or accidentally contaminated grain products.

The most important of the toxic plant alkaloids are the pyrrolizidine alkaloids.[118] More than 350 species of plants in 10 botanical families contain these alkaloids, including *Heliotropium,* which grows widely throughout the southwestern United States and Mexico, and *Senecio* species, common in the Caribbean. Illness commonly starts with fever, vomiting, and abdominal pain followed by jaundice and acute ascites. Liver cell necrosis may progress to chronic or fatal veno-occlusive disease (Chapter 169) or may resolve completely.

Lathyrus

Lathyrus poisoning results from eating the *Lathyrus sativus* species of sweet pea, consumed in Africa and Asia especially during food shortages.[119] The toxic agent appears to be beta-aminoproprionitrile. The principal characteristic of *Lathyrus* poisoning is a slowly progressive spastic paraplegia simulating amyotrophic lateral sclerosis. No effective treatment is known.

Fava Beans

Fava beans, the seeds of a common ornamental vine sometimes grown as food, cause an acute hemolytic anemia when ingested by individuals with glucose-6-phosphate dehydrogenase deficiency.[120] Favism is most common in Mediterranean countries, where this enzyme deficiency is common and fava beans are popular. Extracts of fava beans contain at least 2 agents that oxidize glutathione. However, ingestion by enzymatically susceptible hosts is not invariably followed by hemolysis. Fever and anemia usually begin 1 to 3 days after eating raw or cooked beans and resolve spontaneously over 1 to 3 weeks. The case-fatality rate is about 5%. Supportive treatment, including blood transfusions, may be necessary. Corticosteroids have been recommended.

Miscellaneous Plants

Assorted other plants are occasional causes of food poisoning. These include the accidental ingestion of the wrong part of food plants, such as rhubarb leaves, and the use of plant products as tonics, such as Jimson weed or apricot pit tea. A detailed food and home remedy history is required to identify such cases.

Monosodium Glutamate

Despite the large number of food additives used today, only one, monosodium glutamate (MSG), has been reported as a common cause of acute illness in man. First described as the "Chinese restaurant syndrome" in 1968,[120] the disorder was subsequently attributed to MSG, an agent commonly used in Asian cuisine.[121,122] The mechanism of action of MSG is unknown.[123] Doses above 2 g produce symptoms within 30 minutes in susceptible individuals. Symptoms include headache, orbital pain, dizziness, flushing, paresthesias of the mouth or face, and diaphoresis. Illness usually subsides within an hour of onset, but persistent edema of the lips or upper respiratory tract and asthma of delayed onset (11 to 14 hours after ingestion) have been reported.

Differential Diagnosis

The major clues to the specific cause of food poisoning are: (1) the incubation period; (2) the nature of the suspect food; and (3) the clinical picture. When the meal has not been identified, the incubation period can often be inferred from the time span over which cases occur. When most patients become ill within minutes, hours, or days of each other, the incubation period is usually of comparable duration, i.e., minutes, hours, or days.[4] Table 119–1 shows the usual incubation period for the major types of food poisoning. Identification of the suspect food may provide an important clue to etiology inasmuch as certain foods are more likely to transmit certain food-borne diseases. Table 119–2 shows the major agents associated with selected vehicles. Finally, the clinical picture often reduces the number of possibilities, although it is rarely pathognomonic. The presence or absence of fever, the relative amount of vomiting as contrasted with diarrhea, and the presence or absence of gross or microscopic blood in the stools serve to subdivide most food-borne gastroenteritis into a manageable number of diagnostic possibilities (Table 119–3).

Table 119–1. INCUBATION PERIODS OF FOOD-BORNE ILLNESS BY AGENT

Usual Incubation Period	Agents
Less than 2 hours	Fish/shellfish toxins: Scombrotoxin Tetrodotoxin Saxitoxin Mushroom toxins: Gastrointestinal Muscarine Muscimol Monosodium glutamate Heavy metals: Cadmium Lead Tin
2 to 7 hours	*S. aureus* *B. cereus* Fish/shellfish toxins: Ciguatoxin *Gy. breve* toxin
7 to 14 hours	*C. perfringens* *B. cereus* Mushroom toxins: Amatoxin Gyromitrin
14 hours or longer	*Salmonella* spp. *Shigella* spp. *C. jejuni* *E. coli* *V. cholerae* *V. parahaemolyticus* *C. botulinum* *Y. enterocolitica*

In combination, these clues often afford a presumptive diagnosis. Illness with an incubation period of less than 1 hour is usually of chemical origin, caused by fish toxins, mushroom toxins, or heavy metals; with the exception of the heavy metals, all of these illnesses can be differentiated by their vehicle and by their extra-gastrointestinal symptoms. Illness with an incubation period of 2 to 7 hours is usually caused by *S. aureus* or *B. cereus*, particularly when upper gastrointestinal tract symptoms are prominent. The most common causes of food-borne illness with an incubation period of 8 to 14 hours and primarily lower gastrointestinal tract symptoms are *C. perfringens* and *B. cereus*. Food-borne illness with an incubation period of more than 14 hours and predominantly extra-gastrointestinal symptoms is usually caused by *C. botulinum*. When the symptoms are primarily gastrointestinal and the incu-

Table 119–2. COMMON VEHICLES FOR FOOD-BORNE ILLNESS BY AGENT

Beef	*Salmonella* spp. *C. perfringens* *S. aureus*
Ham/pork	*S. aureus* *Salmonella* spp.
Poultry	*C. perfringens* *Salmonella* spp. *C. jejuni* *S. aureus*
Eggs	*Salmonella* spp. *S. aureus*
Cheese	*E. coli* *Salmonella* spp.
Fish/shellfish	*C. botulinum* *V. cholerae* *V. parahaemolyticus* *Salmonella* spp. Fish and shellfish toxins
Mixed salads	*Shigella* spp. *S. aureus* *Salmonella* spp. *B. cereus*
Fried rice	*B. cereus*
Mushrooms	Mushroom toxins *C. botulinum*

bation period exceeds 14 hours, definitive diagnosis requires laboratory tests, although the presence of dysentery would suggest shigellosis or campylobacteriosis.

Investigation of an Outbreak of Food Poisoning

The following elements should be included in the workup of a possible food poisoning outbreak. They are presented as steps to improve diet recall, to identify exposed but asymptomatic patients for whom early treatment may be useful, and to identify food practices that must be changed to prevent additional illness. Most are in actuality performed in parallel as soon as possible after the outbreak has been recognized.

1. *Verify the diagnosis.* This may involve examination of medical records and results of microbiologic or chemical tests or may be based entirely on the clinical picture before definitive laboratory confirmation is available. However, everything possible should be done to obtain appropriate clinical and food specimens.

2. *Specify the definition of a case.* It is useful to develop a set of clinical characteristics (e.g., fever, vomiting, diarrhea, neurologic abnormalities) that can be used for a presumptive diagnosis in the absence of laboratory results, since laboratory confirmation is often not possible for all or most cases. Clinically defined cases can be used to determine the size of the outbreak and to select groups from whom a detailed food history should be obtained.

3. *Specify whether an outbreak has occurred.* An outbreak of food poisoning is defined as 2 or more cases of the same illness associated with the same food or meal and usually

Table 119–3. USUAL SYMPTOMS OF FOOD-BORNE ILLNESS BY AGENT

	Symptoms			
Agent	*Fever*	*Vomiting*	*Diarrhea*	*Neurologic Abnormalities*
C. botulinum	0	±	±	+
S. aureus	0	+	±	0
C. perfringens	0	±	+	0
B. cereus	±	+	+	0
Salmonella spp.	+	+	+	0
Shigella spp.	+	±	+	0
E. coli	±	±	+	0
V. cholerae	0	±	+	0
V. parahaemolyticus	±	±	+	0
C. jejuni	±	±	+	0
Y. enterocolitica	±	±	+	0
Ciguatoxin	0	+	+	+
Scombrotoxin	0	+	0	+
Shellfish toxins	0	+	0	+
Amanita spp. and related mushroom toxins	0	+	±	+
Other mushroom toxins	0	+	±	0

clustered in time and place. Exceptions are botulism and chemical food poisoning, in which a single case constitutes an outbreak.

4. *Ascertain and characterize the cases.* The minimum information that should be collected includes name, address, and telephone number; age and sex; time of onset of illness; and description of illness.

5. *Obtain a food history.* It is frequently possible to conduct a personal or telephone survey of the population or a sample of it that has been exposed to a suspect meal. Alternatively, a history of sources of food consumed during an appropriate interval before the illness should be obtained; the duration of the interval is suggested by the possible clinical diagnoses. When a suspect meal has been identified, it is important to obtain food histories from representative samples of both affected and nonaffected persons. This will allow calculation of estimated relative risks for each food item.

6. *Identify the cause.* In contrast to clinical diagnosis, in which the clinical picture and isolation of an agent or toxin from the patient may suffice for diagnosis, determination of the cause of an outbreak includes identification of the vehicle and, in the case of bacterial food poisoning, the food-handling practices that led to its contamination. The implicated vehicle can be identified by recovery of bacteria or toxins, but often specimens of the suspect food are no longer available by the time the investigation of the outbreak is initiated. In this instance, the probable cause can be determined by calculating the attack rates according to consumption or nonconsumption of the food items served at the suspect meal. Attack rates of less than 50% are often observed for an item that is the sole source of an outbreak; low attack rates reflect, in part, differences in quantity eaten and distribution of the agent in the food. Although the attack rate in persons exposed to a responsible item may be low, it is almost always significantly higher than the rate in persons who did not eat the responsible food. Cross-contamination of foods may result in some cases among persons who did not eat the responsible food or in the inability to pinpoint a single item of food as the source of the outbreak.

7. *Intervention.* The workup of a food poisoning outbreak is not complete until the food practices responsible for the outbreak have been identified and corrected, circumventing future outbreaks.

References

1. Riemann H, Bryan FL, eds. Food-Borne Infections and Intoxications, 2nd Ed. New York: Academic Press, 1979.
2. Bryan FL. Diseases Transmitted by Foods (A Classification and Summary). Atlanta: Centers for Disease Control, Department of Health, Education and Welfare, 1976.
3. Kazal HL. Laboratory diagnosis of foodborne diseases. Ann Clin Lab Sci 1976; 6:381–99.
4. Horwitz MA. Specific diagnosis of foodborne disease. Gastroenterology 1977; 73:375–81.
5. Foster EM. Foodborne hazards of microbial origin. Fed Proc 1978; 37:2577–81.
6. Meyer KF. The rise and fall of botulism. Calif Med 1973; 118:63–4.
7. Horwitz MA, Hughes JM, Merson MH, Gangarosa EJ. Food-borne botulism in the United States, 1970–1975. J Infect Dis 1977; 136:153–9.
8. Terranova WA, Breman JG, Locey RP, Speck S. Botulism type B: Epidemiologic aspects of an extensive outbreak. Am J Epidemiol 1978; 108:150–6.
9. Sugiyama H. *Clostridium botulinum* neurotoxin. Microbiol Rev 1980; 44:419–48.
10. Lewis GE Jr, Angel PS, eds. Biomedical Aspects of Botulism. New York: Academic Press, 1981.
11. Kao I, Drachman DB, Price DL. Botulinum toxin: Mechanism of presynaptic blockade. Science 1976; 193:1256–8.
12. Hughes JM, Blumenthal JR, Merson MH, Lombard GL, Dowell VR Jr, Gangarosa EJ. Clinical features of types A and B food-borne botulism. Ann Intern Med 1981; 95:442–5.
13. Duchen LW. Motor nerve growth induced by botulinum toxin as a regenerative phenomenon. Proc R Soc Med 1972; 65:196–7.
14. Mann JM, Martin S, Hoffman R, Marrazzo S. Patient recovery from Type A botulism: Morbidity assessment following a large outbreak. Am J Public Health 1981; 71:266–9.
15. Dowell VR, McCroskey LM, Hatheway CL, Lombard GL, Hughes JM, Merson MH. Coproexamination for botulinal toxin and *Clostridium botulinum*. A new procedure for laboratory diagnosis of botulism. JAMA 1977; 238:1829–32.
16. Simpson LL. The action of botulinal toxin. Rev Infect Dis 1979; 1:656–9.
17. Black RE, Gunn RA. Hypersensitivity reactions associated with botulinal antitoxin. Am J Med 1980; 69:567–70.
18. Santos JI, Swensen P, Glasgow LA. Potentiation of *Clostridium botulinum* toxin by aminoglycoside antibiotics: Clinical and laboratory observations. Pediatrics 1981; 68: 50–4.
19. Kaplan JE, Davis LE, Narayan V, Koster J, Katzenstein D. Botulism, Type A, and treatment with guanidine. Ann Neurol 1979; 6:69–71.
20. Pickett J, Berg B, Chaplin E, Brunstetter-Shafer MA. Syndrome of botulism in infancy: Clinical and electro-physiologic study. N Engl J Med 1976; 295:770–2.
21. Arnon SS, Werner SB, Faber HK, Farr WH. Infant botulism in 1931: Discovery of a misclassified case. Am J Dis Child 1979; 133:580–2.
22. Arnon SS, Midura TF, Clay SA, Wood RM, Chin J. Infant botulism: Epidemiological, clinical, and laboratory aspects. JAMA 1977; 237:1946–51.
23. Arnon SS, Damus K, Chin J. Infant botulism: epidemiology and relation to sudden infant death syndrome. Epidemiol Rev 1981; 3:45–66.
24. Moberg LJ, Sugiyama H. Microbial ecologic basis of infant botulism as studied with germfree mice. Infect Immunol 1979; 25:653–7.
25. L'Hommedieu C, Polin RA. Progression of clinical signs in severe infant botulism. Therapeutic implications. Clin Pediatr 1981; 20:90–5.
26. Dack GM. Food Poisoning. Chicago: University of Chicago Press, 1956.
27. Sours HE, Smith DW. Outbreaks of foodborne disease in the United States, 1972–1978. J Infect Dis 1980; 142:122–5.
28. Merson MH. The epidemiology of staphylococcal foodborne disease. Proceedings of the Staphylococci in Foods

Conference. University Park, Pa: Pennsylvania State University, 1973: pp 20–37.
29. Breckinridge JC, Bergdoll MS. Outbreak of foodborne gastroenteritis due to a coagulase-negative enterotoxin producing staphylococcus. N Engl J Med 1971; 284:541–3.
30. Bergdoll MS. The enterotoxins. *In*: Cohen JO, ed: The Staphylococci. New York: Wiley Interscience, 1972: pp 301–33.
31. Hobbs BC, Smith ME, Oakley CL, Warrack GH, Cruickshank JC. *Clostridium welchii* food poisoning. J Hyg 1953; 51:75–101.
32. Loewenstein MS. Epidemiology of *Clostridium perfringens* food poisoning. N Engl J Med 1972; 286:1026–8.
33. Dische FE, Elek SD. Experimental food-poisoning by *Clostridium welchii*. Lancet 1957; 2:71-4.
34. Skjelkvale R, Stringer MF, Smart JL. Enterotoxin production by lecithinase-positive and lecithinase-negative *Clostridium perfringens* isolated from food poisoning outbreaks and other sources. J Appl Bacteriol 1979; 47:329–39.
35. Duncan CL, Strong DH, Sebald M. Sporulation and enterotoxin production by mutants of *Clostridium perfringens*. J Bacteriol 1972; 110:378–91.
36. Duncan CL, Strong DH. Ileal loop fluid accumulation and production of diarrhoea in rabbits by cell-free products of *Clostridium perfringens*. J Bacteriol 1969; 100:86–94.
37. Naik HS, Duncan CL. Detection of *Clostridium perfringens* enterotoxin in human fecal samples and anti-enterotoxin in sera. J Clin Microbiol 1978; 7:337–40.
38. Stringer MF, Turnbull PC, Gilbert RJ. Applications of serological typing to the investigation of outbreaks of *Clostridium perfringens* food poisoning, 1970–1978. J Hyg 1980; 84:443–56.
39. Cooke RA. Pig bel. Perspect Pediatr Pathol 1979; 5:137–52.
40. Rooney J, Shepherd A, Suebu A. *Clostridium welchii* type C antitoxin in the treatment of Pig bel (enteritis necroticans): A controlled trial in Papua, New Guinea. Papua New Guinea Med J 1979; 22:57–9.
41. Lawrence G, Walker PD, Freestone DS, Shann F. The prevention of Pig-bel in Papua, New Guinea. Papua New Guinea Med J 1979; 22:30–4.
42. Hauge S. Food poisoning caused by aerobic spore-forming bacilli. J Appl Bacteriol 1955; 18:591–5.
43. Midura T, Gerber M, Wood R, Leonard AR. Outbreak of food poisoning caused by *Bacillus cereus*. Public Health Rep 1970; 85:45–8.
44. Mortimer PR, McCann G. Food-poisoning episodes associated with *Bacillus cereus* in fried rice. Lancet 1974; 1:1043–5.
45. Terranova W, Blake PA. *Bacillus cereus* food poisoning. N Engl J Med 1978; 298:143–4.
46. Nygren B. Phospholipase C-producing bacteria and food poisoning. An experimental study on *Clostridium perfringens* and *Bacillus cereus*. Acta Pathol Microbiol Scand 1962; 160(Suppl):1–89.
47. Melling J, Capel BJ, Turnbull PCB, Gilbert RJ. Identification of a novel enterotoxigenic activity associated with *Bacillus cereus*. J Clin Pathol 1976; 29:938–40.
48. Turnbull PCB. Studies on the production of enterotoxins by *Bacillus cereus*. J Clin Pathol 1976; 29:941–8.
49. Giannella RA, Brasile L. A hospital food-borne outbreak of diarrhea caused by *Bacillus cereus*: Clinical, epidemiologic, and microbiologic studies. J Infect Dis 1979; 139:366–70.
50. Holmes JR, Plunkett T, Pate P, Roper WL, Alexander WJ. Emetic food poisoning caused by *Bacillus cereus*. Arch Intern Med 1981; 141:766–7.
51. Baine WB, Gangarosa EJ, Bennett JV, Barker WH Jr. Institutional salmonellosis. J Infect Dis 1973; 128:357–9.
52. Horwitz MA, Pollard RA, Merson MH, Martin SM. A large outbreak of foodborne salmonellosis on the Navajo Nation Indian Reservation, epidemiology and secondary transmission. Am J Public Health 1977; 67:1071–6.
53. Rowe B, Hall MLM, Ward LR, deSa JDH. Epidemic spread of *Salmonella hadar* in England and Wales. Br Med J 1980; 19:1065–6.
54. Rout WR, Formal SB, Dammin GJ, Giannella RA. Pathophysiology of salmonella diarrhea in the rhesus monkey: Intestinal transport, morphological and bacteriological studies. Gastroenterology 1974; 67:59–70.
55. Sandefur PD, Peterson JW. Isolation of skin permeability factors from culture filtrates of *Salmonella typhimurium*. Infect Immunol 1976; 23:140–5.
56. Giannella RA. Importance of the intestinal inflammatory reaction on salmonella-mediated intestinal secretion. Infect Immunol 1979; 14:671–9.
57. Anand CM, Finlayson MC, Garson JZ, Larson ML. An institutional outbreak of salmonellosis predominantly due to a lactose-fermenting salmonella newport. Am J Clin Pathol 1980; 74:657–60.
58. Aserkoff B, Bennett JV. Effect of antibiotic therapy in acute salmonellosis on the fecal excretion of salmonellae. N Engl J Med 1969; 281:636–40.
59. Lampert J, Plotkin S, Campos J, Trendler M, Schlagel D, Witte EJ. Shigellosis in a children's hospital—Pennsylvania. Morbid Mortal Wk Rep 1979; 28:498–9.
60. Black RE, Craun GF, Blake PA. Epidemiology of common-source outbreaks of shigellosis in the United States, 1961–1975. Am J Epidemiol 1978; 108:47–52.
61. Weissman JB, Gangarosa EJ, DuPont HL. Changing needs in the antimicrobial therapy of shigellosis. J Infect Dis 1973; 127:611–13.
62. DuPont HL, Hornick RB. Adverse effect of Lomotil therapy in shigellosis. JAMA 1973; 226:1525–8.
63. Merson MH, Morris GK, Sack DA, Wells JG, Feeley JC, Sack RB, Creech WB, Kapikian AZ, Gangarosa EJ. Travelers' diarrhea in Mexico: A prospective study of physicians and family members attending a congress. N Engl J Med 1976; 294:1299–1305.
64. Kudoh Y, Zen-Yoji H, Matsushita S, Sakai S, Maruyama T. Outbreaks of acute enteritis due to heat-stable enterotoxin-producing strains of *Escherichia coli*. Microbiol Immunol 1977; 21:175–8.
65. Taylor WR, Schell WL, Wells JG, Choi K, Kinnunen DE, Heiser PT, Helstad AG. A foodborne outbreak of enterotoxigenic *Escherichia coli* diarrhea. N Engl J Med 1982; 306:1093–5.
66. Tullock EF Jr, Ryan KJ, Formal SB, Franklin FA. Invasive enteropathogenic *Escherichia coli* dysentery. Ann Intern Med 1973; 79:13–17.
67. DuPont HL, Formal SB, Hornick RB, Snyder MJ, Libonati JP, Sheahan DG, LaBrec EH, Kalas JP. Pathogenesis of *Escherichia coli* diarrhea. N Engl J Med 1971; 285:1–9.
68. Gangarosa EJ, Merson MH. Epidemiologic assessment of relevance of the so-called enteropathogenic serogroups of *Escherichia coli* in diarrhea. N Engl J Med 1977; 296:1210–13.
69. Sack RB, Sack DA, Mehlman IJ, Ørskov F, Ørskov I. Enterotoxigenic *Escherichia coli* isolated from food. J Infect Dis 1977; 135:313–7.
70. Blake PA, Rosenberg ML, Costa JB, Ferreira PS, Guimaraes CL, Gangarosa EJ. Cholera in Portugal, 1974. I. Modes of transmission. Am J Epidemiol 1977; 105:337–43.
71. Salmaso S, Greco D, Bonfiglio B, Castellani-Pastoris M, deFelip G, Bracciotti A, Sitzia G, Congiu A, Piu G, Angioni G, Barra L, Zampieri A, Baine WB. Recurrence of pelecypod-associated cholera in Sardinia. Lancet 1980; 2:1124–7.
72. Blake PA, Allegra DT, Snyder JD, Barrett TJ, McFarland L, Caraway CT, Feeley JC, Craig JP, Lee JV, Puhr ND, Feldman RA. Cholera—a possible endemic focus in the United States. N Engl J Med 1980; 302:305–9.
73. Hornick RB, Music SI, Wenzel R, Cash R, Libonati JP, Snyder MJ, Woodward TE. The Broad Street pump revisited: Response of volunteers to ingested cholera vibrios. Bull NY Acad Med 1971; 47:1181–91.
74. Moss J, Vaughn M. Mechanism of action of choleragen. Evidence of ADP-ribosyl transferase activity with arginine as an acceptor. J Biol Chem 1977; 252:2455–7.
75. Francis TI, Lewis EA, Oyediran AB, Okubadejo OA, Montefiore D, Onyewetu II, Mohammed I, Ayoola EA, Vincent R. Effect of chemotherapy on the duration of diarrhoea, and on vibrio excretion by cholera patients. J Trop Med Hyg 1971; 74:172–6.
76. Wilson R, Lieb S, Roberts A, Stryker S, Janowski H, Gunn R, Davis B, Riddle CF, Barrett T, Morris JG Jr, Blake PA. Non-O group 1 *Vibrio cholerae* gastroenteritis associated with eating raw oysters. Am J Epidemiol 1981; 114: 293–8.
77. Dadisman TA Jr, Nelson R, Molenda JR, Garber HJ. *Vibrio*

parahaemolyticus gastroenteritis in Maryland. Am J Epidemiol 1973; 96:414–26.
78. Barker WH Jr. *Vibrio parahaemolyticus* outbreaks in the United States. Lancet 1974; 1:551–4.
79. Lawrence DN, Blake PA, Yashuk JC, Wells JG, Creech WB, Hughes JH. *Vibrio parahaemolyticus* gastroenteritis outbreaks aboard two cruise ships. Am J Epidemiol 1979; 109:71–80.
80. Barker WH Jr, Gangarosa EJ. Food poisoning due to *Vibrio parahaemolyticus*. Ann Rev Med 1974; 25:75–81.
81. King EO. Human infections with *Vibrio fetus* and a closely related *Vibrio*. J Infect Dis 1957; 101:119–28.
82. Blaser MJ, Berkowitz ID, LaForce FM, Cravens J, Reller LB, Wang WL. *Campylobacter* enteritis: Clinical and epidemiologic features. Ann Intern Med 1979; 91:179–85.
83. Blaser MJ, Reller LB. *Campylobacter* enteritis. N Engl J Med 1981; 305:1444–52.
84. Grant IH, Richardson NJ, Bokkenheuser VD. Broiler chickens as potential source of *Campylobacter* infections in humans. J Clin Microbiol 1980; 11:508–10.
85. Bottone EJ. ed. *Yersinia enterocolitica*. Boca Raton, Fla: CRC Press, Inc., 1981.
86. Black RE, Jackson RJ, Tsai T, Medvesky M, Shayegani M, Feeley JC, MacLeod KIE, Wakelee AM. Epidemic *Yersinia enterocolitica* infection due to contaminated chocolate milk. N Engl J Med 1978; 298:76–9.
87. Mäki M, Grönroos P, Vesikari T. In vitro invasiveness of *Yersinia enterocolitica* isolated from children with diarrhea. J Infect Dis 1978; 138:677–80.
88. Boyce JM, Evans DJ Jr, Evans DG, DuPont HL. Production of heat-stable, methanol-soluble enterotoxin by *Yersinia enterocolitica*. Infect Immunol 1979; 25:532–7.
89. Snyder JD, Christenson E, Feldman RA. Human *Yersinia enterocolitica* infections in Wisconsin. Clinical, laboratory and epidemiologic features. Am J Med 1982; 72:768–74.
90. Kadis S, Ciegler A, Ajl S. Microbial Toxins: A Comprehensive Treatise, Vol 8, Fungal Toxins. New York: Academic Press, 1972.
91. Halstead BW. Poisonous and Venomous Marine Animals of the World. Princeton: Darwin Press, 1978.
92. Rumack BH. Poisindex. Denver: Rocky Mountain Poison Center, 1982.
93. Mushroom poisoning among Laotian refugees—1981. Morbid Mortal Wk Rep 1982; 31:287–8.
94. Wieland T, Faulstich H. Amatoxins, phallotoxins, phallolysin, and antamanide: Bioactive components of poisonous *Amanita* mushrooms. CRC Crit Rev Biochem 1978; 5:185–260.
95. Lincoff G, Mitchel DH. Toxic and Hallucinogenic Mushroom Poisoning: A Handbook for Physicians and Mushroom Hunters. New York: Van Nostrand Reinhold, 1977.
96. Rumack BH, Saltzman E. Mushroom Poisoning: Diagnosis and Treatment. Boca Raton, Fla: CRC Press, 1978.
97. Mushroom poisoning. Lancet 1980; 2:351–2 (Editorial).
98. Wauters JP, Rossel C, Farquet JJ. *Amanita phalloides* poisoning treated by early charcoal haemoperfusion. Br Med J 1978; 2:1465.
99. Morris JG Jr, Lewin P, Hargrett NT, Smith CW, Blake PA, Schneider R. Clinical features of ciguatera fish poisoning: A study of the disease in the US Virgin Islands. Arch Intern Med 1982; 142:1090–2.
100. Bagnis R, Kuberski T, Laugier S. Clinical observations on 3,009 cases of ciguatera (fish poisoning) in the South Pacific. Am J Trop Med Hyg 1979; 28:1067–73.
101. Lawrence DN, Enriquez MB, Lumish RM, Maceo A. Ciguatera fish poisoning in Miami. JAMA 1980; 244:254–8.
102. Bagnis R, Chanteau S, Chungue E, Hurtel JM, Yasumoto I, Inoue A. Origins of ciguatera fish poisoning: A new dinoflagellate, *Gambierdiscus toxicus* Adachi and Fukuyo, definitively involved as a causal agent. Toxicon 1980; 18:199–208.
103. Hughes JM, Merson MH. Fish and shellfish poisoning. N Engl J Med 1976; 295:1117–20.
104. Hokama Y, Banner AH, Boylan DB. A radioimmunoassay for the detection of ciguatoxin. Toxicon 1977; 15:317–25.
105. Gilbert RJ, Hobbs G, Murray CK, Cruickshank JG, Young, SEJ. Scombrotoxic fish poisoning: Features of the first 50 incidents to be reported in Britain (1976–9). Br Med J 1980; 2:71–2.
106. Lerke PA, Werner SB, Taylor SL, Guthertz LS. Scombroid poisoning. Report of an outbreak. West J Med 1978; 129:381–6.
107. Senanayake N, Vyravanathan S. Histamine reactions due to ingestion of tuna fish (*Thunnus argentivittatus*) in patients on antituberculosis therapy. Toxicon 1981; 19:184–5.
108. Merson MH, Baine WB, Gangarosa EJ, Swanson RC. Scombroid fish poisoning: Outbreak traced to commercially canned tuna fish. JAMA 1974; 228:1268–9.
109. Earampamoorthy S, Koff RS. Health hazards of bivalve-mollusk ingestion. Ann Intern Med 1975; 83:107–10.
110. Ahles MD. Red tide: A recurrent health hazard. Am J Public Health 1974; 64:807–8.
111. Music SI, Howell JT, Brumback CL. Red tide: Its public health implications. J Florida Med Assoc 1973; 60:27–9.
112. Torda TA, Sinclair E, Ulyatt DB. Puffer fish (tetrodotoxin) poisoning. Clinical record and suggested management. Med J Australia 1973; 1:599–602.
113. Cole RJ, Cox RH. Handbook of Toxic Fungal Metabolites. New York: Academic Presss, 1981.
114. Rodricks JV, Hesseltine CW, Mehlman MA. Mycotoxins in Human and Animal Health. Park Forest South, Ill: Pathotox Publishers, Inc., 1977.
115. Schoental R, Joffe AZ, Yagen B. Cardiovascular lesions and various tumors found in rats given T-2 toxin, a trichothecene metabolite of *Fusarium*. Cancer Res 1979; 39:2179–89.
116. Krishnamachari KAVR, Bhat RV, Nagarajan V, Tilak TBG. Hepatitis due to aflatoxicosis. An outbreak in Western India. Lancet 1975; 1:1061–3.
117. Hardin JW, Arena JM. Human Poisoning from Native and Cultivated Plants. Durham, NC: Duke University Press, 1974.
118. Schoental R. Health hazards of pyrrolizidine alkaloids: A short review. Toxicol Letters 1982; 10:323–6.
119. Somogyi JC. Naturally occurring toxicants in food. Biblthca Nutr Dieta 1980; 29:110–27.
120. Man-Kwoc RH. Chinese Restaurant Syndrome. N Engl J Med 1968; 278:796.
121. Schaumburg HH, Byck R, Gerstl R, Mashman JH. Monosodium L-glutamate: Its pharmacology and role in the Chinese Restaurant Syndrome. Science 1969; 163:826–8.
122. Kenney RA, Tidball CS. Human susceptibility to monosodium L-glutamate. Am J Clin Nutr 1972; 25:140–6.
123. Filer LJ Jr, Garattini S, Kare MR, Reynolds WA, Wurtman RJ, eds. Glutamic Acid: Advances in Biochemistry and Physiology. New York: Raven Press, 1979.

Chapter 120

Intestinal Tuberculosis

Frederick F. Paustian • John B. Marshall

Intestinal tuberculosis is an ancient disease. Hippocrates, who called tuberculosis "phthisis" (from the Greek *phthiein,* meaning to decay), appreciated the severity of tuberculous enteritis as a complication of pulmonary tuberculosis. He noted that "Phthisical persons, the hairs of whose head fall off, die if diarrhea sets in . . . diarrhea attacking a person with phthisis is a mortal symptom."

Since the advent of effective antituberculous chemotherapy in the 1940s, the frequency and severity of intestinal tuberculosis in the United States and Western Europe have markedly decreased. However, intestinal tuberculosis continues to be reported with impressive frequency in developing and/or impoverished areas of the world.

Although now only rarely seen in general clinical or hospital practice, the clinician must nonetheless be cognizant of its existence and varied presentations. The disease may develop secondary to a primary focus elsewhere in the body, usually the lungs, or it may originate within the intestinal tract. Its nonspecific and protean clinical manifestations cause intestinal tuberculosis to be confused with many other diseases, especially Crohn's disease (regional enteritis) and intestinal neoplasms. Many cases go unrecognized until a surgically removed specimen is examined histopathologically, particularly when active pulmonary disease is absent.

Site of Involvement

Tuberculosis may involve any region of the gut, from the esophagus to the anus. Table 120–1 lists the frequency of occurrence of tuberculosis in the various anatomic segments of the gut as compiled from published necropsy[1] and clinical reports.[2–7] There is a striking tendency for enteric tuberculosis to affect the ileum and ileocecal areas preferentially. Other common sites of involvement are the colon (where the frequency decreases segmentally from the ascending colon to the rectum), the appendix, and the jejunum. The location of infection in areas of relative stasis and the apparent affinity of the tubercle bacillus for lymphoid tissue probably account for the predominant occurrence of tuberculosis in the ileocecal region and colon.

Table 120–1. TUBERCULOUS ENTERITIS: ANATOMIC DISTRIBUTION

	Necropsy Reports[1]	Clinical Reports (99 Patients)[2–7]
Duodenum	2.5*	2
Jejunum	24.3	7
Ileum	72.0	80
Ileocecal area	66.1	55
Appendix	25.2	6
Colon	53.8	26
Ascending	30.9	—
Transverse	20.4	—
Descending	22.8	—
Sigmoid	11.1	—
Rectum	11.9	5
Anus	—	4

*Mean values expressed as %.

Tuberculous Enteritis

Epidemiology. Intestinal tuberculosis was recognized as the most common complication of active pulmonary tuberculosis in the first half of this century. Enteric involvement was found in 6% to 90% of patients with pulmonary tuberculosis in necropsy and radiologic series.[8–12] This wide range of occurrence reflected the severity of the related pulmonary tuberculosis and the method and diligence utilized in diagnosing the intestinal aspect of the disease. Thus, Blumberg[13] found roentgenographic evidence of tuberculosis of the intestine in 5% to 8% of early, 14% to 18% of moderately advanced, and 70% to 80% of far advanced cases of pulmonary tuberculosis. A later study by Mitchell and Bristol[12] indicated the association between pulmonary and enteric tuberculosis to be 1% with minimal, 4.5% with moderately advanced, and 24.7% with far advanced pulmonary disease.

With the advent of effective antituberculous chemotherapy, enteric tuberculous disease sharply diminished in frequency to the point that it is now rarely seen and is an uncommon complication of pulmonary tuberculosis.[2,14,15] It is to be noted in this regard that intestinal tuberculosis frequently occurs with minimal or no roentgenographic evidence of pulmonary tuberculosis (Table 120–2).[2–7,16,17] In various reports from the United States, Canada, and England, from 7% to 73% of patients showed no evidence of pulmonary tuberculosis.

The current frequency of occurrence of enteric tuberculosis has not been assessed. Sherman et al.,[2] however, found only 15 cases of intestinal tuberculosis among 4222 patients hospitalized for tuberculosis at the University of Michigan Hospital over the 22-year period from 1956 through 1977.

Studies from the United States and Canada, and particularly from England, have emphasized that immigrants from areas of the world endemic for tuberculosis constitute a large proportion of the patients with intestinal tuberculosis.[4,5,17–21] Intestinal tuberculosis continues to be reported with impressive frequency in developing countries, such as India, Iraq, and South Africa.[22–26] Many publications from these countries report a high frequency of primary intestinal tuberculosis, i.e., tuberculosis of the gut without evidence of extraintestinal tuberculosis (Table 120–2).

Most granulomatous disease of the bowel in the United States and Western Europe is due to Crohn's disease. During the 44-year period extending through 1975, Homan et al.[3] found 31 cases of intestinal tuberculosis at the New York Hospital–Cornell Medical Center in New York City; during this time, 503 patients were diagnosed as having Crohn's disease. Prakash[22] in India, reported 300 cases of intestinal tuberculosis over the 14-year period immediately preceding 1978, during which time Crohn's disease was diagnosed in only 13 patients.

Rigid infectious disease control of dairy herds and pasteurization of milk have virtually eliminated bovine tuberculosis (*Mycobacterium bovis)* in the United States. *Mycobacterium tuberculosis* is the cause of virtually all cases of intestinal tuberculosis in developed countries. There were no culture-proven cases of *M. bovis* intestinal tuberculosis in any of the patients reported in Table 120–1. However, rare examples of *M. bovis* intestinal tuberculosis continue to be reported.[27,28]

Pathogenesis. The pathogenesis of intestinal tuberculosis is incompletely understood. Infection may develop primarily within the intestinal tract or it may occur secondary to a focus elsewhere in the body. Possible routes of infection include direct invasion by ingested organisms, hematogenous seeding, transport by way of infected bile, and extension from adjacent diseased organs or tissues.

Ingestion of tubercle bacilli. Animal studies have shown that intestinal tuberculosis can result from ingestion of food containing tubercle bacilli, especially milk.[11] With widespread pasteurization of milk and the disappearance of bovine tuberculosis in the United States, infected milk is not a significant cause of tuberculosis in this country. Isolated cases of primary tuberculous enteritis, however, have been reported within recent years from England and Japan.[27,28]

Secondary infection of the gut may arise from contamination of enteric chyme by bacteria from another site, usually the lungs, through swallowing of infectious sputum. This mechanism of spread is supported by the strong association between the severity of pulmonary tuberculosis and the frequency of enteric infection. Furthermore, necropsy studies have shown a very high frequency of intestinal tuberculosis in patients who have tuberculous laryngitis.[8]

The factors permitting initiation of intestinal tuberculosis by ingestion of infected material are unclear. Intestinal involvement is probably related to the number and virulence of the ingested organisms and the nutritional status of the patient.[29] Following oral intake of the organism, the tubercle bacillus passes through the stomach (where it is pro-

Table 120–2. RELATIONSHIP BETWEEN ENTERIC AND PULMONARY TUBERCULOSIS

Author	Reporting Date	Country	Period of Study	TBC Enteritis: *No. of Cases*	TBC Enteritis: *Primary (%)*	Pulmonary Tuberculosis: *Active (%)*	Pulmonary Tuberculosis: *Inactive (%)*
Sherman et al.[2]	1980	US	1956–1977	15	20	80*	
Homan et al.[3]	1977	US	1932–1975	31	7	80	13
Abrams and Holden[7]	1964	US	1946–1960	15	73	20	7
Schulze et al.[4]	1977	Canada	—	13	23	23	54
Mandal and Schofield[5]	1976	England	1970–1975	11	45	55	0
Bentley and Webster[6]	1967	England	1955–1965	14	50	29	21
Howell and Knapton[17]	1964	England	1951–1962	12	50	50*	
Novis et al.[25]	1973	South Africa	1962–1971	59	66	15	19
Prakash[22]	1978	India	1959–1977	300	61	0	39
Bhansali[23]	1977	India	1964–1976	196	76	11	14
Das and Skukla[24]	1976	India	1967–1973	93	72	22	6

*No distinction active and inactive.

tected against digestion by its fatty capsule) into the small bowel. The locus of infection is seemingly influenced by: (1) the abundance of lymphoid tissue, (2) increased physiologic stasis, (3) increased rate of electrolyte and water absorption, and (4) minimal digestive activity, permitting greater contact time of the acid-fast bacillus with the mucosal surface.[30,31] In decreasing order of frequency, the organism initiates a focus of infection in the ileum (particularly the ileocecal area), colon, jejunum, rectum, and duodenum; gastric and esophageal tuberculosis are comparatively even less frequent.[1]

Hematogenous spread of the tubercle bacillus from an extraintestinal focus of infection. Blood-borne dissemination and infection are supported by clinical observations. The early intestinal lesion is usually found in the submucosa, with normal overlying mucosa.[32,33] A "silent" bacteremia probably occurs during the primary phase of pulmonary tuberculosis[34] and in patients with miliary tuberculosis.

Bile containing tubercle bacilli. Sequestration of the bacillus by the liver and excretion in the bile are a potential source and route of infection, but this remains unproved.

Extension from contiguous organs. Enteric tuberculosis may occur by direct extension from infected adjacent organs and tissues, e.g., the female adnexa.[35] Invasion of the bowel does not seem to occur, however, when there is tuberculous involvement of the peritoneum. Generalized tuberculous peritonitis is usually not associated with intestinal tuberculosis other than as a consequence of the extension of the infectious process transmurally or from an infected, ulcerating lymph node to the serosal surface.[1]

Histopathogenesis. Whether the infection originates enterogenously or hematogenously, the most active inflammation takes place in the *submucosa*, resulting in marked thickening as a result of edema, cellular infiltration, lymphatic hyperplasia, formation of tubercles, and fibrosis. Later, as the inflammatory process penetrates through the wall to the serosa by way of lymph channels or by direct continuity, *tubercles* may be visualized grossly on the serosal surface. The tubercle bacillus is carried along lymph channels to invade the mesenteric nodes. These lymph nodes show a range of changes from hyperplasia to caseation necrosis and calcification.[1] In the end stage, lymphatic obstruction results and, eventually, the mesentery as well as the involved bowel becomes a thick, fixed mass (Fig. 120–1).

Pathology

Gross Appearance. Tuberculous enteritis is classified on the basis of gross morphologic appearance as ulcerative, hypertrophic, or ulcerohypertrophic.

The *ulcerative* form of the disease is very

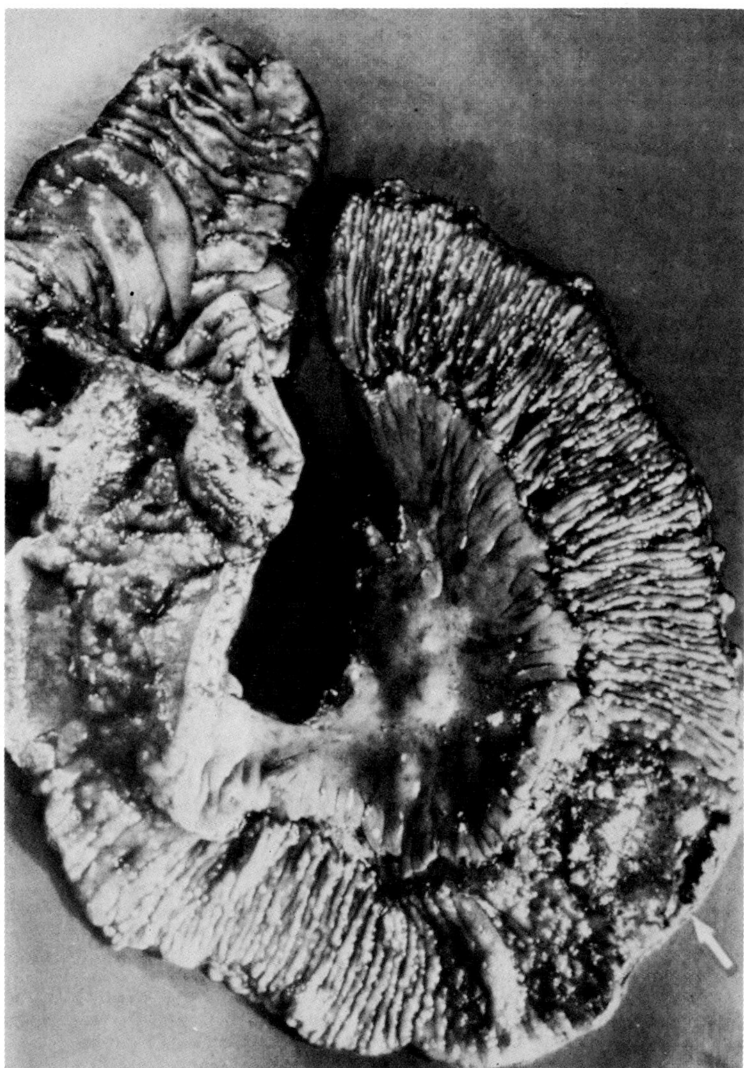

Figure 120–1. Gross specimen of mucosal surface in ileocecal tuberculosis. Arrow points to area of involvement of proximal terminal ileum. Note the myriad of minute nodules over the valvulae conniventes; the hypertrophied, polypoid, stiff terminal ileum and ileocecal valve; and the thick edematous mesentery containing enlarged lymph nodes. (From Paustian FF, Bockus HL. Am J Med 1959; 27:509. Reproduced with permission.)

likely the result of deprivation of blood supply, probably through an endarteritis.[17] Because the process of ulcer formation is relatively slow, an inflammatory wall develops ahead of the advancing ulcer. Most perforations are thus confined. There is an accumulation of collagenous tissue during the process of ulcer healing that subsequently contracts and may cause circumferential stricture of the bowel lumen and obstruction.

The diseased segment is moderately indurated and marked by a conspicuous increase in mesenteric fat; the serosa is studded with nodules.[36] The mesenteric lymph nodes are usually enlarged. The mucosal surface may show single or multiple ulcers, and skip areas may be present with normal-appearing mucosa between involved segments. The ulcers are characteristically transverse and circumferential, but may be round, stellate, or longitudinal and usually do not penetrate the muscularis propria. The margins may be irregular with the bases shaggy or nodular. In the acute phase, there may be a functional stenosis of the involved segment because of spasm. In the more chronic phase, circumferential ("napkin ring") strictures may develop.

The *hypertrophic* form usually occurs in the ileocecal area and the colon. It features a florid inflammatory fibroblastic reaction in the submucosa and subserosa.[29] The mesentery, lymph nodes, and bowel are frequently thickened and matted together by adhesions to form a mass.[36] The mucosal surface may show a large exophytic mass indistinguishable grossly from a neoplasm. Obstruction by the mass and stricturing from contraction of the proliferating collagen tissue may occur.

The *ulcerohypertrophic* form is a combination of the other 2 processes.[35,36] It combines features of ulcers, nodularity, pseudopolyps, hyperplasia, and stenosis.

In the past, the ulcerative type was considered to be secondary to pulmonary tuberculosis and the hypertrophic variety was thought to occur in the absence of pulmonary tuberculosis. This concept no longer obtains because of the poor correlation found to exist between primary tuberculosis and hypertrophy and between the ulcerative form and pulmonary disease.[1,6,17,37] The characteristics of the lesion in human tuberculosis appear to be determined more by the immunologic reaction of the host to the virulence of the tubercle bacillus than to the presence or absence of pulmonary tuberculosis.[1] A relationship seems to exist between the number of tubercle bacilli, their virulence, and the resulting lesion. Thus, a low population density of bacilli with decreased virulence is associated with hypertrophic lesions, whereas a large number of bacilli with enhanced virulence or lack of attenuation are associated with the formation of ulcers.[1,17,38–40]

Microscopic Changes. Caseating granulomas are the histologic hallmark of tuberculosis. Tandon and Prakash[36] emphasize that tuberculous granulomas may be present only in regional lymph nodes, with only non-specific changes in the bowel wall. Careful scrutiny should be made of acid-fast–stained tissue for tubercle bacilli (Fig. 120–2); the organism can occasionally be demonstrated in mesenteric nodes and, less commonly, within the bowel wall.[32]

The microscopic features of the different gross forms are similar. The granulomas tend to be large and confluent. The ulcers usually do not penetrate beyond the muscularis and are lined by non-specific inflammatory granulation tissue. In longstanding lesions, there is a variable degree of fibrosis that extends from the submucosa into the muscularis.

It must be emphasized that the histologic diagnosis of tuberculous enterocolitis may be very difficult in patients who have received antituberculous drugs preoperatively. Tandon and Prakash[36] reported a number of treated patients in whom ulcers had re-epithelialized and who had no active granulomas recognizable in the intestine or lymph nodes.

Differentiation from Crohn's Disease. Since the description of regional enteritis by Crohn et al. in 1932 (Chapter 127), the necessity for absolute proof of tuberculous enteritis has become exceedingly important as regards both treatment and prognosis. Table 120–3 summarizes the important differential features of these 2 diseases.

Clinical Features. Tuberculosis of the gut occurs with approximately equal prevalence in men and women. It has been reported in all age groups but is most frequent between 20 and 75 years of age.

Symptoms. The symptoms of intestinal tuberculosis are non-specific and varied[37,41,42] and a pathognomonic syndrome does not occur in any of its forms. The frequency of the various symptoms in tuberculous enteritis is given in Table 120–4. Abdominal pain, weight loss, fever, weakness, and nausea, it should be noted, are quite frequent. Although radiography of the chest is normal in many patients with intestinal tuberculosis (Table 120–2), the symptoms of anorexia, abdominal pain, and diarrhea in a patient with pulmonary tuberculosis should be viewed as strongly suggestive of tuberculous enteritis.

Because the disease process is commonly located in the lower right quadrant, abdominal pain is most common in this area. The discomfort is often exacerbated by eating and may result in sitophobia. Vomiting and defecation may relieve the distress, which is often cramping or colicky in nature. When partial intestinal obstruction exists, the cramps are extremely severe and generally associated wtih loud borborygmi. At times the pain is dull and diffuse in character, especially when there is involvement of the mesentery or peritoneum. Tuberculous enteritis of the duodenum may produce distress identical to that of duodenal ulcer disease.[43–47] Tuberculous appendicitis may simulate the

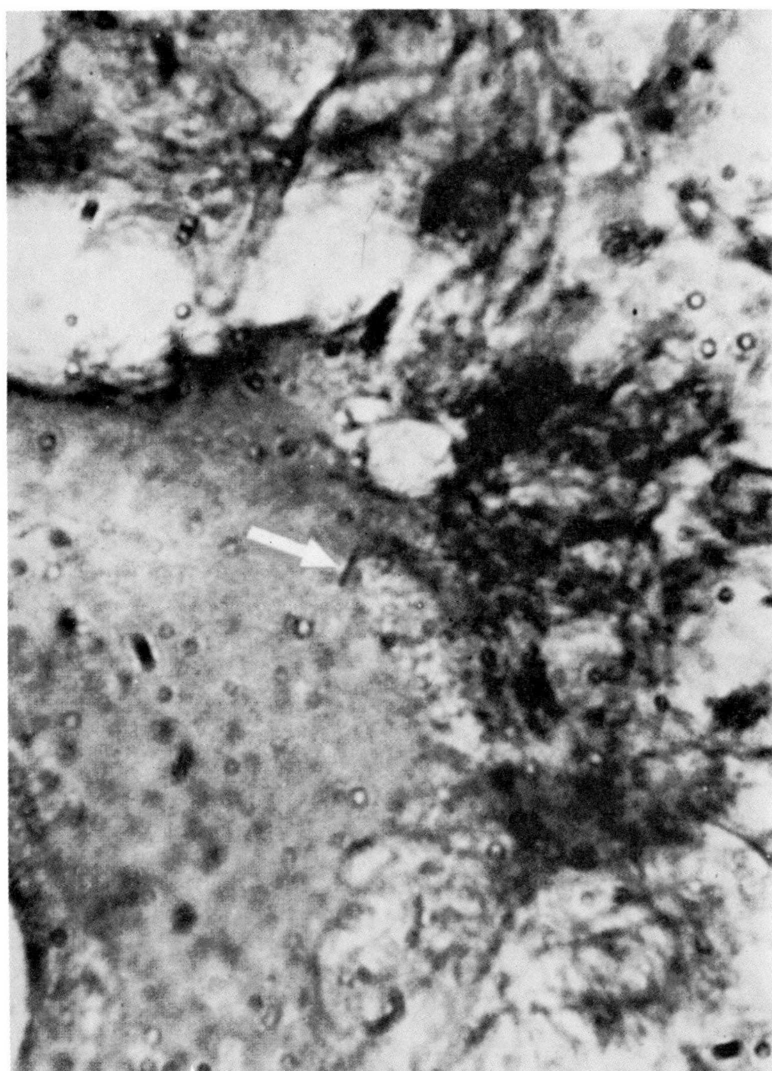

Figure 120–2. Photomicrograph of tubercle in wall of terminal ileum. Arrow points to typical acid-fast staining rod of *Mycobacterium tuberculosis.* (Original magnification × 970.) (From Paustian FF, Bockus HL. Am J Med 1959; 27:509. Reproduced with permission.)

Table 120–3. DISTINGUISHING FEATURES OF ENTERIC TUBERCULOSIS AND CROHN'S DISEASE*

Features	Tuberculosis	Crohn's Disease
Macroscopic		
Anal lesions	Rare	Common
Miliary nodules on serosa	Conspicuous and common	Rare
Length of strictures	Generally less than 3 cm	Usually long
Internal fistulas	Very rare	Frequent
Perforation	Uncommon	Rare
Ulcers:		
Location	Circumferential	More prominent along mesenteric attachment
Direction in relation to long axis	Generally transverse	Longitudinal or serpiginous
Microscopic		
Granulomas:		
Presence	Always present	Absent in at least 25% patients
Incidence in intestine in relation to lymph nodes	May be absent in the intestine but usually present in mesenteric nodes	Not seen in lymph nodes when absent in the intestine
Size	Often large	Usually small
Caseation	Usually present	Absent
Shape	Often confluent	Usually discrete
Surrounding fibrosis	Common	Rare
Hyalinization	Common	Rare
Peripheral collar of inflammatory cells	Usually present	Usually absent
Associated paramyloid	May be present	Absent
Other Features		
Submucosal widening	Generally absent	Generally present
Fissures	Generally absent: do not penetrate the muscularis	Common: penetrate deep
Transmural follicular hyperplasia	Absent	Usually present
Fibrosis of muscularis propria	Prominent	Uncommon
Pyloric gland metaplasia	Common, extensive	Less common, patchy
Epithelial regeneration	Common	Uncommon

*From Tandon HD, Prakash A.[36] Reproduced with permission.

symptom pattern of ordinary acute appendicitis, but more commonly suggests a chronic relapsing disorder with intermittent lower quadrant abdominal pain.[48]

Diarrhea occurs less often than might be expected in view of the inflammatory nature of the disorder. The characteristics are similar to those of non-specific Crohn's disease, daily occurrence of diarrhea with associated cramping pain. The number of stools rarely exceeds 3 to 6 per 24 hours. They are semi-solid to liquid in consistency, and gross blood or pus is seldom noted. Depending upon the extent and location of the inflammatory process in the small bowel, a secondary type of malabsorption may develop, giving rise to steatorrhea.

Table 120–4. SYMPTOM FREQUENCY IN TUBERCULOUS ENTERITIS

Symptom	Frequency*
Abdominal pain	60.1
Weight loss	59.3
Fever	47.2
Weakness	44.8
Nausea	43.8
Borborygmi	43.6
Anorexia	38.4
Vomiting	38.1
Postprandial distress	35.7
Distention	24.4
Night sweats	23.1
Constipation	20.6
Diarrhea	18.4
Amenorrhea	18.0
Hemorrhage	3.7

*Mean values expressed as %. (From Paustian FF, Monto GL.[1] Reproduced with permission.)

Multiple factors contribute to *weight loss* in tuberculous enteritis. Anorexia and sitophobia (due to food-induced distress) are responsible for a marked diminution of food intake. In addition, obstruction of the lymphatic system by the inflammatory process and bacterial overgrowth secondary to stasis from partial obstruction or impaired motility interfere with digestion and absorption.[37,49–51]

Physical Findings. In the moderate to advanced states of the disease, the patient appears malnourished and chronically ill. Vigorous peristaltic activity and distended bowel

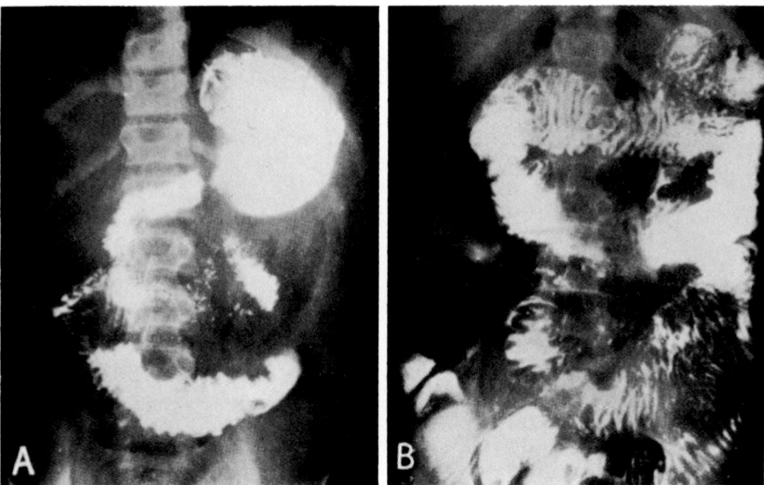

Figure 120–3. Small bowel study of tuberculous enteritis. *B,* Taken 2 hours after *A.* Note the irregularity and prominence of the Kerckring folds and the variability in intestinal caliber, suggesting edema and disturbed motility. (From Bockus HL et al. Ann Intern Med 1940; 13:1461. Reproduced with permission.)

loops may be noted when obstruction exists. Tenderness is most frequently elicited in the right lower abdominal quadrant. Muscle guarding is present in patients with involvement of the peritoneum. In classic ileocecal tuberculosis, a tender, fixed mass is palpable in about 50% of patients.[1,37,52] The abdomen may feel "doughy" in patients with an extensive or diffuse intra-abdominal inflammatory process.[37] Perianal complications, including anusitis, fissures, and perianal abscesses, are notable, especially when there is persistent diarrhea.

Laboratory Aids. Hematologic and biochemical determinations reflect the disturbances of specific organ function and the severity of the disease process, but do not establish a diagnosis of tuberculous enteritis. A negative tuberculin skin test reduces the likelihood of tuberculosis but does not exclude it. Some patients are immunologically hyporesponsive because of the severity of the illness and malnutrition. A positive skin test indicates tuberculous infection but does not establish an active disease process. Culture of acid-fast bacilli from sputum, gastric contents, pleural fluid aspirate, urine, excretions from fistulas, and stool is helpful in establishing the presence of an active tuberculous process; however, it does not in itself provide a diagnosis of tuberculous enteritis.

Radiographic Findings. Although there are no pathognomonic roentgenographic signs for tuberculous enteritis, certain roentgen features suggest the possibility of this disease.[1,29,32,53]

The earliest small bowel manifestations are disturbances in motility resulting in accelerated transit time and hypersegmentation and flocculation of barium. Involved segments of the small bowel may show scalloping and spicule formation with thickening of the mucosal folds (Figs. 120–3 and 120–4). In more

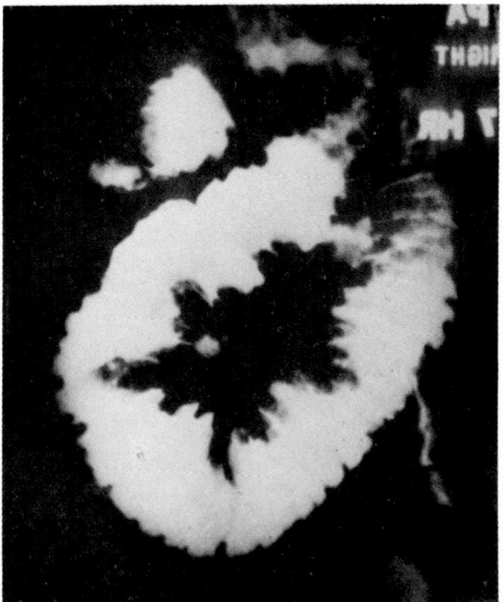

Figure 120–4. Jejunal loop in secondary ulcerative enteric tuberculosis. The involved segment is stiffened owing to a thickened mesentery. The features of marginal crenation and spiculation are well illustrated. A sinus tract leading into a confined perforation is seen in the center of the field.

advanced disease states, linear or stellate ulcers may be present.

Stierlin's sign is characterized by a lack of barium retention in an inflamed segment of ileum, cecum, or ascending colon, with a normally configured column of barium on either side (Fig. 120–5). The sign is not specific but is reflective of extreme irritability due to inflammation, often in association with ulceration. A persistent narrow stream of barium in the small bowel (*"string sign"*) (Fig. 120–6) indicates sustained hypertonicity or stenosis and is commonly seen in both ulcerative tuberculous enteritis and Crohn's disease.

Partial small bowel obstruction is manifested by dilation and stasis proximal to short stenotic segments with irregularity of the bowel silhouette and the mucosal markings. These findings differ from the comparatively smooth mesenteric border outline of similar stenotic segments in Crohn's disease.

The ileocecal area, the most common site of tuberculous involvement, may show a variety of changes.[1,53,54] The Stierlin's sign, already mentioned, is frequently seen in ileocecal tuberculosis. Single filling defects in the cecum, due either to thickening of the ileocecal valve or to an inflammatory cecal mass, cannot be differentiated from other granulomatous disorders or from malignant lesions. However, there is usually an associated shortening of the ascending colon in tuberculosis that is not evident with malignant disease (Fig. 120–5).[55]

The ileocecal valve may show a tendency to gapping because of ulceration or granulation that progresses to fibrosis and results in retraction of the valve lips.[1,54] Roentgenographically, the abnormality is known as *Fleischner's sign* and is manifested by a broad-based triangular appearance of the terminal ileum with the base toward the cecum. Such a configuration is uncommon in Crohn's disease.

Healing of the ileocecal lesion results in shortening and narrowing of the cecum with stiffening of the ileocecal valve leaflets and

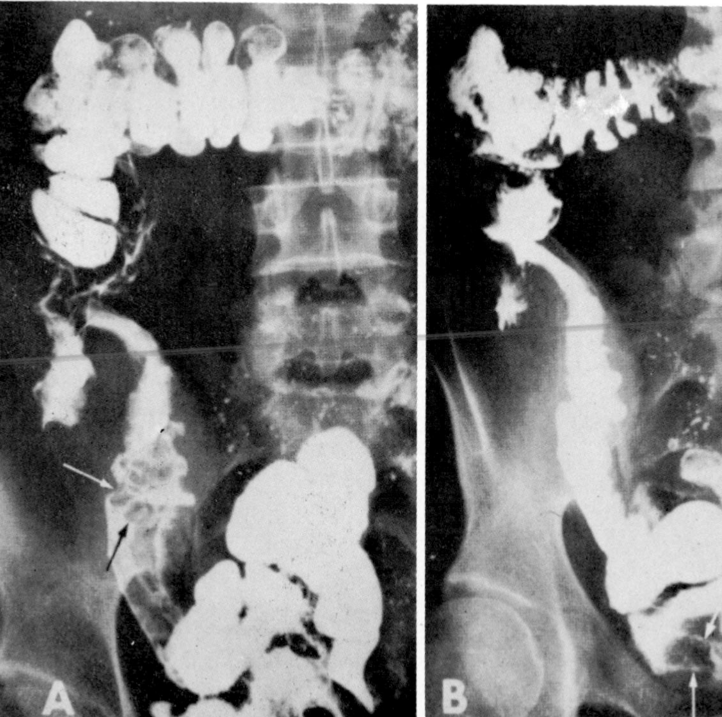

Figure 120–5. Ileocecal tuberculosis. *A,* Ileocecal junction at 2 hours. Note well-filled ileal loops proximal to poorly filled ileocecal area followed by normal-appearing colon—Stierlin sign. Arrows point to subtraction defects in terminal ileum, suggesting polypoid or hypertrophic mucosa. *B,* Shortening of ascending colon disorders, with distorted cecum. These features differentiate inflammatory from malignant disorders, as does the abnormal pattern of terminal ileum with skip area *(arrows).* (From Paustian FF, Bockus HL. Am J Med 1959; 27:509. Reproduced with permission.)

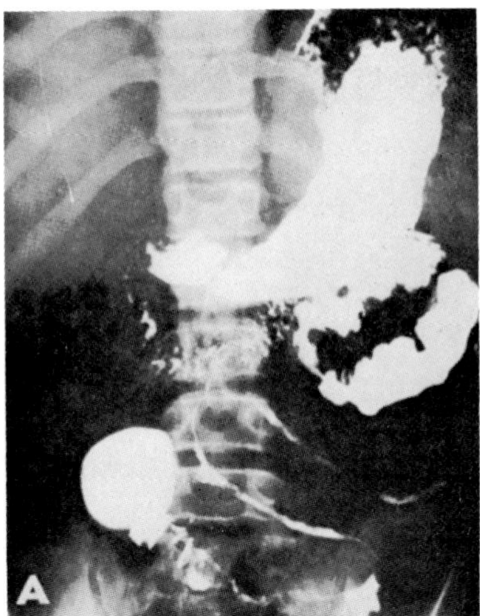

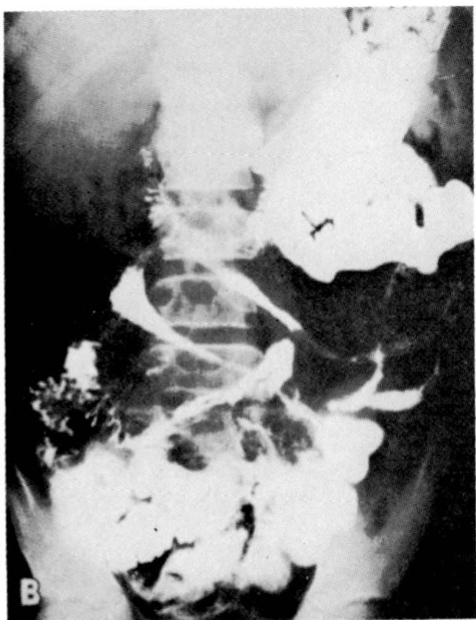

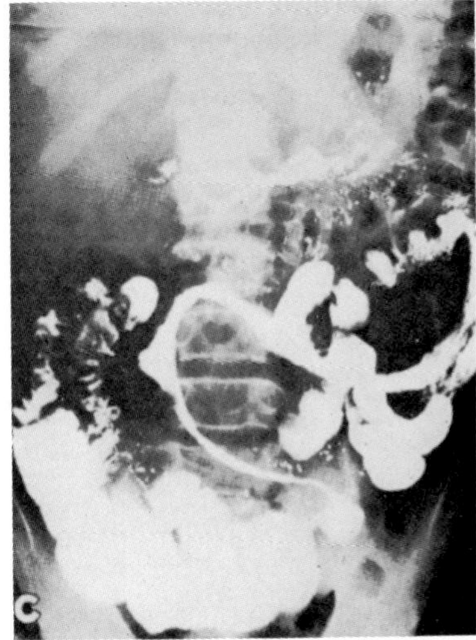

Figure 120–6. *A,* Film exposed 10 minutes after meal taken by mouth shows long narrow jejunal loops, the typical string sign. The distal end of the "string" communicates with a markedly dilated pouch of ileum. *B,* Thirty minutes after the meal the ileal loops in the lower abdomen are filled. Some show an irregular and grossly distorted margin and mucosal pattern, others appear somewhat dilated, indicating stasis. *C,* One hour and 45 minutes after the meal the terminal ileal loops are dilated and appear to be matted together.

stenosis in the prevalvular segment of ileum. The roentgen configuration of the cecum assumes a purse shape with pronounced contraction, especially opposite the ileocecal valve. The latter appears as a broad, deep indentation (Figs. 120–7 and 120–8). As the process continues, the ascending colon becomes shortened and retracts cephalad, straightening the ileocecal junction (Fig. 120–9). The ileocecal valve appears rigid and incontinent and the terminal ileum pear-shaped as the result of preterminal stenosis or kinking.

In the colon the disease tends to be segmental and is manifested morphologically by masses, annular constrictions, and ulcerations (Fig. 120–10). Diffuse tuberculous colitis is rare (Fig. 120–11).

Angiographic studies by Herlinger[56] of 2 patients with tuberculous enteritis revealed hyperemic mesenteric lymph nodes adjacent to localized transmural inflammatory disease of the cecum, a feature not seen in the arteriographic studies of 9 patients with ileocecal Crohn's disease. The vascular features of hypertrophic tuberculous enteritis and malig-

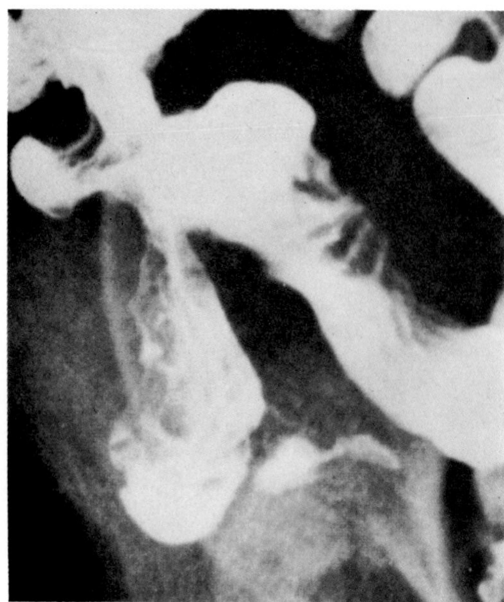

Figure 120–7. Ileocecal tuberculosis. Healing ulcer is illustrated in terminal ileum, with star configuration of converging folds and purse-shaped cecum with broad contraction of wall opposite ileocecal valve. (From Brombart M, Massion J. Am J Dig Dis 1961; 6:589. Reproduced with permission.)

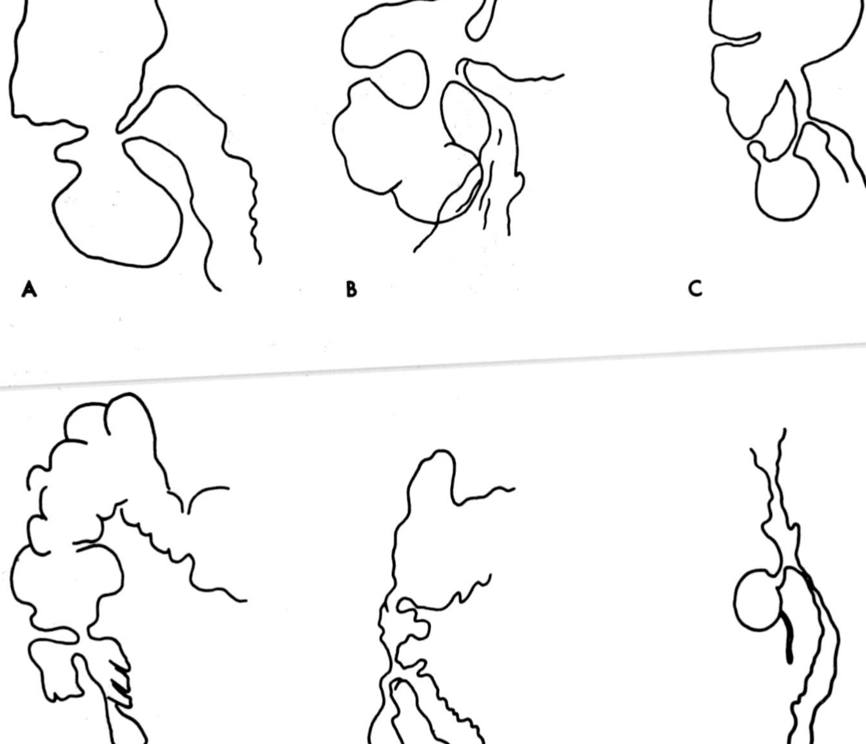

Figure 120–8. Characteristic diagrams from barium contrast studies of the terminal ileum and cecum of patients with ileocecal tuberculosis showing progressive stages of contraction of cecal wall opposite the ileocecal valve resulting in purse-shaped cecum. (From Brombart M, Massion J. Am J Dig Dis 1961; 6:589. Reproduced with permission.)

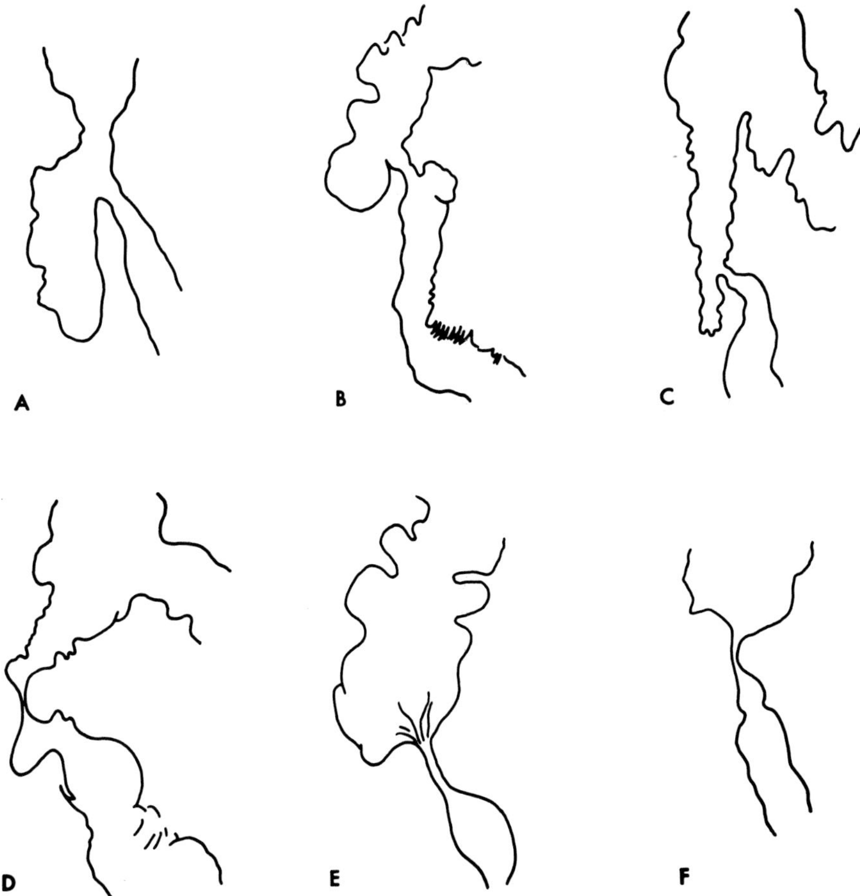

Figure 120–9. Diagrams from barium contrast studies of the terminal ileum and cecum of patients with ileocecal tuberculosis representing progressive stages of cecal contraction and retraction cephalad resulting in straightening of ileocecal junction. (From Brombart M, Massion J. Am J Dig Dis 1961; 6:589. Reproduced with permission.)

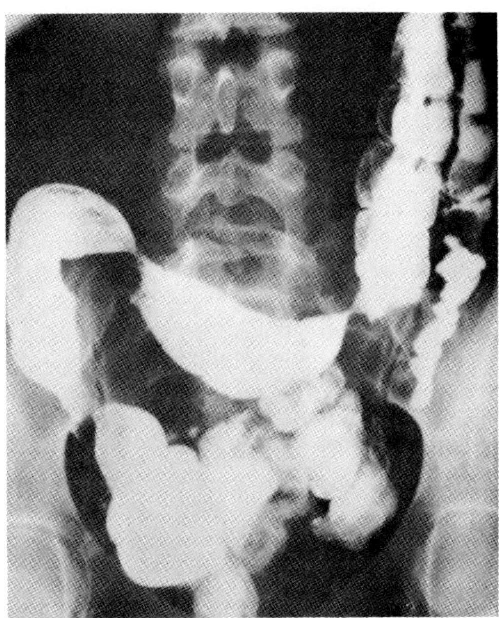

Figure 120–10. Chronic ileocolic tuberculosis. The cecum and terminal ileum are stenotic. Two areas of stenotic narrowing are shown in the transverse colon. (Used through the kindness of Professor Juan Allende of Cordova, Argentina.)

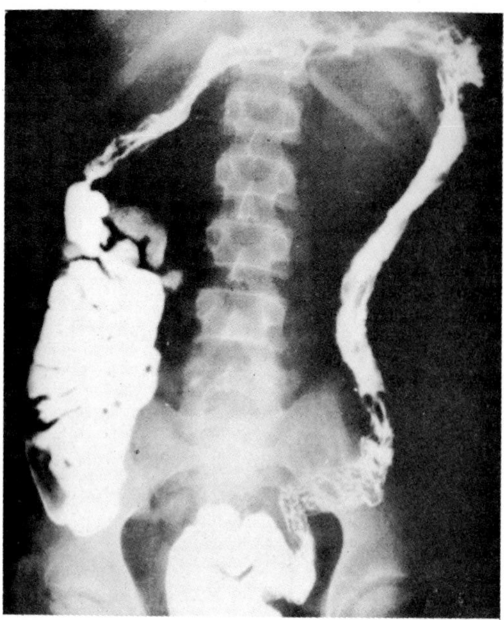

Figure 120–11. Film made after partial evacuation of a barium enema in a boy 15 years of age with primary enterocolic tuberculosis, showing extensive involvement of the entire colon. (From Bockus HL et al. Ann Intern Med 1940; 13:1461. Reproduced with permission.)

nancy are very similar, with both showing pooling of the contrast media and tumor-like capillary blush.[57]

Endoscopy. Colonoscopy may be helpful in the diagnosis of intestinal tuberculosis in some patients. Diagnostic material may be obtained by means of fiberoptic colonoscopy,[28,58–62] thereby foregoing the surgical biopsy or resection previously required for specific diagnosis. The biopsy specimen may reveal caseating granulomas or acid-fast bacilli, or, on appropriate culture, the specimen may be positive for *M. tuberculosis.* Sakai[28] reported obtaining positive cultures from 9 patients with ileocecal and colonic tuberculous ulcers. Granulomas and acid-fast bacilli were not seen in any of the biopsy specimens in these cases. Franklin et al.[58] described a patient with a constricting, ulcerating midtransverse colonic lesion resembling carcinoma from which biopsy specimens showed acid-fast bacilli identified as *M. tuberculosis.* Bretholz et al.,[59] described a patient with an ulcerated polypoid cecal mass from which biopsy of specimens demonstrated caseating granulomas and were positive on culture for *M. tuberculosis.*

Culture of transcolonoscopic biopsy material for acid-fast bacilli should be obtained whenever there are clinical features suggesting the possibility of tuberculosis and when patients with suspected Crohn's disease do not respond to conventional treatment. Caution must be exercised concerning the interpretation of mucosal biopsy cultures that are positive for tubercle bacilli because of contamination with luminal acid-fast organisms. Further studies are required before the sensitivity of colonoscopy in the diagnosis of intestinal tuberculosis can be fully assessed and its potential for transmission of the disease determined.

Diagnosis and Differential Diagnosis. The diagnosis of tuberculous enteritis is not necessarily difficult in the presence of known pulmonary tuberculosis; however, establishment of the diagnosis in the absence of evident pulmonary disease may be a problem of considerable magnitude. It is important to stress that a negative chest roentgenogram does not exclude intestinal tuberculosis from the differential diagnosis. Also to be underscored is that a specific diagnosis may not be possible when the patient has received antituberculous therapy; such drug therapy has an inhibitory effect on culture of the tubercle bacillus from suspected tissue and alters the characteristic histopathologic features of the disease.[35,36,52,63]

The complex of studies from the results of which a specific diagnosis of tuberculous enteritis may be made include: (1) roentgenograms of the chest; (2) tuberculous skin testing; (3) roentgenographic contrast studies of the intestinal tract; (4) culture of all excreta, appropriate body fluids, and suspicious tissue; and (5) histologic study of resected tissue.

Awareness that tuberculous enteritis still exists and may occur in the absence of obvious pulmonary involvement should prompt its inclusion in the differential diagnosis of chronic inflammatory and apparent neoplastic disorders of the small bowel and colon. In North America and Western Europe, the diagnosis of enteric tuberculosis should be given specific consideration when evaluating patients with inflammatory bowel disease who have emigrated from regions where the disease is endemic.

Disease entities that by their symptoms, signs, and radiographic, morphologic, and histologic features must be differentiated from tuberculous enteritis relative to geographic location include:

1. Small bowel: Crohn's disease, lymphoma, vascular insufficiency, and fungal infection.

2. Ileocecal junction and colon: Crohn's disease, ulcerative colitis, cancer, lymphoma, vascular occlusive disease, sarcoidosis, periappendiceal abscess, fungal infection, actinomycosis, and ameboma.

3. Rectosigmoid: Crohn's disease, ulcerative colitis, cancer, ischemic proctocolitis, fungal infection, actinomycosis, ameboma, schistosomiasis, lymphogranuloma venereum, diverticulitis, foreign body, and endometriosis.

Criteria for Diagnosis. Rigid criteria are necessary for establishing the diagnosis of tuberculosis of the intestinal tract. At the present time at least one of the following criteria must be met: (1) animal inoculation or culture of suspected enteric (exclusive of the mucosal layer), mesenteric; or regional lymph node tissue resulting in growth of the tubercle bacillus; (2) histologic demonstration of typical acid-fast staining rods of *M. tuberculosis* in the lesion; (3) histologic evidence of tubercles with caseation necrosis; or (4) typical gross description of operative findings with biopsy of a mesenteric lymph node showing histologic evidence consistent with tuberculosis. A non-laboratory fifth criterion providing evidence for what Logan[64] classifies as "probable tuberculosis" is the response to antituberculosis therapy of a concurrent tuberculosis elsewhere. The validity of such a diagnosis is further supported when the favorable response to chemotherapy is followed by no recurrence of disease.[65]

Complications. Complications of tuberculous enteritis include obstruction, fistula formation, confined perforation with abscess, hemorrhage, enterolithiasis, traction diverticula, and, infrequently, free perforation with generalized peritonitis.

Obstruction of the small or large bowel is common and has been reported in 10% to 60% of cases.[2,3,23,29] Obstruction may develop in several ways: (1) contraction of collagenous tissue following healing of circumferential tuberculous ulcers, (2) encroachment of the thickened bowel wall upon the lumen as a consequence of hypertrophy, (3) kinking or constriction of the intestine by intraperitoneal adhesions, and (4) retraction of the mesentery and shortening of the right colon by scar tissue with resultant kinking and obstruction at the ileocecal junction (due to changing the angle of entrance of the ileum into the colon from 90° to nearly 180°.

Fistulas develop in 1% to 33% of patients.[2,3,25,66,67] They may develop between loops of bowel or between bowel and the abdominal wall, urinary bladder, or female adnexal organs. Usually they are the consequence of secondary bacterial invasion of a necrotic area causing a penetrating abscess.

Free perforation with peritonitis develops in 1% to 26% of patients, with most occurring in the 2% to 7% range.[2,3,23,68] Over 90% are located in the distal 100 cm of ileum or in the appendix.

Confined perforation with abscess formation is an occasional complication of tuberculous enteritis, although its frequency is uncertain.[69] Intra-abdominal abscess may also be caused by rupture of caseous lymph nodes.[23,25] Massive hemorrhage,[2,70,71] enterolithiasis,[67,72] and traction diverticula[73] are rare complications.

Malnutrition is a frequent problem. Multiple factors can contribute to protein-calorie malnutrition, including anorexia, inadequate food intake (often in a background of poverty), and malabsorption. Malabsorption has multiple possible mechanisms and may result from: (1) decreased small intestinal mucosal surface, (2) lymphatic obstruction, (3) fistula formation between the small and large intestine, (4) deconjugation of bile salts secondary to bacterial overgrowth, and (5) decreased bile salt pool because of impaired active absorption in the distal ileum.[51]

Treatment. Intestinal tuberculosis is treated non-operatively, with surgery reserved for specific complications. Although there are relatively few studies of drug therapy for intestinal tuberculosis,[1] most of the well-established principles of treatment for pulmonary tuberculosis[74–76] are applicable as well to intestinal tuberculosis:

1. Drug susceptibility studies should be performed and drugs chosen to which the tubercle bacillus is likely to be susceptible. In the United States, most strains are responsive to the first-line drugs. If the infection is contracted in an area where drug resistance is common (e.g., Southeast Asia) or if the patient has received antituberculous treatment previously, it must be assumed that the bacillus will be resistant to isoniazed (INH). The regimen in such circumstances

should include at least 2 other drugs until results of susceptibility studies are known.

2. At least 2 effective drugs should always be given to avoid multiplication of drug-resistant mutants.

3. Bactericidal drugs, such as INH and rifampin, are preferred.

4. When treatment appears to be failing, therapy should be changed to an entirely new regimen of at least 2 drugs, susceptibility studies rechecked, and accuracy of diagnosis reassessed.

Conditions necessary for effective drug therapy include the use of appropriate drugs in adequate dosage for sufficient periods of time. The first-line antituberculous drugs are INH, rifampin, ethambutol, and streptomycin. Their recommended dosages and possible toxicities are listed in Table 120–5. Second-line drugs are somewhat less effective and generally more toxic. They include pyrazinamide, ethionamide, cycloserine, para-aminosalicylic acid, kanamycin, and capreomycin.[74–78]

Although the published experience for antituberculous therapy of intestinal tuberculosis is limited, the 2-drug combination of INH (300 mg/day) and rifampin (600 mg/day) is the regimen of choice (as with pulmonary tuberculosis) when there is no reason to suspect resistance to INH.[74,78] Prior to the introduction of this bactericidal combination, the most widely used regimen was a combination of INH (300 mg/day) and ethambutol (15 to 25 mg/kg/day). When large numbers of tubercle bacilli were indicated by a positive sputum smear, it was common practice to add streptomycin, 1 g/day, for the first 2 to 3 months in order to reduce further the risk of selection of INH-resistant mutants.[74]

The treatment period for intestinal tuberculosis is 18 to 24 months. There is as yet no basis for short-course treatment of intestinal tuberculosis, as there is for pulmonary tuberculosis.[79]

The indications for *surgery* in intestinal tuberculosis are for the most part limited to the complications of the disease: (1) free perforation of an ulcer; (2) confined perforation with abscess or fistula formation; (3) obstruction caused by stenosis or kinking of the bowel; and (4) massive hemorrhage. Complications requiring surgical intervention may occur during treatment with antituberculous drugs.[12,80]

An additional indication for operation is diagnostic uncertainty, as exemplified by an ileocecal lesion or colonic mass without associated pulmonary tuberculosis and with non-diagnostic endoscopic biopsy studies.

Use of the current antituberculous drugs in well-planned treatment regimens, together with appropriate and timely surgery, will provide therapeutic success in 90% of patients with tuberculous enteritis.[1,3]

Tuberculosis of the Appendix

In the early part of this century, 0.1% to 3% of all appendices removed in general hospitals, and 1.5% to 30% of appendices excised from patients with pulmonary tuberculosis, were affected by tuberculosis.[48,81] Clinical tuberculous appendicitis, however, is rare (Chapter 144), and isolated tuberculosis of the appendix without involvement of the cecum or ileum is unusual.[82–84] The pathogenesis of tuberculosis of the appendix is similar to that of tuberculous enteritis.

The clinical picture of tuberculous appendicitis is variable and non-specific.[47,85–87] It may be that of an acute or chronic appendicitis with attacks of distress in the right lower abdominal quadrant, or the clinical expressions may be very vague, with the disease found only on abdominal exploration.

If the disorder is localized to the appendix, the treatment is appendectomy followed by antituberculous drug therapy. Complications are the result of secondary bacterial infection with abscess and fistula formation.[48] All excised appendices must be examined histologically to avoid error in specific diagnosis.

Tuberculosis of the Colon and Rectum

In the absence of ileocecal tuberculosis, the diagnosis of colonic tuberculosis is difficult. Because of the rarity of the disease today, it is seldom considered in the differential diagnosis of large bowel lesions simulating malignancy or segmental, non-specific granulomatous colitis. Whether hypertrophic or ulcerative, the lesion tends to be segmental. Balthazar and Bryk,[88] in 1980, found reports to that time of 100 cases of segmental tuberculosis of the colon (distal to the cecum) in the English-speaking literature. Chawla et al.,[89] 9 years earlier, were able to find only 10 cases of segmental tuberculosis of the

Table 120–5. FIRST-LINE ANTITUBERCULOUS DRUGS

Drug	Daily Dose (Adult)	Most Common Side Effects	Tests For Side Effects	Remarks
Isoniazid (INH)	300 mg orally	Peripheral neuritis Hepatitis Hypersensitivity: fever, skin rash, arthralgias	Liver tests monthly if high risk for developing toxic hepatitis	Pyridoxine 10–50 mg as prophylaxis for neuritis Discontinue if symptomatic hepatitis or 3-fold elevation of AST
Rifampin	600 mg orally	Hepatitis Thrombocytopenia Fever Orange urine, increased tears and saliva	Liver tests Platelet count	Discontinue if jaundice or 3-fold elevation of AST Negates effect of birth control pills
Ethambutol	15–25 mg/kg orally	Optic neuritis (very rare at 15 mg/kg) Skin rash	Periodic test of visual acuity and red-green color discrimination	Use with caution in presence of renal insufficiency
Streptomycin	0.75–1.0 g IM first 90 days or until the sputum becomes culture negative	Eighth cranial nerve damage Nephrotoxicity Hypersensitivity: skin rash, anaphylaxis	Audiograms Vestibular function BUN/serum creatinine	Use with caution in older patients or those with renal disease

colon among 750 patients with tuberculous enteritis.

The segment of colon involved by tuberculosis is generally of short length (less than 5 to 7 cm), and any segment of the colon may be affected, including the rectum. Skip areas may be present. The morphology varies from masses to annular constricting lesions to ulcerations.[88–95] The clinical manifestations are non-specific and include diarrhea, rectal bleeding, weight loss, fever, and a palpable mass; obstructive symptoms are common.

Segmental colonic tuberculosis is commonly confused with colorectal neoplasms and with Crohn's disease of the colon. To further complicate the problem, carcinoma and tuberculosis of the large bowel may occur simultaneously.[1,96–98] A malignant lesion may facilitate invasion by the tubercle bacillus. However, there is no evidence to indicate a greater frequency of colonic cancer in patients with tuberculosis.

Bockus et al.[99] and others[100,101] have reported the rare occurrence of diffuse tuberculous colitis, a form of colonic tuberculosis closely resembling ulcerative colitis. There have also been reports of concurrent ulcerative colitis and tuberculosis of the colon, the acid-fast bacillus in each instance being an opportunistic invader.[102] Tuberculous adenitis can result in distortion of colonic segments with fixation, traction diverticula, and sinus tracts.[60,88]

Diagnosis of colonic tuberculosis is usually not made until tissue is obtained at surgery. Colonoscopy may be of value, several reports having appeared that describe obtaining specific diagnostic material (caseating granulomas, acid-fast bacilli, and positive cultures) in colonoscopic biopsy specimens.[28,58,59,61] Balthazar and Bryk[88] recommend that a segmental colonic lesion should be considered suspicious for tuberculosis when: (1) it is demonstrated in a young adult between 20 and 45 years of age, (2) it is associated with (a) radiographic changes in the chest that are compatible with active or inactive tuberculosis and/or (b) a positive tuberculin skin test, or (3) the patient originally comes from an area where tuberculosis is endemic.

The segmental hypertrophic form of colonic tuberculosis is generally treated by surgical resection because the lesion cannot be differentiated grossly from malignancy. To differentiate the two, even after resection, it is important to search for caseation in granulomas, and this may be found only in the regional lymph nodes. In the presence of active pulmonary tuberculosis or when endoscopic biopsy specimens reveal features diagnostically supportive of tuberculosis, non-obstructive segmental lesions of the colon and rectum may be treated with antituberculous drugs alone. As in other areas of the intestine, obstruction can occur during the healing phase of the hyperplastic form of the disease and necessitate surgical resection.

Tuberculosis of the Anal Canal

Logan[64] reported in 1969 that at St. Mark's Hospital in London tuberculous fistula-in-ano had declined in frequency from 11.7% in the period from 1935 to 1945 to 0.85% in the

Table 120–6. DIFFERENTIAL DIAGNOSIS OF ANORECTAL CROHN'S DISEASE AND TUBERCULOSIS*

	Crohn's Disease	Tuberculosis
Age	Adolescence or older	Usually over 30 years
Appearance	Non-specific or typical	Usually non-specific
Chest radiograph	Usually no tuberculosis	Frequent
Tuberculin skin test	No relation	Usually positive
Proximal gastrointestinal disease	Usual	No
Histology	Non-caseating granulomas *or* Non-specific inflammation	Caseating granulomas Non-caseating granulomas, *or* Non-specific inflammation (acid-fast bacilli very rare)
Culture for tuberculosis	Negative	Sometimes positive
Response to antituberculous chemotherapy	None	Improvement
Follow-up	May recur locally May develop proximal gastrointestinal disease	Remains healed

*Adapted from Logan VSD.[64]

period from 1958 to 1967. In a series of cases seen from 1958 to 1967, 11 of 12 patients had evidence of pulmonary tuberculosis on chest radiographs.

Tuberculosis of the anal canal manifests itself as ulcers and fissures, fistulas, abscesses, and various hypertrophic exophytic growths.[72,103–105] Crohn's disease is the disorder most likely to be confused with anal tuberculosis; venereal infections, neoplasms, foreign bodies, and traumatic lesions must also be considered. Table 120–6 summarizes contrasting features useful in the differential diagnosis of Crohn's disease of the anorectum and tuberculosis. The possibility of anorectal tuberculosis must be considered when a patient has a chronic anal or perianal lesion that fails to heal in response to the usual simple modes of therapy.[102] Chemotherapy is the treatment of choice for tuberculous lesions.

References

1. Paustian FF, Monto GL. Tuberculosis of the intestines. *In:* Bockus HL, ed. Gastroenterology. Volume 2. 3rd Ed. Philadelphia: WB Saunders, 1976: 750–77.
2. Sherman S, Rohwedder JJ, Ravikrishan KP, Weg JG. Tuberculous enteritis and peritonitis: report of 36 general hospital cases. Arch Intern Med 1980; 140:506–8.
3. Homan WP, Grafe WR, Dineen P. A 44-year experience with tuberculous enterocolitis. World J Surg 1977; 1:245–50.
4. Schulze K, Warner HA, Murray D. Intestinal tuberculosis: experience at a Canadian teaching institution. Am J Med 1977; 63:735–45.
5. Mandal BK, Schofield PF. Abdominal tuberculosis in Britain. Practitioner 1976; 216:683–9.
6. Bentley G, Webster JHH. Gastrointestinal tuberculosis: a 10-year review. Br J Surg 1967; 54:90–6.
7. Abrams JS, Holden WD. Tuberculosis of the gastrointestinal tract. Arch Surg 1964; 89:282–93.
8. Crawford PM, Sawyer HP. Intestinal tuberculosis in 1400 autopsies. Am Rev Tuberc 1934; 30:568–83.
9. Granet E. Intestinal tuberculosis: a clinical, roentgenological and pathological study of 2086 patients affected with pulmonary tuberculosis. Am J Dig Dis 1935; 2:209–14.
10. Cullen JH. Intestinal tuberculosis: a clinical pathological study. Q Bull Sea View Hosp 1940; 5:143–60.
11. Kornblum SA, Zale, C, Aronson W. Surgical complications of intestinal tuberculosis as seen at necropsy. Am J Surg 1948; 75:498–501.
12. Mitchell RS, Bristol LJ. Intestinal tuberculosis: an analysis of 346 cases diagnosed by routine intestinal radiography on 5529 admissions for pulmonary tuberculosis, 1924–49. Am J Med Sci 1954; 227:241–9.
13. Blumberg A. Pathology of intestinal tuberculosis. J Lab Clin Med 1928; 13:405–12.
14. Fraki, O, Paltokallio P. Intestinal and peritoneal tuberculosis. Dis Colon Rectum 1975; 18:685–93.
15. Davies PDO et al. National survey of tuberculosis notifications in England and Wales, 1978–9. Br Med J 1980; 281:895–8.
16. Dillman RO, Graham DY. Primary tuberculous enteritis: forgotten but not gone. Tex Med 1979; 75:48–52.
17. Howell JS, Knapton PJ. Ileo-caecal tuberculosis. Gut 1964; 5:524–9.
18. Findlay JM, Stevenson DK, Addison NV, Mirva ZA. Tuberculosis of the gastrointestinal tract in Bradford, 1967–77. J R Soc Med 1979; 72:587–90.
19. Croker J, Record CO, Wright JT. Ileo-cecal tuberculosis in immigrants. Postgrad Med J 1978; 54:410–2.
20. Wales JM, Mumtaz H, MacLeod WM. Gastrointestinal tuberculosis. Br J Dis Chest 1976; 70:39–57.
21. Tabrisky J, Lindstrom RR, Peters R, Lachman RS. Tuberculous enteritis: review of a protean disease. Am J Gastroenterol 1975; 63:49–57.
22. Prakash A. Ulcero-constrictive tuberculosis of the bowel. Int Surg 1978; 63:23–9.
23. Bhansali SK. Abdominal tuberculosis: experiences with 300 cases. Am J Gastroenterol 1977; 67:324–37.
24. Das P, Shukla HS. Clinical diagnosis of abdominal tuberculosis. Br J Surg 1976; 63:941–6.
25. Novis BH, Bank S, Marks IN. Gastrointestinal and peritoneal tuberculosis: a study of cases at Groote Schuur Hospital, 1962–1971. S Afr Med J 1973; 47:365–72.
26. Hamandi WJ, Thamer MA. Tuberculosis of the bowel in Iraq: a study of 86 cases. Dis Colon Rectum 1965; 8:158–64.
27. Venables GS, Rana PSJB. Colonic tuberculosis. Postgrad Med J 1979; 55:276–8.
28. Sakai Y. Colonoscopic diagnosis of intestinal tuberculosis. Mater Med Pol 1979; 11:275–8.
29. Thoeni RF, Margulis AR. Gastrointestinal tuberculosis. Semin Roentgenol 1979; 14:283–94.
30. Hoon JR, Dockerty MB, Pemberton JDeJ. Ileocecal tuberculosis including a comparison of this disease with nonspecific regional enterocolitis and noncaseous tuberculated enterocolitis. Int Abst Surg 1950; 60:417–30.
31. Rankine JA. Tuberculosis of the ileocecal area. J Int Coll Surg 1952; 18:202–9.
32. Carrera GF, Young S, Lewicki AM. Intestinal tuberculosis. Gastrointest Radiol 1976; 1:147–55.
33. Palmer ED. Tuberculosis of the stomach and the stomach in tuberculosis. Am Rev Tuberc 1950; 61:116–30.
34. Stead WW, Bates JH. Evidence of a "silent" bacillemia in primary tuberculosis. Ann Intern Med 1971; 74:559–61.
35. Paustian FF, Bockus HL. So-called primary ulcerohypertrophic ileocecal tuberculosis. Am J Med 1959; 27:509–18.
36. Tandon HD, Prakash A. Pathology of intestinal tuberculosis and its differentiation from Crohn's disease. Gut 1972; 13:260–9.
37. Lewis EA, Kolawole TM. Tuberculous ileo-colitis in Ibadan: a clinico-radiological review. Gut 1972; 13:646–53.
38. Lurie MB. Native and acquired resistance to tuberculosis. Am J Med 1950; 9:591–600.
39. Hawley PR, Wolfe HRI, Fullerton JM. Hypertrophic tuberculosis of the rectum. Gut 1968; 9:461–5.
40. Recio PM. Tuberculosis of the large bowel. Dis Colon Rectum 1961; 4:439–41.
41. Prakash A, Sharma LK, Koshal A, Poddar PK. Ileocecal tuberculosis. Aust NZ J Surg 1975; 45:371–5.
42. Das P, Kumar P, Gupta CK, Indrayan A. Clinical patterns of abdominal tuberculosis. Am J Proctol 1975; 26:75–86.
43. Jachna JS, Peck H, Davis JG. Tuberculosis of the duodenum. Calif Med 1961; 94:37–9.
44. Lockwood CM, Forster PM, Catto JVF, Stewart JS. A case of duodenal tuberculosis. Am J Dig Dis 1974; 19:575–9.
45. Tandon RK, Pastakia B. Duodenal tuberculosis as seen by duodenoscopy. Am J Gastroenterol 1976; 66:483–6.
46. Tishler JMA. Duodenal tuberculosis. Radiology 1979; 130:593–5.
47. Gleason T, Prinz RA, Kirsch EP, Jablokow V, Greenlee HB. Tuberculosis of the duodenum. Am J Gastroenterol 1979; 72:36–40.
48. Bobrow ML, Friedman S. Tuberculous appendicitis. Am J Surg 1956; 91:389–93.
49. Tandon RK, Bansal R, Kapur BML, Shriniwas O. A study of malabsorption in intestinal tuberculosis: stagnant loop syndrome. Am J Clin Nutr 1980; 33:244–50.
50. Pimparker DD, Donde UM. Intestinal tuberculosis: gastrointestinal absorption studies. J Assoc Phys India 1974; 22:219–28.
51. Desai HG, Zaveri MP, Antia FP. Bile salt metabolism in intestinal tuberculosis. Ind J Med Res 1975; 63:1767–73.
52. Wig KL, Chitkara NL, Gupta SP, Kishore K, Manchanda RL. Ileocecal tuberculosis with particular reference to isolation of *Mycbactarium tuberculosis.* Am Rev Resp Dis 1961; 84:169–78.

53. Brombart M, Massion J, Bodart P, Dive C, Van Trappen G. Radiologic differences between ileocecal tuberculosis and Crohn's disease. Am J Dig Dis 1961; 6:589–622.
54. Gershon-Cohen J, Kremens V. X-ray studies of the ileocecal valve in ileocecal tuberculosis. Radiology 1954; 62:251–4.
55. Anscombe AR, Keddie NC, Schofield PF. Caecal tuberculosis. Gut 1967; 8:337–43.
56. Herlinger H. Angiography in the diagnosis of ileocecal tuberculosis. Gastrointest Radiol 1978; 2:371–6.
57. Kinkhabwala M, Dziadiw R. Arteriographic manifestations of tuberculosis of the splenic flexure and the stomach. Br J Rad 1971; 44:384–7.
58. Franklin GO, Mohapatra M, Perrillo RP. Colonic tuberculosis diagnosed by colonoscopic biopsy. Gastroenterology 1979; 76:362–4.
59. Bretholz A, Strasser H, Knoblauch M. Endoscopic diagnosis of ileocecal tuberculosis. Gastrointest Endosc 1978; 24:250–1.
60. Hiatt GA. Miliary tuberculosis with ileocecal involvement diagnosed by colonoscopy. JAMA 1978; 240:561–2.
61. Tishler JMA. Tuberculosis of the transverse colon. AJR 1979; 133:229–32.
62. Breiter JR, Hajjar J. Segmental tuberculosis of the colon diagnosed by colonoscopy. Am J Gastroenterol 1981; 76:369–73.
63. Campbell EJM. Difficulties in the diagnosis and management of unsuspected tuberculous enteritis and colitis. Gut 1961; 2:202–9.
64. Logan VSCD. Anorectal tuberculosis. Proc R Soc Med 1969; 62:1227–30.
65. Moss JD, Knauer CM. Tuberculous enteritis. Gastroenterology 1973; 65:959–66.
66. Lambrianides AL, Ackroyd N, Shorey BA. Abdominal tuberculosis. Br J Surg 1980; 67:887–9.
67. Vaidya MG, Sodhi JS. Gastrointestinal tract tuberculosis: a study of 102 cases including 55 hemicolectomies. Clin Radiol 1978; 29:189–95.
68. Sweetman WR, Wise RA. Acute perforated tuberculous enteritis: surgical treatment. Ann Surg 1959; 149:143–8.
69. Porter JM, Snowe RJ, Silver D. Tuberculous enteritis with perforation and abscess formation in childhood. Surgery 1972; 71:254–7.
70. Verma P, Kapur BML. Massive rectal bleeding due to intestinal tuberculosis. Am J Gastroenterol 1979; 71:217–9.
71. Goudarzi HA, Mason LB. Fatal rectal bleeding due to tuberculosis of the cecum. JAMA 1982; 247:667–8.
72. Bery K, Virmani P, Chawla S. Enterolithiasis with tubercular intestinal strictures. Br J Radiol 1964; 37:73–5.
73. Nolan DJ, Norman WJ, Airth GR. Traction diverticula of the colon. Clin Radiol 1971; 22:458–61.
74. Stead WW, Bates JH. Tuberculosis. *In:* Isselbacher KJ, Adams RD, Braunwald E, Petersdorf RG, Wilson JD, eds. Harrison's Principles of Internal Medicine. 9th Ed. New York: McGraw-Hill, 1980: 700–11.
75. Vanscoy RE, Wilkowske CV. Antituberculous agents. Mayo Clin Proc 1983; 58:233–40.
76. Bailey WC. Chemotherapy of tuberculosis. *In:* Schlossberg D, ed. Tuberculosis. New York: Praeger, 1983: 65–87.
77. Yoshikawa TT, Fujita NK. Antituberculous drugs. Med Clin North Am 1982; 66:209–19.
78. Glassroth JG, Robins AG, Snider DE Jr. Tuberculosis in the 1980's. N Engl J Med 1980; 302:1441–50.
79. Stead WW, Dutt AK. What's new in tuberculosis? Am J Med 1981; 71:1–4.
80. Jordan GL Jr, DeBakey ME. Complications of tuberculous enteritis occurring during antimicrobial therapy. Arch Surg 1954; 69:688–93.
81. Morrison H, Mixter CG, Schlesinger MJ, Ober WB. Tuberculosis localized in the vermiform appendix. N Engl J Med 1952; 246:329–31.
82. Rose TF. Primary tuberculosis of the vermiform appendix. Med J Aust 1955; 1:756–9.
83. Bhasin V, Chopra P, Kapur BML. Acute tubercular appendicitis. Int Surg 1977; 62:563–4.
84. Mittal VK, Khanna SK, Gupta NM, Aikat M. Isolated tuberculosis of appendix. Am Surg 1975; 41:172–4.
85. Patel PA. Tuberculous appendicitis. Br J Clin Pract 1975; 29:87–90.
86. Jaffe FA. Tuberculous appendicitis: a clinicopathologic study of 17 cases. Am Rev Tuberc 1951; 64:182–91.
87. Braastad FW, Dockerty MB, Waugh JM. Tuberculous appendicitis. Surgery 1950; 27:790–802.
88. Balthazar EJ, Bryk D. Segmental tuberculosis of the distal colon: radiographic features in 7 cases. Gastrointest Radiol 1980; 5:75–80.
89. Chawla S, Mukerjee P, Bery K. Segmental tuberculosis of the colon: a report of ten cases. Clin Radiol 1971; 22:104–9.
90. Hancock DM. Hyperplastic tuberculosis of the distal colon. Br J Surg 1958; 46:63–8.
91. Aronson AR, Slattery LR. Tuberculosis of the transverse colon: report of a case simulating carcinoma. Gastroenterology. 1959; 36:698–701.
92. Gadwood KA, Bedetti CD, Herbert DL. Colonic tuberculosis mimicking annular carcinoma: report of a case. Dis Colon Rectum 1981; 24:395–8.
93. Hoshino M, Shibata M, Goto N, and 11 others. A clinical study of tuberculous colitis. Gastroentest Jpn 1979; 14:299–305.
94. Brenner SM, Annes G, Parker JG. Tuberculous colitis simulating nonspecific granulomatous disease of the colon. Am J Dig Dis 1970; 15:85–92.
95. Davis JW. Hyperplastic tuberculosis of the rectum. Am J Surg 1957; 93:490–2.
96. Randall KJ, Spalding JE. Simultaneous carcinoma and tuberculosis of the colon: report of a case and review of the literature. Br J Surg 1946; 33:372–5.
97. Sane SY, Nimbkar SA. Carcinoma of the colon with tuberculosis. J Postgrad Med 1980; 26:199–200.
98. Tandon HD, Kapoor BML. Carcinoma of the colon associated with tuberculosis: report of a case. Dis Colon Rectum 1974; 17:777–81.
99. Bockus HL, Tumen H, Kornbloom K. Diffuse primary tuberculous enterocolitis: a report of two cases. Ann Intern Med 1940; 13:1461–82.
100. Ahuja SK, Gaiha M, Sachdev S, Maheshwari HB. Tubercular colitis simulating ulcerative colitis: a case report. J Assoc Phy India 1976; 24:617–9.
101. Balikian JP, Uthman SM, Kabakian HA. Tuberculous colitis. Am J Proctol 1977; 28:75–9.
102. Glenn PM, Read HS. Tuberculous ulcerative colitis or ulcerative colitis with superimposed tuberculous infection. Gastroenterology 1946; 6:9–20.
103. Nepomuceno OR, O'Grady JF, Eisenberg SW, Bacon HE. Tuberculosis of the anal canal: report of a case. Dis Colon Rectum 1971; 14:313–6.
104. Ahlberg J, Bergstrand O, Holmstrom B, Ullman J, Wallberg P. Anal tuberculosis: a report of two cases. Acta Chir Scand 1980; Suppl 500:45–7.
105. Alankar K, Rickert RR, Sen P, Lazaro EJ. Verrucous tuberculosis of the anal canal: report of a case. Dis Colon Rectum 1974; 17:254–7.

Chapter 121

Venereal Diseases of the Intestine

Sidney Neimark

The *"gay bowel syndrome,"* a term coined by Sohn and Ribilotti[1] in 1977, describes a group of colonic and rectal diseases occurring in high frequency in homosexual populations and sharing a common mode of sexual transmission. This syndrome is not limited to the homosexual population and may be sexually spread to and by bisexuals and heterosexuals. Males with multiple, often anonymous, partners appear to be at greatest risk. Homosexuality *per se* does not appear to be a major risk factor, but the number and anonymity of the sexual partners increase the risk of sexually transmitted diseases (STDs) and create an environment in which breaking the cycle of STDs through contact tracing and treatment is nearly impossible.

Sexually transmitted diseases are a major and growing public health problem. In 1980, over 1 million cases of gonorrhea and 30,000 cases of syphilis were reported in the United States. The Venereal Disease Division of the Centers for Disease Control estimates that the actual incidence is more than twice that reported. The diseases traditionally considered to be sexually transmitted—syphilis, gonorrhea, lymphogranuloma venereum, and granuloma inguinale—account for only part of all STDs. Sohn and Ribilotti included amebiasis, shigellosis, condyloma acuminatum, fissures, polyps, fistulas, rectal abscesses, hepatitis, non-specific proctitis, foreign bodies, and trauma under the broad term "gay bowel syndrome." Epidemiologic evidence supports sexual transmission of these diseases and an increased prevalence in homosexual populations. Pathogens new to the bowel, such as *Chlamydia trachomatis* and the herpes viruses, have now clearly been implicated as well.

The term "gay bowel syndrome," therefore, collectively refers to proctologic complications of oral-anal, oral-genital, or procto-genital intercourse and pathologic conditions occurring in high frequency in homosexuals but not exclusive to that group.

Gonorrhea

Epidemiology. Gonorrhea is the leading reported venereal disease in the United States. Anorectal infections caused by *Neisseria gonorrhoeae* are common in women and homosexual men. Rectal infections occur in 20% to 60% of women with genital gonorrhea.[2] The prevalence rate in homosexual men has been reported to vary between 12% and 55% in patients seen in STD clinics. Stratified squamous epithelium is resistant to invasion by the gonococcus, but columnar and transitional epithelium are more easily penetrated. Direct inoculation by rectal intercourse is the most obvious route of infection. Pariser and Marino[3] reported that 75% of women with anorectal gonorrhea admitted to having rectal intercourse. Several other studies,[4, 5, 6] however, failed to demonstrate a significant difference in the frequency of rectal intercourse in women with genital gonorrhea, with or without rectal involvement. The role of anal intercourse in women with rectal gonorrhea is therefore still inconclusive. Auto-inoculation of the rectum by vaginal secretions may be an alternative mode of transmission. The role of such urogenital extension, however, is difficult to support.[7]

In men, anorectal gonorrhea occurs almost exclusively in homosexuals or bisexuals practicing anal intercourse. More than 90% of men with anorectal gonorrhea admit to practicing anal receptive intercourse.[8] Over 10% of patients seen at venereal disease clinics have homosexually acquired gonorrhea, and of all homosexual men with gonorrhea, about 45% will have rectal involvement.[3, 4]

Homosexual men appear to be at much greater risk of acquiring venereally transmitted diseases than are their female homosexual counterparts. Lesbians account for only 1% to 2% of reported cases of venereal diseases, whereas homosexual men account for about 25% to 30%.[9] This difference probably reflects the different nature of the male and female homosexual lifestyle. Lesbians are less often promiscuous and tend to have monogamous relationships. On the other hand, male homosexuals have an average of 6 to 8 different sexual contacts per month.[9, 10, 11] This extreme promiscuity and the high occurrence rate of asymptomatic infection provide a common reservoir and a mode of spread for gonococcal infections.

Clinical Manifestations. Two-thirds of patients with anorectal gonorrhea are asymptomatic.[12, 13] When symptoms do occur, they are non-specific and cannot differentiate gonococcal proctitis from other inflammatory lesions of the rectum. Rectal itching and burning, tenesmus, mucoid discharge, and constipation are the most frequently encountered complaints.

Owens and Hill[12] demonstrated that symptoms in the majority of patients with gonococcal proctitis were non-specific and were probably related to trauma or other proctologic disorders. They showed that the range and prevalence of symptoms were no different in a group of homosexual men with and without rectal gonorrhea. Lebedeff and Hochman[14] reported that 71% of symptomatic patients had mucus in the stool and 62% had rectal discomfort. These symptoms were of low diagnostic yield, since 72% of culture-positive symptomatic patients reported mucoid stools, while 65% of culture-negative patients had similar complaints. Sixty-two per cent of culture-positive and 59% of culture-negative patients complained of rectal discomfort. Acute severe symptoms suggestive of rectal gonorrhea, such as hematochezia, severe rectal pain, copious mucopurulent discharge, or ischiorectal abscesses, occur in less than 5% of patients with acute gonorrheal proctitis. In most cases, symptoms rapidly subside and patients become asymptomatic carriers of the gonococcus.

Symptomatic anorectal gonorrhea may simulate a variety of disorders, including ulcerative colitis, ischemic or radiation proctitis, Crohn's colitis, lymphogranuloma venereum, amebiasis, and syphilis. The only sure means of diagnosis is anorectal culture.

Serious complications of anorectal gonorrhea are rare today. Rectal strictures,[15] perianal abscesses, fistulas, and fissures are uncommon since the advent of effective antibiotics; however, disseminated gonococcemia has been reported after anorectal gonorrhea.[13, 16] Septicemia usually presents as a mild febrile illness with malaise, arthralgias, and petechial or pustular skin lesions. The proctitis is often asymptomatic, but rectal cultures will reveal the gonococcus. In addition, the organism may also be recovered from the blood stream and skin lesions. Subacute presentation is most common. However, an acute illness marked by endocarditis, pericarditis, meningitis, hepatitis, or septic arthritis has also been reported.[16]

Diagnosis. Anoscopic examination is normal in 20% of patients with culture-positive gonococcal proctitis.[14] Generalized erythema with friability of the mucosa, mucopurulent discharge, and superficial erosions limited to the anal canal and rectum may be seen. The distal stratified squamous epithelial mucosa of the anal canal is usually spared. In milder subacute cases, proctoscopic findings may be limited to the proximal anal canal, showing only patchy erythema, granularity, and pus that is expressible from the anal crypts and columns of Morgagni.[4] Brunet and Salberg[17] reported that only 5% of patients complained of mucoid discharge, but erythema, edema, and pus in the crypts were present in 63%. The susceptibility of transitional and columnar epithelium in this area and the lack of easy drainage from these blind-end crypts facilitate infection.

Biopsy may show infiltration with neutrophils, lymphocytes, plasma cells, and monocytes, as well as vascular engorgement. Patchy disorganization of the columnar mucous cells and mucosal destruction may also be present.

Bhattacharyya and Jephcott[18] showed that only 30% of rectal smears for gonococcus were positive in patients with culture-positive anorectal gonorrhea. A positive smear in a symptomatic patient or an asymptomatic high-risk patient may be an indication for immediate therapy. Definitive diagnosis of gonococcal proctitis, however, should be based on culture results. A Gram-stained smear alone is likely to miss the diagnosis of anorectal gonorrhea in 70% of patients.[18]

The symptoms, signs, and the results of a Gram stain on a rectal swab are non-specific or too unreliable to formulate a diagnosis of anorectal gonorrhea. Anorectal cultures using modified Thayer-Martin medium have improved the positive yield over a non-selective medium or a selective medium without trimethoprim.[18, 19]

The Centers for Disease Control suggest that cultures can be obtained blindly without the use of the anoscope. Deheragoda[20] failed to show a significant difference in the number of positive cultures for the gonococcus using a blind technique compared with using a swab through a proctoscope. A cotton swab is placed 1 cm into the anal canal and rotated side to side. If fecal material is obtained, the swab should be discarded and the procedure repeated. Immediate inoculation will yield the best results; if delay is anticipated, the use of commercially available Transgrow medium (Difco Laboratories, Detroit, Michigan) is recommended. If plates can be inoculated immediately but transportation to the laboratory for incubation will be delayed, the inoculated agar plates should be held in a CO_2-rich environment. Multiple sites, including the urethra, pharynx, and cervix, should be cultured whenever anorectal gonorrhea is suspected. False-negative cultures may be as high as 6% to 8% during the initial evaluation,[21] especially in women. In highly suspicious cases, cultures should be repeated.

The use of fluorescein-conjugated antigonococcal antibodies[22, 23] is a rapid and sensitive method of identifying *Neisseria gonorrhoeae* isolated on the surface of a selective medium after overnight incubation. False-negative results are uncommon except for cross-reactions with *Neisseria meningitidis*. This combination of fluorescent antibody and routine culture techniques is more sensitive and rapid than conventional biochemical confirmation of subcultured colonies.

Treatment. The Centers for Disease Control's recommendations for the treatment of anorectal gonorrhea are aqueous procaine penicillin G, 4.8 million units IM, with 1 g of probenecid orally or spectinomycin hydrochloride, 2 g IM.[24, 28] Either regimen gives consistently good results, with failure rates of only 2% to 3%. Treatment with penicillin and probenecid has the additional advantage of being more effective against pharyngeal gonorrhea,[12] a common problem in homosexual men, as well as being effective against incubating syphilis.[29]

Alternative treatment regimens consisting of 3.5 g of oral ampicillin with 1 g of probenecid,[30, 31] or 4 to 6 g of tetracycline taken orally,[30] appear to be equally effective in women with anorectal gonorrhea, but are less effective in homosexual men.[12, 27] Gonococci isolated from homosexual men with anorectal disease appear to be more resistant than those isolated from heterosexuals. Auxotyping also tends to show differing types of infecting gonococci in homosexuals and heterosexuals.[32] Agents such as spectinomycin, tetracycline, kanamycin, and trimethoprim-sulfamethoxazole are best reserved for patients in whom penicillins are contraindicated or ineffective.

Of utmost importance are careful post-treatment cultures taken 7 to 14 days after therapy. Patients should be advised to abstain from sexual activities until the post-treatment culture results are known. True treatment failures require determination of antibiotic sensitivities and retreatment regimens tailored to gonococcal sensitivity. Persistent symptoms after therapy despite evidence of bacteriologic post-treatment cure should prompt further evaluation for other possible agents such as herpes virus, chlamydiae, enteric bacterial pathogens, or protozoans.

The enormous dimensions of the public health problem represented by gonorrhea stimulate an active search for an effective vaccine. A protein filament on the outer surface of virulent gonococci, gonococcal pilus, is a likely antigen. The pili are the mediators of gonococcal attachment to the cell surface and may also function to resist phagocytosis. Investigators have prepared and are testing a purified pilus vaccine.[33] Much more work needs to be done, but the initial results are promising.

***Neisseria meningitidis* Infection.** In addition to being at high risk for infections caused by the gonococcus, homosexuals are also at increased risk for oral, genital, and anorectal infections with *Neisseria meningitidis*. Judson et al.[34] speciated 100 consecutive anal isolates of Neisseria organisms in homosexual men and found 15% to be *N. meningitidis*. In homosexual men, meningococcal infections of the anal canal were significantly more prevalent than urethral infections. In anogenital isolates of Neisseria, recovery of the meningococcus was greater from the anal canal in homosexual men than from the urethra (15% vs. 3.5%) or from the anal canal of women (15% vs. 2.5%).

Oral-genital transmission by fellatio or cunnilingus is the probable mode of transmission of the meningococcus from the pharynx to the urethra, cervix, or anus. Direct support of this hypothesis, however, is lacking. The preferential localization of the meningococcus to the anal canal of homosexuals may be due to a largely unique homosexual practice of oral-anal contact (i.e., "rimming"). Pharyngeal isolates in homosexual men are nearly double the reported frequency in the general population (60% to 70% vs. 30% to 35%). In addition to proctitis, *N. meningitidis* has been reported to cause salpingitis, neonatal meningococcal meningitis, postpartum infections, pelvic inflammatory disease, urethritis, and epididymitis.

Like anorectal gonorrhea, meningococcal proctitis is usually asymptomatic. Judson et al.[34] reported that only 3 of 17 patients with anorectal meningococcal infection had symptoms. The symptoms consisted of mild perianal discomfort and mucopurulent discharge that were non-specific and indistinguishable from symptoms produced by *N. gonorrhoeae*.

Based on limited information,[35, 37] currently recommended treatment regimens for gonococcal proctitis appear to be effective also for meningococcal proctitis. As with gonococcal infection, post-treatment proof of cure is necessary. *N. meningitidis* infection must be added to the growing list of sexually transmitted diseases that have a high frequency of occurrence in the homosexual population.

Syphilis

Epidemiology. Syphilis is again increasing in frequency in the United States and is presently the third most commonly reported sexually transmitted disease.[38] Over only a 3-year period, the number of reported cases increased 33% from 20,399 in 1977 to 27,204 in 1980. In addition, a 50.8% increase in the number of men infected with *Treponema pallidum* has been observed and is thought to be due largely to an increased number of reported cases in homosexuals.[39] In acknowledged homosexuals, the occurrence rate has increased over 100%.[40] The reasons for this major health problem in homosexual men include anonymity and the multiplicity of sexual contacts, lack of physician awareness, and the frequency of asymptomatic syphilitic infections.

Primary anal and rectal syphilis is a well-recognized disease. Reports previously indicated that only 2% to 4% of extragenital chancres occurred in the anal canal.[41, 44] More recently, however, the anus and rectum have been reported to be the primary location for extragenital chancres, and at least 50% of all extragenital chancres occur in homosexual men.[45] In both primary and secondary syphilis, a significant number of patients present with anorectal disease.

Clinical Manifestations

Primary Syphilis. No single feature is pathognomonic for anorectal syphilis. The primary chancre usually appears at the site of sexual contact within 4 weeks of infection, but the incubation period may vary from 10 to 90 days. The primary chancre may be situated at the anal verge or within the anal canal and is usually in the midline. Chancres of the rectal mucosa are rare. There is no truly characteristic appearance of the primary syphilitic chancre. Single or multiple ulcers, indistinguishable from typical genital chancres[41, 42, 46] or ulcerations of anal fissures, may be noted.

In addition, other anorectal lesions associated with early syphilis include polyps,[47, 50] rectal masses,[44, 51, 52] ulcerations,[49, 53, 54] and mucosal friability.[55, 56] The lesion of primary anorectal syphilis may be confused with cryptitis, fistulas, fissures, trauma, or carcinoma.[43, 51, 54, 57] Most often, ulcerations are superficial. The classic indurated painless ulcer seen in primary genital syphilis is found less commonly in anorectal disease.[54] Atypical, bizarre-appearing ulcers may sometimes be confused with Crohn's disease, basal cell and squamous cell carcinomas of the anal canal, and adenocarcinoma of the rectum. The primary anorectal lesion may appear to be trivial and may be overlooked or misdiagnosed. Inguinal adenopathy occurs in the majority of cases and presents as painlessly enlarged, rubbery, discrete, indolent, nontender nodes.

Primary anorectal syphilis may be asymptomatic or produce mild non-specific rectal irritation, soreness, itching, discharge, or painful defecation. Constipation, bleeding, and tenesmus may also be presenting symptoms. It is uncertain to what extent secondary infections or trauma contributes to symptoms in anorectal syphilis.

Diagnosis of anorectal syphilis is based primarily on serology, anoscopy, and dark-field examination of anal lesions. These procedures call for experience and skill in specimen collection and examination. Serologic tests for syphilis do not become positive until a few weeks after the appearance of the primary chancre, and anorectal syphilis will heal spontaneously in 2 to 4 weeks. Primary anorectal syphilis must be differentiated from anal fissures, hemorrhoids, herpes simplex, Crohn's disease, ulcerative colitis, basal and squamous cell carcinomas, and erosions occurring in secondary syphilis.

Secondary Syphilis. The characteristic anorectal lesions of secondary syphilis are condylomata lata. These are multiple, oval, flat, hypertrophic grayish papules frequently found in association with a maculopapular rash of the trunk, extremities, palms, and soles; generalized lymphadenopathy; and pharyngeal and palatal ulceration. Condylomata lata are usually asymptomatic, but on occasion the mucous membranes of the anal canal may become eroded, forming circular patches of grayish color surrounded by an inflamed, erythematous areola (so-called mucous patches). Non-specific perianal irritation or itching may be present. These lesions are teeming with treponemes and diagnosis can be confirmed by dark-field examination of material obtained from the lesions. Serologic tests for syphilis should be positive in almost all cases of secondary syphilis. Anorectal ulcerations, especially when inguinal lymphadenopathy is present, should always suggest the possibility of syphilis.

Tertiary Syphilis. Anorectal involvement in tertiary syphilis is rare. When involvement occurs, it usually takes the form of gummas of the rectum.

Diagnosis. History and physical examination may suggest the possibility of syphilis. Physical examination should include a search for extragenital chancres in the mouth, anus, and rectum, and material from all lesions should be collected for dark-field examination. The diagnosis of anorectal syphilis can be supported by a positive serologic test for syphilis, exclusion of other anorectal infections, demonstration of *T. pallidum* by dark-field examination or in rectal biopsy specimens, the occurrence of a Jarisch-Herxheimer reaction after initiation of therapy, and clinical response to treatment within 1 week to 10 days.[58]

Standard silver stain examination of rectal tissue may demonstrate spirochetes,[56] but difficulty in interpretation may yield false-positive results. Immunofluorescent staining using rabbit anti–*T. pallidum* antiserum to demonstrate the presence of the spirochete in tissue may be useful, especially when dark-field examination is negative.[59, 62] Several studies have shown that immunofluorescent stains for *T. pallidum* yield excellent sensitivity.[63, 65] Fluorescein-conjugated antiserum to *T. pallidum* is commercially available and may be useful when examining tissue scrapings from suspected syphilitic lesions, particularly when dark-field examination is equivocal or negative.

Treatment. Once confirmed, patients with syphilis should avoid all sexual contact until follow-up examinations confirm non-infectivity. Examination and serologic testing of all sexual contacts, with the assistance of the Public Health Department, are essential in the management of all cases of syphilis. Sexual contacts must be traced for at least the previous 3 months in cases of primary syphilis and for 1 year in patients with secondary syphilis.

Penicillin is the antibiotic of choice. For primary and secondary syphilis, benzathine penicillin, 2.4 million units IM as a single injection, is given. For tertiary syphilis or secondary syphilis of greater than 1 year's duration, benzathine penicillin, 2.4 million units IM, should be given weekly for 3 injections. Patients who are allergic to penicillin may be treated with tetracycline hydrochloride, 500 mg 4 times a day for 15 days, or erythromycin in the same dosage and schedule. The possibility of a Jarisch-Herxheimer reaction should be explained to the patient, and careful follow-up is necessary to document eradication of the infection and to detect early reinfection. Examination and serologic testing should be repeated at 3- to 4-month intervals for 2 years.

Herpes

Epidemiology. *Herpes simplex genitalis* is a commonly recognized sexually transmitted disease, with descriptions of herpes proctitis dating back to Jean Astruc, physician to King Louis XV of France in 1736. Herpes infections of the anorectal area are being increasingly recognized, particularly in homosexual men, and are a major public health concern. Although the exact prevalence rate of anorectal herpes virus infections is unknown, Goldmeire[66] reported that herpes virus was responsible for 6% of proctitis occurring in homosexual men. In addition, Quinn et al.[67] reported that after gonorrheal proctitis, herpes virus was the leading cause of symptomatic anorectal disease, occurring in 29% of homosexual men with proctitis.[67]

Most cases of anorectal herpes virus infections are acquired by anal coitus. Oral-anal contact may also be a means of spreading herpes virus infections, and several cases of herpes simplex type I virus causing proctitis have been reported.[67]

Herpes virus infections may be caused by 2 types of herpes simplex virus: (1) *type I* causes fever blisters, conjunctivitis, and encephalitis, but may also be isolated in occasional cases of proctitis; (2) *type II* infections are usually spread by sexual activity. Differentiation of type I and type II herpes virus hominis can be made on epidemiologic, clinical, and biologic characteristics.

An incubation period of from 4 to 20 days[69, 71] will elapse between the time of sexual contact and the appearance of herpetic lesions. A carrier state, in which the patient is asymptomatic but infectious, has been clearly shown for genital herpes infections,[68] but not for anorectal disease.

Clinical Manifestations. Itching and soreness appear around the anus 2 to 7 days after sexual contact and progress rapidly. Often only a few hours elapse before severe anal and rectal pain develops. The pain may radiate to the groin, buttocks, and thighs and may be particularly severe with ambulation. Constipation, tenesmus, and rectal discharge often accompany constitutional symptoms of malaise, fever, chills, and headache. These systemic symptoms are more pronounced in initial herpes virus infections and tend to be mild or absent with recurrences. Acute urinary retention and severe constipation are not infrequent and may be due to a pain-induced reflex spasm of anal and bladder sphincters or to herpes virus infection of the sacral ganglia causing a radiculomyelopathy.

Quinn et al.[67] described 15 patients with anorectal herpes. All 15 experienced anorectal pain, 12 complained of constipation, 11 had rectal discharge, 10 had tenesmus, and 7 experienced constitutional symptoms. Similarly, Jacobs[72] noted the frequency of symptoms as follows: pain in 94%, anal itching in 50%, anal discharge in 31%, and systemic symptoms (chills, fever, malaise) in 19%.

Examination of the perianal area and anal canal reveals clusters of small vesicles or ulcerations (Fig. 121–1). In one-third of the lesions, the perianal skin alone will be affected, one-third will involve the anal canal, and one-third will involve both the perianal skin area and the anal canal.[72] Within a few days, the erythema-encircled vesicles rupture and erode, exposing superficial aphthous ulcerations. These ulcerations may become confluent and form large, irregular ulcers surrounded by erythematous, edematous mucosa. Friability of the distal 10 cm of rectal mucosa with discrete ulcerations may be observed on proctoscopic examination. Histologic examination of the rectal mucosa will reveal non-specific inflammation with ulcerations. Bilateral tender inguinal lymphadenopathy is common, particularly in primary infections (up to 70% of patients with anorectal herpes infections).

Anorectal herpes infections are usually self-limiting. Disseminated disease or severe local complications of anorectal herpes can occur in immunodeficient or malnourished patients.[71] Generally, however, the lesions will start to heal spontaneously in 1 to 3 weeks. Secondarily infected lesions, particu-

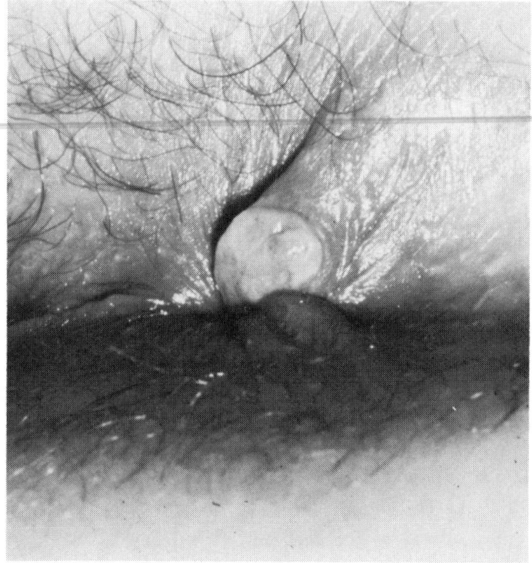

Figure 121–1. Perianal herpetic ulcer. This large confluent ulcer, surrounded by erythema, was markedly painful and tender.

larly those in the anal canal, may take up to 6 weeks to heal. The lesions may become crusted, but healing occurs without scarring. Recurrence is common and may be precipitated by a variety of factors. Although two-thirds of patients with herpes genitalis will have a recurrence within the first year,[73] the relapse or reinfection rate in anorectal herpes infections is unknown. Prior infections do not confer immunity.

Diagnosis. Clinical diagnosis can be confirmed by inoculating appropriate tissue culture material, such as human embryo lung cells, and observing for a characteristic cytopathic effect produced by the virus within 24 to 48 hours.

Scrapings from the base of an unroofed vesicle or ulcer can be stained with Giemsa, hematoxylin and eosin, or by the Papanicolaou method and observed for intranuclear inclusion bodies (Cowdry type A) within multinucleated giant cells.

Antibodies to the herpes virus usually appear 1 to 4 weeks after acute infection. Unless the patient has been previously infected with the herpes virus, serologic tests during the acute infection will be negative. A negative serologic test followed by a positive convalescent phase test is indicative of primary infection. Both microneutralization and a complement fixation test can be used to detect antibodies to the herpes virus.[74, 75]

Treatment. Symptomatic treatment with sitz baths, analgesics, and suppositories is the mainstay of therapy. In patients with perianal skin lesions, sitz baths may aggravate the lesion by causing increased maceration and tissue breakdown. Steroid-containing lotions and suppositories are *best avoided*, since they may *potentiate* the infection. Lesions should be kept clean by applying normal saline or taking sitz baths. Analgesics should be prescribed to relieve pain.

Trials of 5-iodo-2′-deoxyuridine (IDU), vaccines, and autoimmunization have been disappointing.[71] The use of acyclovir, which has proved beneficial in genital and labial herpetic lesions, still awaits confirmation of value in anorectal infections. Lesions on exposed perianal surfaces can be treated by photoinactivation using neutral red or proflavine heterotricyclic dye solutions.[70, 77] These solutions are painted onto unroofed vesicles and then exposed to a 15-watt fluorescent light for 10 minutes. Light exposures are repeated a few hours later and again 24 hours later. Symptomatic relief will usually occur within 24 hours. The major drawback to this technique is that many perianal and all anal canal lesions are inaccessible to photoinactivation.

The likelihood of recurrent attacks should be explained to the patient. Since herpes virus infections and syphilis frequently occur together,[78] each patient must be examined carefully to exclude the possibility of syphilis and other sexually transmitted diseases.[67]

Lymphogranuloma Venereum

Lymphogranuloma venereum (LGV) (lymphogranuloma inguinale, lymphopathia venereum, Nicolas-Favre disease, poradenitis nostras, granulomatous lymphomatosis, Frei's disease) is a rare disorder in the United States. It is caused by *Chlamydia trachomatis*, immunotypes L_1, L_2, and L_3. These obligate intracellular microorganisms are closely related to bacteria. Other immunotypes are known to cause trachoma, psittacosis, and inclusion conjunctivitis in addition to genital and perinatal infections. Anogenital LGV infection has been recognized since 1932[79] but is still infrequently diagnosed.

Clinical Manifestations. After an incubation period of 5 to 28 days, either a small single or multiple painless vesicular lesions appear at the site of inoculation. These resolve quickly and often go unnoticed. Primary lesions are most often vaginal or cervical in women and on the foreskin, meatus, or urethra in men. The initial vesicular lesions may rupture, leaving a grayish ulcer. Three to 6 weeks following the appearance of the initial lesion, tender, fluctuant adenopathy, often with overlying superficial cellulitis, will develop ("buboes"). Frequently, systemic symptoms of fever, malaise, headaches, arthralgias, and anorexia occur. The organism spreads by way of the pelvic and perirectal lymphatics, often causing pelvic pain. Chronic inflammation may result in lymphatic blockage, edema, fistulas, and rectal strictures. Anorectal involvement with LGV is more common in women, but is also being reported in increasing frequency in homosexual men.[80, 81]

A history of direct exposure or spread from a primary genital source followed by tender inguinal adenopathy is common. Rectal and vaginal discharge, perirectal fistula or abscess, cryptitis, and hematochezia are frequent complaints. Change in bowel habits and abdominal pain are uncommon unless a rectal stricture develops. However, progressive rectal stricture, a late stage of LGV infection, can occur in the absence of symptoms.

Physical examination may reveal inguinal adenopathy, left lower abdominal tenderness or pelvic tenderness, perianal granuloma, fistulas, rhagades, and local or dependent edema.

Diagnosis. Digital rectal examination may be normal in the early stages of infection. After the disease is well established, however, stenosis may be easily detected with the examining finger. The strictures that develop are fixed, firm, and unyielding but are not characteristically as hard as carcinomatous strictures.

On proctosigmoidoscopy, acute proctitis due to LGV is marked by a friable, ulcerated, bleeding mucosa with characteristic macular, papular, and vesicular lesions appearing together. Purulent exudate may be noted with secondary infections. Cicatricial changes may involve the lumen circumferentially, causing strictures.

Three characteristic radiographic appearances of LGV are described: (1) low strictures within a few centimeters of the anus with narrowing of the anorectal region, often resulting in eradication of the rectal ampulla; (2) irregular conical constriction with ulcerations and fistulas and non-distensible rectal walls; and (3) long (5 to 15 cm) strictures with the mucosa above the stricture appearing normal.

The Frei test will become positive 7 to 40 days after the onset of adenitis. Once positive, it will remain so for life. Its usefulness in diagnosing proctitis due to LGV is limited by its cross-reactivity with other non–LGV chlamydial strains that are also capable of causing acute proctitis.

A complement fixation test greater than 1:32 is positive in 80% of patients with LGV infections.[82] A 4-fold rise in serum titers is considered evidence of recent infection. Radiation proctitis, ulcerative proctitis, and granulomas from amebic and tuberculous rectal infection may simulate LGV proctitis. These can usually be differentiated by serologic, proctoscopic, and histologic means. Confusion may arise in differentiating *Crohn's disease with isolated rectal involvement* from LGV because both may histologically reveal granulomas, crypt abscesses, and giant cells. Response to a therapeutic trial of absorbable antibiotics may be of some help in establishing a diagnosis of LGV over Crohn's disease.

Treatment

Medical. LGV infections may spontaneously resolve without therapy or sequelae. General supportive measures, including bowel rest, low residue diet, analgesics for pain, and relief of constipation, may be necessary. Antibiotics, particularly tetracyclines, erythromycin, and chloramphenicol, are useful to control symptoms.[83] Fluctuant buboes should be aspirated, not incised.

Surgical. Surgical intervention is employed less often than in the past. Early administration of antibiotics appears to prevent or significantly reduce the frequency of stricture formation.[83] Moreover, rectal strictures may be mechanically dilated, further decreasing the need for their surgical correction. Hence, surgery should be reserved for: (1) impassable rectal strictures not responsive to medical treatment; (2) abscess formations; (3) persistent fistulas; (4) gross destruction of the anal channel, anal sphincter, and perineum; and (5) complicating carcinoma.[84]

Sexual contacts of all patients with lymphogranuloma venereum should be screened.

Non-LGV Chlamydial Infections

Homosexual men appear to be at increased risk for both LGV and non-LGV chlamydial infections. It is now recognized that the latter strains can cause a proctitis that tends to be mild and self-limited and is often asymptomatic.

Epidemiology. In a study by Quinn et al.,[85] *Chlamydia trachomatis* was isolated from 11 of 96 symptomatic homosexual men with proctitis and from 3 of 75 asymptomatic homosexual men. Fecal leukocytes were present in all patients with positive cultures. The diagnosis of *Chlamydia trachomatis* proctitis is based primarily on isolation of the organism from the rectum. Similarity in antibody response in patients infected with LGV and with non-LGV chlamydial strains and the high prevalence (35%) of these antibodies in the homosexual population render serologic diagnosis inaccurate. However, seroconversion or a 4-fold rise in titer in paired serum samples are useful diagnostic indices.

Clinical Manifestations. The spectrum of rectal infections caused by *Chlamydia trachomatis* ranges from asymptomatic to chronic severely ulcerated granulomatous proctitis. The clinical presentation and histologic appearance depend on the infecting strain, with non-LGV chlamydial strains causing asymptomatic or mild proctitis. Rectal infections due to *Chlamydia trachomatis* appear to have a high occurrence rate in homosexual and bisexual men practicing anal-receptive intercourse.[85,86]

Treatment. Treatment with 2- to 3-week courses of tetracycline may be expected to dissipate symptoms and restore the lower bowel to normal, as observed on proctosigmoidoscopic examination.

Condylomata Acuminata

Condylomata acuminata (anal warts) were described by physicians of the ancient world and believed to be caused by anal intercourse (Fig. 121–2). Anal warts are caused by a papilloma virus and usually appear as minute pink papules that rapidly grow into grouped, pedunculated, filiform lesions. These "cauliflower-like" lesions may encircle the anus and extend into the anal canal to the pectinate line. Rarely, lesions appear on the rectal mucosa. Diagnosis is simple because of the classic appearance of the lesions, but these must be differentiated from condylomata lata of secondary syphilis. Also, anal warts may occasionally simulate carcinoma.

The relationship between anal warts and homosexuality is unclear. There is a tacit belief that anal warts are common in homosexuals, but published data refer to small numbers of patients. Still, 80% of men and 50% of women admit to anal intercourse preceding the appearance of anal warts.[87, 88] In a small percentage of men and in 20% of women, anal warts appear to be a consequence of genital warts.[87, 88] The relationship between anal and skin warts is obscure, but 15% of patients presenting with anal warts have warts elsewhere.[87]

Contact tracing of patients with anal warts does not support the concept of sexual transmissibility. The pathophysiology of anal warts remains ill-defined, but trauma in the form of anal intercourse in the presence of a wart virus appears necessary in most cases.

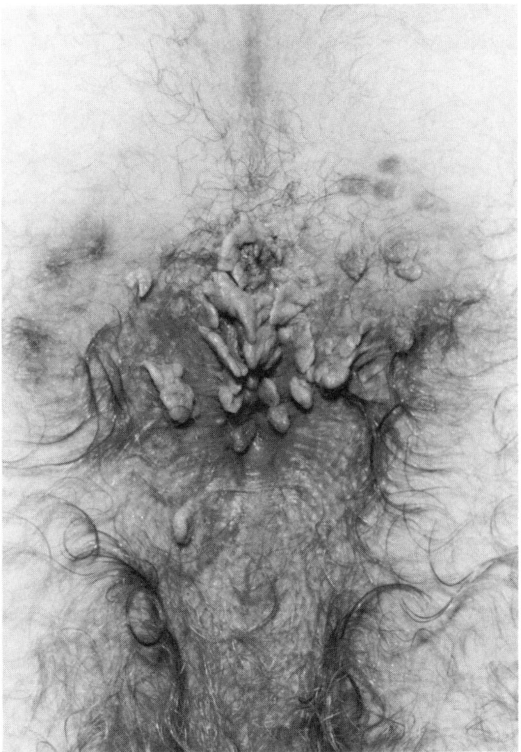

Figure 121–2. Condylomata acuminata. These cauliflower-like lesions encircle the anus. An area of superficial ulceration is also present in the midline above the anus.

Treatment. Warts that are localized or small are best treated by a solution of 25% podophyllin applied on alternate days. Good hygiene is important to prevent secondary infections and damage to surrounding normal tissue. Extensive warts or warts in the anal canal not accessible to topical treatment should be surgically removed using electrocauterization. There is a strong tendency for warts to recur, and regular follow-up may be needed.

Miscellaneous Infections

In addition to the classic sexually transmitted diseases, homosexuals appear to be at increased risk for a variety of enteric infections including amebiasis, giardiasis, Shigella enteritis, Campylobacter enteritis and proctitis, and both type A and type B viral hepatitis.[89–98] The morbidity of these infections does not appear to be any greater in homosexuals than in the heterosexual population.

Acquired Immune Deficiency Syndrome (AIDS)

An acquired cellular immunodeficiency (Chapter 243), expressed in various ways, has been noted to develop in homosexuals.[99–105] Opportunistic infections develop that rarely occur in the absence of immunodeficiency states. *Pneumocystis carinii* pneumonia,[99, 100, 104, 105] extensive mucosal candidiasis,[99] and chronic perianal ulcerative herpes simplex infections,[101] all previously thought to occur predominantly in immunosuppressed states, have been reported in homosexuals with T-cell defects. In addition, an increased frequency of autoimmune thrombocytopenic purpura has been observed in homosexual men.[106] This clinical constellation has been termed *acquired immune deficiency syndrome* (AIDS).

It is possible that a sexually transmitted infection may play a critical role in the pathogenesis of the immunodeficiency. To date, however, spontaneous recovery of cellular immunocompetence has not been described, and recurrent opportunistic infections are not uncommon. In addition, the appearance of Kaposi's sarcoma in large numbers of young homosexual men[102, 103] has raised new concerns regarding the immunocompetence exhibited.

In 1981 the Centers for Disease Control (CDC) alerted the medical community to the unexplained outbreak of *Pneumocystis carinii* pneumonia and Kaposi's sarcoma in homosexual men. By 1983, more than 1900 cases of AIDS were reported to the CDC.[107] Over 750 patients died, resulting in a case-fatality ratio exceeding 60% 1 year after diagnosis.[108]

The salient features of AIDS have simultaneously become clearer. The patients are typically (more than 70%) young homosexual men living in large cities, many of whom have histories of drug use. A prodrome, lasting weeks to months, of weakness, anorexia, lassitude, and generalized non-specific lymphadenopathy often progresses to specific opportunistic infections or the discovery of Kaposi's sarcoma. Multiple simultaneous infections that respond poorly to treatment and have a high tendency to relapse are common. The major populations that appear to be at greatest risk are: (1) homosexual or bisexual men with multiple sexual partners (75% of the reported AIDS cases); (2) IV drug abusers (15%); (3) recent Haitian immigrants (6%); and (4) hemophiliacs using factor VIII products (less than 1%). In somewhat less than 5% of AIDS cases no apparent associated risk factors can be identified.[109–109b] Sexual contacts of AIDS patients and sexual contacts of high risk populations should also be considered at increased risk for developing AIDS.[108]

AIDS should be suspected in high risk patients presenting with unexplained weakness, anorexia, weight loss, lassitude, lymphadenopathy, or (in patients under 60 years of age) Kaposi's sarcoma. Characteristic of AIDS are opportunistic infections or infections caused by unusual pathogens or pathogens of low-grade virulence. More than a dozen microbial species causing serious life-threatening infections in AIDS patients have been identified. These include disseminated cytomegalovirus or herpes simplex virus infections, *Mycobacterium avium-intracellulare, Pneumocystis carinii, Toxoplasma gondii,* and Cryptosporidium.[99, 105]

Several microbial infections affect the gastrointestinal tract in patients with AIDS. One is *candidiasis* (Chapter 57). Oral and esophageal involvement by Candida organisms in patients with AIDS is frequent and often prolonged and refractory to treatment. Another disturbance seen in AIDS patients that affects the gastrointestinal tract is *cryptosporidiosis* (Chapter 232). Of all the gastrointestinal disorders associated with AIDS, cryptosporidiosis is the most ominous in its effects on morbidity and mortality. Other gastrointestinal infections include *giardiasis, amebiasis, coccidiosis, perianal herpes virus infections,* and *herpes proctitis*. In some AIDS patients with these infections, apparent resistance to therapy may actually be reinfection from sexual contacts.

Etiology. Cellular immunodepression causes a "breach" in the host defenses and results in opportunistic infection and altered immune surveillance (see Chapter 243). Clinical evidence in support of a cellular defect is demonstrated by lymphopenia, T-lymphocyte depletion, reversal of the T-helper to T-suppression cell ratio, cutaneous anergy, decreased lymphocyte proliferative responses to mitogens and antigens, and a defect in the natural killer cell activity.[110–110b] In contrast, humoral immunity remains intact, and often hypergammaglobulinemia is noted. Complement levels are also normal.

The cause of the cellular immune dysfunction is unknown. Most evidence points toward a transmissible agent requiring either intimate direct contact involving mucosal surfaces (as by sexual contact) or parenteral spread (as may occur among drug abusers or hemophiliacs receiving factor VIII). Direct transmission other than by sexual contact or contact with blood products has not been documented. The disease has not been reported to spread to health care personnel; however, this should be interpreted with caution since the period between contact and clinical symptoms may exceed 2 years. The CDC has initiated a study of health care personnel who have had documented parenteral or mucous membrane exposure to blood of confirmed or suspected AIDS patients.

Evidence of previous or current cytomegalovirus (CMV) infection is common in reported AIDS cases. Giraldo et al.[111–113] have demonstrated a serologic association between Kaposi's sarcoma and CMV infections. In AIDS patients with *Pneumocystis carinii* pneumonia, CMV is often concomitantly found in lung biopsy specimens.[114] CMV also causes immunosuppression in mice and humans and can persist for months in high titers in the semen.[115] In renal transplant recipients, Rubin et al.[116] have shown that CMV is associated with leukopenia and opportunistic infections. In addition, CMV has been shown to induce transient abnormalities in cellular immunity.[117] Homosexual men have higher rates of serologic evidence of CMV infections than their heterosexual counterparts.[118]

Despite the impressive array of suggestive evidence represented by the foregoing observations, other studies have failed to support an association between AIDS and CMV infection.[100] The major shortcoming of the CMV hypothesis is its failure to explain why this syndrome is apparently new. Homosexuality dates back to antiquity. Why the emergence of AIDS now?

Additional hypotheses regarding the etiology of AIDS have implicated the common use of nitrite inhalants ("*poppers*") by homosexual men to intensify orgasm. A new or mutant unidentified transmissible agent or multiple infections causing "immune overload" have also been proposed as underlying causes. A report has identified evidence of *human T-cell leukemia virus* (HTLV) infection in 19 of 75 patients (25%) with AIDS and in 6 of 23 patients (26%) with lymphadenopathy syndrome alone.[122] These HTLV agents have been associated with certain types of adult T-cell lymphoproliferative disorders and are known to be transmissible by close contact.[123]

Human T-cell leukemia lymphoma virus III (HTLV-III)[123a–d] has been isolated from T cells (Chapter 99) of patients with AIDS or pre-AIDS and appears to be the specific etiologic agent in AIDS. The virus has been grown in cell culture, and at least 90% of AIDS or pre-AIDS patients have antibodies to it. Neither the virus nor antibodies to it are present in homosexual or heterosexual men without AIDS. Another group at the Pasteur Institute in Paris has also isolated a virus from AIDS patients, but it is not known if this is the same virus.[123e]

HTLV-III is a retrovirus (Chapter 100, Viruses). Retroviruses have their genetic information in the ribonucleic acid fraction (RNA) and they contain the enzyme reverse transcriptase connecting RNA to deoxyribonucleic acid (DNA). Many retroviruses depress immune function.

The original HTLV virus, HTLV-I, has been repeatedly isolated from a form of human leukemia and lymphoma that affects mature T cells. HTLV-I is epidemiologically associated with this type of malignancy in certain areas of the world, including southern Japan, parts of the Caribbean, South America, and Africa. A similar virus, HTLV-II, has been isolated in rare instances from patients with hairy cell leukemia.

The HTLV-III virus specifically attacks and kills the helper T cells in blood that are known to be destroyed by AIDS. Its biochemical and immunologic properties are consistent with the predicted characteristics of an AIDS virus and with evidence suggesting that AIDS is a sexually transmitted disease or transmitted by way of blood products from AIDS or pre-AIDS patients.

The HTLV-III antibody in blood recognizes the envelope of the virus. High levels of antibody almost certainly indicate infection with the virus with reproduction in individual T cells. Elevated antibody levels, however, do not necessarily mean active disease; such levels may signify past infection.

HTLV-III virus in the initial reports[123a–d] was isolated from 26 of 72 adult and juvenile patients with AIDS, 18 of 21 pre-AIDS patients, and 3 of 4 normal mothers of juveniles with AIDS. In the controls, none of 115

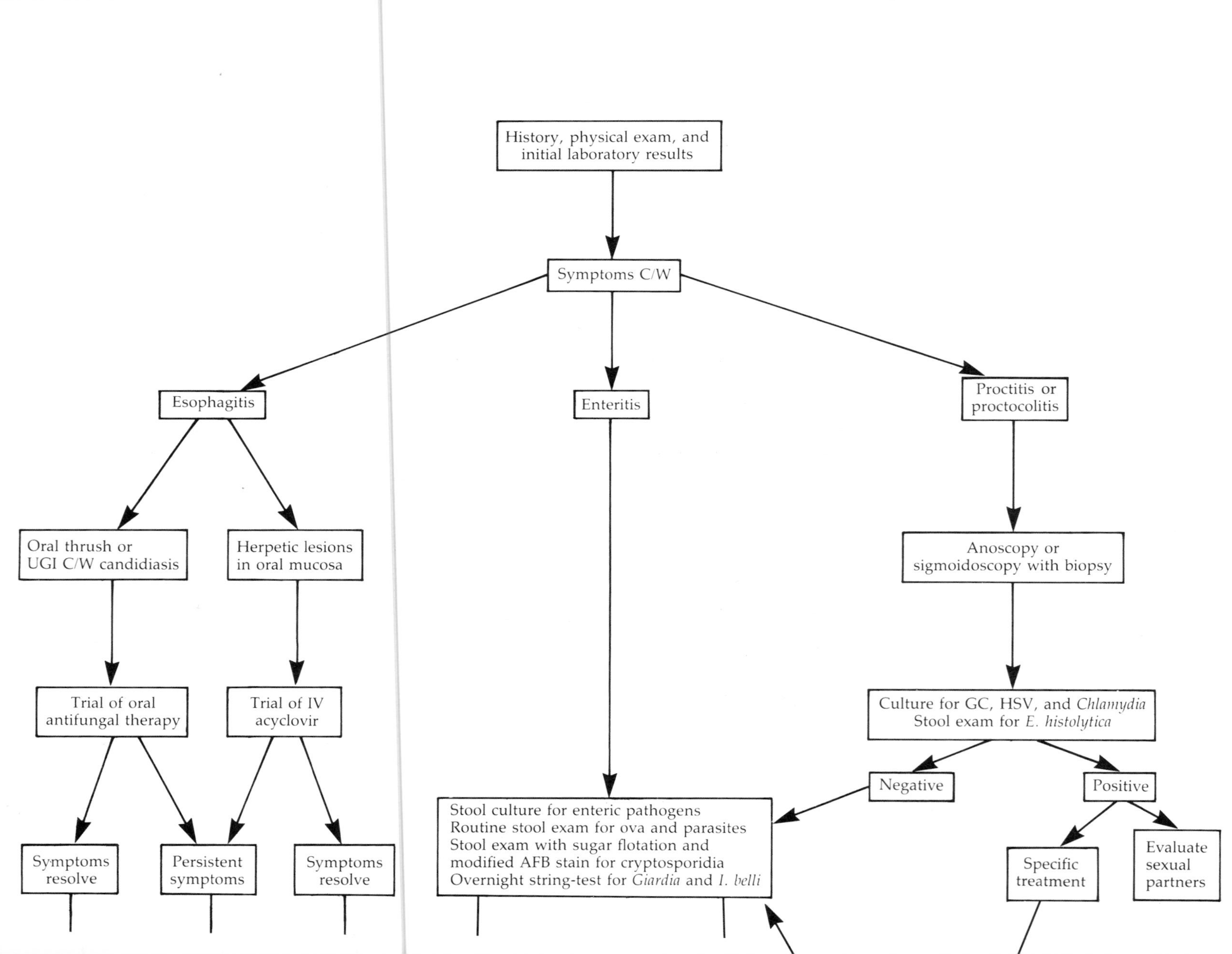
History, physical exam, and initial laboratory results
Symptoms C/W
Esophagitis
Enteritis
Proctitis or proctocolitis
Oral thrush or UGI C/W candidiasis
Herpetic lesions in oral mucosa
Anoscopy or sigmoidoscopy with biopsy
Trial of oral antifungal therapy
Trial of IV acyclovir
Culture for GC, HSV, and Chlamydia
Stool exam for E. histolytica
Negative
Positive
Stool culture for enteric pathogens
Routine stool exam for ova and parasites
Stool exam with sugar flotation and modified AFB stain for cryptosporidia
Overnight string-test for Giardia and I. belli
Symptoms resolve
Persistent symptoms
Symptoms resolve
Specific treatment
Evaluate sexual partners

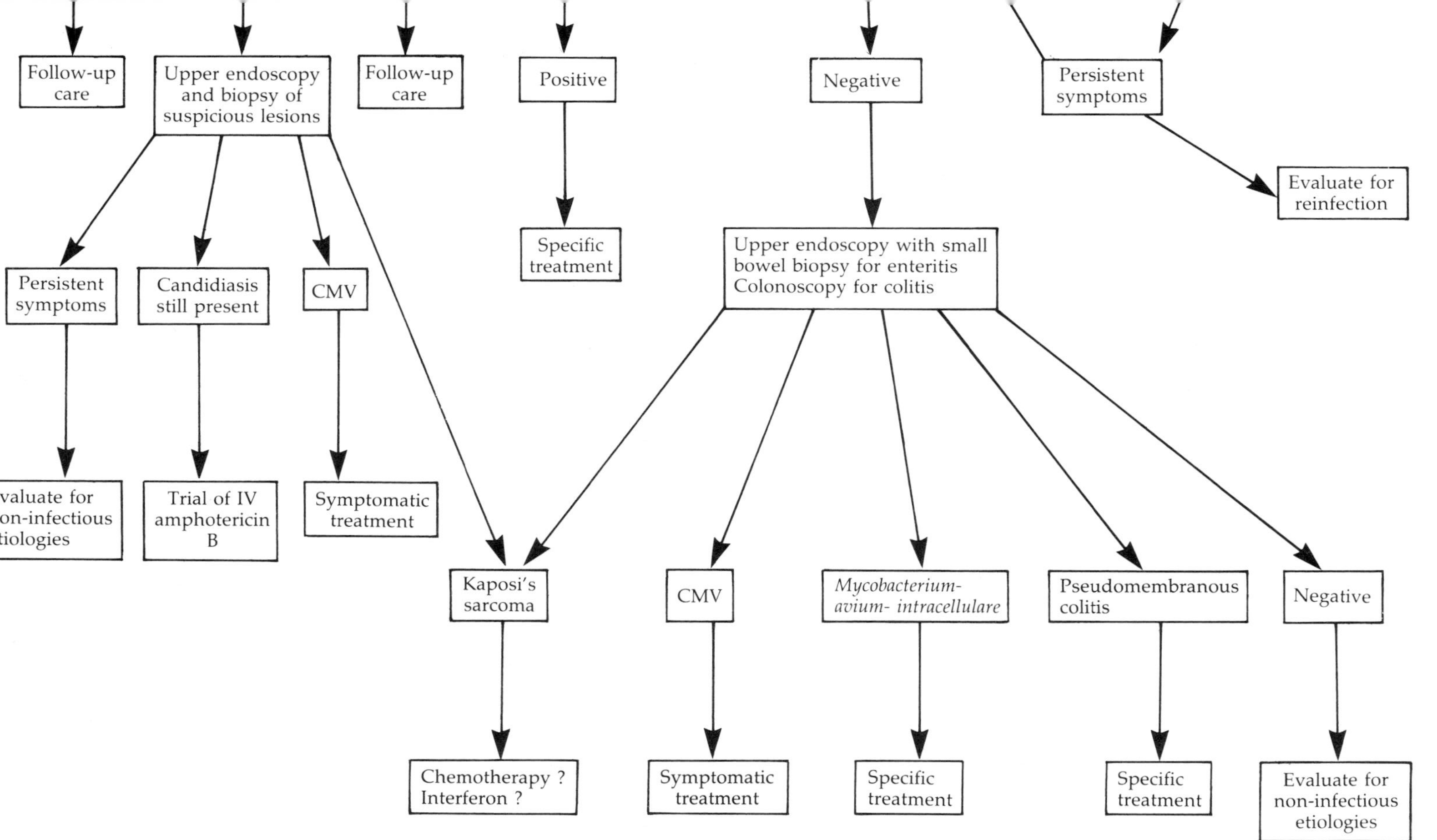

Figure 121–3. Algorithm for the diagnosis and management of intestinal infections in AIDS patients. (Prepared by J. Chan, M.D., University of Miami School of Medicine and partially adapted from Quinn TC et al. N Engl J Med 1983; 309:576–82.)

heterosexual men and only one of 22 homosexual men had this virus in their blood. While antibodies are present in at least 90% of patients with AIDS or pre-AIDS, normal subjects have very low levels of this antibody or lack the antibody altogether.

A method for growing HTLV-III virus in the laboratory in bulk amounts has been developed as a consequence of the finding of a special cell strain of T cells that can produce this virus in large amounts and not be killed by it. This has enabled the biochemical and immunologic characteristics of the proteins and genes of the virus to be determined. It has also provided a basis for detecting antibody to the virus and for large-scale testing for the antibody in suspect populations.[123a,c,d] At present, it has yet to be established what proportion of individuals at high risk for development of AIDS (IV drug abusers, hemophiliacs, blood transfusion recipients, and close heterosexual contacts of high risk subjects) have antibodies to this virus.

Development of a specific vaccine is a distant possibility with the availability now of bulk quantities of the HTLV-III virus.

Approach to Evaluation of Intestinal Infections. Since gastrointestinal lesions in patients with AIDS may result from a variety of pathogens and can involve the alimentary tract from the mouth to the anus, a systematic and comprehensive evaluation is always desirable and often is necessary. The algorithm presented in Figure 121–3 is one approach that has been found to be helpful at the University of Miami.

Esophagitis. Since the most common infectious causes of esophagitis in this patient population are either Candida or herpes simplex, an empiric trial of therapy is acceptable if suggestive lesions are found in the oral mucosa. Oral antifungal therapy can be either nystatin, liquid mouthwash with swallow, or ketoconazole, 200 mg twice daily. Mucocutaneous herpes simplex virus (HSV) infection usually responds to a 7- to 10-day course of IV acyclovir in a usual dose of 250 mg every 8 hours.

Upper gastrointestinal endoscopy and biopsy of suspicious lesions are necessary for those patients who fail to respond to the empiric therapy, or for those who have no suggestive lesions. Barium esophageal or upper gastrointestinal radiographic study may reveal abnormal mucosa but the findings are often non-specific. If persistent candidiasis is shown by endoscopy, a trial of IV amphotericin B in a dose of 30 mg daily for 10 days may be indicated. Cytomegalovirus (CMV) infection can be diagnosed histopathologically by the presence of one or more cells with typical nuclear or cytoplasmic inclusions. CMV culture or serologic studies are not helpful.

Enteritis. Attempts to isolate or identify pathogens from stool by both culture and examination should precede all contrast radiography. Recognition of pathogens is more difficult with the presence of barium in the stool. Stool samples should be examined microscopically for ova and parasites, both directly and after formalin concentration. Special procedures, such as sugar flotation, centrifugation, and modified acid-fast (AFB) stain are required to detect the oocyst of the protozoan cryptosporidium. Many pathogens that involve the duodenum and upper jejunum can best be detected by examining the mucosal contents removed from a nylon string left overnight in the upper intestinal tract (the so-called "string test" or "Enterotest"). Pathogens, such as *Giardia lamblia, Isospora belli,* and occasionally Strongyloides, are better detected with this method.

Infection by *Mycobacterium-avium-intracellulare* (MAI) in the AIDS patient is usually diffuse and overwhelming. The organism has been isolated from blood or bone marrow cultures; however, its association with intestinal symptoms can be established only by demonstrating the organism in biopsy of the intestine.

Proctitis or Proctocolitis. Biopsy of any suspicious perianal or anorectal lesion should be performed together with anoscopy or sigmoidoscopy. Histopathologic examination is the only reliable method for establishing the diagnosis of CMV proctitis or granuloma inguinale. The latter diagnosis is made by the demonstration of Donovan bodies (large macrophages that contain large numbers of *Calymmatobacterium granulomatis*). Painless ulcers that are accessible should be examined under dark-field microscopy. Culture for gonococci (GC), HSV, and lymphogranuloma venereum (LGV) strain of *Chlamydia trachomatis* should be obtained from suspicious lesions. If cultures for Chlamydia are not available, determination of antibodies to *C. trachomatis* may be helpful. Evaluation and treatment of sexual partners are required to prevent reinfection.

Kaposi's Sarcoma. In 1872, Kaposi[124] described "idiopathic multiple pigmented sarcoma of the skin," since eponymously designated *Kaposi's sarcoma*. Classic Kaposi's sarcoma affects elderly males, often of Jewish or Italian descent, causing dark blue or purple-brown plaques or nodules that commonly appear on the extremities (Chapter 18). The disease follows an indolent course, although in a small percentage of patients early dissemination occurs. Extracutaneous involvement most frequently is found in the lymph nodes, the gastrointestinal tract, and the lungs. Early visceral involvement occurs more commonly in an aggressive form of Kaposi's sarcoma seen in young Africans and renal transplant recipients.[125–127]

The natural history of this tumor in patients with AIDS differs from the classically described dermatologic disease, appearing similar instead to the aggressive form seen in Africans and renal transplant patients.[128] Widespread dermatologic involvement, early visceral and lymph node involvement, and a rapidly progressive course resistant to therapy are characteristic of Kaposi's sarcoma in AIDS patients.

Gastrointestinal tract involvement can be demonstrated in 40% to 60% of AIDS patients with Kaposi's sarcoma.[129–130a] Often the initial lesions will develop in the gastrointestinal tract, where they may be detected by contrast roentgenography (Fig. 121–4) or endoscopy (Fig. 121–5).[131, 131a] Any area of the gastrointestinal tract may be involved, but lesions in

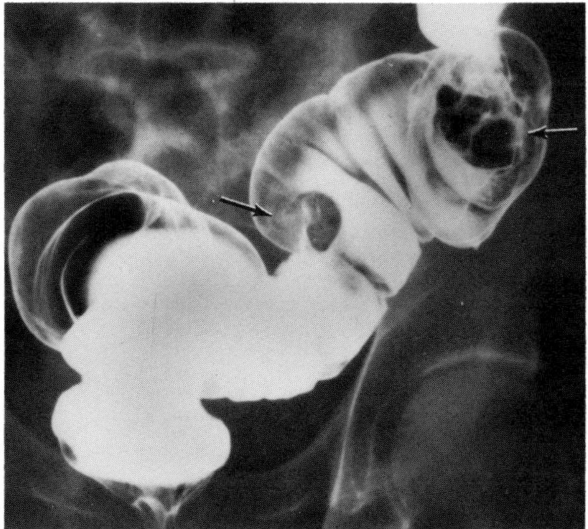

Figure 121–4. Double contrast barium enema in a patient with AIDS and Kaposi's sarcoma. Note the multiple locations of tumor *(arrows)*.

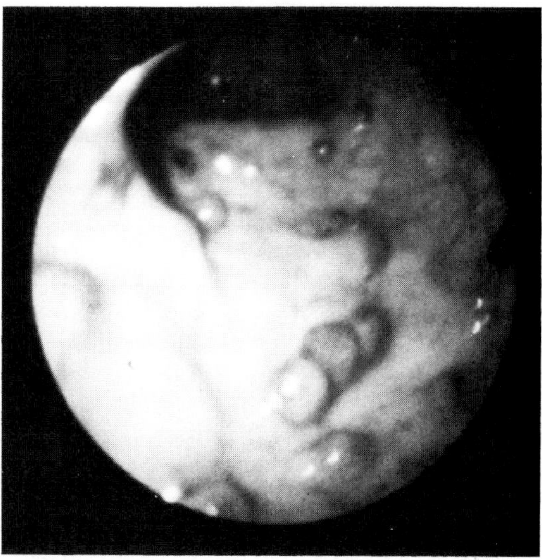

Figure 121–5. Colonoscopic view of Kaposi's sarcoma.

the stomach, small bowel, and distal colon occur most often.[130, 131a–133] Bleeding, perforation, diarrhea, protein-losing enteropathy, and intussusception may occur.[134–136] Generally, however, gastrointestinal lesions are asymptomatic.

The histology of the lesion varies, depending on the stage of evolution. In early stages, the lesion resembles a hemangioma and may be mistaken for any vascular abnormality. Later stages of the lesion show local necrosis and areas of fibrosis. The presence of spindle-shaped cells, demonstrating different degrees of differentiation, in a matrix of vascular structures is the typical histologic finding. Hemorrhage into the surrounding tissue and infiltration by lymphocytes, histiocytes, and mitotic figures may also be present.

The association of Kaposi's sarcoma with a second primary malignancy has been reported in up to 20% of cases.[137] These second primary tumors are frequently lymphosarcoma, Hodgkin's disease, lymphatic leukemia, or adenocarcinoma of the gastrointestinal tract.

Diagnosis. *Barium roentgen studies* may demonstrate abnormalities compatible with Kaposi's sarcoma, but frequently show nonspecific abnormalities or abnormalities similar to those seen in granulomatous colitis or adenocarcinoma.[129] Small flat lesions or small submucosal nodules are more likely to be detected by endoscopy than by radiologic examination. A characteristic abnormality detected on upper gastrointestinal roentgenograms is multiple random submucosal nodules ranging in size from a few millimeters to several centimeters. In larger lesions, central umbilication, described as "bulls-eye lesions" may occasionally be noted. Large gastric lesions may radiologically resemble sessile or occasionally pedunculated polyps. Thickened, nodular, irregular rugal folds are frequently encountered. The duodenal mucosa may also demonstrate submucosal nodules or plaque-like lesions.

Double contrast barium enema examinations demonstrate nodular submucosal defects ranging in size from 2 to 3 mm to 3 to 5 cm (Fig. 121–4). Occasionally, these nodules may coalesce and infiltrate circumferentially to form a narrowed, nodular, rigid segment simulating adenocarcinoma. The presence of skip areas of neoplastic infiltration may result in a radiographic presentation consistent with granulomatous colitis.

Computed tomography is likely to demonstrate retroperitoneal adenopathy, hepatomegaly, splenomegaly, or increased thickness of the rectal wall caused by tumor infiltration.

Endoscopic examination (Fig. 121–5) and *biopsy* are the most accurate and sensitive means of establishing gastrointestinal tract involvement in Kaposi's sarcoma.[129] Endoscopy appears to be a relatively safe procedure in this patient population, but some reservations do apply. First, Kaposi's sarcoma is a vascular tumor. It appears, however, that endoscopic biopsies do not carry an undue risk of hemorrhage. Second, patients with AIDS who develop Kaposi's sarcoma are immunocompromised hosts. Endoscopy in this population may carry a significant risk of infection. Third, and perhaps most significant, is the transmissibility of AIDS. Can endoscopy be a source of person-to-person transmission of AIDS? Are standard endoscopic cleansing techniques and gas sterilization sufficient to prevent possible transmission? Does the endoscopic procedure represent a risk to health care personnel? These questions are unanswered. Certainly, caution dictates that unnecessary or marginally indicated procedures should not be performed.

Endoscopy Precautions. The CDC has formulated interim guidelines for hospital personnel caring for patients with AIDS.[138] These interim guidelines include precautions that should be exercised in the endoscopy suite. In general, procedures appropriate for patients known to be infected with hepatitis B virus are advised when caring for patients known or suspected to have AIDS. Specifically, patient care and laboratory personnel should take precautions to avoid direct contact of skin and mucous membranes with blood, blood products, excretions, secretions, and tissues of such persons. In addition, gloves and gowns and goggles should be worn during the endoscopic procedure to avoid direct skin contact and clothing soilage by body fluids. No definitive statement can be made regarding care of endoscopes. The CDC has outlined precautions for employing reusable items.[138] Cleansing, decontamination, and gas sterilization are clearly advisable.

References

1. Sohn N, Ribilotti JG Jr. The gay bowel syndrome. Am J Gastroenterol 1977; 67:478–84.
2. Klein EJ, Fisher LS, Chow AW, Guz LB. Anorectal gonococcal infection. Ann Intern Med 1977; 86:340–6.
3. Pariser H, Marino AF. Gonorrhea—frequently unrecognized reservoirs. South Med J 1970; 63:198–201.
4. Scott J, Stone AH. Some observations on the diagnosis of rectal gonorrhea in both sexes using a selective culture medium. Br J Vener Dis 1966; 42:103–6.
5. Heimans AL. Culture of gonococci from the rectum on Thayer-Martin selective medium. Dermatologica 1966; 133:319–24.
6. Dans PE. Gonococcal anorectal infection. Clin Obstet Gynecol 1975; 18:103–19.
7. Odegaard K. Trichomonas vaginalis infection and rectal gonorrhea in women. Acta Derm Venereol 1972; 52:326–8.
8. Pariser H. Asymptomatic gonorrhea. Med Clin North Am 1972; 56:1127–32.
9. Ekstrom K. Patterns of sexual behavior in relation to venereal disease. Br J Vener Dis 1970; 46:93–5.
10. Webster B. Venereal disease control in the United States of America. Br J Vener Dis 1970; 46:406–11.
11. Harnisch JP, Wiesner PJ, Holmes KK. Clinical epidemiology of VD: The role of the homosexual. Cutis 1972; 9:221–4.
12. Owens RL, Hill JL. Rectal and pharyngeal gonorrhea in homosexual men. JAMA 1972; 220:1315–8.
13. Harkness AH. Anorectal gonorrhoea. Proc R Soc Med 1948; 41:476–8.
14. Lebedeff DA, Hochman EB. Rectal gonorrhea in men: Diagnosis and treatment. Ann Intern Med 1980; 92:463–6.
15. Hayes HT. Gonorrhea of the anus and rectum. JAMA 1929; 93:1878–81.
16. Holmes KK, Counts GW, Beaty HN. Disseminated gonococcal infection. Ann Intern Med 1971; 74:979–93.
17. Brunet WM, Salberg JB. Gonococcus infection of the anus and rectum in women: Its importance, frequency, and treatment. Am J Syph 1936; 20:37–44.
18. Bhattacharyya MN, Jephcott AE. Diagnosis of gonorrhea in women: Role of the rectal sample. Br J Vener Dis 1974; 50:109–12.
19. Riddell RH, Buck AC. Trimethoprim as an additional selective agent in media for the isolation of *N. gonorrhoeae.* J Clin Pathol 1970; 23:481–3.
20. Deheragoda P. Diagnosis of rectal gonorrhoea by blind anorectal swabs compared with direct vision swabs taken via a proctoscope. Br J Vener Dis 1977; 53:311–3.

21. Schmale JD, Martin JE Jr, Domescik G. Observations on the culture diagnosis of gonorrhea in women. JAMA 1969; 210:312–4.
22. Phillips I, Humphrey D, Middleton A, et al. Diagnosis of gonorrhoea by culture on a selective medium containing vancomycin, colistin, nystatin and trimethoprim (VCNT). A comparison with gram-staining and immunofluorescence. Br J Vener Dis 1972; 48:287–92.
23. Jephcott AE, Morton RS, Turner EB. Use of transport-and-culture medium combined with immunofluorescence for the diagnosis of gonorrhoea. Lancet 1974; 2:1311–3.
24. Duncan WC, Holder WR, Roberts DP, et al. Treatment of gonorrhea with spectinomycin hydrochloride: Comparison with standard penicillin schedules. Antimicrob Agents Chemother 1972; 1:210–4.
25. Fiumara NJ. The treatment of gonococcal proctitis: An evaluation of 173 patients treated with 4 g of spectinomycin. JAMA 1978; 239:735–7.
26. Catterall RD. Anorectal gonorrhoea. Proc R Soc Med 1962; 55:871–3.
27. Kilpatrick ZM. Gonorrheal proctitis. N Engl J Med 1972; 287:967–9.
28. Centers for Disease Control, Public Health Service. Gonorrhea: Recommended treatment schedules. Ann Intern Med 1975; 82:230–3.
29. Schroeter AL, Turner RH, Lucas JB, et al. Therapy for incubating syphilis. Effectiveness of gonorrhea treatment. JAMA 1971; 218:711–3.
30. Schroeter AL, Reynolds G. The rectal culture as a test of cure of gonorrhea in females. J Infect Dis 1972; 125:499–503.
31. Bro-Jorgensen A, Jensen T. Single-dose oral treatment of gonorrhea in men and women, using ampicillin alone and combined with probenecid. Br J Vener Dis 1971; 47:443–7.
32. Evans AJ. Relapse of gonorrhea after treatment with penicillin or streptomycin. Br J Vener Dis 1966; 42:251–62.
33. Tramont EC. Gonococcal pilus vaccine: Studies of the antigenicity and inhibition of attachment. J Clin Invest 1981; 68:881–90.
34. Judson FN, Ehret JM, Eickhoff TC. Anogenital infection with *Neisseria meningitidis* in homosexual men. J Infect Dis 1978; 137:458–63.
35. Faur YC, Wilson ME, May PS. Isolation of *Neisseria meningitidis* from the genito-urinary tract and anal canal. Am J Public Health 1981; 71:53–5.
36. Givan KF, Keyl A. The isolation of Neisseria species from unusual sites. Can Med Assoc J 1974; 111:1077–9.
37. Givan KF, Thomas BW, Johnston AG. Isolation of *N. meningitidis* from the urethra, cervix and anal canal. Br J Vener Dis 1977; 53:109–12.
38. Centers for Disease Control. Annual summary 1980: Reported morbidity and mortality in the United States. Morbid Mortal Weekly Rep 1980; 28:79–83.
39. Centers for Disease Control. Syphilis trends in the United States. Morbid Mortal Weekly Rep 1981; 30:144–9.
40. Henderson RH. Improving sexually transmitted disease health services for gays: A national perspective. Sex Transm Dis 1979; 4:58–62.
41. Downing JG. Incidence of extragenital chancres. Arch Dermatol Syph 1939; 39:150.
42. Wile J, Holman HH. A survey of sixty eight cases of extragenital chancres. Am J Syph 1941; 25:58.
43. Smith D. Infectious syphilis of the anal canal. Dis Colon Rectum 1963; 6:7.
44. Lieberman W. Syphilis of the rectum. Rev Gastroenterol 1951; 18:67.
45. Kvorning SA. Clinical comments on the start of an epidemic of syphilis. Br J Vener Dis 1963; 39:261.
46. Martin EG, Kallet HI. Primary syphilis of the anorectal region. JAMA 1925; 84:1556–8.
47. Jones AJ, Janis L. Primary syphilis of the rectum and gonorrhea of the anus. Am J Syph 1944; 28:453–7.
48. Wells BT, Kierland RR, et al. Rectal chancre: Report of a case. AMA Arch Dermatol 1959; 79:719–20.
49. Gluckman JB, Kleinman MS, May A. Primary syphilis of the rectum. NY State J Med 1974; 74:2210–1.
50. Smith D. Infectious syphilis of the rectum. Dis Colon Rectum 1965; 8:57–8.
51. Tarr JD, Lugar NR. Early infectious syphilis. Male homosexual relations as a mode of spread. Calif Med 1960; 93:35.
52. Haburchale DJ, Davidson H. Anorectal lesions and syphilitic hepatitis. West J Med 1978; 128:64–7.
53. Marino AWM. Proctologic lesion observed in male homosexuals. Dis Colon Rectum 1964; 7:121–8.
54. Samenius B. Primary syphilis of the anorectal region. Dis Colon Rectum 1968; 11:462–6.
55. Akdamar K, Martin RJ, et al. Syphilitic proctitis. Am J Dig Dis 1977; 22:701–4.
56. Nazemi MM, Musler DM, et al. Syphilitic proctitis in homosexuals. JAMA 1975; 231:389.
57. Drusin LM, Homan WP. The role of surgery in primary syphilis of the anus. Ann Surg 1976; 184:65–7.
58. Quinn TC, Lukehart SA, Goodell S, et al. Rectal mass caused by *Treponema pallidum*: Confirmation by immunofluorescent staining. Gastroenterology 1982; 82:135–9.
59. Sachar DB, Klein RS, et al. Erosive syphilitic gastritis: darkfield and immunofluorescent diagnosis from biopsy specimen. Ann Intern Med 1974; 80:512–5.
60. Yobs AR, Clark JW, et al. Further observations on the persistence of *Treponema pallidum* after treatment in rabbits and humans. Br J Vener Dis 1968; 44:116–30.
61. Yobs AR, Brown L, Hunter EF. Fluorescent antibody technique in early syphilis. Arch Pathol 1967; 77:220–5.
62. Jue R, Puffer J, et al. Comparison of fluorescent and conventional darkfield methods for detection of *Treponema pallidum* in syphilitic lesions. Am J Clin Pathol 1967; 47:809–11.
63. Elsas FJ. Comparison of direct and indirect fluorescent antibody methods for staining *Treponema pallidum*. Br J Vener Dis 1971; 47:255–8.
64. Wilkinson AE, Cowell LP. Immunofluorescent staining for the detection of *Treponema pallidum* in early syphilis. Br J Vener Dis 1971; 47:252–4.
65. Daniels KC, Ferneyhough HS. Specific direct fluorescent antibody detection of *Treponema pallidum*. Health Lab Sci 1977; 14:164–7.
66. Goldmeire D. Proctitis and herpes simplex virus in homosexual men. Br J Vener Dis 1980; 56:111–4.
67. Quinn TC, Corey L, et al. The etiology of anorectal infection in homosexual men. Am J Med 1981; 71:395–406.
68. Nahmias AJ, Dowdle WR, et al. Genital infections with type 2 herpes virus hominis—a commonly occurring venereal disease. Br J Vener Dis 1969; 45:294–9.
69. Kaufman RH, Gardner HL, et al. Clinical features of herpes genitalis. Cancer Res 1973; 33:1446.
70. Poste G, Hawkins DF, Thomlinson J. Herpes virus hominis infections of the female genital tract. Obstet Gynecol 1972; 40:871.
71. Nahmias AJ, Roizman B. Infections with herpes simplex viruses 1 and 2. N Engl J Med 1973; 289:667–73, 719–25, 781–9.
72. Jacobs E. Anal infection caused by herpes simplex virus. Dis Colon Rectum 1976; 19:151–7.
73. Chang TW, Fiumara NJ, Weinstein L. Genital herpes: Some clinical and laboratory observations. JAMA 1974; 224:129.
74. Lennette EH, Schmidt NJ, eds. Diagnostic Procedures for Viral, Rickettsial and Chlamydial Infections. 5th Ed. New York: American Public Health Assoc., Inc., 1979.
75. Wentworth BB, Bonin P, Holmes KK, et al. Isolation of viruses, bacteria and other organisms from venereal disease clinic patients: methodology and problems associated with multiple isolations. Health Lab Sci 1973; 10:75–81.
76. Felber TD, Smith EB, et al. Photodynamic inactivation of herpes simplex: Report of a clinical trial. JAMA 1973; 223:289–90.
77. Kaufman RH, Gardner HL, et al. Herpes genitalis treated by photodynamic inactivation of the virus. Am J Gynecol 1973; 117:1144.
78. Catterall RD. Sexually transmitted diseases of the colon and rectum. Clin Gastroenterol 1975; 4:659–69.
79. Bensaude R, Lambling A. Discussion on the etiology and treatment of fibrous strictures of the rectum. Proc R Soc Med 1936; 29:1441–6.
80. Levine JS, Smith PD, Brugge WR. Chronic proctitis in male homosexuals due to lymphogranuloma venereum. Gastroenterology 1980; 79:563–5.

81. Palmer WL, Kirsner JB, Rodaniche EC. Studies on lymphogranuloma venereum infections of the rectum. JAMA 1942; 118:517.
82. Schacter J, Smith DE, Dawson CR, et al. Lymphogranuloma venereum. I. Comparison of the Frei test, complement fixation test, and isolation of the agent. J Infect Dis 1969; 120:372.
83. Annamunthodo H. Rectal lymphogranuloma venereum in Jamaica. Dis Colon Rectum 1961; 4:17.
84. Guzman L. Co-existence of chronic lymphogranuloma venereum and cancer. Radiology 1943; 41:151.
85. Quinn TC, Goodell SE, Mkrtichian PAC, et al. *Chlamydia trachomatis* proctitis. N Engl J Med 1981; 305:195.
86. McMillian A, Sommerville RG, McKie PMK. Chlamydial infection in homosexual men: Frequency of isolation of *Chlamydia trachomatis* from the urethra, ano-rectum and pharynx. Br J Vener Dis 1981; 57:47.
87. Oriel JD. Anal warts and anal coitus. Br J Vener Dis 1971; 47:373.
88. Oriel JD. Natural history of genital warts. Br J Vener Dis 1971; 47:13.
89. Blaser MJ, Parsons RB, Wang WL. Acute colitis caused by *Campylobacter fetus ss. jejuni*. Gastroenterology 1980; 78:448–53.
90. Blaser MJ, Berkowitz ID, La Force FM, et al. Campylobacter enteritis: Clinical and epidemiologic features. Ann Intern Med 1979; 91:179–85.
91. Quinn TC, Corey L, Chaffee RG, et al. Campylobacter proctitis in a homosexual man. Ann Intern Med 1980; 93:458–9.
92. Corey L, Holmes KK. Sexual transmission of hepatitis A in homosexual men. N Engl J Med 1980; 302:435–8.
93. Schmerin MJ, Gelston A, Jones TC. Amebiasis: An increasing problem among homosexuals in New York City. JAMA 1977; 238:1386–7.
94. Mildvan D, Gleb AM, Williams D. Venereal transmission of enteric pathogens in male homosexuals. JAMA 1977; 238:1387–9.
95. Schmerin MJ, Jones TC, Klein H. Giardiasis: Association with homosexuality. Ann Intern Med 1978; 80:801–3.
96. Dritz SK, Ainsworth TE, Back A, et al. Patterns of sexually transmitted enteric diseases in a city. Lancet 1977; 1:3–4.
97. Phillips SC, Mildvan D, Williams DC, et al. Sexual transmission of enteric protozoa and helminths in a venereal disease clinic population. N Engl J Med 1980; 305:603–6.
98. Fawaz KA, Matloff DS. Viral hepatitis in homosexual men. Gastroenterology 1981; 81:537–8.
99. Gottlieb MS, Schroff R, Schanker HM, et al. *Pneumocystis carinii* pneumonia and mucosal candidiasis in previously healthy homosexual men: Evidence of a new acquired cellular immunodeficiency. N Engl J Med 1981; 305:1426–31.
100. Masur H, Michelis MA, Greene JB, et al. An outbreak of community acquired *Pneumocystis carinii* pneumonia: Initial manifestations of cellular immune dysfunction. N Engl J Med 1981; 305:1431–7.
101. Siegal FP, Lopez C, Hammer GS, et al. Severe acquired immunodeficiency in male homosexuals, manifested by chronic perianal ulcerative herpes simplex lesions. N Engl J Med 1981; 305:1439–44.
102. Centers for Disease Control. Kaposi's sarcoma and Pneumocystis pneumonia among homosexual men—New York City and California. Morbid Mortal Weekly Rep 1981; 30:305–7.
103. Friedman-Kien AE, Laubenstein LJ, Rubinstein P, et al. Disseminated Kaposi's sarcoma in homosexual men. Ann Intern Med 1982; 96:693–700.
104. Mildvan D, Mathur U, Enlow RW, et al. Opportunistic infections and immune deficiency in homosexual men. Ann Intern Med 1982; 96:700–4.
105. Follansbee SE, Busch DF, Wofsy CB, et al. An outbreak of *Pneumocystis carinii* pneumonia in homosexual men. Ann Intern Med 1982; 96:705–13.
106. Morris L, Distenfeld A, Amorosi E, et al. Autoimmune thrombocytopenic purpura in homosexual men. Ann Intern Med 1982; 96:714–7.
107. Centers for Disease Control. Update: Acquired immunodeficiency syndrome (AIDS)—United States. Morbid Mortal Weekly Rep 1983; 32:389–91.
108. Centers for Disease Control. Prevention of acquired immune deficiency syndrome (AIDS): Report of inter-agency recommendations. Morbid Mortal Weekly Rep 1983; 32:101–3.
109. Editorial. Acquired immunodeficiency syndrome. Lancet 1983; 1:162–4.
109a. Jaffe HW, Chol K, Thomas PA, et al. National case control study of Kaposi's sarcoma and *Pneumocystis carinii* pneumonia in homosexual men: Part I, epidemiologic results. Ann Intern Med 1983; 99:145–51.
109b. de Shazo RD, Andes WA, Nordberg J, et al. An immunologic evaluation of hemophiliac patients and their wives: Relationships to the acquired immunodeficiency syndrome. Ann Intern Med 1983; 99:159–64.
110. Fauci AS. The syndrome of Kaposi's sarcoma and opportunistic infections: An epidemiologically restricted disorder of immunoregulation. Ann Intern Med 1982; 96:777–9.
110a. Stal RE, Friedman-Kien A, Dubin R, Marmor M. Immunologic abnormalities in homosexual men. Relationship to Kaposi's sarcoma. Am J Med 1982; 73:171–8.
110b. Rogers MF, Morens DM, Stewart JA, et al. National case control study of Kaposi's sarcoma and *Pneumocystis carinii* pneumonia in homosexual men: Part II, laboratory results. Ann Intern Med 1983; 99:151–8.
111. Giraldo G, Beth E, Huang ES. Kaposi's sarcoma and its relationship to cytomegalovirus (CMV). III. CMV DNA and CMV early antigens in Kaposi's sarcoma. Int J Cancer 1980; 26:23–9.
112. Giraldo G, Beth E, Kourilsky FM, et al. Antibody patterns to herpes viruses in Kaposi's sarcoma: Serological association of Europeans with cytomegalovirus. Int J Cancer 1975; 15:839–48.
113. Giraldo G, Beth E, Henle W, et al. Antibody patterns to herpes viruses in Kaposi's sarcoma. II. Serological association of American Kaposi's sarcoma with cytomegalovirus. Int J Cancer 1978; 22:126–31.
114. Ryning FW, Mills J. *Pneumocystis carinii*, *Toxoplasma gondii*, cytomegalovirus, and the compromised host. West J Med 1979; 130:18–34.
115. Lang DJ, Kummer JF, Hartley DP. Cytomegalovirus in semen: Persistence and demonstration in extra cellular fluids. N Engl J Med 1974; 291:121–3.
116. Rubin RH, Cosimi AB, Tolkoff-Rubin NE, et al. Infectious disease syndromes attributable to cytomegalovirus and their significance among renal transplant recipients. Transplantation 1977; 24:458–64.
117. Rinaldo A Jr, Carney WP, Richter BS, et al. Mechanisms of immunosuppression in cytomegaloviral mononucleosis. J Infect Dis 1980; 141:488–95.
118. Drew WL, Mintz L, Miner RC, Sands M. Prevalence of cytomegalovirus infection in homosexual men. J Infect Dis 1981; 143:188–92.
119. Marmon M, Friedman-Kien AE, Laubenstein L, et al. Risk factors for Kaposi's sarcoma in homosexual men. Lancet 1982; 1:1083–7.
120. Jorgenson KA. Amyl nitrite and Kaposi's sarcoma in homosexual men. N Engl J Med 1982; 307:893–4.
121. Goedert JJ, Newland CY, Wallen WC, et al. Amyl nitrite may alter T lymphocytis in homosexual men. Lancet 1982; 1:412–6.
122. Centers for Disease Control. Human T-cell leukemia virus infection in patients with acquired immune deficiency syndrome: Preliminary observations. Morbid Mortal Weekly Rep 1983; 32:233–4.
123. Reitz MS Jr, Kalyanaraman VS, Robert-Guroff M, et al. Human T-cell leukemia/lymphoma virus: The retro virus of adult T-cell leukemia/lymphoma. J Infect Dis 1983; 147:399–405.
123a. Popovic M, Sarngadharan MG, Read E, Gallo RG. Detection, isolation and continuous production of cytopathic retroviruses (HLTV-III) from patients with AIDS and Pre-AIDS. Science 1984; 221:497–500.
123b. Gallo RL, Sacahudd SZ, Popovic M, Shearer GM, Kaplan

M, Haynes BP, Parker TJ, Redfeld R, Oleske J, Safai B, White G, Foster P, Markham PD. Frequent detection and isolation of cytopathic retroviruses (HTLV-III) from patients with AIDS and at risk for AIDS. Science 1984; 224:500–3.

123c. Schupbach J, Popovic M, Gilden RV, Gonda MA, Sarngadharan MG, Gallo RC. Serologic analysis of a subgroup of human T-lymphotropic retroviruses (HTLV-III) associated with AIDS. Science 1984; 224:503–5.

123d. Sarngadharan MG, Popovic M, Bruch L, Schupbach J, Gallo RC. Antibodies reactive with human T-lymphotropic retroviruses (HLTV-III) in the serum of patient with AIDS. Science 1984; 224:506–8.

123e. The Cancer Letter 1984; 10:7.

124. Kaposi M. Idiopathisches multiples Pigmentsarkom der Haut. Arch Dermatol Syphil 1872; 4:265–73.

125. Taylor JF, Templeton AC, Vogel CL, et al. Kaposi's sarcoma in Uganda: A clinicopathological study. Int J Cancer 1971; 8:122–35.

126. Myers BD, Kessler E, Levi J, et al. Kaposi's sarcoma in kidney transplant recipients. Arch Intern Med 1974; 133:307–11.

127. Penn I. Kaposi's sarcoma in organ transplant recipients: A report of 20 cases. Transplantation 1979; 27:8–11.

128. Safai B, Good RA. Kaposi's sarcoma: A review and recent developments. CA 1981; 31:2–12.

129. Rose HS, Balthazar EJ, Megibow AJ, et al. Alimentary tract involvement in Kaposi sarcoma: Radiographic and endoscopic findings in 25 homosexual men. AJR 1982; 139:661–6.

130. Reed WB, Kamath HM, Weiss L. Kaposi's sarcoma with emphasis on the internal manifestations. Arch Dermatol 1974; 110:115–8.

130a. Gottlieb MS, Groopman JE, Weinstein WM, Fahey JL, Detels R. The acquired immunodeficiency syndrome. Ann Intern Med 1983; 99:208–20.

131. Hano R, Owen L, Callen J. Kaposi's sarcoma with extensive silent internal involvement. Int J Dermatol 1979; 9:718–21.

131a. Derezin M, Lewis KJ, Groopman J, Weinstein WM. Gastrointestinal involvement with Kaposi's sarcoma in epidemic acquired immune deficiency syndrome. Gastrointest Endosc 1983; 29:178–9 (Abstract).

132. Roth JA, Schell S, Panzarino S, Coronato A. Visceral Kaposi's sarcoma presenting as colitis. Am J Surg Pathol 1978; 2:209–14.

133. Calenoff L. Gastrointestinal Kaposi's sarcoma: Roentgen manifestations. AJR 1972; 114:525–8.

134. White JA, King MH. Kaposi's sarcoma presenting with abdominal symptoms. Gastroenterology 1964; 46:197–201.

135. Mitchell N, Feder IA. Kaposi's sarcoma with secondary involvement of the jejunum, perforation and peritonitis. Ann Intern Med 1949; 31:324–9.

136. Novis BH, King H, Bank S. Kaposi's sarcoma presenting with diarrhea and protein-losing enteropathy. Gastroenterology 1974; 67:996–1000.

137. Safai B, Mike V, Giraldo G, et al. Association of Kaposi's sarcoma with second primary malignancies. Cancer 1980; 45:1472–9.

138. Centers for Disease Control: Acquired immune deficiency syndrome (AIDS): Precautions for clinical and laboratory staffs. Morbid Mortal Weekly Rep 1982; 31:577–80.

Chapter 122

Intestinal Obstruction

Isidore Cohn, Jr.

Intestinal obstruction is one of the commoner problems facing the gastroenterologist and the gastrointestinal surgeon. Intestinal obstruction is defined as "any hindrance to the passage of the intestinal contents," a definition that gives almost infinite variation to the possible causes, effects, symptoms, and modes of therapy. Ileus is also defined in the dictionary as "obstruction of the intestines," but is almost always used in conjunction with some modifier, such as "adynamic." Many misuse the word to describe a specific form of intestinal obstruction, namely "adynamic ileus."

Classification

The very broad definition of intestinal obstruction makes it obvious that a classification is necessary. One may classify intestinal obstruction on the basis of types or varieties (Table 122–1) and on the basis of mechanisms (Table 122–2).

Table 122–1 is an oversimplified classification and does not take into account the variety of etiologic factors. A *simple obstruction* is one in which the interference with the passage of intestinal contents is the only problem. *Strangulation obstruction* is a form in which there is interference with the blood supply to some or all of the obstructed segment in addition to obstruction of the intestinal lumen.

High and *low small bowel obstructions* have differing causes, different clinical manifestations, and significant biochemical differences related to the loss of different gastrointestinal secretions. Early determination of whether the obstruction is located in the large or small bowel, therefore, is essential because management and prognosis are not identical.

A *closed loop obstruction* is one in which both ends of a segment of bowel are occluded with resulting complete isolation of the segment and a secondary form of obstruction at the proximal end of the closed loop. Common examples of this form of obstruction are volvulus, a loop of small bowel trapped by an adhesive band, and an obstruction of the large bowel in a patient with a competent ileocecal valve. The patient with a closed loop obstruction may not have any interference with the blood supply to the closed loop. By contrast, the obstruction may begin or progress toward the point where the internal pressure in the loop interferes with its circulation. The obstructing agent may also interfere with the blood supply to the closed loop. The net result is a simultaneous strangulated and closed loop obstruction.[1]

Table 122–1. TYPES OF INTESTINAL OBSTRUCTION

I. Simple intestinal obstruction
  A. High small bowel
  B. Low small bowel
  C. Colonic
II. Closed loop obstruction
III. Strangulation obstruction

Table 122–2. MECHANISMS OF OBSTRUCTION

I. Mechanical obstruction
  A. Narrowing of lumen, intrinsic lesions
    1. Congenital
      a. Atresia
      b. Stenosis
      c. Imperforate anus, malformations of anus and rectum
      d. Malrotations
      e. Cysts and reduplications
      f. Meckel's diverticulum
    2. Acquired
      a. Inflammatory
        (1) Enteritis
        (2) Granulomatous disease, specific and nonspecific
        (3) Diverticulitis
      b. Traumatic
      c. Vascular
      d. Neoplastic
        (1) Benign tumors, small or large bowel
        (2) Malignant tumors, small or large bowel
        (3) Endometriosis
  B. Adhesive bands
    1. Congenital
    2. Inflammatory
    3. Traumatic
    4. Neoplastic
  C. Hernia
    1. External
    2. Internal
  D. Extraintestinal masses or structures
    1. Abscess
    2. Tumor
    3. Pregnancy
    4. Annular pancreas
    5. Superior mesenteric artery
  E. Stomal or anastomotic obstruction
    1. Edema
    2. Stricture
  F. Volvulus
  G. Intussusception
  H. Obturation
    1. Gallstones
    2. Foreign bodies
    3. Worms
    4. Bezoars
    5. Meconium
    6. Fecal impaction
  I. Congenital defects, Hirschsprung's disease
  J. Radiation stenosis

II. Physiologic, neurogenic, toxic, chemical imbalance obstruction
  A. Paralytic or adynamic ileus
    1. Peritonitis
    2. Toxic
      a. Pneumonia
      b. Uremia
      c. Generalized infection
    3. Electrolyte imbalance
    4. Neurogenic
      a. Spinal cord lesion
      b. Fracture of spine, pelvis, femur, etc.
      c. Plumbism
      d. Retroperitoneal hematoma or operation
  B. Spastic or dynamic ileus
  C. Toxic megacolon
  D. Drugs*
    1. Within the lumen
      a. Barium sulfate
      b. Cholestyramine
      c. Potassium salts
    2. Within the wall
      a. Anticoagulants
      b. Drugs affecting smooth muscle (antihistamines, opiates)
      c. Drugs interfering with parasympathetic nerve transmission (autonomic ganglion)
      d. Blockers, muscarinic antagonists (tricyclic antidepressants)
    3. Outside the wall
      a. Drugs causing mesenteric vascular occlusion (contraceptive pill, adrenal corticosteroids)
      b. β-adrenoceptor antagonists
      c. Irradiation (thorium, ^{198}Au)

III. Vascular obstruction
  A. Thrombosis of mesenteric vessels
  B. Embolism of mesenteric vessels
  C. Low flow syndromes

*Data from George.[47]

Etiology

The 2 major causes of small bowel obstruction are *hernias* and *adhesions*.[2–7] Over the years from 1930 to 1980, there has been a progressive increase in the frequency of adhesions and a relative decrease in the frequency of hernias as a cause of small bowel obstruction. This trend has now reached the point where these two disorders have reversed their positions in terms of relative frequency (Table 122–3). The increasing frequency of adhesions and the comparative decline in hernias as causes for intestinal obstruction are doubtless a reflection of both the tendency for hernias to be repaired at the time the diagnosis is made and the general increase in abdominal surgery with its attendant increase in postoperative adhesions.

Carcinoma is the most common cause of large bowel obstruction, but is rarely responsible for small bowel obstruction.

Table 122–3. FREQUENCY RATES (%) OF THE VARIOUS CAUSES OF INTESTINAL OBSTRUCTION

Period	Number of Cases	Hernia	Adhesions and Bands	Intussus-ception	Volvulus	Cancer	Foreign Bodies	Congen-ital	Inflam-matory	Other
Prior–1930	9956	46.9	10.7	16.7	2.5	12.8	1.0	0.4	0	8.8
1931–1950	7431	46.4	8.9	14.4	3.2	12.6	1.1	0.6	0	12.4
1951–1970	4709	22.1	33.3	5.0	5.0	18.0	2.3	0.8	2.4	11.1
1971–1980	2212	21.0	50.0	1.7	2.9	13.2	0.7	0.9	1.3	6.2

The changes in relative frequency of the major causes of intestinal obstruction are shown in Table 122–3. Incorporated are specific case reports, which include all types of obstruction seen in the institution concerned. The importance of the increasing frequency of operative procedures is emphasized even further by a comparison of the reports from India and Africa, where the major cause of obstruction remains hernia rather than adhesions (Table 122–4).

Pathophysiology

Clinical and experimental studies have contributed significantly to our understanding of the pathophysiology of intestinal obstruction.[1,8–14,16–19,21–23] The literature is so voluminous, and the disagreements along the way to our current appraisal of the problem are so wide, it was deemed prudent to discuss the current approach without specific reference to the many individuals who contributed to its evolution.[24]

Two of the first findings to be noted in intestinal obstruction are distention of the bowel and fluid and electrolyte losses. The extent of these changes depends to some degree upon the level of the obstruction in the bowel, changes being noted later in large bowel than in small bowel obstruction. The presence and effects of distention take progressively longer to be noted as the obstruction moves down the small bowel. All features are altered in a closed loop obstruction, which most commonly occurs in a patient with a competent ileocecal valve. The development of strangulation adds further complications. Most of the discussion that follows will refer to simple obstruction, except where strangulation is specifically mentioned.

Distention. This begins immediately in simple small bowel obstruction as a result of continuing secretion by the bowel, failure of peristalsis to carry away secretions and ingested material from above, diminution or cessation of normal absorption, and the frequently exaggerated presence of swallowed air. The intestine has amazing properties of distensibility. Indeed, the small bowel can reach proportions that make it difficult to distinguish from the large bowel. The pressures reached within obstructed loops of bowel have little effect until they reach the level of arterial pressure.[15,22] At this point there is interference with arterial circulation to the bowel. If this persists, it probably will result in gangrenous changes in the bowel and lead to an entirely different problem—*strangulation*. As long as the obstruction remains a simple obstruction and as long as perforation does not result from the distention, an animal—and presumably a human—can be kept alive indefinitely by IV feedings if no other complications ensue. Distention itself is not life-threatening but is detrimental because of its secondary effects on the patient's comfort, interference with respiration, sequestration of large quantities of fluid that are lost to the circulatory system, and the opportunity for strangulation to develop.

Table 122–4. ADHESIONS AND HERNIA AS CAUSES OF OBSTRUCTION IN INDIA AND AFRICA*

Country	Number of Cases	% of Total Cases	
		Adhesions	*Hernia*
India	147	15	27
Uganda	794	4	75
Zimbabwe	172	17	36
Nigeria	316	11	65
Nigeria	436	10	35
Ghana	782	10	78

*Adapted from Ellis.[4]

The distended bowel is likely to be edematous, boggy, and heavy and does not function normally in terms of either secretion or absorption. There is no absorption from the distended bowel and therefore the collection of stagnant, bacteria-laden, noxious fluid in the obstructed segment presents no threat to the patient as the source of a lethal toxin. However, if the bowel becomes gangrenous, the strangulated bowel will permit passage of these contents into the peritoneal cavity even though no gross perforation is seen. The development then of toxicity is a very real hazard.[1,8–10] Absorption of this fluid and its toxic products does not occur from normal intestinal mucosa distal to the point of obstruction owing to the very fact of the obstruction and to detoxification by intestinal mucosa. Absorption from the peritoneal cavity after passage of these substances through an intact or damaged bowel wall in strangulation is very rapid and is one of the reasons for early removal of the cause of the obstruction and of the nonviable bowel.

Distention plays a very different role in the *closed loop obstruction*. In this case, the danger is that there is no outlet, either by intubation or by proximal emptying of the intestinal contents, that will relieve the obstruction.[2,8,11,13] As a result, the patient with a closed loop obstruction is quite likely to quickly develop gangrene and strangulation. Experimentally, the sterile closed loop is harmless.[11] While patients are unlikely to develop a sterile closed loop obstruction, the experimental observations are one more demonstration of the importance of bacteria in the lethal effects of intestinal obstruction.

Fluid and Electrolyte Losses. Animals can be kept alive indefinitely with proper replacement of fluids and electrolytes if a simple obstruction is the only problem. The early recognition of the importance of fluid and salt replacement was one of the first major steps leading to increased survival of patients with intestinal obstruction.[9,13,15,18] The level at which the obstruction occurs determines more than any other factor whether the predominant loss will be acid or base. "Pure" acid loss is restricted almost totally to pyloric obstruction. Proper appreciation of this, as well as measurement and replacement of the various electrolytes lost when the lesion is below this level, contributes most importantly to successful management in the preoperative, operative, and postoperative periods. In the patient who has had an appreciable period of obstruction with attendant fluid and electrolyte imbalance, appropriate fluid replacement prior to any operative procedure may make the difference between survival and death. Even in the patient who presents with some complicating emergency, it is rarely necessary or safe to perform an operative procedure without restoring some fluids and electrolytes.[2–7,22,24–27] The patient who presents with markedly dilated bowel and with multiple air-fluid levels visible on plain roentgenograms has lost large quantities of fluid into the gastrointestinal tract and these must be replaced. Early, vigorous fluid replacement of these losses is essential.

The patient with longstanding obstruction, or with obviously mishandled obstruction, may be suffering from varying degrees of inanition. Proper replacement of nutrients may require parenteral hyperalimentation. (Chapter 235).

If distention, fluids, and electrolytes are the keys to intestinal obstruction, why do we still lose some patients with intestinal obstruction even after proper surgical management? The answer may lie in the failure to appreciate some phase of the problem in a particular patient, e.g., inadequate replacement of blood or electrolytes, a too hurried trip to the operating room for the patient who is not properly prepared, the possibility that some area of strangulation has been overlooked, failure to control aspiration during or after induction of anesthesia, the presence of other complicating diseases, the age of the patient, or the unavoidable development of some other complication in the postoperative period.

Strangulation. Strangulation brings with it an entirely new set of problems. *Blood loss* is a major problem, and its extent will depend partly on the length of the strangulated segment.[1,8,14,19,20,22,27,28] In some, the blood loss alone can be fatal. In these situations, only early surgery and massive blood replacement can be expected to have any beneficial result. In the more usual situation in which the strangulated segment is not as long, blood loss can be a major factor but usually will not be fatal by itself. Blood is lost into the lumen of the bowel, in the wall of the bowel, and, eventually, into the peritoneal cavity; the total loss from all these areas can be sizable. The quantity of blood lost will also depend to some extent on whether there is arterial, venous, or combined involvement, with blood loss being greater with only venous obstruction.

Bacteria. Strangulation obstruction sets in motion a series of other detrimental changes. The enormous bacterial population [29] of the stagnant intestinal contents receives a further growth stimulus from the influx of blood with its content of red cells and plasma proteins. In this ideal anaerobic environment, bacterial growth reaches its peak within a few hours. Chemical and bacteriologic studies have demonstrated that intestinal contents can be detected in the peritoneal fluid within 12 to 24 hours after strangulation. Even though no break can be found in the bowel wall by either gross or microscopic examination, examination with a scanning electron microscope may show structural defects in the bowel wall of sufficient size to permit egress of bacteria and bacterial products.

Once these agents are in the peritoneal cavity, their absorption into the circulation is rapid and their distribution and effects are widespread. The fluid in the lumen of a strangulated bowel has been demonstrated to have lethal properties.[1,10,16,17,20,23] Similarly, the fluid in the peritoneal cavity of an experimental animal with a strangulated obstruction has properties that are lethal for a normal animal. The lethal agents have their origin in the strangulated, obstructed segment. Thus, the treatment for strangulation obstruction should be the earliest possible elimination of the strangulated bowel, the removal of any of its products in the peritoneal cavity, and the elimination of any routes of absorption for these contents.

The importance of bacteria in the production of toxicity and the fatal outcome in strangulation obstruction has been established by several different studies.[1,10,16,17,20] The ability of antibiotics to convert an otherwise fatal experimental strangulation obstruction into a nonfatal condition indicates that bacteria probably are the major factor in death from strangulation obstruction when the animal is properly treated for blood loss and fluid and electrolyte imbalance. Successful antibacterial therapy could even be limited to intraluminal administration into the strangulated segment of bowel. The final, definitive experiments are those conducted in germ-free animals given only fluids for replacement. These animals may survive an episode of strangulation obstruction that is lethal to conventional animals. Inasmuch as the test animals were germ-free, it may be concluded that death in otherwise treated strangulation obstruction is the result primarily of bacterial action. Debate continues as to whether the ultimate effects are directly due to the bacteria or to their products. The importance of bacteria, however, cannot be doubted.

Clinical Manifestations

The symptoms and physical findings in a patient with intestinal obstruction will depend to a large extent upon the cause and location of the obstruction. A careful and detailed history is the most important part of making a diagnosis. While historical factors will change somewhat with different types of obstruction, certain basic questions must be answered in each case: Is the patient obstructed? Is the obstruction complete or partial? How long has obstruction been present? What is the level of obstruction? Is strangulation present? Has fluid and electrolyte imbalance become a problem? How urgently can or should the obstruction be relieved? Answers to these questions will permit the physician to initiate appropriate therapy and to minimize subsequent problems.

Symptoms. The key symptoms in any patient with obstruction are *pain, vomiting,* and *obstipation.*[30] *Pain,* the most characteristic feature of intestinal obstruction, is likely to be the first thing the patient notes and may be quite severe. The pain, which is *episodic* and *colicky,* is a result of distention of the bowel and the efforts of peristalsis to push the bowel contents past the obstructing point. A careful history of any similarity to previous episodes may help diagnose some chronic condition that has led to gradual constriction of some part of the gastrointestinal tract. If the pain becomes constant, it suggests the development of strangulation or perforation and peritonitis. Pain related to colonic obstruction may be localized to the lower abdomen or may follow the specific colonic location of the obstruction. Pain of small bowel obstruction is more often localized to the upper or mid-abdomen and may not be as specific in its location.

Vomiting is another key feature of obstruction. The time of onset will be determined by the location of the obstruction. The lower the obstruction, the later the vomiting will occur. In colonic obstruction, vomiting may be absent or late in appearance, depending to some extent upon the competence of the ileocecal valve. The nature of the vomitus may give information about the location of the obstruction. Thus, the vomitus in the presence of pure pyloric obstruction will consist of clear gastric contents. If the obstruction is lower than this, there will be bilious vomitus because of the entrance of bile proximal to the point of obstruction. This differential feature is of considerable importance in infants and children, but is of lesser importance in older individuals because of the relative rarity of pure pyloric obstruction from any cause other than ulcer disease. When the obstruction is in the mid- or low small intestine, the vomitus will have a foul odor and dark appearance and hence is often called "feculent vomiting." The character of the vomitus is due to stasis, rapid bacterial overgrowth, and decomposition of intestinal contents; it does not represent feces, and the term "fecal" vomiting is in reality a misnomer.

Obstipation is another prime factor in intestinal obstruction, and the exact time at which discharge of intestinal contents ceases often can be fixed by the patient. Obstipation, like obstruction, may be partial or complete, depending on the level of the obstruction and the amount of gastrointestinal contents in the bowel distal to the point of obstruction. If the passage of all fecal contents and gas stops completely, there should be little doubt about the diagnosis. Continuing passage of small amounts of fecal matter is common in partial obstruction.

The history should include information about previous operations, previous gastrointestinal symptoms, changes in bowel habit, presence of blood in the stool, weight loss, previous identification of Crohn's disease (regional enteritis), tuberculosis, or other lesions, and use of drugs that might affect the gastrointestinal tract.

Physical Examination. The most important points to note on physical examination are *distention*, the *quality of peristaltic sounds*, and the extent of *dehydration*.[2,22,26,31] *Distention* may be quite marked late in any form of obstruction, and certainly will be if peritoneal irritation has occurred from any cause. In sigmoid volvulus, the degree of distention is out of proportion to the duration of the obstruction. Distention will also be pronounced in any unrelieved form of low small bowel obstruction and in longstanding large bowel obstruction with a competent ileocecal valve. By contrast, distention may be minimal, absent, or intermittent in pyloric obstruction, high small bowel obstruction in which decompression is achieved rapidly and frequently by vomiting, in some cases of large bowel obstruction, and early in strangulation obstruction. Distention of the epigastrium is suggestive of gastric dilatation or obstruction. Distention of the large or small bowel may sometimes be distinguished by the part of the abdomen that is distended.

Auscultation of the abdomen is one of the most important features of the physical examination. More can be learned from determining the presence or absence of peristalsis and the *quality of the peristaltic sounds* than almost any other single physical finding. A silent abdomen, except in the postoperative period, suggests the presence of peritoneal irritation. Almost the only other cause of a silent abdomen in a patient with distention would be a form of adynamic ileus. The usual auscultatory findings in intestinal obstruction are: (1) hyperactive, high-pitched peristaltic rushes, the sound of fluid in the bowel resembling that of water being poured from a bottle; (2) a high, metallic, tinkling sound. Associated with the peristaltic activity will be obvious signs of increasing pain as the waves of peristalsis increase. In addition to the change in intensity of the sounds is an increase in frequency of peristaltic waves as the bowel attempts to push its contents past the point of obstruction.

Dehydration can be detected by the usual findings and would have the expected significance in a patient with intestinal obstruction. Dehydration is not likely to be a serious problem in the early stages of a simple obstruction. However, one should keep in mind that fluid is lost to the outside by vomiting, into the lumen and wall of the bowel proximal to the point of obstruction, and may also be lost into the free peritoneal cavity. In the patient with strangulation obstruction, blood and fluid losses into the bowel lumen, bowel wall, and free peritoneal cavity can be sufficient to cause shock through diminution of circulating fluid volume. Even after the obstruction is relieved, the fluid lost into the lumen of the bowel is effectively lost to the circulation since it rarely is reabsorbed; therefore, this additional amount of fluid must be replaced to bring the patient into balance.

The *pulse rate* is likely to be normal in the early stages of intestinal obstruction unless it is taken during a momentary spasm of pain related to a wave of peristalsis or in the presence of the shock of strangulation obstruction. If pulse rate rises later on, the onset of peritonitis or some other complication may be suspected.[31] The *blood pressure, temperature,* and *respiratory rate* likewise do not provide any definitive information in the early stages of simple intestinal obstruction.

Muscle guarding or *tenderness* of the abdomen or both suggest the presence of strangulation and usually are not found in simple obstruction. If these findings are accompanied by elevated temperature, pulse, and white blood cell count, the presence of a complicating strangulation must be considered.

A *mass* palpated within the abdomen is likely to be another sign of strangulation, suggestive of a coil of intestine protected by other loops of bowel or by omentum. Occasionally, a mass may be palpated in large bowel obstruction when a carcinoma is sufficiently large, has spread to other loops of bowel, or has begun to penetrate the bowel wall and caused adhesions to the omentum.

Visible peristalsis will be present only when there is sufficient distention, peristalsis is sufficiently vigorous, and the abdominal wall is sufficiently thin to permit transmission of this abnormality. It is usually indicative of a later stage of obstruction.

Rectal and *pelvic examinations* may disclose unsuspected lesions capable of producing obstruction or secondary to the obstructing lesions and should never be omitted in anyone suspected of having intestinal obstruction.

Highly important to keep in mind are 2 critical observations in any patient in whom intestinal obstruction is suspected: (1) a careful search for abdominal operative scars; and (2) a diligent search for any external hernias. The omission of such a careful search can be disastrous because, as noted, adhesions and hernias are the cause for over 50% of all cases of intestinal obstruction.

Roentgen Findings*

Radiologic examination of the abdomen is the most important single study after an adequate history and physical examination have been completed. *Plain films of the abdomen* should never be omitted in the patient suspected of having intestinal obstruction. The initial films should include recumbent and erect views of the abdomen to demonstrate any unusual abdominal gas patterns, as well as the possible presence of air under the diaphragm. The patient who is too ill for an upright film can be turned on the side and similar results obtained. Contrast media should not be used in the early roentgenologic evaluation of the patient with small bowel obstruction. If the early films indicate the presence of an obstructing lesion in the large bowel, a barium enema examination may be obtained, provided the radiologist is informed of the suspected clinical diagnosis and uses the proper precautions.

A plain film of the abdomen in a patient with suspected intestinal obstruction may answer several important questions about that patient: Is intestinal obstruction present? Does the obstruction involve the small or large bowel, or both? Is the obstruction of mechanical or paralytic origin? What is the cause of the obstruction? Since much of this needed information may be available from a few simple roentgenograms, diligent study of these films is necessary.

When obstruction occurs, gas in the small bowel separates from the fluid, and gas shadows rapidly become detectable within the small bowel. Shortly thereafter, air-fluid levels appear (Figs. 122–1 and 122–2). These 2 findings are almost always diagnostic of intestinal obstruction. Part of the gas was mixed with the fluid intestinal contents prior to the moment of obstruction, and part represents swallowed air, which continues to contribute to the distention. By the time the patient sees the physician, there has usually been a sufficient time lapse for both air and air-fluid levels to be visible in the small bowel. Plain films should be taken before any enemas are given, since these tend to introduce additional air and confuse the picture. Roentgenograms should include views of the diaphragm to detect free air subsequent to the rupture of any viscus. They should also include the pelvis to detect hernias that may have been missed on physical examination. A chest film should additionally be part of the total roentgen study.

A small bowel distended with air may be distinguished from the colon by the smaller size of the distended loops, the central location of the distended loops, the stepladder

*Dr. Walter McDowell, former Chief of Radiology at the Veterans Administration Hospital, New Orleans, selected all roentgenograms appearing in this section.

pattern that is formed, and the appearance of the valvulae conniventes in the small bowel in contrast to the haustral markings in the colon (Fig. 122–1). Only in the presence of massive distention of the small bowel may differentiating small from large bowel obstruction be difficult.

If there is insufficient clinical and roentgen evidence to establish the diagnosis of small bowel obstruction, and if the patient's condition is not critical or strangulation is not suspected, it is prudent to repeat the study in a few hours to determine if there has been sufficient progression to permit a more definitive diagnosis. Increasing size of the small bowel loops, or failure of abnormal gas to move, would suggest the presence of some obstructing lesion.

If the distention is restricted to the colon, it is fair to assume that both colonic obstruction and a competent ileocecal valve are present. When there is no reflux of air or fluid into the small bowel, the problem is one of a closed loop large bowel obstruction. If the exact location of the obstruction or its etiology is uncertain, a *barium enema study* can be done, provided the radiologist is properly informed of the suspected diagnosis. When there is distention of both the small and large bowel, it may be presumed that the ileocecal valve is patent, and a barium enema study may be performed under the same conditions just outlined. Barium enema examination should provide exact information about the site of the obstruction, its characteristics, and frequently even a specific diagnosis.

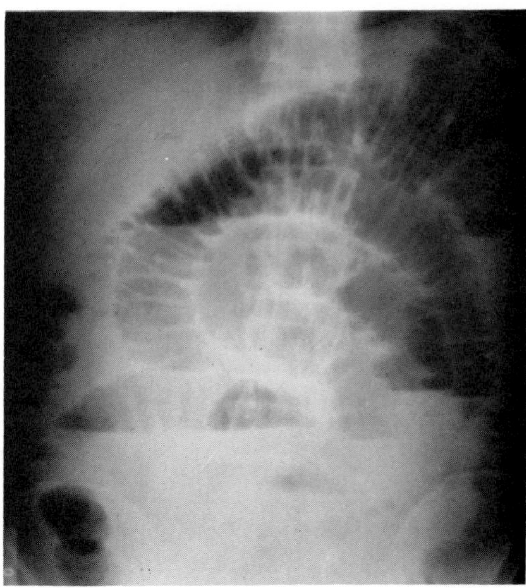

Figure 122–2. Erect film of the same patient as in Figure 122–1. The multiple fluid levels giving the typical stepladder effect are characteristic of intestinal obstruction.

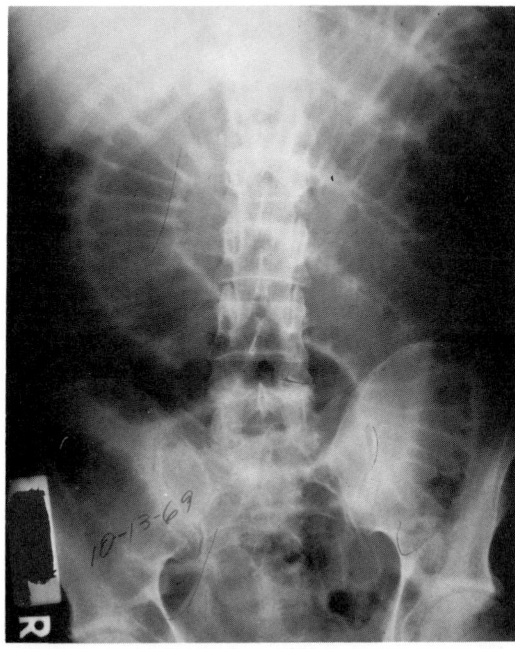

Figure 122–1. Roentgenogram of abdomen in patient with simple mechanical obstruction of the small bowel caused by adhesions. In this film there is marked distention of the small bowel as identified by the linear densities traversing the bowel. These are the valvulae conniventes and identify the distended loops as small bowel and not colon.

If distention is restricted to the small bowel, the level of obstruction may be approximated by the length of distended bowel. If a long intestinal tube is in place, a *water-soluble contrast medium may be instilled through the tube* to outline the obstructing lesion in the small bowel.

Mechanical obstruction may be distinguished from paralytic obstruction by the type of distention seen on the plain roentgenogram. If only specific areas of distention are visible, a mechanical etiology can be suspected. In contrast, distention throughout the alimentary tract would be more in line with a paralytic etiology. If distention extends to the rectum and digital rectal examination is negative, a paralytic basis for the obstruction would be likely.

The roentgen diagnosis of strangulation is very difficult[32,33] (Fig. 122–3). Mellins and Rigler[33] found 2 fairly reliable roentgen signs suggesting strangulation obstruction. The first is the so-called *pseudotumor sign*, consisting of a segment of bowel containing fluid. This is particularly suggestive if dilated bowel

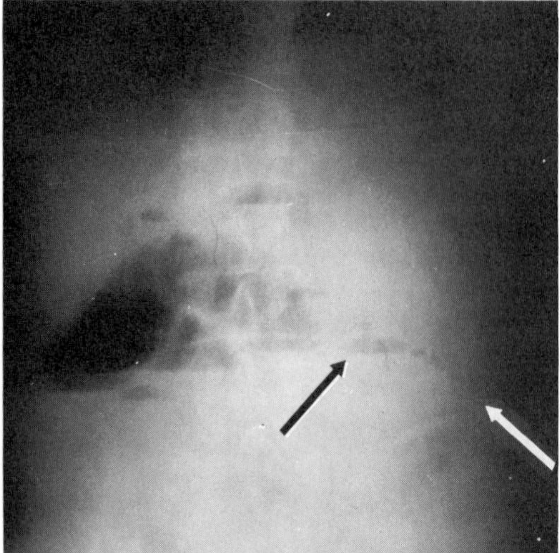

Figure 122–3. Erect film of the abdomen in a patient with small bowel obstruction due to adhesions. The curvilinear collection of small air bubbles in the left abdomen represents the so-called string of beads sign. It is useful in the diagnosis of distended fluid-filled loops of small bowel and also suggests the possibility of strangulation.

is seen proximal to the soft tissue mass. The second finding is the *coffee-bean sign*, consisting of a localized, dilated, fixed loop of intestine distended by gas. *Perforation*, which indicates strangulation of at least some portion of the bowel, can be detected by the presence of *free air under the diaphragm* with the patient in the erect or lateral position.

For additional details regarding the use and value of plain films of the abdomen and barium enema study, the reader is referred to Chapters 32 and 33.

Laboratory Procedures

The basic diagnosis of intestinal obstruction will not be made as a result of any one or any combination of laboratory studies. Once the diagnosis has been made, however, certain laboratory studies are of great value in patient management. The differential diagnosis between a simple and a strangulating obstruction cannot be made on the basis of laboratory examination. There are now sufficient studies to show that the overlap between simple and strangulating obstructions precludes laboratory studies as a reliable means of distinguishing them, except in far advanced cases when other observations simplify the distinction (Fig. 122–4).

In the early stages of intestinal obstruction, laboratory abnormalities will probably not be present because there has not been sufficient change in any of the physiologic parameters to be mirrored in the body chemistry. Dehydration will be apparent in the later stages of obstruction, regardless of the cause. An elevation of the *white blood cell count* may be found as a corollary of hemoconcentration or it may be indicative of some irritative process, such as strangulation or vascular occlusion. However, it is not infallible under these circumstances and may be present in some patients with simple obstruction. An elevation of *serum amylase activity* may result from irritative action on the pancreas as a result of strangulation obstruction of a loop of bowel in contact with this gland, the passage of some toxic component of the strangulated loop into the peritoneal cavity and its contact with the pancreas, increased pressure within the bowel transmitted to the pancreatic duct, or amylase released from other parts of the alimentary tract or elsewhere. The *blood urea nitrogen level* may provide helpful information concerning the presence of dehydration, poor renal function, or blood in the gastrointestinal tract. It may also reflect the very late stages of intestinal obstruction when normal body responses have failed.

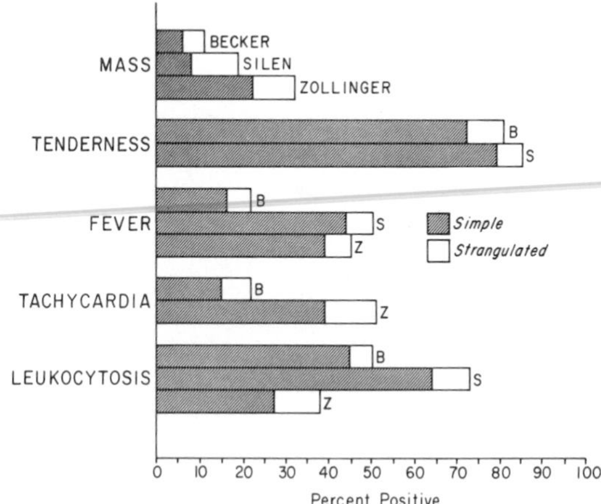

Figure 122–4. Comparative frequency of various signs of strangulation obstruction in simple and strangulation obstruction in 3 different institutions. Becker's figures are from Charity Hospital in New Orleans, Silen's from the University of California in San Francisco, and Zollinger's from the University of Ohio. The results of the 3 studies are amazingly close. Each one indicates the similarity of the results in simple and strangulation obstruction, emphasizing the unreliability of these classic findings as evidence of the presence of strangulation.

Urinalysis may give some clues about the degree of dehydration. This study may also be useful in the detection of diabetes mellitus or some coexisting renal condition.

Although all the foregoing studies may aid in determining the condition of the patient, the really critical values to determine in anyone with intestinal obstruction are those of the serum electrolytes. These values can be most helpful in deciding upon proper fluid replacement therapy prior to, or in conjunction with, any surgical procedure. *Sodium, potassium, chloride, blood gases, and pH* are the critical studies. They should be obtained in any patient with intestinal obstruction who has had symptoms for longer than a few hours. Determination of the *serum potassium level* is highly important in the patient who has been losing gastrointestinal secretions for any length of time. Although a deficiency in *magnesium* is uncommon in intestinal obstruction, lowered magnesium levels occur in the occasional patient and require correction by administration of magnesium.

Substantial loss of chloride (acid) with resultant alkalosis in the patient with pyloric obstruction is the most clear-cut example of electrolyte loss and need in intestinal obstruction. There are electrolyte losses in other forms of obstruction as well, but lower sites of obstruction are likely to be associated with a more balanced loss of electrolytes than is the loss of gastric secretions. In small bowel obstruction well below the ligament of Treitz, losses of gastric secretions and those of the pancreas, liver, and small bowel tend to partially counterbalance each another. Biochemical studies usually show a loss of all electrolytes, with a tendency toward metabolic acidosis.

Special Examinations

Proctosigmoidoscopy may be diagnostic and should be employed whenever appropriate. *Abdominal paracentesis* may reveal bloody fluid suggesting the presence of strangulation. Demonstration of white blood cells and bacteria in a stained preparation of the sediment would reinforce suspicion of strangulation, bowel necrosis, or transmigration of bacteria through an ischemic bowel wall. Failure to find any of these changes, while weighing against strangulation, would not conclusively exclude it. The procedure may be especially useful in patients in whom diagnostic problems exist and in whom a positive finding might speed the decision to perform a definitive operation.

Differential Diagnosis

A careful history and physical examination should do more to establish the diagnosis than any other studies except, of course, a plain roentgenogram of the abdomen showing the classic features of intestinal obstruction.[31] Nevertheless, some conditions may require differential consideration and cause diagnostic concern.

Air and air-fluid levels in the small bowel are ordinarily the result of obstruction. However, peritonitis, peritoneal irritation, dysentery, inflammatory bowel disease, morphine administration, and responses from disease of the kidneys, pelvic organs, vertebral injury, and retroperitoneal operations can all lead to distention and simulate the radiologic picture of obstruction. The differential diagnosis usually can be made on the basis of the history, physical examination, and proper correlation of all available information.

Acute gastroenteritis may be suspected from the history, the more pronounced role of diarrhea, the more generalized abdominal discomfort, the absence of abdominal distention, and the lack of correlation between peristalsis and abdominal pain.

Acute appendicitis is likely to have some localizing signs in the right lower quadrant and to be associated with less distention and vomiting, a younger age distribution, more elevation of the white blood cell count, and more abdominal guarding or tenderness. If for some reason the differentiation cannot be made, early operation and appropriate correction of the basic problem may be required (Chapter 144).

Acute pancreatitis may be suspected from a history of alcohol abuse or gallbladder disease, previous episodes of pancreatitis, the acute onset, and the severity and character of the pain (Chapter 216). High serum and urinary amylase activities would also point more to acute pancreatitis, but it should be remembered that strangulation obstruction may be accompanied by some elevation of amylase. The presence of pancreatic calcification, or scattered areas of calcium deposits throughout the abdomen, would also help in the differential diagnosis.

Perforated peptic ulcer would be characterized by an antecedent history of ulcer symptoms, sudden onset, severe abdominal pain and rigidity, shoulder tip pain, possibly roentgen evidence of free air under the diaphragm, and an earlier rise in white blood cell count and temperature (Chapter 69).

Acute cholecystitis can be distinguished by an antecedent history of biliary colic, localization of pain to the right upper quadrant with tenderness and muscle spasm in that area, perhaps a palpable mass in the right upper quadrant, elevation of the serum bilirubin level, sonographic evidence of calculi, and failure of the gallbladder to be visible on biliary scintigraphy.

Renal colic might be considered, but urinary findings, localization of the pain, presence of an x-ray-opaque stone in the kidney, and the total lack of correlation between pain paroxysms and peristaltic sounds should be of value here.

Peritonitis due to any cause may cause confusion, but a prompt surgical approach will resolve the dilemma. Moreover, peritonitis would be a late sequela if due to untreated intestinal obstruction, and it may not be possible at this stage to determine the initial cause of the peritonitis.

The critical differentiation is between *simple* and *strangulation obstruction*. Unfortunately, this is frequently difficult or impossible. Even more unfortunate is the clinician who is not adequately aware of this difficulty until too late in the patient's course. For years textbooks have iterated the "classic signs" of strangulation. More critical analysis of several large series from various institutions has demonstrated that these signs do not clearly differentiate the 2 types of obstruction. The classic signs are unreliable except in the late stages of strangulation[2,7,26–28,34,35] (Fig. 122–4). A prospective study conducted at Johns Hopkins Hospital[34] comparing 97 different parameters in patients with obstruction demonstrated that neither any one observation nor any combination of studies was capable of making the differential diagnosis with sufficient accuracy to be acceptable. Thus, the clinician who awaits the development of these signs may be delaying fatally. The safer way is to assume that the patient with obstruction may have strangulation and to proceed on this basis.

Treatment

Acute intestinal obstruction constitutes an emergency, strangulation obstruction even more so. The longer the delay between diagnosis and correction, the higher the mortality. These simple and obvious observations should be the cornerstones of the management of any patient with obstruction. The objectives of management should be equally clear: (1) correction of any fluid and electrolyte abnormalities; (2) relief and/or removal of the obstruction; and (3) deflation of the bowel to prevent any sequelae of its distention. Therapy should be directed at correcting all these problems, even though correcting one may alleviate the others. Often it will be necessary to correct the fluid and electrolyte problems before it is either wise or safe to attempt any operative procedure.

The basic need for almost every patient with intestinal obstruction is surgical correction of the obstructive lesion. Exceptions are adhesion obstruction and Crohn's disease, which are often corrected by intubation (Chapter 127, Surgical Management). Uncontrolled rush to the operating room, however, without proper evaluation of the fluid and electrolyte deficits, and without some attempt to decompress the upper gastrointestinal tract, may lead to disaster.

Operative Care. The decision about when to operate is almost as important as the decision to operate. The surgeon should see the patient as soon as possible after the diagnosis of intestinal obstruction is suspected and, together with the internist, plan appropriate therapy. The plan must include proper restoration of fluids and electrolytes, judicious use of intestinal suction, appropriate diagnostic studies, and ultimately surgical intervention to remove the cause of the obstruction with a minimum of other operative maneuvers.

An adhesion causing small bowel obstruction should be lysed.[36–38] If the abdomen is clear, the remainder of the abdomen should be explored. If there are multiple adhesions, nothing further should be done. The specific adhesion that is the cause of the difficulty and that can be recognized as the point where the distended and collapsed bowel meet should be divided without attempting to divide all the other adhesions.

If a previously unrecognized external or internal hernia is present, the bowel in the hernia should be reduced and the hernia defect repaired. A volvulus should be reduced and the point around which the bowel twisted should be eliminated if possible. If some iatrogenic condition has made this condition possible, e.g., an ileostomy or colostomy with an opening between its mesentery and the abdominal wall, this defect should be closed after the bowel has been reduced and untwisted.

In an occasional patient, the degree of distention will make it difficult or impossible to close the abdomen. If a long intestinal tube is in place, it should be possible to aspirate most of the intestinal contents through the tube and thereby obviate the need for an enterotomy. Should the obstruction be in the colon, some immediate decompressive procedure can be life-saving, as discussed in the section on colonic obstruction. However, if the obstruction is small bowel in origin, and if aspiration through the long tube does not relieve the distention quickly enough to permit proper closure of the abdomen, operative decompression should be done. A suction trocar, inserted into the collapsed section of the bowel, should remove as much intestinal contents as needed to permit subsequent closure of the abdomen. This should be done as aseptically as possible. A number of different devices have been designed to assist in this regard. Some surgeons advocate accordion-pleating the bowel on the trocar for maximum decompression of the bowel. This procedure can cause shock in the patient, and it should not be done unless necessary. Multiple insertion of needles to aspirate gas at different levels is to be condemned, since this opens additional avenues for leakage from the bowel.

Aspiration of the bowel should be done only to permit closure of the abdomen and not to prevent absorption of "toxins" formed in the obstructed intestine. Bacterial multiplication and toxin production are dangers only when the bacteria remain in a segment of bowel with damaged viability; neither bacteria nor their toxins are absorbed through the normal mucosa above and below the obstruction. A segment of bowel whose viability is questionable should be resected. The real danger exists only when the organisms and their products get into the peritoneal cavity. The fluid in the bowel is lost to the circulation and should not be considered available for reabsorption.

Parenteral *antibiotics* should be administered to any patient whose bowel is decompressed during the operative procedure. In addition, it is our practice to place kanamycin in the peritoneal cavity immediately after the bowel is decompressed.[11] The antibiotic is used during the operative procedure or instilled intraperitoneally through a small plastic catheter when the patient recovers from anesthesia. This use of an antibiotic will combat the unavoidable bacterial spillage that accompanies operative decompression of the obstructed bowel.

The actual or suspected presence of strangulation is an indication for urgent operation. Replacement of lost blood, removal of the strangulated bowel, antibiotic administration, and fluid resuscitation are the only measures that will improve the condition of such a patient.

Intubation. Every patient with intestinal obstruction should be intubated. Gastric decompression alone is valuable in terms of relief from the distress of distention. Furthermore, preoperative decompression of the stomach minimizes the risk of aspiration during anesthesia. Nasogastric suction using a Levin or similar tube, followed by a longer tube of the Miller-Abbott type, together with proper replacement of fluids and electrolytes, has permitted more orderly and less urgent management of the obstructed patient. Indeed, the successful and intelligent use of intestinal intubation has completely changed the approach to intestinal obstruction. It has permitted detailed study of the patient, frequently making it possible to locate with some accuracy the cause and point of obstruction.

The principal use of the Miller-Abbott–type tube is in small bowel obstruction. Familiarity with the technique of passage of the tube on the part of clinician, radiologist, and ancillary personnel is essential. Utilization of the long tube by inexperienced personnel is fraught with danger. Under these circumstances it is better to use the short tube for decompression of the stomach only. Persistent attempts to pass the long tube when it does not progress lead to the danger of imminent strangulation.

The long tube in experienced hands is most

helpful in the relief of adhesion obstruction. Many of these patients have had one or more operations previously for relief of adhesion obstruction, and further surgery is to be avoided whenever possible.[2–7,22,25,37,38] If an operation cannot be avoided, the tube may serve as an internal "splint" while the adhesions are lysed to allow the bowel to lie in relatively large gentle curves and thereby prevent acute angulation and subsequent obstruction. In all cases, careful monitoring is essential to avoid leaving the tube in too long while irreversible changes take place within the bowel or in fluid and electrolyte balance.

Whenever a patient is being followed with gastrointestinal intubation, it is essential to make observations at frequent intervals to determine the extent of abdominal distention, degree of pain, character of the peristalsis, progression of the tube, amount of suction drainage, and general condition of the patient. If the patient is improving with suction, continuation of this management may be justified. But should the patient's condition deteriorate, or if there is no further improvement, immediate operative intervention is indicated.

In those patients operated on during the obstructive phase and in whom the Miller-Abbott tube has reached the point of obstruction, the surgeon is able to fix the location of the obstruction more rapidly. The tube can also be used in the postoperative period to maintain decompression of the bowel and to splint the bowel in a position permitting "controlled" formation of postoperative adhesions. The tube should be left in place postoperatively until normal peristalsis has returned, inasmuch as it is difficult to replace the tube following its removal.

Long intestinal tubes have no real place in the management of a patient with large bowel obstruction other than to help decompress the proximally distended small bowel. The real problem in the patient with large bowel obstruction is the urgent need for decompression of the colon, and the long tube cannot accomplish this.

Antibiotics. The most recent advance in the care of patients with obstruction has been the demonstration that antibiotics favorably alter the pathologic process of strangulation obstruction. Antibiotics play no significant role in the management of patients with simple obstruction except insofar as they may alter the mortality associated with complications in elderly patients operated on for obstruction. The patient with strangulation obstruction is quite likely to have other complicating factors and also may arrive at the hospital at a time when antibiotics may no longer be effective. Nevertheless, it is well to administer antibiotics systemically as soon as possible to the patient with known or suspected strangulation obstruction.

When the abdomen is opened and the diagnosis confirmed, the peritoneal cavity should be aspirated of all bloody fluid, lavaged completely, and kanamycin instilled.[11] This will reduce still further the risk of bacterial contamination during operation, including that from bacteria that may have permeated a grossly intact bowel wall. Antibiotics will not combat the deleterious effects of bacterial toxins already absorbed from the peritoneal cavity, but lavage of the cavity will eliminate or minimize the toxins present. Hence, the combination of lavage and antibiotic instillation should be effective in diminishing the toxic effects of bacteria, no matter how these effects may be exerted. Antibiotics notwithstanding, the prime need in the patient with strangulation obstruction is *resection of the strangulated segment of bowel*, removal of the cause of both the obstruction and the strangulation, and the restoration of intestinal continuity.

Fluids and Electrolytes. Administration of appropriate kinds and quantities of fluids to replace those lost is the third part of the cornerstone in the management of patients with intestinal obstruction. Fluid replacement can be placed in proper perspective by recognizing that its combination with control of distention may permit indefinite control of the patient with simple obstruction.

The fluid and electrolyte requirements of the patient with intestinal obstruction can be determined from the following observations: (1) the presence of simple or strangulation obstruction; (2) the level of the obstruction in the gastrointestinal tract; (3) the duration of the obstruction; (4) the clinical evidences of dehydration; and (5) the quantities of fluid lost both through gastrointestinal suction and into the distended loops of bowel proximal to the obstruction.

The patient with a strangulation obstruction needs replacement of blood lost into the hemorrhagic bowel wall, the bowel lumen, and the peritoneal cavity. An additional need for blood will be shock from spillage of intestinal contents into the peritoneal cavity. In the patient with an unrecognized strangulation, the loss of blood may not be obvious until operative procedure reveals the extent of the disorder. Loss of blood and the need for replacement increase directly with the length of the strangulated segment; in the patient with a very long loop of strangulated bowel, there may be shock directly related to the loss of blood into the strangulated loop.

In the patient with small bowel obstruction, the loss of gastric, biliary, pancreatic, and small intestinal secretions determines the replacement needs. It is to be emphasized that fluid accumulated in distended loops of bowel is effectively lost to the body. The initial assays of electrolyte levels may be deceptive because the dominant loss may be either acid or alkaline. Fluid replacement can be accomplished with normal saline or a balanced salt solution and should include potassium. The quantity of fluid to be administered, as noted, is determined by the evidence of dehydration, the extent of the loss through suction, and the estimates of the amount lost into the gastrointestinal tract. The patient who arrives at the hospital in the late stages of small bowel obstruction may well require prolonged rehydration prior to any attempted surgical correction in order to avoid irreversible shock during the operative procedure. Good indications of response by the patient are return of a normal urine volume, appearance of hydration, and restoration of an adequate pulse, blood pressure, and central venous pressure.

When obstruction occurs in the large bowel, fluid and electrolyte disturbance is less likely. The urgent need in these cases is for relief of the large bowel distention to prevent perforation of the cecum. Fluid replacement can be accomplished while the operating room is being prepared and probably should not delay decompression except in the unusual case.

The patient with a chronic obstruction will have alteration in serum proteins as well as serum electrolytes. In such patients, it may be necessary to correct protein deficits before extensive surgical maneuvers can be accomplished safely. Under these circumstances evidences of anemia may also become manifest after rehydration.

Nutrition will be impaired during the development of any but the acute obstruction, as well as during recovery when the return of peristalsis is delayed by the changes in bowel wall physiology. Intravenous hyperalimentation has been effective in providing positive nitrogen balance and is particularly useful in the patient with a protein deficit from chronic obstruction, postoperative ileus, adynamic ileus, or ileus related to an acute toxic or infectious process (Chapter 235).

Prognosis

Successive figures from any one of several institutions for which accurate information has been available indicate that the mortality from intestinal obstruction has dropped significantly from the first recording in that particular institution (Table 122–5). Mortality has decreased to at least half its original value in each institution, reaching an amazingly low rate of 4% in one institution.

The presence of strangulation is one of the most important factors determining mortality (Table 122–6). In almost every major series there is a higher mortality for strangulation than for simple obstruction.[5] The major problems of peritoneal inflammation that accompany strangulation obstruction, and the possibility of peritonitis, are factors that cannot be ignored in considering the risks associated with intestinal obstruction.

Recognition of the importance of fluid and electrolyte replacement, blood gases, and an adequate circulating blood volume, together with the more careful monitoring that is so much more common today, has improved the outlook for these patients. Current anesthetic techniques must also be given credit for improving the safety of operative procedures for intestinal obstruction. The widespread and intelligent use of intubation to overcome adhesion obstruction, to improve the patient's preoperative status, and to simplify procedure has likewise done much to lower mortality.

The *age* of the patient is a factor in the outcome of intestinal obstruction. Chronologic age is not as important as physiologic age and the presence of complicating disease processes. In any case, the needs of older patients must receive special care.

The *duration* of the obstruction also plays a role in the ultimate mortality. The longer the obstruction has been present, the greater the chance of strangulation, serious electrolyte imbalance, perforation, or other compli-

Table 122–5. CHANGE IN MORTALITY IN INDIVIDUAL INSTITUTIONS

First Author	Year	Mortality (%)	Institution
MacFee	1940	33	St. Luke's Hospital (New York)
West	1939–1949	16	
Coletti	1952–1959	15	
Richardson	1908–1917	42	Massachusetts General Hospital
McIver	1918–1927	31	
Scudder	1938	35	
McKittrick	1924–1939	20	
Brill	1922–1928	36	Hospital of the University of Pennsylvania
North	1905–1928	31	
Eliason	1934–1943	11	
Nemir	1940–1950	10	
Miller	1924–1929	61	Charity Hospital (New Orleans)
Moss	1930–1932	32	
Boyce	1933–1935	36	
Becker	1940–1949	19	
Turner	1929	27	Mayo Clinic
	1939–1940	21	
	1949–1950	4	

cation. It is for these reasons that intubation should not be prolonged unduly.

The *cause* of the obstruction contributes to the risk, as do the associated complications that may arise from the obstructing agent. Thus, the patient with early obstruction from an incarcerated hernia usually is a better risk than the one with obstruction from carcinoma; the patient with carcinoma is likely to be a better risk than the one with carcinoma and perforation.

Location of the obstruction influences mortality, as is seen from Table 122–7. In general, large bowel obstruction has a higher mortality rate than small bowel obstruction. This probably is related to the high frequency of carcinoma in large bowel obstruction, the significant bacterial content of the large bowel, the difference in the surgical approach to large and small bowel obstruction, and the surgical sequelae of large bowel obstruction.

Special Forms of Intestinal Obstruction

Gallstone Ileus. Gallstones are the most frequently encountered foreign bodies that cause intestinal obstruction.[39–42] Other agents are listed in Table 122–8. Gallstone obstruction has been reported in from 0.3%

Table 122–6. MORTALITY IN SIMPLE AND STRANGULATION OBSTRUCTION

		Simple Obstruction		Strangulation Obstruction	
First Author	Year	*Number*	*Mortality (%)*	*Number*	*Mortality (%)*
MacFee*	1940	108	34	106	32
McKittrick*	1940	91	12	45	36
Nemir*	1952	267	9	91	13
Becker*	1955	728	14	279	31
Smith*	1955	901	6	283	11
Davis*	1956	84	19	70	23
Bendeck*	1957	133	11	151	6
Waldron*	1961	413	11	80	29
Silen*	1962	368	7	112	21
Leffall	1965	1648	3	52	31
Brooks*	1966	133	11	117	5
Davis*	1969	143	3	9	22
Kaltiala	1972	415	5	80	30
Bizer	1981	364	6	41	15

*Data from Cohn.[12]

Table 122–7. COMPARATIVE MORTALITY OF LARGE AND SMALL BOWEL OBSTRUCTION*

First Author	Year	Large Bowel (%)	Small Bowel (%)
Ellison	1947	16	8
Troell	1954	19	12
Becker	1955	33	15
Smith	1955	6	9
Davis	1958	27	18
Waldron	1961	37	12
Zollinger	1963	13	10

*Data from Cohn.[12]

to 5.3% of all cases of obstruction. Thus, it must be considered in a patient with obstruction, but is certainly not a common occurrence.

Pathogenesis. The accepted pathogenesis of gallstone ileus assumes a series of episodes of inflammation in a gallbladder containing stones, the formation of adhesions between the gallbladder and the intestine (most often the duodenum), and the erosion of a large stone through the gallbladder wall into the intestine (Chapter 202). The stone causing obstruction may traverse the common bile duct, although this is unusual. Fistula formation into the duodenum is the usual antecedent to gallstone ileus, since a fistula into the stomach rarely results in obstruction, and a fistula into the colon will deliver the stone into a segment of bowel with a lumen too large to be obstructed by a stone. The stone most often causes obstruction in the distal ileum, but not at the ileocecal valve. The critical size of a stone that will cause obstruction is 2.5 cm. It is wise to search for other stones in the intestine to prevent recurrent bouts of obstruction. Some patients with cholecysto-enteric fistulas have passed stones into the intestine without having an episode of intestinal obstruction.

Table 122–8. CAUSES OF OBTURATION OBSTRUCTION*

- I. Gallstones
- II. Parasites
  - A. *Ascaris*
  - B. *Taenia*
  - C. *Trichocephalus (Trichuris)*
  - D. *Oxyuris*
- III. Fecaliths
- IV. Enteroliths
  - A. Cholesterol and bile acids
  - B. Calcium carbonate and phosphate
- V. Concretions
  - A. Shellac
  - B. Casein
  - C. Bismuth and magnesium carbonate
- VI. Bezoars
- VII. Food boli
- VIII. Miscellaneous
  - A. Metal
  - B. Glass
  - C. Bone
- IX. Meconium

*Adapted from Storck et al.[48]

Diagnosis. The usual patient is a woman in middle or late life who presents with symptoms of small bowel obstruction with abdominal distention and probably has a history of episodes of biliary colic. These attacks may have been relatively mild, but one may have been more severe than the others. Subsequent to that time there may have been additional episodes, which are difficult to distinguish as being due to early partial small bowel obstruction or recurrent biliary colic. Indeed, the patient may not have been aware of the changing symptoms until questioned in greater detail in the postoperative period. Jaundice is not ordinarily a feature, since the most severe attack probably was associated with development of the fistula, and this would act to prevent jaundice. The history may be no more specific than that, and on the basis of the history and physical examination, it seems unlikely that the diagnosis will be made preoperatively except under unusual circumstances.

Radiologic examination is the key to diagnosis. The following findings can lead to a proper preoperative diagnosis: (1) air or contrast medium in the biliary tree; (2) demonstration of a radiopaque stone in the intestine, or a stone in the intestine outlined by contrast medium; (3) change in location of the stone shadow in the intestine; and (4) dilated loops of small intestine. The demonstrated presence of air in the biliary tree in a patient suspected of having intestinal obstruction is almost always diagnostic of gallstone obstruction, and no further study is necessary in most such cases.

Treatment. If the diagnosis can be made preoperatively, the patient should be prepared for operation as soon as possible. In general, this means restoration of fluid and electrolyte balance if seriously impaired, gastrointestinal intubation, administration of antibiotics to help control the inflammatory reaction around the fistula, and early operation. Additional studies of the biliary tree are neither indicated nor desirable.

Since the operative procedure is designed to relieve an acute condition, it should be limited to that objective. At the time of operation, the point of obstruction should be identified and the obstructing gallstone removed from the intestine. If the stone has caused sufficient damage to the intestinal wall to compromise its viability, the affected bowel should be resected and a primary anastomosis accomplished. Usually there is no significant damage to the bowel wall, and it is necessary only to gently remove the stone from the bowel through an enterotomy proximal to the obstruction in a relatively normal portion of the bowel. In the vast majority of patients, this should be all that is done at the time of the emergency procedure. The gallbladder should not be handled at the time of the original operation because of the high mortality rate associated with one-stage procedures, the increased risk of infection, and the unnecessary prolongation of a procedure in a patient who is quite ill.

At a later date, the cholecysto-enteric fistula should be resected along with the gallbladder and the intestinal end of the fistula closed. In recent years, however, a number of surgeons have advocated one-stage repair. I believe that the hazards of the combined procedures do not justify their use.

Some thought has been given to allowing the cholecysto-enteric fistula to close spontaneously so that further surgery would be unnecessary. This is an unwarranted assumption for which there is little evidence. In addition to the possibility of further stone formation, the persistent fistula is an open avenue for the development of ascending cholangitis. Therefore, the patient who recovers from gallstone ileus should be scheduled for removal of the gallbladder and the fistula at some early date.

Prognosis. The improved mortality of recent years (Table 122–9) probably is a result of the combination of better diagnosis, with heightened awareness of the radiologic signs, better anesthesia, better fluid control, antibiotic administration, and the repeated teaching that emergency surgical attacks on the fistula are contraindicated.

Table 122–9. MORTALITY OF GALLSTONE ILEUS

Date	Source	Mortality (%)
Prior–1925*	Moore (334 cases)	75.0
1925–1940*	Foss et al. (150 cases)	57.4
1940–1955*	Deckoff (73 cases)	33.3
1955–1960*	Raiford (112 cases)	27.7
1961–1970	Collected (129 cases)	9.3
1971–1980	Collected (177 cases)	16.3

*Data from Cohn.[12]

Intussusception. Intussusception is the invagination of one part of the intestinal tract into another. Its symptoms are those of acute complete intestinal obstruction or partial and recurrent obstruction. It may involve the small bowel or the large bowel exclusively or the small and large bowel together. Basically there are 2 forms of intussusception, one occurring in the infant and the other in the adult. It is necessary to consider each separately, since etiology, symptoms, and therapy are different.

Frequency. The greatest frequency of intussusception is in the first year of life.[43,44] In Orloff's[44] collected series, 69% of 1814 cases in children occurred during this period. Gross[43] reported an experience with 702 cases prior to 1950 at Children's Hospital in Boston, as contrasted with a collected experience in the English literature of approximately 1300 cases in adults from the turn of the century until recently. The precise occurrence rate is difficult to determine, but 123 adult cases were seen in one hospital during a 36-year period when the institution treated approximately one million patients[44a] and 55 adult cases at Charity Hospital in New Orleans during a period when there were 287 cases in children.[44b]

Forms. Intussusception may involve only the small bowel (*ileo-ileal intussusception*) or only the colon (*colo-colic intussusception*). In Orloff's[44] collected series, 80% of intussusceptions in children were of the ileo-ileal variety. Review of experience in adults showed that 48% were of the enteric type and 52% were of the colonic type.

Invagination can extend for unusual lengths; some cases are described in which the intussuscepting small bowel presents in the rectum. The danger always lies in the possible interference with the blood supply to that portion of the bowel invaginated into another segment of bowel. The longer the intussusception becomes, the longer it remains in place, and the greater the degree of swelling of the bowel, the greater the chance of interference with circulation to the bowel.

Etiology. The difference in etiology is one of the main distinguishing features between the condition in infants and adults. In infants, the cause is unknown for as many as

95% of the cases. By contrast, 80% of adult intussusceptions have an organic cause, with benign or malignant tumors accounting for approximately 65% of these. The frequency of malignant tumors is even higher in those cases that involve only the colon. Thus, cases of intussusception in adults must be treated as though a malignant tumor were present.

There has never been a completely satisfactory explanation for the high frequency of intussusception in infants. Factors such as changes in diet, increase in lymphoid tissue in the intestine, alterations in peristalsis, inflammatory changes in the bowel, and the obvious presence of a Meckel's diverticulum have been described as possible causes. At the moment, greatest favor is given to a correlation with a viral infection that produces enlargement of intestinal wall lymphoid tissue.

Clinical Aspects. The clinical picture and the presenting symptoms of intussusception in an infant are so characteristic as to make the diagnosis almost automatic.[45] *Pain* is the most characteristic and most constant finding. There is sudden onset of severe spasms of abdominal pain, which increase to a maximum intensity and then disappear completely. The pain is related to the passage of the intussusception. Between episodes of pain, the infant (or adult) may be completely symptom-free. In addition to pain, there may be *vomiting*, passage of *blood per rectum*, and the presence of a *palpable abdominal mass*, which represents the segment of intussusception. The extent of vomiting will be related to the level of the bowel involved in the intussusception; the higher the obstruction, the greater the amount of vomiting. Hematochezia is related to interference with the return of circulation from the bowel involved in the intussusception. While some blood is characteristic, significant amounts of bleeding are unusual. In Orloff's[44] collected series, pain was present in 90%, vomiting in 84%, blood in the stool in 80%, an abdominal mass in 73%, and an abdominal or rectal mass in 82%.

In adults there may be a much longer history, with repeated unsuccessful attempts at diagnosis by radiology and other means. Recurrent bouts of intestinal obstruction should alert the clinician to the possibility of intussusception, but the failure to confirm this radiologically may deter him from accepting the diagnosis. Roentgen examination fails to confirm the diagnosis very often because intussusception may not be present at the specific time examination is made as a result of spontaneous reduction. Thus, the diagnosis of intussusception should at least be considered in any adult who has repeated bouts of obstruction without positive roentgen or other findings.

Diagnosis. The diagnosis may be established on the basis of the characteristic history and physical findings. In those patients in whom the intussusception involves the colon, barium enema may confirm the diagnosis (Fig. 122–5). There will be obstruction to the flow of barium at the leading point of the intussusception and a cup-shaped appearance to the barium at this point; as pressure is increased, the intussusception may be reduced partially or completely. If barium passes the point of obstruction, a coil-spring appearance is diagnostic. If any or all of these signs are present, and if a mass can be palpated at the point of obstruction, diagnosis is fairly secure.

Treatment. The treatment for most intussusceptions in the *adult* is surgical resection of the involved segment of bowel. In the

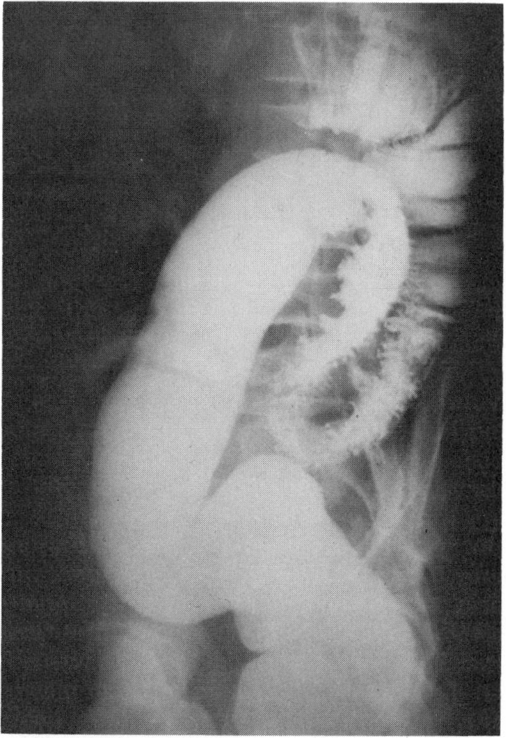

Figure 122–5. Intussusception of the left transverse colon due to a polypoid carcinoma of the colon. There is a faint suggestion of the coiled-spring appearance in the barium-filled colon.

hands of experienced radiologists who work in close conjunction with pediatric surgeons, hydrostatic reduction of the intussusception by barium enema under direct observation is the preferred method of treating some *infants*. This technique cannot be recommended, however, if the radiologist is inexperienced, if the surgeon is unfamiliar with the technique or unwilling to operate urgently if it becomes obvious that barium enema treatment is not successful, or for any patient in whom there is a question of the viability of the bowel. Hydrostatic reduction has no place in the treatment of a patient with recurrent intussusception and should not be used in anyone over 5 years of age.

In *children*, if barium enema reduction is not successful, or is not tried, operative relief of the intussusception is indicated. If the lesion is completely confined to the small bowel and can be manually reduced, this should be accomplished. If no lesion is found leading the intussusception, prophylactic appendectomy is an acceptable procedure because it removes a structure that could later become diseased and that also may provide a point of fixation to prevent recurrent intussusception. Gangrenous bowel must be resected, with proper protection against soilage and adequate antibiotic therapy in the postoperative period.

Treatment of the adult is exclusively surgical. Even if the intussusception can be reduced manually when completely confined to the small bowel, increasing recognition of the frequency of associated and underlying malignant lesions makes resection preferable. If the intussusception involves the colon, the prevalence of malignant disease leading to the intussusception is so high that the entire problem is that of colon cancer and entails performance of an appropriately wide resection.

Prognosis. The mortality of intussusception has been reduced dramatically since the earliest reports of this condition. The current mortality for large or collected series is approximately 5% to 10%. The mortality with irreducible intussusception is considerably higher, with figures reported since 1934 ranging from 40% to 90%.[44]

Volvulus. Volvulus is a form of intestinal obstruction that results from a twisting of the bowel upon itself. The twisting action results in a closed loop obstruction within the limits of the twisted bowel and an open loop obstruction proximal to the twist. In the earliest stages of volvulus there may be only obstruction to intestinal continuity. As the twist persists, or as it twists to an even greater degree, there will be interference with the blood supply to all the bowel involved in the process. Regardless of whether the blood supply is blocked by twisting of the mesentery, the circulation will be interfered with by the distention of the bowel. Thus, the ultimate effect will be the same whether there is actual interference with the vessels themselves or merely counterpressure from the increased intraluminal pressure if the obstruction is not relieved relatively early. The amount of distention within the segment of bowel in the volvulus is out of proportion to the duration of the obstruction and to what might be anticipated for a segment of bowel of this length. In fact, the enormous distention is one of the characteristic features of volvulus that helps to make the diagnosis.

Volvulus can occur only in a segment of bowel that has a mesentery sufficiently long to permit it to twist in this fashion. Therefore, the usual locations for volvulus are highly predictable, although in unusual situations where there is some congenital abnormality or some change in the normal intestinal anatomy, volvulus can occur in any segment of bowel that has sufficient freedom to permit its twisting. The sigmoid is the area most commonly involved because of its normally longer mesentery. Other areas that may be involved include the cecum; the entire small bowel or a portion of it, particularly when there are adhesions; the stomach; and even, in most unusual circumstances, the transverse colon. The twist may occur in the long axis of the involved segment of intestine, or it may occur at right angles to this axis.

Etiology. The etiology of volvulus has never been established. In addition to the long mesentery, which is a sine qua non of volvulus, various authors have suggested the importance of chronic constipation, a diet high in roughage (thought to play a role in the higher frequency of volvulus in some European countries), and the tendency of the bowel to move in response to its heavy contents, thus causing torsion. Interestingly, the occurrence rate of the disorder is higher in men than in women and in inmates of mental institutions than in the population at large.

Clinical Aspects. Symptomatically, the patient with volvulus usually has a sudden onset of severe abdominal *pain* followed quickly by rapidly increasing and marked *abdominal distention*. The continuous abdominal pain is a result of pull on the mesentery from the twisting of the bowel. There will be superimposed intermittent pain related to the distention of the involved loop and to the rushes of peristalsis in the proximal segment. Previous episodes of constipation would have been painless, but the patient is aware that something is different because of the complete obstipation and the associated pain and distention. *Vomiting* will not be significant in the early stages of the disease. *Blood passed per rectum* may be in small amounts and may be missed by the patient.

Tremendous abdominal distention is the hallmark of the disease and should give the clinician his first major clue to the diagnosis. Plain films of the abdomen, recumbent and erect, or the even more impressive barium enema, will clinch the diagnosis. The films (Figs. 122–6 and 122–7) disclose abnormal distention, displacement of the bowel from its normal location, double air-fluid levels, and a sharp cut-off at the point of torsion with distended loops of bowel proximal to this point. Barium enema confirms the sharp point at which barium stops and may give evidence of the spiral pattern of the colon as some of the barium enters the twisted bowel. The absence of bowel from its normal location (left lower quadrant for sigmoid volvulus and right lower quadrant for cecal volvulus) is an additional feature confirming the diagnosis. In volvulus of the small bowel, contrast medium confirmation is not as easy to obtain and usually will be positive only if it is possible to get barium to the proximal point of obstruction following oral administration of the contrast agent (Fig. 122–8). Under these circumstances, it may be possible to see the twist in the mucosa and even to get some barium into the distended segment to outline its distention and abnormal location.

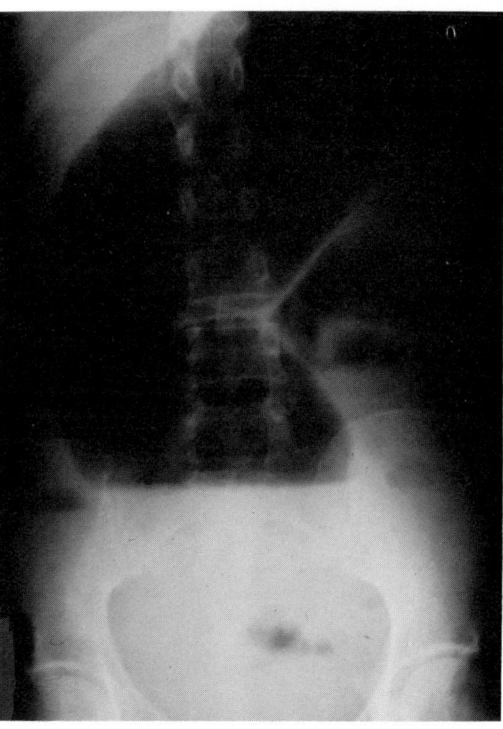

Figure 122–7. Sigmoid volvulus. Erect film of same patient as in Figure 122–6. There is a single fluid level and massive distention of the bowel.

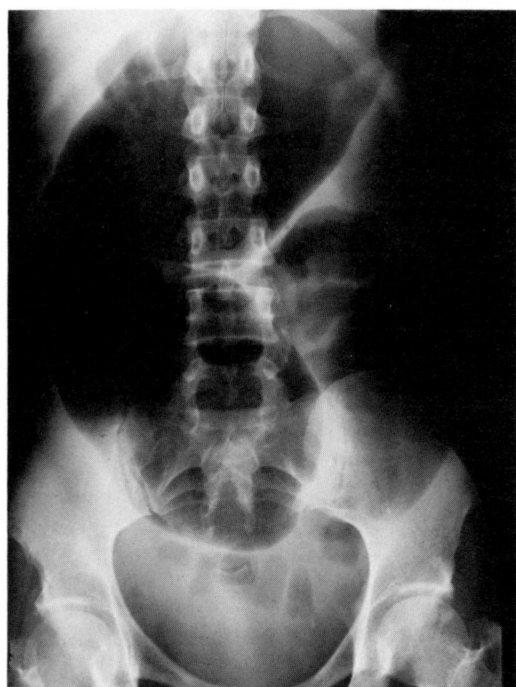

Figure 122–6. Supine film of a patient with sigmoid volvulus. There is a greatly distended loop of sigmoid rising out of the pelvis and practically filling the abdomen.

Treatment. Once the diagnosis ot volvulus has been made, therapy is needed urgently. For sigmoid volvulus, an attempt should be made at nonoperative reduction by insertion of a proctosigmoidoscope, a flexible colonoscope, or a long rectal tube to deflate the bowel. Caution must be employed to prevent rupture of the bowel by forcing the instru-

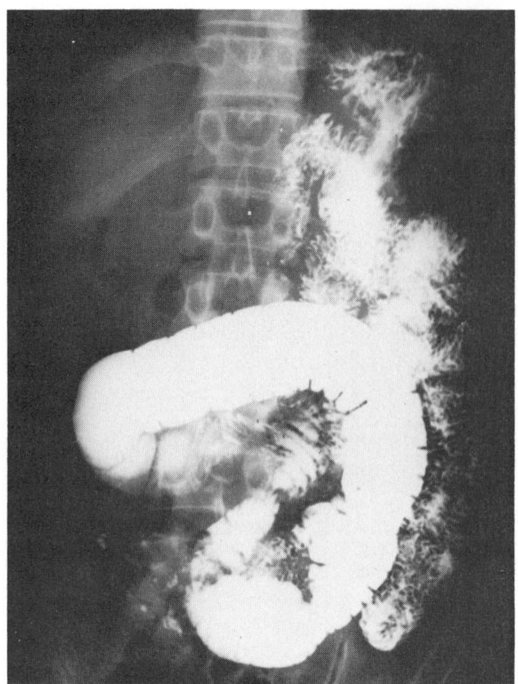

Figure 122–8. Volvulus of the small bowel due to adhesions. In this supine view of the abdomen taken after oral administration of barium, it is easy to see the point of fixation and the axis of rotation, with twisting of the small bowel about this point.

ment through the point of torsion. If the tube successfully enters the twisted segment, there will be an immediate expulsion of gas and feces and the patient will experience prompt relief. Should the nonoperative approach be unsuccessful, immediate surgical correction is necessary. Even in the patient who responds to tube decompression, a careful watch must be maintained to be sure that some portion of the bowel in the volvulus has not become necrotic and gone unrecognized. Such a development would lead to a fecal peritonitis that could be fatal.

When a surgical approach is indicated, the specific procedure will depend upon the operative findings. If the bowel is distended but clearly viable, detorsion is all that is necessary. If there is any question about the viability of the twisted bowel, both the operative procedure and the risk take on significantly different proportions. For a volvulus with gangrene of the small bowel, immediate resection and primary end-to-end anastomosis of the bowel should be accomplished. This should have no more risk than ordinary small bowel resection in the presence of gangrenous bowel. If the right colon is involved, the same procedure should be carried out, but the risk will be greater because of the inherently greater bacterial population in the colon and the differences in blood supply to the right colon and small bowel. If the bowel involved is the transverse colon or sigmoid, resection of the necrotic bowel is mandatory; primary anastomosis is so fraught with danger that it should not be considered. If a double-barrel colostomy can be established, this would be the procedure of choice. If the bowel must be resected so low that it cannot be brought out as a mucous fistula, it should be closed and dropped back into the peritoneal cavity. Closure of the colostomy can be accomplished at a later date as an elective procedure when the patient can be properly prepared.

After multiple attacks of volvulus involving the sigmoid or the cecum, consideration may be given to elective resection to prevent further recurrences. If necessary, the redundant bowel can be resected as an emergency measure, but a primary anastomosis should not be attempted for the reasons just enumerated.

Adynamic Ileus. Adynamic or paralytic ileus, a form of "functional obstruction",[46] is characterized by failure of normal peristalsis to move contents down the gastrointestinal tract with coordinated relaxation of the bowel. Since almost every abdominal operative procedure is followed by varying periods of paralytic ileus, it is obviously a problem of great magnitude. Loss of peristaltic activity is so common following abdominal operations that it is considered a normal part of the postoperative course, and many surgeons use some type of gastrointestinal intubation as part of the therapy after every abdominal operation in an attempt to minimize the associated distention and discomfort. Many believe that the duration of the ileus will be associated with the manner in which the bowel is handled, prolonged ileus being a sequela of rough handling. Others discount this factor. Some think that exposure of the bowel to the normal atmosphere, permitting the bowel to become dry while it is outside the peritoneal cavity, excessive traction on the bowel or its mesentery, and a variety of other factors common to any abdominal procedure are responsible for postoperative ileus.

In addition to cases following abdominal operations, the long list and variety of causes

Table 122–10. CAUSES OF ADYNAMIC ILEUS*

- I. Intra-abdominal
  - A. Peritoneal irritation
    - 1. Traumatic
      - a. Postoperative
      - b. Penetrating wounds
    - 2. Bacterial
      - a. Peritonitis
    - 3. Chemical
      - a. Extravasation of blood
      - b. Perforated peptic ulcer
      - c. Bile peritonitis—early
      - d. Acute pancreatitis—early
  - B. Vascular changes
    - 1. Strangulation
      - a. Intramural
        - (1) Distention following mechanical ileus
      - b. Extramural
        - (1) Compression of the mesenteric vessels
    - 2. Mesenteric thrombosis
  - C. Extraperitoneal irritation
    - 1. Hemorrhage
    - 2. Infection
    - 3. Renal
- II. Extra-abdominal
  - A. Toxic
    - 1. Pneumonia
    - 2. Uremia
    - 3. Empyema
    - 4. Systemic infection
  - B. Neurogenic
    - 1. Injuries and diseases of the spinal cord
    - 2. Lead poisoning
    - 3. Fracture of the lower ribs
      - a. Irritation of the splanchnic nerves

*From Ochsner and Gage.[46]

given in Table 122–10 provide some idea of the frequency of adynamic ileus.

Clinical Aspects. The dominant feature of adynamic ileus is the *abdominal distention* and the *absence of peristaltic sounds* on careful auscultation of the abdomen. Since ileus has so many different causes, it is well to note any pre-existing conditions and to determine how much of the present problem may be related to a known diagnosis. Distention may occur quite rapidly and may be of an extreme degree. There may or may not be *vomiting*. Any oral intake, however, is usually regurgitated so that food and fluid by mouth should not be given.

Abdominal distention is uniform when all segments of bowel are involved. Palpation will reveal neither masses nor tenderness in the absence of some other specific lesion. The silent abdomen is the striking and classic feature.

Roentgenographic examination will confirm the diagnosis after the foregoing observations have been made (Fig. 122–9). The presence of distended loops of bowel throughout the abdomen is characteristic, and the presence of air extending all the way to the rectum makes the diagnosis certain.

Treatment. Therapy for the patient with paralytic ileus is mainly symptomatic, unless there is some specific etiologic agent that can be identified and eliminated. Whenever possible, this should be done as quickly as feasible. If no direct cause can be found, therapy should consist of the measures used for the patient with intestinal obstruction—intubation, fluid and electrolyte support, and prevention of infection. Patience is the major requirement for both patient and physician, since most cases will resolve with time and appropriate therapy. Insertion of a long tube into the small bowel is most helpful. Unfortunately, this is not possible in most cases because of the lack of peristaltic activity needed to propel the tube through the small bowel. Fluid support is essential and has been simplified with the advent of IV hyperalimentation. Enemas probably are of minimal value in stimulating return of peristalsis. A great variety of drugs have been employed in an attempt to stimulate peristalsis, but in my experience most of these drugs do not work. Some of the drugs will help to prevent

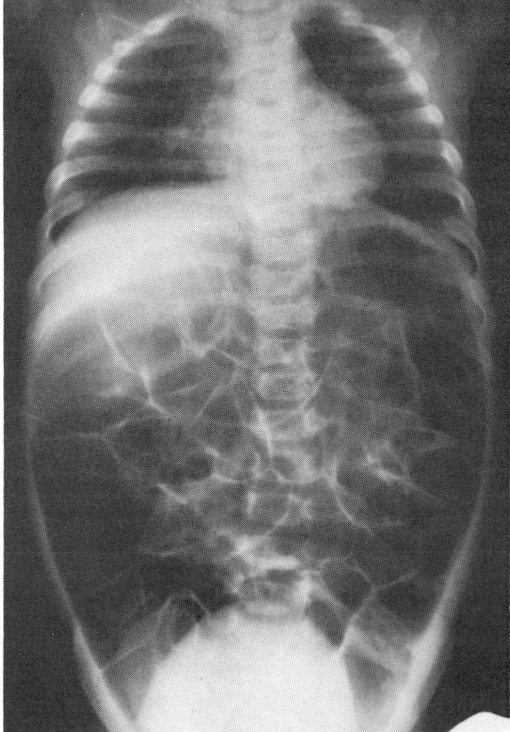

Figure 122–9. Adynamic ileus with generalized distention of both small and large bowel.

loss of peristalsis in the postoperative period, but once peristalsis has ceased, few medications, if any, will initiate the needed peristalsis in the patient with adynamic ileus. The suggestion that peristalsis can be stimulated by a gastrointestinal "pacemaker" has not been accepted widely.

In the patient with massive distention in whom rupture of the bowel is feared, some decompressive procedure may be necessary. Such procedures should be employed with great caution because they: (1) may produce a greater degree of ileus in connection with the additional trauma to the bowel; (2) may not relieve the distention since there is no propulsive force to drive the accumulated gas through the intestine; (3) may be associated with all the complications that might be anticipated from operating upon a patient with massive abdominal distention; and (4) may, in general, lead to further deterioration of an already critical situation. Operative relief should be sought only under most unusual circumstances.

Thus, therapy is mainly dependent on intubation and fluid support with continuing careful search for some specific factor that might be relieved. Throughout, both the physician and the patient must exercise an unusual degree of patience.

Spastic Ileus. "Spastic ileus" is a term that has been used to describe a true obstruction secondary to intense spasm of the gut. This has never been completely documented, and it is highly unlikely that such a phenomenon occurs.

Large Bowel Obstruction. Common causes of obstruction of the large bowel include diverticulitis, volvulus, intussusception, and hernia, but carcinoma is by far the most common.[2,4,6,12,26] Indeed, carcinoma is so much more frequently the cause of obstruction that any other lesion or abnormality must be a secondary consideration. Adhesions are almost nonexistent as a cause of large bowel obstruction, in contrast to their great frequency in the small bowel. The preponderance of cancer among the causes of large bowel obstruction alone mandates management that differs from that of the patient with obstruction of the small bowel.

Diagnosis. The diagnosis of large bowel obstruction is often made on the basis of the history and physical examination. Progressive constipation, abdominal pain, and distention are prominent features. Once the diagnosis is suspected, proctosigmoidoscopy followed by a barium enema is imperative. The radiologist must be given full information about the suspected diagnosis so that he can avoid undue pressure on the head of the column of barium as it reaches the point of obstruction. Forcing barium past the point of obstruction may convert a partial obstruction into a complete one, and thereby convert an elective procedure into an emergency one with entirely different morbidity and mortality rates and duration of hospitalization. Once the radiologist has demonstrated the location and character of the lesion, further therapy can be planned rationally.

Treatment. In the presence of a competent ileocecal valve, a closed loop obstruction of the large bowel will exist, and the danger of perforation of the cecum will dominate any considerations of therapy. Decompression of the large bowel is urgent when the cecum begins to show signs of distention; the rapid performance of a satisfactory decompressive procedure should take precedence over all other therapeutic plans in this situation. If the ileocecal valve is not competent, there will be progressive distention of both the small and large bowel. Here, the management depends on the presence of distention in both areas, rather than primary concern about perforation of the cecum.

For the usual patient with an obstructive neoplasm of the large bowel, management must include care of both the obstruction and the cancer. Since the urgent need is for decompression, the method for achieving decompression is the key to further therapy. When the obstructing lesion is in the right colon, an immediate primary resection with restoration of intestinal continuity and without any type of proximal decompression is appropriate. Choice of a one-stage procedure would be based on the presence of a resectable lesion, a patient who can be gotten into proper condition in a relatively short time by rehydration, return of adequate urinary output, restoration of electrolyte balance, and transfusions if necessary. Gastric intubation should be instituted, but additional time should not be wasted in an attempt to thread the tube down the small bowel, inasmuch as the tube will not decompress the large bowel. Neither mechanical preparation nor antibacterial intestinal antisepsis is possible in the acutely obstructed patient.

When the obstructing lesion is on the left side, an entirely different approach should be employed. An emergency proximal colostomy, preferably in the tranverse colon and preferably away from the planned site of resection, should be performed. Both limbs of the colostomy should be opened immediately to decompress the entire colon. The primary lesion should not be manipulated, lest the bowel be perforated even by the gentlest palpation. The only exception would be those patients in whom the only way to make a critical differential diagnosis is by palpation or visualization of the lesion. The colostomy can be closed at a second operation; it can be removed at that time or left for closure at a third stage, depending on the condition of the patient and the preference of the surgeon.

Some surgeons practice one-stage resection and anastomosis of the colon even in the face of complete obstruction on the left side. Most surgical thinking and practice is opposed to this because of the increased dangers of such a procedure.

Obstruction due to diverticulitis should be handled in a fashion similar to that of the obstructive phase of a patient with carcinoma. The additional dangers in the patient with diverticulitis relate to the possible problems arising from perforation or abscess. Either of these should be handled in an appropriate fashion, including some form of drainage for the perforated area.

Prognosis. In spite of the improvements in mortality in small bowel obstruction, the mortality rate for colonic obstruction still remains in the range of 30%, probably related to the primary disease, the age of the patient, the duration of the obstruction, and its location. Once strangulation supervenes in large bowel obstruction, the mortality may double.

References

1. Cohn I Jr. Strangulation Obstruction. Springfield, Ill: Charles C Thomas, 1961.
2. Becker WF. Intestinal obstruction. An analysis of 1007 cases. South Med J 1955; 48:41–6.
3. Bizer LS, Liebling RW, Delany HM, Gliedman ML. Small bowel obstruction. The role of nonoperative treatment in simple intestinal obstruction and predictive criteria for strangulation obstruction. Surgery 1981; 89:407–13.
4. Ellis H. Intestinal Obstruction. New York: Appleton-Century-Crofts, 1982.
5. Kaltiala EH, Lenkkeri H, Larmi TKI. Mechanical intestinal obstruction. An analysis of 577 cases. Ann Chir Gynaecol Fenn 1972; 61:87–93.
6. Smith GA, Perry JF Jr, Yonahiro EG. Mechanical intestinal obstructions. A study of 1,252 cases. Surg Gynecol Obstet 1955; 100:651–60.
7. Stewardson RH, Bombeck CT, Nyhus LM. Critical operative management of small bowel obstruction. Ann Surg 1978; 187:189–93.
8. Aird I. Morbid influences in intestinal obstruction and strangulation. Ann Surg 1941; 114:385–414.
9. Brooks B, Schumacher HW, Wattenberg JE. Intestinal obstruction: An experimental study. Ann Surg 1918; 67:210–214.
10. Cohn I Jr. Strangulation obstruction: A critical review. Surg Gynecol Obstet 1956; 103:105–37.
11. Cohn I Jr. Intestinal Antisepsis. Springfield, Ill: Charles C Thomas, 1968.
12. Cohn I Jr. Intestinal obstruction. *In*: Bockus HL, ed. Gastroenterology, 3rd Ed, Vol 2. Philadelphia: WB Saunders, 1976; 481–509.
13. Dragstedt LR, Moohead JJ, Burcky FW. Intestinal obstruction. An experimental study of the intoxication in closed intestinal loops. J Exp Med 1917; 25:421–39.
14. Foster WC, Hausler RW. Studies on acute intestinal obstruction. II. Acute strangulation. Arch Intern Med 1924; 34:697–713.
15. Gatch WD, Trusler HM, Ayres KD. Causes of death in acute intestinal obstruction. Clinical applications and general principles of treatment. Surg Gynecol Obstet 1928; 46:332-7.
16. Haerem S, Dack GM, Dragstedt LR. Acute intestinal obstruction. II. The permeability of obstructed bowel segments of dogs to *Clostridium botulinum* toxins. Surgery 1938; 3:339–50.
17. Haerem S, Dack GM, Wilson H. Acute intestinal obstruction. I. The role of bacteria in closed jejunal loops. Surgery 1938; 3:333–8.
18. Hartwell JA, Hoguet JP. Experimental intestinal obstruction in dogs with especial reference to the cause of death and the treatment by large amounts of normal saline solution. JAMA 1912; 59:82–7.
19. Hausler RW, Foster WC. Studies of acute intestinal obstruction. I. Different types of obstruction produced under local anesthesia. Arch Intern Med 1924; 34:97–107.
20. Nemir P Jr, Hawthorne HR, Cohn I Jr, Drabkin DL. The cause of death in strangulation obstruction: An experimental study. I. Clinical course, chemical, bacteriologic and spectrophotometric studies. Ann Surg 1949; 130:857–73.
21. Stone HB, Bernheim BM, Whipple GH. The experimental study of intestinal obstruction. Ann Surg 1914; 59:714–26.
22. Wangensteen OH. Intestinal Obstructions. Physiological, Pathological and Clinical Considerations with Emphasis on Therapy, Including Description of Operative Procedures. Springfield, Ill: Charles C Thomas, 1955.
23. Wangensteen OH, Waldron GW. Studies in intestinal obstruction. IV. Strangulation obstruction: A comparison of the toxicity of the intestine and other tissues autolyzed in vivo and in vitro. Arch Surg 1928; 17:430–9.
24. Wangensteen OH. Understanding the bowel obstruction problem. Am J Surg 1978; 135:131–49.
25. Peetz DJ Jr, Gamelli RL, Pilcher DB. Intestinal intubation in acute, mechanical small-bowel obstruction. Arch Surg 1982; 117:334–6.
26. Zollinger RM, Kinsey DL, Grant GN. Intestinal obstruction. Postgrad Med 1963; 33:165–71.
27. Leffall LD Jr, Quander J, Syphax B. Strangulation intestinal obstruction. A clinical appraisal. Arch Surg 1965; 91:592–6.
28. Shatila AH, Chamberlain BE, Webb WR. Current status of diagnosis and management of strangulation obstruction of the small bowel. Am J Surg 1976; 132:299–303.
29. Sykes PA, Boulter KH, Schofield PF. The microflora of the obstructed bowel. Br J Surg 1976; 63:721–5.
30. Tumen H. Intestinal obstruction. *In*: Bockus HL (ed). Gastroenterology, 2nd Ed, Vol 2. Philadelphia: WB Saunders, 1963; 296.
31. Silen W. Cope's Early Diagnosis of the Acute Abdomen. New York: Oxford University Press, 1979.
32. Bryk D. Strangulating obstruction of the bowel: A reevaluation of radiographic criteria. AJR 1978; 130:835–43.
33. Mellins HZ, Rigler LG. The roentgen findings in strangulation obstructions of the small intestine. AJR 1954; 71: 404–15.
34. Sarr MG, Bulkley GB, Zuidema GD. Preoperative recognition of intestinal strangulation obstruction. Prospective evaluation of diagnostic capability. Am J Surg 1983; 145:176–82.
35. Silen W, Hein MF, Goldman L. Strangulation obstruction of the small intestine. Arch Surg 1962; 85:121–9.

36. Brightwell NL, McFee AS, Aust JB: Bowel obstruction and the long tube stent. Arch Surg 1977; 112:505–11.
37. Hofstetter SR. Acute adhesive obstruction of the small intestine. Surg Gynecol Obstet 1981; 152:141–4.
38. Quatromoni JC, Rosoff L Sr, Halls JM, Yellin AE. Early postoperative small bowel obstruction. Ann Surg 1980; 191:72–4.
39. Day EA, Marks C. Gallstone ileus. Review of the literature and presentation of thirty-four new cases. Am J Surg 1975; 129:552–8.
40. Kasahara Y, Umemura H, Shiraha S, Kuyama T, Sakata K, Kubota H. Gallstone ileus. Review of 112 patients in the Japanese literature. Am J Surg 1980; 140:437–40.
41. Raiford TS. Intestinal obstruction due to gallstone (gallstone ileus). Ann Surg 1961; 153:830–8.
42. Way LW, Dunphy JE. Gallstone ileus. Bull Soc Int Chir 1975; 34:647–51.
43. Gross RE. The Surgery of Infancy and Childhood: Its Principles and Techniques. Philadelphia: WB Saunders, 1953.
44. Orloff MV. Intussusception in children and adults. Surg Gynecol Obstet 1956; 102:313–29.
44a. Ponka A. Intussusception in infants and adults. Surg Gynecol Obstet 1967; 124:99–105.
44b. Cotlar AM, Cohn I Jr. Intussusception in adults. Am J Surg 1961; 101:114–20.
45. Peck DA, Lynn HB, DuShane JW. Intussusception in children. Surg Gynecol Obstet 1963; 116:398–404.
46. Ochsner A, Gage IM. Adynamic ileus. Am J Surg 1933; 20:378–404.
47. George CF. Drugs causing intestinal obstruction: A review. J R Soc Med 1980; 73:200–4.
48. Storck A, Rothschild JE, Ochsner A. Intestinal obstruction due to intraluminal foreign bodies. Ann Surg 1939; 109:844–61.

Chapter 123

Chronic Idiopathic Intestinal Pseudo-obstruction

Howard D. Manten • Albert M. Harary

Intestinal pseudo-obstruction is a syndrome characterized by failure of the intestine to propel its contents, leading to signs and symptoms of bowel obstruction in the absence of a demonstrable obstructing lesion. An acute form ("ileus" or "paralytic ileus") is subsumed in the discussion on Intestinal Obstruction that appears in Chapter 122. Consideration here is confined to the chronic form.

In 1939, Weiss[1] described a family in Germany with idiopathic pseudo-obstruction, and Maldonado et al.,[2] in 1970, described a group of 5 patients in detail. Important reviews have since been published by Faulk et al.,[3] Schuffler,[4] and Snape.[5] In addition to sporadic cases, at least 11 families have been described[3, 6–12] although only some were analyzed histologically.[3, 8–12]

Classification

The syndrome of chronic idiopathic intestinal pseudo-obstruction represents a heterogeneous group of disorders that vary in extent of gastrointestinal tract involvement, histologic appearance, and involvement of other organs. Furthermore, both familial and sporadic forms have been described. Small bowel involvement is usually the most prominent aspect of the syndrome, but there is often involvement of the entire alimentary tract or even other visceral musculature, such as the urinary bladder. Even when the syndrome appears to be localized to an isolated loop of bowel, there may be subtle evidence of abnormality in other parts of the gastrointestinal tract.

Secondary intestinal pseudo-obstruction occurs in the presence of conditions affecting the intestinal musculature or innervation, including diseases such as primary systemic sclerosis, diabetes mellitus, amyloidosis, and Chagas' disease, and certain drugs, such as the phenothiazines and tricyclic antidepressants.[4] Table 123–1 lists the secondary causes of pseudo-obstruction. These diseases will be discussed later in the section on Differential Diagnosis, and certain of them are also touched on in other chapters dealing with related disorders (Chapters 76, 90, 111, and 244).

Pathology and Pathophysiology

Idiopathic pseudo-obstructions may be separated into 3 subtypes on the basis of their intestinal histopathologic features: (1) neuropathic, (2) myopathic, and (3) a form in which no discernible pathologic changes are found. Schuffler[4] has stated "intestinal propulsion is regulated by a complex interplay of intestinal smooth muscle, the myenteric plexus, the autonomic nervous system extrinsic to the intestine, and hormones. Theoretically, any disorder interfering with one or more of these regulatory mechanisms could produce chronic idiopathic pseudo-obstruction." Presumably, the defects in cases that appear normal histologically relate to

Table 123–1. CAUSES OF CHRONIC INTESTINAL PSEUDO-OBSTRUCTION*

Disease-associated	Drugs:
Diseases involving smooth muscle:	Tricyclic antidepressants
Collagen vascular disease:	Anti-parkinsonian drugs
Scleroderma	Ganglionic blockers
Dermatomyositis/polymyositis	Phenothiazines
Systemic lupus erythematosus	Clonidine
Periarteritis nodosa	Opiates
Amyloidosis	
Primary muscle disease:	Celiac disease
Myotonic dystrophy	Jejuno-ileal bypass
Progressive muscular dystrophy	Mesenteric vascular insufficiency
	Ceroidosis
Endocrine disorders:	Radiation enteritis
Hypothyroidism	Alcoholism
Hypoparathyroidism	Psychosis
Diabetes mellitus	Cathartic colon
Pheochromocytoma	Neoplasm with or without celiac plexus invasion
	Malrotation
Neurologic diseases:	*Strongyloides* infection
Parkinson's disease	Azotemia
Hirschsprung's disease	Porphyria
Intestinal hypoganglionosis	*Amanita* mushroom poisoning
Chagas' disease	Lead poisoning
Familial autonomic dysfunction	
Spinal cord injury	**Idiopathic**
Pseudo-Hirschsprung's disease	Visceral myopathy
Multiple sclerosis	Visceral neuropathy
Ganglioneuroma of the intestine	Other forms, undefined

*Modified from Faulk et al.[3]

undefined regulatory or physiologic changes that are not manifest histologically. No disorder of gut hormones has yet been implicated in intestinal pseudo-obstruction. Defective function of the muscarinic acetylcholine receptor of smooth muscle was suggested in one case without significant myopathic or neuropathic changes.[13]

In 1977, Schuffler et al.[14] described a family with intestinal pseudo-obstruction, dysphagia, esophageal aperistalsis, and bladder motor dysfunction. Intestinal smooth muscle obtained from the propositus revealed an abnormal histologic appearance with degeneration and vacuolization of the fibers in both the longitudinal and the circular muscle layers and almost complete absence of external longitudinal muscle in some areas. Electron microscopy revealed destruction of smooth muscle cells and disorganization of the contractile filaments of the muscle. Similar abnormalities of the smooth muscle were later described in 3 other families.[9, 10, 15] (Fig. 123–1). The family described by Faulk and coworkers[9] also had involvement of the iris of the eye. In this family and in one described by Jacobs,[16] the predominant site of muscle degeneration was in the longitudinal muscle layer, with atrophy and replacement of muscle by collagen and very little vacuolization of smooth muscle cells. The disease in these patients has been termed "familial visceral myopathy"[9] or "hereditary hollow visceral myopathy."[14] A sporadic case of visceral myopathy has also been described.[17]

In contrast to these idiopathic forms, when pseudo-obstruction is due to progressive systemic sclerosis (Fig. 123–2), the circular muscle is usually more involved than the longitudinal muscle, and, despite significant fibrosis, the residual smooth muscle cells show none of the degenerative changes seen in visceral myopathy.[3]

In another histologic subtype of idiopathic pseudo-obstruction, the primary abnormality is in the myenteric nerve plexus of the bowel (Fig. 123–3). Dyer and Smith[11] were the first to describe this finding. Smith[11, 18] developed a histologic technique in which thin serial sections are cut parallel to the intestinal wall, and the plexus is silver-stained to obtain an *en face* view of neurons, axons, dendrites, and nerve fibers.[8, 18] In some patients, the neuropathic changes (degeneration and

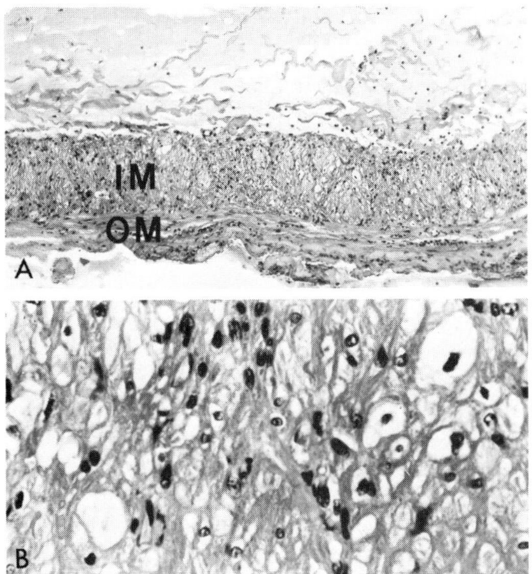

Figure 123–1. Myopathic pseudo-obstruction. *A,* Duodenal wall in familial hollow visceral myopathy. Note thinning, vacuolations, and fibrosis in both inner (IM) and outer (OM) muscle layers. (Hematoxylin and eosin, × 144.) *B,* Vacuolar degeneration of inner muscle with fragmented and indistinct muscle cells. (Hematoxylin and eosin, × 960.) (Photomicrographs kindly provided by Dr. Michael D. Schuffler.) (From Schuffler MD et al. Medicine 1981; 60:173–96. Copyright 1981, The Williams & Wilkins Co., Baltimore. Reproduced with permission.)

swelling of neurons and neuronal processes) are restricted to the myenteric plexus. In others, however, other parts of the nervous system are involved. Cockel and associates[12] reported 4 mentally retarded siblings with calcifications of the basal ganglia and intestinal pseudo-obstruction associated with degeneration of myenteric plexus neurons. Schuffler and associates[19] described 2 siblings with ataxia, abnormal pupillary and deep tendon reflexes, dysarthria, mild autonomic dysfunction, and pseudo-obstruction, but who were not mentally retarded. Histologic specimens revealed widespread degeneration of the myenteric plexuses with a distinctive eosinophilic intranuclear inclusion body seen in neurons of the myenteric plexuses, brain, celiac ganglia, and spinal cord (Fig. 123–3C).

Sporadic visceral neuropathy can be distinguished from *familial* neuropathy by the absence of eosinophilic inclusions on hematoxylin and eosin staining in the former and by the observation of Schwann cell proliferation in areas of marked plexus injury on silver staining.[11, 19]

In order to understand the underlying physiologic derangements in pseudo-obstruction more completely, several investigators have performed jejunal manometric studies in these patients. The data are conflicting, perhaps reflecting the heterogeneous nature of the syndrome. Summers et al.[20] noted the absence of the migrating motor complexes (MMCs) in 2 of their 3 patients; the other patient demonstrated a pattern of clustered contractions more typical of mechanical obstruction, in which there is a cluster of 3 to 10 high-amplitude contractions occurring 5 seconds apart and preceded and followed by at least 1 minute of motor quiescence. In contrast, Sarna et al.[21] reported the presence of MMCs in pseudo-obstruction, which occurred with an abnormally high frequency.

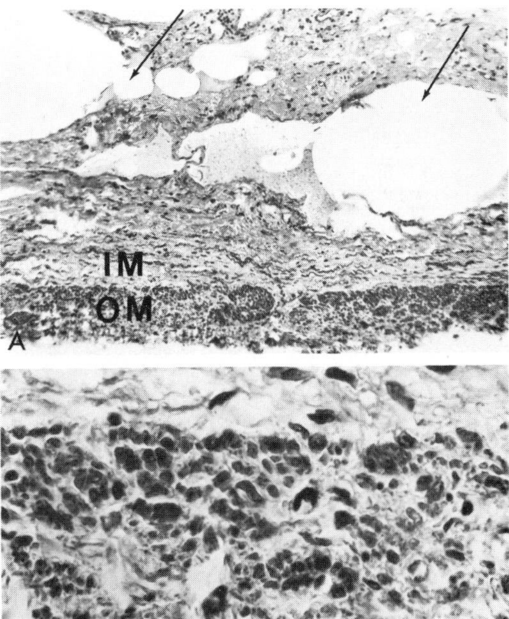

Figure 123–2. Pseudo-obstruction in primary systemic sclerosis. *A,* Duodenal wall in primary systemic sclerosis with pneumatosis cystoides intestinalis. There is extreme thinning of inner (IM) and outer (OM) muscle layers, with almost complete replacement of the inner muscle by collagen. The submucosal cystic spaces represent pneumatosis cystoides *(arrows).* (Masson's trichrome, × 144.) *B,* Higher power view showing normal residual darkly staining muscle cells embedded in a matrix of lighter staining collagen. (Masson's trichrome, × 960.) (Photomicrographs kindly provided by Dr. Michael D. Schuffler.) (From Schuffler MD et al. Medicine 1981; 60:173–96. Copyright 1981, The Williams & Wilkins Co., Baltimore. Reproduced with permission.)

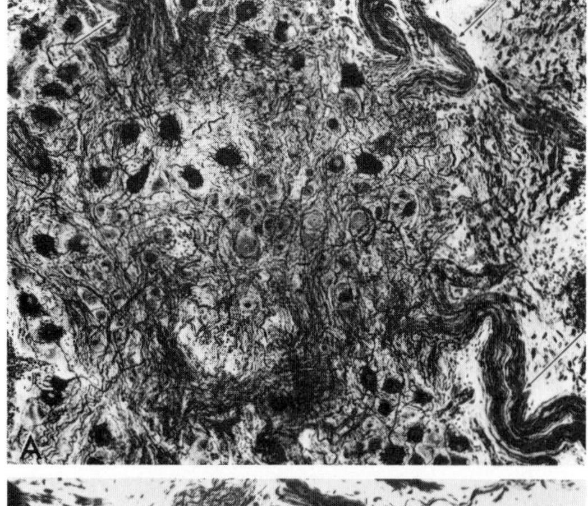

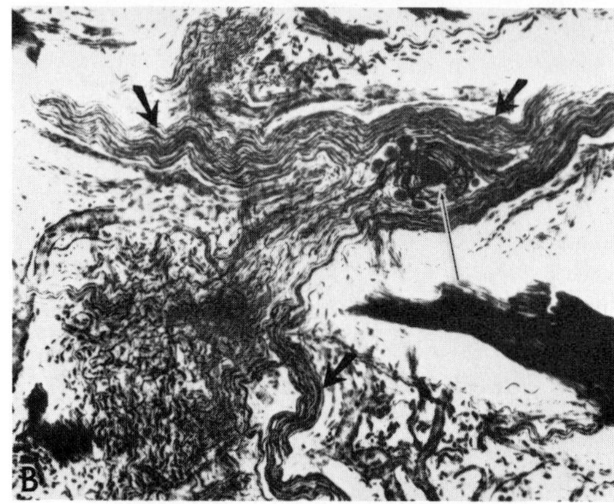

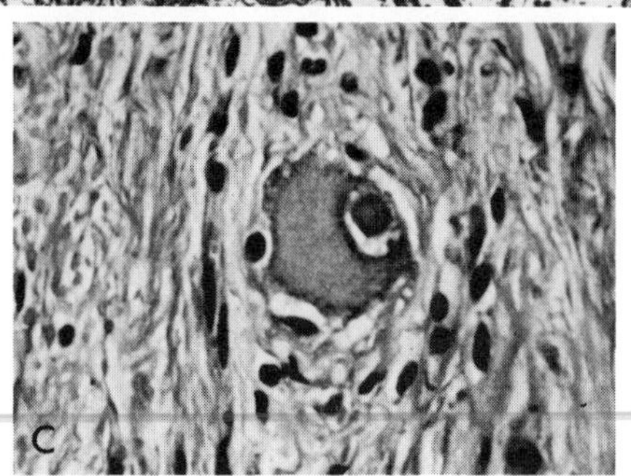

Figure 123–3. Myenteric plexus. *A,* A ganglion of the myenteric plexus of a normal control esophagus. There are a large number of dark- and light-staining neurons and several connecting nerve fiber tracts *(arrows).* (Silver, × 115). *B,* An esophageal ganglion from a patient with familial visceral neuropathy. Only one neuron is present *(long arrow),* surrounded by several smaller dark staining bodies, which are swollen dendrites. The broad arrows point to nerve fiber tracts. (Silver, × 115.) *C,* Single intranuclear inclusion body within a neuron involved with familial visceral neuropathy. (Hematoxylin and eosin, × 460.) (Photomicrographs kindly provided by Dr. Michael Schuffler.) (From Schuffler MD et al. Medicine 1981; 60:173–96. Copyright 1981, The Williams & Wilkins Co., Baltimore. Reproduced with permission.)

The manometric patterns that have been described may correspond to the hypomotility noted in visceral myopathy and the uncoordinated hypermotility of neuropathic pseudo-obstruction. Duodenal myoelectrical studies in patients with pseudo-obstruction whose histologic appearance is normal have revealed abnormally high basal electrical spike activity with normal motor activity. While direct smooth muscle stimulation increased myoelectrical activity, distention did not cause the expected increase. These findings suggest a disturbance in the function of the myenteric plexus.[22] In the same group of patients, colonic myoelectrical activity, which was normal in the basal state and appropriately increased following cholinergic stimulation with neostigmine, did not show the expected increase postprandially. These observations suggest a disruption in the mechanism linking gastroduodenal receptors and the colonic myenteric plexus.[22]

Clinical Manifestations

Symptoms. Symptoms of pseudo-obstruction may be indistinguishable from the symptoms of organic obstruction (Chapter 122). Pseudo-obstruction may affect the total alimentary tract or isolated segments of it (esophagus, stomach, small intestine, or colon). Generally, when there is diffuse involvement, the initial presentation is that of a disorder of the small bowel resembling obstruction.[5] When isolated segments of the gut are involved, symptoms may be referable only to these regions.

Symptoms usually occur in childhood and adolescence, although occasional patients may not develop symptoms until the third or fourth decade of life. Patients with secondary forms of intestinal pseudo-obstruction tend to have their initial presentation somewhat later than those with the primary idiopathic forms.[3]

The symptoms usually appear, subside, and reappear in recurring episodes. Between major attacks, there may be no symptoms or only minor ones. The usual presentation includes visible, pronounced abdominal distention, abdominal pain, and altered bowel habit. When abdominal pain is present, it is usually diffuse and crampy in nature and may be severe. The pain is generally related to abdominal distention and may be relieved by vomiting or passing stool and gas. The chronic nature of the pain may lead to narcotic dependence, which, in turn, may further confuse the diagnosis or increase the intestinal stasis.

Nausea and vomiting are frequently present. The vomitus may be of a large volume and may contain partially digested food if there is delayed gastric emptying. Weight loss of 30 to 60 pounds is common. The most common bowel pattern is diarrhea, due to bacterial overgrowth caused by stasis of small bowel contents. Steatorrhea may result. Constipation occurs less frequently and reflects greater involvement of the large bowel. Other reported defecation patterns include normal bowel habit or alternating diarrhea and constipation, suggestive of the irritable bowel syndrome.

Heartburn is rare and dysphagia is uncommon in idiopathic pseudo-obstruction (compared with their presence in about half the patients with progressive systemic sclerosis).[10] Urinary retention may occur in occasional patients with visceral myopathy, and the cystometrogram in these patients shows a flaccid bladder.[2]

Genetic Aspects. Familial involvement is present in about 30% of patients with idiopathic pseudo-obstruction. Any part of the gastrointestinal or urinary tract may be involved. Some family members may be asymptomatic yet have involvement of the esophagus or small or large bowel observed radiographically or manometrically. The mode of transmission appears to be autosomal dominant with incomplete penetrance in most families, but autosomal recessive inheritance has also been noted.[6, 7] Black, German, Scottish, Mexican, and Italian ancestries have been noted in involved families.[6, 7]

Megaduodenum. Megaduodenum is a variant of chronic idiopathic pseudo-obstruction in which disease is localized to the duodenum (Chapter 83). This does not occur in the neuropathic variant of pseudo-obstruction. The major clinical manifestations are related to delayed gastric emptying; abdominal distention and steatorrhea are not part of the clinical picture.[10] The duodenum may remain the only affected bowel segment, or involvement may eventually progress to involve more of the small bowel.[23] As pointed out in Chapter 83, some patients diagnosed as having superior mesenteric artery syndrome may, in fact, have idiopathic megaduodenum.[24]

Isolated Colonic Involvement. In some cases, the colon may be the most overtly involved part of the bowel. Constipation, recurrent fecal impactions, and dilated segments of the colon are seen on plain films of the abdomen.[25] Watier et al.,[26] in studies made in a group of patients with severe chronic constipation and delayed transit throughout the large intestine ("colonic inertia"), found that some of them also had motor disturbances of the esophagus and bladder. Histopathologic findings in this group of patients included hyperganglionosis, granulomatous-like inflammation around nerve plexuses, loss of neurons, and proliferation of Schwann cells.[25] No familial associations were noted. These patients may well represent a part of the spectrum of patients with the idiopathic pseudo-obstruction syndrome.

Jejunal Diverticulosis. Some patients with intestinal pseudo-obstruction are found to have jejunal diverticulosis (Fig. 123–4) (Chapter 111). In 62 patients with jejunal diverticulosis, Altemeier et al.[27] found 16 with symptoms of obstruction; radiographic evaluation disclosed no mechanical obstruction. Baskin and Mayo[28] detected symptoms of obstruction in 9 of 87 patients with jejunal diverticulosis; 60% of the remainder had no symptoms referable to diverticulosis or obstruction, and 30% had only vague abdominal complaints and dyspepsia. The relationship of diverticulosis and pseudo-obstruction is not clear. It is possible that the diverticula interfere with normal peristalsis; on the other hand, smooth muscle degeneration or uncoordinated peristalsis may cause the diverticula to form. Pathologic specimens in 7 patients with jejunal diverticulosis and intestinal pseudo-obstruction revealed 4 with the smooth muscle histologic pattern of progressive systemic sclerosis, 2 with the pattern seen in familial visceral myopathy, and 1 with myenteric plexus neuropathy.[29] These findings suggest that the diverticula develop as a consequence of an underlying abnormality in intestinal motility or of the intestinal wall.

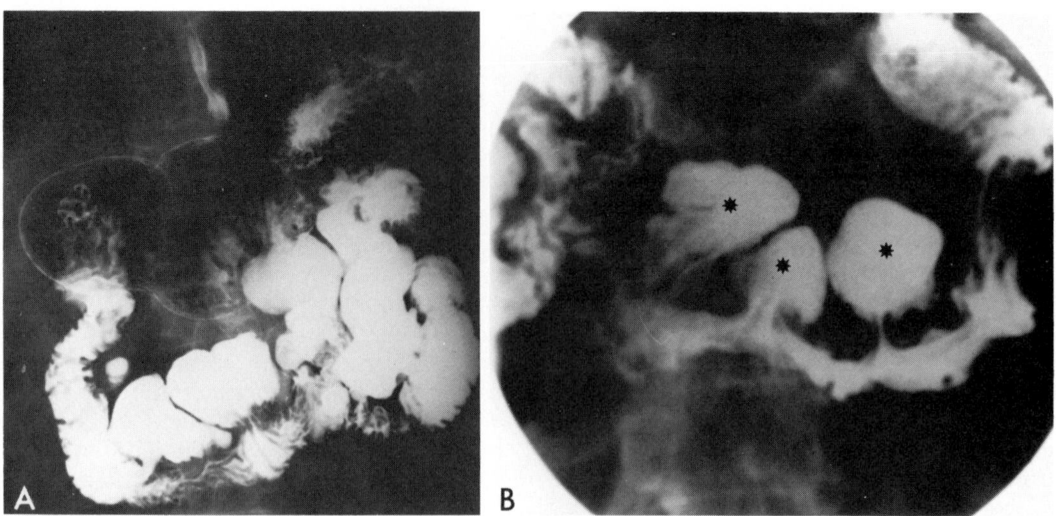

Figure 123–4. *A,* Diverticulosis of the duodenum and jejunum in a patient with pseudo-obstruction. *B,* Spot film showing 3 diverticula in duodenum *(asterisks).*

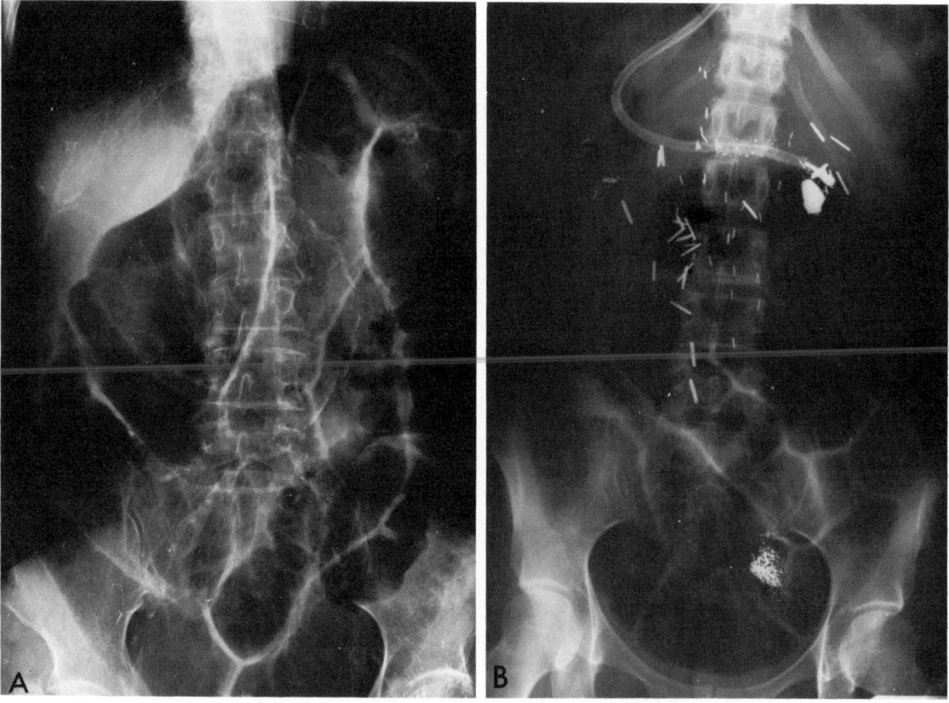

Figure 123–5. *A,* Abdominal plain film of a patient presenting with acute exacerbation of her chronic pseudo-obstruction. There are dilated loops of both small bowel and colon. *B,* Plain film of another patient with an acute exacerbation of chronic pseudo-obstruction. The presence of surgical clips is a frequent finding in these patients. This patient underwent 5 laparotomies for intestinal obstruction before the diagnosis of pseudo-obstruction was made.

Laboratory Findings

No laboratory findings are specific for chronic idiopathic pseudo-obstruction.[3] Laboratory studies may show evidence of poor nutrition, such as anemia, hypocalcemia, hypocholesterolemia, folic acid deficiency, iron deficiency, or hypoalbuminemia. These abnormalities are due to malabsorption caused by bacterial overgrowth, avoidance of eating to reduce symptoms, or both.

Radiologic Features

Radiographic patterns noted in pseudo-obstruction depend on the area of bowel affected. Most cases of pseudo-obstruction involve the alimentary tract diffusely. In some cases, however, only isolated organs are involved. In general, the neuropathic type of pseudo-obstruction tends to have less dilatation of the bowel.[3] When the more distal aspects of the bowel are involved, proximal dilatation may occur. Plain films of the abdomen obtained during acute episodes may show distention of the stomach, small intestine, and colon (Fig. 123–5). This pattern of air throughout the small bowel and colon is different from that noted in mechanical obstruction, in which no air is seen beyond the point of obstruction. A few patients have pneumatosis intestinales or even pneumoperitoneum[3]; thus, the finding of free air should not automatically lead to laparotomy for suspected perforation.

Barium studies usually reveal abnormal esophageal patterns. In myopathic forms of pseudo-obstruction, the esophagus may be dilated and lack peristalsis, as observed fluoroscopically. In the neuropathic form, the esophagram may show multiple, chaotic, local contractions and delayed esophageal emptying. A pattern resembling achalasia may also be seen. Esophageal strictures have not been described in idiopathic pseudo-obstruction, and their presence would suggest scleroderma.[3] If roentgenograms are obtained after ingestion of barium, gastric distention and dilatation may be seen. Schuffler[4] has noted that one-third of his patients with pseudo-obstruction have gastric enlargement. The duodenum is frequently markedly

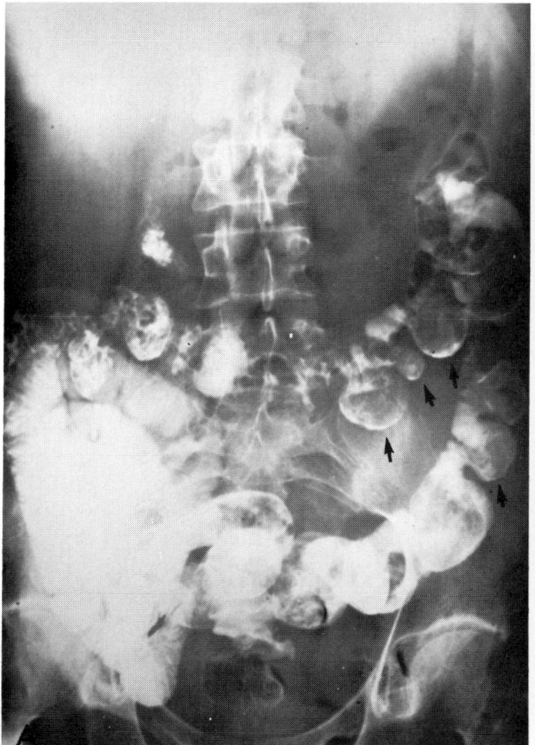

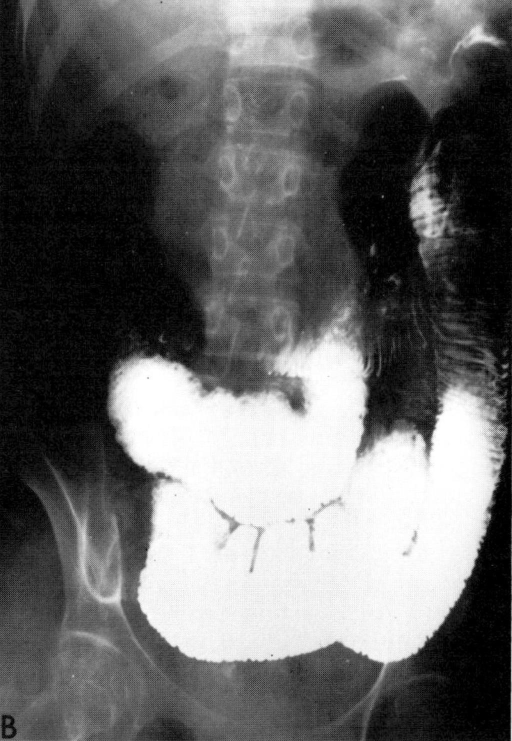

Figure 123–6. *A,* Wide-mouth diverticula noted on barium enema examination of a patient with progressive systemic sclerosis and chronic pseudo-obstruction. *B,* Small bowel series of patient with progressive systemic sclerosis and pseudo-obstruction; note the "packed" accordion-like appearance of the valvulae. (Courtesy of Dr. A. Weinfeld.)

dilatated, especially in patients with visceral myopathy. In visceral myopathy also, peristalsis is minimal in the small bowel and the barium moves very slowly. In visceral neuropathy there is active but uncoordinated peristalsis; thus, although part of the ingested barium may reach the cecum in a normal period of time, some barium still remains in the small bowel 24 hours later. Jejunal diverticulosis may be noted. In visceral myopathy, the barium enema study usually shows a redundant, dilated colon with absent haustra and incomplete evacuation of barium. Wide-mouthed diverticula are seen in instances of scleroderma (Fig. 123–6) In familial visceral neuropathy, there is often extensive diverticulosis and normal emptying of barium.[3]

Esophageal Manometry

Esophageal manometry is generally abnormal in idiopathic pseudo-obstruction.[30] Two different patterns occur that distinguish visceral myopathy and neuropathy. In visceral myopathy, contractions in the lower portion of the esophagus are of low amplitude, primary peristalsis is absent, and there is no increased response to methacholine (Mecholyl). The lower esophageal sphincter usually functions normally in these patients.[14] In contrast, in visceral neuropathy, the lower esophageal sphincter relaxes incompletely, peristalsis is usually absent from the body of the esophagus, repetitive waves are often seen, and the Mecholyl test is usually positive.[19] An achalasia-type pattern has also been seen in some patients.[22]

Diagnosis and Differential Diagnosis

In both acute and chronic presentations of pseudo-obstruction, the diagnostic evaluation must first be directed toward excluding mechanical causes of partial obstruction, such as adhesions, strictures, tumors, or intussusception. Symptoms are similar in pseudo-obstruction and partial mechanical obstruction. In mechanical obstruction, however, the pain tends to be more severe and crampy in nature. Obstipation, constipation, or failure to pass flatus points to mechanical obstruction, while diarrhea is more common in pseudo-obstruction. Other features suggesting pseudo-obstruction are evidence of esophageal or urinary tract involvement, cachexia, a positive family history, onset during childhood or adolescence, failure of symptoms of distention to resolve totally between acute episodes, the presence of systemic conditions that may affect intestinal motility, and jejunal diverticulosis.

Enteroclysis and manometry are very accurate in differentiating mechanical obstruction and pseudo-obstruction. Enteroclysis, or small bowel enema, is a technique of small bowel radiography in which a Bilbao-Dotter tube is passed nasally into the duodenum and used to introduce barium into the small bowel.[31] This test is very sensitive (98%) for structural lesions of the small bowel, in contrast to a 25% to 35% false-negative rate for standard small bowel series or barium enema examination with ileal reflux.[31] Esophageal manometry will be abnormal in at least 80% of patients with pseudo-obstruction, whereas it is normal in patients with small bowel obstruction.[4] Intestinal manometry has been employed as means of identifying asymptomatic cases of visceral myopathy with manifestations elsewhere.[7]

Even with the aid of these relatively accurate tests, the diagnosis may still be unclear in some patients, and exploratory laparotomy may be required. Schuffler[4] urges barium studies of the entire gastrointestinal tract together with IV pyelography, advancing the rationale that "the greater the number of sites involved, the greater will be the physician's confidence in a diagnosis of pseudo-obstruction and the less likely will he want to undertake exploratory laparotomy." In addition, these tests may allow categorization of the pseudo-obstruction as to subtype or relationship to systemic diseases.

A diagnosis of pseudo-obstruction can usually be made on the basis of radiographic studies and esophageal manometry alone.[4] Thus, there is generally no need for biopsy confirmation of the diagnosis. However, if exploratory laparotomy is done and no obstructing lesions are found, full-thickness biopsies of dilated and non-dilated small bowel segments should be obtained. In the case of visceral neuropathy, even full-thickness biopsies may not demonstrate the histologic lesion unless a segment several centimeters long is removed and processed by Smith's technique.[8, 11, 17, 32] Mucosal biopsy of the small bowel is of no value, since neither the myenteric plexus nor the smooth muscle layers are included; these superficial biopsies may, in fact, be misleading, as the bacterial overgrowth associated with pseudo-obstruction may cause secondary mucosal changes simulating celiac disease.[33]

Acute intestinal pseudo-obstruction, or ileus, may be seen in a variety of extraintestinal conditions (Table 123–2). Although acute exacerbations are typical in uncomplicated chronic pseudo-obstruction, these extraintestinal causes of acute ileus must also be considered in the patient with known chronic pseudo-obstruction who presents with an acute exacerbation. Patients with pseudo-obstruction are also at risk of developing volvulus (4 cases out of Schuffler's 35 patients[4]; the presentation of the volvulus may be indistinguishable from the typical acute exacerbation.

Table 123–2. ETIOLOGY OF ACUTE ILEUS

Infections:
Peritonitis
Acute appendicitis
Acute cholecystitis
Diverticulitis
Systemic infections (pneumonia, septicemia)
Retroperitoneal processes:
Spinal fracture
Retroperitoneal hematoma
Renal colic, pyelonephritis
Peritoneal irritation:
Perforated viscus
Acute pancreatitis
Intraperitoneal hemorrhage
Bile peritonitis
Vasculitis
Familial Mediterranean fever
Bowel ischemia:
Arterial insufficiency
Mesenteric venous thrombosis
Strangulation of the bowel
Vasculitis
Thoracic processes:
Myocardial infarction
Rib fracture
Abdominal disruption:
Postoperative
Penetrating wounds
Drug-induced:
Opiates
Anticholinergics
Clonidine
Metabolic abnormalities:
Electrolyte imbalance (especially hypokalemia)
Porphyria
Lead poisoning
Uremia
Chronic illness (e.g., congestive heart failure)

Once a diagnosis of chronic pseudo-obstruction is established, it is important to search for any systemic diseases or conditions that may be affecting the intestine. Schuffler[4] and Faulk et al.[3] stress that the onset of the pseudo-obstruction syndrome may precede the recognition of systemic disease by many years.

Secondary forms of pseudo-obstruction are much more common than primary or idiopathic pseudo-obstruction (Table 123–1), the most common secondary form being progressive systemic sclerosis (PSS). Thorough reviews of other less common secondary forms of pseudo-obstruction have been published by Faulk et al.[3] and Golladay and Byrne.[34]

Search for causes of secondary pseudo-obstruction should begin with a history focused on drug intake, travel to areas of South America where Chagas' disease is endemic, and features suggesting collagen vascular or endocrine disorders. The physical examination should include attention to possible stigmata of the CREST syndrome (*C*alcinosis, *R*aynaud's phenomenon, *E*sophageal dysmotility, *S*clerodactyly, and *T*elangiectasia) and an evaluation of autonomic function—sweating, lacrimation, pupillary reflexes—and cardiovascular responses to orthostasis, deep inspiration, Valsalva maneuver, and cold immersion of the hand.[35, 36] Blood tests should include rheumatoid factor and antinuclear antibody (for collagen vascular diseases), creatine phosphokinase (for myositis and muscular dystrophies), fasting glucose, thyroid function tests, and serologic tests for *Trypanosoma cruzi* (if Chagas' disease is suspected). Urinary porphobilinogens should be checked to exclude porphyria. Chest radiographs may reveal cardiomegaly or fibrotic changes suggesting PSS or an occult malignancy with pseudo-obstruction as a paraneoplastic manifestation.[37] Rectal biopsy is generally of no value, but occasionally may be helpful in the diagnosis of amyloidosis or to demonstrate the eosinophilic intranuclear inclusions of familial visceral neuropathy.[3, 38]

The pseudo-obstruction that occurs in PSS is clinically identical to that in idiopathic pseudo-obstruction, except that the former seems to be more rapidly progressive. Also, the duration of symptoms prior to diagnosis is shorter and the age of onset is later.[10] The best available data on the frequency of pseudo-obstruction in patients with PSS are provided by Schuffler and his associates,[10] who observed 14 patients with pseudo-obstruction in a group of 97 patients with PSS. In most patients, gastrointestinal symptoms developed in the 12 months preceding the diagnosis of PSS.[39] In 3 of the 14 patients studied by Schuffler and associates,[10] pseudo-obstruction symptoms antedated skin manifestations—by 28 years in 1 patient, by 17 years in 1 patient, and by 1 year in the third.[10] Thus, some cases of pseudo-obstruction clinically classified as idiopathic may, in fact, turn out to be due to PSS. The bowel wall biopsies in scleroderma are sufficiently specific to prevent this type of misclassification in those patients with available biopsy material.[4] The histologic changes (Fig. 123–2) feature focal atrophy of both circular and longitudinal smooth muscle layers with replacement by a densely hyalinized fibrosis; no degenerating muscle cells are seen (in contrast to familial visceral myopathy), and the myenteric plexus is not involved.[3] In addition to the radiographic changes described in all types of pseudo-obstruction, barium radiography may reveal certain abnormalities suggestive of PSS: esophageal stricture, wide-mouthed sacculations in both the small and large bowel (Fig. 123–6), and a "packed" (accordioned) appearance of the valvulae.[10] Esophageal manometry shows low pressure in the lower esophageal sphincter and either absent or low-amplitude peristaltic activity.[4]

Treatment

The medical treatment of primary idiopathic pseudo-obstruction has been disappointing to date. Cholinergic agents and metoclopramide have been found to be ineffective.[2, 9, 10, 12, 23, 40, 41] However, Snape[35] has speculated that the subset of patients who have an abnormal smooth muscle muscarinic acetylcholine receptor[13] might respond to drugs that inhibit acetylcholinesterase (e.g., pyridostigmine or neostigmine), thus providing a greater concentration of acetylcholine at the receptor. In patients with intestinal pseudo-obstruction who have diarrhea and presumed bacterial overgrowth, antibiotics may be useful. The initial attempt is usually with tetracycline at a dose of 1 to 2 g/day for 2 weeks. If this is ineffective, other antibiotics should be tried (Chapter 107). About half the patients initially respond, but only one-third continue to respond during multiple courses of antibiotics. In a few patients, the resolution of the diarrhea is accompanied by obstipation and an exacerbation of obstructive symptoms, suggesting that the diarrhea allowed decompression of the hypomotile intestine.[10] In patients with pseudo-obstruction with constipation or predominantly obstructive symptoms, the use of antibiotics is not warranted.

Dietary manipulations may also be beneficial. Schuffler[4] has advocated the use of a low-fat, lactose-free, low-fiber diet. A high load of dietary fat may worsen the steatorrhea and diarrhea of these patients. Additionally, if there is an element of lactase deficiency, the ingestion of lactose will lead to increased gas formation by intestinal bacteria and consequent worsening of distention. In such instances, therefore, lactose intake should be sharply curtailed. A low-fiber diet has been advocated to eliminate the potential for true mechanical obstruction due to bezoar formation.[4] The patient should also be given multivitamins, calcium, vitamin D, monthly vitamin B_{12} injections, and, if indicated, vitamin K, folate, and iron. Dietary manipulations are beneficial in only a minority of patients; they are ineffective when obstructive symptoms are severe.[10] Home parenteral nutrition may be warranted in patients with marked weight loss and intractable symptoms.[10, 42]

As a general rule, surgery should be avoided in diffuse forms of pseudo-obstruction, although when there is isolated segmental involvement, surgery may be beneficial. The results of surgical treatment; however, are unpredictable.[43] In patients with gastroparesis and a dilated stomach, symptomatic improvement has been obtained with a partial gastrectomy with Roux-en-Y gastrojejunostomy.[44] In patients with megaduodenum, symptomatic relief can be obtained from a side-to-side duodenojejunostomy, resection of the dilated duodenum, or partial gastrectomy with Roux-en-Y gastrojejunostomy.[43] None of the patients of Schuffler and his group[10] improved after resection of the jejunum or ileum. In cases in which colonic involvement predominates, subtotal colectomy may be helpful.[45] When surgery is performed because of presumed mechanical obstruction or to correct an isolated segment of dilated bowel, pathologic examination of any resected specimen should be done and full-thickness intestinal biopsies taken and examined.

It perhaps deserves emphasis that there is considerable risk from surgery in these chronically ill, malnourished patients. For example, the overall mortality from surgery for megaduodenum has been reported to be as great as 18%.[17] Furthermore, once laparotomy is done, it becomes very difficult to determine whether future obstructive attacks are due to pseudo-obstruction or to mechanical obstruction caused by postoperative adhesions.

Prognosis and Natural History

The typical patient with chronic idiopathic pseudo-obstruction has had symptoms for more than 10 years before a correct diagnosis is made. Not infrequently, the patient will have had multiple operations for presumed mechanical obstruction during this period. The course is characterized by exacerbations and remissions, which may be spontaneous or may relate to a therapeutic maneuver.[4] In the series of 27 patients studied by Schuffler et al.,[10] 18 patients had documented periods of improvement, usually temporally related to one or more of the therapeutic measures earlier discussed. Of the other 9 patients, 4 had no definite improvement, 3 died within a year of diagnosis, and 2 were lost to follow-up. These observers found that patients generally survive for many years with the syndrome; in their series, death occurred 9 to 50 years after the onset of symptoms, at a mean age of 57 years. Complications, such as aspiration of intestinal contents, volvulus, and surgery, rather than malnutrition are the most frequent causes of death in these patients.[10]

References

1. Weiss W. Zur Etiologie des Megaduodenums. Dtsch Z Chir 1938; 251:317–30.
2. Maldonado JE, Gregg JA, Green PA, et al. Chronic idiopathic intestinal pseudo-obstruction. Am J Med 1970; 49:203–12.
3. Faulk DL, Anuras S, Christensen J. Clinical trends and topics: chronic intestinal pseudo-obstruction. Gastroenterology 1978; 74:922–31.
4. Schuffler MD. Chronic intestinal pseudo-obstruction syndrome. Med Clin North Am 1981; 65:1331–58.
5. Snape WJ. Pseudo-obstruction and other obstructive disorders. Clin Gastroenterol 1982; 11:593–608.
6. Anuras S, Shaw A, Christensen J. The familial syndromes of intestinal pseudo-obstruction. Am J Hum Genet 1981; 33:584–91.
7. Anuras S, Novak T, Ionasescu V, Christensen J. A new familial visceral myopathy with external ophthalmoplegia with intestinal manometry to identify asymptomatic cases. Clin Res 1981; 29:303A.
8. Schuffler MD, Jonak Z. Chronic idiopathic intestinal pseudo-obstruction caused by a degenerative disorder of the myenteric plexus. The use of Smith's method to define the neuropathology. Gastroenterology 1982; 82:476–86.
9. Faulk DL, Anuras S, Gardner D, et al. A familial visceral myopathy. Ann Intern Med 1978; 89:600–6.
10. Schuffler MD, Rohrmann CA, Chaffee RG, et al. Chronic intestinal pseudo-obstruction. A report of 27 cases and review of the literature. Medicine 1981; 60:173–96.
11. Dyer NH, Dawson AM, Smith BF, et al. Obstruction of bowel due to lesion in the myenteric plexus. Br Med J 1969; 1:686–9.
12. Cockel R, Hill EE, Rushton DI, et al. Familial steatorrhea with calcification of the basal ganglia and mental retardation. Q J Med 1973; 42:771–83.
13. Bannister R, Hoyes AD. Generalized smooth-muscle disease with defective muscarinic-receptor function. Br Med J 1981; 282:1015–18.
14. Schuffler MD, Lowe MC, Bill AH. Studies of idiopathic intestinal pseudo-obstruction: I. Hereditary hollow visceral myopathy: Clinical and pathological studies. Gastroenterology 1977; 73:327–38.
15. Shaw A, Shaffer H, Teja K, et al. A perspective for pediatric surgeons: chronic idiopathic intestinal pseudo-obstruction. J Pediatr Surg 1979; 14:719–27.
16. Jacobs E, Ardichvili D, Perissino A, et al. A case of familial visceral myopathy with atrophy and fibrosis of the longitudinal muscle layer of the entire small bowel. Gastroenterology 1979; 77:745–50.
17. Schuffler MD, Dutch EA. Chronic idiopathic intestinal pseudo-obstruction. A surgical approach. Ann Surg 1980; 192:752–61.
18. Smith BE. Changes in the myenteric plexus in pseudo-obstruction. Gut 1969: 9:726.
19. Schuffler MD, Bird TD, Sumi SM, et al. A familial neuronal disease presenting with intestinal pseudo-obstruction. Gastroenterology 1978; 75:889–98.
20. Summers RW, Anuras S, Green J. Jejunal manometry patterns in health, partial intestinal obstruction and pseudo-obstruction. Gastroenterology 1983; 85:1290–1300.
21. Sarna SK, Daniel EE, Waterfall WE, et al. Postoperative gastrointestinal electrical and mechanical activities in a patient with idiopathic intestinal pseudo-obstruction. Gastroenterology 1978; 74:112–20.
22. Sullivan MA, Snape WJ, Matarazzo SA, et al. Gastrointestinal myoelectrical activity in idiopathic intestinal pseudo-obstruction. N Engl J Med 1977; 297:233–80.
23. Erskine JM. Acquired megacolon, megaesophagus and megaduodenum with aperistalsis. A case report. Am J Gastroenterol 1963; 40:588–600.
24. Byrne WJ, Cipel L, Ament ME, Gyepes MT. Chronic idiopathic intestinal pseudo-obstruction syndrome: Radiologic signs in children with emphasis on differentiation from mechanical obstruction. Diag Imag 1981; 50:294–304.
25. Poisson J, Devroede G. Severe chronic constipation as a surgical problem. Surg Clin North Am 1983; 63:193–217.
26. Watier A, Devroede G, Dugvay C, et al. Mechanism of idiopathic constipation: colonic inertia. Gastroenterology 1979; 76:1267.
27. Altemeier WA, Bryant LR, Wulsin JH. The surgical significance of jejunal diverticulosis. Arch Surg 1963; 86:732–44.
28. Baskin RH, Mayo CW. Jejunal diverticulosis: a clinical study of 87 cases. Surg Clin North Am 1952; 32:1185–96.
29. Krishnamurthy S, Kelly MM, Rohrmann CA, et al. Jejunal diverticulosis: a heterogeneous disorder caused by a variety of abnormalities of smooth muscle or myenteric plexus. Gastroenterology 1983; 85:538–47.
30. Schuffler MD, Pope CE. Esophageal motor dysfunction in idiopathic intestinal pseudo-obstruction. Gastroenterology 1976; 70:677–82.
31. Gurian L, Jendrzejewski J, Katon R, et al. Small bowel enema: an underutilized method of small bowel examination. Dig Dis Sci 1982; 27:1101–8.

32. Smith B. The neuropathology of pseudo-obstruction of the intestine. Scand J Gastroenterol 1982; 71(Suppl 7).
33. Schuffler MD, Kaplan LR, Johnson L. Small intestinal mucosa in pseudo-obstruction syndrome. Am J Dig Dis 1978; 23:821–8.
34. Golladay ES, Byrne WJ. Collective review of intestinal pseudo-obstruction. Surg Gynecol Obstet 1981; 153:257–72.
35. Snape WJ. Take the idiopathic out of intestinal pseudo-obstruction. Ann Intern Med 1981; 95:646–7.
36. Ewing DJ, Clarke BF. Diagnosis and management of diabetic autonomic neuropathy. Br Med J 1982; 285:916–8.
37. Schuffler MD, Baird HW, Fleming CR, et al. Intestinal pseudo-obstruction as the presenting manifestation of small-cell carcinoma of the lung. Ann Intern Med 1983; 98:129–34.
38. Kyle RA, Bayrd JA. Amyloidosis: Review of 236 cases. Medicine 1975; 54:271–99.
39. Poirier TJ, Rankin GB. Gastrointestinal manifestations of progressive systemic scleroderma based on a review of 364 cases. Am J Gastroenterol 1972; 58:30–44.
40. Lipton AB, Knaver CM. Pseudo-obstruction of the bowel. Therapeutic trial of metoclopramide. Am J Dig Dis 1977; 22:263–5.
41. Anuras S, Christensen J. Recurrent or chronic intestinal pseudo-obstruction. Clin Gastroenterol 1981; 10:177–89.
42. Faulk DL, Anuras S, Freeman JB. Idiopathic chronic intestinal pseudo-obstruction: Use of central venous nutrition. JAMA 1978; 240:2075–6.
43. Anuras S, Shirazi S, Faulk D, et al. Surgical treatment in familial visceral myopathy. Ann Surg 1979; 189:306–10.
44. Lander RL, Morgan KG, Kruelen DL, et al. Human gastric atony with tachygastria and gastric retention. Gastroenterology 1978; 75:497–501.
45. Melzig EP, Terz JJ. Pseudo-obstruction of the colon. Arch Surg 1978; 113:1186–90.

Bockus

GASTROENTEROLOGY

INDEX

Index

Note: Page numbers in *italics* refer to illustrations; those followed by (t) refer to tables.

Vol. 1—pp. 1–665
Vol. 2—pp. 666–1438
Vol. 3—pp. 1439–2092
Vol. 4—pp. 2093–2624
Vol. 5—pp. 2625–3448
Vol. 6—pp. 3449–4176
Vol. 7—pp. 4177–4730